PROGRESS IN BRAIN RESEARCH

VOLUME 131

CONCEPTS AND CHALLENGES IN RETINAL BIOLOGY
A TRIBUTE TO JOHN E. DOWLING

PROGRESS IN BRAIN RESEARCH

VOLUME 131

CONCEPTS AND CHALLENGES IN RETINAL BIOLOGY
A TRIBUTE TO JOHN E. DOWLING

EDITED BY

HELGA KOLB

John Moran Eye Center, University of Utah, 75 North Medical Drive, Salt Lake City, UT 84132, USA

HARRIS RIPPS

Department of Ophthalmology and Visual Sciences, University of Illinois, College of Medicine, 1855 West Taylor Street, Chicago, IL 60612, USA

SAMUEL WU

Cullen Eye Institute, Baylor College of Medicine, 6565 Fannin Street, NC-205, Houston, TX 77030, USA

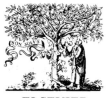

ELSEVIER

AMSTERDAM – LONDON – NEW YORK – OXFORD – PARIS – SHANNON – TOKYO

2001

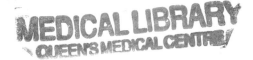
ELSEVIER SCIENCE B.V.
Sara Burgerhartstraat 25
P.O. Box 211, 1000 AE Amsterdam, The Netherlands

First edition 2001

Library of Congress Cataloging in Publication Data
A catalog record from the Library of Congress has been applied for.

ISBN (Volume): 0-444-50677-2
ISBN (Series): 0-444-80104-9
ISSN: 0079-6123

10 0303 078588

♾ The paper used in this publication meets the requirements of ANSI/NISO Z39.48-1992 (Permanence of Paper). Printed in The Netherlands.

List of Contributors

G. Aguirre, James A. Baker Institute for Animal Health, College of Veterinary Medicine, Cornell University, Ithaca, NY 14853, USA

P. Ahnelt, Department of Physiology, University of Vienna, Vienna, Austria

K.A. Andersen, Department of Medicine, University of Chicago, 5841 S. Maryland Avenue, MC 6094, Chicago, IL 60637, USA

W.H. Baldridge, Retina and Optic Nerve Laboratory, Department of Anatomy and Neurobiology and Ophthalmology, Dalhousie University, Halifax, NS B3H 4H7, Canada

D. Balya, Department of Molecular and Cell Biology, Division of Neurobiology, University of California at Berkeley, Berkeley, CA 94720, USA

R. Barlow, Center for Vision Research, Department of Ophthalmology, Upstate Medical University, 750 Adams Street, Syracuse, NY 13210, USA

T.N. Behar, Laboratory of Neurophysiology, National Institute of Neurological Disorders and Stroke, NIH, Bethesda, MD 20892-4066, USA

S.A. Bloomfield, Departments of Ophthalmology, Physiology and Neuroscience, New York University School of Medicine, 550 First Avenue, New York, NY 10016, USA

S.E. Brockerhoff, Department of Biochemistry, Box 357350, University of Washington, Seattle, WA 98195, USA

D.A. Burkhardt, Departments of Psychology and Physiology, University of Minnesota, n218 Elliott Hall, 75 E. River Road, Minneapolis, MN 55455, USA

B. Burnside, Department of Molecular and Cell Biology, University of California, Berkeley, 335LSA #3200, Berkeley, CA 94720-3200, USA

R.L. Chappell, Department of Biological Sciences, Hunter College of the City University of New York, 695 Park Avenue, New York, NY 10021, USA

J. Chen, Doheny Eye Institute, BMT-401, University of Southern California, Los Angeles, CA 90033, USA

E.D. Cohen, Department of Molecular and Cellular Biology, Harvard University, 16 Divinity Avenue, Cambridge, MA 02138, USA

V.P. Connaughton, Department of Biology, The American University, 4400 Massachusetts Avenue, NW, Washington, DC 20016, USA

N. Cuenca, Department of Biotechnology, University of Alicante, Alicante, Spain

T. Darland, Department of Molecular and Cellular Biology, Harvard University, 16 Divinity Avenue, Cambridge, MA 02138, USA

J. De Juan, Departamento de Biotecnología, Facultad de Ciencias, Universidad de Alicante, Apdo. Correos 99, Alicante 03080, Spain

J.E. Dowling, Department of Molecular and Cellular Biology, Harvard University, 16 Divinity Avenue, Cambridge, MA 02138, USA

U.C. Dräger, Eunice Kennedy Shriver Center, Waltham, MA 02452, USA

H. Dreyfus, Laboratoire de Physiopathologie Cellulaire et Moléculaire de la Rétine, EMI 9918 INSERM, Université Louis Pasteur and Clinique Médicale A, Hôpitaux Universitaires de Strasbourg, 1 Place de l'Hôpital, 67091 Strasbourg Cedex, France

B. Ehinger, The Wallenberg Retina Center, Department of Ophthalmology, Lund University Hospital, SE-221 85 Lund, Sweden

W.D. Eldred, Department of Biology, Boston University, 5 Cummington Street, Boston, MA 02215, USA

J.M. Fadool, Department of Biological Sciences, Florida State University, 235 Biomedical Research Facility, Tallahassee, FL 32306-4340, USA

G.L. Fain, Departments of Physiological Science and Ophthalmology, University of California, Los Angeles, Los Angeles, CA 90095-1527, USA

S.-F. Fan, Department of Neurobiology and Behavior, SUNY, Stony Brook, NY 11794-5230, USA

S.K. Fisher, Neuroscience Research Institute and Department of Molecular, Cellular and Developmental Biology, University of California at Santa Barbara, Santa Barbara, CA 93106, USA

F. Gao, Cullen Eye Institute, Baylor College of Medicine, 6565 Fannin Street, NC-205, Houston, TX 77030, USA

M. García, Departamento de Biotecnología, Facultad de Ciencias, Universidad de Alicante, Apdo. Correos 99, Alicante 03080, Spain

R.D. Glickman, Department of Ophthalmology, University of Texas Health Science Center at San Antonio, 7703 Floyd Curl Drive, San Antonio, TX 78229-3900, USA

J. Gottesman, Department of Neuroscience, University of Minnesota, 6-145 Jackson Hall, Minneapolis, MN 55455, USA

M.-H. Han, Institute of Neurobiology, Fudan University and Shanghai Institute of Physiology, Chinese Academy of Sciences, Shanghai 200433, China

D. Henderson, Department of Neuroscience, University of Minnesota, 6-145 Jackson Hall, Minneapolis, MN 55455, USA

D. Hicks, Laboratoire de Physiopathologie Cellulaire et Moléculaire de la Rétine, EMI 9918 INSERM, Université Louis Pasteur and Clinique Médicale A, Hôpitaux Universitaires de Strasbourg, 1 Place de l'Hôpital, 67091 Strasbourg Cedex, France

W. Hoppenstedt, FB7 Neurobiology, University of Oldenburg, D-26111 Oldenburg, Germany

J.B. Hurley, Department of Biochemistry, 375350, University of Washington, Seattle, WA 98195, USA

A.T. Janis, Laboratory of Neurophysiology, National Institute of Neurological Disorders and Stroke, NIH, Bethesda, MD 20892-4066, USA

U. Janssen-Bienhold, FB7 Neurobiology, University of Oldenburg, D-26111 Oldenburg, Germany

K. Johansson, The Wallenberg Retina Center, Department of Ophthalmology, Lund University Hospital, SE-22185 Lund, Sweden

H. Kolb, Department of Ophthalmology, John Moran Eye Center, University of Utah, Salt Lake City, UT 84132, USA

E.M. Lasater, Moran Eye Center, University of Utah Health Sciences Center, 50 North Medical Drive, Salt Lake City, UT 84132, USA

M.M. LaVail, Beckman Vision Center, University of California San Francisco, San Francisco, CA 94143-0730, USA

K.N. Leibovic, 105 High Park Boulevard, Buffalo, NY 14226, USA

T. Léveillard, Laboratoire de Physiopathologie Cellulaire et Moléculaire de la Rétine, EMI 9918 INSERM, Université Louis Pasteur and Clinique Médicale A, Hôpitaux Universitaires de Strasbourg, 1 Place de l'Hôpital, 67091 Strasbourg Cedex, France

G.P. Lewis, Neuroscience Research Institute, University of California at Santa Barbara, Santa Barbara, CA 93106, USA

H. Li, Department of Psychiatry, Harvard Medical School, Boston, MA 02115, USA and Eunice Kennedy Shriver Center, Waltham, MA 02452, USA

L. Li, Department of Physiology, University of Kentucky, 800 Rose Street, Lexington, KY 40536, USA

P. Li, Institute of Neurobiology, Fudan University and Shanghai Institute of Physiology, Chinese Academy of Sciences, Shanghai 200433, China

K.A. Linberg, Neuroscience Research Institute, University of California at Santa Barbara, Santa Barbara, CA 93106, USA

B.A. Link, Department of Molecular and Cellular Biology, Harvard University, 16 Divinity Avenue, Cambridge, MA 02138, USA

S.A. Lipton, The Burnham Institute, Center for Neuroscience and Aging, 10901 North Torrey Pines Road, La Jolla, CA 92037, USA

Y. Liu, Department of Ophthalmology, University of Texas Health Sciences Center, 7703 Floyd Curl Drive, San Antonio, TX 78284, USA

T. Lu, Institute of Neurobiology, Fudan University and Shanghai Institute of Physiology, Chinese Academy of Sciences, Shanghai 200433, China

R.P. Malchow, Departments of Biological Sciences and Ophthalmology and Visual Sciences, University of Illinois at Chicago, M/C 067, 840 West Taylor Street, Chicago, IL 60607, USA

S.C. Mangel, Department of Neurobiology, University of Alabama School of Medicine, CIRC 425, 1719 6th Avenue South, Birmingham, AL 35294-0021, USA

B.R Maple, Cullen Eye Institute, Baylor College of Medicine, 6565 Fannin Street, NC-205, Houston, TX 77030, USA

D.W. Marshak, Department of Neurobiology and Anatomy, University of Texas Medical School, Houston, TX 77225-0708, USA

P. McCaffery, Department of Psychiatry, Harvard Medical School, Boston, MA 02115, USA and Eunice Kennedy Shriver Center, Waltham, MA 02452, USA

D.G. McMahon, Department of Physiology, University of Kentucky, Lexington, KY 40436-0084, USA

I.A. Meinertzhagen, Neuroscience Institute, Life Sciences Centre, Dalhousie University, Halifax, NS B3H 4J1, Canada

R.F. Miller, Department of Neuroscience, University of Minnesota, 6-145 Jackson Hall, Minneapolis, MN 55455, USA

S. Mohand-Said, Laboratoire de Physiopathologie Cellulaire et Moléculaire de la Rétine, EMI 9918 INSERM, Université Louis Pasteur and Clinique Médicale A, Hôpitaux Universitaires de Strasbourg, 1 Place de l'Hôpital, 67091 Strasbourg Cedex, France

C. Mora-Ferrer, Institut für Zoologie III, J. Gutenberg Universität, 55099 Mainz, Germany

R. Nelson, Laboratory of Neurophysiology, National Institute of Neurological Disorders and Stroke, NIH, Building 36 Room 2C02, 36 Convent Dr. MSC 4066, Bethesda, MD 20892-4066, USA

J.M. Ogilvie, Fay and Carl Simons Center for Biology of Hearing and Deafness, Central Institute for the Deaf and Department of Ophthalmology and Visual Sciences, Washington University School of Medicine, 4560 Clayton Avenue, St. Louis, MO 63110, USA

S.E. Ostroy, Department of Biological Sciences, Purdue University, West Lafayette, IN 47907-1392, USA

D.R. Pepperberg, Department of Ophthalmology and Visual Sciences, University of Illinois at Chicago, College of Medicine, 1855 W. Taylor St., Chicago, IL 60612, USA

I. Perlman, Bruce Rappaport Faculty of Medicine, Technion-lsrael Institute of Technology, Haifa, Israel

S. Picaud, Laboratoire de Physiopathologie Cellulaire et Moléculaire de la Rétine, EMI 9918 INSERM, Université Louis Pasteur and Clinique Médicale A, Hôpitaux Universitaires de Strasbourg, 1 Place de l'Hôpital, 67091 Strasbourg Cedex, France

L. Ponomareva, Department of Physiology, University of Kentucky, Lexington, KY 40436-0084, USA

M. Pottek, Department of Neurobiology, University of Oldenburg, D-26111 Oldenburg, Germany

H. Qian, Department of Ophthalmology and Visual Sciences, University of Illinois College of Medicine, 1855 West Taylor Street, Chicago, IL 60612, USA

T.S. Rex, Department of Molecular, Cellular and Developmental Biology, University of California at Santa Barbara, Santa Barbara, CA 93106, USA

H. Ripps, Department of Ophthalmology and Visual Sciences, University of Illinois College of Medicine, 1855 West Taylor Street, Chicago, IL 60612, USA

B. Roska, Department of Molecular and Cell Biology, Division of Neurobiology, University of California at Berkeley, Berkeley, CA 94720, USA

J.A. Sahel, Laboratoire de Physiopathologie Cellulaire et Moléculaire de la Rétine, EMI 9918 INSERM, Université Louis Pasteur and Clinique Médicale A, Hôpitaux Universitaires de Strasbourg, 1 Place de l'Hôpital, 67091 Strasbourg Cedex, France

K. Schultz, Department of Neurobiology, FB7, University of Oldenburg, D-26111 Oldenburg, Germany

Y. Shen, Institute of Neurobiology, Fudan University and Shanghai Institute of Physiology, Chinese Academy of Sciences, Shanghai 200433, China

M. Sikora, Department of Neuroscience, University of Minnesota, 6-145 Jackson Hall, Minneapolis, MN 55455, USA

E. Solessio, SUNY Upstate Medical University, Syracuse, NY, USA

K.E. Sorra, Ortho-McNeil Pharmaceuticals, 1000 Rt 202, Box 300, Raritan, NJ 08869, USA

J. Stone, NSW Retinal Dystrophy Research Center, Department of Anatomy and Histology, University of Sydney F13, Sydney, NSW 2006, Australia

K.M. Studholme, Department of Neurobiology and Behavior, SUNY, Stony Brook, NY 11794-5230, USA

W. Thoreson, Departments of Ophthalmology and Pharmacology, University of Nebraska Medical Center, Omaha, NE 68198-5540, USA

D. Tranchina, Department of Biology and Mathematics, New York University, 100 Washington University Square East, New York, NY 10003, USA

L. Wachtmeister, Department of Clinical Sciences/Ophthalmology, Umeå University, SE-901 85 Umeå, Sweden

E. Wagner, Department of Psychiatry, Harvard Medical School, Boston, MA 02115, USA and Eunice Kennedy Shriver Center, Waltham, MA 02452, USA

T. Wagner, Department of Physiology, University of Kentucky, Lexington, KY 40436-0084, USA

R. Weiler, Department of Neurobiology, University of Oldenburg, D-26111 Oldenburg, Germany

F. Werblin, Department of Molecular and Cell Biology, Division of Neurobiology, University of California at Berkeley, Berkeley, CA 94720, USA

P. Witkovsky, Departments of Ophthalmology and Physiology, New York University School of Medicine, 550 First Avenue, New York, NY 10016, USA

S.M. Wu, Cullen Eye Institute, Baylor College of Medicine, 6565 Fannin Street, NC-205, Houston, TX 77030, USA

X.-L. Yang, Institute of Neurobiology, Fudan University and Shanghai Institute of Physiology, Chinese Academy of Sciences, 220 Han-Dan Road, Shanghai 200433, China

S. Yazulla, Department of Neurobiology and Behavior, SUNY, Stony Brook, NY 11794-5230, USA

D.-Q. Zhang, Department of Physiology, University of Kentucky, Lexington, KY 40436-0084, USA

Z. J. Zhou, Departments of Physiology and Biophysics and Ophthalmology, University of Arkansas for Medical Sciences, Little Rock, AR 72205, USA

C.L. Zucker, Boston University School of Medicine, Department of Anatomy and Neurobiology, 715 Albany Street, Boston, MA 02118, USA

Preface

In late August 2000 a Festschrift was held at the Marine Biological Laboratory, Woods Hole, Massachusetts, to celebrate the career of Professor John E. Dowling on the occasion of his 65th birthday. The fact that John's 65th coincided with the dawn of the new millennium made it a particularly propitious time to take stock of the remarkable advances that have been made in retinal biology, many of which we owe to John, his students and his co-workers. In addition, it provided an opportunity to consider the directions one might anticipate retinal research will take in the future. Thus, this special event was notable not only as a celebration of a fine scientist and wonderful human being, but also because it brought together an outstanding group of individuals whose careers were shaped and enhanced through their interactions with John Dowling. The list of about 150 researchers who worked at his side, whether as undergraduate, grad student, post-doc or co-investigator, is not merely impressive, it constitutes the Who's Who of the vision research community, representing institutions in every corner of the globe. All have benefited from John's guiding hand, and his incredible foresight in identifying avenues of investigation where significant advances were to be made. Although there was time to hear from only a limited number of John's many colleagues in attendance, more than 50 of them have contributed chapters to this volume. The appropriateness of the Marine Biological Laboratory as the venue for the meeting is also noteworthy. John has been associated with the MBL for more than 35 years, during which time he has been a member of the Corporation, and a Neurobiology course director. He has served on advisory councils and numerous committees, was a member of the Board of Trustees, and he is currently the President of the MBL Corporation.

The impact of John's research on the field of visual neuroscience has been monumental, and he has championed virtually every aspect of this remarkably diverse discipline. Indeed, there is a striking correlation between the areas of investigation that John pioneered, and those that remain among the most intensively studied to this day. For example, while still a medical student, John was awarded the Soma Weiss prize for his studies on "The biological activity of retinoic acid," a molecule that continues to grow in interest because of its key role in ocular development and intercellular signaling, not to mention its widespread use in dermatology and the cosmetic industry. Thereafter, as a junior investigator in George Wald's laboratory, he described the exchange of retinoids between the visual cells and the retinal pigment epithelium, a vital and seemingly simple process that is still not fully understood. His innovative work on the identification of retinal cell types and their electrical signatures, the structural and functional organization of the retina, and the neuroactive substances that transmit and modulate neuronal signals, provide the foundation upon which we continue to attempt to build a better understanding of the retina and the means by which it analyzes and extracts meaningful information from a complex visual environment. John rightfully refers to the retina as an "approachable part of the brain," and through his exemplary research has set the stage for the subject of this meeting: "Concepts and Challenges in Retinal Biology."

In his charming little volume *Imagined Worlds*, Freeman Dyson makes mention of a rule formulated by his war-time associate, Reuben Smeed. Smeed's Rule says that "you can either get something done, or get the credit for it, but not both." As we know, there are exceptions to every rule, and John is clearly that exception. He has accomplished much, and he has been showered with the accolades and awards he so richly deserves. Among them are the coveted Friedenwald Award of the Association for Research in Vision and Ophthalmology, the Award of Merit of the Retina Research Foundation, and most recently the Helen Keller Prize for Vision Research. In 1976, about the time of his 40th birthday, John was elected to the National Academy of Sciences, and in 1992 to the American Philosophical Society. In the intervening years, John, who chose to abandon medical school for a career in research, was given the title of honorary Doctor of Medicine by the Faculty of Medicine of the University of Lund, Sweden, and in 1987 he was appointed Maria Moors Cabot Professor of the Natural Sciences at Harvard University.

But honors and awards do not reflect fully the influence John has had on young men and women in every walk of life. During his 18-year tenure as Master of Leverett House, John and his lovely wife Judy, who served with equal responsibility as Co-Master, have helped to guide, nurture and counsel thousands of Harvard undergrads. The organization of this Festschrift and the scientific contributions incorporated in this volume are a tribute to John, and they have afforded his colleagues and former students the opportunity to express their admiration and gratitude.

In addition to providing a memento of the occasion, we hope this book will serve as a fund of basic reference material for future researchers in retinal biology. The volume is divided somewhat arbitrarily into seven areas of retinal research containing chapters that present in some cases a broad overview of a particular topic, and in others an account of current research and studies in progress. Although we have attempted to unify each section in terms of the scientific question being addressed, not all chapters fit neatly into one or another of the selected categories, whereas others bridge more than one field of research. Nevertheless, the chapters that follow exemplify the richness, diversity, and excitement of contemporary retinal research. They also remind us of how much more needs to be done before we understand fully the interrelationship between retinal neurons, the complex interactions between neurons and glial cells, and the mechanisms that govern retinal development.

Cellular Organization and Synaptic Circuitry: This section deals with the organization and synaptology of retinal neurons, and includes the classification of their multiple subtypes, the synaptic connections and neural circuits that underlie signal processing within the retina, and the microcircuitry subserving ON–OFF and directionally-selective pathways. Comparative studies of the structure and function of retinas in diurnal vs. nocturnal animals are presented, and some of the interesting parallels that can be drawn between invertebrates and vertebrates regarding strategies for feedforward and feedback interactions are considered. In addition, the specialized neural chains that allow neuromodulators such as dopamine to influence the retinal message are discussed, and recent studies on gap-junctional channels and the effects of nitric oxide and other agents on junctional communication are described.

Functional Organization: The chapters in this section summarize current views on the mechanisms of synaptic transmission, the formation of discrete functional pathways, and the processes by which visual information is encoded into neural signals. The calcium-dependent chemical synapses that regulate signal transmission from photo-receptors to second-order retinal cells are discussed, and a description is provided of the parallel pathways through which various cell types segregate rod- vs. cone-mediated signals, and sustained versus transient responses. Also included in this section is an account of the responses to complex patterns of light stimuli, suggesting how different sublaminae of the inner retina represent selective aspects of the visual image.

Neurotransmission and Neuromodulation: This section considers the physiological and pharmacological properties of retinal neurotransmitters and their postsynaptic receptors, as well as the uptake mechanisms by which transmitter action is terminated. The effects on neuronal responses of several neurotransmitters and neuromodulators that play key functional roles in signal processing are presented, with emphasis on the three amino acids, glutamate, GABA and glycine, that are used at the vast majority of chemical synapses in the vertebrate retina. The special functions of individual synapses are analyzed in terms of the multiple types of postsynaptic receptors through which these neurotransmitters exert their action.

Photoreceptors, Visual Adaptation and the ERG: The chapters in this section address some of the fundamental issues in photochemistry, describe components of the photoreceptor machinery that regulate light- and dark-adaptation, and describe novel approaches in the use of the electroretinogram for the non-invasive study of retinal disorders. Other chapters consider the ambient light levels that determine the adaptive state of the eye, postreceptoral mechanisms governing contrast sensitivity and network adaptation, and the action of Müller cells in regulating the potassium concentration of the neuronal environment.

Circadian Rhythms: Both structural and functional changes in retinal organization are mediated by circadian oscillators that modulate sensitivity in anticipation of daily changes in ambient illumination. This section deals with the nature of these events in vertebrate and invertebrate retinae, the purported loci from which they originate, and the chemical agents that induce and modulate the periodicity of this behavior. Of considerable interest are the functional consequences of the circadian clock on metabolic activity, and its influence in determining the dominance of pathways mediating rod versus cone signals.

Retinal Development and Genetics: The zebrafish is rapidly becoming the animal model of choice for the study of retinal development and genetically-mediated visual system abnormalities. Several chapters in this section discuss gene regulation of development and differentiation in this teleost, and others describe the techniques of screening for visual abnormalities, the molecular approach being utilized to study the various mutants that are identified, and the cellular mechanisms that have been implicated in disease processes. Development of the vertebrate retina can also be studied in mammals, particularly in rodents and rabbits, and included in this section are recent advances on the roles of neurotransmitter systems and cellular activity in early retinal development, and on the regulation by retinoic acid of ocular development and the expression of important retina-specific proteins.

Retinal Degenerations: The genetic basis of retinal degenerations has long been a topic of intensive study. Chapters in this section describe proteins of the phototransduction cascade that have been associated with various forms of retinitis pigmentosa, and the use of animal models as well as organ culture for the analysis of defective retinal function. Evidence is presented of rod–cone interaction as a cause of cell death induced by rod-specific mutations, and trophic factors and other agents that inhibit the degenerative process are discussed. Other chapters deal with the merits of studying canine models of photoreceptor degenerations, novel approaches toward understanding the sequence of cell biological reactions that lead to the pathological changes associated with retinal detachment, and the origins of free radical-mediated oxidative stress in the aging eye and its relation to age-related macular degeneration. The final chapter in this section considers a mechanism by which elevated intraocular pressure causes ganglion cell death presumably by overstimulation of the NMDA subtype of glutamate receptor; the resultant rise in intracellular calcium and its effect on mitochondria can lead, in turn, to the production of free radicals and cytotoxicity.

Reflections and Comments: A final chapter contributed by John Dowling provides an overview of past accomplishments, and offers some future perspectives on retinal research in the 21st century.

There are two appendices in this volume. The first documents all graduate students, postdoctoral fellows, visiting scholars, collaborators, staff and undergraduate senior thesis students of John Dowling's laboratory during the past 35 years. The second appendix shows a collection of historical and recent photographs of retinal researchers.

We are saddened by the loss of three members of the Dowling "family" earlier last year, Brian Boycott, Pat Sheppard and Geoff Gold. This book is dedicated to the memory of these three individuals.

Helga Kolb,
Harris Ripps and
Samuel Wu
October 2000

Acknowledgments

The organization of the volume has been expedited in large part by the cooperation of the contributors, each of whom submitted manuscripts of high quality, and met the stringent deadlines required for rapid publication. We thank Gus Aguirre, Bob Barlow, Dwight Burkhardt, Jim Fadool, Steve Fisher, Bob Miller and Frank Werblin for assistance in editing the chapters, and the Marine Biological Laboratory for providing the lecture theater, technical assistance and ancillary services that contributed importantly to the meeting's success. We wish to express our gratitude to other members of the organizing committee, which included Steffie Levinson, Bob Barlow, Bob Miller and Frank Werblin, and to the many individuals who assisted with the program and ancillary events, in particular Joseph Dowling and other members of the Dowling family, John Burris, Ken Fulton, Phyllis Keller, Judith Murciano, Henry Rosovsky and Art Silverstein. We are especially grateful to Research to Preventing Blindness and Foundation Fighting Blindness and the Marine Biological Laboratory for sponsoring publication of this book. Tom Merriweather, Paul Carton and Maureen Twaig of the Elsevier Press and Alan Hunt of Keyword Publishing Services Ltd have given their invaluable help and enthusiasm throughout its production.

Contents

Introduction

An historical perspective by Robert Miller and Harris Ripps

The chapters in this volume deal with a broad array of topics, representing the remarkable number of research areas to which John Dowling contributed his insight and interpretive powers during his highly productive scientific career. The volume also commemorates the single most creative and productive historical period in biological research, attributable in large measure to the strong postwar support for research funded by the federal government and private foundations. In the past 40 years we have achieved an unparalleled level of understanding about the structural and functional organization of the retina, the principles of sensory transduction, and the cellular and subcellular mechanisms mediating neuronal communication. Perhaps more than any other scientist in the latter half of the twentieth century, John Dowling helped to create this new level of knowledge and forge it into our contemporary views about retina and brain function. Because this compilation of papers documents John's influence on our present understanding of retinal biology, it seems appropriate to provide a brief historical survey of the key events in visual science that set the stage for John's entry into the field, and place in context the range of investigative science he promoted.

John was an undergraduate at Harvard when, in 1956, he elected to do a research project in the laboratory of George Wald, an inspirational teacher and superb scientist. This experience ignited his interest in science, and led him to abandon medicine eventually and enter graduate school, where he obtained his Ph.D. with Wald in 1961. During the early Harvard years he had the opportunity to work with Ruth Hubbard and Richard Cone on photochemical mechanisms of visual adaptation, with Richard Sidman on inherited retinal dystrophy in rats, and with Ian Gibbons on retinal electron microscopy. With each of these co-workers he acquired new skills that he would utilize to the fullest in these and related areas of research.

The discoveries made in his very first studies in Wald's laboratory almost immediately propelled John's reputation into a position of leadership in retina research. Although the basic biochemistry of visual pigments was fairly well known by that time, there was no information as to the role these pigments played in determining visual sensitivity during light- and dark-adaptation. One common assumption was that Weber's Law, the relationship between the level of background (ambient) illumination and the magnitude of the light stimulus necessary to reach visual threshold, was simply a function of the reduced amount of available photopigment as the background light intensity increased. On this view, a two-fold rise in threshold occurred when 50% of the visual pigment had been bleached. But John showed that this was patently wrong. By raising rats on a vitamin A deficient diet, and feeding them vitamin A acid (retinoic acid) to maintain them in reasonably good health, John was able to relate retinal sensitivity, using the electroretinogram, to the rhodopsin concentration in the eye.

What John discovered was that pigment concentration was correlated with the *logarithm* of the visual threshold, indicating that the rise in visual threshold is far greater than can be accounted for by the loss of quantal absorption. In other experiments, John discovered that if the rhodopsin content of the normal eye was substantially depleted by a bright adapting light, the recovery of log visual sensitivity followed the regeneration of rhodopsin over its full time course, thereby accounting for the classic dark adaptation curve first reported in humans. On the other hand, if the eye had first been exposed to a weak background light that significantly raised visual threshold but bleached a trivial amount of photopigment, the dark adaptation curve showed a rapid fall in threshold with no detectable change in visual pigment concentration. This phenomenon was termed "neural" adaptation to distinguish it from the "photochemical" adaptation observed following intense light stimulation that bleaches a significant fraction of the visual pigment. The two different components of visual adaptation would continue to interest Dowling and his colleagues throughout his career, and some of his work with Harris Ripps, done in the summers at the MBL, was devoted to the mechanisms of adaptation and their role in retinal function. Today, we understand that at least part of the neural adaptation process occurs in the photoreceptors themselves, but there are clearly post-receptor adaptation mechanisms, some of which are only now beginning to be elucidated.

Although John's initial studies dealt primarily with visual photochemistry, his love of the history of science led him to the monumental work of Ramón y Cajal published more than a century ago. Using the silver staining technique described earlier by Camillo Golgi, Cajal was the first to appreciate that the retina is a true nervous center, and a tissue from which one could learn fundamental concepts of brain organization and function. He identified the major cell types in the retina, formulated ideas about the functional polarization of nerve cells, and appreciated the fact that in the retina one knew in which direction the information was moving, something that you could not intuit when looking, for example, at the Purkinje cells of the cerebellum. Cajal also identified amacrine cells as axonless cell types, but was unable to speculate on their role in retinal processing. In Dowling's early exploration of the ultrastructure of the retina, he identified the numerous dendrodendritic synapses which amacrine cells make, as well as their feedback, feedforward, and serial synaptic connections.

Retinal research from the time of Cajal up to the 1960s focused largely on the biochemistry of visual pigments pioneered by George Wald, the electroretinographic studies of Ragnar Granit, and the single unit recordings from the *Limulus* lateral eye performed by H.K. Hartline. The work of these three vision researchers, who later shared the Nobel Prize, and the innovative psychophysical studies of Selig Hecht on the quantum sensitivity of the retina, and those of W.S. Stiles on light- and dark-adaptation greatly advanced the field of retina research. During this period, Hartline recorded the impulse activity of the single fibers he painstakingly dissected from the frog's optic nerve, Barlow and Kuffler discovered that ON- and OFF-center cells have antagonistic surrounds, and later work by Enroth-Cugell and Robson showed that in the cat retina these can be segregated into X and Y subtypes based on whether the response is sustained (X) or transient (Y). The elucidation of the complexities in the center-surround organization of ganglion cell receptive fields points to a spatial organization that cannot be accounted for by a simple wiring structure of the retina, confirming Cajal's contention that the retina is a processing nerve center and does not treat visual space as would a simple camera.

Many other important studies emerged during the latter part of this period. J.Y. Lettvin and his colleagues at M.I.T. were the first to demonstrate that stimuli which would be of behavioral interest to a frog, such as a moving fly, strongly activated a subset of ganglion cells in the animal's retina. These findings prompted other workers to study receptive field properties using more varied stimuli, including moving targets and differently shaped objects. Indeed, this concept led to studies by Barlow and Levick that first revealed the presence of directionally-selective cells in the rabbit retina, and the approach that Hubel and Weisel would later take in studying receptive fields in the cortex of the cat and primate. It was already well established from earlier anatomical and psychophysical work that the photoreceptor population was species-variant; some animals had rich color vision capabilities, while for others with less well-developed cone systems, color was a less important visual cue. However, the physiological data argued for species differences in retinal processing as well. In animals like the frog, which lack binocular vision, the retina handles a great deal of visual information processing, whereas in primates a comparatively greater proportion of their visual processing machinery resides in the visual cortex. Thus retinal processing in primates consists mainly of mechanisms for contrast enhancement and the segregation of rod–cone pathways; binocularity and more demanding discriminations are dealt with by the complex and hypercomplex cells of the visual cortex.

In 1964, as these new lines of investigation were emerging, John joined the Ophthalmology Department at Johns Hopkins, and it was there that John's research career gathered momentum. He was given spacious laboratory facilities where he could accommodate a number of trainees, and he quickly acquired a national reputation for excellence in research. His easy-going manner, leadership qualities, and productive research program began to attract an outstanding group of students and postdoctoral fellows, among them Gus Aguirre, Dwight Burkhardt, Richard Chappell, Mark Dubin, Robert Frank, Helga Kolb, Robert Miller, George Weinstein, Frank Werblin and Paul Witkovsky.

At about this time John shifted his attention from photoreceptor mechanisms to an analysis of retinal structure and function, and he began a lifelong, fruitful collaboration with Brian Boycott, whose work with the Golgi technique had provided new insights into the organization of the retina at the level of the light microscope. Although the Golgi method enabled one to visualize the fundamental cell types of the retina, their interactions through chemical synapses and gap junctions required ultrastructural identification and classification. This involved the use of high resolution electron microscopy, just emerging as a powerful method for interpreting the structural features and synaptology of the nervous system. The light- and electron-microscopic studies of Dowling and Boycott, and their subsequent work with Helga Kolb, remain to this day among the most definitive accounts of the structural organization of the primate retina. John's move to Hopkins also marked the beginning of a new phase in his research career, which included summer trips to Woods Hole, where he began a fruitful and productive collaboration with Harris Ripps. They produced a significant body of work on the adaptive properties of the all-rod skate retina and forged a working relationship that continues to this day. John also did electrophysiological work on *Limulus* in Woods Hole and produced new findings related to the transduction mechanism of the *Limulus* lateral eye. Interest in the invertebrate visual system would continue to capture his attention, particularly when he worked with Richard Chappell and later Ian Meinertzhagen on the dragonfly eye.

Comparative studies of the retina and the need to account for species differences in the degree of retinal processing continued to be of great interest to John. In collaboration with Max Cowan, he identified by electron microscopy the centrifugal fibers in the pigeon retina and showed that they terminated primarily on amacrine cells, and with his student Mark Dubin, John compared the synaptic neuropil of the frog with that of primates. They concluded that the additional complexity of retinal processing in the frog could be accounted for by the relatively greater ratio of amacrine to bipolar synapses; i.e., the simple retina of the primate had relatively few amacrine cell synapses, whereas the retina of the frog achieved its greater complexity with more amacrine synapses. This idea remains as viable today as when it was first stated, and with the discovery of inhibition in the retina, attributed largely to amacrine cells, this view continues to provide a plausible basis for species differences in retinal processing. However, more recent observations, suggesting that ribbon synapses of bipolar cells have multiple active zones for synaptic vesicle release compared to amacrine synapses, may impact on the ultimate interpretation of this observation.

Our understanding of how the retina processes information lagged far behind our knowledge of the outcome of these interactions (ganglion cell output) for many years. The reasons for this were simple. Among the retinal neurons, only ganglion cells could be reliably studied with extracellular electrophysiological techniques. To study preganglionic neurons, the more difficult technique of intracellular recording was required, and reliable methods for obtaining cell penetration and stable recordings from retinal cells had not yet been achieved. All that was to change in the decade of the 1960s. Svaetichin had earlier produced the first intracellular recordings from fish horizontal cells, and Tomita, using superfine microelectrodes and the ingenious "jolting" technique he had developed, accomplished the feat in the cones of the carp retina. It was now clear that some neurons in the distal retina generate slow, graded potentials, but no one had yet described in a systematic way the response patterns of the full complement of neurons in a vertebrate retina. Recordings from the smaller retinal neurons seemed unattainable until the landmark studies of Werblin and Dowling in the mudpuppy, a beast with a tiny eyeball containing a retina with relatively large neurons. Not only did they record from every cell type in this vertebrate retina, they incorporated within the electrode a visible dye so that the cell from which a recording was made could be filled and later identified microscopically to verify the cell type, its anatomical characteristics, and its location within the retinal laminae.

This achievement typifies John's attitude and approach to science. Rather than focus on the difficulty of a research problem, which can sometimes be paralytic, John's approach has been to focus on the solution, and determine the most likely road to a successful outcome. If the problem seems intractable, John takes the view that it has not been tackled with sufficient intensity, or conceivably, in the right species. So if the cells of the retina are too small, find an animal with large cells, and the retina of *Necturus* seemed ideally suited for this approach. The results reported in two 1969 publications with his graduate student Frank Werblin are widely considered the most defining work in retinal neurocircuitry of the last half of the twentieth century. In these two papers, the basic outline of the functional anatomy and neurophysiology of the retina was established, and a plausible model of the interactions which formed the receptive fields was established. In addition to having recorded from and marked every basic cell type, they identified two types of bipolar cells (hyperpolarizing and depolarizing) which, logically, formed the basis of the ON- and OFF-center responses of ganglion cells; they demonstrated the presence of an antagonistic surround in the bipolars, implying that their connections with ganglion cells would provide the center-surround organization that Kuffler had described; and they showed the transient spike activity of amacrine cells, most of which responded both to the onset and offset of illumination. Although nothing was known about the neurotransmitters which were utilized by the different cell types, and the distinction between excitation and inhibition was yet to be discovered, the work of Werblin and Dowling provided the single most important advance in our understanding of the structural and functional organization of the vertebrate retina.

A few years after the Werblin and Dowling work, Müller and Dowling, who continued to work on the mudpuppy retina, published their observations suggesting that the b-wave of the ERG was generated by the Müller cells of the retina, the prominent, radial glial cells that are similar to astrocytes. Although this general conclusion has recently been challenged, these early observations elevated the Müller cells to a research status equivalent to that of the neurons and served to stimulate a great deal of fruitful insights into the many roles which we now understand the Müller cells to play in retinal function and homeostasis.

In 1971, John was given the opportunity to return to Harvard, and eager to return to his roots and engage in undergraduate teaching as George Wald had done before him, he accepted a full professorship in the Department of Biology. The decade of the 1970s ushered in a new era in retinal physiology and anatomy. While many details of retinal neurocircuitry would continue to be filled in, attention shifted to the mechanisms by which neurons communicate. At the time, little was known about synaptic transmission in the retina and brain. Two inhibitory neurotransmitters, γ-aminobutyric acid (GABA) and glycine, had been associated with inhibition in the CNS, but inhibition in the retina was not discovered until the mid-1970s and virtually nothing was known about excitatory neurotransmitters or other substances that would be identified subsequently as "modulators." One of the first key steps towards understanding intercellular signalling between retinal neurons was to determine the nature of the photoreceptor neurotransmitter and its effect on second-order neurons. An important contribution came from Dowling and Ripps in their *Nature* paper of 1973, where they showed that blocking synaptic transmission with high Mg^{++} caused the horizontal cell to hyperpolarize and lose its ability to respond (hyperpolarize) to light. Since both transmitter blockade and photic stimulation cause the cell to hyperpolarize, the only possible explanation for their finding was that the photoreceptor released an excitatory transmitter in the dark that depolarized the horizontal cell: light reduced the rate of transmitter release and caused the horizontal cell to hyperpolarize. In a similar way, the photoreceptor transmitter caused one bipolar tissue to hyperpolarize (OFF) and the other to depolarize (ON) on stimulation with light. The basis for the two channels of OFF and ON bipolar pathways was discovered to be a result of ionotropic and metabotropic receptor channels respectively, by one of John's first postdoctoral students Robert Miller with his colleague, Malcolm Slaughter. In this work, the first metabotropic glutamate receptor in the whole central nervous system was characterized and later identified as mGluR6.

Immunohistochemistry now provided a new way of identifying neurotransmitters, and in a relatively short time, a large array of transmitter candidates, including many peptides, were localized to different neurons and proposed as possible neurotransmitters. As the search for neurotransmitters emerged as a central topic, Dowling began a collaboration with Berndt Ehinger, in which dopamine-containing interplexiform cells were identified in the goldfish and *Cebus* monkey retinas. The discovery of the interplexiform cell, which provided a feedback pathway from the inner to the outer retina, added to the level of complexity in retinal processing. However, dopamine is not confined to interplexiform cells. It is also present in a subtype of amacrine cell, and showing its presence in the retina proved to be one of the most important discoveries of the 1970s, helping to establish the concept of neuromodulation. Accordingly, neuromodulation was served by substances which did not form the main transmission pathway through retinal circuits, but could modulate the activities of these cells and pathways. The numerous ways in which neuromodulation effects are mediated has helped to open an entire branch of cellular physiology of second messenger systems collectively known as cellular transduction. John also demonstrated that dopamine was coupled to adenylate cyclase in the retina in work with Keith Watling and Leslie Iversen in 1979, a finding which opened up an entire new field of inquiry as to the action of dopamine in retinal neurocircuitry. And with Van Buskirk, Dowling showed that isolated horizontal cells show a dopamine-dependent accumulation of cAMP.

At about this time, the search for more conventional neurotransmitters was underway and evidence that glutamate was the transmitter of photoreceptors and bipolar cells emerged. In addition, inhibition was discovered in the 1980s and both glycinergic and GABAergic inhibitory mechanisms were shown to be present in the retina, which distinguished the retina from many other CNS sites where typically one or the other tends to dominate. Work with Ariel, Lasater and Mangel showed that isolated horizontal cells in the fish retina were sensitive to glutamate and aspartate and their agonists, and work with Bloomfield in the rabbit revealed that glutamate and/or aspartate played a role in both outer and inner retinal processing in the rabbit retina.

In another seminal finding, Lasater and Dowling showed in the mid-1980s that electrical coupling between isolated pairs of fish horizontal cells was modulated by dopamine and cAMP. This work revealed how gap junctions could be synaptically modified, and the modulator concept for dopamine went into high gear. Later, in a paper with Knapp, Dowling found that dopamine enhanced excitatory amino acid-gated conductances in cultured horizontal cells, which was the first demonstration of the modulation of ligand-gated channels, and thus provided another important link between dopamine and the control of cellular mechanisms. Additional studies by Knapp, Schmidt and Dowling demonstrated that dopamine altered the kinetics of ion channels gated by excitatory amino acids in horizontal cells, and thus provided a functional link between dopamine and its effect on ion channel conductance. Work with Mangel and later with Yang and Tornqvist showed that dark adaptation led to an uncoupling of horizontal cells and implicated dopamine as playing an important role in postreceptoral light–dark mechanisms.

In the 1990s, as the work on neurotransmitters and neuromodulators intensified, John shifted his research into a new phase incorporating molecular biology and animal behavior. Taking advantage of the rapid reproductive capacity of zebrafish, John began to study how mutations modified visual sensitivity and behavior in zebrafish, and he and his students began to identify genes that were important in regulating visual behavior. In this approach, sometimes referred to as functional genomics, one attempts to identify genes responsible for behavioral patterns and then analyzes where and how the gene works to affect the behavior of the animal. With Brockerhoff, Li and others, behavioral screening tests for isolating zebrafish mutants with visual defects were developed, based on the oculomotor and escape responses of the animal. An ultraviolet visual pigment in zebrafish was identified in 1993, and with Hyatt, Marsh-Armstrong and Schmitt, the importance of retinoic acid as an essential element for development of the zebrafish retina was established. Today, studies of functional genomics in the zebrafish are forming an important new avenue in physiological research, and undoubtedly, this area of investigation will provide a further venue for fruitful progress in John Dowling's lifetime quest to fully understand the visual system.

SECTION I

Cellular organization and synaptic circuitry

H. Kolb, H. Ripps and S. Wu (Eds.)
Progress in Brain Research, Vol. 131

CHAPTER 1

Cellular organization of the vertebrate retina

Helga Kolb[1,*], Ralph Nelson[2], Peter Ahnelt[3] and Nicolas Cuenca[4]

[1]*John Moran Eye Center, University of Utah, Salt Lake City, Utah 84132, USA*
[2]*National Institute of Neurological Diseases and Stroke, NIH, 36/2CO2, Bethesda, MD 20892, USA*
[3]*Department of Physiology, University of Vienna, Vienna, Austria*
[4]*Department of Biotechnology, University of Alicante, Alicante, Spain*

Introduction

Back in the early 1960s we considered the retina to be composed of just five basic nerve cell types held in place by radial glia. Although we knew that the great spanish anatomist Ramon y Cajal had described many more than these types in his treatise on the vertebrate retina (1892), we were trying to simplify the myriad cell classification and unlock the puzzle of their synaptic connections. It was at this time that John Dowling played a pivotal role in our thinking. He suggested that two major information processing pathways existed in the retina, by recognizing vertically flowing connectivity via ribbon synapses, and lateral interconnections, via local circuitry and conventional synapses. This was at a time when researchers were still arguing about how to tell a rod from a cone synapse and how to distinguish bipolar from amacrine synapses in the neuropils of the plexiform layers. Dowling initiated the concept of "simple retinas" where most of the information was thought to be processed via the former connectivity and "complex retinas" where the latter connectivity was more involved. The simple/complex organization divided species' visual systems into those that did most of the visual processing in the retina (complex retinas) or most of the visual processing in higher brain centers (simple retinas). Although we have discovered the organization of

various retinas to be not quite so simple any more, these concepts have contributed enormously to our present state of knowledge.

So, as we stand at the brink of the new century, we have an extensive understanding of the organization of the retina and this understanding is probably still greater than for any other sensory area of the brain. We realize that there are parallel streams of preprocessed information passing from the retina to the brain for higher perceptual processing. Physiological and pharmacological investigations have revealed the specializations of these parallel pathways for visual contrast, visual adaptation, acuity, color, low light sensitivity and movement detection. The anatomical circuits underlying these information pathways are also largely known and the varieties of morphological types of cells involved is fairly complete. We now understand there to be about 70 different morphological types of nerve cell in the vertebrate retina. Throughout vertebrate phylogeny, a continuous thread of the same neural types are present in all retinas. In some retinas, specialization of cell types for motion and direction detection and color contrast have occurred. In other retinas, the system is perfected for the animal to operate at low light levels: sensitivity is enhanced at the expense of color and high acuity performance. Yet all these species have the same sets of neurons with similar morphologies. The following chapter will attempt to summarize the various neural elements of the retina, the manner in which they are arranged in

* Corresponding author: Helga Kolb, Tel.: 801-585-6510; Fax: 801-585-1295; E-mail: helga.kolb@hsc.utah.edu

mosaics often related to the topography of the retina, and the significance of stratification to allow specialized pathways of information transfer to the final common pathways, ganglion cells.

Cell types of the retina

First order neurons: Photoreceptors

The photosensitive cells of the retina are rods and cones. Most retinas are considered duplex in that they exhibit both types of photoreceptor. Cone photoreceptors were probably the first photoreceptor types in evolutionary history (Walls, 1942), and the rods are later-developed, transmuted cones, a sequence still present in embryonic development. Individual vertebrate species experienced photic selection pressures that led to specializations in photoreceptor populations and mosaics. In highly diurnal visual systems, the cones are dominant with relative lack of rods. Thus in birds and reptiles, 6 different varieties of cones are present and only one type of rod (Fig. 1a). First there are double cones consisting of a long principal member and shorter accessory member. In vitamin A2-based visual pigments typically found in fresh water fishes and turtles the double cones contain the 620 nm pigment but the principal cone houses an orange oil droplet below the outer segment. The presence of this oil droplet pushes the sensitivity of the cone into the far red. Two single cones contain red oil droplets and 620 nm visual pigments and yellow oil droplets and the 540 nm pigment respectively. A single 460 nm short wavelength cone (blue) contains the greenish oil droplet that fluoresces in UV light and an ultra-violet sensitive cone contains a colorless oil droplet (Kolb and Jones, 1987). The cones have short axons and end in synaptic pedicles often stacked in two tiers in the outer plexiform layer (birds and reptiles) (Kolb and Jones, 1982; Mariani, 1987). Rods (500 nm pigment) are rare, and cone-like in morphology but lack an oil droplet (Fig. 1a). Their synaptic region is also cone like in being an enlarged pedicle continuous with the cell body without an axon. Oil droplets are not seen in cone photoreceptors of mammalian retinas except for prototherian mammals, i.e. marsupials, that have retained some oil droplet bearing

cones and double cones in some parts of the retina (Ahnelt et al., 1995).

Fish typically have the 6 cone types including the double or twin cones (depending on species), and short wave cones around which a striking mosaic is organized, often with double cones (usually 625 and 535 nm pigments) at the corners (Marc, 1999). Amphibians also have double cones of different pigment varieties (618 and 520) and two types of single cone (618 and 432). Interestingly, where fish have mixed rod and cone retinas, and rods are small and narrow with small synaptic terminals very like mammalian rods, amphibian rod photoreceptors have become enlarged and dominate in proportions in the retina. These huge rods are further subdivided into two wavelength sensitivity types known as the red rods (520 nm) and green rods (432 nm).

By the time early mammals evolved from their reptilian therapsid ancestry, the visual pigments were vitamin A1-based and varied over a 409–568 nm wavelength sensitivity range. The retina had also become specialized into a rod dominated retina with little differences in topography of the retina from center to periphery, exemplified by rodents and insectivores today. These mammals were almost certainly nocturnal or fossorial and most species have retained that adaptive radiation. Species becoming adapted to diurnal conditions concentrated their cone dominated visual apparatus to central retinal areas such as foveas and visual streaks. Most mammals have two types of cone with visual pigments sensitive to the red/green and blue end of the spectrum. In other words most mammals are deuteranopes with dichromatic color vision. The short wavelength cone with sensitivity at the 450 nm peak is the cone type that runs as a constant thread throughout retinal evolution from fish to trichromatic primate vision (Ahnelt and Kolb, 2000).

Cone photoreceptors in mammalian retinas have a typical morphology of short conical outer segment, large mitochondria-filled ellipsoids of the inner segment and a long axon projecting to a conical flat-based cone pedicle or synaptic terminal in the outer plexiform layer (Figs. 1b, 2a and b). The cone pedicles contain from 8 to 40 synaptic ribbons directing vesicles filled with glutamate, the photoreceptor neurotransmitter, to two horizontal cell dendrites and one invaginating cone bipolar dendrite

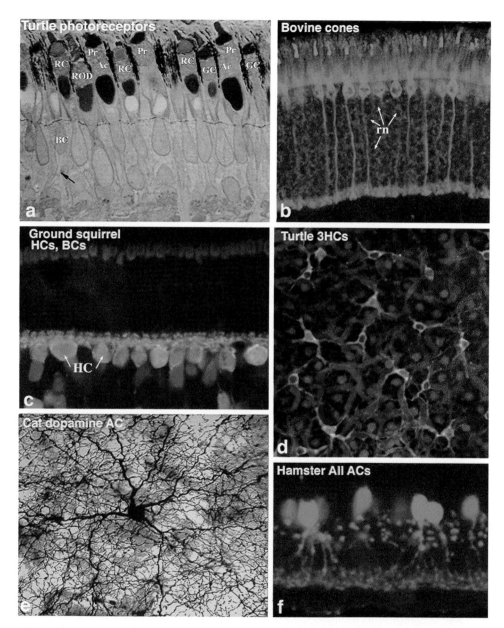

Fig. 1. (a) Toluidine/methylene blue stained 0.5 μm section of turtle retina to show the different photoreceptor types and their distinguishing oil droplets. RC, red single cone; ROD, rod; GC, green cone; Pr, principal member of the double cone; Ac, accessory member of the double cone; BC, blue cone. Arrow shows the oblique axon of the blue cone. (b) Bovine retina to show the cones immunostained with guanylate cyclase activating protein (GCAP1, green). rn, rod nuclei. (c) Double immunostained ground squirrel retina to show the horizontal cells (HC, arrows) colocalizing calretinin (fluorescein/green) and calbindin (rhodamine/red) and bipolar cells stained with one or the other immunostain. (d) Wholemount view of turtle retina double immunostained to calretinin and nNOS. H1 cells and axons contain calretinin (red). H2 cells are double labeled with calretinin and nNOS (orange cells) and H3 cells are single labeled for nNOS (green cells). (e) Cat dopaminergic amacrine cell immunostained for Tyrosine hydroxylase (TOH) as seen in wholemount. The cell is large-bodied and has a plexus of overlapping dendrites from neighboring cells running in S1 of the IPL and forming rings of processes around other varieties of amacrine cell bodies. (f) The AII amacrine is parvalbumin-IR in rodent retinas. This rod pathway amacrine is characterized by lobular appendages in sublamina **a** of the IPL and varicose dendrites in sublamina **b** of the IPL.

6

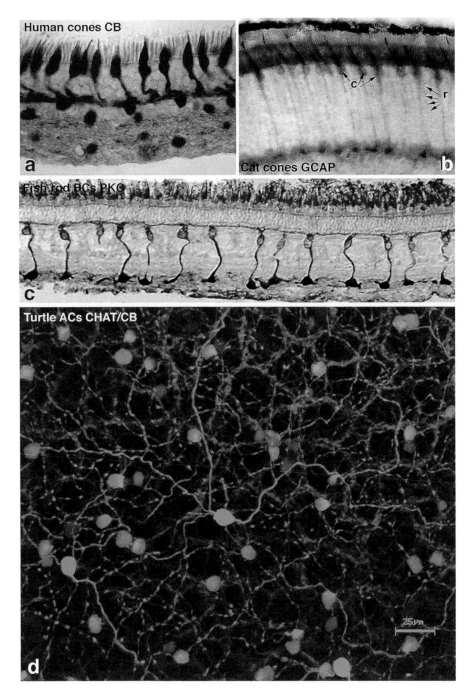

Fig. 2. (a) Section of peripheral human retina immunostained with calbindin (CB). Cones, H2 horizontal cells and amacrine cells are clearly CB-IR. (b) The small thin and infrequent cones of the cat retina are easily seen when immunostained with GCAP1. The inner and outer segments of the rods are less strongly GCAP1-IR. (c) Carp retina stained with antiserum for protein kinase C (PKC) shows intense labeling of the large ON center Mb bipolar cell type. (d) Wholemount of turtle retina immunostained for calbindin (CB) and choline acetyl transferase (CHAT). A wide-field amacrine cell is strongly immunolabeled for CB alone (green cells and dendrites), while the CHAT-IR cells colabel with CB (orange cell bodies) but their dendrites form a plexus of processes in a deeper plane of focus. Scale bar = 25 μm.

(the ribbon triad, Dowling and Boycott, 1966). Other bipolar cell dendrites make flat or basal junctions on the surface of the cone pedicle. The calcium binding protein calbindin is present in all but the blue cones in most retinas (Fig. 2a, human retina). Typically mammalian cones form one layer of cell bodies arranged below the outer limiting membrane. Their size varies from small slender and rod-like, so that they are difficult to distinguish from the overpowering mass of rods in nocturnal species (Fig. 2b, central cat retina), to large and sturdy with clear differences from surrounding rods in diurnal species (Fig. 1b, bovine central retina, 2a, human peripheral retina). In diurnal squirrel retinas the tables are turned so that the rods are scarce and difficult to distinguish from the equally sized and shaped, dominant cone photoreceptor population (Fisher et al., 1976) (see Linberg et al. chapter in this volume).

Rods in most mammalian species (squirrels have exceptional rods, see later chapter by Linberg et al.) are small in cell body and long and slender in inner and outer segment architecture. Their shape is maximized for high density packing in both depth and laterally between the solid and regular spacing of the cone photoreceptors. Their outer segments are particularly long and thin to reach high into the pigment epithelial layer, where in contrast, cone photoreceptors typically allow the long apical pigment epithelial sheath to come down around the outer segment and encapsulate it with a thick glycoprotein layer (Bunt, 1980; Steinberg et al., 1977). Rod axons vary in length dependent on the tier the cell body sits in (Fig. 1b rn, arrows) and end as small rod spherules, stacked up above the cone pedicles at the outer plexiform layer. Each spherule is characterized by 1 to 2 synaptic ribbons directing vesicular output to a small number of postsynaptic dendrites (two horizontal cells and 2 rod bipolar dendrites).

Cones are concentrated at a specialized central temporal area of the retina in many mammalian species, i.e. at an area centralis, or at a linear horizontal specialization of the retina known as a visual streak. These areas of cone and cone pathway concentration push the rod system and low light vision information processing to the peripheral parts of the retina and are instead specialized for high visual acuity, movement detection and form discrimination. When the area centralis is further concentrated and rod photoreceptors and pathways are excluded altogether, a foveal based visual system is developed. This occurs in the highly diurnal primate species where cone vision has evolved high spatial acuity and trichromatic color vision. Foveation follows or results in a large degree of binocular overlap, frontal looking vision and sophisticated eye-hand coordination for the species. Topography of the photoreceptor mosaics in fact establishes the subsequent parallel pathways of information flow to the brain.

Second order neurons: horizontal cells and bipolar cells

The secondary and tertiary pathways of the retina have become specialized for the predominant photoreceptor type. In nocturnal mammals, rods dominate and rod selective secondary neurons are developed at the expense of cone pathway neurons. In diurnal species the cones dominate and second order neurons and pathways specific for color and high acuity are developed.

Horizontal cells are the second order neurons interconnecting photoreceptor terminals laterally across the plane of the retina. They function to modulate the vertical pathways from photoreceptors to bipolar cells in both a feedback and feedforward manner. Horizontal cells have varying morphologies adapted to deal best with particular cohorts of photoreceptors. There are two types of horizontal cells in duplex dichromatic retinas to service rods and cones and in species where color processing is a feature of a retina, they may be further subtypes with color specific connections. Figure 3 illustrates the range of morphologies of horizontal cells across different species and the functional channels with which they are associated. Horizontal cells concerned solely with light intensity changes and shaping adaptational and spatial responses of vertical pathway neurons are Type 1 cells (Fig. 3). They can often be identified with antibodies against calcium binding proteins (Fig. 1c, ground squirrel, Fig. 1d, wholemount turtle retina, Fig. 2a, Human) (Cuenca et al., 2000a). Their bushy dendrites contact all cones in their vicinity and their axon terminals collect

8

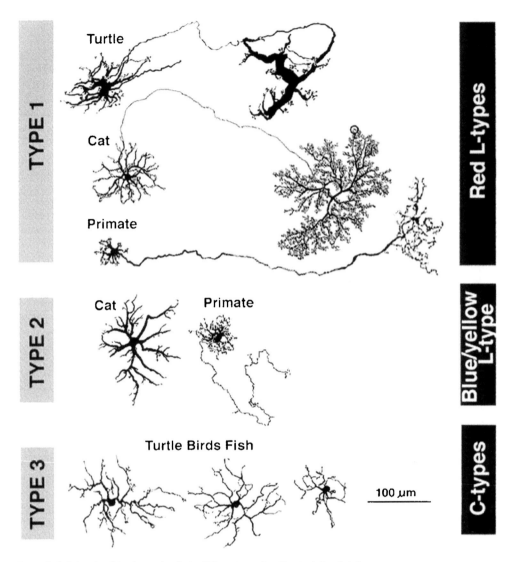

TYPE 1

Turtle

Cat

Primate

Red L-types

TYPE 2

Cat   Primate

Blue/yellow L-type

TYPE 3

Turtle Birds Fish

100 μm

C-types

Fig. 3. Drawings of Golgi stained horizontal cells in different species. See text for details.

information from large numbers of rods in general. The lengths of the axons of luminosity horizontal cells are thought to electrically isolate a cone photoreceptor-involved compartment of the cell from the rod photoreceptor-involved compartment (Nelson et al., 1975). In species where there are few rods (Fig. 3, Turtle) the axon terminal has sparse terminals but is coupled to others with great extents of gap junctions so forming a syncytium of cells influencing huge areas of the outer plexiform layer. Such cells have feedback synapses to rods and feedforward synapses to both their cone dominant

cell body and to other horizontal cell types in turtle (Kolb and Jones, 1984) partially resembling the synaptic contact patterns of H1 cells of other terrestrial vertebrates (Dowling and Werblin, 1969; Lasansky, 1978; Mariani, 1987). Teleost fishes appear to have different patterns of synaptic contacts (Marshak and Dowling, 1984) many of which may be to glycinergic interplexiform cell processes (Marc and Lam, 1981).

GABA is found in Type 1 horizontal cells (Fig. 9a, Turtle H1 cells and axon terminals). GABA is one candidate for the inhibitory feedback or feedforward neurotransmitter to photoreceptors (Marc, 1992; Watt et al., 2000) possibly acting via a calcium independent, reverse transport mechanism (Schwartz, 1999) and at $GABA_A$ receptors on the respective postsynaptic structures (Vardi et al., 1998) (Fig. 5a). An alternate feedback theory involving the gas nitric oxide (NO) has also been suggested recently (Savchenko et al., 1997). NO is thought to have an action on vesicular fusion and enhances calcium influx into cones via cGMP-gated channels in the horizontal cell cone interface. However, it must be emphasized that the actual mechanism for horizontal cell fast feedback still remains a mystery.

Type 2 and Type 3 horizontal cells are typically large, stellate cells, lacking axons, that are concerned solely with cone pathways. In many species with good color vision (but not in primates) such cells respond to color contrast. Thus in turtle (pentachromats) and fish (trichromats), Type 2 and 3 horizontal cells connect to green and blue cones or solely to blue cones (Fig. 3, C-types) (Stell and Lightfoot, 1975; Leeper, 1978). Their physiological responses are biphasic (red/green opponent) and triphasic (blue/green opponent) to spectral stimulation and a cascade feedback model has been postulated to explain their response patterns (Stell and Lightfoot, 1975; Kamermans et al., 1991). The C-type horizontal cells of the turtle can be labeled with antibodies to nitric oxide synthase (Fig. 1d, turtle H2 cells, orange; turtle H3 cells, green) (Cuenca et al., 2000a), again affirming a role for NO in possibly feed-back plasticity (Savchenko et al., 1997) or in regulating the gap junctional complexes that link them in syncytia across the outer plexiform layer (Lu and McMahon, 1997). In mammals, the axonless A-type horizontal cells found in rabbit and cat retinas, and the H2 cell of primates (Fig. 3, Type 2, blue/yellow 1-types) have some attributes of the reptilian and avian Type 3 cells (Peichl and Boycott, 1998). They are axonless or short axon cells and connect with long and short wave cones but with particular selectivity for blue cones in some species (human, monkey: Ahnelt and Kolb, 1994; Dacey et al., 1996; cheetahs: Ahnelt et al., 2000). A neurotransmitter candidate, apart from the NO mentioned above, has not been identified yet for either Type 2 or Type 3 cells, although all horizontal cells are driven by photoreceptor glutamate release via AMPA receptors.

Bipolar cells are the second-order vertical channels of communication between photoreceptors of the outer plexiform layer and ganglion cells of the inner plexiform layer. There are between 9 and 15 different types of bipolar cell depending on the species and the organization of its photoreceptor mosaic (Fig. 4). Non-mammalian species typically have bipolar cells that connect to both rods and cones but some varieties are more rod dominant than others (Fig. 2c Mb rod bipolar cells of the fish retina) (Scholes, 1975). Of the many bipolar types in fish and turtles some may be particularly specialized for color coding and thus, like the Types 2 and 3 horizontal cells, have specific spectral arrangements (Fig. 4 color bipolar cells of fish and turtle) (Scholes, 1975; Ishida et al., 1980; Haverkamp et al., 1999).

The mammalian bipolar cells have split specifically into one rod and 6–7 cone types (Fig. 4, primates). In foveate retinas with high acuity demands on the visual system, a specialized pair of bipolar cells has developed to provide a single cone connectivity to a single ganglion cell (Polyak, 1941; Boycott and Dowling, 1969; Kolb et al., 1969). These are the midget bipolar cells (Fig. 4, acuity cells, primate). Such midget bipolar cells may also be present in birds (Fig. 4, pigeon acuity cells) and ground squirrel retinas (not illustrated, but see Linberg et al. this volume) (Mariani, 1987; Linberg et al., 1996). Midget bipolar and midget ganglion cells will clearly carry a single spectral message to the next stage of color processing in the visual system.

A color opponent message is carried to ganglion cells by one or more cone bipolar cells in the species with good color vision like turtle and fish retinas (Fig. 4) due to contacts with the two spectrally apposed cones (Haverkamp et al., 1999). In primates, midget bipolar cells connecting to red or green cones and blue specific bipolar cells exist (Fig. 4, color, BB) (Mariani, 1984; Kouyama and Marshak, 1992). Primates may also have another truly blue/yellow opponent cell like the turtle and fish retinas (Fig. 4, GBB cell) (Kolb et al., 1997a).

Bipolar axons stratify at different depths of the inner plexiform layer (Fig. 4). In general there is at least one bipolar cell type for every one of the five strata of the inner plexiform layer described by Cajal (1892). In fish and turtle retina the inner plexiform layer is even further laminated to accept more than

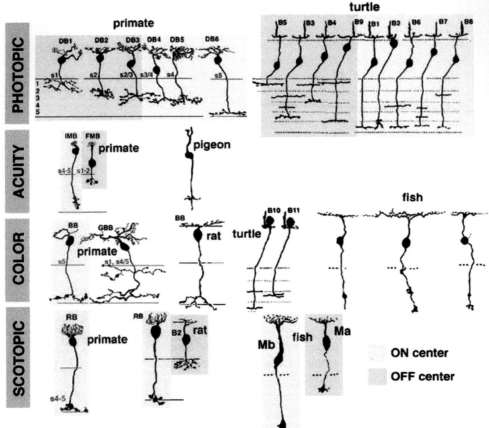

Fig. 4. Golgi stained appearances of bipolar cells in different species' retinas. Lighter shading indicates ON center types, darker shading indicates OFF center types. See text for more details.

one bipolar per stratum and, moreover, such bipolar axons are often bi- or tristratified (Fig. 4) increasing the numbers of ganglion cell types they may interact with.

The multiple strata of the inner plexiform layer, be they 5 or more, are broadly divisible into two functionally different sublaminae a and b. Sublamina a is distal to the ganglion cells and nearest the amacrine cell bodies, and encompasses strata 1 and 2 of Cajal (1892). It is here that OFF center bipolar cells terminate and drive OFF center ganglion cells (Fig. 6, top schematic, as it was demonstrated first in cat retina) (Nelson et al., 1978). Sublamina b includes the proximal 3 strata of Cajal's nomenclature, i.e. S3-5, and this is where ON center bipolar cells end and drive ON center ganglion cells (Fig. 6, top schematic) (cat retina, Nelson et al., 1978). This general

organization of the IPL into the OFF and ON center bipolar to ganglion cell connectivity has been confirmed in all other vertebrate retinas and appears to be a fundamental principle of visual system organization.

Photoreceptors, bipolar cells and ganglion cells are glutamatergic in all vertebrate retinas (Marc et al., 1990; Ehinger et al., 1988). Neuroactive agents such as the calcium binding proteins recoverin, calbindin and calretinin and protein kinases are also found in specific types of bipolar cell (e.g. the large rod/cone mb bipolar of fish retina, Fig. 2c) (Cuenca et al., 1993; Kolb and Zhang, 1997). The ON center (center depolarizing to light) and OFF center (center hyperpolarizing to light) responses of bipolar cells are initiated by sign-inverting and sign-conserving synapses respectively at their dendritic contacts with

11

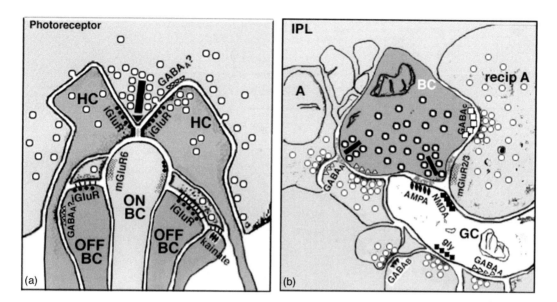

Fig. 5. (a) The organization the photoreceptor synapse to ON bipolar (ON BC), OFF bipolar (OFF BC) dendrites and to horizontal cell dendrites (HC). The distribution of synaptic vesicles, synaptic ribbon and synaptic basal junctions are shown with the present evidence for receptor molecule distributions. (b) The organization of the bipolar cell (BC) axon synapses to amacrine (A) and ganglion cells (GC) in the IPL. The present evidence for the occurrence of receptors at the various synapses is shown. See text for details.

photoreceptors. The present knowledge concerning the types of glutamate and other receptor types occurring at the cone pedicle in the vertebrate retina is shown in Figure 5a. Depolarizing, ON center bipolar cells contact photoreceptors usually at deeply invaginated ribbon related synapses (Kolb et al., 1969) with metabotropic glutamate receptors on their dendrites (Fig. 5a) (Slaughter and Miller, 1981; Nomura et al., 1994; Vardi et al., 1998). OFF center bipolar cells contact photoreceptors at basal junctions (not ribbon related usually) (Kolb et al., 1969) and the postsynaptic receptors are AMPA/ kainate ionotropic types (Fig. 5a) (Slaughter and Miller, 1983; Vardi et al., 1998; Brandstatter et al., 1997; DeVries and Schwartz, 1999). Both ON and OFF bipolar cells drive their respective ON and OFF ganglion cells in the respective **b** and **a** sublaminae of the IPL (Fig. 6, top schematic). Figure 5b also indicates the types of receptor that are involved with cone bipolar axon terminals in the various strata of the IPL, and the manner in which amacrines and ganglion cells are driven via AMPA/Kainate and NMDA glutamate receptors (Wässle, et al., 1998; Qin and Pourcho, 1999a,b; Cai and Pourcho, 1999; Koulen et al., 1998; Fletcher and Wässle, 1999).

Third order neurons: Ganglion cells

Ganglion cells are the final common pathway output neurons of the retina carrying the visual information that has been processed to varying degrees, dependent on species, by the neurons of the retina (i.e. the "simple" versus "complex" retinas). Ganglion cells are spiking neurons that transmit messages by depolarizing spike trains to the next stage of visual processing in the brain. Many physiological and anatomical studies have attempted to understand ganglion cells over the last half century but we are still only brushing the surface of our knowledge concerning their coding of the visual message. We have a near complete understanding of ganglion cell morphology throughout the vertebrate species and their projections to the brain nuclei (Rodieck, 1998, 1999). We begin to understand these cells' coverage of visual space, arrangement in mosaics across the retina (Fig. 6b and c), specific connectivity in OFF center and ON center tiers of the IPL with the neurons that drive them (Fig. 6a) (bipolar cells and amacrine cells) and the synaptic input, channel characteristics and receptors (AMPA, NMDA, GABA_A, GABA_B ionotropic glycine, peptides and

12

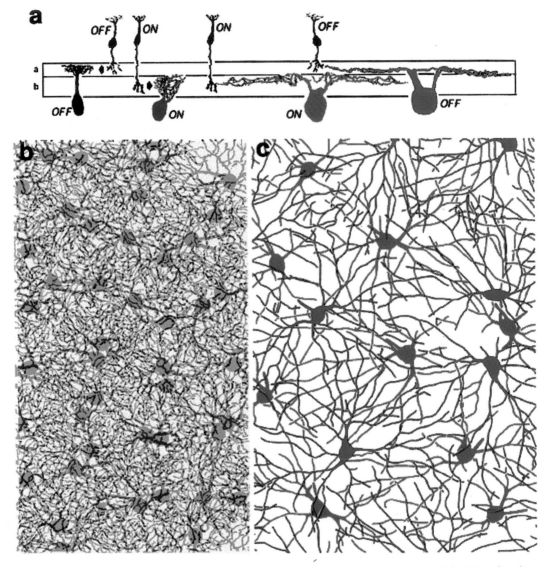

Fig. 6. (a) The organization of the bipolar and ganglion cell contacts segregate into discreet sublaminae of the IPL as first demonstrated in cat retina (Nelson et al., 1978). Thus, OFF center bipolar cells contact OFF center ganglion cells (black beta cell, blue alpha cell) in sublamina **a**, while ON center bipolar cells contact ON center ganglion cells (red beta cell and red alpha cell) in sublamina **b**. (b) The mosaic of overlapping dendrites of OFF center beta cells (grey cells and dendrites) and ON center beta cells (red cells and dendrites) to show dense coverage of visual space by the plexi of dendrites. (c) Similarly the alpha cells of the cat retina are arranged in two plexi of ovelapping dendrites, one consisting of OFF center cells (blue cells) and the other of ON cells (red cells). Modifield from Wässle, Peichl and Boycott, 1981a.

amines) (Fig. 5b) of some of the simplest ganglion cell types.

An important aspect of ganglion cell architecture is the arrangement of their dendrites in the OFF and ON center sublaminae of the IPL so that they will be driven either by OFF center bipolar excitation or ON center bipolar excitation (Fig. 6a). This ensures that they will be preferentially driven by stimuli darker (OFF) or brighter (ON) than the mean background luminance. This fundamental sensory discrimination compensates for the non-linearities in increments and decrements imposed by impulse initiation. In all species, ganglion cells concerned with interpreting fast, transient movements and images coming in from peripheral fields, important as warning signals, are carried by large bodied thick axoned ganglion cells with the fastest conduction velocities. Typically they exhibit huge dendritic trees to cover a lot of visual space (Fig. 7, phasicity cells). Such cells collect from many cone receptors by way of wide-field ON and OFF center bipolar and amacrine cells, the latter often linked by electrical junctions. The rod system also uses intermediate amacrine cells that collect from large numbers of rod bipolar cells for enormous convergences of dim light messages before output to large-field ganglion cells. In contrast ganglion cells that are concerned with high acuity have the narrowest dendritic fields, and collect from the smallest numbers of photoreceptors (even only from one cone in the case of the midget ganglion cell) (Fig. 7, acuity).

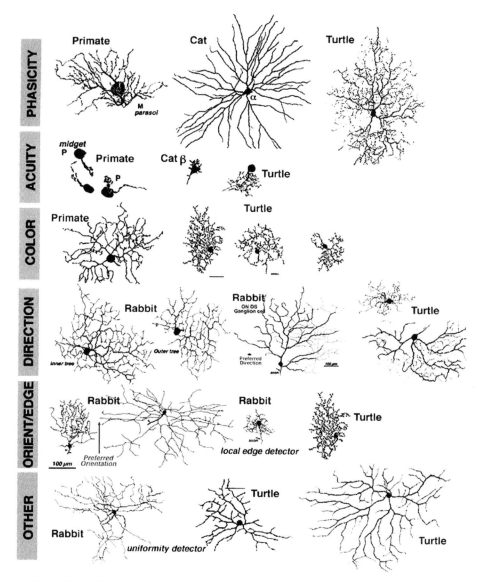

Fig. 7. Drawings of ganglion cells as seen in wholemount view after staining with various techniques such as Golgi and HRP intracellular injections (some of the turtle and rabbit ganglion cells). See text for full description.

Cells such as these are concentrated in the area centrales or foveas of retinas where this important function has evolved (birds, some reptiles, carnivores and primates).

The detection of color requires differential discrimination of signals coming from separate spectral classes of cones. In retinas of species with color vision, double opponent ganglion cells can achieve this (fish, amphibians, birds and reptiles) (Daw, 1967, 1968; Spekreijse et al., 1972; Raynauld, 1972). The color-coded ganglion cell types, that have been identified by intracellular recordings and stainings in non-primate retinas, typically have medium field dendritic tree sizes, and are bistratified to receive ON and OFF center complimentary color specific inputs through cone selective bipolar cells (Fig. 7 color cells, turtle) (Ammermüller et al., 1995; Ammermüller and Kolb, 1996). A blue ON/yellow OFF opponent ganglion cell also occurs in primates (Fig. 7, color cells) (Dacey and Lee, 1994). The midget ganglion cells of the primate retina will, because of connection with a single cone through its midget bipolar cell chain, of necessity also carry a color biased center signal. Furthermore, midget ganglion cells are concentrically organized with color opponent surrounds to their centers (Gouras, 1968). Either horizontal or amacrine cell signals shape the midget ganglion cell surround response, but there is, in fact, no way that the surround can match the center. Midget ganglion cells driven by red cones will always have surround signals that, though probably not pure green, possess spectral weightings shorter that the pure red center and visa versa for the green center driven midget ganglion cell. It appears that the midget ganglion cell chromatic signals remain segregated until they reach the visual cortex where they contribute to spectrally double opponent cortical responses (Gouras, 1991).

Ganglion cells that detect the direction of prey or predator entering the visual field are particularly well developed in retinas that have a visual streak topography (rabbits, frogs, turtles and squirrels). All the neural cell types of the retina are packed closely along a linear area of the retina stretching the length of the horizontal meridian. Second order neurons as well as ganglion cells typically have elongated, elliptical dendritic trees (Fig. 7), have oriented receptive fields and the ganglion cell response is maximally sensitive to orientations or directions of movement orthogonal and parallel to the visual streak. The ganglion cells concerned with directional selectivity (DS) come in ON, OFF or ON–OFF types as seen in their responses to static stimulation (Fig. 7 Rabbit ON DS cell) (Amthor et al., 1984, 1989a; Ammermüller and Kolb, 1996). In most species directional selective ganglion cells are wide-field and known to be driven by special circuitry involving bipolar cells and GABA- and acetylcholine-containing amacrine cells (Famiglietti, 1991; Vaney, 1994; Vaney and Pow, 2000). In the turtle retina more than 50% of the ganglion cells are responsive to motion and direction. Small field types are also included (Fig. 7, Turtle DS cells) (Ammermüller and Kolb, 1996).

One of the goals of retinal research is to find anatomical counterparts of classical feature detection in ganglion cell types such as attempted originally by Lettvin and coauthors (1959) in the frog's eye. We know that orientation- and edge-detector ganglion cells have an oriented morphology along one of the two preferred axes of the eye (Amthor et al., 1989b). Such cells as uniformity and dimming detectors are large field monostratified cells. Some ganglion cells concerned with transmitting information about eye position, circadian rythms and light cycles are also being discovered to have special morphologies (Rodieck, 1998; Pu and Amthor, 1990; Berson et al., 1999; Pu, 1999). Ganglion cells in different species retinas may indeed have strong biases for particular attributes of the visual message, i.e. color, contrast, motion, but recent physiological recordings in turtles and mammals indicate that ganglion cells transmit all of the various attributes to a greater or lesser extent. We now consider that the visual message is better interpreted by the brain from a large, often synchronized set of responses from a consortium of ganglion cells (Brivanlau et al., 1998; Normann et al., 2000).

Third order neurons: amacrine cells

The majority of amacrine cells are inhibitory interneurons. Similar to interneurons in the CNS, amacrines function to control the excitatory pathways of the retinas 'principal neurons' bipolars and ganglion cells. They provide a pathway for both narrow and wide field lateral interactions within the IPL. Inhibitory amacrine cells have been known for a long time to be involved in the formation of directional selectivity (Wyatt and Daw, 1982). Other amacrine cell types may be concerned with spatially constricting the ganglion cells receptive field centers by constructing a strong inhibitory surround (Werblin, 1991; Cook and McReynolds, 1998) and yet others, such as AII cells in mammals, may contribute to ganglion cell centers (Kolb and Nelson, 1996). In the rod pathways through the retina, AII amacrine cells function to increase phasicity and speed up the ganglion cell message to the brain (Nelson, 1982).

Amacrine cells have as diverse a morphology as ganglion cells. The same general types of amacrine cell are found across all the species although in some retinas specific varieties are more numerous and subdivided into multiple subtypes, e.g. birds and turtles have more varieties of radiate wide-field amacrine cells, multiplied because of the thicker substrata of the IPL in such "complex" retinas (Fig. 2d, wide-field amacrine cells immunostained to calbindin, green cells). In mammalian retinas, certain amacrine cells, not seen in non-mammalian retinas, have evolved to take care of the dichotomy of the rod and cone systems (Fig. 1f, AII amacrine cells immunostained to parvalbumin; Fig. 8, AII, A17) (Kolb and Famiglietti, 1974; Kolb, 1997; MacNeil and Masland, 1998).

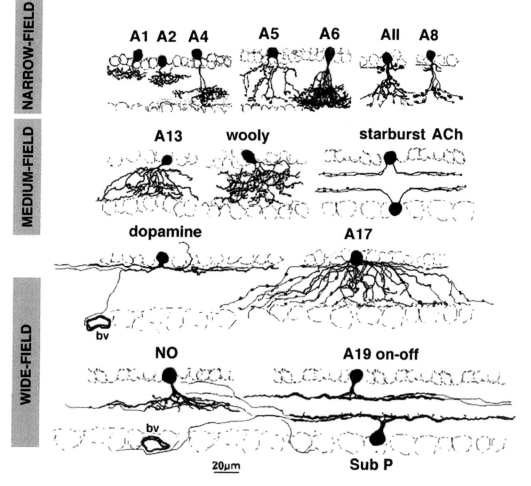

Fig. 8. Drawings of the morphologies of amacrine cells of the mammalian retina. See text for details.

Figure 8 shows some varieties of amacrine cells in the human retina. Very similar appearing types are seen in monkeys, rats, cats and rabbits. Non-mammalian retinas also have similar narrow-field bushy amacrine cells as shown in Fig. 8, usually with rather vertically spread dendrites and complex intertwined dendritic trees (Fig. 10e, Mudpuppy cell, arrow upper right). Such amacrine cells are known to tile the retina rather than overlap their trees (Fig. 1f, AII amacrine cells). They are, thus, extremely numerous in the retina. Most narrow-field amacrine cells are found to contain the inhibitory neurotransmiter glycine (Pourcho and Goebel, 1985; Kolb, 1997; Haverkamp et al., 2000). Two of the narrow-field amacrine cell types are bistratified in the mammalian retina although many bistratified types occur in non-mammalian retinas. The bistratified AII and A8 cells (Fig. 8) are specialized for carrying rod (AII) and cone (A8) signals back and forth between ON and OFF cone bipolar cells and influencing ganglion cells by small-field local circuitry (Kolb and Famiglietti, 1974; Kolb and Nelson, 1996; Dacheux and Raviola, 1986; Strettoi et al., 1992). The medium field amacrine cell types (Fig. 8) are also seen in all species (see example of a medium-field amacrine cell in the mudpuppy retina, Fig. 10e). A13 and starburst amacrine cells contain the inhibitory neurotransmitter GABA. Furthermore the starburst amacrine cells are consistent across all species. We know of no retina that does not contain the mirror-symmetric starburst (Famiglietti, 1983), acetylcholine-containing amacrine cells, the one type arranged in the OFF layer and the other in the ON layer of the inner plexiform layer (Figs. 8, 9d, c and f; and see chapter by Linburg et al. in this volume) (Masland and Tauchi, 1986; Masland, 1988).

Wide-field amacrine cells are common to all vertebrate retinas. Typically, wide-field cells are monostratified to one of the five or more strata of the inner plexiform layer, have tremendous overlap of their dendritic trees between neighbors, are often linked by gap junctions, and have unique axon-like processes extending far across the retina (Figs. 8, A19 cell). Their axons may pass to different layers of the retina (Vaney, 1990). Dopamine cells (Fig. 1e) and interplexiform cells send processes to the OPL. Peptide-containing, substance P (SP) amacrine cells send axons into the nerve fiber cell layer (but not to

the optic nerve) (Kolb et al., 1991; Cuenca and Kolb, 1998) thus causing an erroneous interpretation of them being ganglion cells (Peterson and Dacey, 1998) (Fig. 8). Although a subset of substance P ganglion cells projecting to the accessory optic system does indeed exist in both rabbit and turtle retinas (Brecha et al., 1987; Cuenca and Kolb, 1998). Some wide field amacrines even have axon-like processes that wrap around blood vessels in mammalian vascularized retinas (Fig. 8, dopamine cell, NO cell and Substance P cell). One variety of wide-field amacrine (Fig. 8, A17) cell in the rod dominated mammalian retinas is diffusely branched throughout the IPL but concentrates its synaptic interaction to feedback circuits, through $GABA_C$ receptors, at rod bipolar cell terminals in the ON (sublamina **b**) neuropil of the inner plexiform layer (Fig. 5b) (Nelson and Kolb, 1985). Another variety of wide-field amacrine cell splits into many branches in stratum S4 and has a medium-field dendritic tree away from which radiate many long axon-like processes (Dacey, 1988). It contains NO synthase in the primate retina (Fig. 10b, NADPH-diaphorase cell) (Cuenca, unpublished). Similar large-field morphological varieties of amacrine cells exist in non-mammalian species (Fig. 10d, salamander amacrine cells). Such axon-bearing amacrine cells are invariably GABAergic even where amines, peptides and gases are also present (Pourcho and Goebel 1983; Freed et al., 1996; Haverkamp et al., 2000; Deng et al., 2001). Moreover, amacrine cells in salamander and fish retinas have been demonstrated to contain, both common inhibitory neurotransmitters (GABA and glycine), and several varieties of amines or peptides simultaneously (Marc et al., 1990; Watt et al., 1993; Deng et al., 2001).

Mosaics of cells and plexi of dendrites

Immunostaining techniques or injections of neurons of the retina with Lucifer dyes often reveal complete populations of the same type of neuron distributed in mosaics across the extent of the retina. The first retinal neurons to be revealed as such a population were horizontal cells in fish retina where Procion and Lucifer dyes had spread from neighbor to neighbor through the gap junctions that join such cell types in syncytia (Kaneko, 1971). Since then we have come to

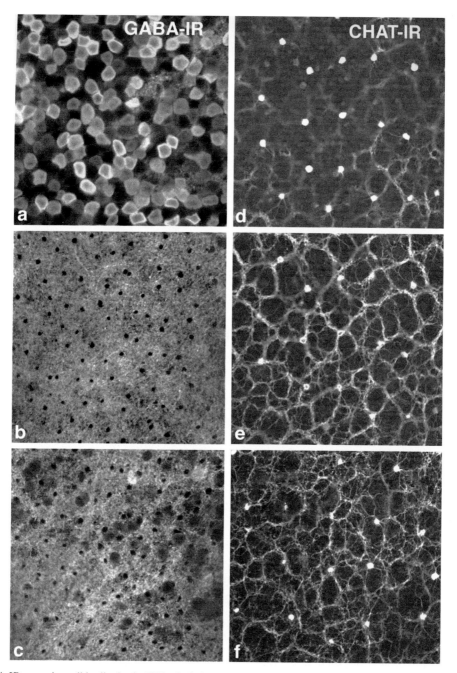

Fig. 9. (a) GABA-IR amacrine cell bodies in the INL of wholemount salamander retina. Many cells are GABA-IR. (b) The first dense plexus of GABA-IR amacrine dendrites are seen at a lower plane of focus in S1 of the IPL. The holes in the plexus are where Muller cell processes pass through the neuropil. (c) The second dense plexus of overlapping dendrites from the GABA-IR cells lies at a deeper plane of focus in S5 of the IPL. Two GABA-IR displaced amacrine cells are visible beneath the plexus in the ganglion cell layer (top right corner). (d) CHAT-IR amacrine cells (starburst cells) are evenly spaced in the INL in turtle wholemount retina. (e) The first CHAT-IR plexus belonging to the cells in (d) are in focus at the S1/2 border of the IPL. (f) The second plexus of displaced starburst cells dendrites at the S3/4 border is visible and the cell bodies of the cells that give rise to these plexi of overlapping dendrites are seen below in the ganglion cell layer.

18

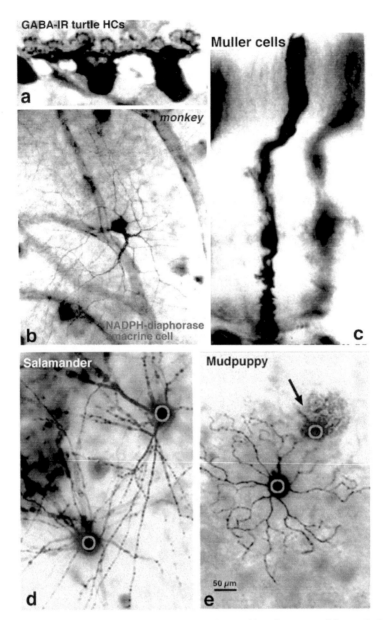

GABA-IR turtle HCs

a

monkey

b

NADPH-diaphorase amacrine cell

Muller cells

c

Salamander

d

Mudpuppy

50 µm

e

Fig. 10. (a) GABA-IR H1 horizontal cells of the turtle retina. HRP-peroxidase immunostaining technique. (b) An amacrine cell is stained by the histochemical reaction to reveal NADPH-diaphorase in the monkey retina. The cell type is a multi-axoned type stratifying in S3 of the IPL. (c) A Golgi stained Muller cell in vertical view of the cat retina. (d) Two wide-field amacrine cells stained with a vital dye and Lucifer yellow in salamander retina. The cell bodies are the size of the white circles and not the bright and enlarged size of the halo. (e) One small-field amacrine cell and one medium-field amacrine cell in the mudpuppy retina stained by the same Lucifer yellow and vital dye technique as in (d). Both (d) and (e) are courtesy of Robert Miller.

understand that horizontal cells in all species are connected by gap junctions between neighbors of the same type only, i.e. homotypic coupling (Vaney, 1991). This circumstance has taught us much about

the manner in which electrical synapses between retinal neurons can be modified by neuroactive agents, such as catecholamines and NO. In addition it has taught a great deal about the arrangement of neurons into regular mosaics with plexi of over-lapping, and perhaps interacting, dendrites contribut-ing uniquely to the different layers of the retina.

The two major ganglion cell types of the cat retina, the alpha and beta ganglion cells, are organized into beautiful mosaics with their dendrites overlapping in the OFF or ON sublaminae of the IPL (Fig. 6b and c) (Wässle et al., 1981a, b). Similar overlapping tiers of dendrites occur for other ganglion cell types like the bistratified directionally selective ganglion cells in rabbit retinas (Amthor et al., 1984). It is into these plexi of ganglion cell dendrites that bipolar cell axons and amacrine cell processes are arranged and make their synaptic contacts.

The dopaminergic cells of mammalian retinas have a striking plexus of overlapping fine dendrites and axonal processes at the outer boundary of the IPL (Fig. 1e). Their dendrites and axons are strategically placed around the bases of AII and A8 amacrine cells primarily, there to make synapses (the "rings" seen in Fig. 11e), probably with release of both dopamine (Jensen and Daw, 1986; Critz and Marc, 1992; Wellis and Werblin, 1995; Kolb et al., 1997b) and GABA. Moreover, the cells release dopamine by volume transmission for diffusion through the inner nuclear layer to the outer plexiform layer (Pourcho, 1982; Wässle and Chun, 1988; Dacey, 1988; Kolb et al., 1991; Witkovsky et al., 1993; Yazulla and Studholme, 1995). Dopaminergic amacrine cells in all species are thought to be driven primarily by GABAergic amacrine input at $GABA_A$ receptors, and commu-nicate at D2 receptors amongst themselves.

Besides revealing the dopamine cells, immuno-cytochemical techniques applied to wholemount retinas coupled with examination by confocal micro-scopy has been able to reveal various other neuro-chemically marked populations of cells in the retina. We know from older techniques and sectioning and imaging techniques (Marc et al., 1978; Marc, 1992) that GABA is the neurotransmitter of approximately 50% of the amacrine cells in all vertebrate retinas and glycine that of the other 50%. Although GABA is found in amacrine cell processes distributed through-out the IPL (Marc and Liu, 2000), frequently two rather prominent bands of GABA-containing processes can be seen running at the outer and inner borders of the IPL, corresponding perhaps to interweaving of many wide-field GABAergic

amacrine processes in these positions. Fig. 9a–c shows these GABAergic plexi of immunostaining in the salamander retina as seen in wholemount views. Many varieties of amacrine contain GABA in salamander (Fig. 9a, GABA-immunoreactive cell bodies in the inner nuclear layer of the salamander retina). Below the cell bodies lies a thick plexus of GABAergic processes leaving only a few holes for passage of Muller cell radial processes (Fig. 9b). Another plexus of GABAergic processes lies above the ganglion cell bodies at the inner border of the inner plexiform layer (Fig. 9c). Amacrine cells such as illustrated in Figure 10d would have the dendritic trees for such plexi. In the rod dominated mammalian retina, the inner GABAergic plexus is constructed primarily of A17 rod amacrine cell processes (also known as indoleaminergic amacrine cells in rabbit retina) (Fig. 8) (Masland, 1988) that make reciprocal synapses at rod bipolar terminals (Fig. 5b) (probably at $GABA_C$ receptors) (Fletcher and Wässle, 1999, and see chapter by Qian, in this volume).

The mirror symmetric cholinergic amacrine cells present in all vertebrate retinas also have tremendous overlap of their dendrites and are organized into two architectural frameworks of the IPL (Fig. 9d, e and f). The normally placed CHAT-immunoreactive amacrine cells (Figs. 2d, 9d) are extremely regularly arranged with little variation in intercell distance and contribute the lacunate plexus of dendrites at the S1/S2 border in the IPL (Fig. 9e). The displaced mirror image group of CHAT immunoreactive amacrine cells (Fig. 9f) contribute a similar lacunate plexus to the S3/S4 border of the IPL. The examples seen in Fig. 9 are from the turtle retina (Cuenca et al., 2000b) but similar arrangements and plexi of CHAT containing dendrites are seen in all other vertebrate retinas and particularly dramatically so in rabbit where these cells were first described (Masland and Tauchi, 1986; Vaney, 1990; Vaney and Pow, 2000). Cholinergic amacrine cells are some of the earliest neurons to appear in the retina during the course of development (Feller et al., 1996; Zhou, 1998). Their influence on establishing the ON/OFF sublamination of the IPL may be pivotal in the formation of retinal and consequent geniculate architecture, because they have taken their place in the neuropil of the IPL at the time that bipolar cell axons are meeting ganglion cell dendrites. The latter are sorting themselves

20

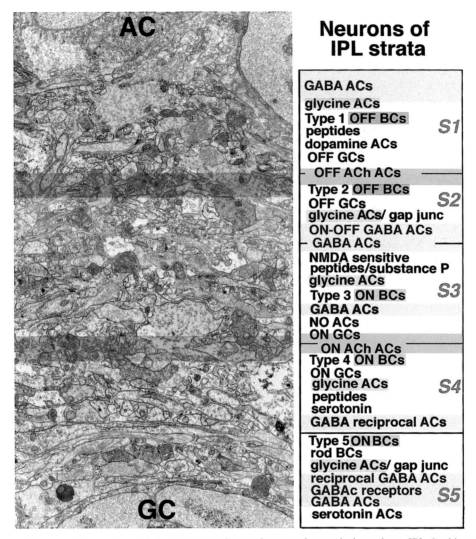

Neurons of IPL strata

GABA ACs	
glycine ACs	
Type 1 OFF BCs	
peptides	**S1**
dopamine ACs	
OFF GCs	
— OFF ACh ACs —	
Type 2 OFF BCs	
OFF GCs	**S2**
glycine ACs/ gap junc	
ON-OFF GABA ACs	
— GABA ACs —	
NMDA sensitive	
peptides/substance P	
glycine ACs	
Type 3 ON BCs	**S3**
GABA ACs	
NO ACs	
ON GCs	
ON ACh ACs	
Type 4 ON BCs	
ON GCs	
glycine ACs	**S4**
peptides	
serotonin	
GABA reciprocal ACs	
Type 5 ON BCs	
rod BCs	
glycine ACs/ gap junc	
reciprocal GABA ACs	
GABAc receptors	**S5**
GABA ACs	
serotonin ACs	

Fig. 11. Summary of the neural elements and their neurotransmitter assignments in a typical vertebrate IPL. In this case the electron micrograph is of salamander IPL, with amacrine cell bodies (AC) at the top and the ganglion cells (GC) at the bottom of the image. To the right is shown the strata of the IPL in the micrograph and the types of processes that are found within these strata. S1 and S2 are OFF center strata where OFF center bipolar axons (OFF BCs) and OFF center ganglion cell dendrites (OFF GCs) make contact. The inner three strata 3–5 are ON center and contain axons and dendrites of bipolar and ganglion cells respectively (ON BCs, ON GCs). OFF acetylcholine-containing amacrine cells (OFF ACh ACs) and ON ACh ACs are shown as pink plexi of processes. Putative glycinergic amacrine dendrites are large lobular processes colored green, occurring throughout the IPL. GABA-IR dendrites are usually arranged in thinner wide-ranging profiles and enlarged beads at bipolar terminals (yellow profiles). Typically ON-OFF ACs are found at the borders of ON and OFF strata and are GABAergic dendrites. Other neurochemical substances contained in various amacrine cell dendrites are shown.

into ON-center and OFF-center stratification levels, pruning their dendritic trees according to synaptic experience and establishing the major lightness and darkness information channels in the brain (Cook and Chalupa, 2000).

Let us not forget the glial cells of the retina

Three basic types of glial cell are found in all vertebrate retinas. They are Muller cells, astrocytes and microglia. All were described originally by

Cajal (1892) but the full realization of their important role in the development, architecture, ionic buffering, scavenging and neurotransmission in the retina in health and disease has only been appreciated in the last 20 years or so (Newman and Reichenbach, 1996, for review). Muller cells are the principal glial cell of the retina, astrocytes are functional components of the nerve fiber layer and microglia are immune system derived elements that react upon nervous system injury or infection. Muller cells are the architectural support glia stretching radially across the thickness of the retina and forming the limits of the retina at the outer and inner limiting membranes. The morphology of the Muller cell is well demonstrated in Golgi staining (Fig. 10c) or immunostaining with antibodies to vimentin, glial fibrillary acidic protein (particularly in diseased states, see chapter by Fisher, this volume) and taurine (Marc et al., 1998). Muller cell processes insinuate themselves between cell bodies of the neurons in the nuclear layers and envelope groups of neural processes in the plexiform layers. Dendrites and axons are only in direct contact, without enveloping Muller cell processes, at their synapses.

Muller cells are important for K+ buffering of the environment surrounding synapses (Newman and Reichenbach, 1996), transporting excess glutamate from the synaptic areas (Brew and Attwell, 1987) and for GABA transport in mammalian retinas (Marc, 1992) thus modulating neural activity (Newman and Zahs, 1998). They have electrical responses to light stimulation in a slow depolarizing manner which suggested originally that they were important components of the electroretinogram recorded from the eye (Miller and Dowling, 1970; Karwosky and Proenza, 1977).

Nor interplexiform cells

Two types of interplexiform cells are present in most vertebrate retinas. They were first discovered in 1969 (Ehinger et al., 1969) and called adrenergic neurons in the fish retina. Later similar cells were seen in cat retina and given the unique name "interplexiform cell" by Antonio Gallego (1971) to denote their dendritic branching in both outer and inner plexiform layers. Other authors characterized the interplexiform

cells (IPCs) more fully (Boycott et al., 1975; Dowling and Ehinger, 1975; Kolb and West, 1977) and assigned neurotransmitter candidates to them: in fish one type of IPC is dopaminergic (Dowling and Ehinger, 1975) and the other glycinergic (Marc, 1995). In cat and most mammals the IPC is GABAergic (Pourcho and Goebel, 1983). There was initially confusion between the dopaminergic and the GABAergic interplexiform cells, until it was discovered that the dopaminergic variety synapses upon horizontal cells in fish OPL, whereas the GABAergic IPC is presynaptic primarily to rod bipolar cell dendrites in mammalian OPL. The dopaminergic cell in most vertebrate retinas is an amacrine cell with few or no processes in the OPL and its major source of synaptic interplay takes place in stratum 1 of the IPL (Fig. 1e) (see also chapters by Linberg et al., Marshak and Yazulla et al., in this volume).

The importance of layering of the IPL

Figure 11 summarizes the present knowledge of the organization of the inner plexiform layer of the vertebrate retina (salamander in this case). This neuropil layer is the culmination of neural processing underlying the visual channels that converge to form the ganglion cell response. A five stratified division of the neuropil was proposed by Cajal (1882) as a result of his morphological studies on different branching levels of bipolar, amacrine and ganglion cell processes. Superimposed on the five strata of organization is a broader subdivision into the neuropil that drives OFF-center ganglion cell responses (sublamina **a**, S1 and S2) and the neuropil that drives ON-center ganglion cell responses (sublamina **b**, S3, S4 and S5) (Fig. 11). The two cholinergic amacrine dendritic plexi lie squarely in the center of sublamina **a** and sublamina **b** forming a consistent framework to the IPL neuropil (Fig. 11, pink bands) on either side of which are arranged various neural profiles that interact with either the OFF or the ON center ganglion cell dendritic trees (Fig. 11). Glycinergic amacrine cells are spread fairly uniformly throughout all strata of the IPL and typically produce large varicose dendritic profiles (Fig. 11, green profiles) making synapses upon bipolar axons and ganglion cell dendrites (Fig. 5b). GABAergic amacrine cell processes are also fairly evenly distributed but occur often in thinner intertwined processes and in varicosities clustered at bipolar axon terminals (Fig. 11 yellow profiles). Dopamine tends to be restricted to amacrine cells that ramify at the inner nuclear/inner plexiform layer border (Fig. 11, in S1), in mammalian species, but in teleosts and reptiles may be tristratified, often with extensive branches to the OPL (Dowling and Ehinger, 1975; Kolb et al., 1997). Their position is strategic for influencing both inner and outer plexiform layers by diffusion of dopamine from their dendrites. Similarly peptidergic and serotonergic amacrine cells are placed at various levels of the IPL usually in combination with GABAergic amacrine cells in the major GABA plexi (Fig. 11). The rod A17 GABAergic amacrine (in mammals) is particularly well developed as a reciprocal amacrine cell with dendritic influence on ON-center bipolar terminals (Fig. 5b) (Fig. 11, S5, yellow).

Summary and future directions

What we have learned about retinal neural circuitry since John Dowling was a student in George Wald's lab, places us at a crossroads of knowledge of the cellular organization of this neural tissue. We understand the morphologies of the neurons comprising the retina, the significance of their branching levels and dendritic characteristics. We are beginning to know all the neurotransmitters that are used by the individual cells and the arrangements of the neurotransmitter receptors that process retinal information. Neurons are arranged in interconnected arrays or mosaics, often with several neurotransmitters per neuron that are released under select conditions. The postsynaptic neurons that work in these arrays are capable of receiving several influences both from neurotransmitters, electrical synapses and a soup of modulators so that each participant in the neural chain can react to stimuli in specific, flexible or even plastic manners. Specific connections are made in specific layers or sublayers of the retina in order to drive the ganglion cell receptive field and provide sensitivity to specialized visual stimuli. Yet neurons must be kept separate by stratification patterns so

that correct connections are made and confusing interactions avoided. Ganglion cells work in concert to provide a cohesive visual message to the brain.

The future lies in a continued honing of this information and learning exactly how the ganglion cell codes this preprocessed retinal information for delivery to the brain and ultimately for perception of the visual image. Perhaps in the future we can design better artificial visual systems constructed on many of the principles that have been elucidated from the biological system. Our knowledge of the multitude of retinal cells' physiology, pharmacology and sensitivity to both physical and chemical environment will aid in therapies to repair or supplant damaged retinal areas after disease and trauma.

John Dowling has often expressed the view that understanding the retina is a basis for understanding the central nervous system in general. The retina is after all, an approachable piece of the brain (Dowling, 1987). Understanding of the retina has in fact proceeded faster that in any other area of the brain in the discipline of neuroscience because of its accessibility for scientific probing. And the giant on whose shoulder sits this ever expanding pyramid of knowledge concerning the retina is John E. Dowling.

Acknowledgments

We dedicate this chapter to Brian B. Boycott who along with John E. Dowling was an inspiration for many of the anatomical studies on the retina reported in this chapter.

References

Ahnelt, P. and Kolb, H. (1994) Horizontal cells and cone photoreceptors in human retina: a Golgi-electron microscopic study of spectral connectivity. *J. Comp. Neurol.*, 343: 406–427.

Ahnelt, P.K. and Kolb, H. (2000) The mammalian photoreceptor mosaic—adaptive design. *Proc. Ret. & Eye Res.*, 19: 711–777.

Ahnelt, P.K., Hokoç, J.N. and Röhlich, P. (1995) Photoreceptors in a primitive mammal, the South American opossum, *Didelphis marsupialis aurita*: characterization with anti-opsin immunolabeling. *Vis Neurosci*, 12: 793–804.

Ahnelt, P.K., Fernández, E., Martinez, O., Bolea, J.A. and Kübber-Heiss, A. (2000) Irregular S-cone mosaics in felid retinas. Spatial interaction with axonless horizontal cells, revealed by cross correlation. *J. Opt. Soc. Am. A*, 17: 580–588.

Ammermüller, J. and Kolb, H. (1996) Functional architecture of the turtle retina. *Prog. Ret. and Eye Res.*, 15: 393–433.

Ammermüller, J., Muller, J.F. and Kolb, H. (1995) The organization of the turtle inner retina. II. Analysis of color-coded and directionally selective cells. *J. Comp. Neurol.*, 358: 35–62.

Amthor, F.R., Oyster, C.W. and Takahashi, E.S. (1984) Morphology of on-off direction-selective ganglion cells in the rabbit retina. *Brain Res.*, 298: 187–190.

Amthor, F.R., Takahashi, E.S. and Oyster, C.W. (1989a) Morphologies of rabbit retinal ganglion cells with concentric receptive fields. *J. Comp. Neurol.*, 280: 72–96.

Amthor, F.R., Takahashi, E.S. and Oyster, C.W. (1989b) Morphologies of rabbit retinal ganglion cells with complex receptive fields. *J. Comp. Neurol.*, 280: 97–121.

Berson, D.M., Isayama, T. and Pu, M. (1999) The eta cell: a new ganglion cell group in cat retina. *J. Comp. Neurol.*, 408: 204–214.

Boycott, B.B. and Dowling, J.E. (1969) Organization of the primate retina: light microscopy. *Phil. Trans. R. Soc.*, B 255: 109–184.

Boycott, B.B., Dowling, J.E., Fisher, S.K., Kolb, H. and Laties, A.M. (1975) Interplexiform cells of the mammalian retina and their comparison with catecholamine-containing retinal cells. *Proc. R. Soc. Lond. B*, 191: 353–368.

Brandstatter, J.B., Koulen, P. and Wässle, H. (1997) Selective synaptic distribution of kainate receptor subunits in the two plexiform layers of the rat retina. *J. Neurosci.*, 17: 9290–9307.

Brecha, N.C., Johnson, J., Bolz, S., Sharma, J.G., Parnavelas, J.G. and Lieberman, A.R. (1987) Substance P-immunoreactive retinal ganglion cells and their central terminals in the rabbit. *Nature*, 327: 155–158.

Brew, H. and Attwell, D. (1987) Electrogenic glutamate uptake is a major current carrier in the membrane of axolotl retinal glial cells. *Nature*, 327: 707–709.

Bunt, A.H. (1980) Comparative studies of 3H-fucose incorporation into vertebrate photoreceptor outer segments. *Vision Res.*, 20: 739–747.

Brivanlau, I.H., Warland, D.K. and Meister, M. (1998) Mechanisms of concerted firing among retinal ganglion cells. *Neuron*, 20: 527–539.

Cai, W. and Pourcho, R.G. (1999) Localization of metabotropic glutamate receptors mGluR1α and mGluR2/3 in the cat retina. *J. Comp. Neurol.*, 407: 427–437.

Cajal, S.R. (1892) The Structure of the Retina. (Translated by S.A. Thorpe and M. Glickstein), Springfield, Ill., Thomas, 1972.

Cook, J.E. and Chalupa, L.M. (2000) Retinal mosaics: new insights into an old concept. *TINS*, 23: 26–34.

Cook, P.B. and McReynolds, J.S. (1998) Lateral inhibition in the inner retina is important for spatial tuning of ganglion cells. *Nature Neurosci.*, 1: 714–719.

Critz, S.T. and Marc, R.E. (1992) Glutamate antagonists that block hyperpolarizing bipolar cells increase the release of dopamine from turtle retina. *Vis. Neurosci.*, 9: 271–278.

Cuenca, N., and Kolb, H. (1998) Circuitry and role of substance P-immunoreactive neurons in the primate retina. *J. Comp. Neurol.*, 393: 439–456.

Cuenca, N., Fernandez, E., Garcia, M. and De Juan, J. (1993) Dendrites of rod dominant ON-bipolar cells are coupled by gap junction in carp retina. *Neurosci. Lett.*, 162: 34–38.

Cuenca, N., Haverkamp, S. and Kolb, H. (2000a) Choline acetyltransferase and nitric oxide synthase are found in horizontal cells of the turtle retina. *Brain Res.*, 878: 228–239.

Cuenca, N., Solessio, E., Anastasopoulos, G. and Kolb, H. (2000b) Spatial relationships of mosaics of neurons in turtle retina as revealed by immunocytochemistry and confocal microscopy. *J. Comp. Neurol.*, Submitted.

Dacey, D.M. (1988) Dopamine-accumulating retinal neurons revealed by in vitro fluorescence display a unique morphology. *Science*, 240: 1196–1198.

Dacey, D.M. (1989) Axon-bearing amacrine cells of the macaque monkey retina. *J. Comp. Neurol.*, 284: 275–293.

Dacey, D.M. and Lee, B.B. (1994) The 'blue-on' opponent pathways in primate retina originate from a distinct bistratified ganglion cell. *Nature*, 367: 731–735.

Dacey, D.M., Lee, B.B., Stafford, D.K., Pokorny, J. and Smith, V.C. (1996) Horizontal cells of the primate retina: cone specificity without spectral opponency. *Science*, 271: 656–659.

Dacheux, R.F. and Raviola, E. (1986) The rod pathway in the rabbit: a depolarizing bipolar and amacrine cell. *J. Neurosci.*, 6: 331–345.

Daw, N.W. (1967) Goldfish retina: Organization for simultaneous color contrast. *Science*, 158: 942–944.

Daw, N.W. (1968) Colour-coded ganglion cells in the goldfish retina: Extension of their receptive fields by means of new stimuli. *J. Physiol.*, 197: 567–592.

Deng, P., Cuenca, N., Doerr, T., Pow, D.V., Miller, R.F. and Kolb, H. (2001) Localization of neurotransmitters and calcium binding proteins to neurons of salamander and mudpuppy retinas. *Vision Res.*, In press.

DeVries, S.H. and Schwartz, E.R. (1999) Kainate receptors mediate synaptic transmission between cones and 'Off' bipolar cells in a mammalian retina. *Nature*, 397: 157–160.

Dowling, J.E. (1987) The Retina: an approachable part of the brain. Belknap Press of Harvard U. Press, Cambridge, Mass.

Dowling, J.E. and Boycott, B.B. (1966) Organization of the primate retina; electron microscopy. *Proc. R. Soc.*, B 166: 80–111.

Dowling, J.E. and Ehinger, B. (1975) Synaptic organization of the amine-containing interplexiform cells of the goldfish and Cebus monkey retinas. *Science*, 188: 270–273.

Dowling, J.E. and Werblin, F.S. (1969) Organization of the retina of the mudpuppy, *Necturus maculosus*. I. Synaptic structure. *J. Neurophysiol.*, 32: 315–338.

Ehinger, B., Falck, B. and Laties, A.M. (1969) Adrenergic neurons in teleost retina. *Z. Zellforsch. Microsk, Anat.*, 97: 285–297.

Ehinger, B., Ottersen, O.P., Storm-Mathisen, J. and Dowling, J.E. (1988) Bipolar cells in the turtle retina are strongly immunoreactive for glutamate. *Proc. Natl. Acad. Sci., USA*, 85: 8321–8325.

Famiglietti, E.V. (1983) 'Starburst' amacrine cells and cholinergic neurons: mirror-symmetric ON and OFF amacrine cells of rabbit retina. *Brain Res.*, 261: 138–144.

Famiglietti, E.V. (1991) Synaptic organization of starburst amacrine cells in rabbit retina: analysis of serial thin sections by electron microscopy and graphic reconstruction. *J. Comp. Neurol.*, 309: 40–70.

Famiglietti, E.V. and Kolb, H. (1976) Structural basis for ON- and OFF-center responses in retinal ganglion cells. *Science*, 194: 193–195.

Feller, M.B., Wellis, D.P., Stellwagen, D., Werblin, F.S. and Shatz, C.J. (1996) Requirement for cholinergic synaptic transmission in the propagation of spontaneous retinal waves. *Science*, 272: 1182–1187.

Fisher, S.K., Jacobs, G.H., Anderson, D.H. and Silverman, M.S. (1976) Rods in the antelope ground squirrel. *Vision Res.*, 16: 875–877.

Fletcher, E.L. and Wässle, H. (1999) Indoleamine-accumulating amacrine cells are presynaptic to rod bipolar cells through GABAc receptors. *J. Comp. Neurol.*, 413: 155–167.

Freed, M.A., Pflug, R., Kolb, H. and Nelson, R. (1996) ON-OFF amacrine cells in cat retina. *J. Comp. Neurol.*, 364: 556–566.

Gallego, A. (1971) Celulas interplexiformes en la retina del gato. *Arch. Soc. Esp. Oftal.*, 31: 299–304.

Gouras, P. (1968) Identification of cone mechanisms in monkey ganglion cells. *J. Physiol. Lond.*, 199: 533–547.

Gouras, P. (1991) Precortical physiology of colour vision. In: *Vision and Visual Dysfunction, Vol. 6: "The Perception of Colour".* Macmillan Press Ltd., England, pp. 163–178.

Haverkamp, S., Möckel, W. and Ammermüller, J. (1999) Different types of synapses with different spectral types of cones underlie color opponency in a bipolar cell of the turtle retina. *Vis. Neurosci.*, 16: 801–809.

Haverkamp, S., Cuenca, N. and Kolb, H. (2000) Morphological and neurochemical diversity of NO positive amacrine cells in the turtle retina, *Cell Tiss. Res.*, 302: 11–19.

Ishida, A.T., Stell, W.K. and Lightfoot, D.O. (1980) Rod and cone inputs to bipolar cells in the goldfish retina. *J. Comp. Neurol.*, 191: 315–335.

Jensen, R.J. and Daw, N.W. (1986) Effects of dopamine and its agonists and antagonists on the receptive field properties of ganglion cells in the rabbit retina. *Neurosci.*, 17: 837–855.

Kamermans, M., Van Dijk, B.W. and Spekreijse, H. (1991) Color opponency in cone-driven horizontal cells in carp retina. *J. Gen. Physiol.*, 97: 819–843.

Kaneko, A. (1971) Electrical connexions between horizontal cells in the dogfish retina. *J. Physiol. (Lond.)*, 213: 95–105.

Karwoski, C.J. and Proenza, L.M. (1977) Relationship between Muller cell responses, a local transretinal potential, and potassium flux. *J. Neurophysiol.*, 40: 244–259.

Kolb, H. (1997) Amacrine cells of the mammalian retina, neurocircuitry and functional roles. *Eye*, 11: 904–923.

Kolb, H. and Famiglietti, E.V. (1974) Rod and cone pathways in the inner plexiform layer of the cat retina. *Science*, 186: 47–49.

Kolb, H. and Jones, J. (1982) Light and electron microscopy of the photoreceptors in the retina of the red-eared slider, *Pseudemys scripta elegans. J. Comp. Neurol.*, 209: 331–338.

Kolb, H. and Jones, J. (1984) Synaptic organization of the outer plexiform layer of the turtle retina: an electron microscope study of serial sections. *J. Neurocytol.*, 13: 567–591.

Kolb, H. and Jones, J. (1987) The distinction by light and electron microscopy of two types of cones containing colorless oil droplets in the retina of the turtle. *Vision Res.*, 27: 1445–1458.

Kolb, H. and Nelson, R. (1996) Hyperpolarizing, small-field, amacrine cells in cone pathways of cat retina. *J. Comp. Neurol.*, 371: 415–436.

Kolb, H. and Zhang, L.L. (1997) Immunostaining with antibodies against protein kinase C isoforms in the fovea of the monkey retina. *Micr. Res. Techn.*, 36: 57–75.

Koulen, P., Brandstätter, J.H., Enz, R., Bormann, J. and Wässle, H. (1998) Synaptic clustering of GABAc receptor r-subunits in the rat retina. *Eur. J. Neurosci.*, 10: 115–127.

Kolb, H., Boycott, B.B. and Dowling, J.E. (1969) A second type of midget bipolar cell in the primate retina, *Appendix Phil. Trans. R. Soc. B (Lond.)*, 255: 177–184.

Kolb, H., Cuenca, N. and DeKorver, L. (1991) Postembedding immunocytochemistry for GABA and glycine reveals the synaptic relationships of the dopaminergic amacrine cell of the cat retina. *J. Comp. Neurol.*, 310: 267–284.

Kolb, H., Goede, P., Roberts, S., McDermott, R. and Gouras, P. (1997a) Uniqueness of the S-conc pedicle in the human retina and consequences for color processing. *J. Comp. Neurol.*, 286: 443–460.

Kolb, H., Netzer, E. and Ammermüller, J. (1997b) Neural circuitry and light responses of the dopamine amacrine cell of the turtle retina. *Mol. Vis.* (http://molvis/v3/kolb), 3: 1–6.

Kolb, H. and West, R.W. (1977) Synaptic connections of the interplexiform cell in the retina of the cat. *J. Neurocytol.*, 6: 155–170.

Kouyama, N. and Marshak, D.W. (1992) Bipolar cells specific for blue cones in the macaque retina. *J. Neurosci.*, 12: 1233–1252.

Lasansky, A. (1978) Contacts between receptors and electrophysiologically identified neurones in the retina of the larval tiger salamander. *J. Physiol. (Lond.)*, 285: 531–542.

Leeper, H.F. (1978) Horizontal cells of the turtle retina II. Analysis of interconnections between photoreceptor cells and horizontal cells by light microscopy. *J. Comp. Neurol.*, 182: 795–810.

Lettvin, J.Y., Maturana, H.R., McCullouch, W.S. and Pitts, E.H. (1959) What the frog's eye tells the frog's brain. *Proc. Inst. Radio Engin.*, 47: 1940–1951.

Linberg, K.A., Suemune, S. and Fisher, S.K. (1996) Retinal neurons of the California ground squirrel, *Spermophilus beecheyi*: a Golgi study. *J. Comp. Neurol.*, 365: 173–216.

MacNeil, M.A. and Masland, R.H. (1988) Extreme diversity among amacrine cells: Implications for function. *Neuron*, 20: 971–982.

Marc, R.E. (1992) The structure of GABAergic circuits in ectotherm retinas. In: Mize, R., Marc, R.E. and Sillito, A. (Eds.), *GABA in the retina and central visual system*. Elsevier, Amsterdam, pp. 61–92.

Marc, R.E. (1995) Interplexiform cell connectivity in the outer retina. In: Djamgoz, M.B.A., Archer, S.N. and Vallerga, S. (Eds.), *Neurobiology and Clinical Aspects of the Outer Retina*. Chapman & Hall, London, pp. 369–393.

Marc, R.E. (1999) The structure of vertebrate retinas. In: Toyoda et al. (Eds.), *The retinal basis of vision*. Elsevier Science B.V., pp. 3–19.

Marc, R.E. and Lam, D.M.K. (1981) Glycinergic pathways in the goldfish retina. *J. Neurosci.*, 1: 152–165.

Marc, R.E. and Liu, W. (2000) Fundamental GABAergic amacrine cell circuitries in the retina: nested feedback, concatenated inhibition, and axosomatic synapses. *J. Comp. Neurol.*, 425: 560–582.

Marc, R.E., Stell, W.K., Bok, D. and Lam, D.M.K. (1978) GABAergic pathways in the goldfish retina. *J. Comp. Neurol.*, 182: 221–246.

Marc, R.E., Liu, W.-L.S., Kalloniatis, M. and Basinger, S.F. (1990) Patterns of glutamate immunoreactivity in the goldfish retina. *J. Neurosci.*, 10: 4006–4034.

Marc, R.E., Murry, R.F., Fisher, S.K., Linberg, K.A. and Lewis, G.P. (1998) Amino acid signatures in the detached cat retina. *Invest. Ophthal. Vis. Sci.*, 39: 1694–1702.

Mariani, A.P. (1984) Bipolar cells in monkey retina selective for cones likely to be blue-sensitive. *Nature*, 308: 184–186.

Mariani, A.P. (1987) Neuronal and synaptic organization of the outer plexiform layer of the pigeon retina. *Am. J. Anat.*, 179: 25–39.

Marshak, D.W. and Dowling, J.E. (1984) Synapses of the cone horizontal cell axons of the goldfish retina. *J. Comp. Neurol.*, 256: 430–443.

Masland, R.H. (1988) Amacrine cells. *TINS*, 11: 405–410.

Masland, R.H. and Tauchi, M. (1986) The cholinergic amacrine cell. *TINS*, 9: 218–223.

Miller, R.F. and Dowling, J.E. (1970) Intracellular responses of the Muller (glial) cells of mudpuppy retina: their relation to b-wave of the electroretinogram. *J. Neurophysiol.*, 33: 323–341.

Nelson, R. (1982) AII amacrine cells quicken the time course of rod signals in the cat retina. *J. Neurophysiol.*, 47: 928–947.

Nelson, R. and Kolb, H. (1985) A17: a broad-field amacrine cell of the rod system in the retina of the cat. *J. Neurophysiol.*, 54: 592–614.

Nelson, R., von Lutzow, A., Kolb, H. and Gouras, P. (1975) Horizontal cells in cat with independent dendritic systems. *Science*, 189: 137–139.

Nelson, R., Famiglietti, E.V. and Kolb, H. (1978) Intracellular staining reveals different levels of stratification for

on-center and off-center ganglion cells in the cat retina. *J. Neurophysiol.*, 41: 427–483.

Newman, E. and Reichenbach, A. (1996) The Muller cell: A functional element of the retina. *TINS*, 19: 307–311.

Newman, E.A. and Zahs, K.R. (1998) Modulation of neuronal activity by glial cells in the retina. *J. Neurosci.*, 18: 4022–4028.

Nomura, A., Shigemoto, R., Nakamura, Y., Okamoto, N., Mizuno, N. and Nakanishi, S. (1994) Developmentally regulated postsynaptic localization of a metabotropic glutamate receptor in rat rod bipolar cells. *Cell*, 77: 361–369.

Normann, R.A., Warren, D.J., Ammermüller, J., Fernandez, E. and Guillory, S. (2001) High spatial-temporal mapping of visual pathways using multielectrode arrays. *Vision Res.*, In press.

Peichl, L. and Boycott, B.B. (1998) Comparative anatomy and function of mammalian horizontal cells. In: Chalupa, L.M. and Finlay, B.L. (Eds.), *Development and Organization of the Retina*. Plenum Press, New York.

Peterson, B.B. and Dacey, D.M. (1998) Morphology of human retinal ganglion cells with intraretinal axon collaterals. *Vis Neurosci.*, 15: 377–387.

Polyak, S.L. (1941) The Retina. University of Chicago, Chicago, Ill.

Pourcho, R.G. (1982) Dopaminergic amacrine cells in the cat retina. *Brain Res.*, 252: 101–109.

Pourcho, R.G. and Goebel, D.J. (1983) Neuronal subpopulations in cat retina which accumulate the GABA agonist (3H) muscimol: a combined Golgi and autoradiographic study. *J. Comp. Neurol.*, 219: 25–35.

Pourcho, R.G. and Goebel, D.J. (1985) A combined Golgi and autoradiographic study of 3(H) glycine-accumulating amacrine cells in the cat retina. *J. Comp. Neurol.*, 233: 473–480.

Pu, M. (1999) Dendritic morphology of cat retinal ganglion cells projecting to the suprachiasmatic nucleus. *J. Comp. Neurol.*, 414: 267–274.

Pu, M. and Amthor, F.R. (1990) Dendritic morphologies of retinal ganglion cells projecting to the nucleus of the optic tract in the rabbit. *J. Comp. Neurol.*, 302: 657–674.

Qin, P. and Pourcho, R. (1999a) Localization of AMPA-selective glutamate receptor subunits in the cat retina; a light- and electron-microscope study. *Vis. Neurosci.*, 16: 169–177.

Qin, P. and Pourcho, R. (1999b) AMPA-selective glutamate receptor subunits GluR2 and GluR4 in the cat retina: an immunocytochemical study. *Vis. Neurosci.*, 16: 1105–1114.

Raynauld, J.-P. (1972) Goldfish retina: sign of the rod input in opponent-color ganglion cells. *Science*, 177: 84–85.

Rodieck, R.W. (1998) *The First Steps in Seeing*. Sinauer Associates Inc., Sunderland, Mass.

Rodieck, R.W. (1999) Retinal ganglion cells: functional roles, receptive field properties, and channels. In Toyoda et al. (Eds.), *The Retinal Basis of Vision*. Elsevier Science, B.V., pp. 151–160.

Savchenko, A., Barnes, S. and Kramer, R.H. (1997) Cyclic nucleotide-gated channels mediate synaptic feedback by nitric oxide. *Nature*, 390: 694–698.

Scholes, J.H. (1975) Colour receptors, and their synaptic connexions in the retina of a cyprinid fish. *Phil. Trans. R. Soc.*, B 270: 61–118.

Schwartz, E.A. (1999) A transporter mediates the release of GABA from horizontal cells. In Toyoda et al. (Eds.), *The Retinal Basis of Vision*, Elsevier Science B.V., pp. 93–101.

Slaughter, M.M. and Miller, R.F. (1981) 2-amino-4-phosphonobutyric acid: A new pharmacological tool for retina research. *Science*, 211: 182–184.

Slaughter, M.M. and Miller, R.F. (1983) An excitatory amino acid antagonist blocks cone input to sign-conserving second-order retinal neurons. *Science*, 219: 1230–1232.

Spekreijse, H., Wagner, H.G. and Wolbarsht, M.L. (1977) Spectral and spatial coding of ganglion cell responses in goldfish retina. *J. Neurophysiol.*, 35: 73–86.

Steinberg, R.H., Wood, I. and Hogan, M.J. (1977) Pigment epithelial ensheathment and phagocytosis of extrafoveal cones in the human retina. *Phil. Trans. R. Soc. B*, 277: 459–474.

Stell, W.K. and Lightfoot, D.O. (1975) Color-specific interconnections of cones and horizontal cells in the retina of the goldfish. *J. Comp. Neurol.*, 159: 473–501.

Strettoi, E., Raviola, E. and Dacheux, R.F. (1992) Synaptic connections of the narrow-field, bistratified rod amacrine cell (AII) in the rabbit retina. *J. Comp. Neurol.*, 325: 152–168.

Vaney, D.I. (1990) The mosaic of amacrine cells in the mammalian retina. *Prog. Ret. Res.*, 9: 49–100.

Vaney, D.I. (1991) Many diverse types of retinal neurons show tracer coupling when injected with biocytin or Neurobiotin. *Neurosci. Lett.*, 125: 187–190.

Vaney, D.I. (1994) Territorial organization of direction-selective ganglion cells in rabbit retina. *J. Neurosci.*, 14: 6301–6316.

Vaney, D.I. and Pow, D.V. (2000) The dendritic architecture of the cholinergic plexus in the rabbit retina: selective labeling by glycine accumulation in the presence of sarcosine. *J. Comp. Neurol.*, 421: 1–13.

Vardi. N., Morigiwa, K., Wang, T.-L., Shi, Y.-J. and Sterling, P. (1998) Neurochemistry of the mammalian cone "synaptic complex". *Vision Res.*, 38: 1359–1369.

Walls, G.L. (1942) The vertebrate eye and its adaptive radiation. Bloomfield Hills, Mich.

Wässle, H. (1998) Glycine and GABA receptors in the mammalian retina. *Vision Res.*, 38: 1411–1430.

Wässle, H. and Chun, M.H. (1988) Dopaminergic and indoleamine-accumulating amacrine cells express GABA-like immunoreactivity in cat retina. *J. Neurosci.*, 8: 3383–3394.

Wässle, H., Peichl, L. and Boycott, B.B. (1981a) Morphology and topography of on- and off-alpha cells in the cat retina. *Proc. R. Soc. Lond. B*, 212: 157–175.

Wässle, H., Boycott, B.B. and Illing, R.-B. (1981b) Morphology and mosaic of on- and off-beta cells in the cat retina and some functional considerations. *Proc. R. Soc. Lond. B*, 212: 177–195.

Watt, C.B., Florak, V.J. and Walker, R.B. (1993) Quantitative analyses of the co-existence of gamma-aminobutyric acid in substance-P amacrine cells of the larval tiger salamander. *Brain Res.*, 603: 111–116.

Watt, C.B., Kalloniatis, M., Jones, B.W. and Marc, R.E. (2000) Studies examining the neurotransmitter properties of horizontal cell populations in the goldfish retina. *Invest. Ophthal. Vis. Sci.*, 41, S943.

Wellis, D.P. and Werblin, F.S. (1995) Dopamine modulates GABAc receptors mediating inhibition of calcium entry and transmitter release from bipolar cell terminals in Tiger salamander retina. *J. Neurosci.*, 15: 4748–4761.

Werblin, F. (1991) Synaptic connections, receptive fields, and patterns of activity in the tiger salamander retina. *Invest. Ophthal. Vis. Sci.*, 32: 459–483.

Witkovsky, P., Nicholson, C., Rice, M.E., Bohmaker, K. and Meller, E. (1993) Extracellular dopamine concentration in the retina of the clawed frog *Xenopus laevis*. PNAS USA 90: 5667–5671.

Wyatt, H.J. and Daw, N.W. (1976) Specific effects of neurotransmitter antagonists on ganglion cells in rabbit retina. *Science*, 191: 204–205.

Yazulla, S. and Studholme, K.M. (1995) Volume transmission of dopamine may modulate light-adaptive plasticity of horizontal cell dendrites in the recovery phase following dopamine depletion in goldfish retina. *Vis. Neurosci.*, 12: 827–836.

Zhou, Z.J. (1998) Direct participation of starburst amacrine cells in spontaneous rhythmic activity in the developing mammalian retina. *J. Neurosci.*, 18: 4155–4165.

H. Kolb, H. Ripps and S. Wu (Eds.)
Progress in Brain Research, Vol. 131

CHAPTER 2

Comparative anatomy of major retinal pathways in the eyes of nocturnal and diurnal mammals

Kenneth Linberg[1,*], Nicolas Cuenca[4], Peter Ahnelt[5], Steven Fisher[1,2] and Helga Kolb[3]

[1]*Neuroscience Research Institute, University of California at Santa Barbara, Santa Barbara, CA 93106, USA*
[2]*Department of Molecular, Cellular and Developmental Biology, University of California at Santa Barbara, Santa Barbara, CA 93106, USA*
[3]*Moran Eye Center, University of Utah School of Medicine, Salt Lake City, UT 84132, USA*
[4]*Department of Biotechnology, University of Alicante, Alicante, Spain*
[5]*Department of Physiology, University of Vienna, Vienna, Austria*

Introduction

One of John Dowling's greatest contributions to our understanding of the retina was the elucidation of the basic synaptic circuitry of the primate retina in a series of light and electron microscope studies (Dowling and Boycott, 1966; Boycott and Dowling, 1969; Kolb et al., 1969). Upon the heels of these studies followed the first intracellular recordings and marking of neurons in the mudpuppy retina that are now classics in the field (Dowling and Werblin, 1969; Werblin and Dowling, 1969). These seminal papers helped us focus back on the older questions of what are the fundamental neural types of the retina, how do they respond to light stimuli and how do they interact to form functional circuits. Cross species comparisons were then begun in the Dowling lab and we began asking questions about how different are the visual systems of various species, and how have such visual systems become adapted to the environment the animal lives in.

From the time of Santiago Ramón y Cajal (1892, 1911) and later Stephen Polyak (1941) we had good descriptions of Golgi impregnated neurons in a variety of vertebrate retinas. Certainly Cajal (1892) recognized the basic similarity of retinal organization across species. All vertebrate retinas contain photoreceptors, horizontal cells, bipolar cells, ganglion cells and the cell class Cajal first named, amacrine cells. But the various species differed remarkably in the numbers and morphologies of cell types within these basic retinal cell classes. Cajal and Polyak's fascinating material has made comparative studies irresistible to many of us, and invites speculation on how such ocular diversity might have evolved.

Gordon Walls published a monumental work in 1942 addressing the evolution of the eye from the standpoint of species-specific retinal specializations with a particular emphasis on photoreceptors. Lettvin et al. (1959) had originally proposed that all the various cell types seen by Cajal in the frog's retina and their numerous stratified interactions in the inner plexiform layer (IPL) were important for coding complex receptive fields of ganglion cells and gave different ganglion cells specific feature detecting

*Corresponding author: Kenneth Linberg, Tel.: 805-893-3611; Fax: 805-893-2005; E-mail: linberg@lifesci.ucsb.edu

capabilities. Dowling (1970) tried to simplify this concept by proposing the idea that species could be divided into those with complex retinas exemplified by the frog and those with simple retinas exemplified by the primate retina. The involvement of numerous amacrine cells in the IPL circuitry as opposed to a simple straight through bipolar and ganglion cell connectivity pattern was considered to be the basic difference between species that processed much of the visual message in the retina over those that were corticate in design. Later Hughes (1977) examined retinal anatomy from the viewpoint of behavioral patterns and environments and Jacobs (1981, 1993) has spent many years giving us an understanding of the spectral characteristics of retinas and ranges of color vision in different species.

So much comparative information has now accumulated from all these studies and in this chapter we would like to summarize our present understanding of the fundamental strategies that some mammals have adopted in their adaptive radiation to process visual information in their retinas. We will compare retinas of species with a nocturnal lifestyle with retinas of species with a diurnal lifestyle.

Retinal circuitry of mammalian retinas: trends, and design characteristics

Mammals have a limited number of photoreceptor cell types when compared with other vertebrates (see chapter by Kolb et al. this volume). Based upon their spectral sensitivity, teleost fish, in general, have at least four types of cone photoreceptors plus rods; reptiles and birds have rods plus one class of double cone and four classes of single cones; while most mammals have only two classes of cone. The exception to the latter occurs in primates where trichromatic color vision appears to have reemerged, arising from three spectrally distinct cone types [short wavelength sensitive (SWS), middle wavelength sensitive (MWS), and long wavelength sensitive (LWS) cones] in addition to the rods (for a brief review of this topic, see Bowmaker, 1998). The evolution of different photoreceptor types, and the pathways that give rise to color vision have been the subject of much speculation (see, for example,

Walls, 1942; Hughes, 1977; Ahnelt and Kolb, 2000), but it is only our recent ability to identify and sequence the various opsin genes that has added much factual information to such speculation (Bowmaker, 1998). In general, the retinas of most mammalian species are dominated by rods, with the interesting exception of those in squirrels (Long and Fisher, 1983; Ahnelt, 1985; Kryger et al., 1998) and tree shrews (Kühne, 1983; Immel and Fisher, 1985; Müller and Peichl, 1989), and it seems generally accepted now that rods evolved relatively late by comparison to cones. This probably occurred due to the evolution of early mammals in a relatively nocturnal environment. Also, during mammalian evolution some of the complexity of color vision seen in fish, birds and reptiles (apparently tetrachromatic in some cases) was replaced by dichromacy in most species (even monochromacy in two species of nocturnal primates (Jacobs et al., 1996)). Trichromacy reemerging in the evolution of certain primate species, again correlated with the environment in which the species was evolving (Bowmaker, 1998).

If a relatively large variety of cone photoreceptor types existed early, and these were used to generate chromatic information about the environment, then the neural pathways within the retina for processing this information must have existed early as well. Thus, a variety of cone pathways must have already existed in the retina at the time at which rods evolved. If cones were specifically connected to second and third-order neurons according to their chromatic sensitivity, then one might expect that a new and separate pathway would have evolved to handle information arising from the highly sensitive rods. Such does not seem to be the case. Instead, it appears that the rod system "plugged into" the existing cone pathways, in a sense "piggy-backing" the information for scotopic vision onto existing photopic pathways in the retina.

In this chapter we compare some specific neural pathways from the retinas of primarily nocturnal species, rats and cats, to that of the "unusual" cone-dominated retina of the diurnal ground squirrel, and make some further comparisons to the primates with their pure cone fovea and rod-dominated periphery. Examples from other species are also used to illustrate specific concepts.

Photoreceptor mosaics

As mentioned previously, virtually all mammals have rod-dominated retinas, with rods outnumbering cones by as much as 1000 : 1. Examples are shown in Figs. 1a and 2 for cat and rat retina. The rods are tightly packed in an extremely thick outer nuclear layer (ONL) consisting of 18 or more ranks of perikarya (Fig. 1a, cat peripheral retina; 3b hamster). The few cones in species like the rat (Fig. 2, <1%; Szél and Röhlich, 1992) or mouse (3%; LaVail, 1976) are slender and rod-like in shape with cell bodies at the outer limiting membrane (Fig. 3b, hamster). In general, dichromatic mammals have two spectral classes of cone, one, being a middle wavelength sensitive cone (MWS) with a λ_{max} between about 500 and 565 nm and the other the short wavelength sensitive (SWS; often referred to as "blue" cones) cone with its λ_{max} ranging from the ultraviolet (rodents) to blue range of the spectrum (365–450 nm; Bowmaker, 1998). The availability of antibodies that recognize these opsins has made it possible to map the distribution of the different cone types in a variety of species. In most species the longer wavelength-sensitive cone is distributed across the whole retina, while the shorter wavelength-sensitive cone is concentrated preferentially in the inferior retina. In some rodents (rat, Szél and Röhlich, 1992;

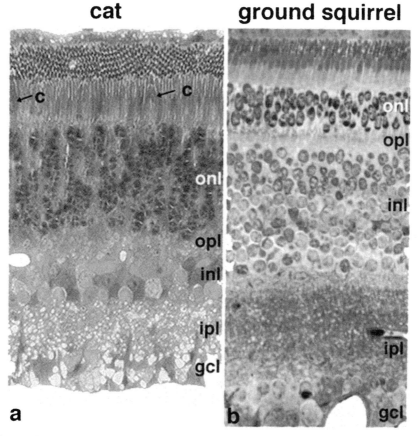

cat   **ground squirrel**

Fig. 1. (a) A light micrograph of a radial section through peripheral cat retina stained with toluidine blue. In this model of a nocturnal retina, only two cones (c, arrows) appear in a field of rods whose nuclei constitute a very thick outer nuclear layer (onl) (from Ahnelt and Kolb, 2000). (b) A similar preparation of ground squirrel retina demonstrates several features of the diurnal retina that differ from the nocturnal type. The short, stout cones of this retina comprise an ONL only 2 to 3 cells thick. In contrast with cat, the ground squirrel INL and IPL are very thick, accommodating many types of bipolar and amacrine cells whose many processes connecting with the dendrites of numerous types of ganglion cell contribute to the thick neuropil. opl = outer plexiform layer; inl = inner nuclear layer; ipl = inner plexiform layer; gcl = ganglion cell layer (from Long and Fisher, 1983).

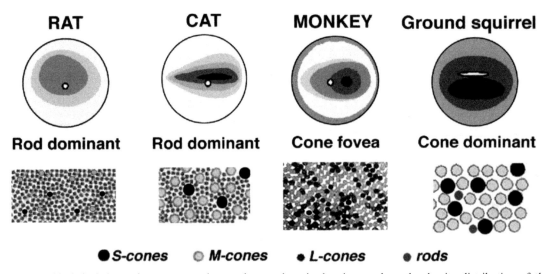

RAT · **CAT** · **MONKEY** · **Ground squirrel**

Rod dominant · **Rod dominant** · **Cone fovea** · **Cone dominant**

● S-cones   ◉ M-cones   • L-cones   • rods

Fig. 2. Topographical depictions of rat, cat, monkey, and ground squirrel retina to show the density distribution of the cone photoreceptors (shading from dark (high density), to pale (low density)). The cone mosaics reflect the retinal specializations such as the *area centralis* (cat), fovea (monkey) or visual streak (ground squirrel) in the different retinas. The optic nerve is the white spot or slit. Below are examples of the photoreceptor mosaics in each species.

mouse, Calderone and Jacobs, 1995; hamster, Calderone and Jacobs, 1999) however, the two types of cone have non-overlapping populations. The cat retina (overall, about 3% cones) differs from that of the rodents by having an *area centralis* where cones reach a peak density (Fig. 2; Steinberg et al., 1973; Linberg et al., 2001), but the overall cone distribution is like that seen in the rodents and even in the *area centralis*, rods predominate over cones by as much as 10 : 1 (Steinberg et al., 1973).

Like most other mammals, ground squirrels are dichromatic, but with a retina dominated by cones (Figs. 1b, 3c). Indeed, for many decades it was thought that the ground squirrel, like the prairie dog (Fig. 3f) had a pure-cone retina, and thus it was regarded as a model system for foveal organization. Cones in these retinas are short and stocky compared to those of rat and cat, and the ONL is only 2–3 layers thick (compare Figs. 1a and 1b). As in the rod-dominated species discussed above, the cones in ground squirrel consist of SWS and MWS types (12% and 88% respectively; Long and Fisher, 1983; Ahnelt 1985; Kryger et al., 1998). The presence of rods was first demonstrated by ERG recordings and then by morphological analyses about 25 years ago (Green and Dowling, 1975; West and Dowling, 1975; Jacobs et al., 1976, 1980; Anderson and Fisher, 1976;

Long and Fisher, 1983; Ahnelt, 1985). Rods and cones appear superficially alike in the ground squirrel retina (Fig. 3c), with the rod outer and inner segments being only slightly longer and thinner. Rods are now easily distinguished in the ground squirrel retina by immunolabeling with antibodies against rhodopsin (Fig. 3d; Kryger et al., 1998), and constitute 14% of the photoreceptor population across the retina. Their highest relative population (30%) is in the deep ventral periphery, while their lowest (5%) occurs in the visual streak. MWS cones contribute 80% to the total photoreceptor population and have their greatest density in the visual streak (Fig. 2); SWS cones constitute only 6% of the total number and have a rather uniform density across the whole retina (Kryger et al., 1998).

In primates trichromacy came about by the addition of a third cone type that evolved separately in the case of New and Old-World monkeys leading to separate MWS and long wavelength sensitive (LWS) cones in addition to the SWS cone (Bowmaker, 1998). Furthermore in catarrhine primates and man, the retina is characterized by a special emphasis on the development of a cone-dominated region, or macula, with its specialized cone-associated pathways (Figs. 2, 3a). In the center of the macula, or fovea, rods are excluded, while in

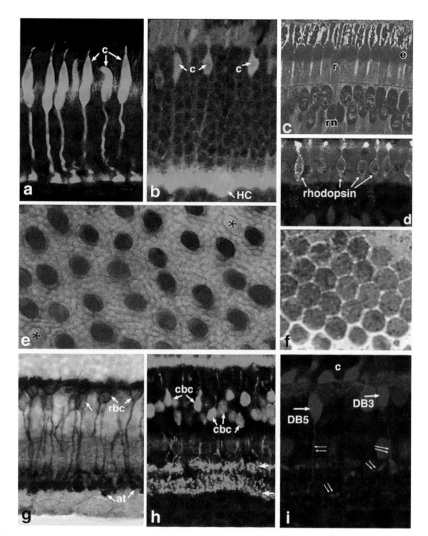

Fig. 3. (a) A confocal image of monkey cones (c, arrows) stained with a fluorescently tagged antibody against GCAP1. Entire cones, labeled from their outer segments to their pedicles, lie amidst unstained rods. (b) A less robust fluorescent image of the few cones (c, arrows) in hamster retina labeled with an antibody against calbindin D. Cone nuclei are restricted to the outermost row of cells in the outer nuclear layer which consists of many ranks of unstained rod nuclei. Horizontal cell nuclei (HC) are also positive for calbindin D. (c) A light micrograph of a radial section, stained with toluidine blue, through the outer retina of a ground squirrel. A single rod (r) lies among the many cones. The ellipsoid region (e) of the photoreceptors, filled with mitochondria, stain darkly. rn = rod nucleus (from Long and Fisher, 1983). (d) A confocal micrograph of a similar region of ground squirrel retina shows that all photoreceptors stain positively for antibodies against recoverin (red) while just the rods (arrows) also colocalize antibodies against rhodopsin (yellow). A type of bipolar cell also appears recoverin-positive. (e) A confocal image of a wholemount of human retina stained with antibodies against calbindin D. The immunoreactive inner segments of the M- and L-cones stand out against the unstained S-cones (*) and the smaller rods. (f) A tangential section of prairie dog retina stained with toluidine blue demonstrates the tight packing of cone inner segments typical of diurnal retinas. (g) A light micrograph of a radial section through rat retina stained with antibodies against protein kinase C known to stain mammalian rod bipolar cells. Rat rod bipolar cells (rbc, arrows) have their nuclei close to the outer edge of the inner nuclear layer while their axon terminals (at, arrows) stratify in the deepest stratum of the IPL adjacent to the ganglion cell layer. (h) In a fluorescent micrograph taken by confocal microscopy, antibodies against recoverin, here shown in green, stain two varieties of cone bipolar cell (cbc, arrows) in the ground squirrel retina, one more intensely than the other. The axon terminals of these cells stratify in two bands in the IPL (thick arrows), the lower thicker than the upper. (i) In another confocal preparation, antibodies against calbindin D label two types of bipolar cell in monkey retina, one (DB5) has axon terminals stratifying in the inner IPL (arrow pairs, left), and the other (DB3) in the outer IPL (arrow pairs, right). A type of amacrine cell also stains, as do the cone pedicles (c).

the perifoveal retina the number of rods gradually increases (Østerberg, 1935), eventually separating the closely packed cones into islands, creating two mosaics (Fig. 3e). In the central 1° of the foveal pit the LWS and MWS cones are packed into a hexagonal mosaic lacking SWS cones (Williams et al., 1981). The SWS cone population distribution has now been determined in a number of primate species (Curcio and Hendrickson, 1991; Wikler and Rakic, 1990) using antibody (Nathans et al., 1986) labeling. With increasing eccentricity the SWS-cone population rises in density to become 14% of the total cone population at the foveal slope (a ring 2 mm or 8° from the foveal center), then tapers to a steady 8% throughout the rest of the peripheral retina. The distribution of LWS and MWS cones has proved impossible to determine by antibody labeling since the molecular structure of the two differs by only a few amino acids. Nevertheless, using microspectrophotometry (Mollon and Bowmaker, 1992) and reflectance photometry (Roorda and Williams, 1999), small patches of these cones in the primate fovea have been mapped. Lacking any apparent regular mosaic, they appear to be packed into various sized arrays of the same type with the LWS cones the more numerous (at least in man; Figs. 2, 10c) (McMahon et al., 2000). Thus, it appears that the central few degrees of the trichromatic primate retina are dominated by red-sensitivity, while the peripheral retina, though still trichromatic psychophysically (G.H. Jacobs, personal communication) is dominated by green-sensitivity but with an additional blue-sensitive component derived from the presence of SWS cones. The latter pattern of dominance by the cones sensitive in the green portion of the spectrum—but with significant input from the SWS cones, is a pattern common to most dichromatic mammals (see Fig. 10b).

Neural pathways for nocturnal living

Specialized rod bipolar and amacrine cells

The predominance of rod photoreceptors and the evolution of specific pathways for processing rod information, must have given the early mammals a tremendous advantage of being able to function well at very low levels of ambient light. Rods, after all, are inherently more sensitive than cones with their ability to respond to the presence of a single photon (Hecht et al., 1942). The purpose of the rod pathway is to gather as much information about the presence of light as possible and this is done by the convergence of many rods onto rod bipolar cells (about 15–50 : 1 in the cat and rat retinas) and then the convergence of information through the bipolar cell pathways onto the ganglion cells (ranging from 100–1 to 5000–1 in central cat retina) (see Sterling et al., 1988). One common feature of most placental mammals is the presence of a separate rod bipolar cell type responding to the light ON signal. This cell is devoted solely to input from rod photoreceptors, which is in contrast to most non-mammalian vertebrates and non-placental mammals where the homologous cell is rod-dominant, but has cone input as well. Figure 3g shows the typical morphology and packing density of ON-rod bipolar cells in the rat retina as revealed by protein kinase C immunostaining (Greferath et al., 1990). Also, there does not appear to be an OFF-bipolar cell devoted solely to the rod pathway. In squirrels, the B4 "rod bipolar" has been shown to have some cone input (West, 1978), while the B3 bipolar cell, an apparent OFF-cone bipolar, also receives its input from rods as well as cones (Fig. 4a, large arrows) (Jacobs et al., 1976; West, 1978; Linberg et al., 1996).

In general, the mammalian rod bipolar cell is much more convergent than any of the cone bipolar subtypes. Each ON-rod bipolar makes dendritic contact with numerous rod spherules [cat: 16–25 (Boycott and Kolb, 1973; Freed et al., 1987; Greferath et al., 1990; Wässle et al., 1991); rabbit: 80–120 (Dacheux and Raviola, 1986; Young and Vaney, 1991); human: 30–45 (Kolb et al., 1992; monkey: 5(fovea)–60(periphery) (Boycott and Dowling, 1969; Boycott and Wässle, 1991; Grünert and Martin, 1991)] high in the outer plexiform layer (OPL) at invaginating, ribbon-related synapses (Fig. 4c). The rod bipolar cell carries the light-on signal to the lower portion of the inner plexiform layer (IPL), specifically to Cajal's strata 4 and 5 (Figs. 3g, 6a). Based upon the demonstration that ON and OFF signals were segregated into two sublaminae of the IPL, these lower-most layers (receiving ON input) were referred to as sublamina "**b**" while

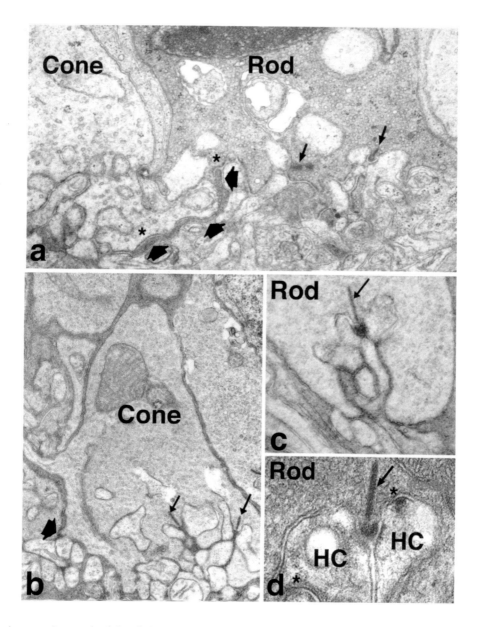

Fig. 4. (a) An electron micrograph of the photoreceptor terminals of the California ground squirrel. Unlike rod spherules in rod-dominant retinas, the cone-like rod terminals in squirrels have several synaptic invaginations with independent synaptic ribbons (small arrows). Note the electron-dense dendritic process (thick arrows) of a bipolar dendrite, that, rising across the OPL makes flat contacts (*) first with a cone pedicle then terminates on the rod terminal (*) (from Jacobs et al., 1976). (b) An electron micrograph of a cone pedicle from the retina of a cat. The multi-invaginated pedicle contains prominently large mitochondria and is presynaptic at ribbons (small arrows) to horizontal cells and ON-center bipolar cell invaginating dendrites. Numerous basal junctions are made by OFF-center bipolar cell dendrites. Note the contact (thick arrow) with a neighboring cone (from Kolb, 1977). (c) An electron micrograph of a rod spherule in the cat retina contains a single invagination at the rod's synaptic ribbon (arrow), where horizontal cell lateral elements and a central ON rod bipolar cell dendrite terminate. (d) An electron micrograph of a rod spherule invagination in peripheral human retina. Two horizontal cell dendrites (HC) form lateral elements in the triad opposing the ribbon synapse (arrow); each contains a small synapse (*) back onto the rod terminal membrane (from Linberg and Fisher, 1988).

the remaining two distal layers (receiving OFF input) were referred to as sublamina "a" by Nelson et al. (1978). Within sublamina **b** of the IPL, the rod signals are channeled into two separate amacrine cell pathways. While undoubtedly many varieties of amacrine cell are involved in the processing of rod signals, it appears that two major types, well-developed in the retinas of rod-dominated, nocturnal mammals, may bear the lion's share of the responsibility for this task. The major amacrine cell type associated with the rod pathway is a narrow-field, bistratified amacrine known as AII (Kolb and Famiglietti, 1974; Famiglietti and Kolb, 1975; Nelson, 1982; Dacheux and Raviola, 1986). In contrast, the A17 cell is an extremely wide-field amacrine with processes that ramify across the IPL, but run for hundreds of microns in stratum 5 (i.e. adjacent to the ganglion cell layer in sublamina **b**) where they create an overlapping plexus of beaded processes (Kolb and Nelson, 1984; Nelson and Kolb, 1985).

The AII amacrine

In species such as the cat (and probably in all rod-dominated retinas as well as the primate peripheral retina), the AII cells are numerous and have a closely packed arrangement tiling the retina (Vaney, 1985; Fig. 5d). They serve to collect rod signals at the rod bipolar axon terminals deep in sublamina **b** of the IPL. They then transmit these signals both in the inner and outer IPL to different types of cone bipolar cell. These cone bipolars synapse onto ganglion cell dendrites. Until the discovery of this pathway, it was assumed that rod bipolar cell axons must be presynaptic to ganglion cell dendrites or even cell bodies, because their large terminals end adjacent to the ganglion cell bodies. It was not until Kolb and Famiglietti (1974) were able to reconstruct the rod bipolar terminals in serial sections by electron microscopy, that this indirect pathway was revealed.

Figures 6a–c summarize the rod pathways of these rod-dominated mammalian species, showing the position of the AII amacrine cell as an intermediary between the rod and cone bipolars. Because the AII cell apparently allowed the rod photoreceptors to utilize already existing cone pathways for transmitting information to the ganglion cells, they are sometimes referred to as "piggy-back" neurons (Strettoi et al., 1992). The AII amacrine is an ON-center cell, and it passes signals from the ON-rod bipolar cell through gap junctions to the terminals of ON-cone (invaginating) bipolar cells in sublamina **b** of the IPL (Fig. 6). It is these cone-bipolars (orange bipolar cell, Fig. 6c) that ultimately pass information from the rod bipolar cell to an ON-center ganglion cells at chemical synapses (Fig. 6c; Kolb, 1979; Sterling et al., 1988). The AII cell (thought to be glycinergic) is also presynaptic to OFF-cone (flat) bipolars in sublamina **a** of the IPL (yellow bipolar, Fig. 6c). The OFF-cone bipolar in turn synapses onto an OFF-center ganglion cell. Just as frequently, the AII cell is directly presynaptic to the OFF-center ganglion cell (Fig. 6c; Kolb and Nelson, 1993). These chemical synapses appear on highly specialized branches off the main dendritic trunk of the AII cell called lobular appendages. The cells probably also integrate additional information from other amacrine cells at these specializations. For example, the lobular appendages are known to be postsynaptic to a dopaminergic amacrine cell (Fig. 10a) whose effect is thought to be the modulation of AII activity depending upon ambient illumination (Pourcho, 1982; Kolb et al., 1990; Voigt and Wässle, 1987; Jensen and Daw, 1986). The physiology of the AII amacrine cell is further complicated by the fact that they are linked to each other by gap junctions. Under scotopic conditions, the coupling of cells through these gap junctions makes the receptive field of any one AII amacrine huge, thus gathering input from large numbers of rods. Under photopic conditions, dopamine released from the dopaminergic amacrine cell apparently uncouples the gap junctions, shrinking the size of the receptive field. Thus, it appears that through their "piggy-back" connectivity onto the cone-system, the rod channel can drive the center responses of both ON- and OFF-center ganglion cells. This seems a parsimonious and clever evolutionary way for the huge numbers of rods in these species to use preexisting cone pathways for providing scotopic input to ganglion cells driven by cones under photopic conditions. Thus, rather than evolve a completely separate pathway, the rod system developed interneurons to take advantage of existing cone pathways which would be inactive in dim light.

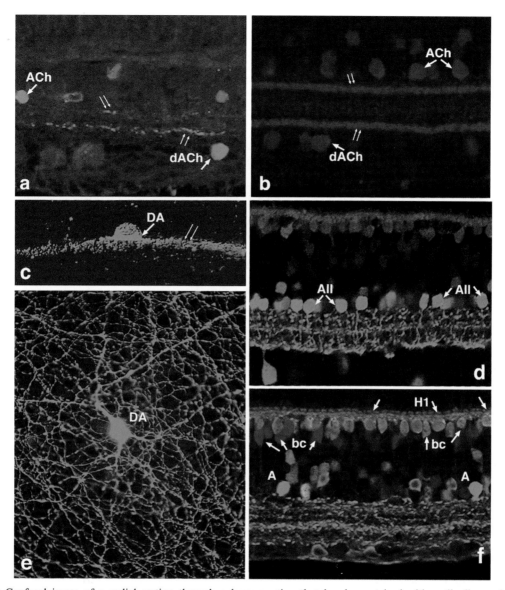

Fig. 5. (a) Confocal image of a radial section through a human retina that has been stained with antibodies against choline acetyltransferase (CHAT) a marker for the cholinergic starburst amacrine cells. Nuclei of one subtype (ACh) reside in the amacrine cell sublayer of the INL and has dendrites running in S2 of the IPL (upper pair of arrows); the other subtype (dACH) resides in the ganglion cell layer and has dendrites running in S4 (lower pair of arrows). (b) In a similar preparation of ground squirrel retina, many more nuclei of CHAT-positive starburst amacrines can be seen (ACh, dACh), contributing to two strongly labeled plexi of dendrites in the IPL (arrow pairs). A second population of amacrine cell nuclei are also faintly positive for CHAT. (c) A dopaminergic amacrine cell (DA, arrow) in the human retina stained with antibodies to tyrosine hydroxylase. The amacrine has a thin layer of dendrites running in S1 (arrow pair) under the amacrine cell bodies. (d) Rod AII amacrine cells are immunostained by antibodies to calretinin. These small-field, bistratified cells (AII, arrows) form a dense distribution tiling the retina with lobular appendages in the OFF layer and distal dendrites in the ON layer. (e) Wholemount view of a dopaminergic amacrine cell in the ground squirrel retina. The cell body (DA) is large and the overlapping dendrites of its and other cells' dendrites form a distinct plexus in stratum 1 of the IPL. (f) Immunostaining of horizontal cells (H1, arrows) in the ground squirrel retina showing that calretinin and calbindin D colocalize in these cells (orange). Many varieties of bipolar (bc, arrows) and amacrine cells (A) label with both calcium binding proteins but rarely colocalize the two.

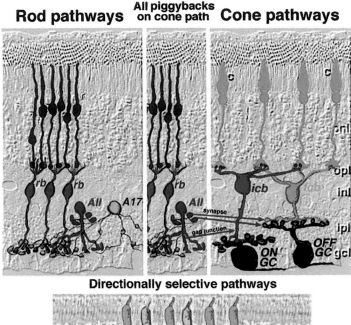

Rod pathways **AII piggybacks on cone path** **Cone pathways**

Directionally selective pathways

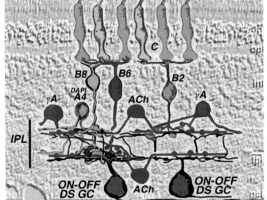

Fig. 6. The major retinal neurons contributing to the main retinal pathways are highlighted against a Nomarski image of unstained retina. (a) The rod pathway starts with hundreds of rods (r, purple) connecting to a single rod bipolar cell type (rb, blue) whose prominent axon terminals stratify in the deepest part of the IPL next to, but not onto, the ganglion cells. The narrow field, bistratified AII amacrine cell (AII, red) is post-synaptic at the rod terminal synapse, as are the beaded processes of the wide field A17 (turquoise) which also make reciprocal synapses back onto the rod bipolar terminal. (b) The AII amacrine carries or "piggy-backs" the rod signals to both ON- and OFF-cone pathways, making gap junctions between its lobular appendages and ON-cone bipolar cells (6c: icb, vermilion) in the inner IPL, and making conventional synaptic output onto the terminals of OFF-cone bipolar cells (6c: fcb, orange) and the dendrites of OFF-ganglion cells (6c: black, right) with its dendrites in the outer IPL. (c) The cone pathways are more numerous with multiple types of bipolar, amacrine, and ganglion cell involved. Unlike the rod pathway, however, cone bipolar cells directly synapse onto their targeted ganglion cells. Therefore this summary diagram is vastly simplified. First of all, the various subtypes of cone (c, green) make the two prominent types of contact with their cone bipolar cells, here represented by diffuse cone bipolar cells. Bipolar cell types whose dendrites make invaginating contacts with cone pedicles (icb, vermilion) have axon terminals in the deeper region of the IPL, called sublamina **b**, presynaptic to ON-ganglion cells (ON GC, black), while bipolar cell types whose dendrites make flat contacts with the cone terminals (fcb, orange), have axon terminals in the upper IPL (sublamina **a**) presynaptic to OFF-ganglion cells (OFF GC, black). (d) The directionally selective pathways involve neurons ramifying in the same strata of the IPL as do the dendrites of the physiologically defined ON–OFF directionally selective ganglion cells (ON–OFF DS GC, black), namely S2 and S4. The ground squirrel retina with its green and blue cones (c) is used as an example. Ramifying in S2 with the outer tier of ON–OFF DS GC processes are the processes of starburst amacrine (ACh, pink) resident in the INL, the terminals of the B2 cone bipolar cell (B2, orange) and certain other amacrines cells (A, red, right), as well as both upper tiers of dendrites of the small field, bistratified, DAPI amacrine cell (DAPI A4, dark green) and the bistratified bipolar cell (B8, salmon). Ramifying with the inner tier of ON–OFF DS GC processes are the major plexus of "displaced" starburst amacrine cells resident in the ganglion cell layer (ACh, pink), the terminals of the B6 bipolar cell (B6, crimson), the dendrites of certain amacrine cells (A, red, left), and both inner tiers of the bistratified A4 amacine (DAPI A4, dark green) and B8 bipolar cell (B8, salmon).

The A17 amacrine

The other well-studied rod pathway-specific inter-neuron is the wide-field A17, or so-called "rod reciprocal" amacrine (Fig. 6a; Kolb and Nelson, 1984; Nelson and Kolb, 1985). This cell is known to be GABAergic, but may also be serotonergic as well (Masland, 1988; Vaney, 1990). The A17 appears to be responsible for integrating and probably amplifying signals of the rod bipolar cells. They are known to interconnect rod bipolar axon terminals over an area of as much as 1 mm in diameter (Kolb et al., 1992). The A17 cells are purely driven by rods, are "ON" cells, and as might be expected from the size of their dendritic trees, have large receptive fields. While their input is from rod bipolar axon terminals, their output is back onto these same terminals in the form of a "reciprocal synapse" (Nelson and Kolb, 1985). The A17 cell is thought to function in a feedback manner with rod bipolar cells through GABAc ρ receptors (Fletcher and Wässle, 1999). Its function is thought to be that of pooling and integrating thousands of small amplitude rod bipolar events to increase the strength of the signal ultimately transmitted through the rod bipolar-AII-ganglion cell pathway.

Horizontal cells

Horizontal cells are the laterally spreading interneurons of the OPL, responsible for integrating information between photoreceptor and bipolar cells in this layer. The horizontal cells seem to play different physiological roles in lower vertebrates where they are probably responsible for providing both antagonistic surround and color opponency information (Werblin and Dowling, 1969; Werblin, 1991; Werblin et al., this volume). Although this is still considered an unresolved issue, the recent evidence of Dacey et al. (1996) seems to indicate that they do not play these roles in the retinas of mammals or primates.

If our two nocturnal species, cats and rats share a commonality of the rod pathway in the inner retina, the same cannot be said of the outer retina. Indeed, there are large variations in horizontal cell structure amongst these and other mammals that make for fascinating, if somewhat complex speculation about

their function (Gallego, 1986; Peichl and González-Soriano, 1994; Peichl et al., 1998). The cat retina contains two types of horizontal cell (Fisher and Boycott, 1974; Kolb, 1974; Boycott et al., 1978), the so-called A-type (Fig. 7), an axonless cell which connects only to cone photoreceptors, and the axon-bearing B-type, structurally one of the most complex neurons described in any retina (Fig. 7), which has connections with both rods and cones. Indeed, defined by the fact that it receives both rod and cone input, the B-type cell is the most common horizontal cell type found in rod-dominated retinas. The A-type cell, however, has apparently been lost in the evolution of the heavily rod-dominated retinas of rats and mice (Peichl and González-Soriano, 1994).

The B-type horizontal cell is not only structurally but also physiologically unusual. The dendrites, arising from the cell body contact only cone photoreceptors, while the elaborate axon terminal branches contact only rod photoreceptors. Because these cells generate only graded potentials, the two ends of the cell are thought to function in isolation from each other due to the length and thinness of the connecting axon (Nelson et al., 1975). The large and elaborate axon terminal can interconnect literally thousands of rod spherules in the OPL. Their axon terminal tips penetrate rod spherules at the synaptic invagination and end as lateral elements slightly more distal than the invaginating rod bipolar dendrites (Fig. 4c). The question of whether horizontal cells influence either the rod itself by a feedback pathway or the rod bipolar by a feed-forward pathway is still open to debate. The only structural correlate of such horizontal cell-to-rod photoreceptor contact is from an ultrastructural study of human retina. Small clusters of synaptic vesicles and associated presynaptic densities were reported in the horizontal cell terminals within the rod invaginations (asterisk, Fig. 4d; Linberg and Fisher, 1988). These apparent synapses are located so that the horizontal cell axon terminal is presynaptic to rod bipolar cell dendrites in the outer OPL and then presynaptic to the rod itself within the synaptic invagination. The rod bipolar cell has been reported to have a weak surround component to its receptive field, but it is not certain if it originates in the OPL or IPL (Dacheux and Raviola, 1986). At the opposite end of the axon-bearing B-type cell, the dendritic tips clustered along

38

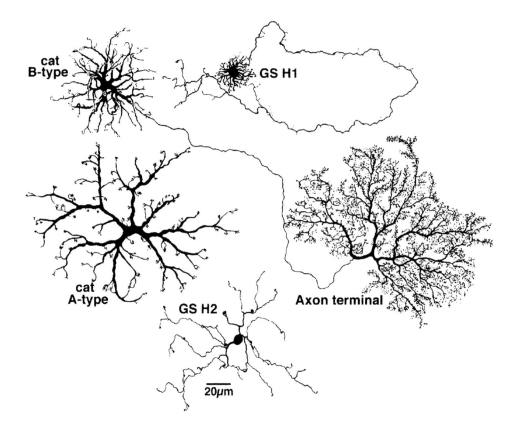

Fig. 7. Examples of Golgi-impregnated horizontal cells from cat and ground squirrel wholemounted retinas are shown at the same scale for purposes of comparison. The axon-bearing or B-type cell for both species has a dendritic end that is cone-connected, and an axon terminal portion contacting rods. The huge number of rods in the nocturnal cat retina can easily be appreciated by the vast number of rods contacted by a single axon terminal (cat B-type) compared with the sparsely branching ground squirrel horizontal cell terminal (GS H1). The axonless A-type horizontal cells are believed to be cone driven with significant S-cone input. The feline example (cat A-type) is sturdier and contacts many more cones than the sciurid example (GS H2). (Cat: from Fisher and Boycott, 1974; squirrel: from Linberg et al., 1996.)

the radiating dendritic branches (Fig. 7) innervate overlying cone pedicles. Specifically, they form the "lateral elements" at each of the many cone ribbon triads (Fig. 4b). In these cone terminal invaginations, Vardi et al. (1998) have reported the presence of $GABA_A$ receptors at the interface of lateral post-synaptic elements and the cone terminal (also see Kolb et al., this volume). Clearly, there is much to learn about the function of these highly complex interneurons.

The GABAergic interplexiform cell

The GABAergic interplexiform cell is found in rod-dominated mammalian retinas. This cell was first described in cat and squirrel monkey retinas (Gallego, 1971; Boycott et al., 1975; Kolb and Famiglietti, 1976; Kolb and West, 1977), and eventually proved to be distinctly different than the dopaminergic interplexiform cell of teleosts and primates (Dowling and Ehinger, 1975; Frederick et al., 1982). Whereas this latter type is presynaptic to cone horizontal cells in the OPL (Dowling and Ehinger, 1975; Frederick et al., 1982), the mammalian GABAergic variety is presynaptic to rod and cone bipolar cells instead (cat, Kolb and West, 1977; human, Linberg and Fisher, 1986). The dopaminergic interplexiform cell is probably concerned with photopic pathways and regulating adaptational changes between light and dark, while the GABAergic interplexiform cell seems devoted to rod-driven circuitry (Marshak, this volume).

Neurons of the cone pathways form the basic circuitry of diurnal retinas

As implied above, the cone pathways consist of a more "direct" relay of information from the photoreceptors to the ganglion cells, in the sense that there is no equivalent to an AII amacrine cell interposed between the cone bipolar cells and the ganglion cells (Fig. 6c). Compared to the rod pathway neurons, there is, in general, also less convergence first between the cones and cone bipolars and then between cone bipolars and ganglion cells.

Two functional classes of cone bipolar cell

Two parallel cone pathways have developed in all vertebrate retinas, one serving to provide information to the brain about brighter than background stimuli (the ON-center channel), and the other about darker than background stimuli (the OFF-center channel). Kuffler (1953) first described these two basic responses of ganglion cell in recordings made from the cat retina. The discovery that all photoreceptors hyperpolarize to the presence of light (Tomita, 1965) raised the question of how these two types of responses arise in the ganglion cells. Later, it was shown in Golgi impregnated tissue studied by electron microscopy, that midget cone bipolar cells in monkey retina consisted of two distinct subtypes, one making invaginating, and the other making flat contacts with cone pedicles (e.g. Fig. 4a, squirrel retina; Kolb et al., 1969). Furthermore, these subtypes of bipolar cell contact different ganglion cell types (Kolb, 1970). These data elucidated the structural basis for the two types of ganglion cell responses. Later it was shown that the invaginating cone bipolar axons branch and contact ganglion cell dendrites in Cajal's strata 3, 4 and 5 of the IPL (next to the ganglion cell layer), and that the flat cone bipolar axons contact ganglion cells whose dendrites branch in the more distal IPL layers (Cajal's strata 1, 2). Intracellular recordings from cat ganglion cell revealed that those branching in the lower portion of the IPL (contacting the invaginating bipolar cells) are of the "ON" variety, while those branching in the upper portion (contacting the flat bipolar cells) are of the "OFF" variety (Nelson et al., 1978; see Fig. 6c).

This effectively divided the IPL into two functional layers corresponding to the "OFF" response (sublamina **a**, Nelson et al., 1978), and ON response (sublamina **b**). This principle has held through each vertebrate species examined (Kolb, 1979; Nelson and Kolb, 1983; Cohen and Sterling, 1990). The ON-(invaginating) bipolars are now known to use metabotropic postsynaptic receptors (Slaughter and Miller, 1981; Nomura et al., 1994; Vardi et al., 1998) and a second messenger system involving a G-protein and calcium (Nawy and Jahr, 1990; Nawy, 2000), while the OFF-(flat) bipolars use the AMP/kainate ionotropic variety of glutamate receptor (Slaughter and Miller, 1983; Vardi et al., 1998; Brandstätter et al., 1997; DeVries and Schwartz, 1999; Kolb et al., this volume). The contact between both types of bipolar and their respective ganglion cell is excitatory, and probably mediated by AMPA or NMDA glutamate receptors (Miller et al., this volume). Although all fall within the "invaginating" or "flat" categories, based upon the branching patterns of their dendrites and axon terminals, as many as 8–10 different subtypes of cone bipolar cell probably exist in all vertebrate retinas (Figs. 3h, i, 5f, 6, 10).

Horizontal cells and the cone pathways

In diurnal species, the A-type (axonless) horizontal cell, with its pure-cone input is usually very well-developed (Fig. 7). In addition, the dendritic end of the axon-bearing horizontal cell (B-type) is also purely cone-connected. A different nomenclature is used for primate and ground squirrel horizontal cells (see Peichl et al., 1998). Both have a horizontal cell that connects only to cones and is called H2. As in the case of the B-type horizontal cell in the cat retina, the sciurid and primate H1 cell connects to cones via its dendrites, and rods through its axon terminals, although their terminal branches are never as elaborate as the cat's. In the ground squirrel the H1 axon is sparse with terminals which match the relatively sparse population of rods (Fig. 7; Linberg et al., 1996). The H2 cell in primates (Ahnelt and Kolb, 1994; Dacey et al., 1996), and probably ground squirrel as well (Linberg et al., 1996) seems to have a particular affinity for the SWS cones. Interestingly, the H2 cell in primates appears to connect only to cones, even along its short, curly, and sparsely branched "axon" (Kolb et al., 1980; Boycott et al., 1987; Wässle et al., 1989). On largely morphological grounds, a third type of horizontal cell (HIII) has recently been identified in human (Kolb et al., 1994) and *Cebus* retina (dos Reis et al., 2000). Whether these truly represent a physiologically separate subclass of horizontal cell remains controversial (Peichl et al., 1998) as does a proposed third type in rabbit retina (Famiglietti, 1990; Hack and Peichl, 1999).

There is physiological evidence for feedback from horizontal cells to photoreceptors. The hyperpolarization of cones by light results in a hyperpolarization of horizontal cells (i.e. sign conserving), which in turn results in a depolarization (i.e. sign inverting) of the cones. The exact nature of this feedback is not understood (for a discussion, see, Rodieck, 1998; p. 109), although there is evidence from non-mammalian species that both GABAergic and nitrogenergic mechanisms may be involved (Marc, 1992; Savchenko et al., 1997). Although searched for by many investigators, in many species, the structural correlates of this feedback synaptic action is lacking. Likewise, presumed synapses between horizontal cells and bipolar dendrites have been the subject of many studies, and yet remain elusive in most species (Dowling et al., 1966; Fisher and Boycott, 1974; Kolb, 1977). Electron microscopy has only shown definite synapses between A-type horizontal cells and bipolar cells in the rabbit retina (Fig. 8a), and only

what has been termed a "rudimentary synapse" lacking vesicles in the cat retina (Fig. 8b). Prominent "desmosomal-like" junctions were identified early in primate OPL between horizontal cell and possible bipolar cell dendrites (Fig. 8c; Dowling and Boycott, 1966). Particle aggregations occur at these junctions (Raviola and Gilula, 1975) as do GluR4 and GABA$_A$ receptors (Haverkamp et al., 2000).

Are specialized neurons of the rod pathway present in cone-dominant retina?

As mentioned previously, there are a few mammalian retinas that are dominated by cones, prominently among them the ground squirrels with only 10–15% of their photoreceptors being rods (Figs. 1b, 2, 3c, d; West and Dowling, 1975; Long and Fisher, 1983). Even so, the ground squirrel photoreceptor mosaic is never free of rods (Long and Fisher, 1983; Ahnelt, 1985; Kryger et al., 1998).The rod terminals in these species are broad and "cone-like," having several invaginations with multiple synaptic ribbons, and receiving many flat as well as invaginating contacts from bipolar cells (Fig. 4a, rod; West and Dowling, 1975; Anderson and Fisher, 1976; Jacobs et al., 1976). While the ground squirrel has an identifiable scotopic system, there has to date been no exclusively rod-driven pathway identified in their retina. Indeed, in this species rods have their input into the cone system early on, because there are gap junctions between

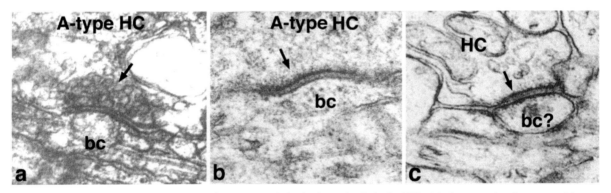

Fig. 8. Electron micrographs of various types of contacts made by horizontal cells in the OPL. (a). A conventional synapse with a pre-synaptic cluster of vesicles (arrow) is made by an A-type horizontal cell dendrite onto a bipolar cell dendrite (bc) in the rabbit OPL (from Fisher and Boycott, 1974). (b). A non-vesicular "synapse" (arrow) is made by an A-type horizontal cell process onto a bipolar cell dendrite (bc) in cat OPL (from Kolb 1974). A desmosome-like contact (arrow) joins horizontal (HC) and bipolar cell (bc?) dendrites in primate OPL (from Dowling and Boycott, 1966).

rods and cones (Jacobs et al., 1976), as well as an OFF- and two types of presumed ON- bipolar cells whose dendrites contact both rods and cones (West, 1978). The closest homologue to a rod bipolar cell in the ground squirrel retina is the so-called B4 bipolar because it has primarily rod input, and has its axon terminal deep the IPL, adjacent to the ganglion cells. This cell type can be immunostained with antibodies against protein kinase Cα (Greferath et al., 1990), a unique marker of rod bipolar cells in other mammals (e.g. Fig. 3g, rat retina). However, two other squirrel bipolar cell types, with exclusively cone input, also stain with this antibody (Cuenca et al., 2001). Furthermore, neither an AII nor A17 amacrine cell has been observed in Golgi impregnation or immunostaining studies of this retina (Linberg et al., 1996; Cuenca et al., 2001). The situation with horizontal cells in the ground squirrel retina is equally curious. The axon-bearing H1 (Linberg et al., 1996) with its sparse terminals spread along and sprouting from its short axon, would seem the obvious candidate for receiving rod input. However, West and Dowling (1975) found only cone input to both the dendrites and axon terminals in the Mexican ground squirrel, and Leeper and Charlton (1985) found no physiological evidence for rod input into a homologous cell type in the retina of the gray (tree) squirrel. The morphology of the axonless cell (H2, Linberg et al., 1996) suggests it to be equivalent to the axonless cells in other species, and thus purely cone driven (see Peichl et al., 1998). Thus, the rod input to horizontal cells in these retinas has not yet been identified. Overall, it seems likely that the rod photoreceptors "piggy-back" onto the cone bipolar system in the ground squirrel retina as in the rat and cat, but instead of utilizing a specialized amacrine cell (AII), the input occurs at the level of the photoreceptor terminal via rod–cone gap junctions and the specialized types of rod–cone bipolar cells. Indeed, DeVries and Baylor (1995) demonstrated in the 13-line ground squirrel that rod signals passed into cones by the gap junctions linking their terminals can be detected in OFF-center sluggish and ON–OFF direction-selective ganglion cells.

Interestingly, the GABAergic interplexiform cell which is associated with the rod pathway in both cat and primate has not yet been identified in the ground squirrel. However, the ground squirrel dopaminergic amacrine (a cell type which in some species is also clearly an interplexiform cell type) is clearly immunostained with tyrosine hydroxylase (Fig. 5e). Like the primate dopaminergic amacrine, this cell has a dendritic tree of overlapping fine dendrites in the upper IPL just beneath the amacrine cell bodies (Fig. 5c, human DA cell). Compared with the cat or primate dopamine cells, however, the rings in the dendritic plexus are not as clearly formed in the ground squirrel retina (compare Fig. 5e with Fig. 2g of cat, in Kolb et al., this volume). Moreover, ground squirrel dopamine cells are especially unusual with some very enlarged dendrites passing to the OPL where they branch and ultimately end in swellings apparently onto cone pedicles (Cuenca et al., 2001).

Neural pathways for complex feature detection such as movement and directional selectivity

The ground squirrel retina is renowned for the complex nature of its ganglion cell responses (Michael, 1968) such as responding to motion in general, and specifically to the directionality of a stimulus. Are there neural pathways in the ground squirrel retina that correlate with these complex ganglion cell properties? One type of amacrine cell, the "starburst," or "cholinergic" amacrine is thought to function in the generation of directionally selective responses in ganglion cells. The starburst amacrine cells occur as mirror-symmetric pairs across the IPL (Famiglietti, 1983; Tauchi and Masland, 1984; Masland and Tauchi, 1986); they are particularly elaborate in rabbit (Vaney, 1984; 1990) and ground squirrel retinas (Linberg et al., 1996). One type of starburst amacrine (a-type) has its cell body in the amacrine cell layer of the INL, with dendrites that stratify specifically to stratum 2 (OFF-sublamina **a**) of the IPL (Figs. 5a, b, 6d, 10). The other type, the "displaced" starburst amacrine (or b-type) has its cell body in the ganglion cell layer and dendrites that branch specifically in stratum 4 (ON-sublamina **b**) of the IPL (Figs. 5a, b, 6d, 10). The starburst cells have medium-sized receptive fields but also have tremendously overlapping dendritic trees. In the peripheral rabbit retina the dendrites from as many as 70 other cells overlap the dendritic field of

42

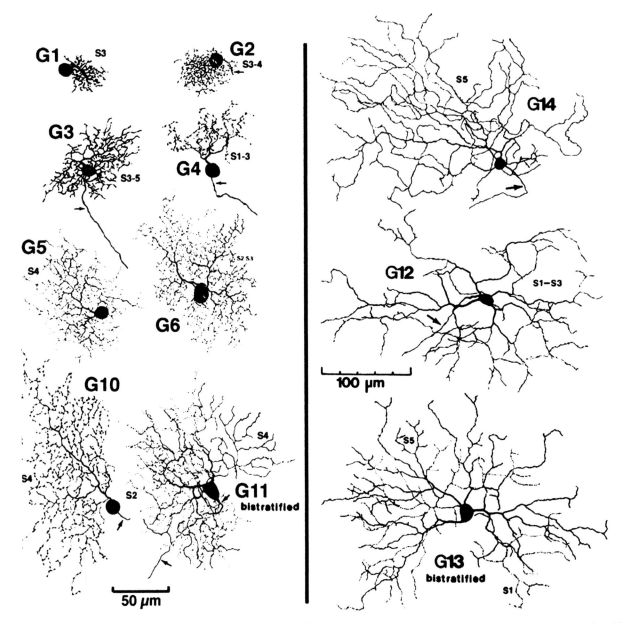

Fig. 9. Examples of several of the many types of ganglion cell in the ground squirrel retina typifies the numerous types of multi-branched and diffusely branching, bi- and tri-stratified ganglion cell seen in cone-dominated diurnal retinas (from Linberg et al., 1996).

a single labeled starburst cell (Tauchi and Masland, 1984; Vaney, 1984). Interestingly, the presence of elaborate starburst amacrines does not correlate with the proportion of cones, but rather the visual behavior of the species. These cells are especially well developed in diurnal species with visual streaks

(Fig. 2), and with large populations of ganglion cells exhibiting complex responses such as ground squirrels, rabbits and turtles (Fig. 9; see Kolb et al., this volume). In nocturnal mammals, or those with foveate retinas, or ganglion cells exhibiting primarily "simple" (e.g. center-surround) properties, the starburst amacrine cells tend to be less numerous, and more sparsely branched (Figs. 5a, 10).

The physiology of the starburst cells has been most thoroughly studied in rabbits. Both types have a center-surround organization with receptive field centers about the diameter of their dendritic fields. The a-type is an OFF-center cell giving a transient burst of small spikes when a light is turned off in the center of its field, while the b-type (displaced) cell gives an ON transient-sustained response (Bloomfield, 1992). The a-type cells receive input primarily from OFF-cone bipolars (Fig. 6d, cell B2), while ON-cone bipolars provide input to the b-type cell (Fig. 6d, cell B6). Bipolar input occurs primarily to spines on the proximal dendrites close to the cell body of both cell types. A distinctive feature of the starburst cells is the presence of beads on their distal dendrites (Fig. 10). At these sites both subtypes are presynaptic to a bistratified ON-OFF, directionally selective ganglion cell (e.g. G11 in ground squirrel, Fig. 9; Amthor et al., 1984; 1989; Famiglietti, 1987; 1991; Tauchi and Masland, 1984; Vaney, 1990; 1994; Vaney and Pow, 2000), while the b-type cell is presynaptic to an monostratified ON-directionally selective ganglion cell (such as G14 in ground squirrel, Fig. 9.; Famiglietti, 1991). Starburst cells themselves are not directionally selective, and, interestingly, removal of the displaced b-type in the ganglion cell layer does not change the response characteristics of the directionally selective cell to which they provide synaptic input (He and Masland, 1997).

Another amacrine cell type found exclusively in these retinas with visual streaks and complex ganglion cell receptive field properties is the "DAPI3" cell (Wright et al., 1997). This is a striking, small-field bistratified amacrine cell in ground squirrel (A4, Linberg et al., 1996), and rabbit. It is known to be glycinergic (Wright et al., 1997; Zucker and Ehinger, this volume). The DAPI3 cell's dendrites branch in strata 2 and 4, the same as those of the cholinergic amacrines and the ON–OFF directionally selective ganglion cells (Figs. 6d, 10c, DAPI/A4 cell in ground squirrel). A bistratified bipolar cell (B8, Linberg et al., 1996) has its axonal endings in these same two strata. Although the essential demonstration of contacts between these cells has not been done, it seems likely that the bistratified bipolar, the starburst cells, and the DAPI3 amacrine cell all participate in forming the receptive field properties of the bistratified ganglion cell.

The foveal pathways of primates

The fovea is a specialized area of retina that perhaps represents the ultimate in diurnal retinal design by excluding rods and rod pathway neurons completely. There are no rod photoreceptors, rod bipolar cells, nor AII amacrine cells within the central 5° of the primate retina (encompassing a diameter of about 0.8 to 1 mm around the point of visual fixation, i.e. the center of the fovea) (Kolb and Zhang, 1997; Kolb et al., 2000). The cone pathways within this region of the retina have the least convergence and represent the greatest resolving capabilities (i.e. highest visual acuity) of all visual systems except those of birds of prey. This is accomplished by the so-called "midget pathways." For comparison, the cone-dominated ground squirrel retina, never achieves a photoreceptor population purely composed of cones, the center of the visual streak having approximately 5% rods (Long and Fisher, 1983; Kryger et al., 1998).

The midget pathways: high acuity and "red–green" color information

Within the fovea, small bipolar cells form a "private line" from a single cone to a single ganglion cell, and hence were given the name "midget" (Polyak, 1941). The midget ganglion cells are also known as "P cells" because they project to individual cells in the parvocellular layer of the lateral geniculate nucleus (Shapley and Perry, 1986). The midget pathway is also organized into ON- and OFF-center channels as described earlier for the "diffuse" cone pathways from peripheral retina. As such, every cone in the fovea will contact one ON- and one OFF-bipolar cell. Thus, the invaginating midget bipolar cells as part of the ON pathway connect to the dendrites of an ON-center midget ganglion cell in sublamina **b** of the IPL, while the flat midget bipolar cells as part of the OFF pathway connect to dendrites of an OFF-center midget ganglion cell in sublamina **a** (Fig. 10b, MGCa, MGCb). Because a single midget bipolar–ganglion cell circuit receives input

44

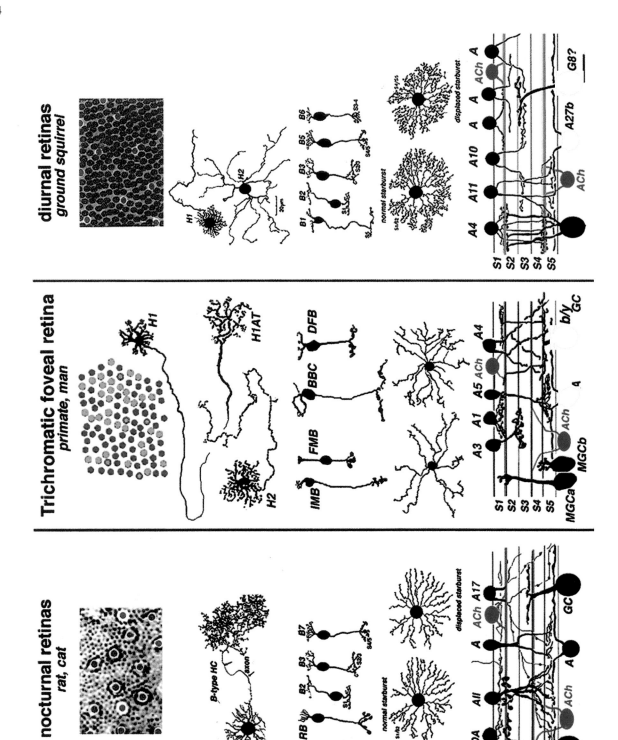

Fig. 10. Three columns summarize the three types of retina discussed in this chapter: diurnal, nocturnal, and primate foveal. The upper panel in each column depicts the photoreceptor mosaics typical for each retinal type. The middle portion of each column contains golgi-stained examples of major neurons in each type of retina, while the lowermost portion of each column recapitulates the neural circuitry central to each retinal type. (a) The nocturnal retina, exemplified here by cat and rat retinas, are populated largely by rods that separate the small population of green cones and even smaller number of blue cones from one another. The rod-connecting, axon-bearing B-type horizontal cell is well developed and its profusely branching axon terminal connects with thousands of rod terminals. The rat lacks the axonless A-type horizontal cell. The uniquely mammalian rod bipolar cell (RB) comprises almost 90% of all bipolar cell types, although several types of cone bipolar (B2, B3, B7) have been identified. The two varieties of starburst amacrine cell are similar to but less elaborate than seen in ground squirrel or rabbit. The two rod-associated amacrine cell types (AII, A17) figure prominently in the circuitry of this retinal type, being the main channel by which rod signals are shunted to the cone pathways and thence to higher visual centers. Nocturnal retinas have fewer varieties of complex ganglion cells; instead the alpha and beta types predominate. (b) The trichromatic foveal retina seen in some primates and humans is essentially rod-free and contains red, green, and some blue cones. At least two types of axon-bearing horizontal cell (B-type, H1, H2) are present, but no axonless type (A-type) has been found. Two types of midget bipolar cells predominate at the fovea (IMB, FMB) although other cone bipolar cell types have been described including several diffuse types (DFB) and a blue cone bipolar cell (BBC). Rod bipolar cells are lacking in the rod-free foveal center. The two types of starburst amacrine cell are sparsely branched, very unadorned and generally not very well developed. The rod associated amacrines AII and A17 do not participate in the foveal circuitry where smaller cone-connecting amacrine cells are seen (A1, A3, A4, A5). The ganglion cell population in the fovea is dominated by the ON- and OFF-midget ganglion cells (MGCa, MGCb) with a small but prominent population of the bistratified blue-ON yellow-OFF ganglion cells (b/y GC). (c) The diurnal retina is exemplified by the ground squirrel retina whose retinal mosaic consists of mostly green cones, a smaller population of blue cones and some rods (not shown). Diurnal retinas have well-developed cone-contacting horizontal cells, including the axonless A types (H2) and axon-bearing horizontal cells (H1) with sparsely branching axon terminals. A number of cone bipolar cells are seen (B1, B2, B3, B5, B6), most having small dendritic fields and non-convergent axon terminals monostratified to various specific strata of the IPL. The two starburst amacrine cell varieties are very elaborate, well developed and numerous. Many amacrine and ganglion cell types are typical of diurnal retinas and their many processes and types of synaptic interactions are reflected in the very thick IPL seen in these retinas.

from a single cone, it is *de facto* also connected in a spectrally specific manner so that each midget bipolar may receive its input from a SWS-, MWS-, or LWS-cone (Fig. 10b). Whether or not midget ganglion cells receive their input from the midget bipolars in a way that makes them spatially and spectrally opponent (Gouras, 1968) is still controversial. For example, a midget ganglion cell that had a center response to long-wavelength stimuli ("red") would have a surround that responded to mid-wavelength stimuli (green). Although not well studied, the more accepted scheme for the organization of such wavelength comparisons by the midget ganglion cells seems to be one in which the cell does not respond to wavelength in a center-surround manner, but would respond antagonistically across its whole field to the presence of "red" or "green" light (see Rodieck, 1998, Ch. 14 for a discussion). Regardless of the exact organization of their receptive fields, it is clear that the midget system carries relatively pure opponent information from the LWS and MWS cones into the brain.

A special pathway for "blue–yellow" color information

The pathway for SWS (blue sensitive) cones is very different from that of the LWS and MWS cones. The SWS cones are absent from the very central 1° of the foveal pit (Williams et al., 1981) but they reach a maximum density on the foveal slope. The synaptic pedicles of these cones have a "simpler morphology" than those of the other two cone types, and lack telodendria (Ahnelt et al., 1987; Kolb et al., 1997). The SWS system has a lower spatial and temporal resolution than those of the other two (Stockman et al., 1991; Humanski and Wilson, 1992). The SWS-cone is contacted by its own subtype of bipolar (Mariani, 1984; Kouyama and Marshak, 1992), which is presumed to be an ON-type since its contacts with the cone are mostly invaginating and ribbon related. The axon of the S-cone bipolar cell ends in the lowermost IPL (ON layer; Fig. 10b, BBC). Its dendrites mostly project to a single SWS cone but occasionally it reaches out to contact another cone of the same type (Mariani, 1984; Kouyama and Marshak, 1992). The S-cone bipolar carries ON

signals to the lower dendrites of the blue-ON–yellow-OFF bistratified ganglion cell (Dacey and Lee, 1994). It is thought that the yellow-OFF response arises from an OFF-diffuse bipolar that contacts primarily the LWS- and MWS-cones with some input from the SWS cones. This bipolar cell would synapse onto the upper dendrites of the bistratified ganglion cell, in the OFF layer of the IPL (Fig. 10b; Dacey and Lee, 1994). As in the case of the other two-wavelength-sensitive systems, it is still unknown if the bistratified ganglion cell represents the sole input into the blue–yellow opponent system. Early electrophysiological investigations of monkey retinal ganglion cells indicated that this information was carried primarily by a SWS cone ON center ganglion cell type with a much larger receptive field than is typical of those in the LWS or MWS systems. This ganglion cell also did not appear to have a spatially antagonistic receptive field structure, but the "blue" and "yellow" opponent responses co-existed within the field. Interestingly, there is no conclusive recording from a "blue-OFF–yellow-ON" type of ganglion cell. The apparent specialized nature of the blue-yellow color system is emphasized by the fact that its ganglion cells are thought to project to a special layer of the lateral geniculate nucleus called the koniocellular (or K) layer (Irvin et al., 1993; Calkins et al., 1998; Calkins and Sterling, 1999).

Other foveal neurons

In the retina of fish and other lower vertebrates it seems fairly clear that horizontal cells are involved in constructing the center/surround organization and that these are specifically connected to the different spectrally sensitive classes of cone (Naka, 1976). There is physiological evidence that horizontal cells in mammalian retina do not function in a similar manner (Dacey et al., 1996). In and near the primate fovea, both horizontal cell types are numerous and closely packed. Interestingly, the rod-connecting axons of human H1 cells project away from the center of the rod-free fovea towards the region where rods first appear, thus avoiding the pure-cone foveal center. Foveal H2 (pure cone-input) cells are small, "bushy," and densely concentrated, reflecting the large density of cones (Fig. 10b). The many varieties of small field amacrine cells are crowded at the fovea (Fig. 10b: A1, A3, A4, A5). Dopamine amacrine cells and starburst amacrine cells are scantily branched, concentrically organized around the fovea, and altogether poorly developed (Fig. 10b). The AII and A17 amacrine cells, with their clearly defined role in the rod pathway are excluded altogether and thus the midget ganglion cells of the fovea carry no signals originating from rods. Other types of ganglion cell, like the large-field phasic M cells (Shapley and Perry, 1986) are present at the fovea but are very small and scantily branched, whereas in comparison, the midget ganglion cells are stacked 8 cell bodies deep and have a great overlap in their dendritic fields. The greatly thickened inner plexiform layer in the fovea reflects the density of the various types of amacrine and ganglion cells in this region.

Summary and future directions

Figure 10 summarizes the characteristic neuronal types in the model retinal systems discussed here: the rod-dominated retinas of largely nocturnal species such as cat; the highly specialized, pure-cone region of the primate fovea; and the cone-dominated retina of the highly diurnal ground squirrel.

The retina of the cat as well as those of other rod-dominated species is characterized by a huge number of rod photoreceptors and convergent neurons for pooling rod signals. The latter are exemplified by horizontal cells with elaborate axon terminals that receive only rod input, a single type of ON rod bipolar cell forming 90% of the bipolar cell population, and the most well developed AII and A17 amacrine cells of any species studied to date. Amacrine cells associated with directional sensitivity (cholinergic starburst cells) are present, but meager, and ganglion cells tend to be of the "simple" center-surround type with large dendritic trees (Fig. 10a).

Understanding retinal circuitry in terms of visual behavior continues to be one of the greatest challenges facing vision scientists. Probably nowhere is this challenge more important than understanding pathways in the human fovea because of our reliance on high acuity vision and color information, and the number of people afflicted with diseases that effect macular vision. The center of the fovea has evolved a system of single, "private" pathways enabling every cone to send their signals to midget ganglion cells that carry information into the brain about acuity and red-green color opponency. Here cone bipolar cells are closely packed and horizontal cells have very small fields with both types interconnecting only a minimum number of cones. Outside the very center, but within the fovea, the SWS-cones are at their highest density as are the unique "blue" cone bipolar cells. Amacrine cells are small-field, and the ganglion cells are almost entirely of the midget types, with the exception being the so-called "blue-yellow" bistratified cell. Cholinergic systems and wide-field amacrine cells are poorly developed (Fig. 10b).

The cone-dominated retinas of diurnal squirrels (and rod-dominated species such as rabbits with a visual streak) tend to have retinas that do much processing of visual information before sending it on to the brain. Cone-devoted bipolar cell types are numerous, as are small-field multistratified amacrine and ganglion cells. Although dominated by cones, these retinas, like those of other non-primate mammals, are dichromatic and the retina seems to be specialized for contrasting opponent color information, detecting movement, and directionality. They have a highly developed cholinergic/starburst and DAPI amacrine cell systems. Rod pathway neurons are ill-developed, or, in some cases, absent (Fig. 10c).

There are many questions remaining about retinal circuitry, and much yet to be learned from studying the retinas of different species. Many questions remain about the functional role of the myriad types of amacrine cell that seem to exist in virtually every species. Is there a specialized OFF-rod bipolar pathway, or a "blue-OFF" pathway homologous to the "blue-ON" pathway? A glance at Fig. 9 shows many morphologically complex ganglion cells about which we know nothing in terms of circuitry or functionality. Whether or not there is a ganglion cell pathway for "red-green" color vision similar to that for the "blue-yellow" system as an alternative to the color-opponent midget system in primates is a hotly debated topic (Rodieck, 1998; Dacey, 2000). While we have learned a tremendous amount about retinal circuitry since the pioneering studies of Dowling et al. (Dowling and Boycott, 1966; Dowling et al., 1966; Boycott and Dowling, 1969; Werblin and Dowling, 1969) there is still much work to be done utilizing comparative morphological and physiological techniques.

References

Ahnelt, P.K. (1985) Characterization of the color related receptor mosaic in the ground squirrel retina. *Vision Res.*, 25: 1557–1567.

Ahnelt, P.K. and Kolb, H. (1994) Horizontal cells and cone photoreceptors in human retina: a Golgi-electron microscopic study of spectral connectivity. *J. Comp. Neurol.*, 343: 406–427.

Ahnelt P.K. and Kolb H. (2000) The mammalian photoreceptor mosaic—adaptive design. *Prog. Ret. & Eye Res.*, 19: 711–777.

Ahnelt, P.K., Kolb, H. and Pflug, R. (1987) Identification of a subtype of cone photoreceptor, likely to be blue sensitive, in the human retina. *J. Comp. Neurol.*, 255: 18–34.

Amthor, F.R., Oyster, C.W. and Takahashi, E.S. (1984) Morphology of on-off direction-selective ganglion cells in the rabbit retina. *Brain Res.*, 298: 187–190.

Amthor, F.R., Takahashi, E.S. and Oyster, C.W. (1989) Morphologies of rabbit retinal ganglion cells with complex receptive fields. *J. Comp. Neurol.*, 280: 97–121.

Anderson, D.H. and Fisher, S.K. (1976) The photoreceptors of diurnal squirrels: outer segment structure, disc shedding, and protein renewal. *J. Ultrastr. Res.*, 55: 119–141.

Bloomfield, S.A. (1992) Relationship between receptive and dendritic field size of amacrine cells in the rabbit retina. *J. Neurophysiol.*, 68: 711–725.

Bowmaker, J.K. (1998) Evolution of colour vision in vertebrates. *Eye*, 12: 541–547.

Boycott, B.B. and Dowling, J.E. (1969) Organization of the primate retina: light microscopy. *Phil. Trans. R. Soc. B*, 255: 109–184.

Boycott, B.B. and Kolb, H. (1973) The connections between bipolar cells and photoreceptors in the retina of the domestic cat. *J. Comp. Neurol.*, 148: 91–114.

Boycott, B.B. and Wässle, H. (1991) Morphological classification of bipolar cells of the primate retina. *Eur. J. Neurosci.*, 3: 1069–1088.

Boycott, B.B., Hopkins, J.M. and Sperling, H.G. (1987) Cone connections of the horizontal cells of the rhesus monkey's retina. *Proc. R. Soc. Lond. B*, 229: 345–379.

Boycott, B.B., Peichl, L. and Wässle, H. (1978) Morphological types of horizontal cell in the retina of the domestic cat. *Proc. R. Soc. Lond. B*, 203: 229–245.

Boycott, B.B., Dowling, J.E., Fisher, S.K., Kolb, H. and Laties, A.M. (1975) Interplexiform cells of the mammalian retina and their comparison with catecholamine-containing retinal cells. *Proc. R. Soc. Lond. B*, 191: 353–368.

Brandstätter, J.B., Koulen, P. and Wässle, H. (1997) Selective synaptic distribution of kainate receptor subumits in the two plexiform layers of the rat retina. *J. Neurosci.*, 17: 9290–9307.

Cajal, S.R. (1892) *The Structure of the Retina.* (Translated by S.A. Thorpe and M. Glickstein) Springfield, Il., Thomas, 1972.

Cajal, S.R. (1911) *Histologie du système nerveux de l'Homme et des Vertébrés.* 2: Paris: A. Maloine.

Calderone, J.B. and Jacobs, G.H. (1995) Regional variations in the relative sensitivity to UV light in the mouse retina. *Vis. Neurosci.*, 12: 463–468.

Calderone, J.B. and Jacobs, G.H. (1999). Cone receptor variations and their functional consequences in two species of hamster. *Vis. Neurosci.*, 16: 53–63.

Calkins D.J. and Sterling, P. (1999) Evidence that circuits for spatial and color vision segregate at the first retinal synapse. *Neuron.*, 24: 313–21.

Calkins D.J., Tsukamoto Y. and Sterling, P. (1998) Microcircuitry and mosaic of a blue-yellow ganglion cell in the primate retina. *J Neurosci.*, 18: 3373–85.

Cohen, E. and Sterling, P. (1990) Demonstration of cell types among cone bipolar neurons of cat retina. *Phil. Trans. R. Soc. Lond. B*, 330: 305–321.

Cuenca, N., Linberg, K., Lewis, G.P., Fisher, S.K., Deng, P. and Kolb, H. (2001) Neurons of the ground squirrel retina: An immunocytochemical and confocal microscope study. *Molecul. Vision*, submitted.

Curcio, C.A. and Hendrickson, A.E. (1991) Organization and development of the primate photoreceptor mosaic. *Prog. Ret. Res.*, 10: 89–120.

Dacey, D.M. (2000) Parallel pathways for spectral coding in primate retina. *Ann. Rev. Neurosci.*, 23: 743–75.

Dacey, D.M. and Lee, B.B. (1994) The 'blue-on' opponent pathways in primate retina originates from a distinct bistratified ganglion cell. *Nature*, 367: 731–735.

Dacey, D.M., Lee, B.B., Stafford, D.K., Pokorny, J. and Smith, V.C. (1996) Horizontal cells of the primate retina: cone specificity without spectral opponency. *Science*, 271: 656–659.

Dacheux, R.F. and Raviola, E. (1986) The rod pathway in the rabbit retina: a depolarizing bipolar and amacrine cell. *J. Neurosci.*, 6: 331–345.

DeVries, S.H. and Baylor, D.A. (1995) An alternative pathway for signal flow from rod photoreceptors to ganglion cells in mammalian retina. *P. N. A. S.*, 92: 10658–10662.

DeVries, S.H. and Schwartz, E.R. (1999) Kainate receptors mediate synaptic transmission between cones and 'Off' bipolar cells in a mammalian retina. *Nature*, 397: 157–160.

dos Reis, J.W.L., Silviera, L.C.L., Carvalho, W.A. and Yamada, E.S. (2000) Are there three classes of retinal horizontal cells in dichromatic Capuchin monkeys? Invest. Ophthalmol. *Vis. Sci.*, 41: S944.

Dowling, J.E. (1970) Organization of vertebrate retinas. *Invest. Ophthalmol.*, 9: 655–680.

Dowling, J.E. and Boycott, B.B. (1966) Organization of the primate retina; electron microscopy. *Proc. R. Soc. Lond. B*, 166: 80–111.

Dowling, J.E. and Ehinger, B. (1975) Synaptic organization of the amine-containing interplexiform cells of the goldfish and Cebus monkey retinas. *Science*, 188: 270–273.

Dowling, J.E. and Werblin, F.S. (1969) Organization of the retina of the mudpuppy, *Necturus maculosus*. I. Synaptic structure. *J. Neurophysiol.*, 32: 315–338.

Dowling, J.E., Brown, J.E. and Major, D. (1966) Synapses of horizontal cells in rabbit and cat retinas. *Science*, 153: 1639–1641.

Famiglietti, E.V. (1983) 'Starburst' amacrine cells and cholinergic neurons: mirror-symmetric ON and OFF amacrine cells of rabbit retina. *Brain Res.*, 261: 138–144.

Famiglietti, E.V. (1987) Starburst amacrine cells in cat retina are associated with bistratified, presumed directionally selective, ganglion cells. *Brain Res.*, 413: 404–408.

Famiglietti, E.V. (1990) A new type of wide-field horizontal cell, presumably linked to blue cones, in rabbit retina. *Brain Res.*, 535: 174–179.

Famiglietti, E.V. (1991) Synaptic organization of starburst amacrine cells in rabbit retina: analysis of serial thin sections by electron microscopy and graphic reconstruction. *J. Comp. Neurol.*, 309: 40–70.

Famiglietti, E. V. and Kolb, H. (1975) A bistratified amacrine cell and synaptic circuitry in the inner plexiform layer of the retina. *Brain Res.*, 84: 293–300.

Fisher, S.K. and Boycott, B.B. (1974). Synaptic connexions made by horizontal cells within the outer plexiform layer of the retina of the cat and the rabbit. *Proc. Roy. Soc. Lond. B*, 186: 317–331.

Fletcher, E.L. and Wässle, H. (1999) Indoleamine-accumulating amacrine cells are presynaptic to rod bipolar cells through GABAc receptors. *J. Comp. Neurol.*, 413: 155–167.

Frederick, J.M., Rayborn, M.E., Laties, A.M., Lam, D.M.K. and Hollyfield, J.G. (1982) Dopaminergic neurons in the human retina. *J. Comp. Neurol.*, 210: 65–79.

Freed, M.A., Smith, R.G. and Sterling, P. (1987) Rod bipolar array in the cat retina: pattern of input from rods and GABA-accumulating amacrine cells. *J. Comp. Neurol.*, 266: 445–455.

Gallego, A. (1971) Celulas interplexiformes en la retina del gato. *Arch. Soc. Esp. Oftal.*, 31: 299–304.

Gallego, A. (1986) Comparative studies on horizontal cells and a note on microglial cells. *Prog. Ret. Res.*, 5: 165–206.

Gouras, P. (1968) Identification of cone mechanisms in monkey ganglion cells. *J. Physiol. Lond.*, 199: 533–547.

Green, D.G. and Dowling, J.E. (1975) Electrophysiological evidence for rod-like receptors in the gray squirrel, ground squirrel and prairie dog retinas. *J. Comp. Neurol.*, 159: 461–472.

Greferath, U., Grünert, U. and Wässle, H. (1990) Rod bipolar cells in the mammalian retina show protein kinase C-like immunoreactivity. *J. Comp. Neurol.*, 301: 433–442.

Grünert, U. and Martin, P.R. (1991) Rod bipolar cells in the macaque monkey: immunoreactivity and connectivity. *J. Neurosci.*, 11: 2742–2758.

Hack, I. and Peichl, L. (1999) Horizontal cells of the rabbit retina are non-selectively connected to the cones. *Eur. J. Neurosci.*, 11: 2261–2274.

Haverkamp, S., Grünert, U. and Wässle, H. (2000) The cone pedicle presents a synaptic microchip in the primate retina. *Invest. Ophthal. Vis. Sci.*, 41: S112.

He, S. and Masland, R.H. (1997) Retinal direction selectivity after targeted laser ablation of starburst amacrine cells. *Nature*, 389: 378–382.

Hecht, S., Schlaer, S. and Pirenne, M.H. (1942) Energy, quanta, and vision. *J. Gen. Physiol.*, 25: 819–840.

Hughes, A. (1977) The topography of vision in mammals of contrasting life style: comparative optics and retinal organization. In: F. Crescitelli, Ed. *Handbook of Sensory Physiology*, Vol. VII/5, *The Visual System in Vertebrates*. Springer-Verlag, Berlin: pp. 613–756.

Humanski, R.A. and Wilson, H.R. (1992) Spatial frequency mechanisms with short-wavelength-sensitive cone inputs. *Vision Res.*, 32: 549–560.

Immel, J.H. and Fisher, S.K. (1985) Cone photoreceptor shedding in the tree shrew (*Tupaia belangerii*). *Cell Tiss. Res.*, 239: 667–675.

Irvin, G.E., Casagrande, V.A. and Norton, T.T. (1993) Center/surround relationships of magnocellular, parvocellular and koniocellular relay cells in primate lateral geniculate nucleus. *Vis. Neurosci.*, 10: 363–373.

Jacobs, G.H. (1981) *Comparative Color Vision*. Academic Press, New York.

Jacobs, G.H. (1993) The distribution and nature of colour vision among the mammals. *Biol. Rev.*, 68: 413–471.

Jacobs, G.H., Neitz, M. and Neitz, J. (1996) Mutations in S-cone pigment genes and the absence of color vision in two species of nocturnal primate. *Proc. Roy. Soc. Lond. B*, 263: 705–710.

Jacobs, G.H., Fisher, S.K., Anderson, D.H. and Silverman, M.S. (1976) Scotopic and photopic vision in the California ground squirrel: physiological and anatomical evidence. *J. Comp. Neurol.*, 165: 209–227.

Jacobs, G.H., Tootell, R.B.H., Fisher, S.K. and Anderson, D.H. (1980) Rod photoreceptors and scotopic vision in ground squirrels. *J. Comp. Neurol.*, 189: 113–125.

Jensen, R.J. and Daw, N.W. (1986) Effects of dopamine and its agonists and antagonists on the receptive field properties of ganglion cells in the rabbit retina. *Neurosci.*, 17: 837–855.

Kolb, H. (1970) Organization of the outer plexiform layer of the primate retina: electron microscopy of Golgi-impregnated cells. *Phil. Trans. Roy. Soc. B. (Lond.)*, 258: 261–283.

Kolb, H. (1974) The connections between horizontal cells and photoreceptors in the retina of the cat: electron microscopy of Golgi preparations. *J. Comp. Neurol.*, 155: 1–14.

Kolb, H. (1977) The organization of the outer plexiform layer in the retina of the cat: electron microscopic observations. *J. Neurocytol.*, 6: 131–153.

Kolb, H. (1979) The inner plexiform layer in the retina of the cat: electron microscopic observations. *J. Neurocytol.*, 8: 295–329.

Kolb, H. and Famiglietti, E.V. (1974) Rod and cone pathways in the inner plexiform layer of the cat retina. *Science*, 186: 47–49.

Kolb, H. and Famiglietti, E.V. (1976) Rod and cone pathways in the retina of the cat. *Invest. Ophthalmol.*, 15: 935–946.

Kolb, H. and Nelson, R. (1984) Neural architecture of the cat retina. *Prog. Ret. Res.*, 3: 21–60.

Kolb, H. and Nelson, R. (1993) Off-alpha and off-beta ganglion cells in the cat retina. II. Neural circuitry as revealed by electron microscopy of HRP stains. *J. Comp. Neurol.*, 329: 85–110.

Kolb, H. and West, R.W. (1977) Synaptic connections of the interplexiform cell in the retina of the cat. *J. Neurocytol.*, 6: 155–170.

Kolb, H. and Zhang, L.L. (1997) Immunostaining with antibodies against protein kinase C isoforms in the fovea of the monkey retina. *Micr. Res. Techn.*, 36: 57–75.

Kolb, H., Boycott, B.B. and Dowling, J.E. (1969) A second type of midget bipolar cell in the primate retina. Appendix Phil *Trans. R. Soc. B. (Lond)*, 255: 177–184.

Kolb, H., Linberg, K.A. and Fisher, S.K. (1992) The neurons of the human retina: a Golgi study. *J. Comp. Neurol.*, 318: 147–187.

Kolb, H., Mariani, A. and Gallego, A. (1980) A second type of horizontal cell in the monkey retina. *J. Comp. Neurol.*, 189: 31–39.

Kolb, H., Cuenca, N., Wang, H.-H. and DeKorver, L. (1990) The synaptic organization of the dopaminergic amacrine cell in the cat retina. *J. Neurocytol.*, 19: 343–366.

Kolb, H., Zhang, L., DeKorver, L. and Cuenca, N. (2000) Amacrine cells that are calretinin-immunoreactive in the monkey retina. *J. Comp. Neurol.* Submitted.

Kolb, H., Goede, P., Roberts, S., McDermott, R. and Gouras, P. (1997). Uniqueness of the S-cone pedicle in the human retina and consequences for color processing. *J. Comp. Neurol.*, 286: 443–460.

Kolb, H., Fernandez, E., Schouten, J., Ahnelt, P., Linberg, K.A. and Fisher, S.K. (1994) Are there three types of horizontal cell in the human retina? *J. Comp. Neurol.*, 343: 370–386.

Kouyama, N. and Marshak, D.W. (1992) Bipolar cells specific for blue cones in the macaque retina. *J. Neurosci.*, 12: 1233–1252.

Kryger, Z., Galli-Resta, L., Jacobs, G.H. and Reese, B.E. (1998) The topography of rod and cone photoreceptors in the retina of the ground squirrel. *Vis. Neurosci.*, 15: 685–691.

Kuffler, S.W. (1953) Discharge pattern and functional organization of mammalian retina. *J. Neurophysiol.*, 16: 37–68.

Kühne, J.-H. (1983) Rod receptors in the retina of *Tupaia belangeri. Anat. Embryol.*, 167: 95–102.

LaVail, M.M. (1976) Survival of some photoreceptors in albino rats following long term exposure to continuous light. *Invest. Ophthalmol. Vis. Sci.*, 15: 64–70.

Leeper, H.F. and Charlton, J.S. (1985) Response properties of horizontal cells and photoreceptor cells in the retina of the tree squirrel, *Sciurus carolinensis. J. Neurophysiol.*, 54: 1157–1166.

Lettvin, J.Y., Maturana, H.R., McCulloch, W.S. and Pitts, W.H. (1959) What the frog's eye tells the frog's brain. *Proc. Inst. Radio. Engrs. NY*, 47: 1940–1951.

Linberg, K.A. and Fisher, S.K. (1986) An ultrastructural study of interplexiform cell synapses in the human retina. *J. Comp. Neurol.*, 243: 561–576.

Linberg, K.A. and Fisher, S.K. (1988) Ultrastructural evidence that horizontal cell axon terminals are presynaptic in the human retina. *J. Comp. Neurol.*, 268: 281–297.

Linberg, K.A., Suemune, S. and Fisher, S.K. (1996) Retinal neurons of the California ground squirrel, *Spermophilus beecheyi*: A Golgi study. *J. Comp. Neurol.*, 365: 173–216.

Linberg, K.A., Lewis, G.P., Shaaw, C., Rex, T.S. and Fisher, S.K. (2001) The distribution of S- and M-cones in normal and experimentally detached cat retina. *J. Comp. Neurol.*, 430: 343–356.

Long, K.O. and Fisher, S.K. (1983) The distributions of photoreceptors and ganglion cells in the California ground squirrel, *Spermophilus beecheyi. J. Comp. Neurol.*, 221: 329–340.

Marc, R.E. (1992) The structure of GABAergic circuits in ectotherm retinas. In: Mize, R., Marc, R.E. and Sillito, A. (Eds), *GABA in the Retina and Central Visual System*. Elsevier, Amsterdam, pp. 61–92.

Mariani, A.P. (1984) Bipolar cells in monkey retina selective for cones likely to be blue-sensitive. *Nature*, 308: 184–186.

Marshak, D.W. and Dowling, J.E. (1987) Synapses of the cone horizontal cell axons of the goldfish retina. *J. Comp. Neurol.*, 256: 430–443.

Masland, R.H. (1988) Amacrine cells. *TINS*, 11: 405–410.

Masland, R.H. and Tauchi, M. (1986) The cholinergic amacrine cell. *TINS*, 9: 218–223.

McMahon, C., Hendrickson, A.E., Dacey, D.M., Neitz, J. and Neitz, M. (2000) L:M cone ratio as a function of eccentricity in primate retina estimated from an analysis of messenger RNA. *Invest. Ophthal. Vis. Sci.*, 1: p. S494.

Michael, C.R. (1968) Receptive fields of single optic nerve fibers in a mammal with an all-cone retina. II. Directionally selective units. *J. Neurophysiol.*, 31: 257–267.

Mollon, J.D. and Bowmaker, J.K. (1992) The spatial arrangement of cones in the primate fovea. *Nature*, 360: 677–679.

Müller, B. and Peichl, L. (1989) Topography of cones and rods in the tree shrew retina. *J. Comp. Neurol.*, 282: 581–594.

Naka, K.-I. (1976) Neuronal circuitry in the catfish retina. *Invest. Ophthal.*, 15: 926–935.

Nathans, J., Thomas, D. and Hogness, D.S. (1986) Molecular genetics of human color vision: the genes encoding the blue, green and red pigments. *Science*, 232: 193–202.

Nawy, S. and Jahr, C.E. (1990) Suppression by glutamate of cGMP activated conductance in retinal bipolar cells. *Nature*, 346: 269–271.

Nawy, S. (2000) Regulation of the On bipolar cell mGluR6 pathway by Ca^{2+}. *J. Neurosci.*, 20: 4471–4479.

Nelson, R. (1982) AII amacrine cells quicken the time course of rod signals in the cat retina. *J. Neurophysiol.*, 47: 928–947.

Nelson, R. and Kolb, H. (1983) Synaptic patterns and response properties of bipolar and ganglion cells in the cat retina. *Vision Res.*, 23: 1183–1195.

Nelson, R. and Kolb, H. (1985) A17: a broad-field amacrine cell of the rod system in the retina of the cat. *J. Neurophysiol.*, 54: 592–614.

Nelson, R., v Lützow, A., Kolb, H. and Gouras, P. (1975) Horizontal cells in cat with independent dendritic systems. *Science*, 189: 137–139.

Nelson, R., Famiglietti, E.V. and Kolb, H. (1978) Intracellular staining reveals different levels of stratification for on-center and off-center ganglion cells in the cat retina. *J. Neurophysiol.*, 41: 427–483.

Nomura, A., Shigemoto, R., Nakamura, Y., Okamoto, N., Mizuno, N. and Nakanishi, S. (1994) Developmentally regulated postsynaptic localization of a metabotropic glutamate receptor in rat rod bipolar cells. *Cell*, 77: 361–369.

Østerberg, G. (1935) Topography of the layer of rods and cones in the human retina. *Acta Ophthal.*, (Suppl.) 6: 1–103.

Peichl, L. and González-Soriano, J. (1994) Morphological types of horizontal cell in rodent retinae: a comparison of rat, mouse, gerbil, and guinea pig. *Vis. Neurosci.*, 11: 501–517.

Peichl, L., Sandmann, D. and Boycott, B.B. (1998) Comparative anatomy and function of mammalian horizontal cells. In: Chalupa, L.M. and Finlay, B.L. (Eds), *Development and Organization of the Retina*. Plenum Press, New York, pp. 147–172.

Polyak, S. L. (1941) *The Retina*. University of Chicago, Chicago, Ill.

Pourcho, R. G. (1982) Dopaminergic amacrine cells in the cat retina. *Brain Res.*, 252: 101–109.

Raviola, E. and Gilula, N.B. (1975) Intramembrane organization of specialized contacts in the outer plexiform layer of the retina: a freeze-fracture study in monkey and rabbits. *J. Cell Biol.*, 65: 192–222.

Rodieck, R.W. (1998) *The First Steps in Seeing*. Sinauer Associates Inc., Sunderland, Mass.

Roorda, A. and Williams, D.R. (1999) The arrangement of the three cone classes in the living human eye (see comments). *Nature*, 397: 520–522.

Savchenko, A., Barnes, S. and Kramer, R.H. (1997) Cyclic nucleotide-gated channels mediate synaptic feedback by nitric oxide. *Nature*, 390: 694–698.

Shapley, R. and Perry, V.H. (1986) Cat and monkey retinal ganglion cells and their visual functional roles. *Trends Neurosci.*, 9: 229–235.

Slaughter, M.M. and Miller, R.F. (1981) 2-amino-4-phosphonobutyric acid: A new pharmacological tool for retina research. *Science*, 211: 182–184.

Slaughter, M.M and Miller, R.F. (1983) An excitatory amino acid antagonist blocks cone input to sign-conserving second-order retinal neurons. *Science*, 219: 1230–1232.

Steinberg, R.H., Reid, M. and Lacy, P.L. (1973) The distribution of rods and cones in the retina of the cat (*Felis domesticus*). *J. Comp. Neurol.*, 148: 229–248.

Sterling, P., Freed, M.A. and Smith, R.G. (1988) Architecture of rod and cone circuits to the *On*-beta ganglion cell. *J. Neurosci.*, 8: 623–642.

Stockman, A., MacLeod, D.I.A. and DePriest, D.D. (1991) The temporal properties of the human short-wave photoreceptors and their associated pathways. *Vision Res.*, 31: 189–208.

Strettoi, E., Raviola, E. and Dacheux, R.F. (1992) Synaptic connections of the narrow-field, bistratified rod amacrine cell (AII) in the rabbit retina. *J. Comp. Neurol.*, 325: 152–168.

Szél, Á. and Röhlich, P. (1992). Two cone types in rat retina detected by anti-visual pigment antibodies. *Exp. Eye Res.*, 55: 47–52.

Tauchi, M. and Masland, R.H. (1984) The shape and arrangement of the cholinergic neurons in the rabbit retina. *Proc. Roy. Soc. Lond. B*, 223: 101–119.

Tomita, T. (1965) Electrophysiological study of the mechanisms subserving color coding in the fish retina. *Cold Spring Harb. Symp. Quant. Biol.*, 30: 559–566.

Vaney, D.I. (1984) "Coronate" amacrine cells of the rabbit retina have the "starburst" dendritic morphology. *Proc. Roy. Soc. Lond. B*, 220: 501–508.

Vaney, D.I. (1985) The morphology and topographic distribution of AII amacrine cells in the cat retina. *Proc. Roy. Soc. Lond. B*, 224: 475–488.

Vaney, D.I. (1990) The mosaic of amacrine cells in the mammalian retina. *Prog. Ret. Res.*, 9: 49–100.

Vaney, D.I. (1994) Territorial organization of direction-selective ganglion cells in rabbit retina. *J. Neurosci.*, 14: 6301–6316.

Vaney, D.I. and Pow, D.V. (2000) The dendritic architecture of the cholinergic plexus in the rabbit retina: selective labeling by glycine accumulation in the presence of sarcosine. *J. Comp. Neurol.*, 421: 1–13.

Vardi, N., Morigiwa, K., Wang, T.-L., Shi, Y.-J. and Sterling, P. (1998) Neurochemistry of the mammalian cone "synaptic complex." *Vision Res.*, 38: 1359–1369.

Voigt, T. and Wässle, H. (1987) Dopaminergic innervation of AII amacrine cells in mammalian retina. *J. Neurosci.*, 7: 4115–4128.

Walls, G.L. (1942) *The vertebrate eye and its adaptive radiation*. Bloomfield Hills, Mich.

Wässle, H., Boycott, B.B. and Röhrenbeck, J. (1989) Horizontal cells in the monkey retina: cone connections and dendritic network. *Eur. J. Neurosci.*, 1: 421–435.

Wässle, H., Yamashita, M., Greferath, U., Grünert, U. and Müller, F. (1991) The rod bipolar cell of the mammalian retina. *Vis. Neurosci.*, 7: 99–112.

Werblin, F. (1991) Synaptic connections, receptive fields, and patterns of activity in the tiger salamander retina. *Invest. Ophthal. Vis. Sci.*, 32: 459–483.

Werblin, F.S. and Dowling, J.E. (1969) Organization of the retina of the mudpuppy, *Necturus maculosus*. II. Intracellular recording. *J. Neurophysiol.*, 32: 339–355.

West, R.W. (1978) Bipolar and horizontal cells of the gray squirrel retina: Golgi morphology and receptor connections. *Vision Res.*, 18: 129–136.

West, R.W. and Dowling, J.E. (1975) Anatomical evidence for cone and rod-like receptors in the gray squirrel, ground squirrel and prairie dog retina. *J. Comp. Neurol.*, 159: 439–460.

Wikler, K.C. and Rakic, P. (1990) Distribution of photoreceptor subtypes in the retina of diurnal and nocturnal primates. *J. Neurosci.*, 10: 3390–3401.

Williams, D.R., MacLeod, D.I.A. and Hayhoe, M. (1981) Punctate sensitivity of the blue-sensitive mechanisms. *Vision Res.*, 21: 1357–1375.

Wright L.L., Macqueen, C.L., Elston, G.N., Young, H.M., Pow, D.V. and Vaney, D.I. (1997) The DAPI-3 amacrine cells of the rabbit retina. *Vis. Neurosci.*, 14: 473–92.

Young, H. and Vaney, D.I. (1991) Rod-signal interneurons in the rabbit retina: 1. Rod bipolar cells. *J. Comp. Neurol.*, 310: 139–153.

H. Kolb, H. Ripps and S. Wu (Eds.)
Progress in Brain Research, Vol. 131

CHAPTER 3

Synaptic organization in the fly's optic lamina: few cells, many synapses and divergent microcircuits

I.A. Meinertzhagen[*] and K.E. Sorra[#]

Neuroscience Institute, Life Sciences Centre, Dalhousie University, Halifax, NS, Canada B3H 4J1

Introduction

In what seems to us a remarkable oversight in the literature on this topic, the authors of most textbook accounts of neurobiology continue to portray the organization of synaptic junctions as one in which a single presynaptic active zone enjoys exclusive rights to synaptic transmission to a single postsynaptic site. And for most of the vertebrate brain this is so. Yet it is patently not so in the vertebrate retina, in which the first widely received report of the synaptic organization of the primate retina by John Dowling and the late Brian Boycott (1966) were to be a remarkable influence on our ideas about retinal microcircuitry. They distinguished two types of chemical synapse, conventional and ribbon, the former resembling synaptic contacts found in most other sites of the vertebrate nervous system. The ribbon synapses differ in having a clear presynaptic ribbon that serves to channel vesicles to the presynaptic plasmalemma prior to exocytosis (Gray and Pease, 1971), an early postulate now supported by recent molecular evidence (Muresan et al., 1999). An architectural feature of ribbon synapses which is

also of great functional significance is that they incorporate multiple postsynaptic elements opposite the site of the presynaptic ribbon, an arrangement that provides the substrate for the retina's rich networks of synaptic microcircuits. In the primate retina, these networks are fed by the triad synapses of cone pedicles (Missotten, 1965), and the dyad synapses of the bipolar terminals (Dowling and Boycott, 1966).

Early reports on the synaptic organization of insect brains (e.g. Lamparter et al., 1969) indicated that synaptic sites incorporating multiple postsynaptic elements are not an accidental discovery of the vertebrate retina, but are also found in insects. Such multiple-contact synapses (Meinertzhagen, 1984) are in fact the main type of structural organization at synaptic contacts in insect brains (Strausfeld and Meinertzhagen, 1998). Even though "Dyade" contacts with two postsynaptic elements in the ant's brain were compared with dyad synapses in the retina quite early on (Lamparter et al., 1969), and such arrangements were simultaneously reported at photoreceptor terminals in flies (Trujillo-Cenóz, 1965; Boschek, 1971; Burkhardt and Braitenberg, 1976), immediate comparison between photoreceptor synapses in insects and vertebrates was not made explicit. Not in fact until an account from Dowling and Chappell (1972) detailed the synaptic contacts at photoreceptor terminals of the simple eye, or ocellus, of the dragonfly were photoreceptor synaptic

---

[*] Corresponding author: I.A. Meinertzhagen, Tel.: (902)-494-2131; Fax: (902)-494-6585; E-mail: IAM@IS.DAL.CA
[#] Present address: K.E. Sorra, Ortho-McNeil Pharmaceuticals, 1000 Rt 202, Box 300, Raritan, NJ 08869, USA

contacts called dyads. That report also identified feedback synapses, and the substrate these provide for reciprocal connections between photoreceptor terminals and their interneurons, although cell identification in the ocellar neuropile was otherwise largely incomplete. Also in the dragonfly, in the first optic neuropile or lamina of the compound eye, a subsequent report from the Dowling laboratory identified the afferent synapses of photoreceptor terminals as triads, and feedback synapses formed back upon those terminals, as dyads (Armett-Kibel et al., 1977). This account provided the first clear terminological union of synaptic contacts found in the insect lamina and the vertebrate retina, endorsing the essential similarity of their organization in the two visual systems. It also took advantage of the compound eye's incredible gift to neuroanatomy, of being constructed from an array of structurally recognizable columns, corresponding to the compound eye's array of ommatidia, each containing a photoreceptor cluster of fixed composition. This repeated structure means that within each neuropile of the optic lobe beneath the compound eye, the columnar neurons (Fischbach and Dittrich, 1989) are also repeated, so as to constitute a population of isomorphic cells.

The fly's lamina cartridge is a precise module of retinal neurons

The structural composition of the optic neuropiles is known comprehensively only in the lamina, in which the cylinder-shaped modules, called cartridges, present an obvious geometrical array. A survey of a number of insect species (reviewed in Strausfeld and Nässel, 1980; Meinertzhagen and Armett-Kibel, 1982) suggests a common architectural plan for the cartridges of different groups. It also reveals that the lamina's cell types are best characterized in the fly's optic lobe, especially in muscoid flies (Figs. lA, 2A–G) and the fruit fly *Drosophila melanogaster* (Figs. 1B. 2F–I). For this reason, recent work emphasizing the fly's lamina, especially in *Drosophila*, using the powerful range of genetic methods accumulated during the last few decades, requires no further advocacy.

The lamina is innervated by six (R1–R6) of the eight photoreceptors from the overlying ommatidia (Braitenberg, 1967), the synaptic terminals of which provide input to groups of second-order interneurons (Trujillo-Cenóz, 1965). These include the lamina's monopolar cell interneurons which number five in all species investigated carefully (Shaw and Meinertzhagen, 1986). In addition to these six classes (R1–R6, L1–L5), within each cartridge are processes of one or more amacrine cells (Am); and three medulla cells—two centrifugal (C2, C3) and one (T1) with a lamina arborisation twinned with Am processes (Campos-Ortega and Strausfeld, 1973). Some cells—L1/L2, L3/L4, C2/C3—form pairs, possibly having arisen during evolution by duplication (Meinertzhagen and Shaw, 1989). As well as these synaptic neurons, the axons of the two central cells of the ommatidium, R7 and R8, bypass the cartridge (Braitenberg, 1967), and three epithelial glia surround it (Boschek, 1971), so bringing to 13 the total number of columnar, amacrine and glial cell classes associated with each lamina cartridge (Fig. 1). Together these constitute a numerically and morphologically determinate network, a visual system in miniature.

The fly's lamina synaptic contacts

Insect synapses resemble the ribbon synapses of the vertebrate retina and various sensory neurons with tonic transmitter release (Juusola et al., 1996), in having a presynaptic organelle at the presumed site of transmitter release. This has been called a presynaptic density or "button" synapse in the dragonfly's photoreceptor terminals (Armett-Kibel et al., 1977), but its shape is actually quite variable across different insect groups, so that in retrospect such descriptive names are not universally valid. In flies, for example, the presynaptic density is shaped like a table and forms a 'T' in fair cross-section (Trujillo-Cenóz, 1965; Boschek, 1971; Fröhlich, 1985). Since their first clear description in fly photoreceptor terminals (Trujillo-Cenóz, 1965), however, most subsequent reports (e.g. Meinertzhagen and O'Neil, 1991) refer to the presynaptic density as a presynaptic ribbon, emphasising the presumed functional similarity of this organelle to the ribbons of the vertebrate retina, as sites of transmitter release through synaptic vesicle exocytosis (Saint Marie and Carlson, 1982). In fact, just as at vertebrate bipolar cells, the organelle is far from ribbon-shaped. Moreover, the shape differs a

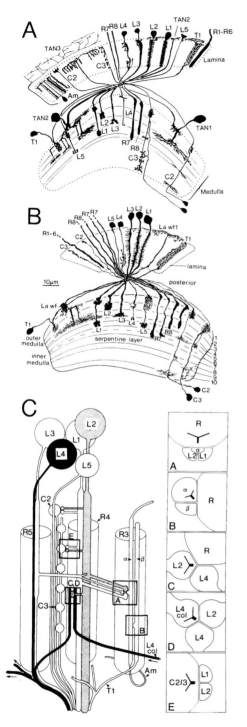

Fig. 1. The classes of neuron in the fly's lamina cartridge. (A), (B) Golgi impregnated cells in: (A) a calliphorid or muscid fly (Shaw, 1984); and (B) *Drosophila melanogaster* (Fischbach and Dittrich, 1989). (A) shows a lamina amacrine cell and two

great deal even among different groups of Diptera, having gradually attained its table shape in flies after an evolutionary progression through intermediate forms (Shaw and Meinertzhagen, 1986).

Higher-order optic neuropiles

The nine identified classes of columnar lamina interneuron (Fischbach and Dittrich, 1989; Meinertzhagen and O'Neil, 1991) are each represented in all cartridges. By comparison, the deeper neuropiles of the optic lobe, the medulla and the two neuropiles of the lobula complex, lobula and lobula plate, are both much more complex and less studied than the lamina (Strausfeld and Nässel, 1980). The cellular composition of the lamina cartridge is numerically determinate, but despite careful reports of Golgi impregnated cell types in the deeper neuropiles (*Musca*: Strausfeld, 1970; *Drosophila*: Fischbach and Dittrich, 1989), and of axon profile counts in the medulla (*Musca*: Campos-Ortega and Strausfeld, 1972), the numbers of neurons within each neuropile column are still unclear. Simple counts of somata, including glia, are available for *Drosophila*, at least for the mid-pupa, and these indicate a total of about 27,000 for the medulla, and 10,500 for the lobula plate and other derivates of the inner optic anlage (extrapolated from Hofbauer and Campos-Ortega, 1990). For an average compound eye having 776 ommatidia (Ready et al., 1976), and assuming a single column in all optic neuropiles for each ommatidium in the compound eye, the mean number of ganglion cells per column must therefore be about 35 for the medulla and 13.5

classes of tangential neuron not shown in (B). (C) Summary diagram of neurons within the *Drosophila* cartridge. For visibility only three R1–R6 terminals are depicted and, ascending R3, only one pair of amacrine and TI processes. Ll–L3 exposed at the cartridge interior are depicted with simplified morphologies. Spines of Ll–L3 reveal the complexity of dendritic arrangements required to accommodate fixed associations of several postsynaptic elements at multiple sites belonging to different synaptic classes. Five of these are shown (boxes), enlarged on the right: **A**, tetrad; **B**, amacrine (α) feedback; **C**, L2 feedback; **D**, input from L4 collateral (col) from adjacent cartridge, either $+x$ or $-y$; **E**, input from C2 or C3. (From Meinertzhagen and O'Neil, 1991.)

56

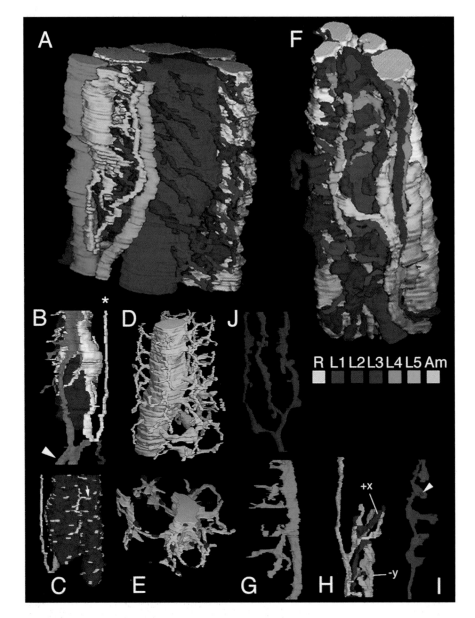

Fig. 2. Three-dimensional reconstructions from serial EM showing images of portions of the cells corresponding to those in Fig. 1. (A) Cartridge in *Musca*, showing R1–R3, R6 and L1–4 in 180 65-nm sections. (B)–(E) Individual elements from the same cartridge as in (A). (B) Proximal portion of R5's terminal with a pair of amacrine and T1 processes, viewed as if from the exterior of the cartridge. The amacrine process arises from an descending fibre (*), T1 from a medulla axon (arrowhead). (C) R5 and R6 and the same amacrine process as in (B) but viewed from the opposite direction, from the cartridge interior, showing tetrad sites, some visited by amacrine spines (arrow). (D) L1, showing the regular arrays of spines in "combs" directed radially between surrounding R1–R6. (E) Portion of L1 viewed axially, showing the distribution of postsynaptic tetrad sites. (F) Cartridge in *Drosophila*, with cells corresponding to, and color-coded as in, (A), from 200 65-nm sections. Cells occupy a mirror-image arrangement within the cartridge cross-section to their counterparts in (A). (G–J) Individual elements from the same cartridge as in (F). (G) L3, with unilateral spines directed to the cartridge interior. (H) The intrinsic axon of L4, accompanied by L4 processes from two adjacent cartridges (+ x, − y) with collaterals extending proximal to this reconstruction. (I) C3, with repeated terminals with output synapses (arrowhead). (J) Three of processes of the basket arborization of T1. (Modified from Hu, 1993.)

for the lobula cortex. Afferent terminals from the retina and lamina, and centrifugal arborizations from the lobula complex, together augment the average number of ganglion cells in each medulla column. The numbers of *types* of neuron are moreover significantly larger than this average number. Golgi impregnations in *Drosophila* reveal at least 57 morphological cell types with somata in the medulla cortex and 26 in the posterior cortex of the lobula plate (Fischbach and Dittrich, 1989), so that many cell types can therefore not occur in each column. In *Musca* similar data indicate about 120 cell types in the medulla, of which 46 occur in every medulla column, and perhaps a further 50 in the lobula complex (Campos-Ortega and Strausfeld, 1972). Although these counts rest on many assumptions, they do indicate, for the medulla at least, that the complement of cells in a medulla column could be several times larger than in a lamina cartridge, and that not all cell types occur in all columns, so that their number in one particular medulla column need not be determinate (Campos-Ortega and Strausfeld, 1972).

The lamina's synapses: some facts and figures

There is extensive documentation of the major afferent synapse of the fly photoreceptor terminal, where, at each site, four postsynaptic elements occupy a stereotypic configuration that invariably includes processes from both L1 and L2 (Burkhardt and Braitenberg, 1976; Nicol and Meinertzhagen, 1982; Fröhlich, 1985). In view of this composition, such synapses have previously been termed tetrads (Burkhardt and Braitenberg, 1976), but it is worth emphasizing that the tetrad composition (Burkhardt and Braitenberg, 1976) and its invariance (Nicol and Meinertzhagen, 1982) were actually overlooked until revealed by serial EM. In addition to morphological studies, tetrads have also been the subject of electrophysiological analysis (Laughlin, 1980; Shaw, 1981; Juusola et al., 1995; Uusitalo et al., 1995). For the remaining synapses in the lamina, little is known however. Based on earlier work in the housefly *Musca domestica* (Strausfeld and Campos-Ortega, 1977; Meinertzhagen, unpublished), and a previous partial enumeration of lamina synapses in the blowfly

Lucilia cuprina (Shaw, 1984), the most comprehensive inventory of synaptic contacts for an insect photoreceptor exists in the lamina of *Drosophila melanogaster* (Meinertzhagen and O'Neil, 1991) as presented in Table 1. This list of synaptic classes from single-section EM gives undue prominence to numerical minorities, however, and fails to indicate the numerical strength of each synaptic connection. Counts of synaptic contacts derived from serial EM address this problem (Table 2), but are based on information from a single cartridge, the small size of which in *Drosophila* has allowed the 13 classes of columnar, amacrine and glial cells to be examined by serial EM using our standard methods (Meinertzhagen, 1996). The stereotypic cellular composition of the cartridge leads us to anticipate that the synaptic organization of this cartridge is an accurate reflection of other cartridges.

Except for one type of junction, all synaptic contacts are of the multiple-contact type (Fig. 1C), formally similar to dyads and triads of the vertebrate retina. The sole monadic contacts are gnarl complexes of amacrine cell processes, which are considered below. There are in total 24 major synaptic classes (Table 1; Meinertzhagen and O'Neil, 1991), each with a different combination of presynaptic neuron and postsynaptic partners; some of these have subtypes, such as the four combinations of postsynaptic partners that include L1 and L2 at tetrad synapses. Of the 24 classes of synapse, the predominant synaptic class is the photoreceptor tetrad synapse. Of the remainder, only four are triad synapses, and these represent combinations of three postsynaptic elements which also appear in pairs at dyads (Table 1), and thus can be construed as imprecision or instability in synaptogenesis. The lamina thus boils down to many tetrads of the same class, and many dyads of different classes: although the number of cells is small, the number of synapses these few cells form is richly diverse.

The complete matrix of synaptic contacts from the single serially-sectioned cartridge indicates a total of 480 synapses, of which 283 are tetrads (Table 2A), with a total of 1187 identifed and 324 unknown postsynaptic contacts (Table 2B). Synaptic numbers are definitive, but the numbers of postsynaptic contacts are slight underestimates, because it is not always possible to trace the full extent of all neurites.

Table 1. Matrix of pre- and postsynaptic cells in a single lamina cartridge of *Drosophila melanogaster*, and their dyad and triad configurations[1]

Postsynaptic partner(s)	Presynaptic cell[2]															Postsynaptic partner(s)
	R1–R6	R7	R8	L1	L2	L3	L4 (intrinsic)	L4 (+x)	L4 (−y)	L5	Amacrine	T1	C2	C3	Ep. Glia	
R1–R6	—	—	—	—	dyad (L4,−y or +x)	—	dyad (L2) / triad (L2, other)	dyad (L2)	dyad (L2, R) / triad (L2, L4 + x) / triad (L2, L4 − y)	—	dyad (T1; L2/3)	—	—	—	—	R1–R6
L1	tetrads (L2; L3, Am/glia)	—	—	—	—	—	—	—	—	—	—	—	—	—	—	L1
L2	tetrads (L1; L3, Am/glia)	—	—	—	—	—	dyad (R)	dyad (L4)	dyad (R, L4 + x)	—	—	—	dyad (L1–3 or R)	dyad (L1)	—	L2
L3	tetrads (L1, L2; Am/glia)	—	—	—	—	—	—	—	—	—	—	—	—	—	—	L3
L4 (intrinsic)	—	—	—	—	dyad (L4 − y/L4 + x)	—	—	—	—	—	—	—	—	—	—	L4 (parent)
L4 (from +x)	—	—	—	—	dyad (L4 − y)	—	—	—	—	—	—	—	—	—	—	L4 (from +x)
L4 (from −y)	—	—	—	—	dyad (L4 + x)	—	—	—	—	—	—	—	—	—	—	L4 (from −y)
L5	—	—	—	—	—	—	—	—	—	—	—	—	—	—	—	L5
Am	tetrads (L1 + L2, Am)	—	—	—	—	—	—	—	—	—	—	—	—	—	—	Am
T1	tetrads (L1, L2, Am)	—	—	—	—	—	—	—	—	—	dyad (L2/3/5) / triad (R; L1/2/3) / monad (at gnarl)	—	dyad (L1–3)	dyad (L2/3)	—	T1
C2	—	—	—	—	—	—	—	—	—	—	—	—	—	—	—	C2
C3	—	—	—	—	—	—	—	—	—	—	—	—	—	—	—	C3
Epithelial glia	tetrads (L1, L2, glia)	—	—	—	—	—	—	—	—	—	monad (gnarl)	—	—	—	—	

[1] Each cell in the matrix gives the synapse (dyad, triad) and lamina cells contributing postsynaptic processes in combination with the postsynaptic cell of that matrix column.

[2] R1–R6: photoreceptor terminals; L1–L5: lamina monopolar cells; Am: amacrine cell; C2, C3: medulla centrifugal cells; Ep. Glia: surrounding epithelial glia.

Table 2A. The numbers of presynaptic sites in each cell of a single cartridge[1]

Presynaptic cell	R1	R2	R3	R4	R5	R6	L1	L2	L3	L4 intrin	L4 (+x)	L4 (−y)	L5	Am	T1	C2	C3	Epith glia	Total identified elements	Other elements	Total all elements
Total number of presynaptic sites	50	50	45	44	42	52	2?	8	0	3	10	10	0	118	0	16	17	0	465	15	480

Table 2B. The numbers of postsynaptic contacts (inputs) upon the cells of the cartridge from presynaptic sites in all other cells[1].

Postsynaptic contact	R1	R2	R3	R4	R5	R6	L1	L2	L3	L4 intr	L4 (+x)	L4 (−y)	L5	Am	T1	C2	C3	Ep. glia	Total
R1	–	–	–	–	–	–	–	1	–	–	3	1	–	11	–	1	–	–	17
R2	–	–	–	–	–	–	–	1	–	1	2	3	–	9	–	–	–	–	16
R3	–	–	–	–	–	–	–	2	–	–	2	1	–	6	–	–	–	–	11
R4	–	–	–	–	–	–	–	–	–	–	2	2	–	10	–	–	–	–	12
R5	–	–	–	–	–	–	–	1	–	–	1	–	–	5	–	1	–	–	7
R6	–	–	–	–	–	–	–	1	–	–	2	1	–	10	–	–	–	–	13
L1	43	44	39	39	38	43	–	1	–	–	1	1	2	7	–	1	2	–	263
L2	48	49	43	39	42	48	–	–	–	1	1	6	1	10	–	8	10	–	314
L3	7	11	5	18	19	14	–	–	–	–	2	–	–	27	–	4	2	–	110
L4 (parent)	–	–	–	–	–	–	–	–	–	3	3	2	–	–	–	–	–	–	7
L4 (from +x)	–	1	–	–	–	1	–	5	–	5	2	3	–	–	–	–	–	–	11
L4 (from −y)	–	–	–	–	–	–	1	5	1	–	4	–	–	–	–	1	–	–	11
L5	–	–	–	–	–	–	–	–	–	–	–	–	–	1	–	1	–	–	1
Am	47	47	43	34	34	46	–	2	–	–	–	–	–	–	–	6	8	–	265
T1	–	–	–	–	–	–	–	2	–	–	–	–	–	76	–	2	–	–	80
C2	–	–	–	–	–	–	–	–	–	–	–	–	–	–	–	–	–	–	0
C3	–	–	–	–	–	–	–	–	–	–	1	–	–	1	–	–	–	–	0
Ep. Glia	0	12	4	3	1	2	–	–	–	–	1	–	–	26	–	–	–	–	49
Totals	145	165	134	133	134	154	2	22	0	5	27	20	0	194	0	30	22	0	1187
Uncertain profiles	55	35	46	43	34	54	0	4	1	0	3	3	0	22	0	20	4	0	324

[1] The terminals of R1–R6, all essentially identical, and the following unique cells: monopolar cells L1–L5, L4 of three types (the intrinsic neuron and invading terminals from two collaterals, one each from the cartridges in the +x and −y directions of the lamina's array); 6 processes from an unknown number of amacrine cells; 6 processes, paired with those of the amacrine cell, from a single medulla T1 cell; 2 medulla centrifugal cells, C2 and C3; and 3 epithelial glial cells surrounding each cartridge. Each postsynaptic contact is counted singly, despite the fact that most form in combinations, most frequently dyads, with 2 postsynaptic elements.

Nevertheless, these numbers do allow us for the first time to see the relative numerical strengths of synaptic pathways, in an approach adopted before only in a partial census of synapses in *L. cuprina* (Shaw, 1984). The 283 tetrads together account for 862 of the 1187 identified postsynaptic contacts in *Drosophila* (Table 2A), so that the remaining 325 identified postsynaptic contacts are allocated among the cartridge's 197 non-tetrad synapses. These are numerically somewhat complex to show here, but as a first step synaptic sites are presented in tabular form in one of two ways. Either the total number of presynaptic sites is listed (Table 2A), or the total number of postsynaptic contacts identified (Table 2B).

Tetrads

The tetrads number about 50 contacts per terminal, providing a total of 283 for our particular cartridge, or 59% of the total number of all synapses for that cartridge (Table 2A). Thin-section and freeze-fracture studies already indicate the invariability of the tetrad's quadripartite organization in *Musca* (Fröhlich, 1985), while serial EM also reveals the strictness with which particular postsynaptic elements associate at one tetrad site (*Musca*: Nicol and Meinertzhagen, 1982; *Drosophila*: Meinertzhagen and O'Neil, 1991). In our *Drosophila* EM series, most postsynaptic elements have been successfully localized for tetrad sites (L1: 87%; L2: 95%). The total input upon processes of L1, L2 and amacrine cells is, respectively, 246, 269 and 251, or to a first approximation roughly equal for all three cell types (amacrine neurites are harder to trace than the spines of L1 and L2, so we assume that we underestimate their total by a somewhat greater margin). If we assume that each tetrad has, indeed, exactly four postsynaptic elements, then the total input from all tetrads occurs at 283 sites for L1 and L2, and possibly as many for amacrine cell processes. That input for the amacrine cells occurs at fewer tetrads, however, because many proximal tetrads contain two amacrine cell processes (*Musca*: Burkhardt and Braitenberg, 1976; Nicol and Meinertzhagen, 1982). By contrast, L3 receives less than 30% of this input, at 74 identified sites.

How does this picture compare with the vertebrate retina? Comparison between insect and vertebrate photoreceptor synapses highlights a surprising number of ultrastructural similarities (Meinertzhagen, 1993), but one rather obvious difference between the counterpart synaptic populations is quantitative. The fly's R1–R6 terminals simply have more tetrads than vertebrate photoreceptors. For example, a primate cone pedicle is much larger than a R1–R6 terminal, yet its triad synapses number only about 25 (e.g. Boycott and Hopkins, 1991), while the rod terminal has but a single active zone (Rao-Mirotznik et al., 1995), compared with 50 tetrads in *Drosophila* or 200 in *Musca* (Nicol and Meinertzhagen, 1982). The reason for this difference is not clear.

Synaptic input upon glia

There are 22 postsynaptic contacts at tetrads, and a further 26 inputs from amacrine processes, upon epithelial glial cells. Fewer than corresponding numbers in *L. cuprina* (Shaw, 1984), these functionally enigmatic inputs continue to defy sensible explanation, despite provoking considerable discussion (e.g. Boschek, 1971; Armett-Kibel et al., 1977; Shaw, 1984). Their location could possibly qualify the glia to participate in the modulation of synaptic transmission between lamina neurons, as has recently been proposed for glia at vertebrate synapses (Araque et al., 1999). However, at tetrads glia are found at only a minority of distal sites, seemingly precluding this role at that synapse. On the other hand, morphologically glia are qualified to fulfill this role at one site, at the characteristic gnarl complexes where the process of a lamina amacrine cell contacts a dendrite of its T1 cell partner from the medulla, with a slender glial sheet interposed between the two (Campos-Ortega and Strausfeld, 1973; Burkhardt and Braitenberg, 1976). Functional evidence for such a role for epithelial glia is lacking on this point, however.

The lamina's synaptic microcircuits

The remarkable extent of synaptic divergence origi-nating at the lamina means that

exclusive throughput pathways are lacking, except for the axons of the two central photoreceptors, R7 and R8, which do not make lamina synapses in any case (Boschek, 1971; Meinertzhagen and O'Neil, 1991; Table 1). Instead, all input pathways are convolved with feedback and feedforward circuits as well as serial connections, all definitively identified in *Drosophila* (Meinertzhagen and O'Neil, 1991). Within this species, L1 and L3 are pure output pathways, lacking presynaptic sites in the lamina, whereas both L2 and L4 are interconnected, both with each other, within and between neighboring cartridges, and with R1–R6. The medulla cell, T1, likewise receives quite abundant input in the lamina but is nowhere presynaptic in this neuropile. L5 is also not presynaptic, but seems to have little in the way of any synaptic input in the lamina, either.

Photoreceptor feedback pathways

Various synaptic inputs received by the photoreceptor terminals, R1–R6, provide direct or indirect feedback pathways. These arise predominantly from amacrine cell processes, and from monopolar cell processes, L2 and L4. Counting a postsynaptic contact at a triad equal to one at a dyad, feedback synapses total about 26% of the number of afferent sites, the tetrads (Table 3). Of these feedback pathways, 54 identified postsynaptic contacts form a direct feedback pathway, either from an amacrine cell process (48) or from L2 (6), which themselves both receive direct photoreceptor terminal input at the tetrads. The overall ratio of these direct feedback synapses to tetrad sites is at least 1:5.2 (54:283, Table 3), and for the amacrine cell this feedback varies between different terminals, from 1:8.4 (for R5) to 1:4.4 (for R4). The overall ratio is thus a bit higher than in the partial sample provided by Shaw (1984) for *L. cuprina*.

Reciprocal connections

Feedback synapses provide for reciprocal connections between a number of neuron pairs, notably R1–R6 and L2 (Strausfeld and Campos-Ortega, 1977); R1–R6 and amacrine cell processes (Meinertzhagen and O'Neil, 1991); L2 and L4 (Braitenberg and Debbage, 1974); and the two neighboring L4 collaterals, $L4_{+x}$ and $L4_{-y}$ (Strausfeld and Campos-Ortega, 1973; Meinertzhagen and O'Neil, 1991). R1–R6 are thus reciprocally connected with both amacrine cells processes and L2. The ratio of afferent to feedback synapses for the amacrine cells for our serially sectioned *Drosophila* cartridge is 5.2:1, while for L2 it is 45:1 (Fig. 3). Pathways for two other reciprocally connected pairs of elements, L2 and L4, and $L4_{-x}$ and $L4_{-y}$, are each represented by only 2–4 synapses, afferent and feedback (Fig. 3).

Centrifugal connections

In addition to inputs from R1–R6, L1–L3 also receive centrifugal inputs from C2 and C3. There are at least 50 postsynaptic sites contributed by 33

Table 3. *Drosophila melanogaster*: Numbers of tetrad and feedback synaptic sites for R1–R6 in a single lamina cartridge.

Terminal	Tetrads	Receptor feedback synapses from:			
		L2 dyads (trials)	L4 (all) dyads (triads)	Amacrine dyads (triads)	Total feedbacks
R1	50	0 (1)	1 (2)	2 (9)	3 (12)
R2	50	1 (0)	4 (2)	2 (7)	7 (9)
R3	45	2 (0)	2 (2)	1 (5)	5 (7)
R4	44	0 (0)	0 (1)	2 (8)	2 (9)
R5	42	1 (0)	1 (0)	3 (2)	5 (2)
R6	52	1 (0)	0 (4)	2 (5)	3 (9)
			Totals		
Dyads (triads)	283	5 (1)	8 (11)	12 (36)	25 (48)
Total synapses	**283**	6	19	48	**73**

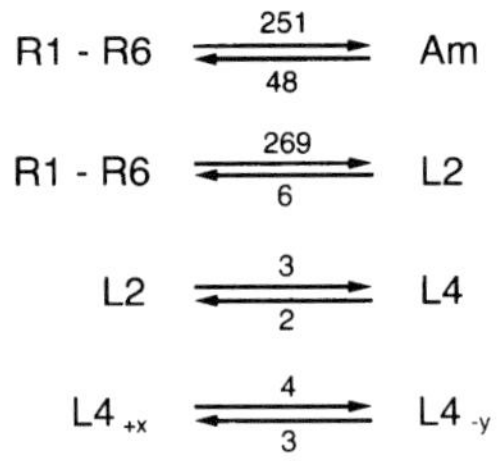

$$R1 - R6 \xrightarrow[48]{251} Am$$

$$R1 - R6 \xrightarrow[6]{269} L2$$

$$L2 \xrightarrow[2]{3} L4$$

$$L4_{+x} \xrightarrow[3]{4} L4_{-y}$$

Fig. 3. Numbers of identified afferent and feedback synaptic sites for four pairs of reciprocally connected *Drosophila* neurons. An individual postsynaptic contact at a triad is counted equal to one at a dyad. Numbers are slight under-estimates, because some neurites cannot be fully traced in the EM series.

centrifugally directed synapses from both medulla cells, in roughly equal number, and predominantly upon L2 (Table 2B).

Pathway strength

Functional correlates of these circuits are still all but impossible to assess except in the broadest of gener-alities. It is also difficult to piece together evidence from different species. From anatomical evidence alone, it is already clear that different species have differing lamina connectivities (Shaw and Moore, 1989). It is also unclear what significance to attach to connections containing very few contacts. Shaw (1984) proposes this may simply reflect the evolu-tionary history of lamina microcircuits in ancestral species. From the comprehensive spreadsheet for *Drosophila* presented here, however, one might dare to make a first cut of pathways having more than, say, 20 contacts. These comprise: the tetrad input upon L1, L2, L3, amacrine and glial cells; the pathway from amacrine to L3 and glial cells; the amacrine feedback pathway to R1–R6; and the amacrine input to T1 (Fig. 4A). If we drop the criterion synaptic strength to only 8+ contacts (Fig. 4B), we add the following pathways: L4 collateral inputs to R1–R6 and to L2; the amacrine pathway to L2; and the inputs from C2 and C3 to L2. To treat the strength of a pathway in such a simple numerate manner takes no account of the weighting assigned to individual synapses or synaptic classes, but may nevertheless be useful. For example, simultaneously recordings from a blue-yellow ganglion cell in the macaque retina while stimulating a single cone input, indicate that the

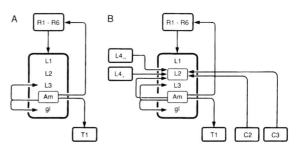

Fig. 4. Lamina pathways represented by significant numbers of synapses. (A) Pathways represented by >20 synaptic sites indicates the prominence of tetrad and amacrine synapses. (B) Pathways represented by >8 synapses, includes pathways in (A) and inputs to L2 from the L4 collaterals (the L4$_{+x}$ pathway has only 6 synapses, however) and the medulla centrifugals, C2 and C3. See Tables 2A,B for numbers of synapses.

strength of the physiological connection within a retinal microcircuit is directly proportional to the number of anatomical synapses (Chichilnisky and Baylor, 1999). Even so, it is not clear whether synaptic contacts in different classes of lamina neuron can have equal gains, nor is it known whether all anatomical synapses function during transmission at any one time or whether some are silent.

The lamina's synapses: maps and patterns

Over the surface of an individual photoreceptor terminal, the distribution of tetrad synapses shows an even dispersion (Fig. 2C), with a minimum spacing distance between neighboring sites (Meinertzhagen and Hu, 1996). This pattern implies the existence of some form of interaction between the tetrads, and it suggests that retinal neurons not only regulate the overall numerical aspects of their synaptic population (Nicol and Meinertzhagen, 1982) but also prescribe the spatial distribution of individual sites.

In contrast, within the depth of the lamina, synapses are not distributed evenly (Fig. 5). The distribution of some synapses simply reflects the varicose terminals that bear them, e.g. synapses of C2 and of two collateral terminals that enter the proximal part of the cartridge from the L4 cells of neighboring cartridges (Strausfeld and Campos-Ortega, 1973; Meinertzhagen and O'Neil, 1991). Other synapses respect partitions which are more cryptic, however, lacking clear structural boundaries.

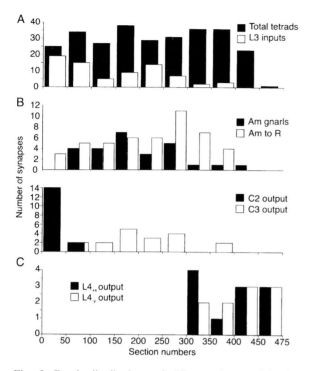

Fig. 5. Depth distributions of different classes of lamina synapse, shown as totals for all R1–R6 terminals in each 50-section stack of 65-nm thick sections of a single *Drosophila* cartridge, from the EM series illustrated but not quantified in Meinertzhagen and O'Neil (1991). Section 1 is distal. All counts are of synapses, not synaptic profiles. (A) Inputs to L3 from R1–R6 at tetrad synapses are localized in the distal lamina. Numbers of tetrad synapses are definitive. No clear peak in their distribution is obvious (cf. Hauser-Holschuh, 1975). Reduced numbers in the proximal lamina (beyond section 400) are because different terminals peter out at different levels. R1–R6 inputs to L3 are received only at tetrads and show a pronounced peak in the very distal lamina, where most synapses incorporate L3 as a single element of the postsynaptic tetrad, as well as a smaller peak in the middle of the lamina. Counts do not include uncertain EM profiles, or those which could not be traced, and so may be slight underestimates. (B) Amacrine synapses, either feedback synapses to R1–R6 or "gnarl" junctions involving T1, show no obvious peak, but are more numerous in the lamina's mid-depth and absent from the proximal lamina. (C) Two types of terminals localized at different depths. C2 has output synapses localized in the most distal part of the lamina, whereas those of C3 are evenly distributed. The collaterals of neighboring L4 cells are exclusively proximal.

For example, tetrad outputs to monopolar cell L3 are localized in the distal lamina, and somewhat in the mid-depth regions (Fig. 5A), even though R1–R6 form tetrads abundantly throughout the entire lamina's depth (Hauser-Holschuh, 1975; Nicol and Meinertzhagen, 1982). Output synapses from L4 collaterals, $L4_{-x}$ and $L4_{-y}$, are localized proximally, providing input upon R1–R6 that is partitioned from amacrine feedback synapses to R1–R6 (Fig. 5B,C). The same is true for inputs to L2 from $L4_{-x}$ and $L4_{-y}$ (proximal) and C2/C3 (distal and mid-depth) (Fig. 5C). These distributions help to define three rather indistinct lamina synaptic strata, distal, mid-depth, and proximal. Further definition of these will need to derive not from observations on a single serially-sectioned cartridge, but from quantitative EM counts on many cartridges (e.g. Hauser-Holschuh, 1975).

In addition to differences in the depth of the lamina, i.e. in a direction parallel to the length of the terminals of R1–R6, there is also some evidence for differences between these terminals (Fig. 6). Such differences are not consistent for all synaptic classes of output and input. There is, however, some evidence for a proximity principle, by which a terminal situated more closely in the cartridge cross-section to its pre- or postsynaptic partner makes more contacts than a more distant terminal (Fig. 6C).

Another feature of the tetrads is that their postsynaptic sites are distributed differently over L1 and L2. L1 is, in general, not postsynaptic over its axon, only on its dendrites, whereas both sites occur in L2. Associated with this difference, and quite unlike the slender dendrites of L1, L2 has dendrites with large swollen bases, over which tetrad sites often cluster (Fig. 2).

Synaptic divergence in retinal microcircuits

The most obvious feature of multiple-contact synapses is that they are divergent. One might ask why retinal circuits, or the microcircuits of much of the insect brain for that matter, have adopted this synaptic design rather than employing a dedicated 1:1 signaling pathway between each presynaptic neuron and its postsynaptic partner, through a network of monads. Here, we suggest three related considerations that bear on this question.

1) *Energy cost.* One possibility is energetic. Available estimates indicate that the metabolic cost

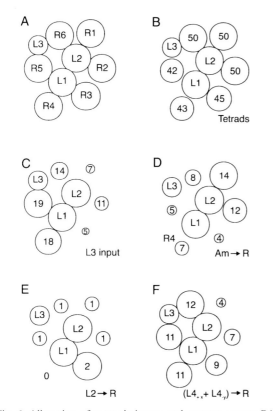

Fig. 6. Allocation of synaptic inputs and outputs among R1–R6, derived from sums presented for different depths in Fig. 5. In each case, the relative allocation of synapses is shown pictorially as the profile area of the corresponding terminal in the cartridge cross-section, and numerically as the number of synapses per terminal, printed within the corresponding terminal. (A) Plan of the cartridge cross-section, shown for a right ventral cartridge viewed as if from the retina looking in (Braitenberg, 1970). (B) Tetrad number varies between 42 (R5) and 50 (R1, R2, R6). (C) L3 inputs from R1–R6 at tetrads is greatest from R5 (45% of all tetrads) and least from R3 (11%). Terminals further from L3 generally donate fewer of its inputs. (D) Feedback synapses from Am cell processes are more numerous upon R1 and R2 than other terminals. (E) As in (D) but for feedback synapses from L2. These appear to be distributed evenly among terminals. (F) As in (E) but for the sum of the indirect feedback synapses from L4 collaterals, L4$_{+x}$ and L4$_{-y}$. The sum of this input apparently complements direct feedback from amacrine cell processes (D), R1 receiving most amacrine input and least from the two L4 collateral, with R5 for example reversing this ratio.

of photoreceptors, in particular of visual transduction, is extremely high, as are the costs of local electrical signals and signal transfer. Energy consumption for synaptic transmission is also not inconsiderable. According to experimentally derived estimates, it costs, for example, 10^4 ATP molecules to transmit 1 bit at the tetrad, approximately 10% of which is paid for by the presynaptic element (Laughlin et al., 1998). Although these costs are small compared with the energy financing of signals in L1/L2, they may be higher for presynaptic neurons that release transmitter tonically, as at photoreceptor and other sensory neurons (Juusola et al., 1996), than at spiking neurons. Multiple-contact synapses are possibly a metabolic economy which cost-shares the secretory apparatus of photoreceptors or other presynaptic neurons to transmit to more than a single interneuron. This energy saving is only possible, however, if the number of postsynaptic elements at individual synaptic sites can be kept within reasonable limits, those set by the need to incorporate postsynaptic elements in particular combinations at single presynaptic sites. This requires that the number of types of visual interneuron be not too large. Energetic considerations likewise dictate that a minimum number of monopolar cells is used to transmit information (Laughlin et al., 1998).

2) *Neuron classes.* The adoption of divergence at individual synaptic sites, as at the tetrad, does indeed seem to occur in networks of relatively few classes of neuron. The fact that divergence at the synaptic site is adopted as an exceptional condition of the retina in vertebrates might perhaps be more a statement about the ability for the rest of the vertebrate brain to elaborate different neuron classes ('equivalence classes': Bullock, 1978). Insects, by contrast, seem to have adopted a design characterized by economy in the number of interneuron classes (Horridge, 1965) for their entire CNS, and they adopt synaptic divergence more widely in their brains. There are a number of possible reasons for this economy, including the obvious genomic cost of programming the differentiation of large numbers of classes of neuron (Miklos, 1993). In *Drosophila*, for example, approximately two thirds of the 5000 or so vital genes participate in forming the compound eye (Thaker and Kankel, 1992), which contains only a handful of cell types, four of them neuronal (Ready et al., 1976). Beneath the compound eye, as we have seen, the story is more complex. But even here, cell numbers are not large, with perhaps 120 or so different cell types (Campos-Ortega and Strausfeld, 1972). Whether this is a large number is a matter of perspective. For

single-cell analysis it is dauntingly large. But, as the sensory substrate of the fly's entire repertoire of sophisticated visual behavior (Heisenberg and Wolf, 1984), it seems relatively few, not so much greater in fact than the numbers of cell classes reported in the vertebrate retina (e.g. Masland and Raviola, 2000). (This line of reasoning assumes however that the genetic costs saved in building few interneuron classes are not offset by the costs expended to programme the developmental assembly of divergent synapses, compared with monadic contacts.) These arguments are necessarily tentative, but we can be sure of one thing, that the extent of this synaptic divergence has probably increased during the course of evolution, by elaborating postsynaptic complexity at multiple-contact synapses, rather than creating new lamina cells. In a specific instance, the tetrads of contemporary species of muscoid fly arose from an ancestral dyadic condition, during a single-step incorporation of amacrine cell elements (Shaw and Meinertzhagen, 1986).

3) *Balancing inputs.* The fact that all photoreceptor tetrads provide input upon each of L1 and L2 (Nicol and Meinertzhagen, 1982) means that transmitter release over the surfaces of these two interneurons is matched at exactly the same sites. The geometry is also symmetrically matched at each site (Fröhlich, 1985). Thus, provided that the number and distribution of postsynaptic receptors (Hardie, 1989) for the transmitter, histamine (Hardie, 1987), are similarly matched between the two cells, their postsynaptic signals can also be matched with perfect precision (Meinertzhagen, 1984; Shaw, 1984). Differences between the light-evoked signals in L1 and L2, as in their response to off-axis illumination (Laughlin and Osorio, 1989) are then the consequence of other factors, such as synaptic inputs from alternative sources which differ between the two cells (Table 1) (Meinertzhagen, 1984). Although anatomical maps define the spatial matching of photoreceptor inputs upon L1 and L2, the organization of the tetrad also ensures the strict temporal synchronization of inputs, needed for high fidelity transmission of spatio-temporal patterns of light activation. It is particularly important that signals in L1 and L2 incorporate the same noise if these signals are to be compared at a later stage in visual signal processing.

Synaptogenesis: the relationship between dendritic growth and temporal and spatial constraints on tetrad formation

Three consecutive phases of photoreceptor innervation of the lamina include: (a) axon ingrowth to the lamina ("axon pathfinding"), which is vertical and establishes the initial array of cartridges; (b) subsequent lateral interchange of photoreceptor axons ("target recognition"), during which growth cones locate and assemble their correct cartridge; and (c) the final stage, synaptogenesis (Meinertzhagen and Hanson, 1993). The location of multiple postsynaptic elements at a single presynaptic release site imposes an important characteristic upon the development of multiple-contact synapses, namely that the motile element during synaptogenesis is not the presynaptic site, as at the neuromuscular junction, but the presumptive postsynaptic dendrites (Meinertzhagen, 1993). Only recently has it been recognized that filopodia of postsynaptic cells may precede the formation of hippocampal cell dendritic spines and synapses (Fiala et al., 1998). In the fly, synaptogenesis is accomplished by small-scale interstitial growth of presumptive dendrites from lamina cells towards presynaptic sites distributed over the photoreceptor terminals (Fröhlich and Meinertzhagen, 1983). Because L1 and L2's spines mostly receive input only from tetrads (Fig. 2E), there is an intimate relationship between the morphogenesis of these dendrites and the formation of tetrads over R1–R6. The patterns of neurite growth are predominantly sculpted by the pattern of synaptic contacts accepted by R1–R6 at presumptive tetrad sites (Meinertzhagen et al., 2000). The number of these sites peaks before the adult fly emerges and then declines during a period of regression and consolidation during which each tetrad progressively incorporates all four of its postsynaptic elements. The pattern of neurites at different stages is consistent with three hypotheses: (a) that neurites from L1 and L2 only survive if they contact a presynaptic site; (b) that a presumptive tetrad only survives if it can progressively acquire not only the appropriate number but also the correct combination of postsynaptic neurites of a concluding tetrad; and (c) that there is an interaction between the neurites of L1 and L2, such that the growth of one respects the pattern of growth of the other (Meinertzhagen et al., 2000). An important omission in our knowledge so far, and the subject of the final section of this review is the role of neural activity in each of these developmental steps.

The role of neural activity in tetrad formation

In the vertebrate visual system, establishing the correct connectivities of cortical neurons during late development is driven by electrical activity originating in the retina (e.g. Shatz, 1996). The direct role of electrical activity in wiring the retina itself is less well established, however. Even less understood is the role of electrical activity in the developing fly's visual system, even though L2 feedback synapses are susceptible to early adult visual experience (Kral and Meinertzhagen, 1989).

The availability in *Drosophila* of neuronal activity mutants allows us to examine the long-term effects of perturbations in neuronal function on the development of photoreceptor terminals. Disrupting many of the functions in neurons involving signaling or transmitter release can all silence electrical activity. One might therefore expect that genetic mutation of such functions in photoreceptors might exert the same action on synaptogenesis, or at least that the synaptic phenotypes of mutants should bear some consistent relationship to each other. This is apparently not the case, however (Hiesinger et al., 2000a). Removing the normal function of molecules of the neurotransmitter release machinery produces, for example, differential results. Photoreceptor terminals which lack neuron-specific Synaptobrevin are enlarged, with increased numbers of synaptic vesicles. By contrast, photoreceptors mutant for the calcium-sensor protein Synaptotagmin, also implicated in vesicle exocytosis, fail to exhibit similar structural defects, and have terminals with fewer vesicles (Hiesinger et al., 2000a). The numbers of tetrad sites themselves are similar both in number and structural composition in these mutants. On the other hand, the mutant *norpA*, which lacks light-evoked potentials (Bloomquist et al., 1988), has more tetrads (Hiesinger et al., 2000a). Thus activity dependence of visual system development has to be qualified, depending on which aspect of activity is perturbed, light-evoked electrogenesis or Ca^{2+}- dependent neurotransmitter release, and which aspect of synaptogenesis is examined.

Discussion and future perspectives

In many ways, the anatomical analysis presented here for the fly is a conclusion to the one embarked on for the dragonfly (Armett-Kibel et al., 1977), which first drew attention to the synapses of the lamina and their multiple-contact organization. What has emerged fully since then is the important role that *Drosophila* has to play in answering questions about synapses and microcircuits, and the paradox that this choice embodies. Electrophysiological studies on lamina cells and their microcircuits are more badly needed than ever, despite recent attempts for example to localize elements of the optic lobe's elementary motion detector circuits (Buchner, 1984) to particular lamina cells (Douglass and Strausfeld, 1995). The technical difficulty of electrophysiological recording in the lamina of *Drosophila* all but deny this approach in such a small fly. However, the genetic advantages of *Drosophila* outweigh the technical difficulties posed by its small size. The recent release of the *Drosophila* genome database (Adams et al., 2000), the ready availability of P-element insertions (e.g. Spradling et al., 1999) to mutate identified genes, and methods to create mutant mosaics comprising the entire eye (Stowers and Schwarz, 1999), make it inevitable that new mutants will soon come on line in a plenitude that neurobiology will be unable to match. Even neuroanatomical analyses at the requisite level do not come easily. It is not a practical prospect to subject mutant flies to the same sort of EM-based analyses as we present here for the wild type. The search for alternative methods using, for example, high-resolution confocal microscopy (Hiesinger et al., 2000b) to image synaptic populations, is therefore of paramount importance. Even so, only data from serial EM provide the unequivocal evidence to authenticate postsynaptic partnerships among neurons. We can be sure that to gain answers to questions about the synaptic organization of even so simple a neuropile as the fly's optic lamina is still going to be a long-term undertaking.

Acknowledgments

Ian Meinertzhagen wishes to thank John Dowling, whose extraordinary generosity of spirit is remembered with much gratitude. Most of the approach to synaptic organization presented in this chapter initially germinated while he was a postdoc in the Dowling lab and has been subsequently nurtured by support from the National Eye Institute (through its grant EY03592) and the National Science and Engineering Research Council of Ottawa (through its grant A000065). Research on insect visual systems has been implemented and supplemented by numerous colleagues and trainees, to all of whom we are deeply indebted. Karin Sorra undertook quantitative work reported in Table 2 and Figs. 3–6, and also acknowledges John Dowling as a mentor while in graduate school. We also thank Ms. Xiangqun Hu for permission to reproduce the reconstructions in Fig. 2, Drs. Simon Laughlin for helpful discussions on tetrad synapses, Dr. Alois Hofbauer for confirmation of optic lobe cell counts, and Ms Jane Anne Horne for help in preparing the figures.

References

Adams, M.D., Celniker, S.E., Holt, R.A., et al. (2000) The genome sequence of *Drosophila melanogaster*. *Science*, 287: 2185–2195.

Araque, A., Parpura, V., Sanzgiri, R.P. and Haydon, P.G. (1999) Tripartite synapses: glia, the unacknowledged partner. *Trends Neurosci.*, 22: 208–215.

Armett-Kibel, C., Meinertzhagen, I.A. and Dowling, J.E. (1977) Cellular and synaptic organization in the lamina of the dragon-fly *Sympetrum rubicundulum*. *Proc. Roy. Soc. Lond. Ser. B*, 196: 385–413.

Bloomquist, B.T., Shortridge, R.D., Schneuwly, S., Perdew, M., Montell, C., Steller, H., Rubin, G. and Pak, W.L. (1988) Isolation of a putative phospholipase C gene of Drosophila, norpA, and its role in phototransduction. *Cell*, 54: 723–733.

Boschek, C.B. (1971) On the fine structure of the peripheral retina and lamina ganglionaris of the fly, *Musca domestica*. *Z. Zellforsch. mikrosk. Anat.*, 118: 369–409.

Boycott, B.B. and Hopkins, J.M. (1991) Cone bipolar cells and cone synapses in the primate retina. *Vis. Neurosci.*, 7: 49–60.

Braitenberg, V. (1967) Patterns of projection in the visual system of the fly. I. Retina-lamina projections. *Exp. Brain Res.*, 3: 271–298.

Braitenberg, V. (1970) Ordnung und Orientierung der Elemente im Sehsystem der Fliege. *Kybernerik*, 7: 235–242.

Braitenberg, V. and Debbage P. (1974) A regular net of reciprocal synapses in the visual system of the fly, *Musca domesfica*. *J. Comp. Physiol.*, 90: 25–31.

Buchner, E. (1984) Behavioural analysis of spatial vision in insects. In: Ali, M.A. (Ed.), *Photoreception and Vision in Invertebrates*. (*NATO Advanced Science Institutes*, Series A Vol. 74, Lennoxville, Quebec). Plenum Press, New York, pp. 561–621.

Bullock, T.H. (1978) Identifiable and addressed neurons in the vertebrates. In: Faber, D.S. and Korn, H. (Eds.), *Neurobiology of the Mauthner Cell*, Raven Press, New York, pp. 1–12.

Burkhardt, W. and Braitenberg, V. (1976) Some peculiar synaptic complexes in the first visual ganglion of the fly, *Musca domestica*. *Cell Tiss. Res.*, 173: 287–308.

Campos-Ortega, J.A. and Strausfeld, N.J. (1972) Columns and layers in the second synaptic region of the fly's visual system: The case for two superimposed neuronal architectures. In: Wehner, R. (Ed.), *Information Processing in the Visual Systems of Arthropods*. Springer-Verlag, Heidelberg, pp. 31–36.

Campos-Ortega, J.A. and Strausfeld, N.J. (1973) Synaptic connections of intrinsic cells and basket arborizations in the external plexiform layer of the fly's eye. *Brain Res.*, 59: 119–136.

Chichilnisky, E.J. and Baylor, D.A. (1999) Receptive-field microstructure of blue-yellow ganglion cells in primate retina. *Nature Neurosci.*, 2: 889–893.

Douglass, J.K. and Strausfeld, N.J. (1995) Visual motion detection circuits in flies: Peripheral motion computation by identified small-field retinotopic neurons. *J. Neurosci.*, 15: 5596–5611.

Dowling, J.E. and Boycott, B.B. (1966) Organization of the primate retina: electron microscopy. *Proc. Roy. Soc. Lond. Ser. B*, 166: 80–111.

Dowling, J.E. and Chappell, R.L. (1972) Neural organization of the median ocellus of the dragonfly. II. Synaptic structure. *J. Gen. Physiol.*, 60: 148–165.

Fiala, J.C., Feinberg, M., Popov, V. and Harris, K.M. (1998) Synaptogenesis via dendritic filopodia in developing hippocampal area CAl. *J. Neurosci.*, 18: 8900–8911.

Fischbach, K.-F. and Dittrich, A.P.M. (1989) The optic lobe of *Drosophila melanogaster*. I. A golgi analysis of wild-type structure. *Cell Tissue Res.*, 258: 441–475.

Fröhlich, A. (1985) Freeze-fracture study of an invertebrate multiple-contact synapse: the fly photoreceptor tetrad. *J. Comp. Neurol.*, 241: 311–326.

Fröhlich, A. and Meinertzhagen, I.A. (1983) Quantitative features of synapse formation in the fly's visual system. I. The presynaptic photoreceptor terminal. *J. Neurosci.*, 3: 2336–2349.

Gray, E.G. and Pease, H.L. (1971) On understanding the organisation of the retinal receptor synapses. *Brain Res.*, 35: 1–15.

Hardie, R.C. (1987) Is histamine a neurotransmitter in insect photoreceptors? *J. Comp. Physiol. A*, 161: 201–213.

Hardie, R.C. (1989) A histamine-activated chloride channel involved in neurotransmission at a photoreceptor synapse. *Nature*, 339: 704–706.

Hauser-Holschuh, H. (1975) Vergleichend quantitative Untersuchungen an den Sehganglien der Fliegen *Musca domestica* und *Drosophila melanogaster*. Ph.D. Thesis, Eberhard-Karls-Universität zu Tübingen, Tübingen.

Heisenberg, M. and Wolf, R. (1984) Vision in *Drosophila*. Springer-Verlag, Berlin, Heidelberg.

Hiesinger, P.R., Meinertzhagen, I.A., Fröhlich, A. and Fischbach, K.-F. (2000a) Vesicle trafficking machinery is essential for activity-independent development of *Drosophila* visual neurons. *Development*, Submitted.

Hiesinger, P.R., Scholz, M., Meinertzhagen, I.A., Fischbach, K.-F. and Obermayer, K. (2000b) Visualization of synaptic markers in the optic neuropils of *Drosophila* using a new constrained deconvolution method. *J. Comp. Neurol.*, 429: 277–288.

Hofbauer, A. and Campos-Ortega, J.A. (1990) Proliferation pattern and early differentiation of the optic lobes in *Drosophila melanogaster*. *Roux's Arch. Dev. Biol.*, 198: 264–274.

Horridge, G.A. (1965) Arthropoda: Physiology of neurons and ganglia. In: Bullock, T.H. and Horridge, G.A. (Eds.), *Structure and Function in the Nervous Systems of Invertebrates*. W.H. Freeman, San Francisco, pp. 1115–1164.

Hu, X. (1993) Three-dimensional reconstruction of optic lobe interneurons and their synapses in the flies *Musca* and *Drosophila*. M.Sc. Thesis, Biology, Dalhousie University.

Juusola, M., Uusitalo, R.O. and Weckström, M. (1995) Transfer of graded potentials at the photoreceptor-interneuron synapse. *J. Gen. Physiol.*, 105: 117–148.

Juusola, M., French, A.S., Uusitalo, R.O. and Weckström, M. (1996) Information processing by graded-potential transmission through tonically active synapses. *Trends Neurosci.*, 19: 292–297.

Kral, K. and Meinertzhagen, I.A. (1989) Anatomical plasticity of synapses in the lamina of the optic lobe of the fly. *Phil. Trans. Roy. Soc. Lond. B.*, 323: 155–183.

Lamparter, H.E., Steiger, U., Sandri, C. and Akert, C. (1969) Zum Feinbau der Synapsen im Zentralnervensystem der Insekten. *Z. Zellforsch. mikrosk. Anat.*, 99: 435–442.

Laughlin, S.B. (1980) Neural principles in the peripheral visual systems of invertebrates. In: Autrum, H. (Ed.), *Handbook of Sensory Physiology, Comparative Physiology and Evolution of Vision in Invertebrates*. Vol. VII/6B, Springer-Verlag, Heidelberg, pp. 133–280.

Laughlin, S.B. and Osorio, D. (1989) Mechanisms for neural signal enhancement in the blowfly compound eye. *J. Exp. Biol.*, 144: 113–146.

Laughlin S.B., de Ruyter van Steveninck R.R. and Anderson J.C. (1998) The metabolic cost of neural information. *Nature Neurosci.*, 1: 36–41.

Masland, R.H. and Raviola, E. (2000) Confronting complexity: strategies for understanding the microcircuitry of the retina. *Ann. Rev. Neurosci.*, 23: 249–284.

Meinertzhagen, I.A. (1984) The rules of synaptic assembly in the developing insect lamina. In: Ali, M.A. (Ed.), *Photoreception and Vision in Invertebrates* (NATO *Advanced Science Institute*, Vol. 74), Plenum Press, New York, pp. 635–660.

Meinertzhagen, I.A. (1993) The synaptic populations of the fly's optic neuropil and their dynamic regulation: parallels with the vertebrate retina. *Progr. Retinal Res.*, 12: 13–39.

Meinertzhagen, I.A. (1996) Ultrastructure and quantification of synapses in the insect nervous system. *J. Neurosci. Methods*, 69: 59–73.

Meinertzhagen, I.A. and Armett-Kibel, C. (1982) The lamina monopolar cells in the optic lobe of the dragonfly *Sympetrum*. *Phil. Trans. Roy. Soc. Lond. Ser. B*, 297: 27–49.

Meinertzhagen, I.A. and Hanson,T.E. (1993) The development of the optic lobe. In: Bate, M. and Martinez, Arias A. (Eds.), *The Development of Drosophila melanogaster*. Cold Spring Harbor Laboratory Press, Plainview, NY, pp. 1363–1491.

Meinertzhagen, I.A. and Hu, X. (1996) Evidence for site selection during synaptogenesis: the surface distribution of synaptic sites in photoreceptor terminals of the flies *Musca* and *Drosophila*. *Cell Molec. Neurobiol.*, 16: 677–698.

Meinertzhagen, I.A. and O'Neil, S.D. (1991) Synaptic organization of columnar elements in the lamina of the wild type in *Drosophila melanogaster*. *J. Comp. Neurol.*, 305: 232–263.

Meinertzhagen, I.A., Piper, S.T., Sun , X.-J. and Fröhlich, A. (2000) Neurite morphogenesis of identified visual interneurons and its relationship to photoreceptor synaptogenesis in the flies, *Musca domestica* and *Drosophila melanogaster*. *Europ. J. Neurosci.*, 12: 1342–1356.

Meinertzhagen, I.A. and Shaw, S.R. (1989) Evolution of synaptic connections between homologous neurons in insects: new cells for old in the optic lobe. In: Erber, J., Menzel, R., Pflüger, H.-J. and Todt, D. (Eds), *Neural Mechanisms of Behavior*. Georg Thieme Verlag, Stuttgart, pp. 124–126.

Miklos, G.L.G. (1993) Molecules and cognition: the latterday lessons of levels, language and *lac*. *J. Neurobiol.*, 24: 842–890.

Missotten, L. (1965) The Ultrastructure of the Human Retina. Arscia Uitgaven N.V., Brussels.

Muresan, V., Lyass, A. and Schnapp, B.J. (1999) The kinesin motor KIF3A is a component of the presynaptic ribbon in vertebrate photoreceptors. *J. Neurosci.*, 19: 1027–1037.

Nicol, D. and Meinertzhagen, I.A. (1982) An analysis of the number and composition of the synaptic populations formed by photoreceptors of the fly. *J. Comp. Neurol.*, 207: 29–44.

Rao-Mirotznik, R., Harkins, A.B., Buchsbaum, G. and Sterling, P. (1995) Mammalian rod terminal: architecture of a binary synapse. *Neuron*, 14: 561–569.

Ready, D.F., Hanson, T.E. and Benzer, S. (1976) Development of the *Drosophila* retina, a neurocrystalline lattice. *Dev. Biol.*, 53: 217–240.

Saint Marie, R.L. and Carlson, S.D. (1982) Synaptic vesicle activity in stimulated and unstimulated photoreceptor axons in the housefly. A freeze-fracture study. *J. Neurocytol.*, 11: 747–761.

Shatz, C.J. (1996) Emergence of order in visual system development. *Proc. Natl. Acad. Sci. USA*, 93: 602–608.

Shaw, S.R. (1981) Anatomy and physiology of identified non-spiking cells in the photoreceptor-lamina complex of the compound eye of insects, especially Diptera. In: Roberts, A. and Bush, B.M.H. (Eds.), *Neurones Without Impulses*. Cambridge University Press, Cambridge, pp. 61–116.

Shaw, S.R. (1984) Early visual processing in insects. *J. Exp. Biol.*, 112: 225–251.

Shaw, S.R. and Meinertzhagen, I.A. (1986) Evolution of synaptic connections among homologous neurons. *Proc. Natl. Acad. Sci. USA*, 83: 7961–7965.

Shaw, S.R. and Moore, D. (1989) Evolutionary remodeling in a visual system through extensive changes in the synaptic connectivity of homologous neurons. *Vis. Neurosci.*, 3: 405–410.

Spradling, A.C., Stern, D., Beaton, A. et al. (1999) The Berkeley *Drosophila* Genome Project gene disruption project: Single P-element insertions mutating 25% of vital *Drosophila* genes. *Genetics*, 153: 135–177.

Stowers, S.R. and Schwarz, T. (1999) A genetic method for generating *Drosophila* eyes composed exclusively of mitotic clones of a single genotype. *Genetics*, 152: 1631–1639.

Strausfeld, N.J. (1970) Golgi studies on insects. Part II: The optic lobes of Diptera. *Phil. Trans. Roy. Soc. Lond. B*, 258: 135–223.

Strausfeld, N.J. and Campos-Ortega, J.A. (1973) The L4 monopolar neurone: A substrate for lateral interaction in the visual system of the fly *Musca domestica* (L.). *Brain Res.*, 59: 97–117.

Strausfeld, N.J. and Campos-Ortega, J.A. (1977) Vision in insects: pathways possibly underlying neural adaptation and lateral inhibition. *Science*, 195: 894–897.

Strausfeld, N.J. and Meinertzhagen, I.A. (1998) The insect neuron: types, morphologies, fine structure and relationship to the architectonics of the insect nervous system. In: Harrison, F.W. and Locke, M. (Eds.), *Microscopic Anatomy of Invertebrates*. Volume 11(B): *Insecta*, Wiley and Sons, New York, pp. 487–538.

Strausfeld, N.J. and Nässel, D.R. (1980) Neuroarchitectures serving compound eyes of Crustacea and insects. In: Autrum, H. (Ed.), *Handbook of Sensory Physiology*, Vol. VII/6B, *Comparative Physiology and Evolution of Vision in Invertebrates*. Springer-Verlag, Heidelberg, pp. 1–132.

Thaker, H.M. and Kankel, D.R. (1992) Mosaic analysis gives an estimate of the extent of genomic involvement in the development of the visual system in *Drosophila melanogaster*. *Genetics*, 131: 883–894.

Trujillo-Cenóz, O. (1965) Some aspects of the structural organization of the intermediate retina of dipterans. *J. Ultrastruct. Res.*, 13: 1–33.

Uusitalo, R.O., Juusola, M. and Weckström, M. (1995) Graded responses and spiking properties of identified first-order visual interneurons of the fly compound eye. *J. Neurophysiol.*, 73: 1782–1792.

H. Kolb, H. Ripps and S. Wu (Eds.)
Progress in Brain Research, Vol. 131

CHAPTER 4

Complexities of retinal circuitry revealed by neurotransmitter receptor localization

Charles L. Zucker[1,*] and Berndt Ehinger[2]

[1]*Department of Anatomy and Neurobiology, Boston University School of Medicine, 715 Albany Street, Boston, MA 02118, USA*
[2]*Department of Ophthalmology, University of Lund, Lund, Sweden*

Nearly all current research on the vertebrate retina, be it focused on normal retinal function and circuitry, aberrant function and circuitry in diseases of the visual system or on the development and genetics of the visual system, is ultimately based on a working knowledge of how the retina is built. By early in the 20th century, largely through the work of Cajal (1892), the main cellular players in the retina had been described. The retina was known to consist of five primary neuronal cell types (photoreceptor, horizontal, bipolar, amacrine and ganglion cells), each with a variety of subtypes. Based on the physical overlap of their respective processes, there was some idea regarding cellular connections and direction of information flow. However, beyond this level of understanding, the retina was pretty much a "black box." Light "went in" via the photoreceptors and the information was sent out to more central parts of the visual system via the axons of the ganglion cells. Through what specific circuits and via what physiological mechanisms did visual processing occur was poorly understood. Much of our current understanding of retinal circuitry and visual function is based on the original studies of Dowling and Boycott (1966) that defined the synaptic organization of the vertebrate retina. Since those studies in the mid 1960s, continuing work performed or inspired by John Dowling has truly provided the backbone of the current state of knowledge about the visual system.

By 1975, a sixth class of retinal neuron, the interplexiform cell, was described by John (Dowling and Ehinger, 1975; Boycott et al., 1975; Dowling and Ehinger, 1978a,b; Hedden and Dowling, 1978). This discovery provided the inspiration for my own doctoral thesis in the laboratory of Steve Yazulla, who incidentally was a post-doctoral fellow with John. John has indeed been the nucleus of an extensive family tree.

Over the last 20 years, much information has been gleaned about retinal structure and function through the use of antibodies directed to neurotransmitters, peptides and their biosynthetic enzymes. In order to get closer to a functional understanding, we have been utilizing localization of neurotransmitter receptor subunits in the retinas of the turtle and rabbit as a tool to probe functionally relevant circuits. We have found that defining a population of amacrine cells (or even an individual cell) based on neurotransmitter content needs to be extended to include a detailed understanding of how those cells interact with their functional partners via a complex admixture of postsynaptic receptors.

Heterogeneous distribution of receptors postsynaptic to individual synaptic boutons

Our first results to suggest multiple levels of interactive complexity came in the turtle retina where we performed ultrastructural localization of gephyrin

---
* Corresponding author: Charles L. Zucker, Tel.: 617-638-4193; Fax: 617-638-4216; E-mail: czucker@bu.edu

(Zucker and Ehinger, 1992, 1993). At the time, the receptor anchoring protein gephyrin was thought to be a reliable marker for the strychnine sensitive glycine receptor. We now know that gephyrin is also associated with at least certain configurations of GABA$_A$ receptors (Yazulla and Studholme, 1991; also see next section). Suffice it to say, that by analyzing gephyrin positive synaptic terminals making more than one synapse, we found that only about one half of the actual synapses were gephyrin immunoreactive. As is shown in Fig. 1, the gephyrin-negative synapse is completely devoid of reactivity. Serial sections through such multi-synaptic profiles confirms that they are either labeled or unlabeled throughout their entire extent. Based on our current understanding, these results would suggest that about 50% of the synapses made by these terminals would

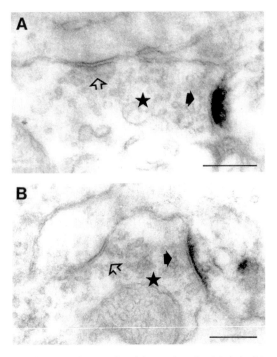

Fig. 1. Electron micrographs of the turtle retina labeled with an antibody to gephyrin visualized using a peroxidase anti-peroxidase technique. So as to not obscure labeling with normally electron dense synaptic membranes, no heavy metal counter staining has been used. These micrographs each show amacrine cell processes (stars) making two synaptic contacts. In each case, one synapse is gephyrin immunopositive (filled arrow) whilst the other is devoid of any immunoreactivity (open arrow). Scale bars = 0.25 μm.

respond via an inhibitory amino acid receptor, likely associated with a chloride channel (which may include both glycine and GABA$_A$ receptors). The remaining synapses would thus contain receptors for an as yet undefined receptor type or neurotransmitter.

The use by a neuron of multiple neuroactive substances is now well established. Typically this is manifested by the corelease of a conventional neurotransmitter along with a neuromodulatory substance such as a peptide. Other recent investigations are showing that two conventional neurotransmitters, such as glycine and GABA or acetylcholine and GABA can also coexist in the same neuron. There are several strategies by which neurons may achieve functional resolution with such a synaptic admixture. One such mechanism described by Sossin and coworkers (1990) involves the differential packaging of neuroactive substances into subsets of synaptic vesicles that are then targeted, and thus transported, to different processes of the same cell. Alternatively, and likely more common, multiple neuroactive substances are localized to, and released by, all of the processes of a neuron. Specificity of neuronal function would reside in the specific complement of postsynaptic receptors rather than specific release sites (Swanson 1983; Eccles 1986). Metabolically, it may be more costly for a cell to separately package, address and release multiple neuroactive substances than to corelease and rely on receptor selectivity to provide resolution of neurotransmitter function.

In light of our findings, we suggest that defining individual synapses as X-ergic based on the biochemical properties of the presynaptic cell as well as the properties of the postsynaptic membrane may be a more useful classification than to define a neuron, in its entirety, as X-ergic. The same argument can be made for all types of neurons, and such a hypothesis may provide a functional explanation for the rapidly growing number of neurotransmitter colocalizations being reported throughout the central nervous system.

Gephyrin: An anchoring protein for multiple inhibitory amino acid receptor types

Localization of gephyrin, which is a 93-kD peripheral membrane glycine receptor associated anchoring protein, has been used in several studies to identify the sites of glycinergic interactions in the retina and other regions of the central nervous system. Recent studies have shown that gephyrin also colocalizes with $GABA_A$ receptors which, like those for glycine, are inhibitory amino acid receptors usually associated with a chloride channel. We have used two antibodies which recognize either gephyrin (mAb7a), or the α and β subunits of the glycine receptor (mAb4a) in order to determine to what extent gephyrin is associated with glycine receptors in the mammalian retina (see Zucker, 1998). Single label studies showed extensive punctate staining throughout most of the inner plexiform layer (IPL) with each antibody. Double-labeling showed that nearly 90% of the glycine receptor sites were also immunoreactive for gephyrin. However, nearly 60% of the total punctae immunoreactive for gephyrin were not stained for glycine receptors. This extensive colocalization of glycine receptors and gephyrin in the inner plexiform layer can be seen by confocal microscopy of double-labeled sections in Fig. 2A–C. Many red punctae, which represent single-labeled gephyrin sites are seen amongst white punctae which are double-labeled for both gephyrin and glycine receptors. A relatively low density of single-labeled glycine receptor immuno-reactive sites (green) is also apparent. This study suggests that although most glycine receptors in the rabbit retina colocalize with the anchoring protein gephyrin, a significant proportion of the gephyrin labeled sites are not associated with glycine receptors. Thus, the localization of gephyrin should be considered indicative of chloride-mediated inhibitory amino acid transmission and not glycinergic in its isolation. Several studies show that bipolar cells express glycine receptors and respond to glycine but do not express gephyrin (Suzuki et al., 1990; Enz and Bormann, 1995). The 10% of glycine receptors not colocalized with gephyrin shown in the present study may represent a novel subtype of glycine receptors found on bipolar cells which do not require gephyrin for the functional clustering of receptor subunits.

DAPI-3 cells and cholinergic transmission

More recently, we have been using receptor localization to study two amacrine cell types in the rabbit retina: the two mirror-symmetric starburst amacrine cell populations and the bistratified DAPI-3 cells. We have studied the distribution of different $GABA_A$ receptor subunit proteins in rabbit retina, taking advantage of the improved resolution attainable with the confocal microscope and the availability of well-characterized monoclonal $GABA_A$ receptor subunit antibodies. Amacrine cells in the inner nuclear and ganglion cell layers of the retina that are stained by intraocular injection of DAPI were classified with the aid of intracellular injections of Lucifer Yellow in the living tissue. Immunohistochemical staining for choline acetyltransferase was also used to identify starburst amacrine cells in rabbit retina.

We have shown that two $\alpha_1/\beta_{2/3}$ subunit containing $GABA_A$ receptor bands in rabbit retina represent the processes of a cell type with morphologically characteristic features, called the DAPI-3 cell (Vaney, 1990; Wright et al., 1997; Zucker and Ehinger, 1998). This cell type has perikarya in the proximal rows of the inner nuclear layer (usually the very innermost) and they send their processes into two sublayers in the inner plexiform layer. These processes juxtapose those of the two mirror symmetric populations of starburst amacrine cells. They occur with roughly the same density as OFF-starburst amacrine cells though the latter have a somewhat wider dendritic field size which ranges from 230–800 µm (compare Fig. 2D and E). The dendritic trees of DAPI-3 cells, which range from about 150 µm up to about 300 µm, exhibit recurvate looping processes, reminiscent of those described for directionally selective ganglion cells (Fig. 2D, E). The DAPI-3 cells form a system of abundant and distinctive cells with the highest $GABA_A$ receptor concentration (subunits α_1 and β_2/β_3) of all retinal cells (Fig. 2F). In contrast to the DAPI-3 cell, we have also shown that the cell bodies and proximal dendrites of starburst amacrine cells exhibit no immunoreactivity for the α_1 $GABA_A$ receptor subunit and only weak immunoreactivity for the $\beta_{2/3}$ subunit (Zucker and Ehinger, 1998). Using triple-labeling for DAPI, $GABA_A$ receptors and glycine transporter, we have also found that the DAPI-3 cells are glycine transporter immunoreactive (Fig. 2G), which along with their high level of glycine immuno-reactivity (Wright et al., 1997), suggests that these cells use glycine as a transmitter.

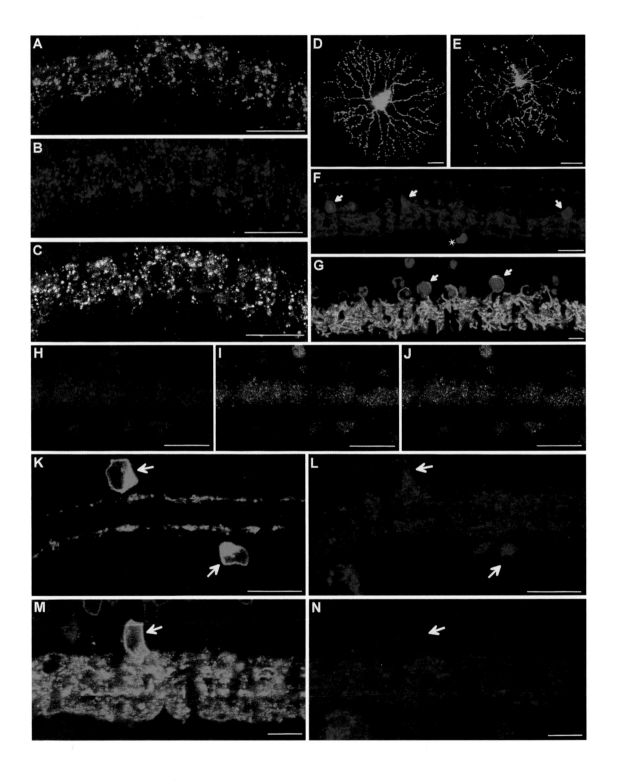

In light of the juxtapositional relationship between the processes of cholinergic starburst amacrine cells and the DAPI-3 cells, we investigated the possibility that DAPI-3 cells possess the appropriate receptors whereby ACh released by starburst amacrine cells can influence them. Indeed, DAPI-3 cells, along with other amacrine and ganglion cell types whose processes ramify further from the sites of acetylcholine release, are rich in both nicotinic and m2 muscarinic ACh receptors (Fig. 3A–F). Muscarinic m2R staining was seen on the cell membrane of several classes of amacrine cells as well as some bipolar and ganglion cells. In the IPL, strong staining was seen to be diffusely distributed within the confines of the two starburst amacrine cell strata with a peak density at about the 50% level (Fig. 3A). Nicotinic receptors were seen on both amacrine and ganglion cell bodies and in processes diffusely distributed throughout most of the IPL (see Fig. 2B). Double-label experiments showed that all strongly GABA$_A$ receptor subunit positive amacrine cells (DAPI-3 cells) were also immunoreactive for both muscarinic (Fig. 3C, D) and nicotinic (Fig. 3E, F) receptors. Starburst amacrine cells labeled with ChAT were invariably m2R immunonegative. Processes from other amacrine and ganglion cell types and possibly bipolar cells, which ramify medially to the starburst amacrine cell strata, are also immunoreactive for muscarinic

and nicotinic acetylcholine receptor proteins. Using the cholinoreceptive DAPI-3 cell as an example, Fig. 3G suggests that acetylcholine may be active over distances greater than that typically defined as a synaptic cleft.

Starburst amacrine cells are known to be the sole source of acetylcholine in the rabbit retina and homologous cells have been found in almost all other vertebrates examined to date. These cholinergic cells clearly interact with ON–OFF directionally selective ganglion cells, other starburst amacrine cells, and bipolar cells (Famiglietti, 1983a, 1991; Brandon, 1987; Vaney, 1990). However, there is evidence that starburst amacrine cells do not make conventional synaptic contacts with other classes of amacrine cells. Using ultrastructural localization of choline acetyltransferase, Brandon (1987) has shown that starburst amacrine cells receive extensive synaptic input from cone bipolar cells and he suggests that this bipolar input may be the sole direct input received by these cells. His study also suggests that the only synaptic output from starburst amacrine cells is onto ganglion cell processes found within the two narrow substrata. In a similar study that also relied on the ultrastructural localization of choline acetyltransferase, Millar and Morgan (1987) showed that starburst amacrine cells contacted other starburst amacrine cells but failed to demonstrate contact

Fig. 2. **A–C:** Confocal micrographs of rabbit retina sections double-labeled for glycine receptor (green) and gephyrin (red). Viewed as separate channels, **A** and **B** show the relative distribution of gephyrin and the glycine receptor in the inner plexiform layer. Both labels are distributed extensively throughout the inner plexiform layer with gephyrin labeled sites being more numerous, especially in the most proximal inner plexiform layer where there are proportionately fewer glycine receptor labeled sites. Viewed simultaneously in **C**, many sites are seen to be labeled for both gephyrin and the glycine receptor. Pixels containing both red and green signals are shown as white to facilitate discrimination. Scale bars = 25 μm. **D, E:** Confocal images of Lucifer Yellow injected starburst and DAPI-3 amacrine cells. Compared to the now classical radiating processes of the starburst amacrine cell, note the undulating, recurvate, asymmetrically distributed varicose processes seen in the DAPI-3 cell. There is some leakage of dye at the cell bodies and along the tracks of the injection capillary. Scale bars = 25 μm. **F:** Fluorescence micrograph of a cryostat section of rabbit retina, injected intravitreally with 60 ng DAPI 26 hours before obtaining the eye and staining for GABA$_{A\alpha1}$ receptor subunit immunoreactivity. In addition to three strongly immunoreactive amacrine cells in the inner nuclear layer (arrows), presumed bipolar and horizontal cells are also weakly stained. Note that the GABA$_A$ receptor subunit positive cells are also strongly DAPI positive. An additional strongly DAPI positive displaced cell is also seen which likely represent an ON starburst amacrine cell (star). Scale bar = 25 μm. **G:** GABA$_A$ receptors (red) and glycine transporter (green) in rabbit retina also labeled with DAPI. Strong GABA$_A$ receptor immunoreactivity is present in two amacrine cells, which also contain GLYT1 immunoreactivity and thus appear orange in color (arrows). These cells are also DAPI positive and are thus DAPI-3 cells. Scale bar = 10 μm. **H–J:** Double-labeling for the GABA$_B$ receptor (**H**, red) and L-baclofen (**I**, green) shows significant colocalization (**J**) within the inner plexiform layer and on ganglion cells. Although amacrine cell body staining for the GABA$_B$ receptor is not well preserved using the fixation required for the L-baclofen labeling, a weakly stained amacrine cell body is also visible. Scale bar = 25 μm. **K – N:** Confocal pairs in **K** and **L** show both OFF- and ON-starburst amacrine cells labeled for choline acetyltransferase (green), both of which are also immunoreactive for GABA$_B$ receptors (red). Scale bars = 25 μm. A similar pair in **M** and **N** shows that GABA$_A$ receptor α_1 subunit labeled DAPI-3 cells (green) are devoid of GABA$_B$ receptors (red). Scale bars = 10 μm.

76

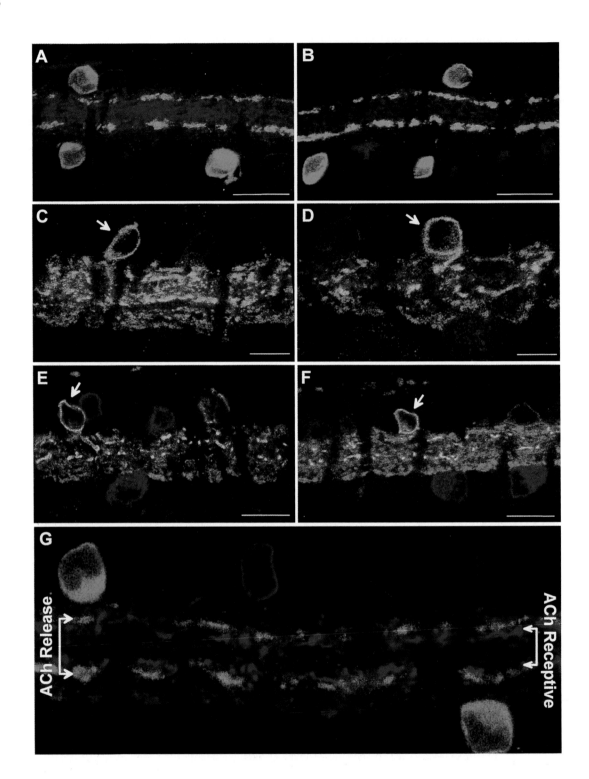

onto any other amacrine cell population. Using Golgi-impregnated material (which labels an individual cell in its entirety), Famiglietti (1983b, 1991) also reported that the major input to starburst amacrine cells was from cone bipolar cells and the primary output was onto ganglion cells. The identification of such interactions is based on the presence of morphologically identifiable "classical" synaptic structures. As a basic principle, cholinergic transmission could occur at any site where acetylcholine is present at a physiologically significant concentration and where cholinergic receptors are both localized and linked in some fashion to either ion channels or some other form of biochemical machinery needed to transduce the cholinergic signal.

Recent studies have suggested that diffuse cholinergic transmission may be a common feature throughout the central nervous system (Descarries et al., 1997). In a variety of brain regions, cholinergic neurons have been shown to display a particularly low density of classical synaptic release sites (Umbriaco et al., 1994, 1995; Contant et al., 1996). These studies showed that only 7–21% of the boutons belonging to cholinergic neurons contained synaptic membrane specializations. This is in stark contrast to GABAergic boutons where one or more synaptic membrane specializations are seen at each terminal (Umbriaco et al., 1994). Other studies in the chick ciliary ganglion have shown that perisynaptic nicotinic acetylcholine receptors, as well as conventional postsynaptic nicotinic acetylcholine receptors, contribute to the responses of postsynaptic cells (Zhang et al., 1997; Ullian et al., 1997). Furthermore, the activity level of the most prevalent form of acetylcholinesterase (the globular G_4 type) does permit physiologically significant levels of acetylcholine to persist well beyond the sites of release (Summers et al., 1994; Taber and Fibriger, 1994). Calculations

suggest that neurotransmitter molecules can diffuse through a dense neuropil up to 10 μm within 50 ms of release (Wightman and Zimmerman, 1990).

Modulation of acetylcholine release by presynaptic GABA_B autoreceptors

The GABA_B type receptor is metabotropic, bicuculline insensitive but baclofen sensitive (Slaughter, 1995; Kaupmann et al., 1997). GABA_B receptors typically act by modulating voltage sensitive calcium channels through a G-protein-coupled mechanism (Zhang et al., 1997; Takahashi et al., 1998). Inhibition of such calcium channels in a presynaptic membrane via GABA binding to a GABA_B autoreceptor is typically thought to effect a negative feedback loop at GABAergic synapses. Although this scheme (of a GABA_B autoreceptor inhibiting further GABA release) has been confirmed by Neal and Shah (1989) in rat cortex, they have also shown that baclofen does not suppress GABA release in the retina. There is growing evidence that retinal GABA_B receptors may be involved in the inhibition of glycine release rather than GABA release. In rabbit retina, it has also been shown by Neal and Cunningham (1995; see also Cunningham and Neal, 1983) that application of the GABA_B agonist baclofen facilitates the light-evoked release of acetylcholine by inhibiting glycine release from a subtype of glycinergic amacrine cell. They have also shown that these glycinergic amacrine cells are themselves stimulated by acetylcholine acting on a muscarinic receptor, thus forming an inhibitory feedback loop onto the cholinergic starburst amacrine cells. The effects of acetylcholine are mimicked by muscarine and blocked by atropine, whereas the glycinergic effects of this circuit are blocked by strychnine. They suggest

---

Fig. 3. **A–B**: Confocal microscopy shows several starburst amacrine cells labeled for choline acetyltransferase (green) double labeled for m2 muscarinic (A—red) and nicotinic (B—red) receptors. For each receptor type, several amacrine and ganglion cells are clearly labeled. The starburst amacrine cells do not show any detectable receptor labeling. Scale bars = 25 μm. **C–D**: Double-labeling of DAPI-3 cells labeled for GABA_A receptor subunits (green) and m2 muscarinic cholinergic receptors (red) shows that each DAPI-3 cell is clearly labeled for the receptors. Scale bars = 25 μm. **E–F**: Again double-labeling of DAPI-3 cells labeled for GABA_A receptor subunits (green) and nicotinic cholinergic receptors (red) shows that each DAPI-3 cell is clearly labeled for the receptors. Scale bars = 25 μm. **G**: Comparison of the sites of acetylcholine release and reception in the rabbit retina. Double-labeling of starburst amacrine cells via ChAT (green) and DAPI-3 cells via GABA_A receptor subunits (red) in the rabbit retina. Most processes from the starburst amacrine cells and the DAPI-3 cells can be seen to juxtapose each other but to not overlap directly. Scale bar = 10 μm.

that an as yet unidentified bistratified glycinergic amacrine cell, which receives both (muscarinic) cholinergic and GABAergic input, feeds back onto the cholinergic cells either directly, or indirectly via bipolar cell terminals which are themselves presynaptic to the starburst amacrine cells. In their model, Neal and Cunningham suggest that one possible location for the GABA$_B$ receptors in this circuit would be on the glycinergic interneuron.

Our recent findings that starburst amacrine cells, which release both acetylcholine and GABA, are immunoreactive for GABA$_B$ receptors (Fig. 2K, L) and that glycinergic amacrine cells, including DAPI-3 cells, do not show GABA$_B$ receptor immunoreactivity (Fig. 2M, N), would suggest an alternative explanation (Zucker et al., 1998). Since the GABA released by starburst amacrine cells has been shown to be via a calcium independent mechanism, presynaptic binding of GABA to a GABA$_B$ autoreceptor would not be expected to effect further release of GABA. On the other hand, the release of acetylcholine from these same cells is calcium dependent. Therefore, GABA$_B$ receptors on starburst amacrine cells would provide an effective mechanism to truncate acetylcholine release, thus effecting a tonic → phasic shift. A common theme that has evolved regarding the role of GABA$_B$ receptors in the retina is the notion that they are involved in an enhancement of transient responses (Ikeda et al., 1990; Müller et al., 1992; Slaughter, 1995 for review). We have also shown that a candidate glycinergic-amacrine cell, the DAPI-3 cell, is acetylcholine-receptive, thus providing a functional circuit consistent with the data of Neal and Cunningham (1995). A schematic diagram is shown in Fig. 4 that incorporates our findings into such a circuit.

In our model, starburst amacrine cell activation consequent to excitatory bipolar cell input would result in an increase in both acetylcholine and GABA release by calcium dependent and independent mechanisms respectively. Acetylcholine would then be available to activate cholinergic receptors on a glycinergic amacrine cell (possibly the DAPI-3 cell which we have shown to be cholinoreceptive) either through direct synaptic or more indirect chemical ephaptic interaction. (Such a "synapse at a distance" mechanism would help explain the apparent dearth of conventional synapses made by

starburst amacrine cells onto non-cholinergic amacrine cells.) Thus activated, the glycinergic interneuron would provide inhibitory glycinergic feedback either directly onto the starburst amacrine cell or indirectly onto the bipolar cell. In parallel to this, GABA released by the starburst amacrine cell would bind to the GABA$_B$ auto-receptors which would then truncate further release of acetylcholine to glycinergic cells by blocking calcium influx. Further GABA efflux from starburst amacrine cells would be maintained (as long as there is bipolar input) since it is not calcium dependent. With acetylcholine release onto the glycinergic amacrine cell inhibited, the starburst amacrine cell would be disinhibited resulting in an increase in acetylcholine release onto the ganglion cell. For that to happen, the GABA$_B$ receptors would have to be relatively far from the ganglion-cell synapse (see Fig. 4). If this assumption holds, then the consequent increase in acetylcholine release suggests that GABA$_B$ receptors underlie the facilitation of responses to motion of extended edges (Grzywacz and Amthor, 1993; Amthor et al., 1996). This is because moving extended edges would cause sustained bipolar inputs onto starburst cells. The same mechanism that causes motion facilitation would be consistent with the general role attributed to GABA$_B$ receptor function in the retina (Slaughter, 1995 for review). This role is converting sustained responses into transient ones, as it would happen with the acetylcholine release. Such a mechanism is also consistent with the data of Neal and Cunningham (1995) that showed an increase in acetylcholine release in the presence of L-baclofen.

Conclusions and future perspectives

From early on, the retina has been attractive for investigation due to its relatively easy access (compared to other regions of the central nervous system) and the inherent elegance of its structure and function. At the most basic level, the retinal lamination that divides it into two plexiform, or synaptic layers, separated by three nuclear layers, has led to a generalized distinction of physiological function. The outer plexiform layer processes visual information in terms of its spatial properties, e.g. edge and contrast enhancement. The inner plexiform layer is involved

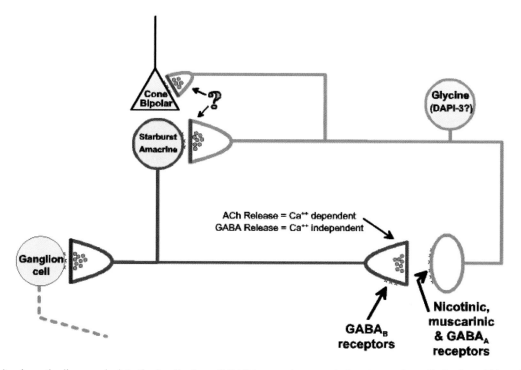

Fig. 4. A schematic diagram depicts the localization of GABA$_B$ receptors on starburst amacrine cells in the rabbit retina. Such localization may suggest a role for presynaptic inhibitory modulation of acetylcholine release in the retina. An acetylcholine receptive glycinergic amacrine cell (possibly the DAPI-3 cell) is also thought to be involved in an inhibitory feedback loop that modulates cholinergic function. Nicotinic, muscarinic and GABA$_A$ receptors that we have shown to be present on the DAPI-3 cells are also shown. The central tenet of our model is that stimulation of the starburst amacrine cell would result in the release of both acetylcholine and GABA via Ca^{++} dependent and Ca^{++} independent mechanisms, respectively. Thus GABA, binding to its presynaptic autoreceptor, could effect a truncation of acetylcholine release through inhibition of an inward Ca^{++} current while at the same time not limiting its own release which is Ca^{++} independent.

in more temporal aspects of vision such as the onset and cessation of light stimuli or its movement across a visual field. Such basic concepts, that have been largely defined, and then greatly expanded on by John Dowling, now provide the foundation upon which most current studies of retinal function are based.

Our most recent studies have been focusing on the DAPI-3 and starburst amacrine cells and the ON-OFF directionally selective ganglion cells. Several lines of evidence suggest that these cell types are potentially functionally related. These include: (1) the known involvement of acetylcholine in directional selectivity; (2) the known synaptic interaction between starburst amacrine cells and ON–OFF directionally selective ganglion cells; (3) a similar (though not identical) stratification of these cells with DAPI-3 cells; (4) the presence of cholinergic receptors

on DAPI-3 cells; (5) the known modulation of acetylcholine release by a cholinoreceptive glycinergic amacrine cell (perhaps the DAPI-3 cell); and (6) physiologically identified glycine receptors on the starburst amacrine cells.

Our aim is to accumulate sufficient data to determine if DAPI-3 cells interact with starburst amacrine cells and/or ON–OFF directionally selective ganglion cells. If so, by deciphering specific details regarding dendritic cofasciculation and synaptic interactions (in both the feedback and feedforward directions), not only will there be increased knowledge regarding the microcircuitry between three relatively well characterized neurons in the mammalian inner plexiform layer, but our incorporation of this circuitry into a working model will also advance our understanding from a functional point of view. If DAPI-3 cells are indeed involved in the

80

circuitry underlying, or modulating directional selectivity, then our models will likely suggest hypotheses that should be tested physiologically. Although there is little evidence to suggest that glycine plays a central role in the actual production of directionally selective properties, other more ancillary functions such as gain control within the directional pathway, cannot be ruled out.

In conclusion, through the use of high resolution neurotransmitter receptor localization and intracellular filling of identified retinal neurons, studies such as those described here are starting to provide the details necessary to allow for the construction of functional circuit models of specific, physiologically defined, visual functions.

Acknowledgments

Supported by NIH grant EY07552 to CLZ, and the Retina Research Foundation, the RP Foundation, the Segerfalk Foundation, the H and L Nilssons Stiftelse, the T and R Söderberg Foundation, the Swedish Medical Research Council (project 14X-2321), the Riksbankens Jubileumsfond and the Faculty of Medicine at the University of Lund to BE.

References

Amthor, F.R., Grzywacz, N.M. and Merwine, D.K. (1996) Extra Receptive Field Motion Facilitation in On-Off Directionally Selective Ganglion Cells of the Rabbit Retina. Vis. Neurosci., 13: 303–309.

Boycott, B.B., Dowling, J.E., Fisher, S.K., Kolb, H. and Laties, A.M. (1975 Dec 2) Interplexiform cells of the mammalian retina and their comparison with catecholamine-containing retinal cells. Proc. R. Soc. Lond. B. Biol Sci., 191(1104): 353–368.

Brandon, C. (1987) Cholinergic neurons in the rabbit retina: dendritic branching and ultrastructural connectivity. Brain Res., 426: 119–130.

Cajal, S.R. (1892) La Retine des vertebrates. Cellule., 9: 119–225.

Contant, C., Umbriaco, D., Garcia, S., Watkins, K.C. and Descarries, L. (1996) Ultrastructural characterization of the acetylcholine innervation in adult rat neostriatum. Neurosci., 71: 937–947.

Cunningham, J.R. and Neal, M.J. (1983) Effect of gamma-aminobutyric acid agonists, glycine, taurine and neuropep-

tides on acetylcholine release from the rabbit retina. J. Physiol., 336: 563–577.

Descarries, L., Gisiger, V. and Steriade, M. (1997) Diffuse transmission by acetylcholine in the CNS. Prog. Neurobiol., 53: 603–625.

Dowling, J.E. and Ehinger, B. (1975) Synaptic organization of the amine-containing interplexiform cells of the goldfish and Cebus monkey retinas. Science, 188(4185): 270–273.

Dowling, J.E. and Ehinger, B. (1978a) Synaptic organization of the dopaminergic neurons in the rabbit retina. J. Comp. Neurol., 180(2): 203–220.

Dowling, J.E. and Ehinger, B. (1978b) The interplexiform cell system. I. Synapses of the dopaminergic neurons of the goldfish retina. Proc. R. Soc. Lond. B. Biol. Sci., 201(1142): 7–26.

Dowling, J.E. and Boycott, B.B. (1966) Organization of the primate retina: electron microscopy. Proc. R. Soc. Lond. B Biol. Sci., 166(2): 80–111.

Eccles, J.C. (1986) Chemical transmission and Dale's principle. In T. Hökfelt, K. Fuxe and B. Pernow (Eds.), Progress in Brain Research, Vol. 68, Elsevier, Amsterdam pp. 3–13.

Enz, R. and Bormann, J. (1995) Expression of glycine receptor subunits and gephyrin in single bipolar cells of the rat retina. Vis. Neurosci., 12(3): 501–507.

Famiglietti, E.V. (1983a) "Starburst" amacrine cells and cholinergic neurons: mirror-symmetric ON and OFF amacrine cells of rabbit retina. Brain Res., 261: 138–144.

Famiglietti, E.V. (1983b) On and off pathways through amacrine cells in mammalian retina: the synaptic connections of "starburst" amacrine cells. Vis. Res., 23: 1265–1279.

Famiglietti, E.V. (1991) Synaptic organization of starburst amacrine cells in rabbit retina: analysis of serial thin sections by electron microscopy and graphic reconstruction. J. Comp. Neurol., 309(1): 40–70.

Grzywacz, N.M. and Amthor, F.R. (1993) Facilitation in ON-OFF directionally selective ganglion cells of the rabbit retina. J. Neurophysiol., 69(6): 2188–2199.

Hedden, W.L. Jr. and Dowling, J.E. (1978 Apr 13) The interplexiform cell system. II. Effects of dopamine on goldfish retinal neurones. Proc. R. Soc. Lond. B Biol. Sci., 201(1142): 27–55.

Ikeda, H., Hankins, M.W. and Kay, C.D. (1990) Actions of baclofen and phaclofen upon ON- and OFF-ganglion cells in the cat retina. Eur. J. Pharm., 190: 1–9.

Kaupmann, K., Huggel, K., Heid, J., Flor, P.J., Bischoff, S., Mickel, S.J., McMaster, G., Angst, C., Bittiger, H., Froestl, W. and Bettler, B. (1997) Expression cloning of GABA$_B$ receptors uncovers similarity to metabotropic glutamate receptors. Nature, 386(6622): 239–246.

Millar, T.J. and Morgan, I.G. (1987) Cholinergic amacrine cells in the rabbit retina synapse onto other cholinergic amacrine cells. Neurosci. Lett., 74(3): 281–285.

Müller, F., Boos, R. and Wässle, H. (1992) Actions of GABAergic ligands on brisk ganglion cells in the cat retina. Vis. Neurosci., 9: 415–425.

Neal, M.J. and Shah, M.A. (1989) Baclofen and phaclofen modulate GABA release from slices of rat cerebral cortex and spinal cord but not from retina. *Br. J. Pharmacol.*, 98(1): 105–112.

Neal, M.J. and Cunningham, J.R. (1995) Baclofen enhancement of acetylcholine release from amacrine cells in the rabbit retina by reduction of glycinergic inhibition. *J. Physiol.*, 482: 363–372.

Slaughter, M.M. (1995) GABA$_B$ receptors in the vertebrate retina. *Pro. Retin. Eye Res.*, 14(1): 293–312.

Sossin, W.S., Sweet-Cordero, A. and Scheller, R.H. (1990) Dale's hypothesis revisited: Different neuropeptides derived from a common prohormone are targeted to different processes. *Proc. Natl. Acad. Sci. USA*, 87: 4845–4848.

Summers, K.L., Cuadra, G., Naritoku, D. and Giacobini, E. (1994) Effects of nicotine on levels of acetylcholine and biogenic amine in rat cortex. *Drug Dev. Res.*, 31: 108–119.

Suzuki, S., Tachibana, M. and Kaneko, A. (1990) Effects of glycine and GABA on isolated bipolar cells of the mouse retina. *J. Physiol.*, 421: 645–662.

Swanson, L.W. (1983) Neuropeptides—New vistas on synaptic transmission. *Trends in Neurosci.*, 6, 294–295.

Taber, M.T. and Fibriger, H.C. (1994) Cortical regulation of acetylcholine release in rat stiatum. *Brain Res.*, 639: 354–356.

Takahashi, T., Kajikawa, Y. and Tsujimoto, T. (1998) G-Protein-coupled modulation of presynaptic calcium currents and transmitter release by a GABA$_B$ receptor. *J. Neurosci.*, 18(9): 3138–3146.

Ullian, E.M., McIntosh, J.M., Sargent, P.B. (1997) Rapid synaptic transmission in the avian ciliary ganglion is mediated by two distinct classes of nicotinic receptors. *J. Neurosci.* 17(19): 7210–7219.

Umbriaco, D., Garcia, S., Beaulieu, C. and Descarries, L. (1995) Relational features of acetylcholine, noradrenaline, serotonin and GABA axon terminals in the stratum radium of adult rat hippocampus (CA1). *Hippocampus*, 5: 605–620.

Umbriaco, D., Watkins, K.C., Descarries, L., Cozzari, C. and Hartman, B.K. (1994) Ultrastructural and morphometric features of the acetylcholine innervation in adult parietal cortex. An electron microscopic study in serial sections. *J. Comp. Neurol.*, 348: 351–373.

Vaney, D.I. (1990) The mosaic of amacrine cells in the mammalian retina. *Prog. Retin. Res.*, 9: 2–39.

Wightman, R.M. and Zimmerman, J.B. (1990) Control of dopamine extracellular concentration in rat striatum by impulse flow and uptake. *Brain Res.*, 15: 135–144.

Wright, L.L., Macqueen, C.L., Elston, G.N., Young, H.M., Pow, D.V. and Vaney, D.I. (1997) The DAPI-3 amacrine cells of the rabbit retina. *Vis. Neurosci.*, 14: 473–492.

Yazulla, S. and Studholme, K.M. (1991) Glycine-receptor immunoreactivity in retinal bipolar cells is postsynaptic to glycinergic and GABAergic amacrine cell synapses. *J. Comp. Neurol.*, 310: 11–20.

Zhang, J., Shen, W. and Slaughter, M.M. (1997) Two metabotropic gamma-aminobutyric acid receptors differentially modulate calcium currents in retinal ganglion cells. *J. Gen. Physiol.*, 110(1): 45–58.

Zucker, C.L. (1998) Localization of gephyrin and glycine receptor subunit immunoreactivity in the rabbit retina. *Vis. Neurosci.*, 15(2): 389–395.

Zucker, C.L., Ehinger, B. and Grzywacz, N.M. (1998) GABA$_B$ receptors and cholinergic function in the rabbit retina. *Soc. Neurosci.*, 24(57.13): 136.

Zucker, C.L. and Ehinger, B. (1992) Heterogeneity of receptor immunureactivity at synapses of glycine-utilizing neurons. *Proc. Roy. Soc. Lond. B*, 249: 89–94.

Zucker, C.L. and Ehinger, B. (1993) Synaptic connections involving immunoreactive glycine receptors in the turtle retina. *Vis. Neurosci.*, 10(5): 907–914.

Zucker, C.L. and Ehinger, B. (1998) Distribution of GABA$_A$ receptors on a bistratified amacrine cell type in the rabbit retina. *J. Comp. Neurol.*, 393(3): 309–319.

H. Kolb, H. Ripps and S. Wu (Eds.)
Progress in Brain Research, Vol. 131
© 2001 Elsevier Science B.V. All rights reserved

CHAPTER 5

Synaptic inputs to dopaminergic neurons in mammalian retinas

David W. Marshak*

*Department of Neurobiology and Anatomy, University of Texas Medical School, Houston,
TX 77225-0708, USA*

Dopaminergic neurons of mammalian retinas

The visual system remains responsive over an enormous range of background light intensities, and virtually all of this adaptation is accomplished within the retina. John Dowling and his coworkers have made enormous contributions to our understanding of this process. They and others have shown that dopamine plays a major role in both light adaptation and dark adaptation, changing the strength of many types of chemical and electrical synapses so that the retina can detect small changes in luminance contrast as the background intensity is changing. John Dowling and his colleagues have also done some of the most important work on the morphology and functions of dopaminergic neurons in the retina. It would require a much longer review than this one to adequately summarize all of their contributions. Instead, I am going to focus on a single question. How does the dopaminergic cell generate a response to the ambient light intensity when all of its input is derived from neurons that are adapting, themselves? I propose an answer to this question that, so far, only applies to the rod-driven responses of dopaminergic neurons in mammalian retinas.

In mammals, there is a single population of dopaminergic cells with dendrites branching in the outermost stratum of the inner plexiform layer (IPL) and axons that also ramify in the same stratum, for the most part. There is also typically a sparse plexus in the outer plexiform layer (OPL) and very few, if any, axons in other strata of the IPL. Dopaminergic neurons labeled with antibody to tyrosine hydroxylase in a whole mount preparation from macaque retina are illustrated in Fig. 1. The plexus in the OPL is particularly extensive in New World Monkeys (Dowling and Ehinger, 1975; Dowling et al., 1980). Figure 2 shows a dopaminergic cell in a vertical section from the macaque retina. These cells have been shown to use dopamine as a neurotransmitter by several techniques. Using aldehyde-induced fluorescence, endogenous dopamine was first localized to amacrine cells in the human retina (Ehinger, 1966) and later in the macaque retina (Ehinger and Falck, 1969a,b; Mariani et al., 1984). These cells are the only neurons that take up dopamine and related amines in human (Ehinger and Floren, 1979; Frederick et al., 1982) and macaque (Ehinger and Floren, 1979; Akagi et al., 1980; Holmgren, 1982) retinas. The rate-limiting enzyme in the pathway for dopamine synthesis, tyrosine hydroxylase, has also been localized to these cells by immunocytochemical techniques (Nguyen-Legros et al., 1984, 1992; Mariani and Hokoc, 1988; Dacey, 1990; Mitrofanis and Provis, 1990; Mills and Massey, 1999).

---

* E-mail: david.w.marshak@uth.tmc.edu

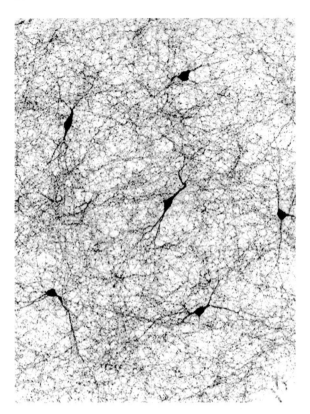

Fig. 1. Dopaminergic amacrine cells from the macaque retina labeled with antibody to tyrosine hydroxylase in a whole mount preparation. Note the rings of terminals in sublamina 1 of the inner plexiform layer that surround the perikarya of AII amacrine cells.

Physiological studies of dopaminergic neurons in mammals

Li and Dowling (2000) have recently reviewed the evidence that dopamine is released during light stimulation and also in total darkness. These apparently contradictory results can be reconciled if there is a U-shaped relationship between dopamine release and light intensity, and there is indirect evidence that this is true in mammalian retinas. The major targets of dopaminergic cells in mammals are the AII amacrine cells, which convey signals from rod bipolar cells to cone bipolar cells (Voigt and Wässle, 1987). The gap junctions between AII amacrine cells are closed by dopamine (Hampson et al., 1992), and AII cells are also uncoupled when the retina is maintained in total darkness or in light at the upper

end of the scotopic range. Light appears to inhibit dopamine release in the low scotopic range because AII amacrine cells are extensively coupled (Bloomfield et al., 1997). Computer modeling studies indicate how these changes in AII coupling might contribute to both light and dark adaptation. The limited coupling of AII cells in total darkness is optimal to detect rare, single-photon signals, and the extensive coupling in low scotopic backgrounds increases the signal to noise ratio in the rod pathway. The reduction of AII coupling again at higher intensities limits the spread of rod signals to the cone bipolar cells because the number of coupled bipolar cells is reduced proportionally (Smith and Vardi, 1995; Vardi and Smith, 1996). The effects of 6-hydroxydopamine lesions and dopamine antagonists on the electroretinogram in cats are also consistent with a U-shaped relationship between dopamine release and light intensity. These treatments have no effect at low scotopic intensities, when dopamine release is normally inhibited. The effects of picrotoxin are maximal in this range, a finding suggesting that the major inhibitory input to the dopaminergic cells is from GABAergic amacrine cells (Naarendorp et al., 1993).

Dopamine release by light stimuli in the entire scotopic range has never been studied systematically in mammals, but we have examined two points at either end of the curve in our work on the release of endogenous dopamine from the macaque retina in vitro (Boelen et al., 1998). The basal level of dopamine released in steady, low photopic light is not different from that in total darkness after 40 min of dark adaptation. On the other hand, many of the earlier experiments that have been interpreted as evidence for inhibition of dopamine release in the dark were conducted in dim, red light, not in total darkness. These early experiments also typically used nocturnal or crepuscular animals, whose retinas are extremely sensitive to light under these conditions (Kramer, 1971; Bauer et al., 1980; Marshburn and Iuvone, 1981; Godley and Wurtman, 1988). The AII amacrine cells and most ON cone bipolar cells probably respond to the red light, inhibiting dopamine release. One group found that dopamine was released from the cat retina during total darkness and at the offset of a steady, photopic background light (Hamasaki et al., 1986). In this

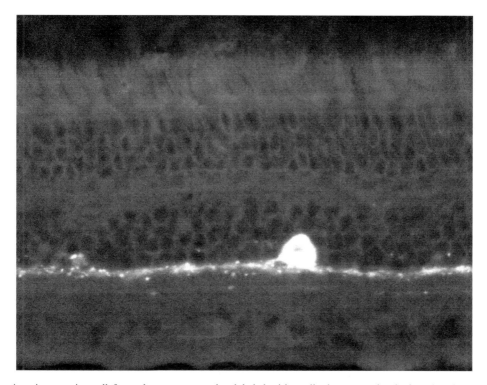

Fig. 2. Dopaminergic amacrine cell from the macaque retina labeled with antibody to tyrosine hydroxylase in a vertical section. A second population of tyrosine hydroxylase-immunoreactive amacrine cells has been described in macaque retina (Mariani and Hokoc, 1988; Mariani, 1991). The sparse, faint labeling in the middle of the inner plexiform layer may be processes from these cells.

and in our experiments conducted in total darkness, the OFF cone bipolar cells are stimulated, instead.

The light responses of dopaminergic cells have not been recorded in the in an intact, mammalian retina, but dopaminergic cells isolated from the mouse retina have been studied using whole-cell voltage and current clamp techniques. Dopaminergic perikarya are capable of generating action potentials, and 80% of the cells sampled did so spontaneously. The dopaminergic cells have hyperpolarizing responses mediated by $GABA_A$ receptors or strychnine-sensitive glycine receptors and depolarizing responses mediated by ionotropic glutamate receptors (Gustincich et al., 1997; Feigenspan et al., 1998).

Synaptic inputs to mammalian dopaminergic neurons

Figure 3 summarizes the major cone (3A) and rod (3B) pathways of mammalian retinas (reviewed by Kolb, this volume). The rods and cones differ in their connections with horizontal cells and contact different sets of bipolar cells. There are two basic types of cone bipolar cells, ON bipolar cells that depolarize when stimulated with light and OFF bipolar cells that hyperpolarize to the same stimuli. Cone bipolar cells make direct, excitatory synapses onto ON and OFF retinal ganglion cells. There is only one type of rod bipolar cell, however, and it has depolarizing responses to light. The rod bipolar cells connect to the retinal ganglion cells indirectly, via the cone bipolar cells, and this pathway is highly sensitive. The rod bipolar cells make excitatory synapses onto AII amacrine cells, which then excite ON cone bipolar cells through gap junctions and inhibit OFF cone bipolar cells via chemical synapses. In a second, less sensitive rod pathway, signals flow directly from rods to cones via gap junctions (Nelson, 1977). In rodents, there is a third rod pathway (not illustrated). One OFF cone bipolar cell subtype receives input directly from rods (Jacobs et al., 1976; West, 1978; Hack et al., 1999).

A.

B.

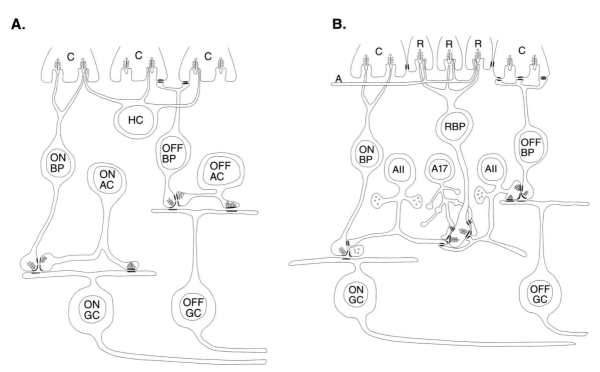

Fig. 3. **A.** Cones (C) provide input to ON and OFF cone bipolar cells (BP) and horizontal cells (HC). Bipolar cells make excitatory, ribbon synapses onto ON and OFF ganglion cells (GC). The bipolar cells also synapse on amacrine cells (AC), which make inhibitory synapses back onto bipolar cells and forward onto amacrine cells and ganglion cells. **B.** Rods (R) provide input to rod bipolar cells (RBP) which synapse onto bistratified AII amacrine cells and A17 amacrine cells. A17 cells make inhibitory, feedback synapses onto rod bipolar cells. AII amacrine cells relay the rod signal to OFF ganglion cells via inhibitory synapses onto OFF cone bipolar cells and to ON ganglion cells via gap junctions with ON cone bipolar cells. Rods also make gap junctions with cones.

In mammalian retinas, dopaminergic cells receive input from the axon terminals of bipolar cells (Hokoc and Mariani, 1987, 1988; Kolb et al., 1990; Gustincich et al., 1997). These bipolar cells have not been identified, but three lines of evidence suggest that they are a distinct type. First, the light-stimulated release of dopamine from the monkey retina is inhibited by 2-amino-4-phosphonobutyric acid (APB; Boelen et al., 1998). Taken with the electrophysiological evidence, this finding suggests that the bipolar cell presynaptic to the dopaminergic cell is an ON type, unlike other bipolar cells ending in the upper half of the inner plexiform layer. Second, there is often only a single postsynaptic process at the ribbon synapses from these bipolar cells onto dopaminergic cells rather than two, as at typical bipolar cell synapses (Hokoc and Mariani, 1987, 1998; Kolb et al., 1990, 1991; Gustincich et al., 1997). This observation also suggests that these bipolar cells are highly selective in

their contacts. One possibility is that these are wide-field or bistratified bipolar cells. These would be particularly well suited to convey a global adaptation signal because they receive input over a wide area of the retina in primates (Mariani, 1983; Hokoc and Mariani, 1988). In rabbits, Jeon and Masland (1995) labeled a similar type of bipolar cell, which they called wide field. Bistratified bipolar cells have also been observed in the squirrel retina using the Golgi method (Linberg et al., 1996). Third, none of the electron microscopic studies of the bipolar cell synapses onto dopaminergic cells in mammalian retinas have reported input to these bipolar cells from AII amacrine cells, and I have seen none in the macaque retina (unpublished observations). This suggests that the bipolar cells presynaptic to dopaminergic cells only get rod input from rod-cone gap junctions, a relatively insensitive pathway (Nelson, 1977). The remainder of the input to dopaminergic cells is from amacrine cells, including GABAergic amacrine cells. The dopaminergic cells make a few synapses back onto bipolar cells that provide their input, but the vast majority of their output is directed to amacrine cells (Holmgren, 1982; Hokoc and Mariani, 1987, 1988; Kolb et al., 1990, 1991). Taken with the results from physiological experiments, these findings led to the model illustrated in Fig. 4.

Model of the neural circuit providing input to dopaminergic cells

In total darkness (Fig. 4A), the dopaminergic cell receives no input and fires spontaneously. In the scotopic range, the neural circuit providing input to the dopaminergic cell essentially computes the difference between the signal from rods via the AII amacrine cells and the signal from rods via the gap junctions between rods and cones. The AII pathway is far more sensitive, and therefore, in the low scotopic range, GABAergic amacrine cells that receive input from AII amacrine cells inhibit the dopaminergic cells (Fig. 4B). In higher scotopic background intensities, the rod signal conveyed to cones via gap junctions depolarizes the bipolar cells presynaptic to the dopaminergic cells, and the activity of the dopaminergic cells reflects a balance between these two inputs (Fig. 4C). Thus, the dopaminergic cells are hyperpolarized when the rod input via the AII pathway predominates but begin to depolarize when the signal from rod-cone gap junctions appears. In photopic backgrounds, APB blocks all input to dopaminergic cells, and they are spontaneously active (Fig. 4D). This explains why there are roughly equal amounts of dopamine released from the macaque retina in total darkness and in steady photopic backgrounds, either with or without APB (Boelen et al., 1998).

The GABAergic amacrine cells presynaptic to the dopaminergic cells are a key element in the model. These amacrine cells receive inhibitory input from OFF amacrine cells and excitatory input from ON cone bipolar cells that, in turn, receive input from AII amacrine cells. GABAergic amacrine cells that might receive input in the proximal half of the inner plexiform layer and terminate on dopaminergic amacrine cells in the most distal stratum have been

described in several mammalian retinas. There are four candidates in ground squirrels, A20 through 23 (Linberg et al., 1996). In rabbits, there are three, including: diffuse multistratifed, wavy multistratified and fountain (MacNeil et al., 1999). In primates, candidates include the wavy multistratified cells of macaques, known as tristratified in humans, wooly diffuse and A13 amacrine cells (Mariani, 1990; Kolb et al., 1992). A13 amacrine cells are also candidates in cats (Kolb et al., 1981). Dopamine is released by blocking tonic inhibitory input from GABAergic amacrine cells (Kamp and Morgan, 1981; Marshburn and Iuvone, 1981; Naarendorp et al., 1993). However, this cannot be the only mechanism for releasing dopamine because it does not include a function for the bipolar cell synapses and ionotropic glutamate receptors on dopaminergic cells.

The most controversial aspect of the model is that the excitatory input to dopaminergic cells is from ON bipolar cells terminating in the distal half of the inner plexiform layer. This is based on the evidence that dopamine release is greatly enhanced by flashing light on a low photopic background, and APB blocks this component. Dopaminergic cells might have receptors for APB, themselves, but this is unlikely because dopaminergic cells have depolarizing responses to glutamate mediated by ionotropic receptors (Gustincich et al., 1997). The APB might act at other Group III metabotropic glutamate receptors, which have been localized in the inner retina of rats (Hartveit et al., 1995). But the effects of APB there are expected to be modulatory. The ON bipolar cells of mammals are the only retinal neurons known to use metabotropic glutamate receptors for their primary signaling pathway, and therefore the ON bipolar cells are the neurons whose light responses are most strongly affected by APB (Thoreson and Witkovsky, 1999). A second possibility is that the dopamine originated from a second population of amacrine cells known to contain small quantities of immunoreactive tyrosine hydroxylase and its messenger RNA (Mariani and Hokoc, 1988; Gustincich et al., 1997). However, these cells do not take up catecholamines, and it would be unprecedented for a cell to use dopamine as a neurotransmitter without an uptake mechanism to recycle it. Third, amacrine cells might transmit a signal from ON bipolar cell axons in the inner half of the IPL to dopaminergic

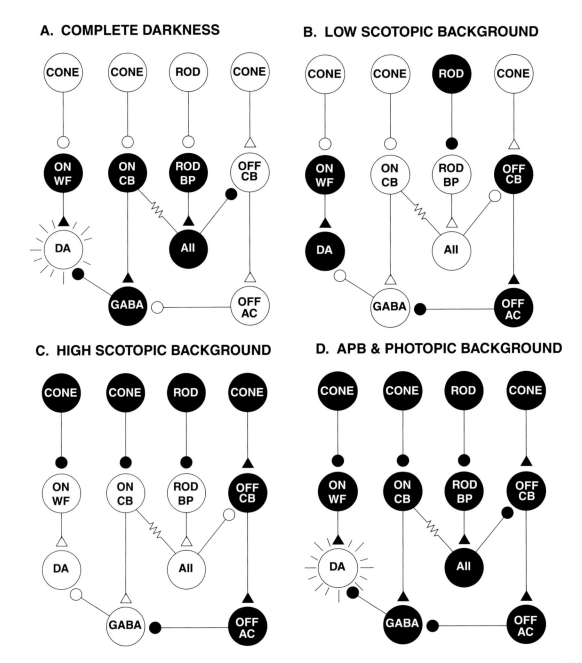

Fig. 4. Model of the neural circuit providing input to the dopaminergic cells. **A.** In total darkness, rods and cones are depolarized. OFF cone bipolar cells (OFF CB) and OFF amacrine cells (OFF AC) are depolarized (white). GABAergic amacrine (GABA) cells are hyperpolarized (black). Dopamine (DA) cells are spontaneously active (lines). AII amacrine (AII) cells are uncoupled and hyperpolarized. **B.** In low scotopic backgrounds, rods are hyperpolarized and cones are depolarized. Rod bipolar cells are depolarized. Therefore, the AII amacrine cells and the ON bipolar cells electrically coupled to them are depolarized. However, the wide field (WF) ON bipolar cells presynaptic to the dopaminergic cells remain hyperpolarized because they do not receive AII input. OFF cone bipolar cells and OFF amacrine cells are hyperpolarized. GABAergic amacrine cells are depolarized, and dopaminergic cells are inhibited. AII cells are coupled and depolarized. **C.** In high scotopic backgrounds, rods are hyperpolarized by light and cones by their gap junctions. Rod bipolar cells and both types of ON cone bipolar cells are depolarized. OFF cone bipolar cells and OFF amacrine cells are hyperpolarized. Dopaminergic cells are depolarized. AII amacrine cells are uncoupled and depolarized. **D.** Photopic light stimulation with APB, an agonist at mGluR6 receptors of rod bipolar cells and ON cone bipolar cells, eliminates all synaptic input to the dopaminergic cells, and they are spontaneously active.

cells branching in the outer half. There is no evidence for a direct, excitatory connection since the cholinergic amacrine cells, the only ones with an excitatory transmitter, are unistratified (Rodieck and Marshak, 1992), and there is no indication that dopaminergic cells make gap junctions except with one another (Vaney, 1994). The fourth, most plausible explanation for the results is that ON bipolar cells contact the dopaminergic cells directly. However, there are no monostratified ON bipolar cells that terminate in the outer half of the IPL in rats, the most thoroughly studied mammalian species, (Euler et al., 1996; Hartveit, 1997), and the same is expected in other mammalian retinas. The blue cone bipolar cells in central macaque retina make a few synapses in the outer half of the IPL (Calkins et al., 1998), but contacts between blue cone bipolar cell axons and dopaminergic dendrites were not observed in a light microscopic double labeling experiment (unpublished observations). This leaves the bistratified or wide field bipolar cells, which costratify with the dendrites of dopaminergic cells (Mariani, 1983; Kolb et al., 1992; Jeon and Masland, 1995; Linberg et al., 1996). The light responses of these bipolar cells are unknown, but they are expected to be depolarizing based on these results.

Conclusions and future perspectives

Dopamine plays a critical role in both light and dark adaptation, and to do that, the dopaminergic neurons must able to detect the absolute, ambient light intensity, despite the fact that the neurons that provide their input are adapting rapidly. To account for this, I have developed a model of the neural circuit that provides input to the dopaminergic neurons in mammalian retinas based on published anatomical and physiological data. The model predicts that dopaminergic cells are spontaneously active in the dark, and under scotopic conditions, they compare the strength of signals in two pathways originating from the rods. In low scotopic intensities, input from the more sensitive pathway, via the AII amacrine cells, drives GABAergic amacrine cells that inhibit the dopaminergic cells. At higher scotopic intensities, the less sensitive pathway, via rod-cone gap junctions, drives the excitatory input from

bipolar cells to the dopaminergic cells. As a result, the dopamine release vs. intensity function is U-shaped and has a larger dynamic range than any of the individual neurons that provide input to the dopaminergic cells. The descending portion of the dopamine release vs. intensity function, in the low scotopic range, is mediated by inhibition driven by the AII pathway. The balance between this inhibition and excitation through rod-cone gap junctions produces the ascending portion of the release vs. intensity function, in the high scotopic range.

A thorough study of dopamine release from a mammalian retina under a wide range of scotopic background intensities is essential to test this model. The results may provide some insight into the etiology of myopia, or near-sightedness, in humans. A recent study showed that sleeping with room lights or a night light on during the first two years of life predisposed children to myopia. These findings suggest that a period of darkness is essential to prevent myopia in some people (Quinn et al., 1999), and the model deals with the regulation of dopamine release from mammalian retinas under comparable conditions. This is important because dopamine has been implicated in the regulation of eye growth in primates. Infant macaque eyes become abnormally elongated after they are occluded with opaque contact lenses, and this effect is blocked by the dopaminergic agonist, apomorphine (Iuvone et al., 1991).

I should point out, however, that the model does not account for the major changes in dopaminergic cells that take place under photopic conditions. In cat retina, more dopamine is released after a bright flash under light-adapted conditions than under dark-adapted conditions (Kramer, 1971). In rats, tyrosine hydroxylase activity increases after photopic light stimulation (Iuvone, 1984; Brainard and Morgan, 1987; Witkovsky et al., 2000). The activity of dopaminergic cells in mammals may also have circadian component that would further extend their dynamic range. There is a circadian rhythm of tyrosine hydroxylase activity in quail retina (Manglapus et al., 1999) and a circadian influence on dopamine release in fish retina (Weiler et al., 1997). I plan to add these elements and a conductance-based model of the dopaminergic cells in order to gain some insight into the behavior of this neural circuit under photopic conditions. Ultimately, the model will have to be dynamic, including the postsynaptic action of dopamine so that it will be possible to predict how the dopamine cell influences its own input and modulates the activity of other retinal neurons.

Acknowledgments

Supported by grants IBN 9223834 from the National Science Foundation and MH38310 from the National Institute of Neurological Diseases and Stroke. I wish to thank Dr. Helga Kolb and Dr. Sally Firth for their comments on the manuscript.

References

Bauer, B., Ehinger, B. and Aberg, L. (1980) [^{3}H]-Dopamine release from the rabbit retina. *Albrecht von Graefes Archiv. Opththalmol.*, 215: 71–78.

Bloomfield, S.A., Xin, D. and Osborne, T. (1997) Light-induced modulation of coupling between AII amacrine cells in the rabbit retina. *Vis. Neurosci.*, 14: 565–576.

Boelen, M.K., Boelen, M.G. and Marshak, D.W. (1998) Light-stimulated release of dopamine from the primate retina is blocked by 1-2-amino-4-phosphonobutyric acid (APB). *Vis. Neurosci.*, 15: 97–103.

Brainard, G.C. and Morgan, W.W. (1987) Light-induced stimulation of retinal dopamine: a dose-response relationship. *Brain Res.*, 424: 199–203.

Calkins, D.J., Tsukamoto, Y. and Sterling, P. (1998) Microcircuitry and mosaic of a blue-yellow ganglion cell in the primate retina. *J. Neurosci.*, 18: 3373–3385.

Dacey, D.M. (1990) The dopaminergic amacrine cell. *J. Comp. Neurol.*, 301: 461–489.

Dowling, J.E., Ehinger, B. (1975) Synaptic organization of the amine-containing interplexiform cells of the goldfish and Cebus monkey retinas. *Science*, 188: 270–273.

Dowling, J.E., Ehinger, B. and Floren, I. (1980) Fluorescence and electron microscopical observations on the amine-accumulating neurons of the Cebus monkey retina. *J. Comp. Neurol.*, 192: 665–685.

Euler, T., Schneider, H. and Wässle, H. (1996) Glutamate responses of bipolar cells in a slice preparation of the rat retina. *J. Neurosci.*, 16: 2934–2944.

Feigenspan, A., Gustincich, S., Bean, B.P. and Raviola, E. (1998) Spontaneous activity of solitary dopaminergic cells of the retina. *J. Neurosci.*, 18: 6776–6789.

Godley, B.F. and Wurtman, R.J. (1988) Release of endogenous dopamine from the superfused rabbit retina in vitro: effect of light stimulation. *Brain Res.*, 452: 393–395.

Gustincich, S., Feigenspan, A., Wu, D.K., Koopman, L.J. and Raviola, E. (1997) Control of dopamine release in the retina: a transgenic approach to neural networks. *Neuron*, 18: 723–736.

Hack, I., Peichl, L. and Brandstätter, H. (1999) An alternative pathway for rod signals in the rodent retina: Rod photoreceptors, cone bipolar cells and the localization of glutamate receptors. *Proc. Nat. Acad. Sci., USA*, 96: 14130–14135.

Hamasaki, D.I., Trattler, W.B. and Hajek, A.S. (1986) Light ON depresses and light OFF enhances the release of dopamine from the cat's retina. *Neurosci. Letts.*, 68: 112–116.

Hampson, E.C.G.M., Vaney, D.I. and Weiler, R. (1992) Dopaminergic modulation of gap junction permeability between amacrine cells in mammalian retina. *J. Neurosci.*, 12: 4911–4922.

Hartveit, E. (1997) Functional organization of cone bipolar cells in the rat retina. *J. Neurophysiol.*, 77: 1716–1730.

Hartveit, E., Brandstätter, J.H., Enz, R. and Wässle, H. (1995) Expression of the mRNA of seven metabotropic glutamate receptors (mGluR1 to7) in the rat retina. An in situ hybridization study on tissue sections and isolated cells. *Eur. J. Neurosci.*, 7: 1472–1483.

Hokoc, J.N. and Mariani, A.P. (1987) Tyrosine hydroxylase immunoreactivity in the rhesus monkey retina reveals synapses from bipolar cells to dopaminergic amacrine cells. *J. Neurosci.*, 7: 2785–2793.

Holmgren, I. (1982) Synaptic organization of the dopaminergic neurons in the retina of the cynomolgus monkey. *Invest. Ophthalmol. Vis. Sci.*, 22: 8–24.

Iuvone, P.M. (1984) Regulation of retinal dopamine biosynthesis and tyrosine hydroxylase activity by light. *Federation Proc.*, 43: 2709–2713.

Iuvone, P.M., Tigges, M., Stone, R.A., Lambert, S. and Laties, A.M. (1991) Effects of apomorphine, a dopamine receptor agonist, on ocular refraction and axial elongation in a primate model of myopia. *Invest. Ophthalmol. Vis. Sci.*, 32: 1674–1677.

Jacobs, G.H., Fisher, S.K., Anderson, D.H. and Silverman, M.S. (1976) Scotopic and photopic vision in the California ground squirrel: physiological and anatomical evidence. *J. Comp. Neurol.*, 165: 209–227.

Jeon, C.-J. and Masland, R.H. (1995) A population of wide-field bipolar cells in the rabbit's retina. *J. Comp. Neurol.*, 360: 403–412.

Kamp, C.W. and Morgan, W.W. (1981) GABA antagonists enhance dopamine turnover in the rat retina in vivo. *Eur. J. Pharmacology*, 69: 273–279.

Kolb, H., Cuenca, N. and DeKorver, L. (1991) Postembedding immunohistochemistry for GABA and glycine reveals the synaptic relationships of the dopaminergic amacrine cell of the cat retina. *J. Comp. Neurol.*, 310: 267–284.

Kolb, H., Cuenca, N., Wang, H.H. and DeKorver, L. (1990) The synaptic organization of the dopaminergic amacrine cells in the cat retina. *J. Neurocytol.*, 19: 343–366.

Kolb, H., Linberg, K.A. and Fisher, S.K. (1992) Neurons of the human retina: a Golgi study. *J. Comp. Neurol.*, 318: 147–187.

Kolb, H., Nelson, R. and Mariani, A. (1981) Amacrine cells, bipolar cells and ganglion cells of the cat retina: a Golgi study. *Vision Res.*, 21: 1081–1114.

Kramer, S.G. (1971) Dopamine: A retinal neurotransmitter. I. Retinal uptake, storage, and light-stimulated release of ^{3}H-dopamine in vivo. *Invest. Ophthalmol. Vis. Sci.*, 10: 438–452.

Li, L. and Dowling, J.E. (2000) Effects of dopamine depletion on visual sensitivity of Zebra fish. *J. Neurosci.*, 20: 1893–1903.

Linberg, K.A., Suemune, S. and Fisher, S.K. (1996) Retinal neurons of the California ground squirrel, *Spermophilus beecheyi*: a Golgi study. *J. Comp. Neurol.*, 365: 173–216.

MacNeil, M.A., Heussy, J.K., Dacheux, R.F., Raviola, E. and Masland, R.H. (1999) the shapes and numbers of amacrine cells: matching of photofilled with Golgi-stained cells in the rabbit retina and comparison with other mammalian species. *J. Comp. Neurol.*, 413: 305–326.

Manglapus, M., Iuvone, P.M., Underwood, H., Pierce, M. and Barlow, R.B. (1999) Dopamine mediates circadian rhythms of rod-cone dominance in the Japanese quail retina. *J. Neurosci.*, 19: 4132–4141.

Mariani, A.P. (1983) Giant bistratified bipolar cells in monkey retina. *Anat. Rec.*, 206: 215–220.

Mariani, A.P. (1990) Amacrine cells of the rhesus monkey retina. *J. Comp. Neurol.*, 301: 318–400.

Mariani, A.P. (1991) Synaptic organization of type 2 catecholamine amacrine cells in the rhesus monkey retina. *J. Neurocytol.*, 20: 332–342.

Mariani, A.P. and Hokoc, J.H. (1988) Two types of tyrosine hydroxylase-immunoreactive amacrine cells in the rhesus monkey retina. *J. Comp. Neurol.*, 276: 81–91.

Mariani, A.P., Kolb, H. and Nelson, R. (1984) Dopamine-containing amacrine cells of the rhesus monkey retina parallel rods in their spatial distribution. *Brain Res.*, 322: 1–7.

Marshburn, P.D. and Iuvone, P.M. (1981) The role of GABA in the regulation of the dopamine/tyrosine hydroxylase-containing neurons of the rat retina. *Brain Res.*, 214: 335–347.

Mills, S.L. and Massey, S.C. (1999) AII amacrine cells limit scotopic acuity in central macaque retina: a confocal analysis of calretinin labeling. *J. Comp. Neurol.*, 411: 19–34.

Mitrofanis, J. and Provis, J.M. (1990) A distinctive soma size gradient among catecholaminergic neurones of human retinae. *Brain Res.*, 527: 69–75.

Naarendorp, F., Hitchcock, P.F. and Sieving, P.A. (1993) Dopaminergic modulation of rod pathway signals does not affect the scotopic ERG of cat at dark adapted threshold. *J. Neurophysiol.*, 70: 1681–1691.

Nelson, R. (1977) Cat cones have rod input: a comparison of the response properties of cones and horizontal cell bodies in the cat. *J. Comp. Neurol.*, 172: 109–136.

Nguyen-Legros, J., Botteri, C., Phuc, L.H., Vigny, A. and Gay, M. (1984) Morphology of primate's dopaminergic amacrine cells as revealed by TH-like immunoreactivity on retinal flat-mounts. *Brain Res.*, 295: 145–153.

Nguyen-Legros, J., Durand, J. and Simon, A. (1992) Catecholamine cell types in the human retina. *Clin. Vision Sci.*, 7: 435–447.

Quinn, G.E., Shin, C.H., Maguire, M.G. and Stone, R.A. (1999) Myopia and ambient lighting at night. *Nature*, 399: 113–114.

Rodieck, R.W. and Marshak, D.W. (1992) Spatial density and distribution of choline acetyltransferase immunoreactive cells in human, macaque, and baboon retinas. *J. Comp. Neurol.*, 321: 46–64.

Smith, R.G. and Vardi, N. (1995) Simulation of the AII amacrine cell of mammalian retina: functional consequences of electrical coupling and regenerative membrane properties. *Vis. Neurosci.*, 12: 851–860.

Thoreson, W.B. and Witkovsky, P. (1999) Glutamate receptors and circuits in the vertebrate retina. *Pro. Retin. Eye Res.*, 18: 765–810.

Vaney, D.I. (1994) Patterns of neuronal coupling in the retina. *Pro. Retin. Eye Res.*, 13: 301–355.

Vardi, N. and Smith, R.G. (1996) The AII amacrine network: coupling can increase correlated activity. *Vision Res.*, 36: 3743–3757.

Voigt, T. and Wässle, H. (1987) Dopaminergic innervation of AII amacrine cells in mammalian retina. *J. Neurosci.*, 7: 4115–5128.

Weiler, R., Baldridge, W.H., Mangel, S.C. and Dowling, J.E. (1997) Modulation of endogenous dopamine release in the fish retina by light and prolonged darkness. *Vis. Neurosci.*, 14: 351–356.

West, R.W. (1978) Bipolar and horizontal cells of the gray squirrel retina: Golgi morphology and receptor connections. *Vision Res.*, 18: 129–136.

Witkovsky, P., Gabriel, R., Haycock, J.W. and Meller, E. (2000) Influence of light and neural circuitry on tyrosine hydroxylase phosphorylation in the rat retina. *J. Chem. Neuroanat.*, 19: 105–116.

H. Kolb, H. Ripps and S. Wu (Eds.)
Progress in Brain Research, Vol. 131
© 2001 Elsevier Science B.V. All rights reserved

CHAPTER 6

Molecular diversity of gap junctions between horizontal cells

Ulrike Janssen-Bienhold*, Konrad Schultz, Werner Hoppenstedt and Reto Weiler

FB 7 Neurobiology, University of Oldenburg, D-26111 Oldenburg, Germany

Introduction

It is well established now that mosaics of electrotonically coupled retinal neurons are acting in concerted patterns during visual information processing. A part of this processing in the outer retina is accomplished by horizontal cells which have become an excellent model system for studying the functional aspects of gap junctional coupling for network formation, plasticity of neuronal networks and information processing (reviewed in Vaney, 1994; Cook and Becker, 1995; Hankins, 1995; Weiler et al., 2000a).

Based on their morphology, connectivity patterns and physiological properties, up to four horizontal cell subtypes have been identified in the retina of different vertebrates (Kaneko, 1970; Kolb, 1974; Stell et al., 1982; Boycott, 1988). The cells of each subtype form a coupled network in the plane of the retina.

The structural correlates of these gap junctions were first described by Yamada and Ishikawa (1965). They observed "fused membrane structures" between horizontal cells of the same morphological type in the teleost and selachian retina, five years before Goodenough and Revel (1970) defined the term "gap junction". Furthermore, Yamada and Ishikawa (1965) noted that such junctions may represent a

device for electrical transmission of stimuli and that horizontal cells in the fish retina are "morphologically separate but functionally a single unit." Support for this hypothesis came from electrophysiological studies by Naka and Rushton (1967). They performed intracellular recordings from fish horizontal cells and showed that light-induced potentials, i.e. "S-potentials" (Svaetichin, 1953), can propagate freely over large distances. They proposed the involvement of electrically coupled elements in the formation of the "S-space". However, it took four more years, before Kaneko (1971) provided direct evidence for electrical and dye coupling in horizontal cells of the dogfish retina by means of dual-recording experiments and injections of Lucifer Yellow.

Numerous studies have since characterized the ultrastructure, physiology and pharmacology of gap junctions connecting horizontal cells. These reveal that the different types of horizontal cells make only homologous gap junctions in all vertebrate retinas and that both, gap junction morphology and horizontal cell coupling can be modulated in a complex fashion by the level of light-adaptation, different neuromodulators, second messengers, pH and voltage (reviewed in Vaney, 1994; Hankins, 1995; Weiler et al., 2000a). Thereby, gap junctions provide a high degree of plasticity to the coupled network of horizontal cells which is essential for their function. Horizontal cells mediate the antagonistic center-surround organization of bipolar and ganglion cell receptive fields and

---

* Corresponding author: Ulrike Janssen-Bienhold, Tel.: 441-7983419; Fax: 441-7983423; E-mail: ulrike.janssen.bienhold @uni-oldenburg.de

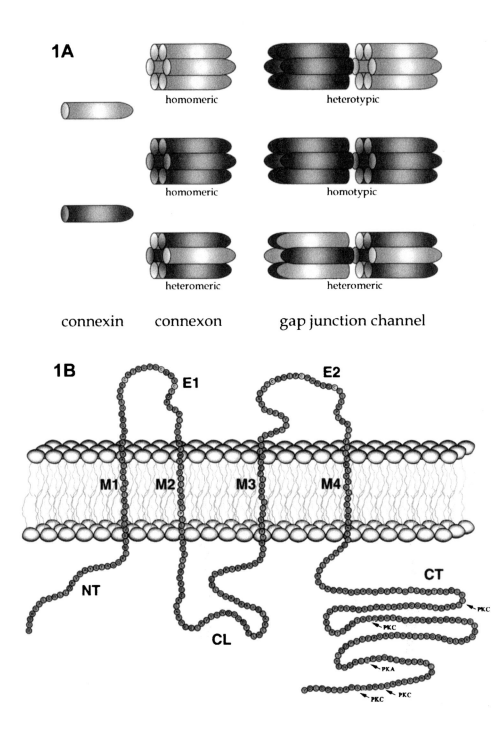

Fig. 1. Schematic representation of the organization of connexins in connexons and intercellular channels (A) and of the topology of a connexin relative to the plasma membrane (B). **A:** A connexon is composed of six protein subunits arranged radially around a central pore. A connexon is termed homomeric, when all six connexins are identical and heteromeric, when it is composed of different connexins. Many types of heteromeric connexons are possible, which differ in either the number, or the spatial organization, of different connexins. A gap junction channel is formed by the head-to-head interaction of two connexons in the extracellular space.

they adjust the synaptic gain at photoreceptor-bipolar synapses (reviewed in Wu, 1994).

In contrast to the extensive knowledge of the morphology and dynamic regulation of horizontal cell gap junctions, information on the characteristics, molecular identity and cellular localization of the gap junctional channel forming proteins (i.e. connexins) is sparse, and studies in this field are just getting into the limelight of retinal research.

Moreover, the efforts towards analyzing the molecular composition of horizontal cell gap junctions is proving to be more complex than previously thought, because the selective nature of horizontal cell coupling, and its differential modifiability by neuromodulators and second messengers, suggests that multiple types of connexins are expressed in the different horizontal cell subtypes and might even exhibit distinct distribution patterns within each cell.

A break through in this field came with the introduction of an isolated cell preparation of retinal cells. John Dowling's group had developed a method to separate and accumulate horizontal cells by means of gravity sedimentation on a Ficoll gradient (Van Buskirk and Dowling, 1981). Pairs of solitary fish horizontal cells and the dual whole-cell patch-clamp technique has been used to study the biophysical properties of single horizontal cell gap junctional channels and hemichannels. These studies provided the first indications in regard to the molecular composition of horizontal cell gap junction channels. Recent progress has been made on the identification of horizontal cell connexins now by using a combination of different techniques, including immunobiochemistry (e.g. Western blotting, immunocytochemistry and immunoelectron microscopy), reverse transcriptase polymerase chain reaction (RT-PCR) with degenerate primers and molecular cloning.

This chapter reviews selected aspects of gap junctions in horizontal cells and summarizes recent data on the molecular identity of connexins expressed in horizontal cells.

Molecular characteristics of gap junctions

Gap junctions were originally characterized as a close apposition separated only by a 2–4 nm gap of the plasma membranes of two neighbouring cells. They have a characteristic septalaminar appearance when viewed under the electron microscope, and consist of clustered channels (hexagons) whose unique design allows a direct intercellular exchange of small ions and molecules, thus giving rise to electrical and metabolic coupling, respectively (reviewed in Bruzzone et al., 1996).

Gap junction channels posses a unique structure (Fig. 1A). They span the plasma membrane of two adjacent cells with each cell contributing one half of the channel, the so-called connexon or hemichannel. Like other membrane channels, gap junction channels are oligomeric assemblies of integral membrane proteins, i.e. connexins. However, these intercellular channels are more complex than oligomeric channels, because connexons, which are composed of six connexins delineating a central pore, contain either a single type of connexin (homomeric) or different connexins (heteromeric) (Fig. 1A). Connexins exhibit a characteristic folded topology with four transmembrane domains, two extracellular loops (E1 and E2) and three cytoplasmic regions (Fig. 1B). The cytoplasmic loop and the carboxy-terminal tail account for most of the differences in connexin molecular size and show the greatest diversity in sequence. In comparison, the transmembrane domains and the two extracellular loops are most highly conserved among the connexin family members.

Gap junction channels require the contribution of two connexons, one from each cell, which can be

---

The interaction of two homomeric connexons yields a homotypic channel with 12 identical connexin proteins. A heterotypic channel is formed by the interaction of two homomeric connexons, each of which is composed of another connexin, and heteromeric channels result from the association of a heteromeric connexon with either a homomeric connexon, or another heteromeric connexon. **B:** Topology of carpCx43 predicted from amino acid sequence alignment with rat Cx43, the topology of which has been verified by hydropathy plots. The four membrane-spanning regions (M1–M4), two extracellular loops (E1 and E2) with the characteristically spaced cysteine (C) residues and the cytoplasmic domains, the amino-terminal (NT) and carboxy-terminal (CT) tails and the cytoplasmic loop (CL) are indicated, together with the putative PKA- and PKC-phosphorylation sites (arrows). The different length of the CL and CT sequences contribute to the variations in the molecular mass among connexins.

either identical or different, thus forming homotypic or heterotypic intercellular channels. Finally, a remarkable variety of heteromeric channels can be constructed from the interaction of a heteromeric connexon with either another heteromeric connexon or a homomeric connexon (Fig. 1A). Thus, with the more than 20 known connexin genes and each connexin possessing distinct physiological properties, the number of physiologically distinct gap junction channel types that could theoretically exist is immense (reviewed in Bruzzone et al., 1996; Simon and Goodenough, 1998).

Functional aspects and ultrastructure of horizontal cell gap junctions

Horizontal cells are second order neurons localized in the distal part of the inner nuclear layer. Their dendrites extend laterally through the outer plexiform layer where they make contacts with synaptic pedicles of cones and spherules of rods within their dendritic field.

Morphology, subtypes and connectivity of horizontal cells vary considerably from one species to another, with individual subtypes exclusively connected to cones or rods, or to a mixture of both (reviewed in Stell et al., 1982; Boycott, 1988). In the teleost retina, four distinct types of horizontal cells have been identified, three of which are connected exclusively to cones (H1–H3) and one type (H4) to rods (reviewed in Stell et al., 1982). In comparison, most mammalian retinas have only two types, termed A-type and B-type horizontal cells, both of which are exclusively connected to cones at their dendrites (Kolb, 1974; Dacheux and Raviola, 1982; Boycott, 1988). One type, the B-type horizontal cells bear a thin axon ending in an extensive terminal arborizations with terminals exclusively connected to rods, serving as a kind of "rod horizontal cell" in the mammalian retina (Nelson, 1977; Dacheux and Raviola, 1982).

Most types of horizontal cells exhibit receptive fields that are significantly larger than their dendritic fields, as revealed in studies which measure light-evoked potentials in single horizontal cells of the intact retina. The large receptive fields have been attributed to electrical coupling at gap junctions,

which thereby permit the formation of vertically separated syncytiums and the transmission of visual information across large areas of the retina (reviewed in Hankins, 1995).

Progress has been made in the analysis of the coupling of horizontal cells using connexon-permeant fluorescent dyes (Procion Yellow and Lucifer Yellow) and small biotynilated tracers (biocytin and Neurobiotin). Both, dye and tracer coupling have demonstrated functional cytoplasmic continuity between adjacent cells via gap junctions and revealed a semiquantitative index of cell coupling by comparing the diffusion of dye/tracer from cell to cell. At present, the combination of the dye-/tracer-coupling techniques with the electrophysiological measurement of receptive-field size is regarded as a reliable approach to monitor intercellular coupling (reviewed in Vaney, 1994, 1996).

Since Kaneko (1971) first demonstrated dye coupling between horizontal cells, numerous studies performed in a variety of vertebrate retinas have shown that each functional horizontal cell subtype is similarly homologously coupled. Even the axon terminals of horizontal cells exhibit homologous coupling. In addition, these studies have shown that the size of the receptive field, and the number of cells showing dye/tracer coupling in such a network, vary among horizontal cell subtypes and between species (reviewed in Vaney 1994, 1996). For example, in the teleost retina all types of horizontal cells (H1–H4) have large receptive fields in the range of 3–4 mm in diameter, but only the cone horizontal cells (H1–H3) show significant spread of Lucifer Yellow or biocytin (Teranishi and Negishi, 1994) and have gap junctions that can be identified by electron microscopy (Witkovsky and Dowling, 1969).

With regard to the molecular characteristics of gap junctions and the gap junction channel forming proteins (see section above), the variations in receptive-field size and tracer coupling among horizontal cell subtypes are thought to reflect differences in (i) the extent of coupling, which is regulated by the size of the homologous gap junctions formed between the cells, and (ii) the biophysical properties of the gap junction channels, which are determined by the molecular composition of the channels.

The presence and different phenotypes of gap junctions between the different types of horizontal

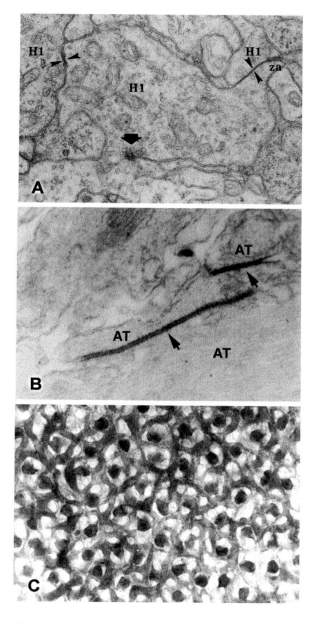

Fig. 2. Horizontal cell gap junctions in the turtle retina. **A:** Gap junctions between dendrites of H1 horizontal cells (arrow heads). A zonula adherens (za) is associated with the gap junction on the right-hand side. ×42,000. **B:** Gap junctions (arrows) between axon terminal processes (AT). The gap junctions reveal the characteristic septalaminar structure, are immunolabeled with anti-Cx26 and have no specializations on either cytoplasmic side. ×33,000. **C:** Photomicrograph of tracer-coupled axon terminals and cell bodies of H1 horizontal cells labeled following injection of Neurobiotin into a single axon terminal. It is proposed that the somata were labeled following retrograde transport of Neurobiotin down the axons.

cells have been confirmed in numerous ultrastructural and freeze-fracture studies. These support the notion that different and even multiple connexins might be expressed in the different types of horizontal cells. In all species, gap junctions appear to be quite numerous among the distinct subtypes of horizontal cells, and show variations in size and appearance, according to their location within the cellular compartments, e.g. dendrites (Fig. 2A), axon terminal (Fig. 2B) or perikaryon (Raviola and Gilula, 1975; Kolb, 1977; Witkovsky et al., 1983; Kolb and Jones, 1984; Baldridge et al., 1989).

The expression of at least two different connexins in one cell type might also be the basis for the different gap junctions and coupling patterns observed between the perikarya and between the axon terminals of horizontal cells in the turtle retina. The perikarya of H1 horizontal cells show a relative weak dye coupling compared to their axon terminals. This different coupling pattern is not only reflected in the size of the receptive field measured for H1 cell bodies and axon terminals (Piccolino et al., 1982), respectively, but also in the different size and phenotypes of their gap junctions. Whereas, gap junctions between perikarya and dendrites of turtle H1 cells are small (0.02–0.07 μm^2) and accompanied by a distinct zonula adherens and clusters of vesicles on both sides of the membrane, neighbouring axon terminal processes make the largest gap junctions (0.1–1 μm^2) that have been observed in the turtle retina, and they lack the associated zonula adherens (Witkovsky et al., 1983; Kolb and Jones, 1984). The notion that turtle H1 horizontal cells express at least two different connexins is further supported by the fact that their dendrites and axon terminals are not coupled to each other, although they intermingle in the outer plexiform layer (Witkovsky et al., 1983; Kolb and Jones, 1984). In this case the connexins forming connexons within the membrane of axon terminals must be different from and incompatible with the connexins assembled into connexons in the membrane of the dendrites and cell bodies. Thereby, two functional independent networks can develop (Fig. 2C).

Axon terminals and dendrites of H1 cells intermingle in the outer plexiform layer (in focus) without making gap junctions with each other. See text for details. (A: refigured from Kolb and Jones, 1984; C: provided by J Ammermüller).

Modulation of horizontal cell gap junctions

An important physiological factor affecting horizontal cell coupling is the state of light adaptation. Several studies in different vertebrate retinas have shown that the receptive-field sizes of horizontal cells decreases in response to an increase of the ambient illumination, consistent with increased gap-junctional resistance and uncoupling of the cells (Baldridge and Ball, 1991; Xin and Bloomfield, 1999). In contrast, studies on teleost horizontal cells have indicated that prolonged darkness reduces the receptive-field size of the cells and their dye coupling (Mangel and Dowling, 1985; Tornqvist et al., 1988). To reconcile this contrast, Baldridge and Ball (1991) suggested a triphasic relationship between the adaptational state of the retina and the degree of horizontal cell coupling. Their model proposes that horizontal cells are coupled maximally under dim, scotopic illumination and that exposure to brighter ambient illumination as well as further dark adaptation will induce uncoupling of the cells. This model has been confirmed by a dye coupling study in the goldfish retina (Wear and Baldridge, 2000) and by a recent study in the rabbit retina, which has shown that the coupling between A-type horizontal cells and between B-type horizontal cells is weak under dark-adapted as well as light-adapted conditions, whereas dim background illumination, within a log unit of rod threshold, leads to dramatic increases in coupling (Xin and Bloomfield, 1999).

A likely candidate that controls horizontal cell coupling is the neuromodulator dopamine. In different vertebrate retinas, the application of dopamine narrows the receptive field of horizontal cells and reduces the spread of Lucifer Yellow or Neurobiotin among them, indicating that dopamine is of functional importance for the regulation of the horizontal cell network (reviewed in Witkovsky and Dearry, 1992; Dowling, 1994; Weiler et al., 2000a). Dopamine levels in the retina are known to vary with changes in the ambient light conditions. However, there has been a controversy about the dark–light adaptational state resulting in an increase of endogenous dopamine levels and the subsequent uncoupling of horizontal cells. A number of studies in the teleost retina performed in John Dowling's lab have suggested that prolonged darkness leads to the uncoupling of cone horizontal cells and that this effect is mediated by an increase in dopamine release (Mangel and Dowling, 1985; Tornqvist et al., 1988; reviewed in Dowling, 1994). In contrast, several other studies have shown that both dopamine synthesis and release are stimulated by light. Taken together, the data supporting the functional role of dopamine as a light mediating signal predominates (reviewed in Witkovsky and Dearry, 1992). However, these differences might be species dependent and dopamine cell-morphology dependent. In teleosts the dopamine cell is an interplexiform cell. In mammals the dopamine cell is an amacrine cell.

In all species so far studied, the uncoupling effect of dopamine on horizontal cells was shown to be mediated by D1 dopamine receptors and to involve the activation of the cyclic adenosine $3',5'$-monophosphate (cAMP)-cascade, most likely leading to the protein kinase A (PKA) mediated phosphorylation of a gap junction channel protein. Thus, dopamine regulates the open probability of single gap junction channels and reduces both the duration and frequency of channel openings (McMahon and Brown, 1994). This results in an impaired electrical coupling between pairs of horizontal cells (Lasater and Dowling, 1985; McMahon et al., 1989; McMahon and Brown, 1994), and the reduction of receptive-field sizes and dye coupling among horizontal cells in the intact retina (reviewed in Hankins, 1995; Baldridge et al., 1998; Weiler et al., 2000a).

Dopamine released in a light-dependent manner may not be the only endogenous modulator affecting horizontal cell coupling, though Baldridge and Ball (1991) reported that background illumination decreases horizontal cell receptive-field size in both normal and 6-hydoxydopamine-lesioned goldfish retinas. The search for another modulator released in the retina during light adaptation has recently implicated retinoic acid (RA). RA is a light-correlated byproduct of the phototransduction cycle and has multiple effects in the retina, including the modulation of horizontal cell coupling. Application of RA to a dark-adapted retina reduces the receptive-field size of horizontal cell somata and impairs dye coupling among them in both fish and mammalian retina. However, coupled axon terminals of fish horizontal cells are not affected by RA, indicating that gap junctions between cell bodies and between axon terminals of cone horizontal cells are composed of different connexins. Moreover, the RA-effect on horizontal cell coupling appears to be dopamine-independent (reviewed in Weiler et al., 2000a).

Most recent studies on coupled horizontal cell pairs isolated from the zebrafish retina have confirmed the uncoupling effect of RA, and demonstrated that RA reduces the open probability of single gap junction channels by only affecting the channel opening frequency (Zhang et al., 2000). Changes in intracellular pH and Ca^{2+}-concentrations do not appear to be involved. Thus, it is possible that retinoic acid either binds directly to the gap junction channel forming proteins, thereby inducing a change in their conformation and affecting channel open frequency, or it exerts its effects via a yet unknown second messenger system.

Another important neurotransmitter affecting horizontal cell coupling is nitric oxide (NO). Nitric oxide is liberated in the L-arginine/L-citrulline metabolic pathway. It activates soluble guanylate cyclase, leading to an increase of cyclic guanosine $3',5'$-monophosphate (cGMP). The nitric oxide producing synthase (NADPH diaphorase) has been localized in several types of retinal neurons, including horizontal cells (Weiler and Kewitz, 1993; reviewed in Goldstein et al., 1996). Studies on both the intact horizontal cell network and isolated pairs of horizontal cells have shown that an increase of the intracellular level of nitric oxide or cGMP significantly affects horizontal cell coupling by increasing gap junction resistance and decreasing receptive-field size, dye coupling and electrical coupling (McMahon, 1994; Pottek et al., 1997). Complementary single-channel recordings performed on hybrid bass horizontal cell pairs demonstrated that the application of the NO donor sodium nitroprusside (SNP), or of cGMP decreases horizontal cell coupling by reducing the frequency of channel openings (Lu and McMahon, 1997). Furthermore, horizontal cell coupling appears to be modulated by intracellular acidification (Negishi et al., 1985), by arachidonic acid (Miyachi et al., 1994) and by transjunctional voltage (Lu and McMahon, 1996).

What is the molecular composition of horizontal cell gap junction channels?

Several connexins have been described in the vertebrate retina at the mRNA level, including Cx43, Cx32, Cx26 and all members of the new γ-class of connexins (i.e. fish Cx34.7, fish Cx35 and its mammalian homologue Cx36). The mRNA level of the three γ-connexins is quite high in the retina (O'Brien et al., 1998; Condorelli et al., 1998). The Cx35 and Cx36 connexins do not appear to be expressed in horizontal cells of the fish and mammalian retina, though. Immunocytochemical labeling in hybrid bass retina showed Cx35 to be present only in the dendrites and axon terminals of bipolar cells and throughout much of the inner plexiform and ganglion cell layers (O'Brien et al., 1998). Using an anti-Cx36 antibody, Weiler et al. (2000b) have observed a Cx36 distribution pattern in AII amacrine processes in the inner plexiform layers of the rat and mouse retina.

The new zebrafish connexins

Three new members of the connexin family, termed zfCx27.5, zfCx44.2 and zfCx55.5, have been cloned from a zebrafish retinal cDNA library (Dermietzel et al., 2000). The multiple alignment of the predicted amino acid sequences of the three zebrafish connexins with a number of mammalian connexins revealed a remarkable conservation of amino acids in the transmembrane domains and both extracellular loops (Fig. 1B, E1 and E2), indicating that the new zebrafish connexins posses the conventional connexin structure. However, the cytoplasmic hinge regions and the carboxy-terminal tails, both of which determine the specificity of a connexin protein, were least well conserved.

Although zfCx27.5 showed a homology score of about 80% with rat Cx26, Dermietzel et al. (2000) assumed that it does not represent the fish ortholog of the mammalian Cx26, because substantial differences occur in the cytoplasmic loop and the carboxy-terminal domain. Moreover, both channels exhibit different channel properties. In contrast to Cx26 channels which display weak voltage sensitivity and unitary conductance of 120–140 pS, unitary conductance of zfCx27.5 channels is in the range of 60 pS and they exhibit a moderate voltage sensitivity. Northern blots and multiple tissue RT-PCR revealed a low level expression of zFCx27.5 mRNA in retina and brain. But at present there are no data available about the cellular distribution of this connexin, because in situ hybridization has failed as yet and an antibody is not available. Nevertheless, according to the biophysical properties of zfCx27.5 channels, it is tempting to speculate that this connexin may be a component of gap junction channels between cone-driven horizontal cells in the teleost retina, because they exhibit a similar unitary conductance of 50–60 pS (McMahon and Brown, 1994; Lu and McMahon, 1996).

The most interesting candidate among the new zebrafish connexins is zfCx55.5 (Dermietzel et al., 2000). This connexin shows a lower degree of amino acid sequence homology to other vertebrate connexins and is exclusively expressed in the retina. Expressing zfCx55.5 in N2A cells produces channels with a unitary conductance of ∼50 pS, which is similar to that recently described for Cx57 (Manthey et al., 1999). The macroscopic voltage sensitivity of zfCx55.5 channels is unique, because they open in response to voltage steps of either polarity. This property makes homomeric zfCx55.5 connexons an ideal partner for the construction of heterotypic polarized or rectifying electrical synapses (Dermietzel et al., 2000). In the teleost retina zfCx55.5 is expressed in a distinct population of horizontal cells. According to their location in the distal part of the inner nuclear layer, these zfCx55.5 positive horizontal cells are likely to be H4 horizontal cells.

Connexin43: a candidate for dendro-dendritic gap junctions between teleost horizontal cells?

Since the connexins forming a gap junction channel determine its biophysical (i.e. permeability, ionic selectivity and unitary conductance) and gating properties, the electrophysiological analysis of these properties is regarded as a useful tool to characterize and identify a yet unknown connexin protein (Spray, 1996).

McMahon et al. (1989) were the first who analyzed the functional properties of individual gap junction channels between pairs of poorly coupled cone-driven horizontal cells of the white perch retina. They identified channels with a unitary conductance of 50–60 pS which exhibit relatively long open times of several tens of milliseconds. The unitary conductance of these channels was not significantly affected by dopamine. But, dopamine reduced the open probability of the channels by decreasing both the open duration and the open frequency. Similar results have been obtained in two different zebrafish retinas (*Brachydanio rerio*, McMahon and Brown, 1994 and *Danio aquipinatus*, McMahon and Mattson, 1996). In both teleosts, the unitary conductance of horizontal cell gap-junction channels was about 50 pS, and dopamine revealed the same effects on their gating properties (e.g. reducing the open duration and open frequency of channel openings).

The unitary conductance of gap junction channels of teleost horizontal cells is most similar to that of channels formed by mammalian Cx43 (reviewed in Spray, 1996), suggesting that they are composed of a homologue of the mammalian Cx43. Support for this notion has been provided by recent studies. Using Western blotting, in vitro phosphorylation and immunoprecipitation Janssen-Bienhold et al. (1998a,b) have demonstrated that a homologue of rat Cx43 is indeed expressed in the carp retina (Fig. 3A), and provable in samples of isolated and enriched horizontal cell fractions (Fig. 3B). Dopamine (200 µM), 8-bromo-cAMP (1 mM) and forskolin (100 µM) had significant effects on the endogenous phosphorylation of horizontal cell proteins of 43–46 kD. Cx43 isolated from membranes of the carp retina appeared to be a dominant target for PKA-mediated phosphorylation. Thus, it is plausible that dopamine might exert its effects on horizontal cell coupling via the PKA-mediated phosphorylation of Cx43, a conclusion that is consistent with electrophysiological data (Lasater and Dowling, 1985; McMahon et al., 1989).

A consensus sequence for PKA-mediated phosphorylation is present in the carboxy-terminal region (aa 343–346) of the carp homologue of Cx43 (Fig. 1B), the cDNA of which has been cloned recently and predicts a protein with a molecular mass of 43,277 dalton (Dermietzel et al., 2000). For the analysis of the biophysical properties of carpCx43 channels, cRNA for carpCx43 was

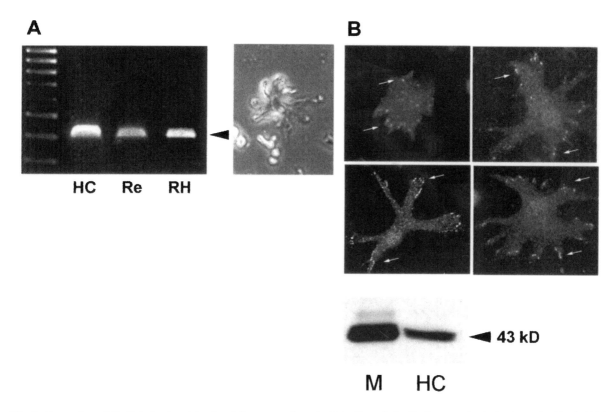

Fig. 3. Expression of Cx43 in horizontal cells of the carp retina. **A:** Detection of the Cx43 transcript in horizontal cells. A 414 bp transcript was amplified from cDNA derived from a single horizontal cell (HC, shown in the right panel), the whole carp retina (Re) or rat heart (RH, positive control). Each horizontal cell was photographed before its cytoplasm was aspirated and used for single cell RT-PCR. An ethidiumbromide stained 2% agarose gel is shown and the 414 bp transcript is indicated by an arrowhead. **B:** Immunolocalization of Cx43 in different types of horizontal cells (upper panel). Cx43 is more restricted to patches in the membrane of horizontal cell dendrites (arrows), indicating that it may be a component of dendro-dendritic gap junctions. On Western blots (lower panel) Cx43 immunoreactive proteins ($\leftarrow$43 kD) are present in samples of retinal membranes (M) and enriched horizontal cell fractions (HC).

injected into oocytes. The protein was efficiently assembled into homotypic channels which did not show significant differences in their biophysical properties from rat Cx43 channels (Dermietzel et al., 2000).

In an attempt to identify the cellular distribution of Cx43 expression in the retina, in situ hybridization studies have been performed on sections of the carp retina with a carpCx43 cRNA (Dermietzel et al., 2000). These studies revealed a prominent expression in the inner nuclear layer and the ganglion cell layer. But, they did not provide unequivocal evidence for the expression of Cx43 in horizontal cells.

We decided to use a multiple approach, including single-cell RT-PCR, in situ hybridization

and immunocytochemistry to look for the specific localization of Cx43.

RT-PCR with carpCx43 specific primers and cDNA derived from single horizontal cells resulted in the amplification of cDNA fragments of the expected size (414 bp, Fig. 3A, HC). Since, a product of the same size was amplified from carp retinal cDNA (Fig. 3A, Re) and a control cDNA derived from rat heart (Fig. 3A, RH), we suggest that horizontal cells of the carp express the ortholog of rat Cx43 (see section above). The expression of Cx43 mRNA in horizontal cells was confirmed by in situ hybridization, using a carpCx43 cRNA anti-sense probe and isolated plated horizontal cells. Cx43 mRNA was localized in a characteristic pattern around the nucleus, which was not observed in horizontal cells probed with the carpCx43 sense-probe (Janssen-Bienhold and Hoppenstedt, unpublished observations).

Although we have not yet verified the localization and distribution of Cx43-immunoreactivity in the outer plexiform layer by immunoelectron microscopy, the pattern of Cx43 immunolabeling, in the dendrites and dendritic tips of isolated horizontal cells, suggests that Cx43 might be a component of dendro-dendritic gap junction channels (Fig. 3B, arrows). In addition, we have seen Cx43-immunoreactivity in the distal outer plexiform layer beneath the photoreceptor terminals where dendro-dendritic gap junctions of horizontal cells occur (Raviola and Gilula, 1975; Witkovsky et al., 1983; Kolb and Jones, 1984).

Connexin26 in horizontal cells of the vertebrate retina

Connexin26 is a unique member among the more than 20 members of the connexin protein family, because it is apparently not a phosphoprotein in vivo and has no pronounced voltage dependence. Cx26 expressed in oocytes forms channels with unitary conductance of about 50–70 pS (Spray et al., 1994), which is in the range of conductance values obtained for Cx43 under phosphorylating conditions and for single channels between teleost horizontal cells (50–60 pS, see section above). Moreover, Cx26 is thought to be involved in neuronal plasticity, because its expression is transiently increased during synaptogenesis and circuit formation in the developing neocortex of the rat (Nadarajah et al., 1997). We therefore hypothesized that Cx26 might be one of the connexins expressed in teleost horizontal cells, because of these neurons neuronal plasticity, in their light-dependent modulation of both their gap junctions (see section above) and their synapses with cone photoreceptors (reviewed by Wagner and Djamgoz, 1993).

Again we used a multiple approach, including fluorescence immunocytochemistry, immunoelectron microscopy, Western blotting and single-cell RT-PCR, to analyze whether Cx26 is expressed in horizontal cells of the carp retina or not.

RT-PCR with cDNA, derived from single horizontal cells, carp retina and mouse liver (positive control), and a specific combination of primers resulted in the amplification of cDNA fragments of the expected size of 248 bp (Fig. 4A). The fragments amplified from horizontal cell cDNAs were purified, subcloned in a plasmid vector and sequenced. Sequence analysis revealed the highest homology of all analyzed horizontal cell Cx26-fragments to rat and mouse Cx26 (98% identities at the amino acid level). Thus, horizontal cells express a homologue of mammalian Cx26 (Janssen-Bienhold et al., 2000, 2001). The expression of Cx26 in horizontal cells was confirmed by Western blotting. Immunofluorescence microscopy revealed a prominent localization of Cx26-immunoreactivity in the outer plexiform layer and in isolated cells. By electron microscopy we showed the presence of Cx26-immunoreactivity in the membrane of the invaginating dendrites of horizontal cells (Fig. 4B, asterisks). There was no septalaminar structure, typical of gap junctions, between the photoreceptors and horizontal cells, and no Cx26 labeling was found at the photoreceptor membrane (Fig. 4B, right), suggesting that Cx26 forms hemichannels instead in the membrane of the dendritic tips of horizontal cells.

Functioning and modifiable hemichannels were shown to be present in the surface membrane of isolated horizontal cells of the catfish retina (DeVries and Schwartz, 1992) and skate retina (Malchow et al., 1993). But, the conductance of these hemichannels is voltage-dependent and can be modulated by distinct mechanisms, such as protons and cyclic nucleotides (e.g. cAMP and cGMP; DeVries and Schwartz, 1992). This suggests that the connexins may be modulated by PKA-mediated phosphorylation, so, it is unlikely that these hemichannels are composed of Cx26. Based on the physiological data and the restricted localization of Cx26 within the membrane of the terminal dendrites of horizontal cells, it seems that teleost horizontal cells express at least two different types of hemichannel-forming connexins, in soma and dendrites. The functional importance of these hemichannels is not yet clear. But, recent studies by Fahrenfort et al. (2000) indicates that the gap-junction channel blocker, carbenoxolone (100 µM), blocks the feedback pathway from horizontal cells to cones. Based on the

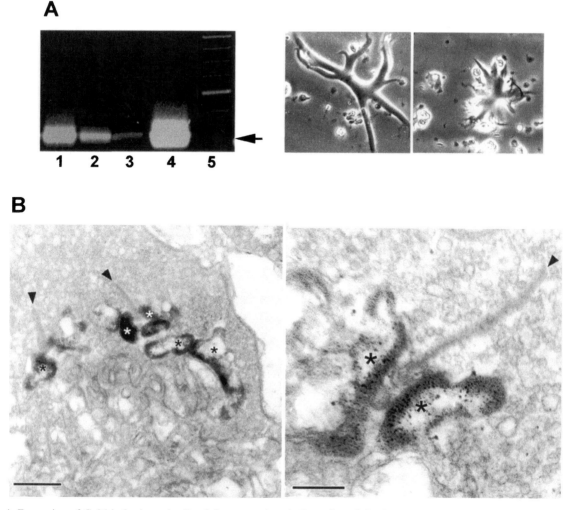

Fig. 4. Expression of Cx26 in horizontal cells of the carp retina. **A:** Detection of the Cx26 transcript in horizontal cells. A 248 bp transcript was amplified from cDNA derived from single horizontal cells (lanes 1 and 2, left-hand panel; the corresponding cells are shown in the right-hand panel), the whole carp retina (lane 3, left-hand panel) or mouse liver (lane 4, positive control, left-hand panel). A sample of a 1000 bp ladder was separated in lane 5. Each horizontal cell was photographed (right-hand panel) before its cytoplasm was aspirated and used for single cell RT-PCR. An ethidiumbromide stained 2% agarose gel is shown and the 248 bp transcript is indicated by an arrow. **B:** Electron micrographs showing prominent Cx26-immunolabeling of the lateral dendrites of horizontal cells (asterisks) invaginating the terminals of the cone photoreceptors. Note the restricted localization of Cx26 to the membrane region of horizontal cell dendrites and the absence of a gap junction characteristic septalaminar membrane arrangement at the corresponding location (right-hand panel). Scale bars: 1 μm (left-hand panel); 0.25 μm (right-hand panel).

presence of Cx26-hemichannels at the tips of the terminal dendrites of teleost horizontal cells, Kamermans (personal communication) proposed an involvement of these hemichannels in the feedback mechanism. Support for this idea comes from a recent immuno-electron-microscopical study performed on the turtle retina. Again Cx26-immunoreactivity is localized at the membrane of the terminal dendrites of horizontal cells deep within the photoreceptor-horizontal cell synaptic complex (Fig. 5A). The labeling is not as prominent as that in teleost horizontal cell dendrites (compare Figs. 5A and 4B right), but it is also restricted to the horizontal cell membrane facing the synaptic ribbon of the

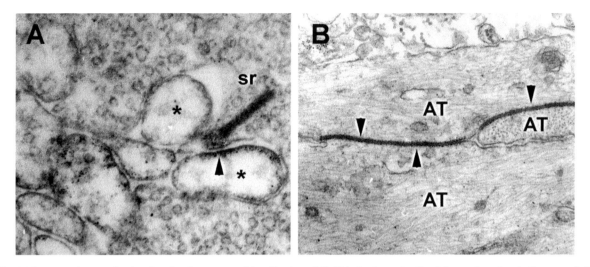

Fig. 5. Electron micrographs showing the ultrastructural localization of Cx26 in horizontal cells of the turtle retina **A:** Punctate Cx26-immunoreactivity is present in the membrane region of the lateral dendrites of horizontal cells (asterisks) adjacent to the membrane of the cone photoreceptors within the photoreceptor-horizontal cell synaptic complex (arrowhead). There is no septalaminar membrane structure at this location and no Cx26-immunolabeling at the photoreceptor membrane. **B:** Cx26-immunolabeling of gap junctions (arrowheads) between axon terminals (AT) of H1 horizontal cells. Note the parallel arrays of neurofilaments in the cytoplasm of two processes (left-hand side).

cone, and indicative of the presence of hemichannels at this location. However, despite these very promising hints, further physiological studies will be needed to see whether hemi-gap junction channels are involved in the feedback mechanism between horizontal cells and photoreceptors.

In the turtle retina Cx26-immunoreactivity is also localized at the membranes of the large gap junctions between axon terminals of H1 horizontal cells (Fig. 5B). In this case, punctate labeling appears on both sides of the gap junction, suggesting that Cx26 is one of the components. We cannot yet decide whether the gap junctions between the axon terminals are exclusively composed of homotypic Cx26-channels, because we have also seen Cx32-immunoreactivity at these gap junctions (Hoppenstedt et al., 2000). However, since the Cx32-antibody used in this study was generated in sheep against the whole Cx32 protein isolated from rat liver, and overall homology of rat Cx32 with rat Cx26 is relatively high (64%), it is conceivable that the Cx32-antibody we used also recognizes Cx26. It is also possible that the axon terminal gap junctions possess both homotypic Cx26-and Cx32-channels, heterotypic Cx26/Cx32-channels and/or heteromeric Cx26/Cx32-channels, respectively, but this has to be verified in future

studies. Taken together, it seems that horizontal cells of the teleost and turtle retina express Cx26, which most likely is not only a component of complete gap junction channels mediating homologous coupling, but also a component of hemichannels that are possibly involved in the feedback pathway from horizontal cells to cones.

Concluding remarks

The plasticity and flexibility of gap junctional coupling between horizontal cells is of physiological importance for the retina and provides it with the potential to optimize vision for ambient light conditions. This plasticity exists at two levels, that of the channel conductance which is mediated by rapid responses to changes in neuronal activity and that of connexin expression which affects longterm changes in the extent of coupling.

Research in John Dowling's lab, and the ongoing work in many groups of his former students and collaborators has contributed remarkably towards our knowledge and understanding of the regulation and modulation of gap junctional coupling among horizontal cells. John and his coworkers have pioneered the electrophysiological analysis of gap-junctional coupling of horizontal cells and, moreover, with their measurement of a single gap-junction channel conductance in 1989 (McMahon et al.,) have provided the first hints for the identity of one of the connexins (Cx43) possibly expressed in cone-driven horizontal cells of the teleost retina. Using a combination of different techniques our group has recently confirmed the expression of Cx43 in teleost horizontal cells and has identified Cx26 as a further connexin expressed in and located at distinct sites of horizontal cells of the teleost and turtle retina. Taken together the success of the previous and recent studies is very promising, and it is hopeful that the different connexins forming gap-junction channels between the subtypes of horizontal cells of the vertebrate retina will soon all be identified.

Acknowledgments

This research was supported by a grant from the Deutsche Forschungsgemeinschaft to U.J.-B. and R.W. and from the German-Israel-Foundation to R.W. We thank Dr. Helga Kolb for critical reading of the manuscript, and U.J.-B. thanks the Alexander von Humboldt Foundation for the Feodor Lynen Fellowship which enabled her to spend a wonderful creative and informative year in John Dowling's lab.

References

Baldridge, W.H., Ball, A.K. and Miller, R.G. (1989) Gap junction particle density of horizontal cells in goldfish retinas lesioned with 6-OHDA. *J. Comp. Neurol.*, 287: 238–246.

Baldridge, W.H. and Ball, A.K. (1991) Background illumination reduces horizontal cell receptive-field size in both normal and 6-hydroxydopamine-lesioned goldfish retinas. *Vis. Neurosci.*, 7: 441–450.

Baldridge, W.H., Vaney, D.I. and Weiler, R. (1998) The modulation of intercellular coupling in the retina. *Cell and Dev. Biol.*, 9: 311–318.

Boycott, B.B. (1988) Horizontal cells of mammalian retinae. *Neurosci. Res.*, (Suppl. 8): S97–S111.

Bruzzone, R., White, T.W. and Paul, D.L. (1996) Connections with connexins: the molecular basis of direct intercellular signaling. *Eur. J. Biochem.*, 238: 1–27.

Condorelli, D.F., Parenti, R., Spinella, F., Trovato Salinario, A., Belluardo, N., Cardile, V. and Cicirata, F. (1998) Cloning of a new gap junction gene (Cx36) highly expressed in mammalian brain neurons. *Eur. J. Neurosci.*, 10: 1202–1208.

Cook, J.E. and Becker, D.L. (1995) Gap junctions in the vertebrate retina. *Microscopy Res. Techn.*, 31: 408–419.

Dacheux, R.F. and Raviola, E. (1982) Horizontal cells in the retina of the rabbit. *J. Neurosci.*, 2: 1486–1493.

Dermietzel, R., Kremer, M., Paputsoglou, G., Stang, A., Zoidl, G., Meier, M., Janssen-Bienhold, U., Weiler, R., Nicholson, B., Bruzzone, R. and Spray, D. (2000) Molecular and functional diversity of neural connexins in the retina. *J. Neurosci.*, 20: 8331–8343.

DeVries, S.H. and Schwartz, E.A. (1992) Hemi-gap junction channels in solitary horizontal cells of the catfish retina. *J. Physiol.*, 445: 201–230.

Dowling, J.E. (1994) The neuromodulatory role of dopamine in the teleost retina. In: Niznik, H.B. (Ed.), *Dopamine Receptors and Transporters. Pharmacology, Structure and Function.* Marcel Dekker Inc., New York, pp. 337–357.

Fahrenfort, I., Sjoerdsma, T. and Kamermans, M. (2000) Low concentrations of cobalt block negative feedback from HCs to cones, using non-GABAergic pathway. *Invest. Ophthalmol. Vis. Sci.*, 41: 943.

Goldstein, I.M., Ostwald, P. and Roth, S. (1996) Nitric oxide: a review of its role in retinal function and disease. *Vis. Res.*, 36: 2979–2994.

Goodenough, D.A. and Revel, J.P. (1970) A fine structural analysis of intercellular junctions in the mouse liver. *J. Cell Biol.*, 45: 272–290.

Hankins, M.W. (1995) Horizontal cell coupling and its regulation. In Djamgoz, M.B.A., Archer, S.N. and Vallerga, S. (Eds.), *Neurobiology and Clinical Aspects of the Outer Retina.* Chapman & Hall, London, pp. 195–220.

Hoppenstedt, W., Janssen-Bienhold, U., Traub, O. and Weiler, R. (2000) Connexin expression in the turtle retina. *Zoology*, 103, (Suppl. III): 67.

Janssen-Bienhold, U., Stachowiak, U., Dermietzel, R. and Weiler, R. (1998a) Isolation of connexin43 from fish retinal membranes and its PKA-mediated phosphorylation. *Invest. Ophthalmol. Vis. Sci.*, 39: 984.

Janssen-Bienhold, U., Dermietzel, R. and Weiler, R. (1998b) Distribution of connexin43 immunoreactivity in the retinas of different vertebrates. *J. Comp. Neurol.*, 396: 310–321.

Janssen-Bienhold, U., Schultz, K., Gellhaus, A., Schmidt, P. and Weiler, R. (2000) Expression of connexin26 in horizontal cells of the fish retina. *Invest. Ophthalmol. Vis. Sci.*, 41: 941.

Janssen-Bienhold, U., Schultz, K., Gellhaus, A., Schmidt, P., Ammermüller, J. and Weiler, R. (2001) Identification and localization of connexin26 within the photoreceptor–horizontal cell synaptic complex. *Vis. Neurosci.*, in press.

Kaneko, A. (1970) Physiological and morphological identification of horizontal, bipolar and amacrine cells in goldfish retina. *J. Physiol.*, 207: 623–633.

Kaneko, A. (1971) Electrical connexions between horizontal cells in the dogfish retina. *J. Physiol.*, (Lond.), 213: 95–105.

Kolb, H. (1974) The connections between horizontal cells and photoreceptors in the retina of the cat: electron microscopy of Golgi preparations. *J. Comp. Neurol.*, 155: 1–14.

Kolb, H. (1977) The organization of the outer plexiform layer in the retina of the cat: electron microscopic observations. *J. Neurocytol.*, 6: 131–153.

Kolb, H. and Jones, J. (1984) Synaptic organization of the outer plexiform layer of the turtle retina: an electron microscopic study of serial sections. *J. Neurocytol.*, 13: 567–591.

Lasater, E.M. and Dowling, J.E. (1985) Dopamine decreases conductance of the electrical junctions between cultured retinal horizontal cells. *Proc. Natl. Acad. Sci. USA*, 82: 3025–3029.

Lu, C. and McMahon, D.G. (1996) Gap junction channel gating at bass retinal electrical synapses. *Vis. Neurosci.*, 13: 1049–1057.

Lu, C. and McMahon, D.G. (1997) Modulation of hybrid bass retinal gap junctional channel gating by nitric oxide. *J. Physiol. (Lond.)*, 499: 689–699.

Malchow, R.P., Qian, H. and Ripps, H. (1993) Evidence for hemi-gap junctional channels in isolated horizontal cells of the skate retina. *J. Neurosci. Res.*, 35: 237–245.

Mangel, S.C. and Dowling, J.E. (1985) Responsiveness and receptive field size of carp horizontal cells are reduced by prolonged darkness and dopamine. *Science*, 229: 1107–1109.

Manthey, D., Bukauskas, F., Lee, C.G., Kozak, C.A. and Willecke, K. (1999) Molecular cloning and functional expression of the mouse gap juncton gene connexin-57 in human HeLa cells. *J. Biol. Chem.*, 274: 14716–14723.

McMahon, D.G., Knapp, A.G. and Dowling, J.E. (1989) Horizontal cell gap junctions: single channel conductance and modulation by dopamine. *Proc. Natl. Acad. Sci. USA*, 86: 7639–7643.

McMahon, D.G. (1994) Modulation of electrical synaptic transmission in zebrafish retinal horizontal cells. *J. Neurosci.*, 14: 1722–1734.

McMahon, D.G. and Brown, D.R. (1994) Modulation of gap-junction channel gating at zebrafish retinal electrical synapses. *J. Neurophysiol.*, 72: 2257–2268.

McMahon, D.G. and Mattson, M.P. (1996) Horizontal cell electrical coupling in the giant danio: synaptic modulation by dopamine and synaptic maintenance by calcium. *Brain Res.*, 718: 89–96.

Miyachi, E-I., Kato, C. and Nakaki, T. (1994) Arachidonic acid blocks gap junction between retinal horizontal cells. *NeuroReport*, 5: 485–488.

Nadarajah, B., Jones, A.M., Evans, W.H. and Parnavelas, J.G. (1997) Differential expression of connexins during neocortical development and neuronal circuit formation. *J. Neurosci.*, 17: 3096–3111.

Naka, K.-I. and Rushton, W.A.H. (1967) The generation and spread of S-potentials in fish (Cyprinidae). *J. Physiol. (Lond.)*, 192: 437–461.

Negishi, K., Teranishi, T. and Kato, S. (1985) Opposite effects of ammonia and carbon dioxide on dye coupling between horizontal cells in the carp retina. *Brain Res.*, 342: 330–339.

Nelson, R. (1977) Cat cones have rod input: a comparison of the response properties of cones and horizontal cell bodies in the retina of the cat. *J. Comp. Neurol.*, 172: 109–136.

O'Brien, J., Bruzzone, R., White, T.W., Al-Ubaidi, M. and Ripps, H. (1998) Cloning and expression of two related connexins from the perch retina define a distinct subgroup of the connexin family. *J. Neurosci.*, 18: 7625–7637.

Piccolino, M., Neyton, J., Witkovsky, P. and Gerschenfeld, H.M. (1982) γ-Aminobutyric acid antagonists decrease junctional communication between L-horizontal cells of the retina. *Proc. Natl. Acad. Sci. USA*, 79: 3671–3675.

Pottek, M., Schultz, K. and Weiler, R. (1997) Effects of nitric oxide on the horizontal cell network and dopamine release in the carp retina. *Vision Res.*, 37: 1091–1102.

Raviola, E. and Gilula, N.B. (1975) Intramembrane organization of spezialized contacts in the outer plexiform layer of the retina. A freeze-fracture study in monkeys and rabbits. *J. Cell Biol.*, 65: 192–222.

Simon, A.M. and Goodenough, D.A. (1998) Diverse functions of vertebrate gap junctions. *Trends in Cell Biol.*, 8: 477–483.

Spray, D.C., Bai, S., Burk, R.D. and Saez, J.C. (1994) Regulation and function of liver gap-junctions and their genes. *Prog. Liver Dis.*, 12: 1–18.

Spray, D.C. (1996) Physiological properties of gap junction channels in the nervous system. In Spray, D.C. and Dermietzel, R. (Eds.), *Gap Junctions in the Nervous System*. RG Landis Company, Austin, Texas, pp. 39–59.

Stell, W.K., Kretz, R. and Lightfoot, D.O. (1982) Horizontal cell connectivity in goldfish. In: Drujan, B.J. and Laufer, M. (Eds.), *The S-potential*. Alan R. Liss Inc., New York, pp. 51–75.

Svaetichin, G. (1953) The cone action potential. *Acta physiol. scand.*, 29 (Suppl. 106): 565–600.

Teranishi, T. and Negishi, K. (1994) Double-staining of horizontal and amacrine cells by intracellular injection with Lucifer Yellow and biocytin in carp retina. *Neurosci.*, 59: 217–226.

Tornqvist, K., Yang, X.-L. and Dowling, J.E. (1988) Modulation of cone horizontal cell activity in the teleost fish retina. III. Effects of prolonged darkness and dopamine on electrical coupling between horizontal cells. *J. Neurosci.*, 8: 2279–2288.

Van Buskirk, R. and Dowling, J.E. (1981) Isolated horizontal cells from carp retina demonstrate dopamine-dependent accumulation of cyclic AMP. *Proc. Natl. Acad. Sci. USA*, 78: 7825–7829.

Vaney, D.I. (1994) Patterns of neuronal coupling in the retina. *Prog. Ret. Res.*, 13: 301–355.

Vaney, D.I. (1996) Cell coupling in the retina. In: Spray, D.C. and Dermietzel, R. (Eds.), *Gap Junctions in the Nervous System*. RG Landis Company, Austin, Texas, pp. 79–101.

Wagner, H.-J. and Djamgoz, M.B.A. (1993) Spinules: A case for retinal synaptic plasticity. *Trends Neurosci.*, 16: 201–206.

Wear, A. and Baldridge, W.H. (2000) Triphasic adaptation of horizontal cells in goldfish retina: A Lucifer Yellow dye coupling study. *Invest. Opthalmol. Vis. Sci.*, 41: 942.

Weiler, R. and Kewitz, B. (1993) The marker for nitric oxide synthase, NADPH-diaphorase, co-localizes with GABA in horizontal cells and cells of the inner retina in the carp retina. *Neurosci. Lett.*, 158: 151–154.

Weiler, R., Pottek, M., He, S. and Vaney, D.I. (2000a) Modulation of coupling between retinal horizontal cells by retinoic acid and endogenous dopamine. *Brain Res. Rev.*, 32: 121–129.

Weiler, R., Feigenspan, A., Teubner, B. and Willecke, K. (2000b) Cellular localization of the murine connexin Cx36 in the mammalian retina. *Invest. Ophthalmol. Vis. Sci.*, 41: 620.

Witkovsky, P. and Dowling, J.E. (1969) Synaptic relationships in the plexiform layers of carp retina. *Z. Zellforsch.*, 100: 60–82.

Witkovsky, P., Owen, W.G. and Woodworth, M. (1983) Gap junctions among the perikarya, dendrites, and axon terminals of the luminosity-type horizontal cell of the turtle retina. *J. Comp. Neurol.*, 216: 359–368.

Witkovsky, P. and Dearry, A. (1992) Functional roles of dopamine in the vertebrate retina. *Prog. Ret. Res.*, 11: 247–292.

Wu, S.M. (1994) Synaptic transmission in the outer retina. *Annu. Rev. Physiol.*, 56: 141–168.

Xin, D. and Bloomfield, S.A. (1999) Dark- and light-induced changes in coupling between horizontal cells in mammalian retina. *J. Comp. Neurol.*, 405: 75–87.

Yamada, E. and Ishikawa, T. (1965) The fine structure of the horizontal cells in some vertebrate retinas. *Cold Spring Harbor Symp. quant. Biol.*, 30: 383–392.

Zhang, D.Q., Stone, J.F. and McMahon, D.G. (2000) Modulation by retinoic acid of electrical synaptic transmission in bass retinal neurons. *Invest. Ophthalmol. Vis. Sci.*, 41: 941.

H. Kolb, H. Ripps and S. Wu (Eds.)
Progress in Brain Research, Vol. 131
© 2001 Elsevier Science B.V. All rights reserved

CHAPTER 7

Real time imaging of the production and movement of nitric oxide in the retina

William D. Eldred*

Department of Biology, Boston University, 5 Cummington Street, Boston, MA 02215, USA

Introduction

Starting in the 1980s, John Dowling was one of the original retinal researchers to investigate the role of neuromodulators in retinal function. In particular, John and his co-workers published the first seminal papers linking dopamine and the second messenger cyclic adenosine monophosphate (cAMP) to horizontal cell function (Young and Dowling, 1989; McMahon et al., 1994) and to specific neurotransmitter systems (O'Brien and Dowling, 1985; Dowling, 1994). John's original results demonstrating that second messenger systems play an important role in many retinal cell types, provided a starting point for my present research on the production and function of nitric oxide (NO) and cyclic guanosine monophosphate (cGMP) in the retina. Our current results build on his initial studies, and show that NO and cGMP may function as neuromodulators in every retinal cell type. However, there is much we do not know about NO and we have just begun to scratch the surface of establishing the role of NO in retinal processing. John Dowling was prophetic, in that second messengers and neuromodulation do form a critical part of retinal function.

In the past few years, there has been an explosion of interest in the role of NO in retinal function, development and pathology. NO represents a new

class of neuroactive substances that serves a wide variety of synaptic and non-synaptic functions that are not characteristic of traditional neurotransmitters. It is not like a classical neurotransmitter, in that it is not stored for vesicular release, but made on demand. The action of NO is not restricted to specific morphologically specialized sites and it can activate soluble guanylate cyclase (sGC) to synthesize cGMP in cells that are not connected synaptically. This cGMP can in turn activate ion channels, protein kinase G or phosphodiesterases (PDEs). NO can also have direct effects on target proteins like NMDA receptors or ADP-ribosyl transferase. This review is not intended to be an exhaustive account of NO in the retina, but it will summarize many recently discovered aspects of NO in the retina and suggest new areas for future research. For a more detailed review of the localization, function, development, biochemistry and molecular biology of the NO–cGMP signal transduction system in retina, please see Eldred (2000).

Function of NO in the retina

NO has been shown to affect the physiology of all neuronal cell types in the retina. For instance, NO increases the gain and extends the voltage range of synaptic exocytosis in cone photoreceptors (Rieke and Schwartz, 1994; Savchenko et al., 1997). In bipolar cells, NO donor produces an inward current accompanied by a rise in dim and bright flash

* Tel.: 617-353-2439; Fax: 617-353-6340; E-mail: eldred@bio.bu.edu

response amplitudes, and an increase in membrane conductance (Shiells and Falk, 1992b). A number of studies have examined the effect of NO on horizontal cells. Miyachi et al. (1990), report that injection of the NO precursor, L-arginine, into H1 luminosity-type horizontal cells in turtle retina, reduces their light responses, dramatically increases their input resistance, and decreases their response to a surround while increasing their response to stimulation of their receptive field centers. McMahon and Ponomareva (1996) report that bath application of L-arginine decreases the responses to kainate in H1 horizontal cells in a manner similar to cGMP and NO. Thus, it is likely that the H1 cells can serve as their own source and target of NO to negatively modulate their gain at photoreceptor-horizontal cell synapses. In amacrine cells, Mills and Massey (1995) conclude that by working through cGMP, the NO released by light stimulation (Koistinaho et al., 1993) decreases the rod input and increases the cone input during light adaptation by uncoupling the AII amacrine cells from the cone bipolar cells.

Wexler et al. (1998) demonstrate that NO can depress the function of $GABA_A$ receptors on amacrine cells. They conclude that NO stimulates sGC to increase cGMP levels, which then increases phosphorylation by PKG to depress GABA currents. The increased cGMP also stimulates a cGMP-activated PDE to decrease cAMP levels and protein kinase A phosphorylation. Thus, activators of adenylate cyclase, like dopamine, enhance $GABA_A$ currents, while activators of guanylate cyclase, like NO, do the opposite. Therefore, cAMP and NO–cGMP function in a push-pull mechanism in GABAergic transmission in these amacrine cells. Finally, by working through cGMP, NO modulates cyclic nucleotide gated channels by activating a NO-sensitive sGC in photoreceptors (Savchenko et al., 1997), bipolar cells (Shiells and Falk, 1992a) and ganglion cells (Ahmad et al., 1994).

Localizations of nitric oxide synthase in the retina

Historically, the first localizations of NOS in the retina were done before the identification of NOS. This is because NADPH-diaphorase histochemistry was first used over 45 years ago (Wislocki and Sidman, 1954) to selectively stain retinal neurons. Only much later (Vincent and Hope, 1992), did the NADPH-diaphorase activity become associated with NOS. In recent years, many commercial antibodies against specific NOS isoforms have become available. When all of these previous anatomical localizations of NOS are examined as a whole, neuronal NOS (nNOS) has been demonstrated in the retina of all species examined. While there are species-specific differences in localization, when all species are considered together, nNOS has been located in members of every retinal cell type. The most complete analysis of the anatomy, physiology and biochemistry of the NO–sGC–cGMP signal transduction pathways has been done in the turtle retina (Miyachi et al., 1990; Blute et al., 1997, 1998, 1999, 2000). Therefore, much of the rest of this chapter will focus on the turtle retina.

Blute et al. (1997) find both NADPH-diaphorase and NOS-like immunoreactivity (-LI) in the ellipsoids and inner segments of photoreceptors, efferents from the brain to the retina, at least three amacrine cell types and in many processes in the IPL. In optimized double-labeled preparations, all cells with NADPH-diaphorase activity also have nNOS-LI, although some somata in the ganglion cell layer only have nNOS-LI. The NADPH-diaphorase positive (ND)1 amacrine cells (Fig. 1) are relatively common. In retinal cross sections, the ND1 cells have large vertically oriented, darkly staining pyriform shaped somata with well-labeled dendritic arborizations. The ND2 amacrine cells (Fig. 2) are the most common of the three NADPH-diaphorase amacrine cell types in the turtle retina. These cells have smallish, moderately stained somata that give rise to several delicate processes, which arborize in both the outer and inner IPL. Finally, the ND3 amacrine cells (Fig. 3) have large, well stained, flattened, oval somata that often give rise to two thick, weakly labeled primary processes that arborize in the outer IPL. The ND1 and ND2 amacrine cell types in turtle are very similar to the ND1 and ND2 (Vaney and Young, 1988) or type 1 and type 2 (Sagar, 1990) NADPH-diaphorase positive amacrine cell types in the rabbit, and to the NDa and NDb NADPH-diaphorase positive amacrine cell types in the guinea pig (Cobcroft et al., 1989). With some nNOS antisera, there are large numbers of somata in the

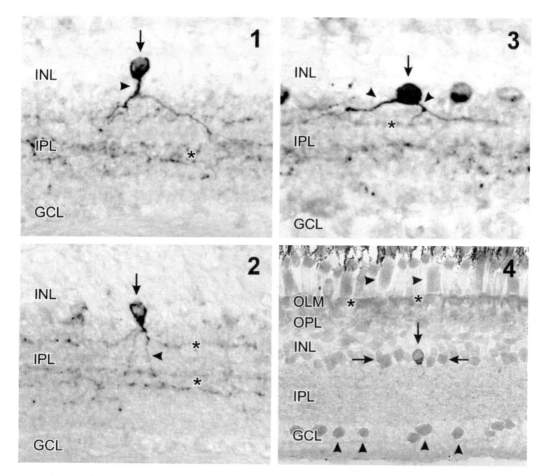

Figs. 1, 2, 3 and 4. In turtle retina, at the light microscopic level, nNOS-LI is present in at least three amacrine cell types and their processes in the IPL (Blute et al., 1997). The ND1 amacrine cells (vertical arrow, Fig. 1) with nNOS-LI, have a thick primary process (horizontal arrowhead) that branches to form processes studded with boutons in the deeper portions of the IPL (asterisk). The ND2 amacrine cells (vertical arrow, Fig. 2) have very delicate processes (arrowhead) that arborize in both the inner and outer regions of the IPL (asterisks). The ND3 amacrine cells (vertical arrow, Fig. 3) often have two well labeled primary processes (arrowheads) that arborize in the outer IPL (asterisk). In Fig. 4 some nNOS antisera label photoreceptor inner segments (horizontal arrowheads), Müller cell processes near the outer limiting membrane (asterisks) and many somata in the GCL (vertical arrowheads). In addition, there are often many faintly labeled somata (horizontal arrows) and some strongly labeled amacrine cells (vertical arrow) in the INL. The presence of nNOS-LI in relatively large numbers of somata in both the INL and GCL is consistent with the somatic NO production seen in stimulated retinal slices. In this and subsequent figures: OLM, outer limiting membrane; ONL, outer nuclear layer; OPL, outer plexiform layer; INL, inner nuclear layer; IPL, inner plexiform layer; GCL, ganglion cell layer; ILM, inner limiting membrane.

GCL with nNOS-LI (Fig. 4), some of which have axons and are ganglion cells.

In addition to amacrine and ganglion cells, NOS-LI and NADPH-diaphorase are also in retinal efferents in the turtle (Blute et al., 1997; Haverkamp and Eldred, 1998a). Blute et al. (1997) used a combination of NOS immunocytochemistry and NADPH-diaphorase histochemistry to label 7–10

efferent fibers that exit the optic nerve head and travel in the ganglion cell axon layer before entering the IPL. Haverkamp and Eldred (1998a) then used cholera toxin B as a retrograde tracer to locate the somata that give rise to these efferents near the locus coeruleus in the turtle brain.

NOS-LI has also been ultrastructurally localized in the OPL in turtle (Haverkamp and Eldred, 1998b).

112

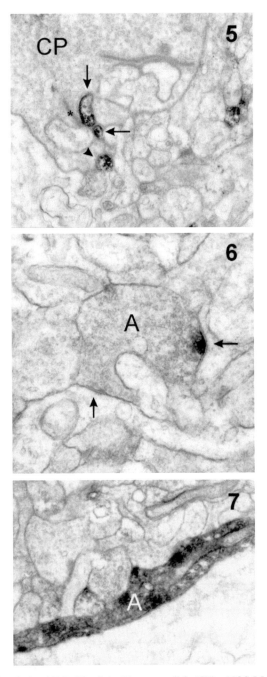

nNOS-LI is found in both invaginating bipolar and in horizontal cell processes at photoreceptor terminals, and in presumptive OFF-bipolar cells that make basal synaptic contacts with photoreceptors (Fig. 5). Thus, NO is potentially produced at all types of synaptic contacts in the outer retina. A similar selective localization of NOS is also seen in the IPL of the turtle retina, where some amacrine cells have NOS-LI only at presynaptic specializations and not in their general cytoplasm (Fig. 6). A single amacrine cell process that lacks diffuse cytoplasmic nNOS-LI can make several conventional synapses, some that have presynaptic nNOS-LI and others that lack nNOS-LI (Fig. 6). In other amacrine cell processes, there is strong NOS-LI found throughout their cytoplasm (Fig. 7). These differences in intracellular localization of NOS suggest that there may be significant differences in NO production in specific cell types. The selective subcellular localization of strong nNOS-LI at synaptic contacts, made by cells with low or undetectable levels of nNOS-LI at the light microscopic level, suggests that NO may be utilized at many more synaptic contacts than previously realized.

Localization of nitric oxide production in the retina

Although a number of studies have examined the localization of NOS and the effects of NO on specific cells or channels, few studies have directly examined the production of NO. To date, there has been only one pharmacological–biochemical study of NO production in the retina. Neal et al. (1998) used continuous and flashing lights to stimulate the retina and an NO-sensitive probe to measure NO production and release in a retinal eyecup. They found that blocking the ON-bipolar cells with APB, blocked the flickering light-stimulated release of NO. They also found that blocking of glutamate receptors with the non-selective glutamate receptor antagonist PDA, blocked the NO release stimulated

Figs. 5, 6 and 7. In Fig. 5, in this cone pedicle (CP), nNOS-LI is present in three different postsynaptic elements. At the photoreceptor ribbon (asterisk), nNOS-LI is clearly visible in one of the lateral horizontal cell processes (vertical arrow), and in the central element (horizontal arrow) which is probably a dendrite from an ON-bipolar cell. In addition, a putative OFF-bipolar cell process with nNOS-LI is making a basal synapse with this same photoreceptor (arrowhead). In Fig. 6, there is an amacrine cell process (A) making two conventional synaptic contacts (arrows). Note that there is no diffuse NOS-LI in the cytoplasm and that there is nNOS-LI found associated with one of the synapses (horizontal arrow), but not the other (vertical arrow). In contrast, the amacrine cell process (A) in Fig. 7 has NOS-LI that diffusely fills its cytoplasm.

by continuous light, but had no effect on the NO release stimulated by flickering light. From these results, Neal et al. (1998) concluded that because PDA blocks all glutamatergic synapses except from the photoreceptors to the ON-bipolar cells, the NO release stimulated by flickering light must be from ON-bipolars or Müller cells. In contrast, because both APB and PDA block the NO release stimulated by continuous light, they concluded it must be from amacrine cells.

Although Neal et al. (1998) did suggest that NO could be released by several retinal cell types, their study did not provide any information about which specific cell types were involved, the kinetics of NO production or about the movement of NO in the retina. Moreover, there is no information about the production of NO at specific subcellular sites, or even if all the immunocytochemically localized nNOS can synthesize NO. Recently, we have applied a newly developed technique that now allows the real time visualization of the production and movement of NO in the retina. A new class of NO-specific fluorescent probes, diaminofluoresceins (DAFs), has been developed that can bind an oxidation product of NO to form highly fluorescent triazolofluoresceins (Kojima et al., 1998a,b,c; Nagata et al., 1999; Igarashi et al., 1999; Goetz et al., 1999). DAF-2 has high specificity for NO and does not react with NO_2^-, NO_3^-, $O_2^{\cdot-}$, H_2O_2 or $ONOO^-$ to give any fluorescent product (Kojima et al., 1998a). In the remainder of this chapter, I will describe how we have used DAF-2 to provide the first detailed images of NO production in specific retinal cells. We have found that NO is produced by all the cell types shown to contain nNOS, and that there are differences in the kinetics of NO production in different cells (Blute et al., 2000).

NMDA stimulated NO production in turtle retina

We have used DAF-2 to image the production and localization of NO in retinal slices stimulated with the glutamate receptor agonist NMDA (Blute et al., 2000). In some but not all photoreceptors, NMDA stimulated increases in NO-induced fluorescence (-IF) throughout the entire inner segment, soma and synaptic terminal (Fig. 8A). These increases in NO-IF are first observed in the ellipsoid, and the strongest overall increases in NO-IF in photoreceptors are in the ellipsoid. Within 30 s, lower levels of increased NO-IF are seen in photoreceptor somata and synaptic terminals. The presence of oil droplets indicates that at least some of these photoreceptors are cones.

In retinal slices stimulated with NMDA, horizontal (Fig. 8B) and bipolar cell (Fig. 8C) somata with increased NO-IF are rarely observed, but fluorescent processes in the OPL are common (Fig. 8B–C). Many amacrine cells have NMDA stimulated NO-IF that is confined to their somata, while in other cases the NO-IF increases in their somata and processes (Fig. 8D–G). Some of the labeled amacrine cells have swellings on their processes that resemble synaptic boutons (Fig. 8D–E), while others do not (Fig. 8F–G). When present, the active boutons have more intense NO-IF than the rest of the adjacent process, although the NO-IF in boutons is still often weaker than the NO-IF in the somata of the same cells (Fig. 8D). There are also activated processes in the IPL that are not associated with labeled somata (Fig. 8I). These isolated processes with NO-IF usually have boutons. The boutons on a given process can display individualized patterns of NO-IF increases, in that the timing, peak levels, and kinetics of NO-IF in a given bouton are independent of other boutons, even those on the same process. In addition, there are isolated boutons with high NO-IF found in the IPL that are not associated with any labeled processes (Fig. 8D). These results suggest that the regulation of NOS activity can occur at the level of individual synapses. Some of these amacrine cells with increased NO-IF closely resemble the type 3 nNOS amacrine cells (Fig. 8F) that have been described previously in turtle retina (Blute et al., 1997).

In response to NMDA, numerous somata in the GCL exhibit strong increases in NO-IF (Fig. 8D, G and I), many of these somata are quite large and are likely to be ganglion cells. The NO-IF in somata in the GCL often reaches some of the highest levels in the retina. The NO-IF is usually seen in somata in the GCL before it is seen in amacrine cell somata, although both populations can be active concomitantly (Fig. 8D and G). After several minutes of NMDA stimulation, there is often considerable NO-IF in Müller cells. The NO-IF in Müller cells frequently begins in their processes near the outer or

114

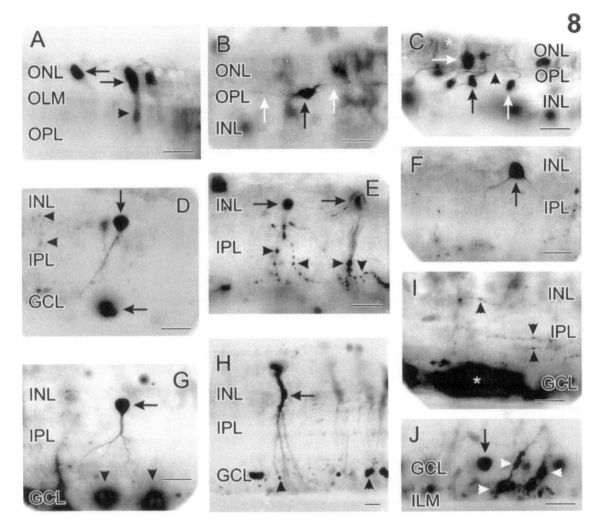

Fig. 8. These are contrast-reversed digital images of NMDA-stimulated increases in DAF-2 fluorescence. Strong NO-IF is concentrated in the following: (A) the ellipsoids (horizontal arrows), somata and synaptic terminals (arrowhead) of many photoreceptors; (B) horizontal cell somata (black arrow) and their dendritic processes (white arrows) in the OPL; (C) apical processes of Müller cells (asterisk) near the OLM, bipolar cell somata (both normally placed, vertical arrows; and displaced, horizontal arrow), some bipolar cell Landolt clubs and in bipolar cell processes in the OPL (arrowhead); (D) amacrine cell somata (vertical arrow) and processes, somata in the GCL (horizontal arrow) and in isolated boutons (horizontal arrowheads); (E) amacrine cell somata (horizontal arrows) and processes with many labeled boutons (arrowheads); (F) amacrine cells that closely resemble type 3 nNOS amacrine cells (vertical arrow); (G) novel amacrine cell types (horizontal arrow), and ganglion cell somata with NO-IF (arrowheads) which appears to diffuse into the surrounding GCL; (H) Müller cell somata (horizontal arrow) and small swellings on their processes (arrowheads); (I) somata in the GCL (asterisk) and amacrine cell processes and their associated boutons (vertical arrowheads); (J) a somata (vertical arrow) and some Müller cell processes with associated swellings (arrowheads) near the GCL and ILM. ONL, outer nuclear layer; OLM, outer limiting membrane; OPL, outer plexiform layer; INL, inner nuclear layer; IPL, inner plexiform layer; GCL, ganglion cell layer; GCAL, ganglion cell axon layer; ILM, inner limiting membrane. Scale bars, 20 μm

inner limiting membranes and spreads centrally to their somata (Fig. 8H). Near the GCL and ganglion cell axon layer, the Müller cells have small varicosities with strong NO-IF (Fig. 8J).

In some cases, it is possible to speculate about the function of the NO produced at certain sites. For instance, cells with primarily somatic NO increases may use NO to modulate gene expression

(Peunova and Enikolopov, 1993). In cells, with extensive cytoplasmic NO-IF, the NO may function as an intracellular signaling molecule to coordinate events throughout the cell, such as the regulation of intracellular calcium levels (Clementi, 1998) or receptor modulation (McMahon and Ponomareva, 1996; Wexler et al., 1998). Finally, the selective production of NO-IF at boutons suggests that NO may function at individual synapses to influence synaptic release (Meffert et al., 1994), intracellular calcium levels (Clementi, 1998) or receptor function (McMahon and Ponomareva, 1996).

Kinetics of NO-IF production in response to NMDA stimulation

All somatic increases in NMDA-stimulated NO-IF have a similar general time course when their intensity levels are plotted against time (Fig. 9). The general time course of all of these responses is more consistent with a biochemical time scale, rather than a synaptic time scale. During the rising phase, the intensity of NO-IF increases exponentially from baseline levels to a transient peak, which is immediately followed by a slower exponential decrease. The kinetic profiles for a given cell type are usually closely correlated, in that ganglion cells resemble other ganglion cells more than amacrine cells, and amacrine cells resemble other amacrine cells more than ganglion cells. The two ganglion cell somata shown in Fig. 9 have nearly identically shaped kinetic profiles, although one response is almost twice as large. Amacrine cell somata have less steeply rising and falling phases than ganglion cells, which results in a longer duration of increased NO-IF. Boutons in the IPL display less stereotypic responses, with a slower, more linear (less exponential) rising phase, a lower relative peak, and often a slower decay (Fig. 9). These results indicate that different retinal cell types may use different signal transduction pathways to produce NOS. For instance, some cells may activate NOS by fluxing calcium into the cell via voltage- or ligand-gated channels, while other cells may release intracellular calcium stores to activate NOS.

Correlation of the localizations of nNOS and NO production

As these are the first detailed images of the cells that can make NO in the retina, it is useful to compare these results to the existing localizations of NOS. In many cases, there is a close correlation. The high levels of NO-IF seen in the ellipsoid in photoreceptors, agrees with the immunocytochemical and histochemical localization of NOS in this organelle (Koch et al., 1994; Blute et al., 1997) in many species. The previous ultrastructural localization of nNOS-LI at specific contacts in the OPL (Haverkamp and Eldred, 1998b) is consistent with the strong NMDA-stimulated increase in NO-IF we see in the OPL. In addition, previous physiological studies support NO production by horizontal cells in the turtle retina (Miyachi et al., 1990) and in the hybrid bass retina (McMahon and Ponomareva, 1996).

Large numbers of amacrine cell somata have prominent nNOS-LI (Blute et al., 1997). These amacrine cells often have nNOS-LI in their dendritic

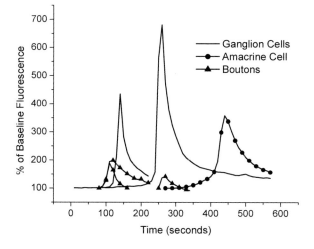

Fig. 9. Kinetics of NMDA-stimulated NO-induced fluorescence (NO-IF) over time, as seen in 2 different ganglion cells, a representative amacrine cell and three boutons in the IPL. The X-axis is the time in seconds following the administration of NMDA. The intensity of fluorescence is baseline corrected and is expressed as the percentage of baseline ($F/F_0 \times 100$). The ranges of t_{rising} and $t_{falling}$ are 8.5–23 s and 15–58 s, respectively.

arborizations in the IPL (Figs. 1–3), but in other cases, it is confined to their somata (Fig. 4). Consistent with the strong nNOS-LI observed in multiple amacrine cell types, we find that NMDA dramatically increases NO-IF in the somata and/or processes of a wide variety of amacrine cells (Fig. 8D–G). As described earlier in turtle, the type 3 nNOS amacrine cell type is characterized by a large soma at the INL–IPL border that gives rise to sparse, weakly immunoreactive processes, which arborize in the outer layers of the IPL (Blute et al., 1997). The nNOS-LI in these cells fades quickly in the more distal portions of these processes, and thus the processes cannot be traced very far in the IPL. There is a close correlation between the relative subcellular levels of nNOS in the type 3 cells and where we see increased NO-IF in these same cells, in that NO-IF is only visible in the soma and proximal processes of these cells. However, in many cases the amacrine cells with NO-IF are novel amacrine cell types, and thus there are clearly other amacrine cells, in addition to the previously described three nNOS containing amacrine cell types (Blute et al., 1997), that can produce NO in the turtle retina. This suggests that isoforms other than conventional nNOS may function in retina. Immunocytochemistry indicates that there is nNOS in many somata in the GCL in turtle (Fig. 4 and Blute et al., 1997), which is consistent with our current localization of NO-IF in large numbers of somata in the GCL.

Ultrastructural analysis in the IPL indicates that in some cases nNOS-LI is found concentrated at specific synaptic contacts in dendritic processes that have little overall cytoplasmic nNOS-LI (Fig. 6), while in other cases a process is filled with cytoplasmic nNOS-LI (Fig. 7). We see a correlation in the production of NMDA-stimulated NO-IF and nNOS-LI in some dendritic processes. In some processes there is an even production of NO-IF throughout the process, which probably corresponds with diffuse cytoplasmic nNOS. In contrast, in other processes, there is more selectivity in the subcellular production of NO-IF, in that the boutons are the foci of NO-IF production. These results indicate that the production of NO at specific subcellular sites of nNOS is selectively and tightly regulated, and that multiple sources within a given cell or dendritic process can be discretely activated.

Finally, previous studies have described the presence of nNOS in Müller cells (Liepe et al., 1994; Kurenni et al., 1995), although they often have much less nNOS-LI than other retinal cell types. In turtle retina, there is frequently little nNOS-LI in Müller cells, even though NADPH-diaphorase histochemistry can produce some labeling in Müller cells. The NO-IF we see in Müller cells may be due to the presence of a NOS isoform other than nNOS, which would be consistent with our NADPH-diaphorase labeling and the localization of eNOS-LI in Müller cells (Haverkamp et al., 1999). It is also possible that Müller cells may not actually make NO, but instead take it up from surrounding cells that release it. This would be consistent with the late appearance of NO-IF in the Müller cells and their common close proximity to retinal neurons with NO-IF.

Movement of NO in the retina

Although the neutral, hydrophobic, non-electrolyte NO is reported to be freely diffusible, the range of NO action is largely unknown. The half-life of NO has been reported to range from several seconds (Ignarro et al., 1993; Lancaster, 1994), up to 70 h in solutions with proteins (Beckman and Koppenol, 1996). Models predicting the diffusion and possible sphere of influence of NO do exist (Lancaster, 1994, Wood and Garthwaite, 1994), but they require several untested assumptions and are based on the physical characteristics of NO measured in artificial in vitro situations. In the complex cellular milieu of the retina, it is likely that NO may behave quite differently. We can now use DAF-2 imaging to directly examine the spread of NO-IF from a variety of identified, actively producing sources. DAF has only a 9.6% trapping efficiency for NO (Nakatsubo et al., 1998), which allows over 90% of the NO produced to interact with its normal cellular targets. By assuming this free NO behaves normally, we can examine the diffusion of NO by analyzing the spread of NO-IF.

In many cells, even cells with very high peak increases in fluorescence (650% of baseline), there is relatively little spread of NO-IF beyond the cell boundary (Fig. 10). In these cells, the NO-IF is largely confined to the site of production and

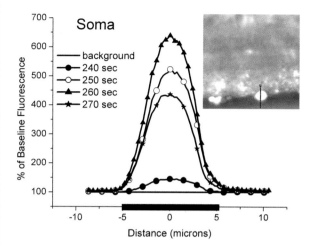

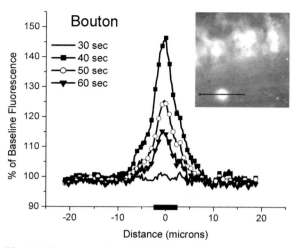

Fig. 10. Line scan profile of a soma in the GCL at four sequential time points after stimulation with NMDA. The image of the NO-IF at the peak level (inset) illustrates the region of the line scan. The intensity of each pixel under the line was measured, then normalized to baseline levels ($F/F_0 \times 100$) and plotted. The background correction produces a background trace that is a flat line at 100% (black line). The first response to NMDA in this cell occurs at 240 s (red line, $\sim$140% of baseline) and the maximum level of NO-IF occurs at 260 s (blue line, $\sim$650% of baseline). Although there is a large increase in NO-IF, it is almost completely contained within the boundaries of the soma. The bar on the X-axis indicates the actual size of the soma.

Fig. 11. Line scan profile of NO-IF in a bouton in the IPL at four sequential time points after NMDA stimulation. The image of the NO-IF at the peak level (inset) illustrates the area of the line scan. The intensity of each pixel under the line was measured, then normalized to baseline levels ($F/F_0 \times 100$) and plotted. The first time point at 30 s (black line) only shows minor deviations from baseline, while 10 s later the NO-IF increases to a maximum of 150% of baseline. In contrast to the soma shown in Fig. 9, although the overall magnitude of NO-IF increase is smaller in this bouton, there is more diffusion from the source. The bar on the X-axis indicates the actual size of the bouton.

does not spread more than 10 μm from the source. However, in other cells, the NO-IF spreads well beyond their cell boundaries (Figs. 8I and 11), as would be predicted by the previous models of NO diffusion. This spread is seen to occur, even from cells with relatively low overall increases in NO-IF (peak of 150% of baseline) (Fig. 11).

These results indicate that the retention or spread of NO from a source is not purely a function of NO concentration, and that other biochemical mechanisms are involved that can be selectively localized in specific subcellular compartments. This apparent retention is probably not due to the selective partitioning of the DAF-2 label, because retinas stimulated with NO-donor indicate that the DAF-2 is evenly loaded in all of the contiguous cells. This retention of NO may be the result of a cytoplasmic sink and/or a membrane barrier. This retention could be mediated by NO binding to thiols or metalloproteins in the cytosol and/or membrane. Cell surface

thiols have been implicated in NO binding and exchange to move NO into cells (Zai et al., 1999), and they may function to provide some membrane barrier. Glutathione, a major thiol, is present at high levels in Müller cells (Pow and Crook, 1995), which may explain the retention and movement of NO-IF in Müller cells from an active source through the rest of the cell. This might also explain the appearance of NO-IF in Müller cells, in that the glutathione they contain could serve as a sink for NO produced in adjacent cells. Alternatively, the cause of NO confinement may result from simple charge interactions between the uncharged NO and the hydrophobic lipid bilayers. Such preferential concentration and lateral motion of NO in membranes is reported in endothelial cells (Malinski, et al., 1993).

Functionally active spatial concentrations of NO

A previous study of NO production by endothelial cells used NO-sensitive porphyrinic electrodes to

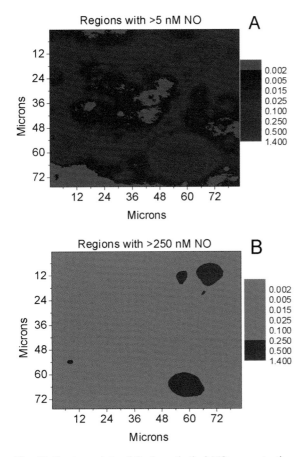

Fig. 12. Contour plots of the hypothetical NO concentrations found in the retina. The maximum NO concentration is based on the actual value of 1.3 µM NO measured at endothelial cells (Malinski et al., 1993). By assuming the fully active somatic sources produce 1.3 µM NO, and the relationship between NO concentration and DAF fluorescence to be linear, we can model the concentrations of NO in this image of NMDA stimulated retina. The pseudocolor scales on the right, indicate the colors corresponding to the calculated concentrations of NO in µM. Note the amacrine somata in the INL, and the soma in the GCL, produce far more NO than the small boutons and processes in the IPL. The threshold for activation of sGC by NO is reported to be as low as 5 nM (Beckman and Koppenol, 1996) or as high as 250 nM NO (Stone and Marletta, 1996). In panel A, we assume a threshold of 5 nM. Regions of the retina with calculated values lower than 5 nM are indicated by gray. Although the majority of the retina has values greater than 5 nM, there are some areas below 5 nM, even in the central IPL. In contrast, in panel B, where we assume a threshold of 250 nM, only regions over or very near the active somata would have activated sGC. In this case, the levels of NO in the somatic sources spreads slightly beyond the somatic boundaries, but extremely high levels are retained locally over the source.

measure the concentration of NO at the surface of an active cell to be 1.3 µM (Malinski et al., 1993). If we assume that a fully active somatic source produces 1.3 µM NO, and that there is a linear relationship between NO and DAF-2 fluorescence (Blute et al., 2000), then we can model the theoretical concentrations of NO seen in a region of a stimulated retinal slice (Figs. 12A and 12B). In this retinal slice stimulated with NMDA, the somatic sources in the INL and the GCL produced higher levels of NO-IF than the small boutons and processes in the IPL.

The threshold for activation of sGC, the main target of NO, is reported to range from 5 nM (Beckman and Koppenol, 1996) up to 250 nM (Stone and Marletta, 1996). Based on the assumption that the most active sources produce 1.3 µM NO, we can plot the regions with NO concentrations above 5 nM (Fig. 12A) and 250 nM (Fig. 12B), respectively. Assuming a 5 nM threshold for sGC activation (Fig. 12A), the majority of the IPL has sufficient NO to activate sGC, although there are some regions in the central IPL with sub-threshold levels of NO. If the threshold for the activation of sGC is 250 nM (Fig. 12B), then the activation of sGC would be dramatically more confined to the somata of NO synthesizing cells and some of their contiguous processes. In Fig. 12B, the majority of the IPL is below the threshold for activation of sGC. In either case, although some NO-IF does spread beyond the cellular boundaries, extremely high levels are still retained, localized over the sources. The true regions of sGC activation are likely to lie between these two extreme situations. Depending on the actual threshold for sGC activation, the levels of NO produced by the spread are likely to be inadequate to stimulate sGC in all cells. The existence of these different concentrations of NO, produced by diffusion gradients in the IPL, may be functionally related to the differences in sensitivity of the activation of sGC by NO that are reported for specific retinal types (Blute et al., 1998).

Conclusions and future perspectives

In summary, our research indicates that NOS can be activated to produce NO in every cell type in the retina, which is consistent with many of the previous anatomical and biochemical localizations of nNOS. The other exciting outcome of our research is that NO is much less diffusible that originally proposed. This alleviates one of our major difficulties in thinking about the function of NO, in that it does not just freely diffuse throughout a given tissue. There can also be significant variability between cell types, in that it is largely retained within some somata and synaptic boutons, while in other cells, it moves out from the cellular source into the surrounding cells. Furthermore, the production of NO can be regulated at the level of individual synaptic boutons. This behavior greatly increases the potential specificity of the NO signal transduction system.

The results described in this chapter have indicated that NO is likely to play a wide variety of roles in the retina. However, many questions remain to be answered. As described previously, it is possible to produce NO-IF in many more cells than have been reported to contain nNOS. Even though endothelial NOS (eNOS) has been reported to exist in Müller cells and some horizontal cells in turtle retina (Haverkamp et al., 1999), it still does not account for all of the NO-IF we see. This raises the possibility that other isoforms of NOS can function in retina. The presence of the inducible NOS (iNOS) isoform has been shown in both normal and pathological retinas (Park et al., 1994; López-Costa et al., 1997). Our unpublished results of Western blots of rat and turtle retinas using a wide variety of nNOS, iNOS and eNOS antisera, indicate that there are potentially some lower molecular weight novel isoforms of NOS in the retina. Furthermore, some of these novel NOS-like proteins can be localized using electron immunocytochemistry at specific synaptic structures. Future studies will be needed to confirm and characterize these potential novel NOS isoforms, and to examine the localization and function of eNOS- and iNOS-like proteins in retina. There is also the possibility that mitochondrial NOS (Bates et al., 1995; Tatoyan and Giulivi, 1998) plays a role in the retina. This would be consistent with the NO-IF we see in photoreceptor ellipsoids, which consist largely of mitochondria.

Although our studies do describe some of the specific cell types that can make NO, many details about these cells remain to be clarified. The production of NO-IF in these various cells seems to be unique to each cell type, in that some have NO-IF at boutons, others have somatic NO-IF, while still others virtually fill with NO-IF. The specific cell types associated with each of these NO production characteristics needs to be clarified, and their anatomy and synaptic connectivity needs to be determined. Moreover, our studies to date have focused primarily on the effects of glutamatergic receptor activation. It will also be very important to examine the role of inhibitory receptors on these same signal transduction systems. Our preliminary results indicate that inhibition of GABAergic receptors can have significant effects on NO and cGMP production, and that these effects are considerably different from the effects of glutamate receptor activation (Eldred and Blute, 2000).

The fact that DAF can label the cells that make NO in a living retinal slice, provides a very unique opportunity to examine the electrophysiology of NO production in specific retinal cell types. It is possible that production of NO at synaptic boutons involves different synaptic connectivity than when somatic NO is produced. It is also possible that activation of cytoplasmic NOS involves mobilization of intracellular calcium stores, while NOS in boutons is activated by calcium fluxing through membrane channels. For instance, do excitatory postsynaptic potentials in ganglion cells produce a different activation of NOS than when the ganglion cells produce action potentials? Finally, it will be necessary to examine the biochemical basis underlying the spread or lack of spread of NO out of specific cells or subcellular regions. Is this control of the spread of NO, a permanent characteristic of a given cell type, or can it be modulated? Perhaps NO produced by one NOS isoform or at a specific subcellular site spreads, while NO at other sites or from other isoforms does not.

Previous studies have indicated that the different cell types that contain sGC can each show unique sensitivities to NO, in that some cells are much more sensitive than others (Blute et al., 1998). This suggests that it will be important to determine the actual concentrations of NO produced by different sources or in different regions of the retina. The use of DAF to image NO production gives excellent spatial resolution down to the subcellular level, and therefore, it would be ideal to develop a way to quantify the DAF imaging to correlate specific image intensities with actual levels of NO. We are currently exploring three methods to accomplish quantitative measurements of NO using DAF imaging. The first uses the fact that the rate of rise of NO-IF can be directly correlated with the concentration of NO (Blute et al., 2000). This suggests that we can use the rate of rise to determine at least the relative concentrations of NO in specific regions within an image. The second method uses the fact that the wavelength of the fluorescent light emitted by DAF is different before and after it binds NO. This raises the possibility that we can use a ratio of these wavelengths to get a measure of the NO concentration. Finally, we are attempting to combine our imaging methods with the use of NO-sensitive microelectrodes (Malinski et al., 1993; Silverton et al., 1999), to actually measure the concentration of NO at a specific site with NO-IF in a retinal slice. Once the concentration at a specific site is known, we can use the linear nature of the reaction of DAF with NO to determine the true concentrations of NO in the rest of the image.

Finally, it will be important to determine the downstream signal transduction pathways activated by NO in specific cells. Our results indicate that NO functions to activate sGC in many retinal cell types. However, little is known about the function of cGMP in these specific cells. For instance, reagents are just becoming available to examine the function and localization of PDEs, cGMP gated channels and PKG in specific retinal cell types. Given the relatively large number of cells and cell types that we have shown can produce NO, it is unlikely that the production of cGMP is the only function of NO in the retina. It will be particularly important to examine the interactions of NO with calcium, in that calcium can activate NOS and NO can modulate intracellular levels of calcium in the retina (Eldred et al., 1999).

Acknowledgments

I wish to thank Felicitas B. Eldred for her excellent technical assistance and Dr. Todd A. Blute for critical reading of the manuscript and doing most of the experiments. This research supported by NIH EY 04785 to W.D.E.

References

Ahmad, I., Leinders-Zufall, T., Kocsis, J.D., Shepherd, G.M., Zufall, F. and Barnstable, C.J. (1994) Retinal ganglion cells express a cGMP-gated cation conductance activatable by nitric oxide donors. Neuron, 12: 155–165.

Bates, T.E., Loesch, A., Burnstock, G. and Clark, J.B. (1995) Immunocytochemical evidence for a mitochondrially located nitric oxide synthase in brain and liver. Biochem. Biophys. Res. Commun., 213: 896–900.

Beckman, J.S. and Koppenol, W.H. (1996) Nitric oxide superoxide and peroxynitrite: The good, the bad and the ugly. Am. J. Psychol., 271: C1424–C1437.

Blute, T.A., DeGrenier, J. and Eldred, W.D. (1999) Stimulation with NMDA or kainic acid increases cGMP-like immunoreactivity in turtle retina: involvement of nitric oxide synthase. J. Comp. Neurol., 404: 75–85.

Blute, T.A., Lee, M.R. and Eldred, W.D. (2000) Direct imaging of NMDA-stimulated nitric oxide production in the retina. Vis. Neurosci., 17: 557–566.

Blute, T.A., Mayer, B. and Eldred, W.D. (1997) Immunocytochemical and histochemical localization of nitric oxide synthase in the turtle retina. Vis. Neurosci., 14: 717–729.

Blute, T.A., Velasco, P. and Eldred, W.D. (1998) Functional localization of soluble guanylate cyclase in turtle retina: Modulation of cGMP by nitric oxide. Vis. Neurosci., 15: 485–498.

Clementi, E. (1998) Role of nitric oxide and its intracellular signalling pathways in the control of Ca^{2+} homeostasis. Biochem. Pharmacol., 55: 713–718.

Cobcroft, M., Vaccaro, T. and Mitrofanis, J. (1989) Distinct patterns of distribution among NADPH-diaphorase neurones of the guinea pig retina, Neurosci. Lett., 103: 1–7.

Dowling, J.E. (1994) The neuromodulatory role of dopamine in the teleost retina. In: Niznik, H.B. (Ed.), Dopamine Receptors and Transporters. Marcel Dekker Inc., New York, pp. 37–57.

Eldred, W.D. (2000) Nitric oxide in the retina. In Steinbusch, H.W.M., de Vente, J. and Vincent, S. (Eds.), Handbook of Chemical Neuroanatomy, Functional neuroanatomy of the nitric oxide system, 17, 111–145.

Eldred, W.D., Lee, M.R. and Blute, T.A. (1999) Modulation of intracellular calcium levels by nitric oxide in the turtle retina. Invest. Ophthal. Vis. Sci., (Suppl. 40): S235.

Eldred, W.D. and Blute, T.A. (2000) Nitric oxide production stimulated by inhibition of GABA receptors in the turtle retina: Quantitative imaging. Invest. Ophthal. Vis. Sci., (Suppl. 41): S247.

Goetz, R.M., Thatte, H.S., Prabhakar, P., Cho, M.R., Michel, T. and Golan, D.E. (1999) Estradiol induces the calcium-dependent translocation of endothelial nitric oxide synthase. Proc. Natl. Acad. Sci. USA, 96: 2788–2793.

Haverkamp, S.H. and Eldred, W.D. (1998a) Localization of the origin of retinal efferents in the turtle brain and the involvement of nitric oxide synthase. J. Comp. Neurol., 393: 185–195.

Haverkamp, S.H. and Eldred, W.D. (1998b) Localization of nNOS in photoreceptor bipolar and horizontal cells in turtle and rat retinas. *NeuroReport*, 10: 2231–2235.

Haverkamp, S., Kolb, H. and Cuenca, N. (1999) Endothelial nitric oxide synthase (eNOS) is localized to Müller cells in all vertebrate retinas. *Vision Res.*, 39: 2299–2303.

Igarashi, J., Thatte, H.S., Prabhakar, P., Golan, D.E. and Michel, T. (1999) Calcium-independent activation of endothelial nitric oxide synthase by ceramide. *Proc. Natl. Acad. Sci. USA*, 96: 12583–12588.

Ignarro, L.J., Fukuto, J.M., Griscavage, J.M., Rogers, N.E. and Byrns, R.E. (1993) Oxidation of nitric oxide in aqueous solution to nitrite but not nitrate: comparison with enzymatically formed nitric oxide from L-arginine. *Proc. Natl. Acad. Sci. USA*, 90: 8103–8107.

Koch, K-W., Lambrecht, H-G., Haberecht, M., Redburn, D. and Schmidt, H.H.H.W. (1994) Functional coupling of a Ca^{2+}/calmodulin-dependent nitric oxide synthase and a soluble guanylyl cyclase in vertebrate photoreceptor cells. *EMBO J.*, 13: 3312–3320.

Koistinaho, J., Swanson, R.A., de Vente, J. and Sagar, S.M. (1993) NADPH-diaphorase (nitric oxide synthase)-reactive amacrine cells of rabbit retina: Putative target cells and stimulation by light. *Neurosci.*, 57: 587–597.

Kojima, H., Nakatsubo, N., Kikuchi, K., Kawahara, S., Kirino, Y., Nagoshi, H., Hirata, Y. and Nagano, T. (1998a) Detection and imaging of nitric oxide with novel fluorescent indicators: diaminofluoresceins. *Anal. Chem.*, 70: 2446–2453.

Kojima, H., Nakatsubo, N., Kikuchi, K., Urano, Y., Higuchi, T., Tanaka, J., Kudo, Y. and Nagano, T. (1998b) Direct evidence of NO production in rat hippocampus and cortex using a new fluorescent indicator: DAF-2 DA. *NeuroReport*, 9: 3345–3348.

Kojima, H., Sakurai, K., Kikuchi, K., Kawahara, S., Kirino, Y., Nagoshi, H., Hirata, Y. and Nagano, T. (1998c) Development of a fluorescent indicator for nitric oxide based on the fluorescein chromophore. *Chem. Pharm. Bull.*, 46: 373–375.

Kurenni, D.E., Thurlow, G.A., Turner, R.W., Moroz, L.L., Sharkey, K.A. and Barnes, S. (1995) Nitric oxide synthase in tiger salamander retina. *J. Comp. Neurol.*, 361: 525–526.

Lancaster, J.R. (1994) Simulation of the diffusion and reaction of endogenously produced nitric oxide. *Proc. Natl. Acad. Sci. USA*, 91: 8137–8141.

Liepe, B.A., Stone, C., Koistinaho, J. and Copenhagen, D.R. (1994) Nitric oxide synthase in Müller cells and neurons of salamander and fish retina. *J. Neurosci.*, 14: 7641–7654.

López-Costa, J.J., Goldstein, J. and Saavedra, J.P. (1997) Neuronal and macrophagic nitric oxide synthase isoforms distribution in normal rat retina. *Neurosci. Lett.*, 232: 155–158.

Malinski, T., Taha, Z., Grunfeld, S., Patton, S., Kapturczak, M. and Tomboulian, P. (1993) Diffusion of nitric oxide in the aorta wall monitored in situ by porphyrinic microsensors. *Biochem. Biophys. Res. Commun.*, 193: 1076–1082.

McMahon, D.G. and Ponomareva, L.V. (1996) Nitric oxide and cGMP modulate retinal glutamate receptors. *J. Neurophysiol.*, 76: 2307–2315.

McMahon, D.G., Rischert, J.C. and Dowling, J.E. (1994) Protein content and cAMP-dependent phosphorylation of fractionated white perch retina. *Brain Res.* 659: 110–116.

Meffert, M.K., Premack, B.A. and Schulman, H. (1994) Nitric oxide stimulates Ca^{2+}-independent synaptic vesicle release. *Neuron*, 12: 1235–1244.

Mills, S.L. and Massey, S.C. (1995) Differential properties of two gap junctional pathways made by AII amacrine cells. *Nature*, 377: 734–737.

Miyachi, E., Murakami, M. and Nakaki, T. (1990) Arginine blocks gap junctions between retinal horizontal cells. *NeuroReport*, 1: 107–110.

Nagata, N., Momose, K. and Ishida, Y. (1999) Inhibitory effects of catecholamines and anti-oxidants on the fluorescence reaction of 4,5-diaminofluorescein, DAF-2, a novel indicator of nitric oxide. *J. Biochem. (Tokyo)*, 125: 658–61.

Nakatsubo, N., Kojima, H., Kikuchi, K., Nagoshi, H., Hirata, Y., Maeda, D., Imai, Y., Irimura, T. and Nagano, T. (1998) Direct evidence of nitric oxide production from bovine aortic endothelial cells using new fluorescence indicators: diaminofluoresceins. *FEBS Lett.*, 427: 263–266.

Neal, M., Cunningham, J. and Matthews, K. (1998) Selective release of nitric oxide from retinal amacrine cells and bipolar cells. *Invest. Ophthal. Vis. Sci.*, 39: 850–853.

O'Brien, D.R. and Dowling, J.E. (1985) Dopaminergic regulation of GABA release from the intact goldfish retina. *Brain Res.*, 360: 41–50.

Park, C.-S., Pardhasaradhi, K., Gianotti, C., Villegas, E. and Krishna, G. (1994) Human retina expresses both constitutive and inducible isoforms of nitric oxide synthase mRNA. *Biochem. Biophys. Res. Commun.*, 205: 85–91.

Peunova, N. and Enikolopov, G. (1993) Amplification of calcium-induced gene transcription by nitric oxide in neuronal cells. *Nature*, 364: 450–453.

Pow, D.V. and Crook, D.K. (1995) Immunocytochemical evidence for the presence of high levels of reduced glutathione in radial glial cells and horizontal cells in the rabbit retina. *Neurosci. Lett.*, 193: 25–28.

Rieke, F. and Schwartz, E.A. (1994) A cGMP-gated current can control exocytosis at cone synapses. *Neuron*, 13: 863–873.

Sagar, S. (1990) NADPH-diaphorase reactive neurons of the rabbit retina: differential sensitivity to excitotoxins and unusual morphological features. *J. Comp. Neurol.*, 300: 309–319.

Savchenko, A., Barnes, S. and Kramer, R.H. (1997) Cyclic-nucleotide-gated channels mediate synaptic feedback by nitric oxide. *Nature*, 390: 694–698.

Shiells, R.A. and Falk, G. (1992a) Properties of the cGMP-activated channel of retinal on-bipolar cells. *Proc. R. Soc. Lond. B Biol. Sci.*, 247: 21–25.

Shiells, R.A. and Falk, G. (1992b) Retinal on-bipolar cells contain a nitric oxide-sensitive guanylate cyclase. *Neuro Report*, 3: 845–848.

Silverton, S.F., Adebanjo, O.A., Moonga, B.S., Awumey, E.M., Malinski, T. and Zaidi, M. (1999) Direct microsensor measurement of nitric oxide production by the osteoclast. *Biochem. Biophys. Res. Commun.*, 259: 73–77.

Stone, J.R. and Marletta, M.A. (1996) Spectral and kinetic studies on the activation of soluble guanylate cyclase by nitric oxide. *Biochemistry*, 35: 1093–1099.

Tatoyan, A. and Giulivi, C. (1998) Purification and characterization of a nitric oxide synthase from rat liver mitochondria. *J. Biol. Chem.*, 273: 11044–11048.

Vaney, D.I. and Young, H.M. (1988) GABA-like immunoreactivity in NADPH-diaphorase amacrine cells of the rabbit retina. *Brain Res.*, 474: 380–385.

Vincent, S.R. and Hope, B.T. (1992) Neurons that say NO. *Trends Neurosci.*, 15: 108–113.

Wexler, E.M., Stanton, P.K. and Nawy, S. (1998) Nitric oxide depresses GABA$_A$ receptor function via coactivation of cGMP-dependent kinase and phosphodiesterase. *J. Neurosci.*, 18: 2342–2349.

Wislocki, G.B. and Sidman, R.L. (1954) The chemical morphology of the retina. *J. Comp. Neurol.*, 101: 53–91.

Wood, J. and Garthwaite, J. (1994) Models of the diffusional spread of nitric oxide: implications for neural nitric oxide signaling and its pharmacological properties. *Neuropharmacology*, 33: 1235–1244.

Young, L.H.Y. and Dowling, J.E. (1989) Localization of cyclic adenosine monophosphate in the teleost retina: Effects of dopamine and prolonged darkness. *Brain Res.*, 504: 57–63.

Zai, A., Rudd, M.A., Scribner, A.W. and Loscalzo, J. (1999) Cell-surface protein disulfide isomerase catalyzes transnitrosation and regulates intracellular transfer of nitric oxide. *J. Clin. Invest.*, 103: 393–399.

Functional organization

H. Kolb, H. Ripps and S. Wu (Eds.)
Progress in Brain Research, Vol. 131

CHAPTER 8

Integration and segregation of visual signals by bipolar cells in the tiger salamander retina

Samuel M. Wu*, Fan Gao and Bruce R. Maple

Cullen Eye Institute, Baylor College of Medicine, 6565 Fannin Street, NC-205, Houston, TX 77030, USA

Introduction

Bipolar cells are the central neurons of the vertebrate retina. Integrating visual signals at both synaptic layers of the retina, they are the first neurons along the visual pathway to exhibit center-surround antagonistic receptive field (CSARF) organization, the basic alphabet for encoding spatial information in the visual system (Kuffler, 1953; Hubel and Wiesel, 1962). Over three decades ago, Frank Werblin and John Dowling made the first intracellular recordings from bipolar cells in the mudpuppy retina, and discovered that these cells could be divided into two types, according to their CSARF organization: the ON-center (OFF-surround) and the OFF-center (ON-surround) bipolar cells (Werblin and Dowling, 1969). Later works on other vertebrate species have confirmed their findings, and it is now widely accepted that ON-center and OFF-center bipolar cells generate the ON and OFF pathways, two important parallel channels for spatial information processing in the visual system (Kaneko, 1970; Hubel and Livingstone, 1987).

The ON and OFF pathways are initiated at the outer plexiform layer (OPL) by postsynaptic receptors at the glutamatergic synapses between photoreceptors and bipolar cell dendrites. In the OFF-center bipolar cells, glutamate binds to AMPA/kainate receptors and activates a cation conductance with a reversal potential near 0 mV (Slaughter and Miller, 1983a, b; Attwell et al., 1987; Maple and Wu, 1996; Wu and Maple, 1998). In the ON-center bipolar cells glutamate generally acts at L-AP4 type glutamate receptors, which close a cation conductance through a cGMP-G protein cascade (Slaughter and Miller, 1981; Nawy and Jahr, 1990; Wu and Maple, 1998). (In the ON-center bipolar cells of some fish, however, the cone inputs are mediated by a glutamate-activated chloride conductance with a reversal potential near −60 mV (Saito et al., 1979; Grant and Dowling, 1995)). At the inner retina, the ON and OFF pathways are segregated by the stratification of bipolar cell axon terminals in the inner plexiform layer (IPL): the OFF-center cells synapse on amacrine and ganglion cells at distal levels of the IPL (sublamina A), and the ON-center cells make synapses at proximal levels of the IPL (sublamina A) (Famiglietti and Kolb, 1976; Nelson et al., 1978).

In the mid 60s, John Dowling and Brian Boycott found that rod and cone photoreceptors in primates make synapses on dendrites of different bipolar cells, and based on the patterns of synaptic contacts, they classified bipolar cells into rod and cone bipolar cells (Dowling and Boycott, 1966; Dowling, 1968). Subsequent studies have shown that there are at least nine morphologically distinguishable types of cone bipolar cells and one type of rod bipolar cell in the mammalian retina (Boycott and Wassle, 1991; Euler and Wassle, 1995). However, the light

---
* Corresponding author: Samuel M. Wu, Tel.: (713) 708-5966; Fax: (713) 798-6457; E-mail: swu@bcm.tmc.edu

responses of these morphologically distinct bipolar cells have not been systematically studied. In lower vertebrates, physiological and anatomical studies have indicated that bipolar cells received mixed inputs from rods and cones (Dowling and Werblin, 1969; Lasansky, 1973, 1978). Recent physiological evidence from the tiger salamander retina, nevertheless, suggests that bipolar cells, both ON-center and OFF-center, fall into two groups: one being rod-dominated and the other cone-dominated (Hensley et al., 1993; Yang and Wu, 1997), so it has been important to correlate the physiology and morphology of these distinctly different types of bipolar cells.

In addition to photoreceptor inputs, bipolar cells also receive inhibitory synaptic inputs from amacrine cells in the inner retina (Wong-Riley, 1974), and in some species from horizontal cells in the outer retina (Naka, 1972). These inputs are commonly referred as lateral or "surround" synapses because horizontal cells and amacrine cells have long lateral processes that convey visual signals to a bipolar cell from cells in surrounding regions (Boycott and Dowling, 1969; Lasansky, 1973). Signals from these lateral processes mediate light responses opposite in sign to those mediated by photoreceptors, thus forming the center-surround antagonism of the cell's receptive field (Werblin and Dowling, 1969; Kaneko, 1970). Moreover, interplexiform cells, which receive synaptic inputs from bipolar cells and amacrine cells in the inner retina, make synapses on bipolar cell dendrites in the outer retina (Dowling and Ehinger, 1975).

Since most studies of bipolar cell light responses have been carried out using intracellular recording techniques in eyecup or isolated whole-mount preparations (Thibos and Werblin, 1978; Hare and Owen, 1996; Yang and Wu, 1997), it has been difficult to routinely stain the cells for morphological identification or to separate ionic current components of light responses under voltage clamp conditions. On the other hand, most voltage clamp studies of bipolar cells have been performed with dissociated cells or light-adapted retinal slices, where light responses were usually absent or weak. In this article, we review some of our recent studies on the light-evoked current responses of voltage-clamped bipolar cells in dark-adapted slices of the tiger salamander retina. The excitatory synaptic inputs from photoreceptors, and inhibitory inputs from horizontal cells, amacrine cells and interplexiform cells are described. Characteristics of these inputs are correlated with bipolar cell morphology, as revealed by fluorescence microscopy. The segregation of visual signals by the stratification of bipolar cell axon terminals in the IPL is discussed.

Synaptic inputs to bipolar cells

Photoreceptor inputs to bipolar cells

ON-center and OFF-center bipolar cells

Figure 1A shows current records from an ON-center bipolar cell (also known as *depolarizing bipolar cell*, or DBC) that was voltage clamped in a dark-adapted tiger salamander retinal slice. Currents were recorded at various holding potentials, and a 500 μm light spot, which covered the bipolar cell's receptive field center (Skrzypek and Werblin, 1983), was presented to the cell at each holding potential. The light response had two components: At −60 mV (E_{Cl}, the equilibrium potential for chloride channels at inhibitory synapses from amacrine cells and interplexiform cells) the cell exhibited a sustained inward current (ΔI_C), mediated predominantly by cation channels at glutamatergic synapses from photoreceptors (Nawy and Jahr, 1990). At 0 mV (near E_C, the equilibrium potential for glutamate-gated cation channels (Wu and Maple, 1998)), light onset and offset gave rise to transient outward currents (ΔI_{Cl}), probably mediated by chloride channels at synapses from amacrine cells (narrow field amacrine cells exhibit light responses with similar waveforms when stimulated by small spots of light (Vallerga, 1981)).

The photoreceptor inputs to bipolar cells can be isolated by using pharmacological agents to block the light-evoked ΔI_{Cl}. Among all antagonists tested, we found imidazole-4-acetic acid (I4AA), a GABA$_C$ receptor antagonist and GABA receptor agonist (Qian and Dowling, 1994; Lukasiewicz and Shields, 1998), to be the most effective in blocking ΔI_{Cl} in bipolar cells. In the presence of 10 μM I4AA (Fig. 1B), the light-evoked current became sustained at all voltages and reversed near 0 mV, indicating it was mediated predominantly by ΔI_C. Under these

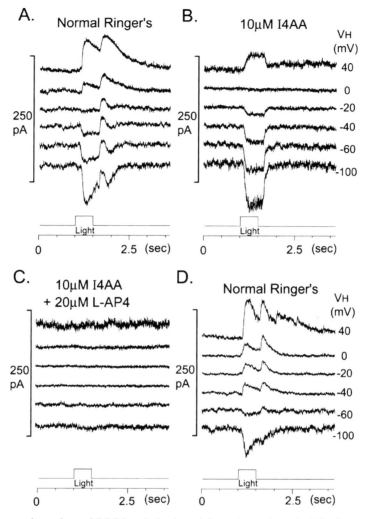

Fig. 1. Current records from a voltage clamped DBC in a dark-adapted tiger salamander retinal slice in normal Ringer's (A), in 10 μM I4AA (B), in 10 μM I4AA + 20 μM L-AP4 (C), and after normal Ringer's wash (D). Currents were recorded at 6 holding potentials (from − 100, − 60, − 40, − 20, 0 and + 40 mV), and a 0.5 s light step (650 nm, − 1 log unit attenuation, 500 μm spot, covering the bipolar cell receptive field center) was delivered to the cell at each holding potential (from Gao et al., 2000).

conditions, the addition of 1–2 μM strychnine did not exert further effects on the light-evoked current (not shown). ΔI_C was completely and reversibly abolished (Fig. 1C and D) by subsequent addition of 20 μM L-AP4, a specific glutamate analogue for the DBC glutamate receptors (Slaughter and Miller, 1981; Nawy and Jahr, 1990). These results demonstrate that the current responses of DBCs to center illumination (500 μm light spots) are mediated by two current components: an L-AP4-sensitive ΔI_C and an I4AA-sensitive ΔI_{Cl}.

Figure 2 shows a similar set of experiments on an OFF-center bipolar cell (or *hyperpolarizing bipolar cell*, HBC). The light-evoked current response of HBCs also had two components. At E_{Cl} this cell exhibited a sustained outward ΔI_C during the light step and a transient inward ΔI_C at light offset, both mediated by photoreceptor inputs (Slaughter and Miller, 1983a, b). Near E_C, the cell gave rise to more slowly developing outward currents (ΔI_{Cl}) during the light step and at light offset, both probably mediated by amacrine cells. Because light elicited a cationic

128

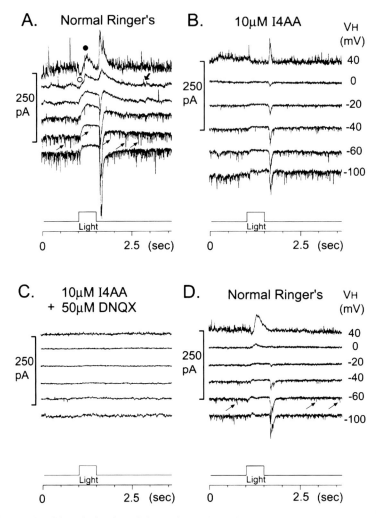

Fig. 2. Current records from an HBC in a dark-adapted tiger salamander retinal slice in normal Ringer's (A), in 10 μM I4AA (B), in 10 μM I4AA + 50 μM DNQX (C), and after normal Ringer's wash (D) with the same voltage clamp protocol and light stimuli as the DBC shown in Fig. 1. Discrete spontaneous excitatory and inhibitory postsynaptic currents (sEPSCs, smaller arrows in A and D, sIPSCs, large arrow in A) are present (from Gao et al., 2000).

conductance decrease and a simultaneous chloride conductance increase, the peak response of this cell to light onset (marked with ● in Fig. 2A) did not exhibit a reversal potential, but both the brief initial response (marked with ○) and the large transient current at light offset reversed near 0 mV, consistent with being generated by a cationic conductance mechanism. Application of 10 μM I4AA also blocked ΔI_{Cl} in HBCs (Fig. 2B), and subsequent addition of 50 μM DNQX, a specific AMPA/kainate receptor antagonist, reversibly blocked ΔI_C (Fig. 2C and 2D). These results suggest that the current

responses of HBCs to center illumination (500 μm light spots) are mediated by two current components: a DNQX-sensitive ΔI_C and an I4AA-sensitive ΔI_{Cl}.

The balance of rod and cone inputs to bipolar cells

In the tiger salamander retina, cones display similar sensitivity to red and green light, while rods are much more sensitive to green light (Yang and Wu, 1989, 1996). Consequently, the relative strength of rod and cone inputs to bipolar cells can be estimated

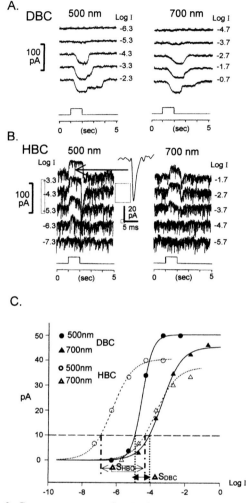

Fig. 3. Current responses of a DBC (A) and an HBC (B) to 500 nm and 700 nm light steps of various intensities (the intensity for each trace is given in log units of attenuation). Inset in B, one of the sEPSCs that contributed to the current noise of this cell. (C) The response-intensity relations for these current responses. The horizontal dashed line indicates the criterion response amplitude (10 pA) used to calculate ΔS (from Wu et al., 2000).

by a measure termed the *spectral difference*: $\Delta S = S_{700} - S_{500}$, where S_{700} and S_{500} correspond to intensities of 700 nm and 500 nm light giving responses of equal amplitude, for a small criterion amplitude (Yang and Wu, 1996). This is demonstrated in Fig. 3C, which shows response-intensity curves for light responses (at E_C) for a DBC (Fig. 3A) and an HBC (Fig. 3B). At a criterion response of 10 pA, the spectral difference (ΔS) was 0.8 for the

DBC and 2.6 for the HBC. Since ΔS is about 0.1 for cones and about 3.4 for rods (Yang and Wu, 1990), we concluded that the DBC of Fig. 3 was relatively cone-dominated, while the HBC was relatively rod-dominated. Overall, a wide range of rod–cone dominance was observed both for DBCs ($\Delta S = 0.2 - 2.9$) and for HBCs ($\Delta S = 0.3 - 3.1$). The relative rod or cone dominance (expressed in ΔS) of various types of bipolar cells will be discussed later in this chapter.

Spontaneous excitatory postsynaptic currents (sEPSCs) in bipolar cells

Glutamate is released from photoreceptors through a calcium-dependent vesicular process (Copenhagen and Jahr, 1988; Ayoub et al., 1989). Calcium entry into photoreceptor synaptic terminals triggers exocytosis of glutamatergic vesicles (Rieke and Schwartz, 1996), releasing packages of glutamate, each of which activate a number of glutamate receptors that initiate transient postsynaptic currents termed miniature excitatory postsynaptic currents (mEPSCs) (Maple et al., 1994). Since one cannot always be certain that these transient postsynaptic events are mediated by single exocytotic events, we have used the term *spontaneous* (instead of *miniature*) excitatory postsynaptic currents, or sEPSCs, to describe the discrete currents observed in bipolar cells. SEPSCs are seen in most HBCs, but analogous (sign inverted) discrete postsynaptic currents are generally not observed in DBCs (Maple et al., 1999; Wu and Maple, 1998) (compare Figs. 1 and 2, 3A and B, for example). This probably reflects a difference in the kinetics of the glutamate receptors in DBCs and HBCs. DBCs utilize L-AP4 metabotropic glutamate receptors, which generate relatively slow conductance changes via a second messenger system (Nawy, 1999). Therefore, the postsynaptic response to transmitter release from a single vesicle, or cluster of vesicles is likely to be heavily filtered in DBCs. HBCs, on the other hand, utilize rapidly activating ionotropic AMPA receptors, and are capable of generating sEPSCs with a rise time of about 1 ms (Smith and Dudek, 1996).

Figure 4 shows data from an experiment where a rod and an HBC were simultaneously voltage clamped in a retinal slice. Depolarization of the rod

130

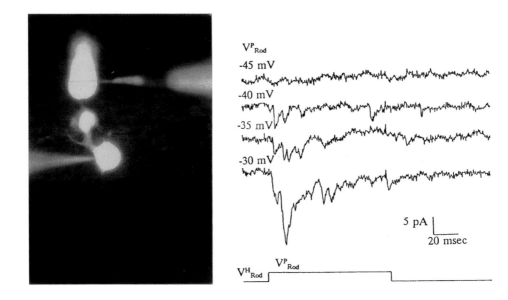

Fig. 4. (A) Fluorescence photograph of a rod and an HBC, both filled with Lucifer Yellow and under simultaneous voltage clamp. (B) Current responses of the HBC to depolarization of the rod. The HBC was held at -40 mV ($= E_{Cl}$) and the rod was stepped from a holding potential (V_{Rod}^{H}) of -50 mV to various pulse potentials (V_{Rod}^{P}). SEPSCs increased in frequency with progressive depolarization of the rod (from Wu and Maple, 1998).

caused an increase of sEPSC frequency in the HBC, consistent with voltage-dependent vesicular release of neurotransmitter from the rods. The sEPSCs in HBCs reversed near 0 mV (Fig. 5Aa), as did responses to focal application of 100 μM glutamate at the HBC dendrites (Fig. 5Ab), suggesting that both involve a similar conductance mechanism. The frequency of sEPSCs decreased about 10 fold when the Ca^{2+} in the Ringer's solution was replaced with Co^{2+} (Fig. 5Bb), consistent with the sEPSCs being mediated by calcium-dependent neurotransmitter release (Weakly, 1973). In Co^{2+} Ringer's the sEPSC frequency increased by about 4 fold when the osmolarity of the solution was increased by the addition of 0.5 M sucrose (Fig. 5Bc), and this is also consistent with vesicular release of neurotransmitter (Fatt and Katz, 1952) from photoreceptors. Finally, the sEPSCs were abolished by 20 μM CNQX, an antagonist for kainate/AMPA type glutamate receptors (Monaghan et al., 1989) (Fig. 5Bd). Taken together, these results suggest that synaptic transmission from photoreceptors to bipolar cells is mediated by sEPSCs that result from Ca^{2+}-dependent, vesicular release of glutamate from photoreceptors.

Horizontal cell inputs to bipolar cells: feedback and feedforward synaptic pathways

Horizontal cells mediate bipolar cell surround responses through a feedback synaptic pathway (horizontal cell → cone → bipolar cell) (Baylor et al., 1971; Burkhardt, 1977; Wu, 1991a) and through feedforward synapses (horizontal cell → bipolar cell) (Dowling and Werblin, 1969; Yang and Wu, 1991; Hare and Owen, 1992; Wu, 1992). Two major synaptic mechanisms have been proposed for the feedback actions of horizontal cells on cones. A long-standing hypothesis is that horizontal cells release an inhibitory neurotransmitter (GABA, in several species) in darkness that binds to receptors on cone synaptic terminals and opens chloride channels in the cone plasma membrane. In this scheme, when illumination of the receptive field surround hyperpolarizes the horizontal cells and suppresses feedback transmitter release, the cones are depolarized, causing depolarization in HBCs and hyperpolarization in DBCs (Murakami et al., 1982; Kaneko and Tachibana, 1986; Wu, 1991a). A second proposed mechanism is that horizontal cells directly modulate calcium currents in cones, resulting in an increase of

A.

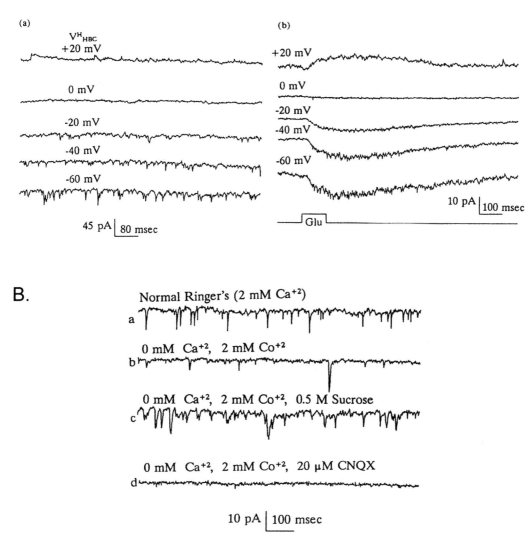

Fig. 5. (Aa) SEPSCs of an HBC, clamped at different potentials. The sEPSCs reversed near 0 mV. (Ab) Current responses of an HBC to focal pressure ejection of 100 μM glutamate near the dendrites. These responses also reversed near 0 mV. (B) SEPSCs from an HBC in (a) normal Ringer's solution, (b) Ringer's with Co^{2+} substituted for Ca^{2+}, (c) hyperosmotic Co^{2+} Ringer's, and (d) Co^{2+} Ringer's containing 20 μM CNQX (adapted from Maple et al., 1994).

the calcium-dependent glutamate release that depolarizes the HBCs and hyperpolarizes the DBCs (Karmermans and Spekreijse, 1999). It is possible that one or the other mechanism is favored in different species or under different conditions. The two mechanisms may also coexist in some feedback synapses in which both $GABA_A$-gated chloride channels and calcium current modulation are involved.

Properties of the feedforward synapses are less well understood. Studies of the salamander retina have suggested that feedforward synapses contribute significantly to the surround antagonism of DBC light responses (Yang and Wu, 1991; Hare and Owen, 1992; Wu, 1992). However, application of GABA to the dendrites of salamander bipolar cells elicits no response (in Co^{2+} Ringer's) (Maple and Wu, 1996), so if horizontal cells make feedforward synapses on bipolar cells in the salamander retina, GABA is probably not the neurotransmitter used at these synapses. Histochemical evidence suggests that only about 50–60% of the horizontal in the salamander retina are GABAergic (Wu, 1986; 1991b), the identity of neurotransmitter(s) used by the rest of the horizontal cells is unknown (but unlikely to be glycine (Wu, 1991b; Wu and Maple, 1998; Yang and Yazulla, 1988a, b)). A feedforward synapse from horizontal cells to DBCs would require an excitatory synaptic conductance mechanism, but no such mechanism has yet been found on the dendrites of salamander DBCs.

Figure 6A summarizes the horizontal cell (HC) feedback (synapses 1 and 2) and hypothetical feedforward (synapse 3) synaptic pathways to the DBCs. Figure 6B shows the input–output relations of the HC → cone → DBC feedback synaptic pathway (solid curve in the lower left quadrant) obtained by combining the input–output relations of the HC → cone synapse (upper left quadrant, (Wu, 1991a)) and the input–output relation of the cone → DBC synapse (lower right quadrant). The input–output relation of the hypothetical HC → DBC feedforward synaptic pathway (dashed curve in lower left quadrant) was obtained by recording the HC and DBC light responses in the presence of L-AP4, which

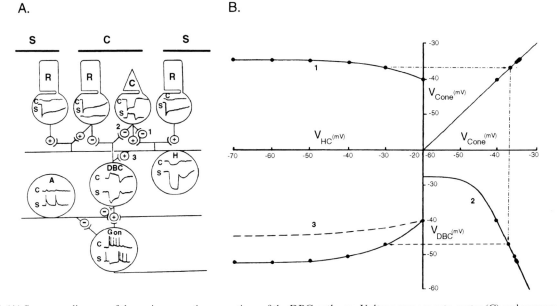

Fig. 6. (A) Summary diagram of the major synaptic connections of the DBC pathway. Voltage responses to center (C) and surround (S) light stimuli are shown in each cell. R, rod. C, cone. H, horizontal cell. A, amacrine cell. G_{on}, ON-center ganglion cell. (+), sign-preserving chemical synapse. (−), sign-inverting chemical synapse. Synapse 1 is the HC-cone feedback synapse, synapse 2 is the cone-DBC synapse, and synapse 3 is the HC-DBC feedforward synapse. (B) Input–Output relation of the HC-DBC feedback synaptic pathway (solid curves) and the feedforward synapse (synapse 3; dashed curve in lower left quadrant). The upper left quadrant shows the input–output relation of the HC-cone feedback synapse (synapse 1) obtained with the truncated cone preparation (Wu, 1991a). The lower right quadrant shows the input–output relation of the cone-DBC synapse (synapse 2; SM Wu, unpublished data). Data points in the lower left quadrant were obtained by projecting data points in the HC-cone feedback input–output relation to the upper-right, lower-right and then lower-left quadrants (broken arrows). This procedure gives rise to the input–output relation of the HC-DBC signals through the feedback pathway (solid curve in lower left quadrant). The voltage gain of the HC-DBC feedback pathway equals the product of the HC-cone feedback synapse and that of the cone-DBC synapse. Near the HC dark potential (− 20 mV), for example, the voltage gain of the HC-DBC feedback pathway = (voltage gain of the HC-cone feedback synapse) × (voltage gain of the cone-DBC synapse) = (− 0.33) × (− 1.75) = + 0.58. The dashed curve in the lower left quadrant was obtained by recording the HC and DBC responses in the presence of 20 μM L-AP4, which selectively blocks the photoreceptor-DBC synapses without affecting the HC responses (Yang and Wu, 1991). Therefore, the dashed curve represents the input–output relation of the HC-DBC feedforward synapse, because one of the synapses (the cone-DBC synapse, 2 in Fig. 6A) in the feedback pathway is blocked by L-AP4. (from Wu, 1992).

selectively blocks the photoreceptor → DBC synapses (Yang and Wu, 1991). It is important to note that the DBC light responses in L-AP4 may not, in fact, be completely mediated by horizontal cell synapses. It is quite possible that inhibitory synapses made by sustained amacrine cells onto bipolar cell axon terminals contribute to this surround antagonism. This point will be addressed again later.

Amacrine cell inputs to bipolar cells

We have already shown (in Figs. 1 and 2) how changes in the illumination of a bipolar cell's receptive field center can elicit chloride conductance increases. Two neurotransmitters, GABA and glycine, are known to activate chloride conductances in bipolar cells. In bipolar cells of the salamander retina, glycine receptors are present on both the dendrites and axon terminals, while GABA receptors are present only on the axon terminals (Wu and Maple, 1998). Since there is no evidence for GABAergic or glycinergic horizontal cell input to salamander

bipolar cells, the chief candidates for the presynaptic neurons mediating ΔI_{Cl} are GABAergic and glycinergic amacrine cells and interplexiform cells. Each of these will now be discussed in turn.

GABAergic amacrine cell inputs to bipolar cells

The majority of amacrine cells use GABA or glycine as their neurotransmitter (Smiley and Yazulla, 1990; Yang and Yazulla, 1988a, b). While the GABA receptors on amacrine cells and ganglion cells are largely GABA$_A$ receptors, those on bipolar cell axon terminals are largely GABA$_C$ receptors (Lukasiewicz, 1996; Koulen et al., 1997; Lukasiewicz and Shields, 1998) (although GABA$_A$- and GABA$_B$-mediated responses have also been observed in bipolar cells (Maguire et al., 1989)). Figure 7 shows that the light-evoked chloride current (ΔI_{Cl}) and the chloride current induced by focal application of GABA at the IPL were suppressed in both DBCs and HBCs by I4AA. Moreover, it has been shown that the primary site of I4AA action is in the inner retina

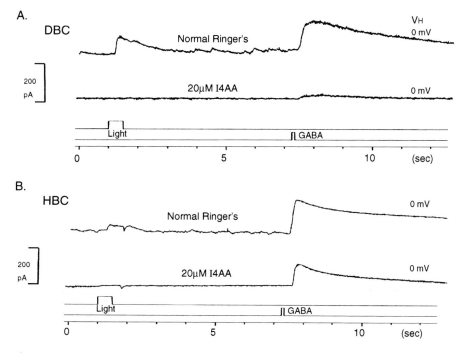

Fig. 7. Effects of 20 μM I4AA on light-evoked and GABA-induced chloride currents in a DBC (A) and an HBC (B). The cells were voltage clamp at 0 mV (near E$_C$), and a 0.5 s light step (650 nm, − 1, 500 μm spot) and a 200 ms puff of GABA (500 μM in puff pipettes at the IPL) were delivered (from Gao et al., 2000).

134

(Gao et al., 2000). These results are consistent with the idea that ΔI_{Cl} in bipolar cells is largely mediated by GABAergic amacrine cells via $GABA_C$ receptors. It is important to note, as we will show later, that not all types of bipolar cells exhibit a large ΔI_{Cl}, suggesting that GABAergic amacrine cells exert different feedback inhibitory actions to different types of bipolar cells.

Glycinergic amacrine cell inputs to bipolar cells

Discrete inhibitory postsynaptic currents (sIPSCs) mediated by glycinergic amacrine cells and interplexiform cells have been observed in bipolar cells (Maple and Wu, 1998; Tian et al., 1998; Gao and Wu, 1998; 1999). In order to determine whether sIPSCs in bipolar cells were of dendritic or axonal origin, we utilized the Ca^{2+} dependence of synaptic

transmission at these synapses. At the IPL, glutamate depolarizes amacrine cells (Maple and Wu, 1996) and interplexiform cells (Maple and Wu, 1998), both of which may release glycine at synapses on bipolar cells. Our experimental strategy was to determine the location of glycinergic synaptic inputs to bipolar cells by applying glutamate to the IPL in Co^{2+} Ringer's (which blocked synaptic transmission (Weakly, 1973)), with simultaneous focal application of Ca^{2+} Ringer's solution at various locations in order to locally reenable synaptic transmission. For the DBC shown in Fig. 8, when synaptic transmission was locally reenabled at the dendrites (A), IPL application of glutamate did not elicit any response, but when synaptic transmission was locally enabled at the axon terminals (B), sIPSCs *were* elicited by IPL glutamate application. We observed glutamate-induced axonal sIPSCs in 69% of forty-two bipolar cells studied with intact axons. Such axonal sIPSCs

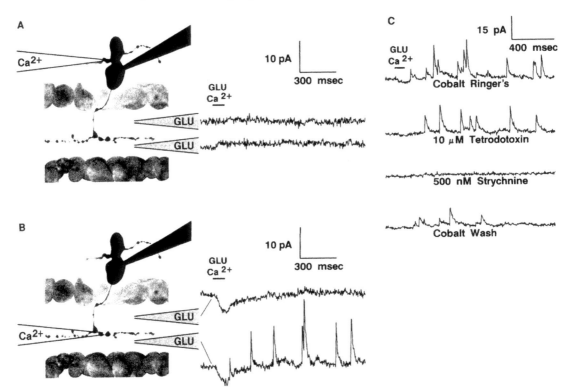

Fig. 8. Characterization of telodendritic glycinergic IPSCs. Responses are shown for a DBC stimulated by simultaneous focal application of glutamate (GLU) and calcium in a Co^{2+} Ringer solution bath. (A) sIPSCs were not elicited when calcium was applied to the dendrites. (B) sIPSCs were observed when calcium was applied to the telodendria, but only when glutamate was also applied at the proximal IPL. (C) The telodendritic sIPSCs were relatively unaffected by 10 μM TTX, but were reversibly abolished by 500 nM strychnine. The holding potential was − 10 mV for all traces (adapted from Maple and Wu, 1998).

were always reversibly abolished by 500 nM strychnine (C), so they appear to be generated by glycinergic synapses. These sIPSCs also persisted in 10 µM tetrodotoxin (TTX), suggesting that they can be generated in the absence of presynaptic sodium spikes. We observed axonal sIPSCs in 69% of 42 bipolar cells with intact axons. These results suggest that most bipolar cells receive synaptic inputs from glycinergic amacrine cells, and that these inputs are mediated by discrete sIPSCs generated at the bipolar cell axon terminals.

Interplexiform cell inputs to bipolar cells

Synaptic inputs from interplexiform cells to bipolar cell dendrites were studied by the same approach as for the glycinergic amacrine cell inputs. Figure 9A shows a spatial profile for responses of a DBC to application of glutamate at different levels of the retina. Discrete IPSCs were weakly elicited when glutamate was applied at the OPL, but much larger responses were elicited by application of glutamate to the IPL. Furthermore, the glycinergic IPSCs were elicited most strongly, and with the shortest latency, when glutamate was applied to the distal IPL (sublamina A), where the HBCs make their output synapses. Application of glutamate at the proximal IPL (sublamina B) near the axon terminals of this cell elicited far fewer glycinergic IPSCs, with a long latency, riding on top of a more graded inhibition (probably GABAergic) that was not obviously composed of discrete IPSCs. Figure 9C shows when Co^{2+} was substituted for Ca^{2+} in the bath, glutamate puffs at the distal IPL elicited IPSCs when calcium was applied near the dendrites, but not when calcium was applied near the axon terminal. This result was consistent with the presence of Ca^{2+}-dependent glycinergic synapses at the bipolar cell dendrites. Calcium sensitivity was definitely restricted

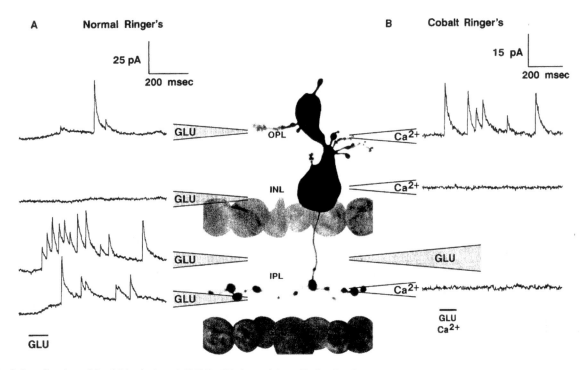

Fig. 9. Localization of dendritic glycinergic IPSCs. (A) A spatial profile for the glutamate (GLU) responses of a DBC. The IPSCs were best elicited by application of glutamate at the distal IPL, although a weaker response was also isolated to the OPL. (B) Responses to application of glutamate at the distal IPL. In this case, the cell was bathed in Co^{2+} Ringer solution and Ca^{2+} Ringer solution was simultaneously applied focally to different regions of the slice. IPSCs were elicited only when calcium was applied at the OPL. The holding potential was -10 mV for all traces (from Maple and Wu, 1998).

A.

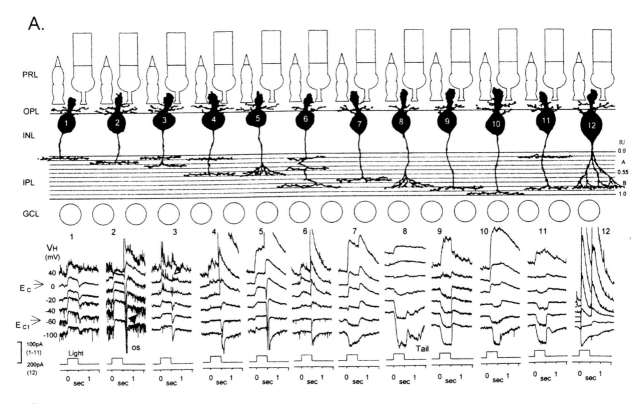

B.

Cell Type		1	2	3	4	5	6	7	8	9	10	11	12
Level of axon termination (IU)	1st	.00-.15	.15-.30	.05-0.15	.10-.35	.35-.55	.05-.15	.55-.70	.70-.80	.80-.90	.90-1.0	.10-.20	.80-.90
	2nd			.25-.40	.45-.55		.30-.40					.80-.90	
	3rd						.60-.85						
ΔS ± S.E. (N)		2.8±0.2 (7)	2.2±0.7 (12)	1.7±0.3 (8)	0.9±0.2 (5)	0.4±0.3 (6)	1.1±0.2 (2)	0.6±0.4 (7)	1.8±0.5 (13)	0.9±0.3 (4)	2.2±0.5 (6)	1.2±0.4 (2)	1.8±0.5 (3)
ΔI_CON±S.E. in pA (N)		+70±9 (8)	+53±5 (14)	+35±5 (10)	+12±3 (6)	+41±7 (7)	+23±7 (2)	-38±4 (7)	-50±7 (13)	-74±8 (4)	-67±9 (8)	-83±6 (2)	-76±11 (3)
ΔI_COFF OS		-.31±.23	-4.9±1.3	-3.8±1.0	-4.8±1.1	-14.5±2.5	-2.8±.7	-.19±.1	.13±.1	-.09±.04	.35±.23	-.02±.14	.63±.02
ΔI_CON Tail		.57±.04	.50±.09	.29±.08	.13±.08	.49±.07	.19±.13	.06±.04	.43±.09	.01±.01	.38±.07	.09±.06	.03±.02
ΔI_{Cl}ON /ΔI_CON		.68±.07	.63±.09	1.04±.24	1.8±.5	1.5±.6	3.7±.1	-2.2±.2	-.91±.31	-.22±.05	-1.18±.26	-.01±.01	-6.3±.3
ΔI_COFF/ΔI_CON		-.18±.06	-.96±.22	-.78±.15	-13.2±2.9	-2.8±.8	-7.9±.9	.8±.2	.28±.07	.26±.07	.31±.13	.23±.07	4.0±.1
sEPSCs		***	***	*	*	**	**	0	0	0	0	**	0
sIPSCs		*	*	***	***	0	***	**	*	**	0	*	**

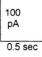

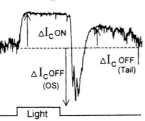

HBC
($V_H = E_{Cl} = -60$mV)

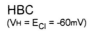

DBC
($V_H = E_{Cl} = -60$mV)

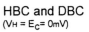

HBC and DBC
($V_H = E_C = 0$mV)

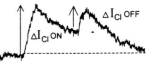

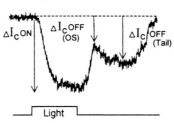

to the OPL, as no responses were obtained when calcium was applied at the mid INL, contrary to what would be expected, if the IPSCs occurred at amacrine cell synapses on the bipolar cell body. Dendritic IPSCs were observed in only 16% (which included both DBCs and HBCs) of the 44 cells studied in this manner, and all dendritic IPSCs could be reversibly abolished by 500 nM strychnine (Maple and Wu, 1998). These results suggest that subpopulations of bipolar cells received synaptic inputs from glycinergic interplexiform cells, which mediate discrete IPSCs by strychnine-sensitive glycine receptors in the OPL.

Segregation of visual signals by stratification of bipolar cell axon terminals in the IPL

We have characterized bipolar cells of the salamander retina according to five physiological parameters associated with the synaptic inputs described in the previous section: (1) the amplitude of light-evoked excitatory inputs (ΔI_C) from photoreceptors; (2) the spectral difference (ΔS), which reflects the relative strengths of rod and cone inputs; (3) the mean amplitude of discrete postsynaptic currents (sEPSCs) generated by vesicular release of glutamate from photoreceptors; (4) the magnitude of light-evoked inhibitory inputs (ΔI_{Cl}) from GABAergic amacrine cells (and possibly other inhibitory neurons); (5) the rate of discrete inhibitory synaptic currents (sIPSCs) generated by glycinergic amacrine cells and/or inter-plexiform cells. In addition, fluorescence microscopy was used to characterize bipolar cell morphology, with emphasis on the shape of the axon terminals and the levels at which the terminals ramified in the IPL. Combining these physiological and morphological data, we were able to define 12 different classes

of bipolar cells, as summarized in Fig. 10. The physiological parameters tabulated in Fig. 10B will now be discussed with respect to how visual signals are mapped in the IPL.

Segregation of ON-center and OFF-center bipolar cell (DBC and HBC) outputs in the IPL

All bipolar cells that ramified exclusively in sub-lamina A of the IPL (types 1–5 in Fig. 10) exhibited an outward light-evoked current (ΔI_C) near E_{Cl}, and thus, they were HBCs. Likewise, all cells that ramified exclusively in sublamina B (types 7–10) were DBCs, exhibiting an inward ΔI_C near E_{Cl}. These results are in agreement with the general observation that the OFF-center and ON-center pathways are segregated into sublamina A and sublamina B, respectively (Famiglietti and Kolb, 1976; Nelson et al., 1978). However, we observed three types of bipolar cells that ramified in both sublamina A and sublamina B. One of these was a class of pyramidally branching cell (type 12), with axonal processes that began branching in sublamina A but terminated at a proximal level of sublamina B (0.8–0.9 IU (inner plexiform units, with the INL margin corresponding to 0.0 IU and the ganglion cell margin to 1.0 IU (Wu et al., 2000)). These cells appeared to be purely DBCs, based on an inward ΔI_C at E_{Cl} and the absence of sEPSCs. Another class of cell (type 11) that stratified in both sublamina A and sublamina B appeared to be a hybrid. These cells exhibited sEPSCs and excitatory responses to dendritic application of glutamate (like HBCs) (Maple and Wu, 1996), also displayed a net inward ΔI_C at E_{Cl} (like DBCs). A tristratified cell (type 6) also appeared to possess both ON and OFF conductance mechanisms. These cells

Fig. 10. **A.** Morphology (sketches of Lucifer yellow filled cells in retinal slices) and light-evoked current responses recorded under voltage clamp conditions at various holding potentials. For all cells, $E_C \approx 0$ mV and $E_{Cl} = -60$ mV, and thus ΔI_C and sEPSCs were measured at -60 mV and ΔI_{Cl} and sIPSCs were measured at 0 mV. Vertical calibration bar at the lower left side of the current responses is 100 pA for type 1–11 bipolar cells and 200 pA for the type 12 bipolar cell. **B.** Summary of the levels of axon terminal ramification in the IPL (in IU), the average $\pm$ standard error (S.E.) values (N: number of cells for the averaging) of the relative spectral difference (ΔS) and the amplitude (in pA) and polarity (+: outward, $-$: inward) of the light-evoked excitatory current at light onset (ΔI_CON), the ratios of excitatory current response at light offset/onset (ΔI_COFF/ΔI_CON) for off overshoot (OS) and tail (Tail) responses, the ratios of light-evoked inhibitory ON and OFF current response/excitatory ON current response (ΔI_{Cl}ON/ΔI_CON, ΔI_{Cl}OFF/ΔI_CON), and the relative amplitude of sEPSCs and frequency of sIPSCs (0: absent, *: low, **: medium, ***: high) for the 12 classes of bipolar cells. The inserts at the bottom of Fig. 5B illustrate how ΔI_CON, ΔI_COFF(OS), ΔI_COFF(Tail), ΔI_{Cl}ON and ΔI_{Cl}OFF of the HBC and the DBC are measured. The values of ΔI_COFF(OS), ΔI_COFF(Tail), ΔI_{Cl}ON and ΔI_{Cl}OFF are normalized relative to the value of ΔI_CON prior to averaging (from Wu et al., 2000).

normally appeared to be HBCs, with sEPSCs and an outward ΔI_C at E_{Cl}, but in the presence of 100 μM picrotoxin these light responses were converted to an inward (DBC-like) current (not shown). Thus, there appeared to be a perfect correlation between the sign of photoreceptor inputs received by bipolar cells and the level(s) at which the bipolar cells' axonal processes *terminated* in the IPL: cells with processes terminating exclusively in sublamina A received excitation in darkness (OFF-center), cells with axons terminating exclusively in sublamina B received excitation in light (ON-center), and cells with axon terminations in both sublamina A and sublamina B received excitation (and simultaneous deexcitation) both in darkness and in light (ON- and OFF-center).

Rod and cone dominance in the IPL

Output synapses of the rod- and cone-dominated bipolar cells are also segregated in the IPL. The spectral difference data presented in Fig. 10 shows a general trend for rod-dominated bipolar cells to ramify near the margins of the IPL and for cone-dominated cells to ramify more centrally in the IPL. This correlation was particularly strong for the HBCs, with the most rod-dominated cells (types 1 and 2) being monostratified in the distal half of sublamina A (sA_1: 0.0–0.3 IU) and the most cone-dominated cells (type 5) being monostratified or pyramidally-branching within the proximal half of sublamina A (sA_2: 0.3-0.55 IU). Even within sA_1 a gradient of rod-cone dominance was observed, with the cells ramifying in the distal half of sA_1 (type 1) being the most rod-dominated of all bipolar cells observed, and with cells ramifying in the proximal half of sA_1 (type 2) being slightly less rod-dominated. Cells that were bistratified within sublamina A displayed intermediate values of ΔS, but these could still be divided into two different classes, based on anatomy and spectral sensitivity. The bistratified HBCs exhibited a wide range of axon terminal morphologies, but spectrally they fell into two groups, which also differed consistently with respect to their more proximal level of ramification. Type 4 cells, with a proximal stratum at a depth of 0.45–0.55 IU, were more cone-dominated than type 3

cells, whose most proximal level of ramification was at 0.25–0.40 IU.

The gradient of rod and cone dominance for the DBCs in the IPL was similar, but less strict than for the HBCs. Following a margin to center organization of rod–cone dominance, the most proximally ramifying DBCs (type 10; 0.9–1.0 IU) were rod-dominated, the most centrally ramifying DBCs (type 7; 0.55–0.7 IU) were cone-dominated, and cells ramifying at intermediate levels were more mixed (types 8 and 9; 0.7–0.9 IU). On the other hand, the mixed cells fell into two different classes that received more or less rod input (types 8 and 9, respectively), and among these there was no simple correlation between ΔS and the level of ramification. It appears that rod and cone information is not segregated as simply for the ON-center pathways of the retina, as it is for the OFF-center pathways.

The kinetics of the photoreceptor inputs at light offset was also consistent with these gradients of rod–cone dominance in the IPL. Cone photoreceptors rapidly depolarize to a steady state dark potential at the cessation of a light stimulus, whereas rod photoreceptors depolarize more slowly, taking seconds to reach a steady state potential (Yang and Wu, 1996). This was reflected in the photoreceptor component of bipolar cell light responses, as visible in Fig. 10A for the traces at − 60 mV (E_{Cl}). At light offset, the responses of cone-dominated cells (those with a small ΔS) were dominated by a rapidly developing, strongly transient inward current (in the case of HBCs) or a slightly less rapidly developing, mildly transient outward current (in the case of DBCs). For HBCs this transient tended to shoot beyond the pre-stimulus dark current level, and the size of this overshoot (ΔI_{COFF}(OS) in figure 10, relative to the size of the response to light onset) was negatively correlated with ΔS. The responses of rod-dominated cells (those with a large ΔS), on the other hand, were dominated by a slowly developing inward current (in the case of HBCs) or outward current (in the case of DBCs). The size of this slow current tail (ΔI_{COFF}(tail) in Fig. 10, given relative to the response at light onset) was positively correlated with ΔS. (The type 5 cone-dominated HBCs, which displayed a sizeable tail, were an exception to this rule. It is not clear why this was so, but perhaps these cells receive particularly strong input from a type of rod, rod$_C$, which is strongly electrically coupled to cones (Wu, 1988; Wu and Yang, 1988)). These observations are consistent with a general tendency for cone-dominated bipolar cells to ramify more centrally in the IPL than rod-dominated bipolar cells.

SEPSCs in HBCs

Rod- and cone-dominated HBCs could also be distinguished by characteristics of the sEPSCs associated with their photoreceptor inputs (Maple et al., 1994; Wu and Maple, 1998). Rod-dominated HBCs (types 1 and 2) were readily identified by the presence of large amplitude sEPSCs. SEPSCs were also observed in the more cone-dominated HBCs (types 3-6), but they appeared to be much smaller in mean amplitude. It is beyond the scope of this review to quantitatively analyze these sEPSCs, so their amplitudes are characterized in an approximate scale (0—***) in Fig. 10B. It is worth to note that the rod-dominated HBCs (types 1 and 2) could be easily and reliably distinguished from more cone-dominated HBCs (types 3-6) based on qualitative examination of the noise associated with ΔI_C. As is visible in the traces of Fig. 10, the rod-dominated HBCs exhibited much more noise (at E_{Cl}) and some much larger sEPSCs (of up to 1 nS peak conductance) than did the cone-dominated HBCs. This difference points to a *functional* segregation of rod and cone information in the IPL. Perhaps it is advantageous for the retina to operate in a more stochastic mode when analyzing dim signals and a less stochastic mode when analyzing bright signals (Ashmore and Falk, 1981). Large voltage fluctuations in rod-dominated HBCs probably play a significant role in generating the high frequency of spontaneous action potentials observed in ganglion cells under dark-adapted conditions (Kuffler et al., 1957).

Inhibitory inputs to bipolar cells

As discussed previously, most bipolar cells, when held near E_C, displayed outward current responses at light onset and light offset. In cases where these inhibitory responses were very transient (e.g. the onset response of cell 12 or the offset response of cell 5

in Fig. 10), they clearly reversed near E_{Cl}, indicating they were generated by a chloride conductance increase. It was more difficult to characterize the I–V properties of more sustained inhibitory inputs, since these were masked by photoreceptor inputs at holding potentials away from E_C. Nevertheless, the overall I–V characteristics of the light responses suggested that a sustained chloride conductance increase contributed to the onset response of many bipolar cells. Consider, for instance, the responses to light onset for HBC types 1, 2, and 5 in Fig. 10. The responses of type 2 cells reversed near $+20$ mV, considerably positive to the reversal potential for glutamate-activated currents in HBCs. This is understandable, if the light-induced cationic conductance decrease occurring at photoreceptor synapses was accompanied by a smaller conductance *increase* to an ion with a negative equilibrium potential (for instance, a *chloride* conductance increase at amacrine cell synapses). In the case of type 1 HBCs, the light responses did not reverse at all, and that is consistent with a chloride conductance increase, that was comparable in magnitude to the cationic conductance decrease at photoreceptor synapses. Finally, for type 5 HBCs the light responses did not reverse, but became *larger* with increasingly positive potentials, and this is consistent with a chloride conductance increase that was larger than the accompanying cationic conductance decrease. Since DBCs undergo a cationic conductance increase at light onset, a simultaneous chloride conductance increase would be expected to make the light response reverse negative to E_C in these cells, and this was, in fact, observed. Where the reversal potential of DBC light responses differed from E_C, it was always negative to E_C (and positive to E_{Cl}).

The table in Fig. 10B summarizes the relative strengths of the inferred chloride currents at light onset ($\Delta I_{Cl}ON$) and light offset ($\Delta I_{Cl}OFF$) for each of the 12 classes of bipolar cells we have defined. Among the 6 classes of HBCs, the mean values of both $\Delta I_{Cl}ON$ and $\Delta I_{Cl}OFF$ (relative to the magnitude of $\Delta I_C ON$) were negatively correlated with ΔS, i.e. the inhibition at both light onset and light offset was stronger for the cone-dominated cells than for the rod dominated cells. Among the DBC's there was not, in general, a strong correlation between either $\Delta I_{Cl}ON$ or $\Delta I_{Cl}OFF$ and ΔS, but both ON and

OFF inhibition were stronger for the most cone-dominated cells (type 7) than for the most rod-dominated cells (type 10). Overall, the strength of these inhibitory inputs appeared to be more closely related to axon morphology than to the value of ΔS per se. The relative magnitude of $\Delta I_{Cl}ON$ and tended to be largest among bipolar cell types 4, 5, 6, 7, and 12, all cells with ramifications near a central region (0.4–0.7 IU) of the IPL. Similarly, $\Delta I_{Cl}OFF$ was largest in cells with ramifications in sublamina A_2 (0.3–0.55 IU).

The receptive field organization of inhibitory inputs to bipolar cells has not yet been investigated, but a few points should be noted with respect to surround antagonism. First, ΔI_{Cl} can not mediate surround antagonism of HBC responses to light onset, because it is synergistic with the photoreceptor inputs. [E_{Cl} is probably near -60 mV in bipolar cells (Maple and Wu, 1998). This is negative to the resting potential of bipolar cells in darkness, and negative to potentials at which bipolar cell synaptic calcium conductances are measurably activated (Heidelberger and Matthews, 1992).] On the other hand, $\Delta I_{Cl}OFF$ *can* antagonize the excitatory OFF overshoots ($\Delta I_{COFF}(OS)$) observed in HBCs. In other words, inhibitory inputs from amacrine cells do not contribute to a static inhibitory surround in HBCs, but they might be important in regulating sensitivity to transient light stimuli. In contrast, a ΔI_{Cl} generated by amacrine cells *could* contribute to an inhibitory surround in DBCs. This is especially a possibility for the type 10, rod-dominated DBCs, which exhibit a relatively large and sustained $\Delta I_{Cl}ON$. As discussed previously, bipolar cell inhibitory surrounds are thought to be largely generated through presynaptic inhibition of cones by horizontal cells, but in the DBC pathway, amacrine cells could conceivably generate an inhibitory surround for rod signals. On the other hand, amacrine cells probably contribute little to the inhibitory surrounds of type 9 and 11 DBCs, since $\Delta I_{Cl}ON$ is very small in these cells.

sIPSCs from glycinergic interneurons

A portion of the inhibition received by bipolar cells was mediated by sIPSCs that, as demonstrated previously, appear to be generated at synapses from glycinergic amacrine and interplexiform cells. Most bipolar cells exhibited some sIPSCs, but, overall, this inhibition accounted for only a small fraction of the total chloride current elicited by light stimuli. This type of inhibition was particularly strong, however, in the type 3 bistratified HBCs. These cells, for which *axonal* glycinergic sIPSCs were particularly strongly driven by IPL glutamate application (Maple and Wu, unpublished observations), displayed strong bursts of sIPSCs both at light onset and offset. On the other end of the spectrum, very few or no light-elicited sIPSCs were observed in type 5 HBCs and type 10 DBCs. Type 7 DBCs, which have been shown to receive a particularly strong *dendritic* input from glycinergic interplexiform cells (Maple and Wu, 1998), varied greatly with respect to sIPSC activity: in some, the sIPSCs contributed greatly to $\Delta I_{Cl}OFF$, but in others very few sIPSCs were observed. Further study of inhibitory inputs to bipolar cells may lead to a division of type 7 cells into different subtypes.

Conclusions and future perspectives

In summary, we have used voltage clamp techniques to characterize synaptic mechanisms mediating the excitatory and inhibitory components of bipolar cell light responses. Based on a comparison of light response characteristics and axon terminal morphology, 12 different types of bipolar cells were defined, each with synaptic processes that terminate at a unique depth (or combination of depths) within the IPL. The stratification of bipolar cell axon terminals leads to an orderly mapping of visual signals within the IPL. In addition to a segregation of visual information into OFF-center and ON-center layers (sublaminas A and B, respectively), there is an overlying mapping of spectral information along the depth of the IPL, with cone signals being transmitted predominantly to the central IPL and rod signals predominantly to the margins of the IPL. Superimposed on these two mappings is a more complex set of inhibitory interactions involving amacrine cells and interplexiform cells. It appears that while the retina represents information about positions within the visual world in two dimensions, it also uses the orthogonal third dimension (the depth of the retina) to represent qualities of visual stimuli. This orderly segregation of visual signals along the depth of the IPL simplifies the integration of visual information in the retina, and it begins a chain of parallel information processing pathways organized in three-dimensions in the visual system (Hubel and Livingstone, 1987; Hubel and Wiesel, 1979).

Further research into the outputs of each type of bipolar cells to amacrine cells (ACs) and ganglion cells (GCs) are crucial for unravel mechanisms of signal integration and segregation in the inner retina. It is important to determine, for example, whether dendrites of various types of ACs and GCs stratify in the IPL in patterns that are complementary to the pattern of bipolar cell axon terminal stratification described in Fig. 10, and if they do, whether the qualities of the AC and GC light responses follow the light response qualities of the bipolar cells with axon terminals stratified at the same IPL levels. It is also important to study inhibitory synaptic interactions in the IPL. Fundamental questions remain concerning mechanisms of surround inhibition and the role of amacrine cells in generating bipolar cell receptive field surrounds. Further study of spontaneous post-synaptic currents in bipolar cells should also prove useful, both as an aid in dissecting retinal circuitry and as a tool for understanding mechanisms of synaptic transmission.

Acknowledgments

This work was supported by grants from NIH (EY 04446, EY 02520), the Retina Research Foundation (Houston), the RGK Foundation (Austin), and Research to Prevent Blindness, Inc.

References

Ashmore, J.F. and Falk, G. (1981) Photon-like signals following weak rhodopsin bleaches. *Nature*, 289: 489–491.

Attwell, D., Mobbs, P., Tessier-Lavigne, M. and Wilson, M. (1987) Neurotransmitter-induced currents in retinal bipolar cells of the axolotl, Ambystoma mexicanum. *J. Physiol.*, 387: 125–161.

Ayoub, G.S., Korenbrot, J.I. and Copenhagen, D.R. (1989) Release of endogenous glutamate from isolated cone photo-receptors of the lizard. *Neurosci. Res.*, (Suppl. 10): S47–55.

Baylor, D.A., Fuortes, M.G. and O'Bryan, P.M. (1971) Receptive fields of cones in the retina of the turtle. *J. Physiol.*, 214: 265–294.

Boycott, B.B. and Dowling, J.E. (1969) Organization of the primate retina: light microscopy. *Philos. Trans. R. Soc. Lond. Biol.*, 255: 109–194.

Boycott, B.B. and Wassle, H. (1991) Morphological classification of bipolar cells in the macaque monkey retina. *Eur. J. Neurosci.*, 361: 1069–1088.

Burkhardt, D.A. (1977) Responses and receptive-field organization of cones in perch retinas. *J. Neurophysiol.*, 40: 53–62.

Copenhagen, D.R. and Jahr, C.E. (1988) Release of endogenous excitatory amino acids from turtle photoreceptors. *Nature*, 341: 536–539.

Dowling, J.E. (1968) Synaptic organization of the frog retina: an electron microscopic analysis comparing the retinas of frogs and primates. *Proc. R. Soc. Lond. B. Biol. Sci.*, 170: 205–228.

Dowling, J.E. and Boycott, B.B. (1966) Organization of the primate retina: electron microscopy. *Proc. R. Soc. Lond. B. Biol. Sci.*, 166: 80–111.

Dowling, J.E. and Ehinger, B. (1975) Synaptic organization of the amine-containing interplexiform cells of the goldfish and Cebus monkey retinas. *Science*, 188: 270–273.

Dowling, J.E. and Werblin, F.S. (1969) Organization of retina of the mudpuppy, Necturus maculosus. I. Synaptic structure. *J. Neurophysiol.*, 32: 315–338.

Euler, T. and Wassle, H. (1995) Immunocytochemical identification of cone bipolar cells in the rat retina. *J. Comp. Neurol.*, 361: 461–478.

Famiglietti, E.V., Jr. and Kolb, H. (1976) Structural basis for ON-and OFF-center responses in retinal ganglion cells. *Science*, 194: 193–195.

Fatt, P. and Katz, B. (1952) Spontaneous subthreshold activity at motor nerve endings. *J. Physiol.*, 117: 109–128.

Gao, F., Maple, B.R. and Wu, S.M. (2000) An I4AA-sensitive chloride current contributes to the center light responses of bipolar cells in the tiger salamander retina. *J. Neurophysiol.*, 83: 3473–3482.

Gao, F. and Wu, S.M. (1998) Characterization of spontaneous inhibitory synaptic currents in salamander retinal ganglion cells. *J. Neurophysiol.*, 80: 1752–1764.

Gao, F. and Wu, S.M. (1999) Multiple types of spontaneous excitatory synaptic currents in salamander retinal ganglion cells. *Brain Res.*, 21: 487–502.

Grant, G.B. and Dowling, J.E. (1995) A glutamate-activated chloride current in cone-driven ON bipolar cells of the white perch retina. *J. Neurosci.*, 15: 3852–3862.

Hare, W.A. and Owen, W.G. (1992) Effects of 2-amino-4-phosphonobutyric acid in the distal layers of the tiger salamander's retina. *J. Neurophysiol.*, 445: 741–757.

Hare, W.A. and Owen, W.G. (1996) Receptive field of the retinal bipolar cell: a pharmacological study in the tiger salamander retina. *J. Neurophysiol.*, 76: 2005–2019.

Heidelberger, R. and Matthews, G. (1992) Calcium influx and calcium current in single synaptic terminals of goldfish retinal bipolar neurons. *J. Physiol.* 447: 235–256.

142

Hensley, S.H., Yang, X.L. and Wu, S.M. (1993) Relative contribution of rod and cone inputs to bipolar cells and ganglion cells in the tiger salamander retina. *J. Neurophysiol.*, 69: 2086–2098.

Hubel, D.H. and Livingstone, M.S. (1987) Segregation of form, color, and stereopsis in primate area 18. *J. Neurosci.*, 7: 3378–3415.

Hubel, D.H. and Wiesel, T.N. (1962) Receptive fields, binocular interaction and functional architecture in the cat's visual cortex. *J. Physiol.*, 160: 106–154.

Hubel, D.H. and Wiesel, T.N. (1979) Brain mechanisms of vision. *Sci. Am.*, 241: 150–162.

Kaneko, A. (1970) Physiological and morphological identification of horizontal, bipolar and amacrine cells in goldfish retina. *J. Physiol.*, 207: 623–633.

Kaneko, A. and Tachibana, M. (1986) Effects of gamma-aminobutyric acid on isolated cone photoreceptors of the turtle retina. *J. Physiol.* 373: 443–461.

Karmermans, M. and Spekreijse, H. (1999) The feedback pathway from horizontal cells to cones, a mini review with a look ahead. *Vision Res.*, 39: 2449–2468.

Koulen, P., Brandstatter, J.H., Kroger, S., Enz, R., Bormann, J. and Wassle, H. (1997) Immunocytochemical localization of the GABAc receptor rho subunits in the cat, goldfish and chicken retina. *J. Comp. Neurol.*, 380: 520–532.

Kuffler, S.W. (1953) Discharge patterns and functional organization of the mammalian retina. *J. Neurophysiol.*, 16: 37–68.

Kuffler, S.W., Fitzhugh, R. and Barlow, H.B. (1957) Maintained activity in the cat's retina in light and darkness. *J. Gen. Physiol.*, 40: 683–702.

Lasansky, A. (1973) Organization of the outer synaptic layer in the retina of the larval tiger salamander. *Philos. Trans. R. Soc. Lond. B. Biol. Sci.*, 265: 471–489.

Lasansky, A. (1978) Contacts between receptors and electrophysiologically identified neurones in the retina of the larval tiger salamander. *J. Physiol.*, 285: 531–542.

Lukasiewicz, P. and Shields, C.R. (1998) Different combinations of GABAa and GABAc receptors confer distinct temporal properties to retinal synaptic responses. *J. Neurophysiol.*, 79: 3157–3167.

Lukasiewicz, P.D. (1996) GABA$_C$ receptors in the vertebrate retina. *Mol. Neurobiol.*, 12: 181–194.

Maguire, G., Maple, B., Lukasiewicz, P. and Werblin, F. (1989) Gamma-aminobutyric type B receptor modulation of L-type calcium channel current at bipolar cell terminals in the retina of the tiger salamander. *Proc. Natl. Acad. Sci. USA*, 86: 10144–10147.

Maple, B.R., Gao, F. and Wu, S.M. (1999) Glutamate receptors differ in rod- and cone-dominated off-center bipolar cells. *Neuroreport*, 10: 1–6.

Maple, B.R., Werblin, F.S. and Wu, S.M. (1994) Miniature excitatory postsynaptic currents in bipolar cells of the tiger salamander retina. *Vision Res.*, 34: 2357–2362.

Maple, B.R. and Wu, S.M. (1996) Synaptic inputs mediating bipolar cell responses in the tiger salamander retina. *Vision Res.*, 36: 4015–4023.

Maple, B.R. and Wu, S.M. (1998) Glycinergic synaptic inputs to bipolar cells in the tiger salamander retina. *J. Physiol.*, 506(3): 731–744.

Monaghan, D.T., Bridges, R.J. and Cotman, C.W. (1989) The excitatory amino acid receptors: their classes, pharmacology, and distinct properties in the function of the central nervous system. *Annu. Rev. Pharmacol. Toxicol.*, 29: 365–402.

Murakami, M., Shimoda, Y., Nakatani, K., Miyachi, E. and Watanabe, S. (1982) GABA-mediated negative feedback from horizontal cells to cones in carp retina. *Jpn. J. Physiol.*, 32: 911–926.

Naka, K.I. (1972) The horizontal cells. *Vision Res.*, 12: 573–588.

Nawy, S. (1999) The metabotropic receptor mGluR6 may signal through G$_o$, but not phosphodiesterase, in retinal bipolar cells. *J. Neurosci.*, 19: 2938–2944.

Nawy, S. and Jahr, C.E. (1990) Suppression by glutamate of cGMP-activated conductance in retinal bipolar cells. *Nature*, 346: 269–271.

Nelson, R., Famiglietti, E.V., Jr. and Kolb, H. (1978) Intracellular staining reveals different levels of stratification for on- and off-center ganglion cells in cat retina. *J. Neurophysiol.*, 41: 472–483.

Qian, H. and Dowling, J.E. (1994) Pharmacology of novel GABA receptors found on rod horizontal cells of the white perch retina. *J. Neurosci.*, 14: 4299–4307.

Rieke, F. and Schwartz, E.A. (1996) Asynchronous transmitter release: control of exocytosis and endocytosis at the salamander rod synapse. *J. Physiol.*, 493: 1–8.

Saito, T., Kondo, H. and Toyoda, J.I. (1979) Ionic mechanisms of two types of on-center bipolar cells in the carp retina. I. The responses to central illumination. *J. Gen. Physiol.*, 73: 73–90.

Skrzypek, J. and Werblin, F.S. (1983) Lateral interactions in absence of feedback to cones. *J. Neurophysiol.*, 49: 1007–1016.

Slaughter, M.M. and Miller, R.F. (1981) 2-amino-4-phosphonobutyric acid: a new pharmacological tool for retina research. *Science*, 211: 182–185.

Slaughter, M.M. and Miller, R.F. (1983a) An excitatory amino acid antagonist blocks cone input to signconserving second-order retinal neurons. *Science*, 219: 1230–1232.

Slaughter, M.M. and Miller, R.F. (1983b) Bipolar cells in the mudpuppy retina use an excitatory amino acid neurotransmitter. *Nature*, 303: 537–538.

Smiley, J.F. and Yazulla, S. (1990) Glycinergic contacts in the outer plexiform layer of the Xenopus laevis retina characterized by antibodies to glycine, GABA and glycine receptors. *J. Comp. Neurol.*, 299: 375–388.

Smith, B.N. and Dudek, F.E. (1996) Amino acid-mediated regulation of spontaneous synaptic activity patterns in the rat basolateral amygdala. *J. Neurophysiol.*, 76(3): 1958–1967.

Thibos, L.N. and Werblin, F.S. (1978) The response properties of the steady antagonistic surround in the mudpuppy retina. *J. Physiol.* 278: 79–99.

Tian, N., Hwang, T.N. and Copenhagen, D.R. (1998) Analysis of excitatory and inhibitory spontaneous synaptic activity in mouse retinal ganglion cells. *J. Neurophysiol.*, 80: 1327–1340.

Vallerga, S. (1981) Physiological and morphological identification of amacrine cells in the retina of the larval tiger salamander. *Vision Res.*, 21: 1307–1317.

Weakly, J.N.C. (1973) The action of cobalt ions on neuromuscular transmission in the frog. *J. Physiol.*, 234: 597–612.

Werblin, F.S. and Dowling, J.E. (1969) Organization of the retina of the mudpuppy, Necturus maculosus. II. Intracellular recording. *J. Neurophysiol.*, 32: 339–355.

Wong-Riley, M.T.T. (1974) Synaptic organization of the inner plexiform layer in the retina of the tiger salamander. *J. Neurocytol.*, 3: 1–33.

Wu, S.M. (1986) Effects of gamma-aminobutyric acid on cones and bipolar cells of the tiger salamander retina. *Brain Res.*, 365: 70–77.

Wu, S.M. (1988) The off-overshoot responses of photoreceptors and horizontal cells in the light-adapted retinas of the tiger salamander. *Exp. Eye Res.*, 47: 261–268.

Wu, S.M. (1991a) Input-output relations of the feedback synapse between horizontal cells and cones in the tiger salamander retina. *J. Neurophysiol.*, 65: 1197–1206.

Wu, S.M. (1991b) Signal transmission and adaptation-induced modulation of photoreceptor synapses in the retina. *Prog. Retinal. Res.*, 10: 27–44.

Wu, S.M. (1992) Feedback connections and operation of the outer plexiform layer of the retina. *Curr. Opin. Neurobio.* 2: 462–468.

Wu, S.M., Gao, F. and Maple, B.R. (2000) Functional architecture of synapses in the inner retina: segregation of visual signals by stratification of bipolar cell axon terminals. *J. Neurosci.*, 20(12), 4462–4470.

Wu, S.M. and Maple, B.R. (1998) Amino acid neurotransmitters in the retina: a functional overview. *Vision Res.*, 38(10), 1371–1384.

Wu, S.M. and Yang, X.L. (1988) Electrical coupling between rods and cones in the tiger salamander retina. *Proc. Natl. Acad. Sci. USA*, 85: 275–278.

Yang, C.Y. and Yazulla, S. (1988a) Light microscopic localization of putative glycinergic neurons in the larval tiger salamander retina by immunocytochemical and autoradiographical methods. *J. Comp. Neurol.*, 272: 343–357.

Yang, C.Y. and Yazulla, S. (1988b) Localization of putative GABAergic neurons in the larval tiger salamander retina by immunocytochemical and autoradiographic methods. *J. Comp. Neurol.*, 277: 96–108.

Yang, X.L. and Wu, S.M. (1989) Modulation of rod-cone coupling by light. *Science*, 244: 352–354.

Yang, X.L. and Wu, S.M. (1990) Synaptic inputs from rods and cones to horizontal cells in the tiger salamander retina. *Science in China—Series B, Chemistry, Life Sciences and Earth Sciences*, 33: 946–954.

Yang, X.L. and Wu, S.M. (1991) Feedforward lateral inhibition in retinal bipolar cells: inputoutput relation of the horizontal cell-depolarizing bipolar cell synapse. *Proc. Natl. Acad. Sci. USA*, 88: 3310–3313.

Yang, X.L. and Wu, S.M. (1996) Response sensitivity and voltage gain of the rod- and cone-horizontal cell synapses in dark- and light-adapted tiger salamander retina. *J. Neurophysiol.*, 76: 3863–3874.

Yang, X.L. and Wu, S.M. (1997) Response sensitivity and voltage gain of rod- and cone-bipolar cell synapses in dark-adapted tiger salamander retina. *J. Neurophysiol.*, 78: 2662–2673.

H. Kolb, H. Ripps and S. Wu (Eds.)
Progress in Brain Research, Vol. 131

CHAPTER 9

Transmission at the photoreceptor synapse

Paul Witkovsky[1,*], Wallace Thoreson[2] and Daniel Tranchina[3]

[1] *Departments of Ophthalmology and Physiology, New York University School of Medicine, 550 First Avenue, New York, NY 10016, USA*
[2] *Departments of Ophthalmology and Pharmacology, University of Nebraska Medical Center, 985540 Nebraska Medical Center, Omaha, NE 68198, USA*
[3] *Departments of Biology and Mathematics, New York University, 100 Washington University Square East, New York, NY 10003, USA*

Introduction

The rod and cone photoreceptors of mature retinas develop from non-motile ciliated cells whose distal endings elaborate membranous disks that house the visual pigments. The biochemical transduction cascade coupling light capture by visual pigment molecules to surface membrane electrical events converges on the gating of a cGMP-dependent cation channel. Light brings about the reduction of [cGMP] and the closing of some cation channels, resulting in a hyperpolarization of the photoreceptor.

Another of the photoreceptor's special features is its slow kinetics. A bright flash delivered in 1 ms initiates voltage changes in rods and cones that can take up to seconds. to complete, and in the more usual case, a constantly changing light pattern of modest intensity induces a continuous modulation of photoreceptor voltages.

The unusual nature of photoreceptor electrophysiology—relative depolarization in darkness changing to a more hyperpolarized level during light—sets the parameters for the functioning of its synapse at which the photoreceptor communicates information about changing light patterns to second order retinal neurons. The synaptic signal is conveyed through a neurotransmitter whose release is a calcium-dependent process; because calcium channels have a higher

open probability as the membrane depolarizes, there is a greater calcium current during darkness than in light. For the photoreceptor to signal time-modulated light signals effectively, its calcium channel has to be non-inactivating.

The effective operating range of rod and cone photoreceptors is from -35 to -40 mV in darkness, grading smoothly to about -60 mV as incident light intensity increases towards saturation, so the calcium current has to be modulated by voltage in this range. In fact, the particular calcium channels found in photoreceptors (discussed in more detail below) are only weakly activated between -35 and -60 mV and the slope of the relation between voltage and Ca channel activation function is shallow over that range of voltages. Corresponding measurements of intracellular calcium concentration, $[Ca]_i$, show that it attains its highest level in darkness, when it is still less than 1 µM, according to some estimates (Krizaj and Copenhagen, 1998; Krizaj et al., 1999), falling to perhaps 0.1 µM in bright light. Thus photoreceptors have evolved mechanisms to control transmitter release with very low levels of calcium, compared to those which gate transmitter release at other, faster, synapses (Neher, 1998). This essay focuses on the special features of transmitter release by rods and cones and the activation of the bipolar and horizontal cells with which photoreceptors communicate. It begins with a survey of the components that are known to participate in signal transfer between photoreceptors and their synaptic targets, or to

* Corresponding author: Paul Witkovsky, Tel.: 212-263-6488; Fax: 212-263-7602; E-mail: pw20@is2.nyu.edu

influence that process. It ends with a quantitative model of the photoreceptor synapse that utilizes some of the described components to describe the kinetics of synaptic transfer.

The photoreceptor transmitter is glutamate

The neurotransmitter in question is glutamate, the most widely encountered excitatory transmitter in the brain. The evidence that both rods and cones utilize glutamate is compelling (Thoreson and Witkovsky, 1999). Immunocytochemical studies show that rods and cones, bipolar cells and ganglion cells concentrate glutamate in synaptic terminals. In contrast, retinal inhibitory interneurons, horizontal and amacrine cells, utilize gaba and glycine, and typically colocalize another monoamine or peptide transmitter. Glutamate release evoked by elevated $[K^+]$ has been measured from individual cones (Copenhagen and Jahr, 1989) and light-gated glutamate release from the photoreceptor layer freed from the inner retina was shown by Schmitz and Witkovsky (1996). Correspondingly, the post-synaptic neurons, horizontal and bipolar cells, possess glutamate receptors in their synaptic endings. These may be ionotropic receptors, usually of the AMPA (Sasaki and Kaneko, 1996; Maple et al., 1999) or KA sub-types (deVries and Schwartz, 1999), but at least in one horizontal cell, also of the NMDA type (O'Dell and Christensen, 1986). And in addition a wide variety of metabotropic glutamate receptors is associated with the photoreceptor synapse, at both pre- and post-synaptic locations (reviewed in Brandstatter et al., 1998).

Glutamate transporters

Removal of glutamate from the synaptic cleft occurs partly by diffusion, but mainly is brought about by glutamate transporters (Arriza et al., 1994). Genetic studies show that the population of glutamate transporters is diverse, while immunocytochemical studies show that they have particular locations, some in neurons and others in glial cells (Rauen et al., 1998). Glutamate transporters have certain common properties, including a high affinity for glutamate and a voltage dependence, which is in the direction of increasing transport rate with hyperpolarization. Gaal et al. (1998) showed that the transporter of the cone cleared glutamate more rapidly when the cone was illuminated, resulting in a hyperpolarization of the horizontal cell. These data suggest a role for neuronal glutamate transporters in shaping the kinetics of post-synaptic responses (Roska et al., 1998).

Glutamate transporters also are electrogenic, the stoichiometry varying with the particular transporter. In photoreceptors (Grant and Werblin, 1996; Eliasof and Jahr, 1996) and at least some ON-bipolar cells (Grant and Dowling, 1995), glutamate transporter activity is associated with Cl flux. The pharmacology and physiological properties of glutamate-activated Cl current suggest an amalgam of a transporter and a channel, and the resultant Cl current can affect transmitter release by influencing the Ca current of rods and cones. One mechanism is a direct action whereby reduction in $[Cl]_i$ inhibits Ca current (Thoreson et al., 1997). Another mechanism is through a voltage change, whose direction and amplitude are hard to assess, since E_{Cl} is close to the membrane potential of the photoreceptor in darkness. Another complication in that connection is that cones have a prominent Ca-dependent Cl current (Maricq and Korenbrot, 1988).

The glutamate transporter of the Mueller glial cell of the retina (Barbour et al., 1991; Derouiche and Rauen, 1995) works in series with those of photoreceptors, horizontal and bipolar cells. Glial processes are excluded from the synapse, but avidly take up any residual glutamate from extracellular space. In darkness, moreover, when transmitter release by rods and cones is at its highest, photoreceptors, horizontal and bipolar cells are relatively depolarized, whereas the Muller glial cell is hyperpolarized. Thus in darkness glial glutamate transport is at a relatively high rate, neuronal glutamate transport at a low rate. The relative contributions of this mix of transporter activity in setting the [glutamate] of the synaptic cleft is still unknown, as are the kinetics of the change in [glutamate] brought about by changing light levels.

Desensitization of ionotropic glutamate receptors

The rate of change of glutamate concentration in the cleft controls the conductance of the receptors on second-order neurons that initiate the post-synaptic potential. Receptor desensitization, which refers to a loss of conductance while the transmitter is still bound to the receptor, may play a role in shaping the post-synaptic response. Both AMPA receptors (AMPARs) and kainate receptors (KARs) in distal retinal neurons show desensitization (Eliasof and Jahr, 1997; deVries and Schwartz, 1999). Eliasof and Jahr (1997) studied AMPAR desensitization in horizontal cells by applying saturating concentrations of glutamate. Their experiments revealed an extremely rapid and profound desensitization. Yang et al. (1998), however, found that cyclothiazide, which blocks AMPAR desensitization, did not change the kinetics of light-evoked responses in horizontal cells. This apparent contradiction might be resolved if [glutamate] in the outer plexiform layer did not achieve the required level for desensitization. In contrast, de Vries and Schwartz (1999) noted an asymmetry in the OFF-bipolar cell currents evoked by imposing a voltage step on a cone from -70 to -35 mV or the reverse. In the former case [glut] at -70 mV is presumed to be too low to induce desensitization, so the depolarizing step elicits a large current. In the reverse case, KA receptors are desensitized at -35 mV by tonic [glut], resulting in a small current in response to the hyperpolarizing step.

Thus KARs appear to undergo desensitization at the glutamate concentrations found in vivo and the differences between AMPARs and KARs in the outer retina in this respect may reflect different inherent affinities for glutamate. AMPARs in horizontal cells which are directly adjacent to the sites of vesicle release have a low affinity for glutamate. KARs in OFF-bipolar cells making flat contacts are farther from the release site, if it turns out, as postulated (deVries and Schwartz, 1999), that photoreceptors release glutamate only at ribbon synapses. And in this case they would be presumed to have a relatively high affinity for glutamate. In the inner plexiform layer, the kinetics of certain amacrine cell and ganglion cell responses to light are affected by cyclothiazide (Tran et al., 1999). Amacrines receive input from ON-bipolar cells whose phasic synapses release glutamate at a much higher rate than that achieved by photoreceptors (von Gersdorff et al., 1996), which suggests that under certain conditions the glutamate concentration in the synaptic cleft will

be much higher than that at the photoreceptor synapse. Much further work is required to define the properties of these synapses and to establish the concentration(s) of glutamate which obtain in the synaptic clefts of different retinal synapses.

Structure of the photoreceptor synapse

Photoreceptor synaptic transmission occurs at sites with a stereotyped but complex geometry (Dowling, 1987). During retinal development, outgrowing neurites of horizontal and bipolar cells approach the rod and cone synaptic terminals. Some neurites penetrate more or less deeply into the rod–cone bases; these are the invaginating contacts. Or, in the case of flat bipolar cell contacts with cones, they array themselves in shallow indentations along the surface of the synaptic terminal. Photoreceptors themselves extend telodendritic processes which form electrical synapses with neighboring photoreceptors, or, more rarely, become one of the post-synaptic processes at a ribbon synapse of a neighboring photoreceptor (Lasansky, 1973). The processes arrayed in the invaginations have a specific geometry in relation to the pre-synaptic specializations associated with the positioning of transmitter-filled vesicles for release. These include a synaptic ribbon, arciform density and paramembranous proteins which form the complex required for vesicle exocytosis. The calcium channels which gate the calcium influx that triggers exocytosis are distributed near the docking sites (Taylor and Morgans, 1998).

The positioning of post-synaptic processes with respect to sites of glutamate release presumably is important in relation to whether their glutamate receptors have high or low affinity for glutamate, because as mentioned above, glutamate released from vesicles is actively taken up by neural and glial transporters. This consideration may be particularly important for flat bipolar contacts on cones in view of the postulate that glutamate is released not adjacent to the site of flat contact, but rather from a more distant ribbon synapse.

The presently available evidence about the composition of naturally occurring gluRs and their locations within post-synaptic terminals is far from complete. In fact, the full subunit composition of any naturally occurring GluR in a retinal neuron is unknown. EM-immunocytochemistry (Vardi et al., 1998; Brandstatter et al., 1998) suggests the presence of certain glutamate receptor (GluR) subunits within terminal dendrites. A number of studies show that immunoreactivity for GluR1, GluR2/3 and GluR4 are found among bipolar and horizontal cell processes in the outer plexiform layer. These are the subunits of AMPA receptors (Hollman and Heinemann, 1994) but there are the inevitable species differences which complicate reaching general conclusions about the make up of AMPA receptors. Immunocytochemical studies provide evidence for the presence of KAR subunits (GluR 5–7, KA1,2) in outer retinal synapses. EM-immunocytochemistry also reveals some unexpected findings, such as the presence of ionotropic gluR subunits in ON-bipolar cells which are known to respond to light through a metabotropic receptor, mGluR6. Brandstatter et al., (1996) have drawn attention to an intriguing finding, which is that only one of the two post-synaptic processes emanating from the same cell type contains a particular mGluR. GluRs typically are clustered with the aid of scaffolding proteins, of which a variety have been identified, and been shown to be specific to the different classes of GluR, including ionotropic and metabotropic types. Recent evidence shows that such scaffolding proteins are present in retinal synapses (Koulen et al., 1998) where they may serve to link GluRs to certain intracellular enzymes, e.g. soluble guanylate kinases, as has been found in brain (Ziff, 1997).

The calcium currents of rods and cones

The advent of voltage clamp methods that could be applied to small cells (Hamill et al., 1981) made it possible to study calcium currents in photoreceptors. The literature is consistent in identifying L-type voltage-gated Ca channels in rods and cones (Bader et al., 1982; Corey et al., 1984; Lasater and Witkovsky, 1991; Wilkinson and Barnes, 1996).

L-Ca channels are characterized by sensitivity to dihydropyridines, half-maximum of the Boltzmann activation function at relatively depolarized voltages (-30 to -15 mV), lack of inactivation in the face of a sustained depolarizing step, and relatively slow

kinetics. An L-Ca current has been shown to underlie glutamate release by rods and cones (Rieke and Schwartz, 1996; Schmitz and Witkovsky, 1997), retinal bipolar cells (Tachibana et al., 1993) and to contribute to catecholamine release from chromaffin cells (Artalejo et al., 1991), whereas N, P, Q and R calcium channels gate transmitter release at fast synapses (Olivera et al., 1994). It has been reported that a cGMP-dependent, Ca current in cones contributes to the control of transmitter release (Rieke and Schwartz, 1994).

Intracellular regulation of calcium in photoreceptors

Photoreceptors experience a steady influx of calcium at both ends, which is greater in darkness than in light. In the outer segment, the plasma membrane is abundantly provided with cGMP-gated channels that have a high relatively permeability to divalent cations, such that ca. 15% of the inward current is carried by Ca^{2+}. In the inner segment and synaptic terminal, the L-Ca channels have a relatively high open probability at the membrane potentials of rods and cones in darkness, permitting a steady calcium influx. Light reduces Ca^{2+} permeability at both ends of the photoreceptor. In the outer segment a Na/K-Ca exchanger restores the low [Ca] of the cytoplasm (McCarthy et al., 1994), whereas in the inner segment, a Ca-ATPase is largely responsible for maintaining cytosolic [Ca] levels (Krizaj and Copenhagen, 1998; Morgans et al., 1998).

Influx of calcium through voltage-gated Ca channels is only one route whereby rods and cones regulate $[Ca]_i$. The intracellular cisternae found in photoreceptor inner segments are calcium stores that can be triggered either to release Ca^{2+} or to sequester it. Ca release from the endoplasmic reticulum is under the control of two types of receptor. The inositol trisphosphate (IP3) receptor is activated through a metabotropic, G protein-linked cascade in which the enzyme phospholipase C is activated to breakdown a membrane lipid, phosphatidyl inositol trisphosphate, into diacylglycerol (DAG) and IP3. DAG remains in the membrane, where it activates PKC, while IP3 diffuses to its receptor, causing a release of Ca and an up-regulation of PKC. Protein kinase C has been found to up-regulate transmitter release by retinal bipolar cells (Minami et al., 1998). The ryanodine receptor, whose structure resembles that of the IP3 receptor, is activated by Ca influx, a phenomenon called calcium induced calcium release (CICR). Besides these receptors, a host of transporter and pumps act both at intracellular sites and at the surface membrane to maintain calcium homeostasis. Ca imaging experiments, using fluorescent Ca sensors, indicate that [Ca] is kept in the range $0.1-1.0$ micromolar as photoreceptors respond to light/darkness.

Krizaj et al. (1999) examined whether Ca released from intracellular stores affected transmitter release by rods. Caffeine was used to stimulate release and changes in $[Ca]_i$ were monitored by fluorescence. Puffs of caffeine evoked a transient $1-2$ s rise in [Ca] followed by a more sustained decay. Parallel measures of glutamate release by the photoreceptor layer showed a caffeine-induced depression. The transient rise in $[Ca]_i$ could not be resolved by the glutamate measures which were averaged over several minutes. However when horizontal cell membrane potential was monitored during exposure of the eyecup to caffeine, a brief depolarization followed by a sustained hyperpolarization was observed, on the time scale which roughly paralleled the changes in [Ca]. These data raise an important question: does the exocytotic machinery of rod photoreceptors respond to the general cytoplasmic level of [Ca], or does it sample [Ca] in a microzone that is part of the local region where exocytosis occurs?

Modulation of photoreceptor calcium currents

Voltage-gated calcium channels in rods and cones are subject to modulation by numerous neuroactive substances and also show a substantial degree of regulation by calcium itself and by pH. Barnes et al. (1993) found that an alkaline shift of pH increased L-channel current. Since retinal pH changes as a function of its metabolic state, which in turn is influenced by light and darkness, the Ca current will be influenced by the metabolic activity of photoreceptors, which is known to be very high (Shichi, 1983). Recently, Verweij et al. (1996) proposed that the feedback influence which horizontal cells exert upon cones is mediated through a leftward shift of the Ca activation function along the voltage axis, an effect which works against the direct hyperpolarizing action of light on cones, hence a "negative" feedback. A similar result was reported for somatostatin (Akopian et al., 2000), which, acting through an sst-2a receptor, increases the delayed rectifying current of rods and cones. However this same peptide had a differential action on Ca currents, increasing that of cones, while diminishing that of rods. The increase results from a leftward shift of the Ca activation function. Koulen et al. (1999) recently identified a metabotropic glutamate receptor (mGluR8) which is coupled to Ca entry. The location of mGluR8 is on the photoreceptor terminal, where it functions as an autoreceptor.

Photoreceptor coupling

Photoreceptor coupling is well documented in the retinas of lower vertebrates and it has been inferred for mammalian retinas based on the transmission of rod signals through the retinal network (Nelson, 1977). In amphibian and turtle eyes, rods are coupled to other rods (Copenhagen and Owen, 1976; Gold and Dowling, 1979), which results in noise reduction and spatial integration that may be important for perception of very dim lights. Studies of dim light responses in primate photoreceptors, however (Schneeweis and Schnapf, 1995) led to the conclusion that the rods were uncoupled from other rods, but were coupled to cones.

Rod–cone coupling also is well documented in amphibian retinas. Physiological evidence suggests that a small fraction of rods are very tightly coupled to cones; such rods have markedly altered kinetics reflecting cone input. Because both rod–cone and rod-rod coupling exist, the cone signal is transmitted with progressive attenuation through the rod network, resulting in inhomogeneity in light-evoked response kinetics among the rod population. Rod–cone coupling is increased by dopamine through a D2 receptor (Krizaj et al., 1998), consistent with the general role of dopamine in promoting light adaptive changes in retinal function (reviewed in Witkovsky and Dearry, 1991). Presumably rod–cone coupling will contribute to the dynamics of transmitter release by rods, but this requires experimental confirmation.

Replenishment of glutamate released at photoreceptor synapses

In their classical study, Heuser and Reese (1973) showed that exocytosing vesicles added vesicular membrane to the synaptic terminal, but that exocytosis was balanced by recovery of membrane (endocytosis) at an adjacent region. There membrane was taken up by coated vesicles and added to intracellular cisternae from which new vesicles were derived. Photoreceptors were shown to conform to this pattern of renewal (Ripps et al., 1976).

The source of the glutamate which is used to fill the vesicles is still not fully determined. An important cycle involves glutamine and the Muller glial cell. Glial cells take up glutamate, converting it to glutamine with an enzyme, glutamine synthetase which is confined to glial cells (Linser and Moscona, 1979). Glutamine is moved out of glia and into photoreceptors by transporters that need to be better characterized. Glutamine is converted to glutamate by glutaminase, which has been shown to be present in rods and cones. Although there is evidence that this system operates for the photoreceptor, Winkler et al. (1999) showed that blocking glutamine synthetase had almost no effect on generation of the electroretinographic b-wave, which is a measure of ON-bipolar cell activity (Stockton and Slaughter, 1989) and hence an indirect monitor of the photoreceptor synapse. On the other hand, blocking a glutamate transporter rapidly eliminated the b-wave.

Glutamate in the synaptic cleft

The concentration and kinetics of extracellular glutamate at the photoreceptor synapse are still subjects of active investigation. The function of other components of the synapse depend on the rise and fall of glutamate in a very direct way. For example, the proximity of the GluR to the release site will have to match its affinity for glutamate and the degree of desensitization and recovery from desensitization of a given GluR will depend directly on the kinetics and magnitude of glutamate concentration changes. Gaal et al. (1998) studied cone to horizontal transfer in the salamander retina. They found that when photoreceptor transmission was blocked with 20 mM Mg^{2+}, horizontal cells hyperpolarized and lost light responsiveness. In this state exogenous glutamate depolarized the HC. A superimposed light flash, to which photoreceptors would still be responsive, induced a horizontal cell hyperpolarization, suggesting that a cone glutamate transporter was more active when hyperpolarized. Supporting evidence came from the findings that the hyperpolarizing response was blocked by DHKA, and that substituting kainate, which is not transported, for glutamate, blocked the phenomenon. Gaal et al. (1998) also found that the plot of horizontal cell depolarization against [glutamate], when the transporter and synaptic transmission were blocked, was fit by a logistic function with a Hill coefficient near 2 and half-activation at 32 μm. This data suggest that [glutamate] varies in the low micromolar range over the functional range of cone light responsiveness.

Modeling transmission at the photoreceptor synapse

The preceding sections outline some of the basic membrane properties of rods and cones that bear on the way they release their transmitter, glutamate. Neither rods, cones, nor the cells with which they communicate produce action potentials, so synaptic transfer is the process whereby slow light-induced potential changes in photoreceptors induce similar slow potentials in bipolar and horizontal cells. When one takes into account that in addition to multiple photoreceptor classes, there exist a variety of postsynaptic receptors for glutamate which are arrayed on various dendritic terminals of horizontal and bipolar cells, it is clear that there are multiple photoreceptor synapses. For example, in photoreceptor to horizontal and OFF-bipolar cell transmission the polarity of the potential changes is the same, i.e. the synapse is sign-conserving. In photoreceptor to ON-bipolar cell transmission, the synapse is sign-inverting. The evidence is very strong that sign inversion results from a metabotropic receptor (mGluR6; Nakajima et al., 1993) on the ON-bipolar cell. Its activation by glutamate leads to a second messenger cascade whose details are still not entirely worked out, but whose end result is to decrease a cyclic nucleotide-dependent cation current

(Nawy and Jahr, 1991). Thus when light hyperpolarizes the photoreceptor, its release of glutamate is reduced, resulting in an opening of cation channels in the ON-bipolar cell and a resulting depolarization.

As a beginning step towards understanding the kinetic properties of synaptic transfer from photoreceptors to second-order retinal neurons, the present authors have developed a quantitative model for transmission at a sign-conserving synapse, i.e. through ionotropic gluRs between rods or cones and horizontal or OFF-bipolar neurons. Although, as discussed above, the glutamate receptors of horizontal vs. OFF-bipolar cells may be different, a fundamental similarity is that glutamate opens a non-specific cation channel, resulting in depolarization of the post-synaptic neuron. Our model has a completely physiological focus in that its components and their behavior have been described in the literature. The point of generating a model is to see whether the interactions of its components that we postulate provide a realistic description of the kinetics of post-synaptic responses. When that is accomplished, the consequences of changing the parameters of model components or of introducing new variables can be evaluated.

At sign-conserving photoreceptor synapses, the sequence of events resulting in synaptic transmission is:

(a) Light activates a transduction cascade in the photoreceptor outer segment resulting in closure of some of its cGMP-dependent channels and a resulting hyperpolarization. Other intrinsic channels help to shape the complex waveform of the photoreceptor's light-evoked voltage.

(b) The photoreceptor's voltage controls Ca influx through L-type channels. The relation between voltage and Ca influx is given by a Boltzmann relation with appropriate slope factor and voltage of half-activation.

(c) Ca influx determines the rate of glutamate release according to a relation described in the next section.

(d) Glutamate diffuses to its post-synaptic targets, but its concentration in the synaptic cleft is lowered by transporters located in both neurons and glia.

(e) Glutamate activates post-synaptic receptors to initiate the conductance changes that mediate post-synaptic currents. The relation between [glutamate] and conductance change is determined by a Michaelis-Menten function with a Hill coefficient near 2.

The following section provides a quantitative description of (b)–(e) above, using data of Corey et al., 1984; Rieke and Schwartz, 1996; Schmitz and Witkovsky, 1996, 1997; Witkovsky et al., 1997 and Thoreson et al., work in progress. Although other workers have dealt with elements of the model outlined above (Attwell et al., 1987; Wu, 1988; Belgum and Copenhagen, 1988), those previous studies did not attempt to account for the kinetics of post-synaptic responses and/or they dealt only with rod transmission.

Glutamate release

A preparation consisting of an isolated layer of photoreceptors developed by Cahill and Besharse (1992) to study circadian rhythms was adapted by Schmitz and Witkovsky (1996) to study glutamate release. The method utilized an enzyme cascade (Fosse et al., 1986) terminating in bacterial luciferase by which photons were generated in proportion to glutamate degradation. The main findings were that glutamate release was higher in darkness than in light by a factor of when glutamate uptake was inhibited with dihydrokainate. The process was calcium-dependent and was inhibited by blockers of L-type Ca channels, but not blockers of N- or P-type calcium channels (Schmitz and Witkovsky, 1997).

Spectral sensitivity measures showed that only glutamate release from rods was being monitored. Light steps of graded intensity induced steady-state plateau voltages in rods and a progressive attenuation of glutamate release. When light was factored out and glutamate release plotted against rod plateau voltage, the data were well fit by a Boltzmann function for the L-Ca current of amphibian rods (Corey et al., 1984 and cf. Fig. 1).

Relation of Ca influx to glutamate release

The goodness of fit illustrated in Fig. 1 implies that glutamate release is a linear function of Ca current.

152

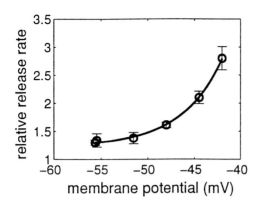

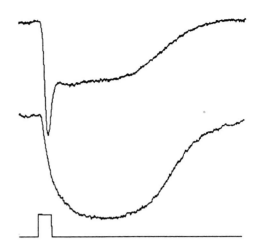

Fig. 1. Relation of rod voltage and glutamate release to calcium current. The data points ±SEM were obtained from plots of rod voltage vs. intensity and glutamate release vs. intensity, then factoring out intensity to yield rod voltage vs. glutamate release (cf. Witkovsky et al., 1997 for more details). The line through the points is the Boltzmann function for the L-type Ca current, with values for half-saturation and slope factor taken from Corey et al. (1984). Reproduced from Witkovsky et al., 1997 with permission of the J. Neuroscience.

Fig. 2. Intracellular dual recordings from a rod-horizontal cell pair under scotopic conditions. The upper record is the rod response. The stimulus marker below the traces indicates the timing of a 200 ms flash of 567 nm light delivering 12.3 log quanta incident $cm^{-2} s^{-1}$. The arrowheads indicate plateau responses of the rod and the horizontal cell.

Similarly, Rieke and Schwartz (1996) determined for salamander rod terminals that changes in capacitance, which are a measure of net [exocytosis–endocytosis] changed in a linear manner with $[Ca]_i$, which was monitored with a fluorescent calcium indicator.

Input–output relation between photoreceptors and second-order neurons

We established conditions that permitted examination of pure rod or pure cone input to either horizontal or OFF-bipolar cells. For rod input, animals were fully dark-adapted and the retinal slices prepared under infra-red illumination. A D2 dopamine antagonist, spiperone, was added to the bath to prevent rod–cone coupling (Krizaj et al., 1998). For cone input, the light-sensitivity of rods was suppressed by a blue background light. The same background illumination reduced cone sensitivity only slightly, but did make cone kinetics more transient. The light-evoked currents of second-order neurons were recorded with perforated patch electrodes under voltage clamp. V_{hold} was -40 mV, i.e. close to the membrane potential of the neuron in darkness.

Our model was developed in two stages. The first stage (Witkovsky et al., 1997) concerns the "steady-state" gain between rods and horizontal cells. That is, when a step of light is imposed, rods reach a maintained membrane potential value—the plateau of the rod's light-evoked response—and horizontal cells do the same (Fig. 2). The model attempts to account for the membrane potential, u, of the HC, as follows:

$$u = \frac{(G_s E_s + G_r E_r)}{(G_s + G_r)}, \qquad (1)$$

where G_s is the synaptic conductance (glutamate-gated), E_s is the equilibrium potential for current through this conductance, G_r is the combined conductance of other currents (mainly K), and E_r is the net reversal potential of those currents.

The post-synaptic conductance G_s, is defined by a Hill function:

$$G_s = G_s^{max} \frac{[glutamate]^n}{K_{glut}^n + [glutamate]^n}, \qquad (2)$$

where n is close to 2 and K_{glut} is the concentration required to half-saturate the receptor population.

Glutamate release from the photoreceptor gives rise to a concentration of glutamate in the synaptic cleft, governed by

$$[\text{glutamate}] = \alpha\, r(v), \qquad (3)$$

where α is a constant, r is the rate of release and v is the rod potential.

The rate of release of synaptic transmitter is given by

$$r(v) = C\left\{1 + \exp\left[\frac{(A - v)}{B}\right]\right\}^{-1} + r_0 \qquad (4)$$

where C is a constant and r_0 is the baseline release rate. A and B are, respectively, the voltage for half activation of the Ca current and the slope factor in the Boltzmann relation. It follows that our model takes glutamate release to be a linear function of $[\text{Ca}]_i$

The justification for this assumption is that, in our study (Witkovsky et al., 1997) we found that the relation between rod voltage and glutamate release was matched perfectly by the activation function for the L-type Ca current of the rod (Fig. 1).

If we define a normalized glutamate conductance, $g_s = G_s/G_r$, we can reconfigure Eq. (1) above as:

$$u = \frac{(g_s E_r + E_r)}{(g_s + 1)}. \qquad (5)$$

This equation provides a very good fit to the data points on a plot of rod voltage vs. horizontal cell voltage (Fig. 3).

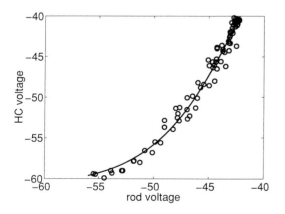

Fig. 3. Steady state model of rod vs. horizontal cell light-induced potential changes. The data points are taken from simultaneous intracellular recordings of rods and horizontal cells. The line through the data is the best fit of Eq. (5) in the text. Reproduced from Witkovsky et al., 1997 with permission of the J. Neuroscience.

In the second stage of the model we extend the above formulation to the generation of post-synaptic currents. We chose to look at post-synaptic currents rather than voltages to avoid the complications of the voltage-dependent conductances present in second-order retinal neurons which contribute to the different kinetics of the light-evoked responses of photoreceptors compared to those of horizontal and bipolar cells (cf. Fig. 2). For this determination we need to consider the dynamics of calcium change, since that governs the rate of glutamate release.

We define $y = [Ca^{2+}]/[Ca^{2+}]_{\text{dark}}$, the normalized free calcium concentration at any point in the cytoplasm. The calcium concentration reflects a balance between calcium influx through voltage-gated Ca channels and efflux which is governed by a Ca transporter (exchange pump). In Eq. (6) below it is assumed that the rate of the transporter is proportional to the free calcium concentration.

$$\tau_{Ca}\frac{dy}{dt} = g(v) - y, \qquad (6)$$

where v = photoreceptor voltage, and the function $g(v)$ is the fractional activation of the voltage-gated Ca current, normalized by its value in darkness. A Boltzmann relation governs

$$g(v) = \left(1 + \exp\left[\frac{A - v_{\text{dark}}}{B}\right]\right) \times \left(1 + \exp\left[\frac{A - v}{B}\right]\right)^{-1} \qquad (7)$$

We define $z = [\text{glut}]/[\text{glut}]_{\text{dark}}$, the normalized glutamate concentration in the synaptic cleft. It increases in direct proportion to $[Ca^{2+}]$ (the term, y, in Eq. 7) and decreases at a rate determined by diffusion and activate re-uptake. If we ignore the voltage-dependence of re-uptake and make the simplifying assumption that the rate of glutamate removal is proportional to [Glut], then we have:

$$\tau_{\text{glut}}\frac{dz}{dt} = y - z \qquad (8)$$

The term, z, determines the fraction of bound glutamate receptors, f, according to:

$$f = \frac{z^n}{z^n + k_{\text{glut}}^n}. \qquad (9)$$

In this equation k_{glut} is the [glutamate] sufficient to bind half the receptors, and n is the Hill coefficient for cooperativity, whose value is near 2.

The glutamate conductance, G, is proportional to the fraction of bound receptors, f. Thus we have:

$$G = G_{max} \frac{z^n}{z^n + k_{glut}^n} = G_{max} \; f. \qquad (10)$$

To this point, receptor desensitization has not been taken into account. Since we find that including desensitization does not improve the fit of the model to data, it is omitted here. The fits to the data were obtained for matched sets of photoreceptor voltages and second-order cell currents generated by a series of 1 s light flashes of different intensities. Equations (6) and (8) were integrated; any choice of free parameters in those equations gave rise to a family of postsynaptic conductance responses. The values of the free parameters were varied and the best-fit values determined by a least squares method, using an iterative computer program. Figure 4 shows how the model matches data from four photoreceptor synapses: rod to HC, rod to OFF-BC, cone to HC, and cone to OFF BC.

The essential finding was that for the four pairs (rod to HC; cone to HC; rod to OFF BC; cone to OFF BC), the relation between peak light-evoked current in the second-order neuron to peak photoreceptor voltage was fit by a Michaelis-Menten function with a slope very close to 1.0. This fixed relation implies a constancy of synaptic transfer over a wide range of illumination levels. Accordingly, we take the photoreceptor voltage change to be the controlling element for a change in calcium current at the photoreceptor synaptic terminal.

The strength of the model is that, with relatively simple assumptions and few free parameters, it captures the essence of post-synaptic kinetics for both rod and cone synaptic transfers mediated through ionotropic glutamate receptors. Another strength is that the components of the model are physiological in nature and accessible to experimentation. Undoubtedly the model is incomplete in the sense that additional components need to be included to achieve a more perfect fit of predicted and real responses. For example, we are currently exploring how making glutamate transport voltage-dependent

(Gaal et al., 1998) will affect the fit of the model to data. Our hope and expectation is that our model will contribute to understanding how photoreceptors faithfully convey information about light stimuli to the retinal network.

Conclusions and future perspectives

The retina arises embryologically from the central nervous system and its cells share many of the properties of neurons in the brain. Yet the retina has a unique role in providing information to the brain about a complex visual world, and certain of its special features have evolved in relation to that task. One of the most compelling is its ceaseless activity: even in complete darkness photoreceptors drip glutamate at a relatively brisk rate, while many ganglion cells fire spikes at a more or less steady pace. Moreover, there can be no "timeout" while the retina reorganizes itself for daytime or nighttime vision. Instead an interconnected set of neuromodulatory mechanisms accomplishes this task on the run.

In this context the photoreceptor and ON-bipolar cell output synapses have become model systems for investigating the properties of tonic neurotransmission. At no other known synapses do non-inactivating, high voltage-activated (HVA) calcium channels play such a dominant role in triggering vesicle release. The HVA calcium currents are subject to multiple controls, including direct neuromodulation of the channels by, e.g. neuropeptides (Akopian et al., 2000), dopamine (Stella and Thoreson, 2000) and by nitric oxide (Kurenny et al., 1994). Many other elements contribute to the regulation of $[Ca]_i$, including intracellular stores (Krizaj et al., 1999), calcium pumps and transporters (Krizaj and Copenhagen, 1998; Morgans et al., 1998) and calcium-dependent currents which contribute to the regulation of membrane voltage and so have an impact on the calcium current (Maricq and Korenbrot, 1988).

The link between Ca entry and exocytosis in photoreceptors and ON-bipolar cells also is poorly understood from a molecular biological perspective. In conventional presynaptic terminals a host of intracellular proteins organize vesicle transport, docking, priming and release (Chapman et al., 1995). There is some indication that photoreceptors may

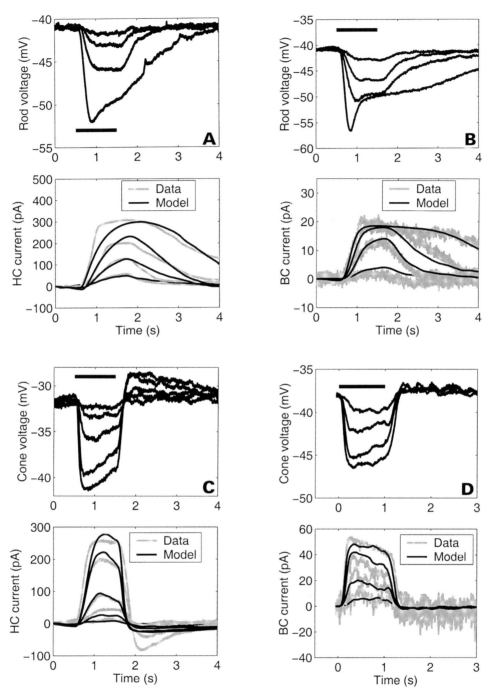

Fig. 4. Dynamic model of photoreceptor to second-order retinal neuron synaptic transfer. Each set of two panels shows light-evoked photoreceptor responses to a set of 1s stimuli of different intensity in the upper panel, whose light-evoked voltages are the input to the model. Stimuli were 580 nm for rods (panels A, B) and 680 nm for cones (C, D). The lower panel illustrates the best fit of the model to photocurrents recorded from horizontal cells (A, C) and OFF-bipolar cells (B, D). All recordings were made using the perforated patch technique. Horizontal and bipolar cells were held at − 40 mV. See text for presentation of the equations underlying the model.

lack certain of these proteins (Mandell et al., 1990) and in any case we lack basic information about their function. In relation to the apparent linear relation between calcium current and release (cf. Fig. 1) we need to know the properties of the calcium sensor. Is it synaptotagmin, which is found at photoreceptor ribbon synapses (Koontz and Hendrickson, 1993) as has been proposed for spiking synapses (Augustine et al., 1994)? Synaptotaginin is thought to require 4 Ca^{2+} to initiate vesicle exocytosis: were this the case for the photoreceptor, then the linear calcium-release relation probably would reflect the independence of calcium microdomains (Augustine et al., 1991).

On the post-synaptic side several crucial question have emerged recently: (1) to what extent does the glutamate transporter control [glutamate] in the synaptic cleft? (2) what is the true extracellular concentration of glutamate and does it cause desensitization of post-synaptic ionotropic glutamate receptors? (3) what is the subunit composition of igluRs in retinal cells? How many different igluRs reside in a given post-synaptic cell and is their relative number fixed or subject to regulation, as has been shown for hippocampal neurons (Hayashi et al., 2000)?

Our intuition, based on a survey of the literature, is that every aspect of synaptic communication in the retina is subject to modulation. Given that the retina has to transmit a coherent statement to the brain about the visual world, either in dim light or in bright light, it is unthinkable that each retinal synapse be subject to modulation without some overarching control, i.e. we suppose that a hierarchical framework of neuromodulatory mechanisms exists. In that context, a primary task for future studies is to examine the interrelations among the more than fifty putative neuromodulators which have been identified in retinal neurons.

A personal note

One of the authors (P.W.) takes this opportunity to pay a personal tribute to John Dowling. Long ago, as a recent PhD and having just finished a post-doctoral year with Gunnar Svaetichin in Caracas, Venezuela, I met John Dowling for the first time at Johns Hopkins University. Together with Brian Boycott he was working out the central principles of the retinal wiring diagram, based on a combination of light and electron microscopy. The retina they studied in greatest detail was that of the primate, but at the time (mid 1960s) the mammalian eye seemed largely inaccessible to microelectrode recording, whereas the fish retina that I and others worked on was more suitable for functional anatomy, i.e. drawing inferences about the responses of individual retinal cells from their synaptic connections. John, who has always shown remarkable prescience about which were the important new directions of research, suggested that I come to Baltimore to study the synaptic organization of the carp retina.

Naively, I imagined that I would carry out neurophysiological studies, while John would do the electron microscopy. But he had another idea: I should learn electron microscopy and related techniques and do the work myself, under his guidance. So with his considerable help, both on questions of technique and of interpretation, I was introduced to the field of retinal synaptic connectivity. We published one paper together in 1969 on the synaptic organization of the carp retina which was well received, and the orientation I received from that brief period in his laboratory has influenced my way of looking at the nervous system ever since. In my view, the papers of John Dowling on the synaptic organization of the retina have played a seminal role in guiding our interpretations of retinal function.

Many other scientists also contributed importantly to our understanding of retinal synapses, among them Helga Kolb, who was in the Dowling laboratory during the period I worked there and Brian Boycott, who was a frequent visitor. Still others, who have gone on to become the leaders in our field, were his students (e.g. Frank Werblin) and collaborators at this same time. John Dowling's ability to attract people to his laboratory and his charismatic persuasiveness as a teacher are two more of his many talents. It is a pleasure to acknowledge John Dowling's pivotal role in bringing retinal neurobiology to the forefront of modern investigations of nervous system function.

Acknowledgments

Supported by the National Eye Institute (EY 03570 and EY 10542), Research to Prevent Blindness, Inc., the Nebraska Lions Foundation and the Hoffritz Foundation.

References

Akopian, A., Johnson, J., Gabriel, R., Brecha, N. and Witkovsky, P. (2000) Somatostatin modulates voltage-gated K and Ca currents in rod and cone photoreceptors of the salamander retina. *J. Neurosci.*, 20: 929–936.

Arriza, J.L., Fairman, W.A., Wadiche, J.I., Murdoch, G.H., Kavanaugh, M.P. and Amara, S.G. (1994) Functional comparisons of three glutamate transporter subtypes cloned from human motor cortex. *J. Neurosci.*, 14: 5559–5569.

Artalejo, C., Mogul, D., Perlman, R.L. and Fox, A.P. (1991) Three types of bovine chromaffin cell Ca2 + channels: facilitation increases the opening probability of a 27 pS channel. *J. Physiol.*, 444: 213–240.

Attwell, D., Borges, S., Wu, S.M. and Wilson, M. (1987) Signal clipping by the rod output synapse. *Nature*, 328: 522–524.

Augustine, G.J., Adler, E.M. and Charlton, M.P. (1991) The calcium signal for transmitter secretion from presynaptic nerve terminals. *NY Acad. Sci.*, 635: 365–381.

Augustine, G.J., Betz, H., Bommert, K., Charlton, M.P., deBello, W.M., Hans, M. and Swandulla, D. (1994) Molecular pathways for presynaptic calcium signaling. In: Stjarne, L., Greengard, P., Grillner, S., Hokfelt, T. and Ottoson, D. (Eds.), *Molecular and Cellular Mechanisms of Neurotransmitter Release.* Raven Press, NY.

Augustine, G.J. and Neher, E. (1992) Calcium requirements for secretion in bovine chromaffin cells. *J. Physiol.*, 450: 247–271.

Bader, C.R., Bertrand, D. and Schwartz, E.A. (1982) Voltage-activated and calcium-activated currents studied in solitary rod inner segments from the salamander retina. *J. Physiol.*, 331: 253–284.

Barbour, B., Brew, H. and Attwell, D. (1991) Electrogenic uptake of glutamate and aspartate into glial cells isolated from the salamander (Amblystoma) retina. *J. Physiol.*, 436: 169–193.

Barnes, S., Merchant, V. and Mahmud, F. (1993) Modulation of transmission gain by protons at the photoreceptor output synapse. *Proc. Natl. Acad. Sci.*, 90: 10081–10085.

Belgum, H.J. and Copenhagen, D.R. (1988) Synaptic transfer of rod signals to horizontal and bipolar cells in the retina of the toad (Bufo marinus). *J. Physiol.*, 396: 225–245.

Brandstatter, J.H., Koulen, P., Kuhn, R., van der Putten, H. and Wassle, H. (1996) Compartmental localization of a metabotropic glutamate receptor (mGluR7): two different active sites at a retinal synapse. *J. Neurosci.*, 16: 4749–4756.

Brandstatter, J.H., Koulen, P. and Wassle, H. (1998) Diversity of glutamate receptors in the mammalian retina. *Vision Res.*, 38: 1385–1397.

Cahill, G.M. and Besharse, J.C. (1992) Light-sensitive melatonin synthesis by Xenopus photoreceptors after destruction of the inner retina. *Vis. Neurosci.*, 8: 489–490.

Chapman, E.R., Hanson, P.I. and Jahn, R. (1995) The neuronal exocytotic fusion machine: some new developments. *Neuropharmacology*, 34: 1343–1349.

Copenhagen, D.R. and Jahr, C.E. (1989) Release of endogenous excitatory amino acids from turtle photoreceptors. *Nature*, 342: 536–539.

Copenhagen, D.R. and Owen, W.G. (1976) Functional characteristics of lateral interactions between rods in the retina of the snapping turtle. *J. Physiol.*, 259: 251–282.

Corey, D.P., Dubinsky, J.M. and Schwartz, E.A. (1984) The calcium current in inner segments of rods from the salamander (Ambystoma tigrinum) retina. *J. Physiol.*, 354: 557–575.

Derouiche, A. and Rauen, T. (1995) Coincidence of L-glutamate/L-aspartate transporter (GLAST) and glutamine synthetase (GS) immunoreactions in retinal glia: evidence for coupling of GLAST and GS in transmitter clearance. *J. Neurosci. Res.*, 42: 131–143.

DeVries, S.H. and Schwartz, E.A. (1999) Kainate receptors mediate synaptic transmission between cones and 'Off' bipolar cells in a mammalian retina. *Nature*, 397: 157–160.

Dowling, J.E. (1987) *The Retina. An Approachable Part of the Brain.* Belknap Press, Cambridge, MA.

Eliasof, S. and Jahr, C.E. (1997) Rapid AMPA receptor desensitization in catfish cone horizontal cells. *Vis. Neurosci.*, 14: 13–18.

Fosse, V.M., Kolstad, J. and Fonnum, F. (1986) A bioluminescence method for the measurement of L-glutamate: applications to the study of changes in the release of L-glutamate from lateral geniculate nucleus and superior colliculus after visual cortex ablation in rats. *J. Neurochem.*, 47: 340–349.

Gaal, L., Roska, B., Picaud, S.A., Wu, S.M., Marc, R. and Werblin, F.S. (1998) Postsynaptic response kinetics are controlled by a glutamate transporter at cone photoreceptors. *J. Neurophysiol.*, 79: 190–196.

Gold, G.H. and Dowling, J.E. (1979) Photoreceptor coupling in retina of the toad, Bufo marinus. I. Anatomy. *J. Neurophysiol.*, 42: 292–310.

Grant, G.B. and Dowling, J.E. (1995) A glutamate-activated chloride current in cone-driven ON bipolar cells of the white perch retina. *J. Neurosci.*, 15: 3852–3862.

Grant, G.B. and Werblin, F.S. (1996) A glutamate-elicited chloride current with transporter-like properties in rod photoreceptors of the tiger salamander. *Vis. Neurosci.*, 13: 135–144.

Hamill, O.P., Marty, A., Neher, E., Sakmann, B. and Sigworth, F.J. (1981) Improved patch clamp technique for high resolution current recording from cell and cell-free membrane patches. *Pflug. Arch.*, 391: 85–100.

Hayashi, Y., Shi, S.-H., Esteban, J.A., Piccini, A., Poncer, J.-C. and Malinow, R. (2000) Driving AMPA receptors into synapses by LTP and CAMKII: requirement for GluR1 and PDZ domain interaction. *Science*, 287: 2262–2267.

Heuser, J.E. and Reese, T.S. (1973) Evidence for recycling of synaptic vesicles membrane during transmitter release at the frog neuromuscular junction. *J. Cell Biol.*, 57: 315–344.

158

Hollman, M. and Heinemann, S. (1994) Cloned glutamate receptors. *Annu. Rev. Neurosci.*, 17: 31–108.

Koontz, M.A. and Hendrickson, A. (1993) Comparison of immunolocalization patterns for the synaptic vesicle proteins p65 and synapsin I in macaque monkey retina. *Synapse*, 14: 268–282.

Koulen, P., Fletcher, E.L., Craven, S.E., Bredt, D.S. and Wassle, H. (1998) Immunocytochemical localization of the postsynaptic density protein PSD-95 in the mammalian retina. *J. Neurosci.*, 18: 10136–10149.

Koulen, P., Kuhn, R., Wassle, H. and Brandstatter, J.H. (1999) Modulation of the intracellular calcium concentration in photoreceptor terminals by a presynaptic metabotropic glutamate receptor. *Proc. Natl. Acad. Sci.*, 96: 9909–9914.

Krizaj, D. and Copenhagen, D.R. (1998) Compartmentalization of calcium extrusion mechanisms in the outer and inner segments of photoreceptors. *Neuron*, 21: 249–256.

Krizaj, D., Gabriel, R., Owen, W.G. and Witkovsky, P. (1998) Dopamine D2 receptor-mediated modulation of rod-cone coupling in the Xenopus retina. *J. Comp. Neur.*, 398: 529–538.

Krizaj, D., Bao, J-X., Schmitz, Y., Witkovsky, P. and Copenhagen, D.R. (1999) Caffeine-sensitive calcium stores regulate synaptic transmission from retinal rod photoreceptors. *J. Neurosci.*, 19: 7249–7261.

Kurenny, D.E., Moroz, L.L., Turner, R.W., Sharkey, K.A. and Barnes, S. (1994) Modulation of ion channels in rod photoreceptors by nitric oxide. *Neuron*, 13: 315–324.

Lasansky, A. (1973) Organization of the outer synaptic layer in the retina of the larval tiger salamander. *Phil. Trans. R. Soc. Lond. B*, 265: 471–489.

Lasater, E. and Witkovsky, P. (1991) The calcium current of turtle photoreceptor axon terminals. *Neurosci. Res.*, (Suppl. 15): S165–S173.

Linser, P. and Moscona, A.A. (1979) Induction of glutamine synthetase in embryonic neural retina: localization in Muller fibers and dependence on cell interactions. *Proc. Natl. Acad. Sci.*, 76: 6476–6480.

Mandell, J.W., Townes-Anderson, E., Czernik, A.J., Cameron, R., Greengard. P. and De Camilli, P. (1990) Synapsins in the vertebrate retina: absence from ribbon synapses and heterogeneous distribution among conventional synapses. *Neuron*, 5: 19–33.

Maple, B.R., Gao, F. and Wu, S.M. (1999) Glutamate receptors differ in rod- and cone-dominated off-center bipolar cells. *NeuroReport*, 10: 3605–3610.

Maricq, A.V. and Korenbrot, J.I. (1988) Calcium and calcium-dependent chloride currents generate action potentials in solitary cone photoreceptors. *Neuron*, 1: 503–515.

McCarthy, S.T., Younger, J.P. and Owen, W.G. (1994) Free calcium concentrations in bullfrog rods determined in the presence of multiple forms of fura-2. *Biophys. J.*, 67: 2076–2089.

Minami, N., Berglund, K., Sakaba, T., Kohmoto, H. and Tachibana, M. (1998) Potentiation of transmitter release by protein kinase C in goldfish retinal bipolar cells. *J. Physiol.*, 512: 219–225.

Morgans, C.W., El Far, O., Berntson, A., Wassle, H. and Taylor, W.R. (1998) Calcium extrusion from mammalian photoreceptor terminals. *J. Neurosci.*, 18: 2467–2474.

Nakajima, Y., Iwakabe, H., Akazawa, C., Nawa, H., Shigemoto, R., Mizuno, N. and Nakanishi, S. (1993) Molecular characterization of a novel retinal metabotropic glutamate receptor mGluR6 with a high agonist selectivity for L-2amino-4-phosphonobutyrate. *J. Biol. Chem.*, 268: 11368–11373.

Nawy, S. and Jahr, C.E. (1991) cGMP-gated conductance in retinal bipolar cells is suppressed by the photoreceptor transmitter. *Neuron*, 7: 677–683.

Neher, E. (1998) Vesicle pools and Ca2 + microdomains: new tools for understanding their roles in neurotransmitter release. *Neuron*, 20: 389–399.

Nelson, R. (1977) Cat cones have rod input: a comparison of the response properties of cones and horizontal cell bodies in the retina of the cat. *J. Comp. Neurol.*, 172: 109–136.

O'Dell, T.J. and Christensen, B.N. (1986) N-methyl-D-aspartate receptors coexist with kainate and quisqualate receptors on single isolated catfish horizontal cells. *Brain Res.*, 381: 359–362.

Olivera, B.M., Miljanich, G.P., Ramachandran, J. and Adams, M.E. (1994) Calcium channel diversity and neurotransmitter release: the ω-conotoxins and ω-agatoxins. *Ann. Rev. Biochem.*, 63: 823–867.

Rauen, T., Taylor, W.R., Kuhlbrodt, K. and Wiessner, M. (1998) High-affinity glutamate transporters in the rat retina: a major role of the glial glutamate transporter GLAST-1 in transmitter clearance. *Cell Tiss. Res.*, 291: 19–31.

Rieke, F. and Schwartz, E.A. (1994) A cGMP-gated current can control exocytosis at cone synapses. *Neuron*, 13: 863–873.

Rieke, F. and Schwartz, E.A. (1996) Asynchronous transmitter release: control of exocytosis and endocytosis at the salamander rod synapse. *J. Physiol.*, 493: 1–8.

Ripps, H., Shakib, M. and MacDonald, E.D. (1976) Peroxidase uptake by photoreceptor terminals of the skate retina. *J. Cell Biol.*, 70: 86–96.

Roska, B., Gaal, L. and Werblin, F.S. (1998) Voltage-dependent uptake is a major determinant of glutamate concentration at the cone synapse: an analytical study. *J. Neurophysiol.*, 80: 1951–1960.

Sasaki, T. and Kaneko, A. (1996) L-glutamate-induced responses in OFF-type bipolar cells of the cat retina. *Vision Res.*, 36: 787–795.

Schmitz, Y. and Witkovsky, P. (1996) Glutamate release by the intact light-responsive photoreceptor layer of the Xenopus retina. *J. Neurosci. Meth.*, 68: 55–60.

Schmitz, Y. and Witkovsky, P. (1997) Dependence of photoreceptor glutamate release on a dihydropyridine-sensitive calcium channel. *Neurosci.*, 78: 1209–1216.

Schneeweis, D.M. and Schnapf, J.L. (1995) Photovoltage of rods and cones in the macaque retina. *Science*, 268: 1053–1056.

Shichi, H. (1983) *Biochemistry of Vision*. Academic Press, NY.

Stella, S. and Thoreson, W.B. (2000) Differential modulation of rod and cone calcium currents in tiger salamander retina by

D2 dopamine receptors and cAMP. *Eur. J. Neurosci.*, 12: 3537–3548.

Stockton, R.A. and Slaughter, M.M. (1989) B-wave of the electroretinogram. A reflection of ON bipolar cell activity. *J. Gen. Physiol.*, 93: 101–122.

Tachibana, M., Okada, T., Arimura, T., Kobayashi, K. and Piccolino, M. (1993) Dihydropyridine-sensitive calcium current mediates neurotransmitter release from bipolar cells of the goldfish retina. *J. Neurosci.*, 13: 2898–2909.

Taylor, W.R. and Morgans, C. (1998) Localization and properties of voltage-gated calcium channels in cone photoreceptors of Tupaia belangeri. *Vis. Neurosci.*, 15: 541–552.

Thoreson, W.B., Nitzan, R. and Miller, R.F. (1997) Reducing extracellular chloride suppresses dihydropyridine-sensitive calcium currents and synaptic transmission in amphibian photoreceptors. *J. Neurophysiol.*, 77: 2175–2190.

Thoreson, W.B. and Witkovsky, P. (1999) Glutamate receptors and circuits in the vertebrate retina. *Prog. Retinal and Eye Res.*, 18: 765–810.

Tran, M.N., Higgs, M.H. and Lukasiewicz, P.D. (1999) AMPA receptor kinetics limit retinal amacrine cell excitatory synaptic responses. *Vis. Neurosci.*, 16: 835–842.

Vardi, N., Morigiwa, K., Wang, T.-L., Shi, Y.-J. and Sterling, P. (1998) Neurochemistry of the mammalian cone 'synaptic complex'. *Vision Res.*, 38: 1359–1369.

Verweij, J., Kamermans, M. and Spekreijse, H. (1996) Horizontal cells feed back to cones by shifting the cone calcium-current activation range. *Vision Res.*, 36: 3943–3953.

Von Gersdorff, H., Vardi, E., Matthews, G. and Sterling, P. (1996) Evidence that vesicles on the synaptic ribbon of retinal bipolar neurons can be rapidly released. *Neuron*, 16: 1221–1227.

Wilkinson, M.F. and Barnes, S. (1996) The dihydropyridine-sensitive calcium channel subtype in cone photoreceptors. *J. Gen. Physiol.*, 107: 621–630.

Winkler, B.S., Kapousta-Bruneau, N., Arnold, M.J. and Green, D.G. (1999) Effects of inhibiting glutamine synthetase and blocking glutamate uptake on b-wave generation in the isolated rat retina. *Vis. Neurosci.*, 16: 345–353.

Witkovsky, P. and Dearry, A. (1991) Functional roles of dopamine in the vertebrate retina. *Prog. Ret. Res.*, 11: 242–292.

Witkovsky, P., Schmitz, Y., Akopian, A., Krizaj, D. and Tranchina, D. (1997) Gain of rod to horizontal cell synaptic transfer: relation to glutamate release and a dihydropyridine-sensitive calcium current. *J. Neurosci.*, 17: 7297–7306.

Wu, S.M. (1988) Synaptic transmission from rods to horizontal cells in dark-adapted tiger salamander retina. *Vision Res.*, 28: 1–8.

Yang, J.-H., Maple, B., Gao, F., Maguire, G. and Wu, S.M. (1998) Postsynaptic responses of horizontal cells in the tiger salamander retina are mediated by AMPA-preferring receptors. *Brain Res.* 797: 125–134.

Ziff, E.B. (1997) Enlightening the postsynaptic density. *Neuron*, 19: 1163–1174.

H. Kolb, H. Ripps and S. Wu (Eds.)
Progress in Brain Research, Vol. 131
© 2001 Elsevier Science B.V. All rights reserved

CHAPTER 10

Organization of ON- and OFF-pathways in the zebrafish retina: neurotransmitter localization, electrophysiological responses of bipolar cells, and patterns of axon terminal stratification

Victoria P. Connaughton*

Department of Biology, The American University, 4400 Massachusetts Avenue, NW, Washington, DC 20016, USA

Introduction

In the vertebrate retina, signals originate in the photoreceptors, propagate proximally through the retinal network via bipolar neurons, and are transmitted to the brain through ganglion cells. All three neurons within this vertical pathway (photoreceptors, bipolar cells and ganglion cells) use glutamate as their neurotransmitter. Lateral inhibitory inputs from GABA-containing horizontal cells in the distal retina and GABA- and glycine-containing amacrine cells in the proximal retina are believed to modify this vertical flow of information (Dowling, 1987).

Bipolar cells are physiologically classified as either OFF- or ON-subtypes based on their response to light and/or glutamate, the photoreceptor neurotransmitter. OFF-bipolar cells are depolarized by glutamate release in the dark. ON-bipolar cells are depolarized by light onset, when glutamate release is *decreased*. These physiological characteristics are correlated with neuronal morphology and glutamate receptor expression. Classically, the axon terminals of OFF-bipolar cells typically ramify within sublamina

*Tel.: 202-885-2188; Fax: 202-885-2182; E-mail: vconn@ american.edu

a of the inner plexiform layer (IPL) (Famiglietti et al., 1977; Stell et al., 1977), though there are some reports of multistratified OFF-type cells with terminals in both sublaminae (Maple and Wu 1996; Connaughton and Nelson, 2000). OFF-type bipolar cells express ionotropic, AMPA/kainate-type glutamate receptors on their dendritic arbors (Sasaki and Kaneko, 1996; DeVries and Schwartz, 1999). ON-bipolar cell axon terminals ramify in sublamina *b* of the IPL (Famiglietti et al, 1977; Stell et al., 1977) or sublaminas *a* and *b*. These cells express metabotropic APB-type receptors (Slaughter and Miller, 1981; Nawy and Jahr, 1990; Nawy, 1999) and/or glutamate receptors linked to chloride channels (Grant and Dowling, 1995, 1996). The present manuscript describes ON- and OFF-pathways in the zebrafish retina.

Bipolar cell characteristics have been documented in a variety of other vertebrates, such as fish (Kaneko and Tachibana, 1985; Lasater, 1988), salamander (Lasansky, 1978; Tessier-Lavigne et al., 1988), rat (Karschin and Wässle, 1990), cat (Nelson and Kolb, 1983), and monkey (Dacey, 1999). As yet, there are few physiological studies of the zebrafish visual system. Zebrafish has been a vertebrate model in genetic and developmental studies for twenty years. Due to their rapid generation time and easy

162

laboratory maintenance, a large number of mutant zebrafish strains have been identified, including (most recently) those characterized by retinal and/or visual system defects (Brockerhoff et al., 1995; Malicki et al., 1996; Chung and Dowling, 1997; Fadool et al., 1997; Neuhauss et al., 1999). While some of these mutations are identified by morphological changes in retinal anatomy (Fadool et al., 1997), others appear morphologically normal, but are behaviorally abnormal, suggesting an underlying physiological defect (Brockerhoff et al., 1995; Chung and Dowling, 1997). In some cases, the characteristics of the visual system defects are analogous to those associated with documented visual problems, such as color blindness (i.e. *pob*, Brockerhoff et al., 1997). Thus, it becomes important to understand retinal physiology and neurotransmitter distribution within the zebrafish model to serve as a basis for later experiments examining the mechanisms underlying retinal mutations.

Physiological experiments have documented the electrical properties of photoreceptors (Fan and Yazulla, 1997), horizontal cell gap junctions (McMahon, 1994; McMahon and Brown, 1994), bipolar cells (Connaughton and Maguire, 1998; Connaughton and Nelson, 2000), and dopaminergic potentiation of ganglion cell responses (Cohen and Dowling, 2000) in the zebrafish. My goal in this chapter is to summarize the existing morphological, electrical, and immunohistochemical data pertaining to bipolar cells, the middle component of the vertical transduction pathway. From such data one can gain insight into the circuitry patterns of the inner retina, which governs ON- and OFF-pathways.

My collaboration with John Dowling began with a study detailing the techniques for culturing adult and larval zebrafish retinal cells (Connaughton and Dowling, 1998). Since then, this work has expanded to include the use of the zebrafish retinal slice preparation (Fan and Yazulla, 1997; Connaughton and Maguire, 1998) to study bipolar cell activity in larval zebrafish with visual system defects.

Bipolar cell morphology

As viewed in the slice (Fig. 1), the zebrafish retina has an ordered structure similar to other vertebrates. All retinal layers can be clearly identified and cell bodies

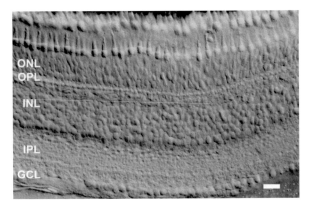

Fig. 1. Light micrograph of the zebrafish retinal slice. Retinal layers are indicated to the left of the photo, with ONL = outer nuclear layer, OPL = outer plexiform layer, INL = inner nuclear layer, IPL = inner plexiform layer, GCL = ganglion cell layer. Bipolar cell somata are located in the mid-distal INL. Bar = 5μm. Photo was taken using a Nikon microscope and DIC optics. (Connaughton et al., 1999b)

distinguished. In general, bipolar cells have flask-shaped or rounded somata within mid to distal inner nuclear layer (INL). A dendritic process extends from the soma into the outer plexiform layer (OPL) and a thinner axonal process, ending in a terminal, extends proximally into the IPL. These neurons are small in size, averaging 5 μm in diameter (Connaughton and Maguire, 1998).

Both voltage- and neurotransmitter-gated current activity has been documented in these cells using whole-cell patch clamp techniques (Hamill et al., 1981) and voltage-clamp protocols in the zebrafish retinal slice (Connaughton and Maguire, 1998; Connaughton and Nelson, 2000; Connaughton et al., 2000). Bipolar cells were identified, prior to whole-cell patch recordings, by soma position in the INL. Intracellular staining of recorded neurons with Lucifer Yellow (present in the patch pipette) typically allowed visualization of the entire neuron, confirming initial identification.

Multiple morphological types of bipolar cells have been identified in other fish retinae (Scholes, 1975; Sherry and Yazulla, 1993). In a recent study documenting glutamate responses in zebrafish bipolar cells, 13 morphological types were identified (Connaughton and Nelson, 2000). These types were classified by axon terminal ramification patterns (Fig. 2), which identified three regions in the IPL: a thick sublamina *a*, with three bands of boutons,

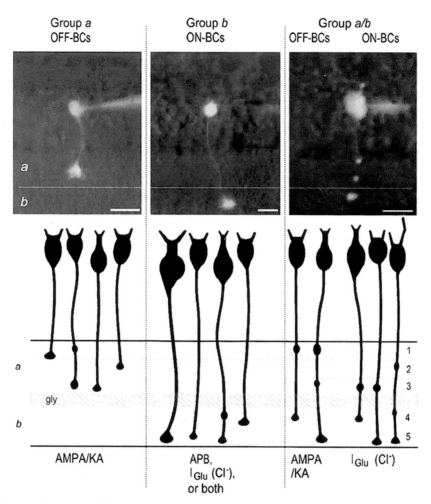

Fig. 2. Schematic diagram showing the different morphological types of bipolar cells identified in the zebrafish retina. ON- and OFF-type bipolar cells were categorized into three morphological Groups, based on axon terminal ramification patterns: Group *a* bipolar cells have axon terminal(s) restricted to sublamina *a*, Group *b* cells have axon terminal(s) only within sublamina *b*, Group *a/b* cells are multistratified with terminals in both sublaminae. A correlation of bipolar cell morphology with glutamate-gated current responses indicates OFF-bipolar cells express kainate/AMPA receptors and are classified within Groups *a* and *a/b*. ON-bipolar cells, expressing a metabotropic APB-type receptor and/or a glutamate receptor linked to a chloride channel, are localized to Groups *b* and *a/b*. Layers 1–5 within the IPL are indicated to the right. The "gly" line within the middle of the IPL denotes a terminal free zone labeling positively with an anti-glycine antibody. (Reprinted with permission from Connaughton and Nelson, 2000.)

a narrow terminal-free zone in the mid-IPL, and a thin sublamina *b*, with two bands of terminals. Bipolar cells were separated into three corresponding groups: cells with axonal boutons exclusively in sublamina *a* (Group *a*), those with terminals in sublamina *b* (Group *b*), and multistratified cells with terminals in both sublaminae (Group *a/b*). Each group contains a number of types, characterized by the particular layers in which the boutons reside

(Connaughton and Nelson, 2000). The separation of bipolar cells into these groups agrees with immuno-cytochemical data showing glutamate-containing bipolar cell axon terminals ramify within a thick OFF-sublamina and/or a thin ON-sublamina, separated by a bouton-free zone staining positively with anti-glycine (Fig. 4; Connaughton et al., 1999b). These morphological groupings were found to correlate with bipolar cell glutamate responses

(Connaughton and Nelson, 2000), but not with voltage-gated current activity (Connaughton and Maguire, 1998).

Electrical properties

Voltage-gated currents

In general, the voltage-gated currents identified in zebrafish bipolar cells are similar to those reported in other species (i.e. Kaneko and Tachibana, 1985; Lasater, 1988; Karschin and Wässle, 1990). Zebrafish bipolar cells express a variety of voltage-gated currents (Fig. 3); however, as reported in white bass (Lasater, 1988), not all zebrafish bipolar cells express the *same* compliment of currents. In fact, the differential expression of potassium currents was used to distinguish between two populations of cells, which do not correspond to ON- and OFF-cell types (Connaughton and Maguire, 1998).

Depolarization-activated outward currents

Two outward potassium currents, identified by sensitivity to internal cesium and external tetraethyl-ammonium (TEA), were elicited in response to membrane depolarizations. Each current was readily distinguished by its kinetics. In the majority of cells, depolarizing voltage pulses elicited a rapidly activating A-current (I_A; Fig. 3A, left) that reached peak amplitude within 5 ms of pulse onset and then decayed with time for the remainder of the stimulus. This current was sensitive to 4-aminopyridine (4-AP), a selective I_A antagonist, and to holding potential. In contrast, bipolar neurons lacking I_A expressed a slowly activating, delayed rectifying potassium current (I_K; Fig. 3B, left). Each type of potassium current was recorded in a separate group of cells; no zebrafish bipolar cells were found to express both I_A and I_K (Connaughton and Maguire, 1998).

In both populations of cells, a calcium-dependent potassium current (K_{Ca}) was also elicited in response to membrane depolarizations. In general, this current comprised < 30% of the total outward current amplitude. K_{Ca} was sensitive to the selective antagonist apamin, as well as to potassium and calcium channel blockers (Connaughton and Maguire, 1998).

Hyperpolarization-elicited inward currents

Hyperpolarizing voltage pulses elicited different responses from the two populations of cells. Neurons expressing I_A appear to lack an inward rectifier (Fig. 3A, right) as a small amplitude, sustained inward current was recorded in response to hyperpolarizing voltage pulses (Connaughton and Maguire, 1998). In contrast, zebrafish bipolar neurons expressing I_K also expressed a time-dependent inward rectifying current (I_H; Fig. 3B, right) in response to membrane hyperpolarizations. H-current amplitude was reduced in Na^+-free Ringer or by the bath application of cesium or barium (Connaughton and Maguire, 1998).

Depolarization-activated inward currents

Zebrafish bipolar cells express an inward calcium current (I_{Ca}) in response to membrane depolarizations (Fig. 3C). A sodium current was not identified in these cells, consistent with findings in other species (Kaneko and Tachibana, 1985; Lasater, 1988; Kaneko et al., 1989, 1991; Karschin and Wässle, 1990). I_{Ca} was typically elicited with membrane depolarizations > −50 mV and reached maximum amplitude at −20 to −10 mV. This current was antagonized by cadmium and cobalt, but not tetrodotoxin, and eliminated in Ca^{+2}-free Ringer.

Similar to findings reported in salamander (Maguire et al., 1989), zebrafish bipolar cells express T- and/or L-type calcium currents (Connaughton and Maguire, 1998). In most cells examined, rapidly activating transient (T-type) currents, sensitive to nickel, were identified. These currents activated at holding potentials ≤ −60 mV. In contrast, depolarizing voltage pulses elicit a slower, more sustained (L-type) current in other cells. The L-current was typically small in amplitude, and blocked by nifedipine. Interestingly, some bipolar cells expressed only one type of Ca^{+2} current (T- or L-type), while others express both T- and L-currents (Connaughton and Maguire, 1998).

Ca^{+2} channel activity is functionally important in the vesicular release of neurotransmitters. The L-type calcium channels identified in goldfish Mb-type ON-bipolar cells (Heidelberger and Matthews, 1992) have

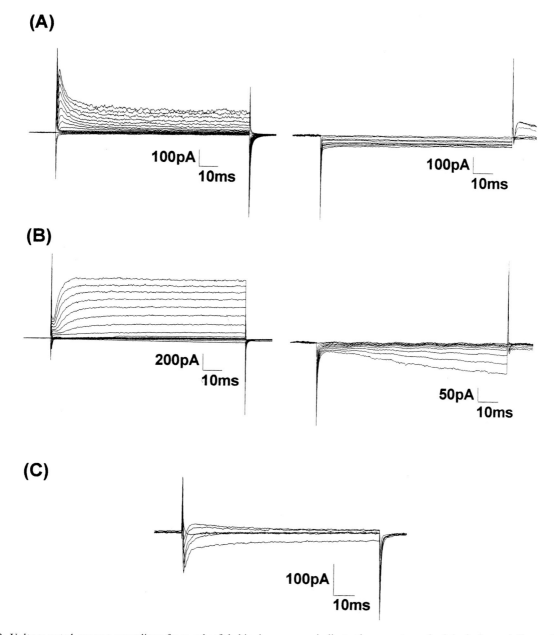

Fig. 3. Voltage-gated current recordings from zebrafish bipolar neurons indicate there are two physiological populations of cells. Whole-cell current traces recorded from one population were characterized by (A) a rapidly activating A-type potassium current in response to membrane depolarizations (left) and a sustained inward hyperpolarizing current (right). In contrast, the other group of cells (B) responded to membrane depolarizations with a slowly activating delayed rectifying potassium current (I_K, left) and a slowly activating H-current (right) in response to membrane depolarizations. Cells within both populations also a expressed calcium-dependent potassium current (not shown) and (C) depolarization elicited calcium currents. All currents were elicited in response to test voltages ranging from -80 to $+60$ mV (10 mV increments, 100 ms step duration, $V_{hold} = -60$ mV). (Modified from Connaughton and Maguire, 1998.)

166

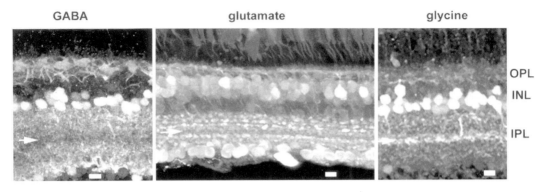

GABA   **glutamate**   **glycine**

OPL

INL

IPL

Fig. 4. Light micrographs showing the distribution of neurotransmitters in the zebrafish retina. GABA (left), glutamate (middle) and glycine (right) distribution patterns were examined using immunocytochemical techniques (Connaughton et al., 1999b). GABA immunoreactivity was observed in horizontal cells and their processes in the OPL and a population of amacrine cells. GABA-containing amacrine cell processes were identified throughout the IPL. Photoreceptors, bipolar cells and ganglion cells labeled strongly with the glutamate antibody. Glycine-positive structures were identified as amacrine cells and interplexiform cells. Glycine labeling was observed throughout the IPL, with the strongly immunoreactive band of processes corresponding to immunonegative regions in GABA and glutamate sections (arrows). All bars = 5 μm. Retinal layers are indicated to the right of the micrographs. (Modified and reprinted with permission from Connaughton et al., 1999b.)

been extensively studied as the large size of the axon terminals allows direct recordings from synaptic boutons. L-type Ca^{+2} channels in these cells mediate neurotransmitter release and vesicle cycling (i.e. Lagnado et al., 1996; von Gersdorff et al., 1996), as well as light-evoked action potentials observed in dark-adapted tissue (Zenisek and Matthews, 1998; Protti et al., 2000). Within zebrafish, intracellular labeling with Lucifer Yellow (Connaughton and Nelson, 2000) and immunocytochemical staining with an anti-glutamate antibody (Connaughton et al., 1999b) have identified Mb-type bipolar cells with large axon terminals, in addition to a diversity of other ON-cell types. Though T- and L-type calcium currents are differentially expressed in zebrafish bipolar cells, the majority of cells expressing L-type currents were morphologically identified ON-bipolars (see below; Connaughton and Maguire, 1998) suggesting that L-type calcium currents may underlie synaptic transmission to postsynaptic amacrine and ganglion cells within the proximal retina.

Correlation of voltage-gated currents with ON- and OFF- morphology

Zebrafish bipolar cells express a diversity of potassium and calcium currents in response to changes in

membrane potential. These currents are not the same in all cell types, but differentiate between two distinct populations. It is logical to hypothesize that these two physiological populations may correspond to ON- and OFF-cell types. To test this, voltage-gated current activity was correlated with axon terminal ramification patterns (Connaughton and Maguire, 1998). Of the cells expressing I_A, 67% were presumed OFF-bipolar neurons (classified within Group *a*), and 33% were presumed ON-cells classified within Group *b*. Similarly, I_K was expressed in cells identified as OFF-cells (46%) or as ON-cells (54%). Ca^{+2} current activity also varied among cells. T-type currents were recorded in most cells, whereas L-type Ca^{+2} currents were found predominantly in cells with a single axon terminal ramifying in sublamina *b* (Connaughton and Maguire, 1998). Taken together, these data suggest that most OFF-bipolar neurons express I_A while the majority of ON-cells express I_K and L-type Ca^{+2} currents. It should be noted, however, that the other current types were also identified within these groups, prompting the conclusion that there is no obligatory correlation between voltage-gated current activity and ON- and OFF-cell types (as determined by axon terminal ramification patterns). This suggests that the complexity of voltage-gated currents expressed in these cells function to maintain the neuron within its operating range (Lasater, 1988) and shape the light responses of these cells and that the requirements of these operations may not differ among ON- and OFF-types.

Excitatory mechanisms

Glutamate distribution patterns

The distribution patterns of the neurotransmitters glutamate, GABA, and glycine were examined using fixed, vibratome sectioned tissue (Connaughton et al., 1999b). In general, cone photoreceptors, bipolar cells and ganglion cells were brightly labeled with a glutamate antibody (Fig. 4, center), as in other species (Marc et al., 1990; Van Haesendonck and Missotten, 1990; Yang and Yazulla, 1994; Jojich and Pourcho, 1996). Horizontal and amacrine cells displayed light-to-moderate labeling. Bipolar cells dominated the observed glutamate immunoreactivity patterns in the inner retina. Bipolar cell somata were localized to a dense (2–3 cell bodies thick) layer in the mid-INL. Punctate labeling, corresponding to axon terminals, was observed throughout the IPL. This labeling occurred in five distinct strata. The three distal layers are mainly OFF-bipolar axon terminals. Two proximal layers contained the terminals of many ON-bipolar cells. Large, bulbous (Mb-type) axon terminals were identified within the innermost IPL (Connaughton et al., 1999b).

Glutamate-gated currents

To examine glutamate-evoked responses in bipolar cells, whole-cell patch clamp and puff pipette techniques were used within the retinal slice. Ligand-gated currents were elicited in response to focal puffs of glutamate or glutamate agonists onto the dendritic arbor (Connaughton and Nelson, 2000). Glutamate elicited four different current responses in zebrafish bipolar cells (Fig. 5): an excitatory AMPA/kainate response (OFF-cells), an inhibitory response generated via an APB-sensitive second messenger system, an inhibitory response mediated through a chloride channel, and the coexpression of APB and chloride mechanisms (ON-cells). Responses to N-methyl-D-aspartate (NMDA) were not observed (Connaughton and Nelson, 2000). Each physiological response was correlated with bipolar cell morphology to identify bipolar cell types comprising the ON- and OFF-pathways within the zebrafish retina.

OFF-bipolar cell responses

Glutamate evoked CNQX-sensitive, AMPA/kainate-like responses in 15% of bipolar neurons (Fig. 5A). Currents were characterized by a conductance increase, a positive reversal potential (E_{rev}), and a peak current of 20–30 pA. Similar responses were obtained with kainate, an ionotropic glutamate receptor agonist. Kainate-elicited currents were recorded from morphologically identified OFF-bipolar cells with axon terminals restricted to sublamina a (Group a) or from cells with terminals in both sublaminae (Group a/b) (Connaughton and Nelson, 2000).

Using a dual puffer technique to apply both glutamate and kainate to the same cell, Connaughton and Nelson (2000) were able to further categorize glutamate responses in OFF-bipolar cells. Interestingly, they found that zebrafish OFF-bipolars do not consistently respond to both glutamate and kainate, but appear to have two conductance mechanisms: one with sensitivity to both glutamate and kainate and another with sensitivity to kainate, but not glutamate. These responses were obtained regardless of the order of agonist application. Cells responding to glutamate but not kainate were observed, but these cells expressed an I_{Glu}-like chloride current later identified in ON-type cells (see below). Thus, there appears to be more than one conductance mechanism present on zebrafish OFF-bipolar cells. Similar findings have been reported in salamander (Maple et al., 1999) and mudpuppy (Kim and Miller, 1993), where the differences in OFF-bipolar cell response kinetics and antagonist sensitivity were found to be indicative of rod vs. cone inputs to these cells.

ON-bipolar cell responses

The three remaining glutamate-gated current types identified in zebrafish were localized to presumed ON-bipolar cells. Four percent of the examined ON-cells were characterized by a glutamate-elicited

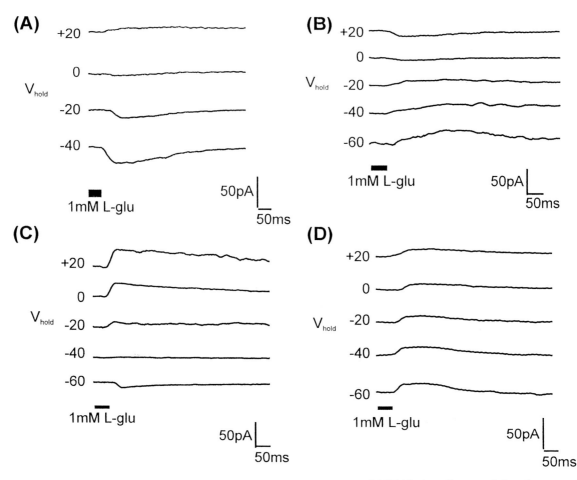

Fig. 5. Four distinct glutamate responses were identified in bipolar neurons. Presumed OFF-bipolar cells responded to glutamate with a conductance increase and a reversal potential (E_{rev}) near 0 mV (A). This response was mimicked by kainate. Three different glutamate conductance mechanisms were recorded from morphologically identified ON-bipolar cells. In 4% of cells, glutamate, or the ON-type agonist APB, elicited a conductance decrease with E_{rev} near 0 mV (B). The majority of bipolar neurons (60%) responded to glutamate with a conductance increase and $E_{rev} = E_{Cl}$ (C). Eleven percent of zebrafish bipolar neurons expressed "all outward" currents in response to glutamate application (D). Currents in (D) were result from the simultaneous expression of APB-type conductance decrease and a glutamate-evoked chloride conductance increase. (modified from Connaughton and Nelson, 2000). For each set of traces, holding potential (V_{hold}) is given to the left of each trace; drug application is indicated by the bar at the bottom of the traces.

conductance decrease, E_{rev} near 0 mV, and a peak current amplitude of 20 pA (Fig. 5B). This response was mimicked by the metabotropic agonists 2-amino-4-phosphonobutyric acid (APB) and *trans*-1-amino-1, 3-cyclopentanedicarboxylic acid (*trans*-ACPD). Bipolar cells responding to these agonists had identifiable axon terminals exclusively in sublamina *b*, placing them within Group *b*, corresponding to the classical morphology of ON-BCs (Connaughton and Nelson, 2000).

In the majority of ON-bipolar cells examined (60%), glutamate elicited a chloride current accompanied by a conductance increase (Fig. 5C). This current is similar to I_{Glu}, the glutamate-mediated chloride channel identified in bass bipolar cells (Grant and Dowling, 1995). I_{Glu} is directly gated by glutamate, sensitive to changes in chloride ion concentration, antagonized by glutamate transporter blockers, and sensitive to changes in external sodium concentration (Grant and Dowling, 1995).

The chloride current in zebrafish was also insensitive to picrotoxin and strychnine, indicating it is elicited directly by glutamate and not indirectly through inhibitory GABAergic or glycinergic inputs. Further, the observed E_{rev} changed in a predicted manner with changing $[Cl]_{in}$ or $[Cl]_{out}$. In contrast to I_{Glu}, however, the current in zebrafish was only partially sensitive to Li^+ substitution for Na^+_{out} (Connaughton and Nelson, 2000). Bipolar cells expressing this current were classified in Groups *a*, *b*, and *a/b* with the majority localized to Group *b*, suggesting most neurons expressing this current are probably ON-bipolar cells. However, the diverse morphology observed in this group was less adherent to classical morphological patterns compared to bipolar cells expressing the metabotropic (APB-type) receptor.

Finally, the third glutamate-elicited response, recorded from 14% of morphologically identified ON-bipolar cells, was characterized by outward currents at all holding potentials tested. No E_{rev} was observe across the range of holding potentials tested (Fig. 5D). This glutamate response was generated by two opposing mechanisms. Evidence for the coexpression of two mechanisms was obtained through the following experiments. First, the "all outward" currents were observed to change over time resulting in a current similar to the chloride current described above. Second, the chloride current was revealed after the bath application of APB (Connaughton and Nelson, 2000). Taken together, these findings suggest that cells expressing "all outward" currents may have two conductance mechanisms to glutamate (i.e. Saito, et al., 1979; Nawy and Copenhagen, 1987): an APB-sensitive conductance decrease, and an APB-insensitive chloride conductance (see also Grant and Dowling, 1996). Bipolar cells expressing this type of glutamate-gated current were consistently classified within Group *b*, like metabotropic ON-BC types.

Correlation of glutamate gated currents with ON- and OFF- morphology

In contrast to voltage-gated current activity, bipolar cell glutamate responses were used to identify ON- and OFF-morphological types (Fig. 2). OFF-bipolar cells, expressing AMPA/kainate type receptors, were found in Groups *a* and *a/b*; whereas, ON-bipolar cells were classified within Group *b* or Group *a/b*. Though these findings are as predicted for monostratified cells, they also provide evidence for the functional role of the diverse multistratified cells consistently identified in teleost retinas (i.e. Scholes, 1975; Sherry and Yazulla, 1993).

Inhibitory mechanisms

GABA distribution patterns

The observed labeling of GABA-positive structures was most intense in the proximal retina, where presumed amacrine cells and their processes within the IPL were positively labeled (Fig. 4, left). Overall, staining of GABA-containing processes within the IPL was either homogeneous or organized into two broad bands, separated by an immunonegative layer. A few cells in the ganglion cell layer were also found to contain GABA; probably representing a population of displaced amacrine cells. In the distal retina, labeling was restricted to horizontal cells and their processes. Similar labeling patterns were also observed with antibodies to glutamic acid decarboxylase (GAD), the synthetic enzyme for GABA. Bipolar cells and photoreceptors were unlabeled (Connaughton et al., 1999b). The observed labeling patterns indicate bipolar cell dendrites and axon terminals are surrounded by GABA-containing structures possibly mediating lateral inhibitory connections.

GABA-gated currents

Consistent with immunocytochemical findings describing the distribution of GABA in the zebrafish retina, inhibitory GABA-evoked currents in bipolar neurons are predominantly localized to the axon terminals. Responses to the focal application of GABA onto bipolar cell dendrites (Fig. 6A, top traces) elicited small (5 pA) responses in < 15% of cells tested, while over half of the cells responded to GABA application onto terminal boutons (Fig. 6A, bottom) with robust responses (30–50 pA). The absence of a response to GABA application onto

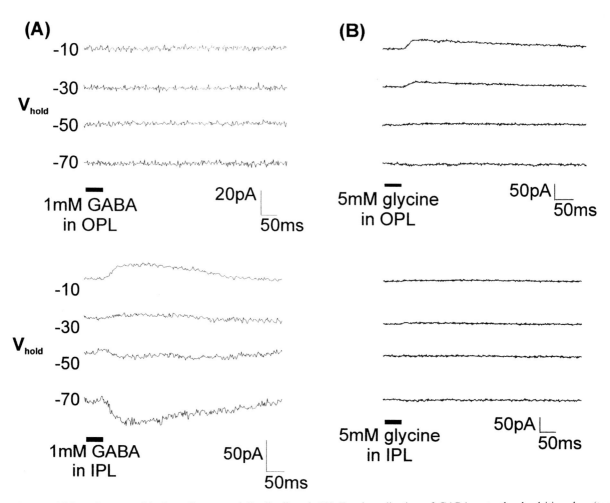

Fig. 6. Inhibitory inputs to bipolar cells are spatially distributed. (A) Focal application of GABA onto the dendritic arbor (top) typically failed to evoke responses from bipolar neurons (95% of cells tested). In contrast, GABA applied to the axon terminal(s) (bottom) elicited robust currents measuring 30–50 pA in most cells. These currents were elicited through the activation of $GABA_C$ and $GABA_A$ receptor types. In contrast, the focal application of glycine (B) onto the dendritic arbor (top) elicited more robust and consistent responses than glycine application onto axon terminals (bottom). Taken together, these findings indicate zebrafish bipolar cells have GABA receptors predominantly localized to the axon terminal region, while glycine receptors provide direct inputs primarily to the dendritic arbor. For each set of traces, holding potential (V_{hold}) is given to the left; drug application is indicated by the bar at the bottom of the traces.

bipolar cell dendrites, observed with or without cobalt in the bath solution, (Connaughton et al., 2000) is a somewhat surprising finding. Anatomical evidence in other species indicates GABAergic horizontal cell input modulating bipolar cell glutamate responses may occur directly, through synapses onto bipolar cell dendrites (Dowling et al., 1966; Werblin and Dowling, 1969; Lasansky, 1973) or indirectly, via a feedback pathway from horizontal

cells onto photoreceptor terminals (Burkhardt, 1977; Kondo and Toyoda, 1983; Wu, 1986; Wu and Maple, 1998). The small amplitude of GABA-evoked responses at bipolar cell dendrites suggests that direct, presynaptic GABA inputs onto bipolar cells is not a major OPL pathway in the zebrafish retina.

GABA-gated currents in zebrafish bipolar cells were examined in the intact retinal slice (using the above protocols) and using voltage probe measurements of isolated cells (Connaughton et al., 2000). Both techniques show GABA application elicits a chloride current agonized by muscimol, blocked by picrotoxin, and partially sensitive to bicuculline. In addition, isolated bipolar cells are sensitive to a wide range of GABA concentrations (10 nM to 20 μM) which are blocked by zinc. Taken together these findings suggest that bipolar cells and their axon terminals express primarily $GABA_C$ receptors, though a minority of $GABA_A$ receptors are also present (Connaughton et al., 2000). A diversity of GABA receptors has also been reported in white bass (Qian and Dowling, 1995) and ferret (Lukasiewicz and Wong, 1997) bipolar cells. GABA responses were obtained from bipolar cells within Groups *a*, *b* and *a/b*, consistent with the immunoreactivity profile of GABA processes surrounding bipolar cell terminals at all depths in the IPL.

Glycine distribution patterns and current activity

Glycine containing structures were observed in the INL, in the ganglion cell layer, and within both plexiform layers (Fig. 4, right). Glycine-positive amacrine cells, located in the proximal INL or in the ganglion cell layer, were more oblate than GABA-positive cells, suggesting they represent a separate population of amacrine cells. Glycine-containing interplexiform cells (IPCs; Marc and Lam, 1981; Kalloniatis and Marc, 1990) were also identified. IPCs were characterized by a positively labeled cell body in the mid-INL and a process extending into the OPL. In addition to the glycine-positive puncta observed throughout the IPL, a prominent band of processes was identified in the mid-IPL. A comparison of glycine and GABA immunoreactivity patterns implies that the glycine-positive band corresponds to the immunonegative region observed in other sections (Fig. 4, arrows). No labeling was observed in the distal INL or in the ONL (Connaughton et al., 1999b). Preliminary physiological data indicates that glycine-evoked currents (Fig. 6B) were more consistently recorded after glycine application onto dendritic arbors (77% of cells tested) than onto the axon terminals (26% of cells tested), in contrast to GABA-evoked current responses. Taken together, these findings suggest

that glycine modulates direct inhibitory connections in the OPL; whereas, GABA provides the major inhibitory input to bipolar cell terminals. Present experiments are examining these differential inhibitory connections.

Applicability of existing data to studies of visual system defects

Recently, zebrafish mutants with visual system defects have been described. Some of these mutants are characterized by obvious morphological and/or developmental abnormalities (i.e. Malicki et al., 1996; Fadool et al., 1997) while other defects are difficult to identify because the animals are morphologically indistinguishable from wildtype siblings. As a result, behavioral screens, such as the optokinetic nystagmus (i.e. Brockerhoff et al., 1995) and the optomotor response (Neuhauss et al., 1999), have been employed to detect animals carrying these recessive mutations. Subsequent techniques, such as electroretinograms (ERGs), can then be used to pinpoint physiological mechanisms underlying the observed defects.

One of the first mutants to be identified using behavioral screens was *noa* (no optokinetic nystagmus a; Brockerhoff et al., 1995). *Noa*'s are characterized by morphologically normal retinal layering, optic nerve structure and retinal cell differentiation in comparison to wildtype siblings. However, their optokinetic response is absent and b-wave of the ERG is both delayed and reduced in amplitude (Brockerhoff et al., 1995). As the b-wave is a reflection of ON-bipolar cell activity (Stockton and Slaughter, 1989), the physiological data collected from *noa* mutants suggests that the mutation is localized to the bipolar neurons. Thus, an examination of voltage- and ligand-gated current activity in mutant and wildtype bipolar cells (Connaughton et al., 1999a) could suggest a possible mechanism underlying the observed behavioral defect.

Whole-cell patch clamp techniques in the larval (6–10 days postfertilization) retinal slice were used to document voltage- and glutamate-gated currents expressed in wildtype and *noa* bipolar neurons. Voltage-gated currents recorded in both wildtype and *noa* (Fig. 7A, B) cells (Connaughton et al., 1999a) appear similar to voltage-gated currents reported in adult

(A)

(B)

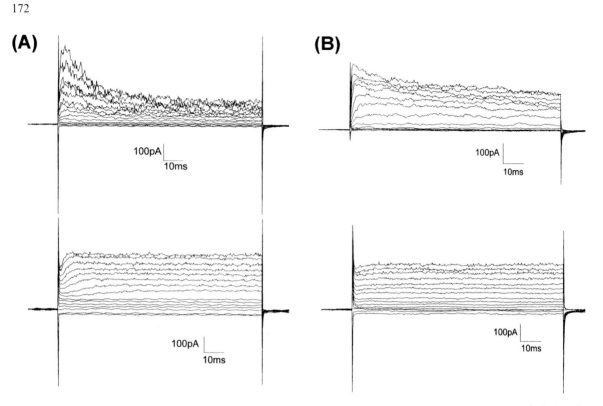

Fig. 7. Bipolar cells in wildtype and *noa* retinas express similar voltage-gated currents. Representative families of whole-cell current traces taken from (A) wildtype and (B) *noa* bipolar cells. In each retina (6–10 day postfertilization), two physiological populations of cells, one expressing I_A (top traces) and the other expressing I_K (bottom) in response to membrane depolarizations, were identified. All currents were elicited in response to test voltages ranging from -80 to $+60$ mV (10 mV increments, 100 ms step duration, $V_{hold} = -60$ mV).

neurons (Connaughton and Maguire, 1998) with two physiological populations identified. Bipolar cells classified within one population expressed I_A in response to membrane depolarizations; while cells in the other population expressed I_K.

Glutamate-gated currents documented in these cells were determined using kainate and APB, the selective agonists for OFF- and ON-type bipolar cells, respectively. In wildtype bipolar cells, kainate application elicited a current characterized by a conductance increase and a positive E_{rev} (Fig. 8A). These responses were blocked by 6-cyano-7-nitroquinoxaline-2, 3-dione (CNQX, Fig. 8C). Neurons expressing these currents were classified within morphological Groups *a* or *a/b*, similar to findings reported for OFF-bipolar cells in adults (Connaughton and Nelson, 2000). APB was an effective agonist (Fig. 8E) of dendritic receptors on presumed ON-bipolar cells (Connaughton et al., 1999a).

Bipolar cells within *noa* retinas also responded to kainate application. Here, as in wildtype animals, kainate-gated currents were accompanied by a conductance increase and a positive E_{rev} (Fig. 8B). However, these responses were distinct with regard to two characteristics. First, CNQX did not block kainate responses elicited in *noa* bipolar cells in the slice (Fig. 8D). Second, kainate-gated currents were expressed in morphologically identified OFF- (classified within Group *a*) and ON-type (Group *b*) cells. At the concentrations tested, no APB responses (Fig. 8F) were recorded from *noa* bipolar cells in the intact slice preparation (Connaughton et al., 1999a). Interestingly, APB application was also found to abolish the a-wave of the ERG (see chapter by Brockerhoff, this volume). Taken together, these findings suggest a possible defect in mGluR expression and/or function in this visual defect. Thus, all cells examined appear to express OFF-type dendritic

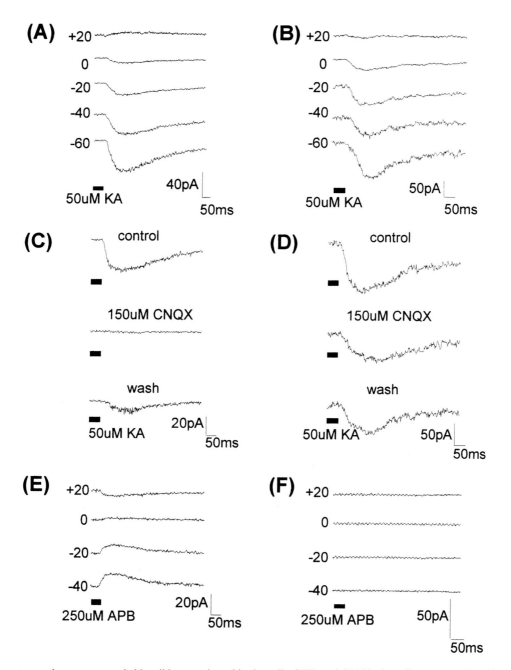

Fig. 8. Glutamate-gated currents recorded in wildtype and *noa* bipolar cells. OFF- and ON-bipolar cell types were identified using the selective glutamate agonists, kainate and APB. (A) Bipolar neurons in wildtype retinas express kainate-elicited currents characterized by a conductance increase and E_{rev} between 0 and +20 mV. These currents were blocked by CNQX (C). These neurons were morphologically identified as OFF-cells. Similar currents were recorded from *noa* bipolar neurons (B), though the kainate-gated currents in these cells were CNQX-insensitive (D). Kainate-evoked currents in *noa* retinas were recorded from morphologically identified OFF- and ON-cell types. (E) APB responses were elicited from a subset of morphologically identified wildtype ON-bipolar neurons; whereas, (F) APB failed to evoke responses in *noa* bipolar cells recorded within the slice preparation. For traces in (A, B, E, F), holding potential is given to the left; all traces in (C) and (D) were recorded at $V_{hold} = -60$ mV). Drug application is indicated by the bar at the bottom of the traces.

glutamate receptors, and the classic metabotropic ON-type receptor appears to be absent. On-going experiments are examining the I_{Glu}-type chloride conductance mechanism in these cells.

Conclusions and future perspectives

Classically, retinal bipolar cells are separated into ON- and OFF-types, each with an associated stratification pattern. OFF-cells arborize in sublamina *a* of the IPL and ON-cells arborize in sublamina *b* (Famiglietti et al., 1977; Stell et al., 1977). This neatly separates the IPL into two regions of opposing polarity, which is maintained in connections with postsynaptic ganglion and amacrine cells.

In zebrafish, ON- and OFF-bipolar cells display an incredible diversity of morphological and physiological responses. This diversity is most apparent in adult retinas, though it is also evident in larval tissue 6 dpf and older. Monostratified cells comprise 62% of the identified bipolar cells; the remaining identified types are multistratified with terminals residing in both sublaminae. What is the response of these multistratified cells? Do they maintain a distinct polarity (OFF or ON) or are they responsive to both light onset and offset, like some populations of multistratified amacrine cells? There are two lines of evidence suggesting that multistratified zebrafish bipolar cells should be exclusively classified as either ON- or OFF-subtypes, but not ON-OFF types. First, dual puffer experiments applying kainate and glutamate onto bipolar cell dendrites indicates OFF-type kainate responses are never found together on the same bipolar cell with ON-type chloride currents. Second, kainate responses were localized to neurons with "classic" OFF morphology (Group *a*); whereas, APB and chloride responses were localized to some neurons with "classic" ON morphology (Group *b*). It also appears that multistratified OFF-bipolar cells in zebrafish tend to have their axon terminals more distally located (layers 1, 2, and 4 of the IPL; Fig. 2) than multistratified ON-cell boutons (layers 3, 4 and 5 of the IPL; Fig. 2), suggesting an ON-/OFF-morphological distinction between multistratified cell types.

In addition to their morphology, OFF- and ON-cells have a diversity of electrophysiological characteristics associated with them. As many as 3 types of glutamate responses have been recorded from both ON- and OFF-cell subtypes. In other studies, the different glutamate responses identified in ON- (Grant and Dowling, 1996) and OFF- (Kim and Miller, 1993; Maple et al., 1999) bipolar cells are attributed to different photoreceptor inputs. In ON-type cells, APB responses are elicited in response to rod inputs and chloride currents evoked by glutamate release from cones (Grant and Dowling, 1996). If this applied to zebrafish, it would suggest that bipolar cells receiving APB inputs are postsynaptic to rods only, those expressing chloride currents (I_{Glu}) are postsynaptic to cones, and a combination of these mechanisms (identified as "all outward" currents) is present in mixed rod-cone neurons. Indeed, multistratified bipolar cells have been identified as cone-connected types in related species (Scholes, 1975). Multistratified ON-types in zebrafish appear to utilize only the cone synapse related to I_{Glu}.

Two different glutamate-gated currents, identified by desensitization kinetics and single channel conductances, have been identified in salamander bipolar cells and correspond to rod- and cone-dominated OFF-bipolar cell types (Maple et al., 1999). Further, rod and cone inputs to OFF-bipolar cells in mudpuppy were found to be differentially sensitive to the antagonist kynurenic acid (Kim and Miller, 1993). In zebrafish, differences in glutamate-gated OFF-bipolar cell currents were identified based on differential agonist (kainate) selectivity, suggesting a difference in subunit composition of the receptors. It is interesting to note that a visual system defect in *noa* bipolar cells appears to involve OFF-bipolar cell kainate receptors, suggesting this receptor type may play a large role in processing light signals in the retina.

This review has summarized current data pertaining to the ON- and OFF-bipolar cell pathways in the zebrafish retina. Overall, the electrical and morphological characteristics identified in these cells are generally similar to those reported in other species, suggesting that zebrafish would be an excellent model system to study synaptogenesis and/or changes or mutations in neurotransmitter distribution, receptor identification, and current activity. The continued identification of strains with visual system defects, and the analysis of the mechanisms underlying these defects, will ultimately enhance our understanding of retinal circuitry and nerve cell function in the vertebrate visual system.

References

Brockerhoff, S.E., Hurley, J.B., Janssen-Bienhold, U., Neuhauss, S.C.F., Driever, W. and Dowling, J.E. (1995) A behavioral screen for isolating zebrafish mutants with visual system defects. Proc. Natl. Acad. Sci., 92: 10545–10549.

Brockerhoff, S.E., Hurley, J.B., Niemi, G.A. and Dowling, J.E. (1997) A new form of inherited red-blindness identified in zebrafish. J. Neurosci., 17: 4236–4242.

Burkhardt, D.A. (1977) Responses and receptive-field organization of cones in perch retina. J. Neurophysiol., 40: 53–62.

Chung, S.C. and Dowling, J.E. (1997) Isolation and characterization of a motion sensitive-defective mutant in zebrafish. Invest. Ophthal. Vis. Sci., 38: S619.

Cohen, E.D. and Dowling, J.E. (2000) Dopamine potentiates synaptic transmission from bipolar cells in the cyprinid retina. Invest. Ophthal. Vis. Sci., 41: S936.

Connaughton, V.P. and Dowling, J.E. (1998) Comparative morphology of distal neurons in larval and adult zebrafish retina. Vision Res., 38: 13–18.

Connaughton, V.P. and Maguire, G. (1998) Differential expression of voltage-gated K$^+$ and Ca^{+2} currents in bipolar cells in the zebrafish retinal slice. Eur. J. Neurosci., 10: 1350–1362.

Connaughton, V.P., Allwardt, B. and Dowling, J.E. (1999a) Defective glutamate receptors in bipolar cells of zebrafish noa mutants. Invest. Ophthal. Vis. Sci., 40: S441.

Connaughton, V.P., Behar, T.N., Liu, W.-L.S. and Massey, S.C. (1999b) Immunocytochemical localization of excitatory and inhibitory neurotransmitters in the zebrafish retina. Vis. Neurosci., 16: 483–490.

Connaughton, V.P., Bender, A.M. and Nelson, R. (2000) GABA-evoked responses in zebrafish retinal bipolar cells. Invest. Ophthal. Vis. Sci., 41: S621.

Connaughton, V.P. and Nelson, R. (2000) Axonal stratification patterns and glutamate-gated conductance mechanisms in zebrafish retinal bipolar cells. J. Physiol., 524: 135–146.

Dacey, D.M. (1999) Primate retina: cell types, circuits and color opponency. Progr. Ret. Eye Res., 18: 737–763.

DeVries, S.H. and Schwartz, E.A. (1999) Kainate receptors mediate synaptic transmission between cones and 'off' bipolar cells in a mammalian retina. Nature, 397: 157–160.

Dowling, J.E., Brown, J.E. and Major, D. (1966) Synapses of horizontal cells in rabbit and cat retinas. Science, 30: 1639–1641.

Dowling, J.E. (1987) The Retina, an Approachable Part of the Brain. The Belknap Press of Harvard University Press, Cambridge, MA.

Fadool, J.M., Brockerhoff, S.E., Hyatt, G.A. and Dowling, J.E. (1997) Mutations affecting eye morphology in the developing zebrafish (Danio rerio). Developmental Genetics, 20: 288–295.

Famiglietti, E.V. Jr., Kaneko, A. and Tachibana, M. (1977) Neuronal architecture of On and Off pathways to ganglion cells in carp retina. Science, 198: 1267–1269.

Fan, S.-F. and Yazulla, S. (1997) Electrogenic hyperpolarization-elicited chloride transporter current in blue cones of zebrafish retinal slices. J. Neurophysiol., 77: 1447–1459.

Grant, G.B. and Dowling, J.E. (1995) A glutamate-activated chloride current in cone-driven ON bipolar cells of the white perch retina. J. Neurosci., 15: 3852–3862.

Grant, G.B. and Dowling, J.E. (1996) ON bipolar cell responses in the teleost retina are generated by two distinct mechanisms. J. Neurophysiol., 76: 3842–3849.

Hamill, O.P., Marty, A., Neher, E., Sakmann, B. and Sigworth, F.J. (1981) Improved patch-clamp techniques for high resolution current recording from cells and cell-free membrane patches. Pflüegers Arch., 391: 85–100.

Heidelberger, R. and Matthews, G. (1992) Calcium influx and calcium current in single synaptic terminals of goldfish retinal bipolar cells. J. Physiol., 447: 235–256.

Jojich, L. and Pourcho, R.G. (1996) Glutamate immunoreactivity in the cat retina: a quantitative study. Vis. Neurosci., 13: 117–133.

Kalloniatis, M. and Marc, R.E. (1990) Interplexiform cells of the goldfish retina. J. Comp. Neurol., 297: 340–358.

Kaneko, A., Pinto, L.H. and Tachibana, M. (1989) Transient calcium current of retinal bipolar cells of the mouse. J. Physiol., 410: 613–629.

Kaneko, A., Suzuki, S., Pinto, L.H. and Tachibana, M. (1991) Membrane currents and pharmacology of retinal bipolar cells: a comparative study on goldfish and mouse. Comp. Biochem. Physiol., 98C: 115–127.

Kaneko, A. and Tachibana, M. (1985) A voltage-clamp analysis of membrane currents in solitary bipolar cells dissociated from Carassius auratus. J. Physiol., 358: 131–152.

Karschin, A. and Wässle, H. (1990) Votlage- and transmitter-gated currents in isolated rod bipolar cells of rat retina. J. Neurophysiol., 63: 860–876.

Kim, H.G. and Miller, R.F. (1993) Properties of synaptic transmission from photoreceptors to bipolar cells in the mudpuppy retina. J. Neurophysiol., 69: 352–360.

Kondo, J. and Toyoda, J.-I. (1983) GABA and glycine effects on the bipolar cells of the carp retina. Vision Res., 23: 1259–1264.

Lagnado, L., Gomis, A. and Job, C. (1996) Continous vesicle cycling in the synpatic terminal of retinal bipolar cells. Neuron, 17: 957–967.

Lasansky, A. (1973) Organization of the outer synaptic layer in the retina of the larval tiger salamander. Philos. Trans. R. Soc. Lond., B., 265: 471–489.

Lasansky, A. (1978) Contacts between receptors and electrophysiologically identified neurones in the retina of the larval tiger salamander. J. Physiol., 285: 531–542.

Lasater, E.M. (1988) Membrane currents of retinal bipolar cells in culture. J. Neurophysiol., 60: 1460–1480.

Lukasiewicz, P.D. and Wong, R.O.L. (1997) GABA$_C$ receptors on ferret retinal bipolar cells: a diversity of subtypes in mammals? Vis. Neurosci., 14: 989–994.

Maguire, G., Maple, B., Lukasiewicz, P. and Werblin, F. (1989) γ-amino butyrate type B receptor modulation of L-type calcium channel current at bipolar cell terminals in the retina of the tiger salamander. *Proc. Natl. Acad. Sci.*, 86: 10144–10147.

Malicki, J., Neuhauss, S.C.F., Schier, A.F., Solnica-Krezel, L., Stemple, D.L., Stainier, D.Y.R., Abdelilah, S., Zwartkruis, F., Rangini, Z. and Driever, W. (1996) Mutations affecting development of the zebrafish retina. *Development*, 123: 263–273.

Maple, B.R., Gao, F. and Wu, S.M. (1999) Glutamate receptors differ in rod- and cone-dominated off-center bipolar cells. *Neuroreport*, 10: 3605–3610.

Maple, B.R. and Wu, S.M. (1996) Synaptic inputs mediating bipolar cell responses in the tiger salamander retina. *Vision Res.*, 36: 4015–4023.

Marc, R.E. and Lam, D.M.K. (1981) Glycinergic pathways in the goldfish retina. *J. Neurosci.*, 1: 152–165.

Marc, R.E., Liu, W.-L.S., Kalloniatis, M., Raiguel, S.F. and Van Haesendonck, E. (1990) Patterns of glutamate immunoreactivity in the goldfish retina. *J. Neurosci.*, 10: 4006–4034.

McMahon, D.G. (1994) Modulation of electrical synaptic transmission in zebrafish retinal horizontal cells. *J. Neurosci.*, 14: 1722–1734.

McMahon, D.G. and Brown, D.R. (1994) Modulation of gap-junction channel gating at zebrafish retinal electrical synapses. *J. Neurophysiol.*, 72: 2257–2268.

Nawy, S. (1999) The metabotropic receptor mGluR6 may signal through Go, but not phosphodiesterase, in retinal bipolar cells. *J. Neurosci.*, 19: 2938–2944.

Nawy, S. and Copenhagen, D.R. (1987) Multiple classes of glutamate receptor on depolarizing bipolar cells in retina. *Nature*, 325: 56–58.

Nawy, S. and Jahr, C.E. (1990) Suppression by glutamate of cGMP-activated conductance in retinal bipolar cells. *Nature*, 346: 269–271.

Nelson, R. and Kolb, H. (1983) Synaptic patterns and response properties of bipolar and ganglion cells in the cat retina. *Vision Res.*, 23: 1183–1195.

Neuhauss, S.C.F., Biehlmaier, O., Seeliger, M.W., Das, T., Kohler, K., Harris, W.A. and Baier, H. (1999) Genetic disorders of vision revealed by a behavioral screen of 400 essential loci in zebrafish. *J. Neurosci.*, 19: 8603–8615.

Protti, D.A., Flores-Herr, N. and von Gersdorff, H. (2000) Light evokes Ca^{+2} spikes in the axon terminal of a retinal bipolar cell. *Neuron*, 25: 215–227.

Qian, H. and Dowling, J.E. (1995) $GABA_A$ and $GABA_C$ receptors on hybrid bass retinal bipolar cells. *J. Neurophysiol.*, 74: 1920–1928.

Saito, T., Kondo, H. and Toyoda, J.-I. (1979) Ionic mechanisms of two types of On-center bipolar cells in the carp retina. *J. Gen. Physiol.*, 73: 73–90.

Sasaki, T. and Kaneko, A. (1996) L-glutamate-induced responses in OFF-type bipolar cells of the cat retina. *Vision Res.*, 36: 787–795.

Scholes, J.H. (1975) Colour receptors, and their synaptic connexions, in the retina of a cyprinid fish. *J. Physiol.*, 270: 61–118.

Sherry, D.M. and Yazulla, S. (1993) Goldfish bipolar cells and axon terminal patterns: a Golgi study. *J. Comp Neurol.*, 329: 188–200.

Slaughter, M.M. and Miller, R.F. (1981) 2-amino-4-phosphonobutyric acid: a new pharmacological tool for retina research. *Science*, 211: 182–185.

Stell, W.K., Ishida, A.T. and Lightfoot, D.O. (1977) Structural basis for On- and Off-center responses in retinal bipolar cells. *Science*, 198: 1269–1271.

Stockton, R.A. and Slaughter, M.M. (1989) B-wave of the electroretinogram, a reflection of ON bipolar cell activity. *J. Gen. Physiol.*, 93: 101–122.

Tessier-Lavigne, M., Attwell, D., Mobbs, P. and Wilson, M. (1988) Membrane currents in retinal bipolar cells of the axolotl. *J. Gen. Physiol.*, 91: 49–72.

Van Haesendonck, E. and Missotten, L. (1990) Glutamate-like immunoreactivity in the retina of a marine teleost, the dragonet. *Neurosci. Lett.*, 111: 281–286.

Von Gersdorff, H., Vardi, E., Matthews, G. and Sterling, P. (1996) Evidence that vesicles on the synaptic ribbon of retinal bipolar neurons can be rapidly released. *Neuron*, 16: 1221–1227.

Werblin, F.S. and Dowling, J.E. (1969) Organization of the retina of the mudpuppy, *Necturus maculosus* II. Intracellular recording. *J. Neurophysiol.*, 32: 339–355.

Wu, S.M. (1986) Effects of gamma-aminobutyric acid on cones and bipolar cells of the tiger salamander retina. *Brain Res.*, 365: 70–77.

Wu, S.M. and Maple, B.R. (1998) Amino acid neurotransmitters in the retina: a functional overview. *Vision Res.*, 38: 1371–1384.

Yang, C.Y. and Yazulla, S. (1994) Glutamate-, GABA- and GAD-immunoreactivities colocalize in bipolar cells of tiger salamander retina. *Vis. Neurosci.*, 11: 1193–1203.

Zenisek, D. and Matthews, G. (1998) Calcium action potentials in retinal bipolar neurons. *Vis. Neurosci.*, 15: 69–75.

H. Kolb, H. Ripps and S. Wu (Eds.)
Progress in Brain Research, Vol. 131
© 2001 Elsevier Science B.V. All rights reserved

CHAPTER 11

Retinal information processing and ambient illumination

Richard L. Chappell*

*Department of Biological Sciences, Hunter College, City University of New York, 695 Park Avenue, New York, NY 10021, USA
and Ph.D. Program in Biology, The Graduate Center, City University of New York, New York, NY 10016, USA*

I began working in John Dowling's laboratory at the Wilmer Institute of Ophthalmology of the Johns Hopkins University Medical Center as a doctoral student in the late 1960s. As I began my summer project, I was fortunate to be in the company of a fine group of young scientists working in John's lab, including Dwight Burkhardt, Mark Dubin, Helga Kolb, Bob Miller, and Frank Werblin, to name a few. With John's insight and guidance, I embarked on a study which attempted to address the question, "where are the action potentials in retinal neurons?"

At the time there was concern regarding the absence of action potentials in recordings from neurons of the outer retina of vertebrates, including the retinal bipolar cells which provide the afferent interplexiform pathway for visual information. Was it possible that visual information could be conveyed between plexiform layers electrotonically and neurotransmitters released at the terminals of these elongated cells without action potentials? Or were the intracellular electrodes used for recording their responses simply injuring the cells so that impulses, normally present, were not being recorded?

John suggested the dragonfly ocellus might provide a useful preparation with which to address this issue. Considering Ruck's (1961a,b,c) classical studies of

extracellular recordings from this hearty preparation, it appeared that intracellular recordings might reveal responses exhibiting both action potentials and slow potentials from its photoreceptor cells with their elongated, axon-like terminal processes.

Intracellular recordings had not been made from an ocellar retina and dragonflies could not be ordered from a supply house. Collecting dragonflies from ponds around Baltimore became an interesting avocation. The median ocellus (Fig. 1) of an *Anax junius* dragonfly provided the first intracellular recording from a photoreceptor in the ocellar retina. As it turned out, there was a single, tetrodotoxin sensitive, action potential at the start of the photoreceptor's depolarizing response followed by a sustained tonic depolarization (Chappell and Dowling, 1972).

John's suggestion had led to a viable preparation and my summer project had the makings of a thesis. It took longer to obtain recordings from second order neurons in the dragonfly ocellar retina but this was also accomplished. Blocking the photoreceptor spikes with tetrodotoxin, I could show that a second order response survived. In this way, I was able to demonstrate that action potentials were not necessary there for synaptic transmission, even for these elongated photoreceptor axons (Chappell, 1970; Chappell and Dowling, 1972). The result supported the possibility that this might also be the case for bipolar cells of vertebrate retinas as is now generally believed to be the case.

* Tel.: 212-772-5294; Fax: 212-772-5227;
E-mail: rchappell@gc.cuny.edu

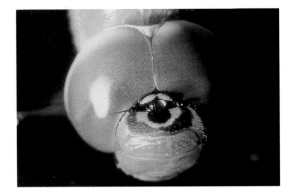

Fig. 1. Dragonfly eyes. This close-up of the head of the large "green darner" (*Anax junius*) dragonfly shows the clear lens of the median ocellus located in the center of the dark line between the two antennae and in front of the yellow vertex which protrudes just below the juncture of the two elaborate compound eyes. The ocellus is a simple eye without facets. Closer inspection may also reveal one of the dragonfly's two lateral ocelli located at the lateral tip of the vertex just above the base of the antenna on the left side of the picture. The other small lateral ocellus is hidden in the shadow on the other side. [Modified from Chappell, 1970]

Morphological evidence for photoreceptor feedback

At about this time, the Fuortes lab was providing electrophysiological evidence for feedback onto photoreceptors in the turtle retina (Baylor et al., 1971). Morphological evidence for such feedback onto photoreceptors had not been established although reciprocal synapses were commonly observed elsewhere in the retina. Electron micrographs of the dragonfly ocellar retina provided direct morphological evidence for synaptic feedback onto photoreceptors from second order neurons (Dowling and Chappell, 1972). Subsequent electrophysiological studies provided pharmacological evidence supporting this observation (Klingman and Chappell, 1978; Stone and Chappell, 1981).

Decremental sensitivity and ambient illumination

What role might feedback play in such a simple eye? Impulses, recorded extracellularly from the intact ocellar nerve, provide some insight regarding this question. Over the remarkable range of the five log units in mean intensities examined, the ocellar nerve responded to any decrement in intensity by a factor of two with a brief burst of impulses. Intracellular recordings showed that this coincided with conditions which were just sufficient to bring the potential of the second order cells (L-neurons) back briefly to the cell's resting potential at light 'off' (Fig. 2). In addition to meaning this 'off' response is very Weber-Fechner-like over this range, the finding suggests that the ocellus is elegantly suited to the role of a shadow detector since a volley of impulses can be expected to reach the brain any time a shadow passing over the ocellus reduces intensity by 50%, independent of the mean intensity of the surroundings over a range of five log units.

Feedback onto the photoreceptor terminal is well suited as a mechanism which can "re-set" the gain of the photoreceptor-to-second-order synapse such that the decrement (shadow) response becomes almost invariant over a wide range of intensities. In this way the dynamic range of the system is extended dramatically even though the sustained "slow potential" of the photoreceptor might otherwise reach saturation. Instead, its changes are compensated by the feedback system it drives and this system, in turn, tends to re-set the system nearer the mean of the ambient intensity. These are, after all, the conditions (ambient illumination over a broad range of intensities) under which the visual task must be performed. The more the features of a response remain Weber-Fechner-like as mean intensity changes, the simpler the system's analysis task becomes over that broad range of intensities. That is to say that at the cost of information about the absolute intensity of illumination, information concerning incremental changes in intensity (contrast) around any particular mean intensity of illumination becomes relatively similar over many log units once the system becomes adapted to that particular level of ambient light intensity. Thus stimuli which modulate the mean intensity, such as increments and decrements, as opposed to light 'on' and light 'off', may provide a better test for the study and understanding of visual processing than the classical flash of light in the dark, a point to which I will return.

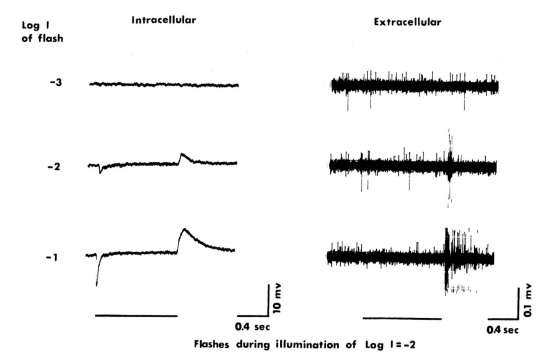

Fig. 2. Dragonfly ocellar responses to incremental stimulation. Intracellular responses recorded from a second order neuron (L-neuron) of the retina of a dragonfly median ocellus using a glass capillary electrode are shown on the left. Ocellar nerve impulses recorded extracellularly using a metal electrode placed in the median ocellar lens under corresponding conditions of illumination are shown on the right. Only a low level of background firing of impulses is observed during steady illumination which induces a sustained hyperpolarization in the L-neuron of several millivolts. A flash of light 10 times dimmer than the background light (upper traces, Log I of flash = −3) elicits no noticeable response in either the L-neuron or the ocellar nerve recordings. A flash of light of equal intensity (Log I = −2) causes a brief hyperpolarizing transient at light "on" and a brief depolarization to the level of the cell's original resting potential at light "off". Extracellularly, there is no noticeable "on" response recorded from the ocellar nerve but a brief burst of impulses is seen at light "off" (middle traces). For a flash ten times as bright as the background illumination, the brief hyperpolarization of the L-neuron at light "on" is much larger and there still is no "on" response recorded from the ocellar nerve while both the intracellular and the extracellular "off" responses are more pronounced (lower traces). [Modified from Chappell, 1970]

GABA studies and photoreceptor feedback

In the early 1980's, studies of coupling modulation in the turtle retina (Gerschenfeld et al., 1982; Piccolino et al., 1982) demonstrated that γ-aminobutyric acid (GABA) antagonists decreased junctional conductances between its large field horizontal cells as evidenced by increased coupling resistance between them and a narrowing of their receptive fields. This mechanism was suggested as an alternative hypothesis to explain the GABA antagonist effects observed by Lam et al. (1978) in catfish horizontal cells which they ascribed to the removal of GABAergic feedback onto catfish photoreceptors. To address this issue, I suggested to Ken Naka that we compare the effect

of the $GABA_A$ antagonist bicuculline on the responses of turtle and catfish horizontal cells under similar stimulus conditions. Catfish horizontal cell responses were dramatically changed by even 10 μM bicuculline: the 'on' phase of the flash response became very slow to peak and the incremental and white noise stimuli responses were substantially reduced or absent (Chappell et al., 1985), consistent with the findings of Lam et al. (1978). For the turtle horizontal cell response, however, we did not find a significant bicuculline effect on response dynamics even at doses up to 200 μM bicuculline. An example is provided in Fig. 3. While the first order Wiener kernel (the impulse response, calculated by a cross-correlation of a horizontal cell's response with the

180

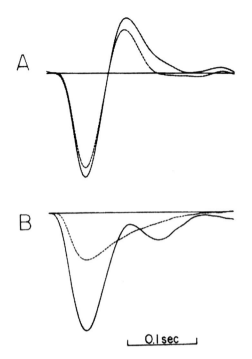

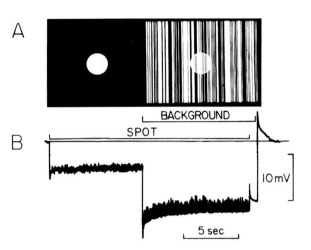

Fig. 3. Effects of bicuculline on turtle and catfish horizontal cell responses. (A) The first-order kernel (impulse response) obtained by cross-correlation of a white-noise stimulus with the response of a turtle horizontal cell bathed in normal Ringer solution (solid line) showed little change when the preparation was superfused with Ringer containing 200 μM bicuculline (dotted line). (B) Under the same conditions of illumination, during superfusion with only 10 μM bicuculline, the catfish horizontal cell response became more tonic and the peak amplitude of its first-order response (solid line) was reduced by more than 50% (dotted line). [Chappell and Naka, unpublished results]

Fig. 4. Enhancement of a turtle horizontal cell response to an intensity-modulated spot of light. The intracellular response recorded from a turtle horizontal cell during stimulation of the retina with a white-noise modulated spot is shown in B, before and after steady background illumination in the form of the random grating (A, right side) was turned on. Although the cell was hyperpolarized an additional ten millivolts by turning on the steady background grating and the amplitude of modulation of the spot intensity remained unchanged, the amplitude of the horizontal cell response to the modulated spot more than doubled (B, right side). [Chappell and Naka, unpublished results]

varying intensity of a pseudo white noise modulated light source) showed essentially no change for turtle even in the presence of 200 μM bicuculline (Fig. 3A), 10 μM bicuculline reduced the amplitude of a catfish horizontal cell's impulse response by over 50% (Fig. 3B). From this we concluded that the GABA$_A$ antagonist bicuculline does not alter the dynamics of the turtle horizontal cell response as it does for catfish. Consequently, the coupling resistance changes observed between turtle horizontal cells may not be the mechanism involved in the conversion from faster, more differentiating responses to slower, more tonic responses observed in the catfish retina in the presence of bicuculline (Chappell et al., 1985).

Surround enhancement effect

In the course of these studies, it was noticed that addition of a stationary random grating background illumination increased the amplitude of turtle horizontal cell responses to white-noise modulated spot illumination (Fig. 4). This is the opposite of what one might have predicted based on knowledge of lateral inhibition of spot responses in the retina by surround illumination. Further investigation showed that the same effect could be demonstrated also by adding steady annular surround illumination around the white-noise modulated spot (Chappell et al., 1985). The same was true for both the turtle and the catfish horizontal cell response as shown in Fig. 5 for the case of frequency-swept, sinusoidal intensity modulation of a light source in the presence or absence of surround illumination. Interestingly, an enhancement effect in the response of some mudpuppy horizontal cells had been reported a decade earlier by Burkhardt (1974).

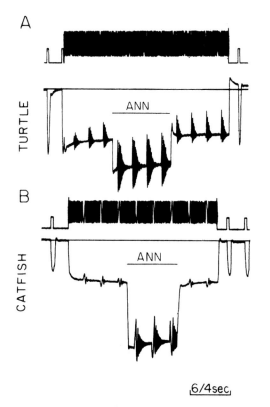

Fig. 5. Steady surround illumination enhances horizontal cell response to a sinusoidally modulated spot of light. Intracellularly recorded responses of both turtle (A, lower trace) and catfish (B, lower trace) horizontal cells to a spot of light modulated by a frequency-swept sinusoid (A and B, upper traces) was substantially enhanced by the addition of steady annular illumination (ANN). Note time scale is 6 s for A and 4 s for B. [Chappell and Naka, unpublished results]

The enhancement effect on rapid flicker reported in amphibian retinas (Frumkes and Eysteinsson, 1987), cat (Pflug et al., 1990; Nelson et al., 1990) and human (Frumkes et al., 1992) is thought to involve a suppressive rod–cone interaction. We were interested, therefore, in examining whether the enhancement effect we observed in recordings from turtle and catfish horizontal cells could be related to rod–cone interaction and/or feedback onto photoreceptors. The skate retina provided a valuable preparation on which to test these possibilities. On the one hand, it has no cones (Szamier and Ripps, 1983) so that presence of the effect would suggest that, at least for the skate, a rod–cone interaction was not involved. On the other hand, current evidence suggests that feedback onto vertebrate photoreceptors occurs onto cones and not rods so that in the all-rod retina of the skate, the feedback would also be an unlikely mechanism to explain the effect. The skate horizontal cell response to a sinusoidally modulated spot of light was dramatically enhanced by the addition of annular surround illumination. Even so, the size of the cell's response to 'on/off' flashes of light of increasing intensities and the same spot diameter were greatly reduced by the addition of the same steady surround, as one would predict on the basis of the presence of the classical inhibitory surround (Naka et al., 1988). Clearly, rod–cone interaction is not necessary for this effect in the skate since its retina has no cones, but what about feedback?

Experiments providing pharmacological evidence for independent 'on' and 'off' interplexiform pathways in the skate retina have revealed a picrotoxin-sensitive component of the electroretinogram (ERG) of the skate (Chappell and Rosenstein, 1996). In addition, interesting effects of GABA$_A$ antagonists on response dynamics of amphibian horizontal cells have been reported (Stone and Witkovsky, 1984). Although turtle response dynamics were not altered by picrotoxin (Chappell et al., 1985), the absence of GABAergic feedback onto skate rods had not been tested. Since studies on isolated skate retinal cells had shown the presence of GABA receptors on its bipolar (Qian et al., 1997) and Müller cells (Qian et al., 1996) but not its horizontal cells (Malchow and Ripps, 1990), it was possible to use the intracellular horizontal cell response as a glutamate electrode to monitor the transmitter release from skate rods in the eyecup preparation before and after picrotoxin-induced changes in the simultaneously recorded ERG. When this was done, no change in the horizontal cell response was observed despite the substantial changes observed in the ERG, confirming the assumption that in the skate, as is believed to be the case in other vertebrate retinas, there is no GABA feedback onto rods (Chappell et al., 2001).

Conclusions and future perspectives

A thesis problem concerning slow potential modulation of synaptic transmission in an invertebrate retina led to the first morphological evidence for feedback onto photoreceptors. Pharmacological

182

studies concerning feedback in a vertebrate retina led to the observation of surround enhancement of horizontal cell responses to a modulated spot of light. Examining the importance of rod-cone interactions to surround enhancement by looking for its presence in an all-rod retina deomonstrated it is not necessary for the effect but left open the possibility that feedback onto photoreceptors might play a role. Knowledge of GABA receptor distribution from patch-clamp studies of isolated retinal neurons allowed the interpretation of simultaneous ERG and intracellular horizontal cell recordings in the intact skate retina in order to rule out the possibility of GABAergic feedback onto rod photoreceptors in this all-rod retina and its role in surround enhancement. The mechanism for surround enhancement, therefore, remains an important question to resolve.

There are two points I would like to address in considering future perspectives for vision research. First, it seems reasonable that the retinal system is optimized toward the visual task it must perform—the extraction of contrast and movement information from a scene in which most objects are illuminated at an intensity within a log unit of the mean intensity of the scene's ambient illumination. Therefore, studies designed to consider the processing of incremental and/or decremental changes in illumination and other dynamic stimuli under conditions of ambient (background/surround/mean) illumination will add much to our knowledge of the processing of visual information. An example of the importance of studies under light adapted conditions is provided by the dynamic response of an extracellularly recorded "off" ganglion cell in the skate retina shown in Fig. 6. The frequency-swept sinusoidal stimulus used elicited no response for the first 10 min after the dynamic stimulus having a mean intensity of 0.1 $\mu W/cm^2/s$ was turned on following 45 min of dark adaptation. It took 40 min to reach the fully light-adapted response level of the cell (Chappell and Glynn, 1993).

The importance of conducting retinal studies under conditions comparable to ambient illumination is a point which Ken Naka and I addressed some time ago (Naka and Chappell, 1984). At the time, the computational capacity necessary to deal with dynamic stimuli was not readily available. Today, computational capacity is no longer limiting, although analysis remains complex. Clinically,

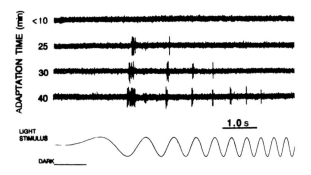

Fig. 6. Light adaptation of a skate ganglion cell response. Following 45 min of dark adaptation, a frequency-swept sinusoidal stimulation illuminating the entire retina with light having a mean intensity of 0.1 $\mu W/cm^2/s$ was turned on (LIGHT STIMULUS, bottom trace). Responses recorded extracellularly from a decrementally responding skate ganglion cell continued to adapt over the period of 40 min before the final steady-state level of response sensitivity was reached. [Modified from Chappell and Glynn, 1993]

however, the electroretinogram's capabilities have already been extended by the increased availability of multifocal ERG recording systems which provide both first and second order correlations of patterned stimuli. For example, multifocal ERG recording has already proven useful in describing the preipheral vision loss found recently to be associated with use of the important antiepileptic drug vigabatrin (Ponjavic et al., 2000). Now that a practical clinical tool for a dynamic form of clinical assessment is in use in conditions approximating ambient illumination, knowledge of visual processing under ambient conditions becomes even more relevant.

The second point is simply that the ability to apply the knowledge from studies of the pharmacology of isolated neurons obtained using patch-clamp recording techniques to the interpretation of data from intact retinal circuitry may provide new opportunities to understand the processing of visual information as it did for our studies of picrotoxin-induced changes in the skate ERG using the eyecup preparation. In our case, the knowledge from studies of isolated skate horizontal cells (Malchow and Ripps, 1990), suggested the viability of the approach of using its horizontal cells as electrodes to monitor photoreceptor transmitter release in evaluating evidence for GABAergic feedback onto the photoreceptors. Thus a new technology has come full circle in allowing us to approach questions in more classical intact retinal preparations armed with knowledge of specific classes of receptors on particular types of retinal cells to assist us in the interpretation of our results. Such studies will hold relevance for the further interpretation of the clinically important ERG and its relation to visual disorders and, presumably, the study of genetic manipulations induced in animal models as well.

Acknowledgments

I wish to express my appreciation to Drs. Harris Ripps, Frank Werblin and Helga Kolb for their assistance with the manuscript. This work has been supported in part by NEI/NIH grant EY00777, NSF grant BNS-8304932 and ONR grant N00014-92-J-1954. "Research Centers in Minority Institutions" award RR-03037 from the National Center for Research Resources of the National Institutes of Health, which supports the infrastructure of the Biological Sciences Department at Hunter College, is also acknowledged. The contents are solely the responsibility of the author and do not necessarily represent the official views of the NCRR/NIH.

References

Baylor, D.A., Fuortes, M.G.F. and O'Bryan, P.M. (1971) Receptive fields of cones in the retina of the turtle. *J. Physiol. (Lond.)*, 214: 265–294.

Burkhardt, D.A. (1974) Sensitization and centre-surround antagonism in *Necturus* retina. *J. Physiol. (Lond.)*, 236: 593–610.

Chappell, R.L. (1970) Intracellular responses in the Anisopteran ocellus. *Ph.D. Thesis*. Johns Hopkins University, Baltimore, MD, pp. 1–123.

Chappell, R.L. and Dowling, J.E. (1972) Neural organization of the median ocellus of the dragonfly. I. Intracellular electrical activity. *J. Gen. Physiol.*, 60: 121–147.

Chappell, R.L. and Glynn, P. (1993) Equivalent sine wave frequency for interpretation of responses to frequency-swept sinusoids defined: an algorithm from studies of skate ganglion cells. *Biol. Bulletin*, 185: 308–310.

Chappell, R.L., Naka, K.-I. and Sakuranaga, M. (1985) Dynamics of turtle horizontal cell response. *J. Gen. Physiol.*, 86: 423–453.

Chappell, R.L. and Rosenstein, F.J. (1996) Pharmacology of the skate electroretinogram indicates independent ON and OFF bipolar cell pathways. *J. Gen. Physiol.*, 107: 535–544.

Chappell, R.L., Schuette, E., Anton, R. and Ripps, H. (2001) GABA$_C$ receptors modulate the rod-driven ERG b-wave of the skate retina. *Doc. Ophthalmol.* In press.

Dowling, J.E. and Chappell, R.L. (1972) Neural organization of the median ocellus of the dragonfly. II. Synaptic structure. *J. Gen. Physiol.*, 60: 148–165.

Frumkes, T.E., Lange, G., Denny, N. and Beczkowska, I. (1992) Influence of rod adaptation upon cone responses to light offset in humans: I. Results in normal observers. *Vis. Neurosci.*, 8: 83–89.

Frumkes, R.E. and Eysteinsson, T. (1987) Suppressive rod-cone interaction in distal vertebrate retina: Intracellular records from *Xenopus* and *Necturus*. *J. Neurophysiol.*, 57: 1361–1383.

Gerschenfeld, H.M., Neyton J., Piccolino, M. and Witkovsky, P. (1982) L-horizontal cells of turtle: network organization and coupling modulation. *Biomed. Res.*, (Suppl. 3): 21–34.

Klingman, A. and Chappell, R.L. (1978) Feedback synaptic interaction in the dragonfly ocellar retina. *J. Gen. Physiol.*, 71: 157–175.

Lam, D.M.-K., Lasater, E.M. and Naka, K.-I. (1978) Gamma-aminobutyric acid: a neurotransmitter candidate for cone horizontal cells of the catfish retina. *Proc. Natl. Acad. Sci. USA*, 75: 6310–6313.

Malchow, R.P. and Ripps, H. (1990) Effects of gamma-amino butyric acid on skate horizontal cells: evidence of an electrogenic uptake mechanism. *Proc. Natl. Acad. Sci.*, 87: 8945–8949.

Naka, K.-I. and Chappell, R.L. (1984) Seeing in the Light. In: Aoki K. et al. (Eds.), *Animal Behavior: Neurophysiological and Ethological Approaches*. Springer-Verlag, Berlin, pp. 125–135.

Naka, K.-I., Chappell, R.L., Sakuranaga, M. and Ripps, H. (1988) Dynamics of skate horizontal cells. *J. Gen. Physiol.*, 92: 811–831.

Nelson, R., Pflug, R. and Baer, S.M. (1990) Background-induced flicker-enhancement in cat retinal horizontal cells. II. Spatial properties. *J. Neurophysiol.*, 64: 326–340.

Pflug, R., Nelson, R. and Ahnelt, P.K. (1990) Background-induced flicker-enhancement in cat retinal horizontal cells. I. Temporal and spectral properties. *J. Neurophysiol.*, 64: 313–325.

Piccolino, M., Neyton, J., Witkovsky, P. and Gerschenfeld, H.M. (1982) γ-Aminobutyric acid antagonists decrease junctional communication between L-horizontal cells in the turtle retina. *Vision Res.*, 14: 119–123.

Ponjavic, V., Gränse, L., Andréasson, S. and Ehinger, B. (2000) Multifocal-ERG and full-field ERG in patients on vigabatrin. *Invest. Ophthalmol. and Vis. Sci.*, 41: S242.

Qian, H., Li, L., Chappell, R.L. and Ripps, H. (1997) GABA receptors of bipolar cells from the skate retina: actions of zinc on GABA-mediated membrane currents. *J. Neurophysiol.*, 78: 2402–2412.

Qian, H., Malchow, R.P., Chappell, R.L. and Ripps, H. (1996) Zinc enhances ionic currents induced in skate Müller (glial) cells by the inhibitory neurotransmitter GABA. *Proc. Roy. Soc. (Series B)*, 263: 791–796.

184

Ruck, P. (1961a) Electrophysiology of the insect dorsal ocellus. I. Origin of the components of the electroretinogram. *J. Gen. Physiol.*, 44: 605–627.

Ruck, P. (1961b) Electrophysiology of the insect dorsal ocellus. II. Mechanisms of generation and inhibition of impulses in the ocellar nerve of dragonflies. *J. Gen. Physiol.*, 44: 629–639.

Ruck, P. (1961c) Electrophysiology of the insect dorsal ocellus. III. Responses to flickering light of the dragonfly ocellus. *J. Gen. Physiol.*, 44: 641–657.

Stone, S.L. and Chappell, R.L. (1981) Synaptic feedback onto photoreceptors in the ocellar retina. *Brain Res*, 221: 374–381.

Stone, S.L. and Witkovsky, P. (1984) The actions of gamma aminobutyric acid, glycine and their antagonists upon horizontal cells of the *Xenopus* retina. *J. Physiol.*, 353: 249–264.

Szamier, R.B. and Ripps, H. (1983) The visual cells of the skate retina: structure, histochemistry, and disc-shedding properties. *J. Comp. Neurol.*, 215: 51–62.

H. Kolb, H. Ripps and S. Wu (Eds.)
Progress in Brain Research, Vol. 131
© 2001 Elsevier Science B.V. All rights reserved

CHAPTER 12

Plasticity of AII amacrine cell circuitry in the mammalian retina

Stewart A. Bloomfield*

Departments of Ophthalmology, Physiology and Neuroscience, New York University School of Medicine, 550 First Avenue, New York, NY 10016, USA

Overview

As first described in the seminal work of Boycott and Dowling (1969), visual signals generated in the rod and cone photoreceptors are segregated into different second-order bipolar cells, thus forming two parallel, vertical streams within the mammalian retina. Under photopic light conditions, cone-mediated signals are carried by two physiological types of bipolar cell, ON- and OFF-center, that show opposite polarity responses to light (Werblin and Dowling, 1969; Kaneko, 1970). In turn, the axon terminals of these cone bipolar cell types stratify in separate sublamina within the inner plexiform layer (IPL), thereby differentially innervating the ON- and OFF-center ganglion cells (Famiglietti and Kolb, 1976; Bloomfield and Miller, 1986).

In contrast, only a single physiological type of bipolar cell, displaying exclusively ON-center response activity, appears to be postsynaptic to rods. Interestingly, the axon terminals of these rod bipolar cells rarely make synaptic connections directly with ganglion cells but, instead, provide excitatory inputs to two types of ON-center amacrine cells: the AII and S1 cells (Kolb and Famiglietti, 1974; Famiglietti and Kolb, 1975; Kolb, 1979; Dacheux and Raviola, 1986; Sandell et al., 1989; Strettoi et al., 1990).

* Tel.: 212-263-5770; Fax: 212-263-8072;
E-mail: blooms01@med.nyu.edu

The wide-field S1 amacrine cells make mainly reciprocal inhibitory synapses back onto the axon terminals of rod bipolar cells and thus serve as a feedback pathway providing lateral inhibition (Sandell et al., 1989; Strettoi et al., 1990). The narrow-field, bistratified AII cells form the most numerous subtype of amacrine cell and partake in a number of different synaptic circuits. The AII cells form sign-inverting, glycinergic chemical synapses with axon terminals of OFF-center cone bipolar cells in sublamina *a* of the IPL and sign-conserving electrical synapses, in the form of gap junctions, with axon terminals of a number of subtypes of ON-center cone bipolar cell in sublamina *b* (Famiglietti and Kolb, 1975; Strettoi et al., 1992, 1994). By way of these two circuits, rod-mediated ON- and OFF-center signals utilize cone circuitry in the IPL to reach the ganglion cells.

Based on this synaptic circuitry, it is clear that AII cells are essential elements in the rod pathways in that most, if not all, signals must pass through them first before being output to central brain structures. Kolb and Famiglietti (1974) first posited, based on the morphological evidence, that AII cells subserve simple rod-driven receptive field properties of dark-adapted ganglion cells. Subsequent electrophysiological studies lent support to this idea, showing that AII cells have response thresholds, saturation levels and spectral sensitivities virtually identical to rods (Nelson, 1982; Dacheux and Raviola, 1986;

Bloomfield et al., 1997). The AII cells thus became frequently referred to simply as the "rod amacrine cells".

Although AII cells are clearly part of the rod pathways in the retina, the purely rod-driven nature of their responses is curious considering that they make numerous contacts with cone bipolar cells. Although the AII–cone bipolar cell gap junctions are thought to provide a pathway for rod-mediated ON-center signals to reach ganglion cells, in the transition from rod to cone vision the direction of signal flow should change whereby cone signals would be conducted to AII cells. In addition to these electrical synapses, AII cells also receive a sizeable synaptic input from OFF-center cone bipolar cells (Sterling, 1995; Strettoi et al., 1992, 1994). This input accounts for nearly 40% of the chemical synaptic input from bipolar cells with the remainder received from rod bipolar cells. Thus, AII cells are clearly positioned to receive and transmit both rod and cone signals, suggesting that they should be capable of a wide dynamic range of activity extending over both dark- and light-adapted conditions.

In addition to the junctions formed with cone bipolar cells, neighboring AII cells also show extensive homologous coupling via gap junctions (Famiglietti and Kolb, 1975; Vaney, 1991; Strettoi et al., 1992). Recent studies have shown that the permeabilities of these two sets of gap junctions can be modulated by different pharmacological mechanisms (Hampson et al., 1992; Mills and Massey, 1995). Coupling between AII cells is diminished by dopamine and cyclic AMP, whereas nitric oxide (NO), acting through its intracellular messenger cGMP, reduces the permeability of AII–cone bipolar cell junctions. There is now abundant evidence that both dopamine and NO levels in the retina, as well as that of their intracellular messengers, are regulated by changes in ambient light conditions, suggesting that the gap junctional conductances of AII cells may be modulated with changes in adaptational state (reviewed by Witkovsky and Dearry, 1992). For example, endogenous dopamine levels are increased by light, suggesting that AII–AII cell coupling should be maximal under dim light conditions. Similarly, increases in stimulus brightness results in an increase in cGMP levels in cone bipolar cells and enhanced release of NO by amacrine cells, suggesting that the coupling between AII amacrine cells and cone bipolar cells should diminish in the transition from night to day.

Clearly, then, the wide variety of synaptic inputs to AII cells should afford these neurons the ability to display a number of different response properties. Moreover, these circuits appear dynamically regulated whereby the spatial organization and content of AII cell activity should be modified under changing ambient light conditions. The sections below review recent work aimed at elucidating the different light-evoked activities of AII amacrine cells and their modulation related to altered adaptational states of the retina.

Receptive field organization of dark-adapted AII amacrine cells

In the dark-adapted retina, AII amacrine cells display a stereotypic ON-center–OFF-surround receptive field organization (Fig. 1A). The light-evoked response consists of a transient depolarization at light onset followed by a sustained component and a large, oscillating hyperpolarization. Dark-adapted AII cells show relatively small ON-center receptive fields extending only approximately 60–80 μm across with the OFF-surround receptive fields extending 100–130 μm (Fig. 1B). The small receptive field of a dark-adapted AII cell is thus comparable to that of its narrow dendritic arbor. This correspondence is inconsistent with fact that neighboring AII cells show numerous, prominent gap junctions suggesting that signals could propagate laterally across the IPL. To determine the actual extent of coupling between AII cells, we turned to the biotinylated tracer, Neurobiotin, that was shown first by Vaney (1991) and then subsequently by numerous investigators to effectively pass through gap junctions, thereby allowing visualization of coupled neuronal groups (Vaney, 1994; Goddard et al., 1991; Hidaka et al., 1993; Bloomfield et al., 1995, 1997; Xin and Bloomfield, 1997). Injection of a single dark-adapted AII cell with Neurobiotin typically labels only a small array of 7–10 darkly labeled AII cells surrounded by a more lightly labeled array of 10–15 AII cells (Fig. 2A). A group of 30–40 smaller cell bodies identified as cone bipolar cells are also visable,

A

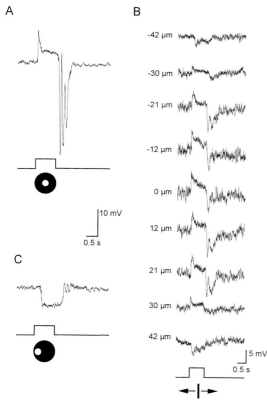

B

-42 μm

-30 μm

-21 μm

-12 μm

0 μm

12 μm

21 μm

30 μm

42 μm

10 mV

0.5 s

C

5 mV

0.5 s

Fig. 1. **A.** Typical response of a dark-adapted AII cell in the rabbit retina consisting of a transient at light onset, a sustained depolarization and a large oscillating hyperpolarization at light offset. Stimulus was a 75 μm diameter spot of light centered over the cell. Stimulus intensity $= \log - 5.5$. Trace below response indicates onset and offset of the light stimulus. **B.** Response of same cell as in **A** after the small spot of light was tranlated laterally by about 100 μm. Translated spot evokes an OFF-surround response. **C.** Light-evoked responses of an AII amacrine in a well dark-adapted retina. This is the same cell injected with Neurobiotin, resulting in the coupling pattern illustrated in Fig. 2. Stimulus is a 50 μm-wide/6.0 mm-long rectangular slit of light which was moved in discrete steps across the retinal surface. At 0 μm the slit was centered over the cell. The values to the left of each trace represent how far OFF-center the slit was positioned; polarity of number indicates direction of movement. Stimulus trace is presented at the bottom of the figure. Stimulus intensity $= \log - 5.5$. Maximum intensity $(\log 0.0) = 2.37 \text{ mW/cm}^2$.

presumably labeled by tracer movement across the AII–cone bipolar cell gap junctions (Fig. 2B). These results indicate that the relatively constrained network formed by coupled AII amacrine cells in the dark-adapted retina corresponds well to the size of their ON-center receptive fields.

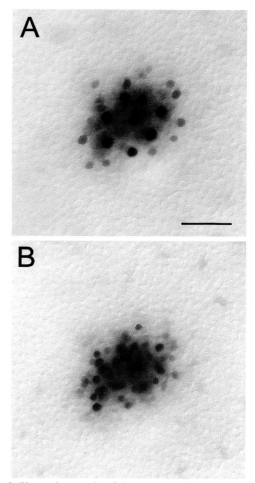

Fig. 2. Photomicrographs of the tracer coupling pattern of AII amacrine cells and cone bipolar cells in a well dark-adapted retina following in jection of Neurobiotin into a single AII cell. The visual streak lays along the horizontal axis. **A.** Plane of focus on AII amacrine cell bodies. An inner ring of eight darkly labeled AII cells and an outer ring of 10–15 lightly labeled AII cells are visible. Calibration bar $= 25$ μm. **B.** Plane of focus of somata of cone bipolar cells laying distal to the AII somata in the INL.

In a series of experiments, we used different background intensities to examine how adaptation of the retina within the scotopic and mesopic ranges alters the receptive field organization of AII cells. Fig. 3 shows the response profile of an AII cell under a constant adapting light of $\log -5.5$ intensity, approximately 1.5 log units above rod threshold. Under these conditions, the response waveform remains quite similar to that seen under dark-adapted conditions. However, the ON-center receptive field measures approximately 400 μm across, some

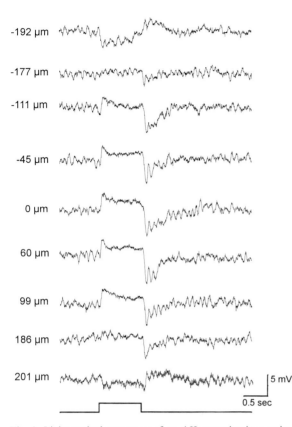

-192 μm

-177 μm

-111 μm

-45 μm

0 μm

60 μm

99 μm

186 μm

201 μm

5 mV

0.5 sec

Fig. 3. Light-evoked responses of an AII amacrine in a retina maintained under constant background illumination of − 5.5 log intensity. Stimulus is a 50 μm-wide/6.0 mm-long rectangular slit of light which was moved in discrete steps across the retinal surface. Conventions the same as in Fig. 1B. The center-receptive field of this cell was measured at 399 μm along the axis parallel to the visual streak. Stimulus intensity = log −4.5. Maximum intensity (log 0.0) = 2.37 mW/cm^2. [From Bloomfield et al., 1997]

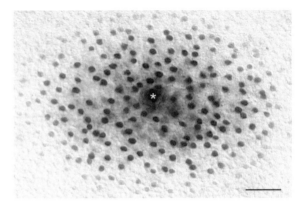

Fig. 4. Photomicrograph providing a flatmount-view of a group of tracer-coupled AII amacrine cells following injection of one cell (star) with Neurobiotin. retina was exposed to a log −5.5 intensity fullfield illumination for 1 h prior to the tracer injection. Plane of focus is on the AII cell somata in the proximal inner nuclear layer. Bipolar cell somata in the more distal inner nuclear layer were also labeled by the injection but are not visible in this photomicrograph. Calibration bar = 50 μm. [From Bloomfield and Xin, 2000]

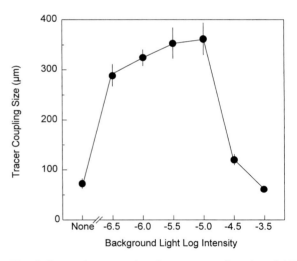

Fig. 5. Scatterplot comparing the tracer coupling size of AII cells injected with Neurobiotin across a range of background light intensities corresponding to the scotopic and mesopic levels. Each data point illustrates the average and standard error of multiple injections. Well dark-adapted retinas are represented by data point corresponding to 'none' background light intensity. [From Bloomfield et al., 1997]

6–7 times the size of the center receptive fields of AII cells in dark-adapted retinas. Consistent with the increase in receptive fields seen for AII cells adapted with dim background lights, there is also a significant increase in the extent of the tracer-coupling following injection of Neurobiotin. For example, Fig. 4 illustrates the coupling pattern of an AII adapted with a background light of log −6.0 consisting of 201 labeled AII cells and an additional 243 cell bodies of cone bipolar cells within the more distal INL.

Figure 5 summarizes the change in tracer coupling pattern of AII cells seen under different intensity background light illumination. Under dark-adapted conditions, AII cells are coupled in relatively small groups, but following exposure to dim background lights there is a dramatic increase in tracer coupling reflected in labeling of upwards of 700 AII cells and 1200 cone bipolar cells. This increase in coupling between light-sensitized AII cells was found to correspond to a proportional increase in the size of their ON-center and OFF-surround receptive fields. Further light adaptation of the retina with more intense background illumination results in a decrease in the extent of tracer coupling to levels similar to those seen in dark-adapted retina. These robust concomitant changes in tracer coupling and receptive field size of AII cells indicate a clear modulation of AII–AII coupling under different adaptational states. Although there was also a change in the number of cone bipolar cells labeled under different adapting conditions, this appears to be an epiphenomenon of changes in AII–AII coupling rather than a direct effect of light on AII–cone bipolar cell coupling (Bloomfield et al., 1997).

Pathways underlying the center–surround responses of dark-adapted AII cells

Bipolar cells are first in the visual pathways to display antagonistic center–surround receptive field organization. Their surrounds are believed to be generated by reciprocal feedback synapses from horizontal cells to photoreceptors (Werblin and Dowling, 1969; Baylor et al., 1971; Miller and Dacheux, 1976). Extrinsic polarization of horizontal cells has been shown to mimic the effects of surround illumination on both bipolar and ganglion cells, suggesting that surround inhibition displayed at all levels of the retina is ultimately derived from the lateral interactions in the OPL (Naka and Nye, 1971; Naka and Witkovsky, 1972; Marchiafava, 1978; Toyoda and Tonosaki, 1978; Mangel, 1991). Following this scheme, then, the ON-center responses of dark-adapted AII cells should reflect the excitatory inputs from rod bipolar cells. The glutamatergic synapses between rod bipolar and rods express postsynaptic mGluR6 receptors for which L-APB is a potent agonist (Slaughter and Miller, 1981; Yamashita and Wässle, 1991; Nakajima et al., 1993). It is well known that, via this site of action, APB blocks the ON-center responses of bipolar cells and all downstream neurons (Slaughter and Miller, 1981, 1985; Massey et al., 1983; Bloomfield and Dowling 1985a,b). Application of APB reversibly blocks both the ON-center and OFF-surround

responses of AII amacrine cells, consistent with the idea that these response components are derived from the rod bipolar cell input (Fig. 6). However, in addition to the direct inputs from rod bipolar cells, there is an alternative pathway for rod-mediated signals to reach AII amacrine cells. Rod signals may be communicated directly to cones via gap junctions that link the two types of photoreceptors; indeed, rod signals have been recorded in cat cone photoreceptors

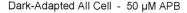

Dark-Adapted AII Cell - 50 µM APB

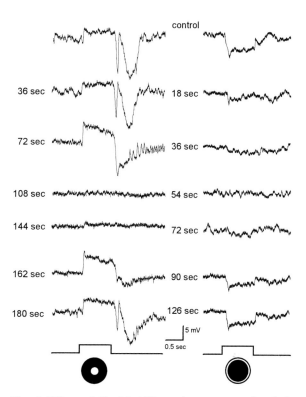

Fig. 6. Effects of 50 µM APB on the responses of a dark-adapted AII cell. Prior to drug application (control), the cell responded to the 75 µm-diameter spot of light (left panel) with the typical ON-center response components. Presentation of an annular light stimulus (inner diameter = 75 µm, outer diameter = 350 µm) evoked a clear OFF-surround response. The values to the left of each trace indicates time from the beginning of the 40 s long application of APB; for example, the response at 72 s corresponds to 32 s after return to the control superfusate APB produced an approximate 10 mV hyperpolarization and reversibly blocked both the ON-center and OFF-surround responses. Intensity of both spot and annular stimuli = log −5.5. Traces at bottom indicate presentation of light stimuli. [From Bloomfield and Xin, 2000]

(Nelson, 1977). These rod signals can then be passed on to ON-center cone bipolar cells and, in turn, to AII cells via the gap junctional contacts in the IPL. It is thus possible that at least a portion of the ON-center responses in AII cells derives from both rod and cone bipolar cells. APB does not differentiate between the two routes in that both types of bipolar cell express mGluR6 receptors on their dendrites in the OPL (Nakajima et al., 1993; Akazawa et al., 1994; Nomura et al., 1994; Vardi and Morigiwa, 1997). However, as aforementioned, nitric oxide (NO), acting via activation of a guanylate cyclase, reduces the coupling between AII cells and ON-center cone bipolar cells and so these substances can be used to differentiate between the two pathways. Application of the NO donor, SNAP, or the membrane permeant analog, 8-bromo-cGMP has no effect on the ON-center responses of dark-adapted AII cells (Bloomfield and Xin, 2000). Coupled with the results from the APB experiments, these findings suggest that rod-mediated signals in AII cells are derived from rod bipolar cell inputs and argue against signal transmission to AII cells via the gap junctions formed ON-center cone bipolar cells. Thus, under dark-adapted conditions, the AII–cone bipolar cell junctions appear to transmit information effectively in only one direction.

Again, the abolition of AII cell center- and surround-mediated responses by APB suggest that these components derive from inputs of rod bipolar cells showing similar physiology. Unfortunately, recordings from mammalian bipolar cells are extremely difficult to obtain and so the receptive organization of these cells have been inferred to a large extent from recordings made in lower vertebrates retinas. Over the years, however, we have been able to compile recordings from rod bipolar cells in the rabbit retina, identified morphologically following injections with HRP or Neurobiotin via the recording microelectrode. A review of these data show that rod bipolar cells display robust ON-center responses with both transient and sustained components. However, rod bipolar cell consistently fail to show OFF-surround activity following exposure to annular, displaced spots or slits of light which were effective in evoking surround activity of AII amacrine cells (Fig. 7). In contrast, surround responses could easily be evoked from cone bipolar cells,

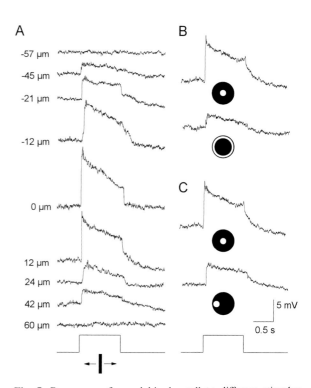

Fig. 7. Responses of a rod bipolar cell to different stimulus configurations. **A.** Responses to a 50 µm-wide/6.0 mm-long rectangular slit of light moved in discrete steps across the retinal surface. Conventions are the same as in Fig. 2A. ON-center receptive field was measured to be about 100 µm across. Stimulus intensity = log −5.5. **B.** Responses to a 75 µm-diameter spot of light and an annulus of light (inner diameter = 75 µm, outer diameter = 350 µm). Conventions are the same as in Fig. 3. Both stimuli produced an ON-center response with the annulus failing to produce an OFF-surround. Stimulus intensity = log −5.5. **C.** Responses to a 75 µm-diameter spot of light first centered over the cell and then displaced laterally by 100 µm. In both cases the spot evoked an ON-center response with the displaced stimulus failing to produce an OFF-surround. Stimulus intensity = log −5.5. Taken together, these data indicate that rod bipolar cells do not express OFF-surround receptive fields. [From Bloomfield and Xin, 2000]

suggesting that the negative result from rod bipolar cells was not due to technically related problems.

Clearly, then, the surround activity of AII cells cannot be derived from rod bipolar cells since the latter apparently do not express surround receptive fields. Supporting evidence for this idea was provided by results of experiments that examined the effects of CNQX (or DNQX), a non-NMDA glutamate receptor antagonist, on the responses of dark-adapted AII cells. It was reasoned that if the center–surround responses of AII cells were, in fact, derived from rod bipolar cells, than they should be reduced or abolished by CNQX at the glutamatergic rod bipolar to AII cell synapses (Boos et al., 1993; Brandstätter et al., 1997). However, application of CNQX had opposite effects on the center- and surround-mediated activity of AII amacrine cells (Bloomfield and Xin, 2000). Whereas CNQX reversibly blocked the surround responses of AII cells, it surprisingly increased the ON-center responses. These opposing effects of CNQX effects suggest actions on different circuits and are thus inconsistent with the idea the both the center- and surround-mediated responses arise from signals passing through the same synapses connecting rod bipolar to AII cells.

If the surround responses of dark-adapted AII cells do not reflect inputs from rod bipolar cells, they must be generated in the inner retina. The most obvious mechanism is lateral inhibition from neighboring amacrine cells. To explore this possibility, we examined the effects of antagonists of glycine and GABA, the two most common inhibitory transmitters utilized by amacrine cells. Application of the glycine antagonist, strychnine, had only minor and varied effects on the surround responses of AII cells. In contrast, application of the different GABA blockers reversibly enhanced the ON-center responses of AII cells but reduced or completely blocked the OFF-surround responses (Fig. 8). Specifically, the selective GABA$_A$ blocker bicuculline and the selective GABA$_C$ blocker TPMPA had approximately equivalent effects on the response activity of AII cells, whereas the non-selective blocker picrotoxin was about twice as effective. These data indicate that in the generation of AII cell surround activity, both GABA$_A$ and GABA$_C$ receptors are activated to an approximate 60:40 ratio.

Taken together, the pharmacological studies implicate GABAergic inhibition from amacrine cells as the source of the surround responses of AII cells. Many amacrine cells show sodium-mediated action potentials that play a role in propagating signals laterally across the IPL. It is likely, then, that the lateral inhibitory signals underlying AII surround inhibition are propagated actively, to at least some extent, along amacrine cell dendrites. Recently, Cook and

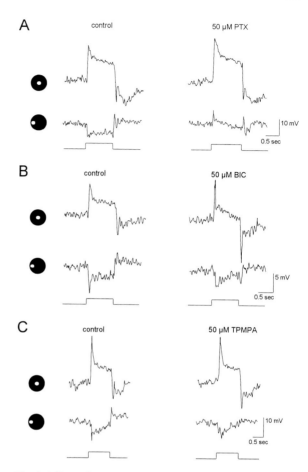

Fig. 8. Effects of GABA blockers on the ON-center and OFF-surround responses of dark-adapted AII cells. **A.** Application of 50 μM picrotoxin (PTX) increased the amplitude of the ON-center response and abolished the OFF-surround response, replacing the latter with a small depolarization; this depolarization is an ON-center response evoked by light scatter into the center receptive field. **B.** Bicuculline (BIC) produced only a modest increase in the ON-center response and reduction in the OFF-surround. **C.** TPMPA also had modest effects on the response activity of AII cells, similar to those of BIC.

McReynolds (1998) and Taylor (1999) showed that blocking amacrine spiking with TTX reduces lateral inhibition in certain ganglion cell types. Application of TTX produces an enhancement of the ON-center responses but abolishes the OFF-mediated surround of dark-adapted AII amacrine cells (Fig. 9). Overall, then, the effects of TTX, CNQX and the GABA antagonists have qualitatively similar, differential actions on the ON-center and OFF-surround responses of AII amacrine cells.

192

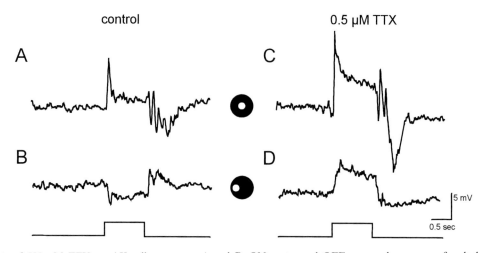

control   0.5 µM TTX

A   C

B   D

5 mV

0.5 sec

Fig. 9. Effects of 500 nM TTX on AII cell responses. **A** and **B**. ON-center and OFF-surround response of a dark-adapted AII cell to a 75 µm-diameter spot of light centered over the cell and displaced laterally by 100 µm. Traces at bottom indicate presentation of light stimuli. **C** and **D**. A 3 min application of TTX produced a 5 mV depolarization of the membrane and enhanced the ON-center response. TTX also reduced the OFF-surround response, replacing it with a depolarization with waveform similar to that of the ON-center response, albeit smaller in amplitude. Analogous to the effects of CNQX, we believe that the depolarizing response is an ON-center response, evoked by light scatter into the center receptive field, that was revealed after reduction or abolition of the OFF-surround.

Combining the results of the pharmacological studies, we can propose circuit diagram for the pathways responsible for the different response components of dark-adapted AII cells (Fig. 10). The finding that APB reversibly blocks the ON-center response is consistent with the idea that these signals arise from inputs from presynaptic rod bipolar cells. However, the results indicate that an ON-center, spiking, GABAergic amacrine cell(s) underlies the surround inhibition of AII cells. There are two possible sources of this inhibition. First, the dendrites of AII cells stratifying in sublamina *b* receive a rich chemical-mediated inhibitory input from a homogeneous population of as yet unidentified amacrine cells (Strettoi et al., 1992). Second, rod bipolar cell axon terminals receive a GABAergic feedback synapse from the S1 (A17) subtype of amacrine cell (Dacheux and Raviola, 1986; Strettoi et al., 1990). We suggest that this feedback synapse is most likely responsible for the surround responses of AII cells (cf. Bloomfield and Xin, 2000). First, the S1 amacrine cells receive excitatory inputs from rod bipolar cells and are thus operational under scotopic conditions when AII cells show surround responses. Second, the GABAergic feedback synapse to rod bipolar cells form the only output synapse for S1 cells. Third, the

S1 cells are ON-center and have expansive receptive fields indicating wide lateral propagation of their signals across the IPL. Fourth, S1 amacrine cells display sodium-mediated action potentials. Thus, the S1 cells show all the necessary physiological and morphological criteria of the neuron responsible for generating the surround of AII cells. Interestingly, the feedback synapse from S1 to rod bipolar cells is analogous to the horizontal cell-to-cone photoreceptor feedback synapses believed to underlie the surround responses of bipolar cells under photopic light conditions. The S1 feedback synapse may thus reflect an analogous scotopic pathway in the inner retina.

Following our model, then, stimulation of the surround receptive field of an AII cell gives rise to activation of peripheral rod bipolar cells that excite S1 amacrine cells. Signals within the S1 cell are then propagated laterally across their extensive dendrites via both passive and active processes. These surround signals activate GABAergic feedback synapses which then shunt the membrane of central rod bipolar cell axon terminals resulting in a decreased release of glutamate from the rod bipolar cells and a hyperpolarization of AII cells. One caveat to this scheme is that rod bipolar cells must tonically release glutamate

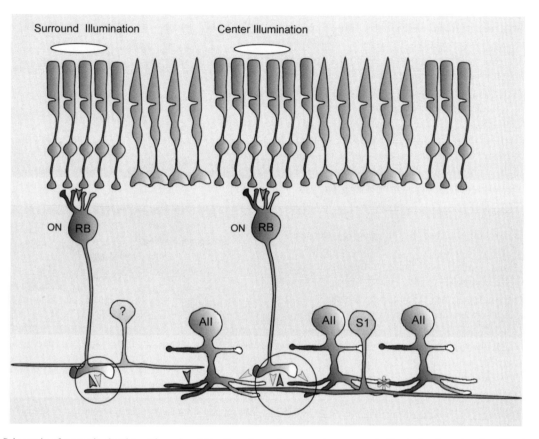

Fig. 10. Schematic of synaptic circuitry subserving AII cell center and surround responses in the dark-adapted retina. Illumination of the center receptive field of an AII cell produces an ON-center responses via the rod → rod bipolar cell → AII amacrine cell pathway (large circle). Illumination of the surround receptive field produces an OFF-surround response by the pathway rod → rod bipolar cell → S1 amacrine cell (small circle) which carries the signal centrally and feeds back via a GABAergic inhibitory (sign inverting) synapse to central rod bipolar cell axon terminals (large circle). Activation of this "surround-generating" circuit shunts the signal in the rod bipolar cell axon terminal thereby reducing the glutamate release onto AII cells and producing the hyperpolarizing OFF-response. An alternative, but less likely, pathway for surround inhibition may be from unidentified amacrine cells (?) which provide direct inhibitory inputs onto AII amacrine cell dendrites. Asterisks, gap junctions; light arrowheads, sign-conserving synapse; dark arrowheads, sign-inverting synapse; AII, AII amacrine cell; RB, rod bipolar cell; S1, S1 amacrine cell; ON, ON-center.

onto the postsynaptic AII and S1 amacrine cells that, in turn, provides for a basal release of GABA from S1 cells back onto the axon terminals of rod bipolar cells. A tonic release of glutamate from rod bipolar cells would provide a requisite level that could then be decreased following activation of the S1 feedback synapses by surround stimulation. Again, our data suggest that both $GABA_A$ and $GABA_C$ receptors play a role in the inhibitory circuits responsible for AII surround responses. This is consistent with the clustering of both receptor types at rod bipolar cell axon terminals (Euler and Wässle, 1998; Fletcher et al., 1998).

Receptive field organization of light-adapted AII cells

As aforementioned, several electrophysiological studies reported that AII cells show ON-center responses similar to those of presynaptic rod bipolar cells and response threshold and saturation levels virtually identical to rods. These findings reinforced the idea that AII cells function to convey rod-mediate signals and are thereby operational exclusively under scotopic light conditions. However, the exclusive rod-mediated responsiveness of AII cells is curious in that, as discussed above, AII cells receive

194

a formidable input from OFF-center cone bipolar cells. Further, cone-mediated signals could be received by AII cells via the gap junctions formed with ON-center cone bipolar cells in a reversal of signal flow across the junctions in the transmission from dark to light adapted conditions. Although it had been suggested that these junctions close with light adaptation (Mills and Massey, 1995; Sterling, 1995), ON-center cone-mediated signals, albeit small in amplitude, were recorded in AII cells following presentation of bright light stimuli which saturated rod responses (Nelson, 1977; Dacheux and Raviola, 1986).

As discussed above, we found no light-induced changes in the conductance of AII–cone bipolar cell gap junctions under scotopic to mesopic light conditions (Bloomfield et al., 1997). However, the possibility remained that the gap junctions could be modulated under brighter photopic conditions. In a series of experiments, we examined the movement of Neurobiotin between AII and ON-center cone bipolar cells under bright light conditions. Because previous studies had shown that AII cells saturate within 3 log units of rod threshold, we designed our experiments to record AII cells under dark-adapted conditions and then to light adapt the retina prior to intracellular injection of Neurobiotin. Figure 11 shows the results of one such experiment in which we impaled an AII cell in the dark-adapted retina. Presentation of a dim light stimulus (log −6.0) produced an ON-center response with the stereotypic transient and sustained components. However, 24 sec after presentation of an extremely bright stimulus (log −1.0) the intense stimulus produced a sustained hyperpolarization; in fact, we first thought that the microelectrode had shifted from the AII cell and into a horizontal cell! However, over the next 1–2 min, the hyperpolarizing response gradually declined in amplitude and the ON-center response returned. This sequence in which rapid light adaptation of retina produced an OFF-response which was replaced with an ON-center response over 1–4 min was seen in numerous AII cells following this protocol or one in which stimuli were superimposed on bright background lights. The ON-center response to intense stimulation then typically remained stable as long as the impalement was maintained.

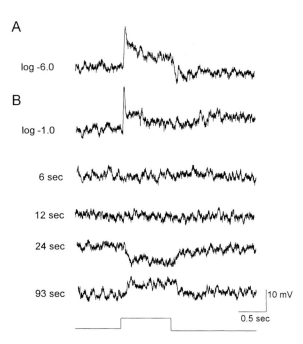

Fig. 11. Responses of a dark-adapted AII amacrine cell following rapid light adaptation. **A**: Response to a relatively dim (log − 6.0) 75 μm diameter spot of light. **B**: Responses of cell to an intense (log −1.0) 75 μm diameter spot of light at various times after initial presentation. Initial presentation of the intense stimulus evoked a depolarizing response which was more transient that that evoked by the dim stimulus. Presentation of the intense stimulus 6 and 12 s later produced no response. However, presentation of the intense stimulus 24 s after the initial presentation produced a hyperpolarizing OFF-center response. This OFF-response gradually declined in amplitude and was replaced at 63 s after initial stimulus presentation by a depolarizing ON-center response. Trace at bottom indicates onset and offset of light stimulus. Maximum light intensity (log 0.0) = 2.37 mW/cm^2. [From Xin and Bloomfield, 1999]

In contrast to previous reports, these results suggested that AII cells continue to respond under photopic light conditions, warranting a reexamination of the operating range of AII cells. Figure 12 compares the operating range of a dark-adapted and a light-adapted AII cell. Dark-adapted AII cells show response thresholds similar to those of rod photoreceptors (log −7.0) and display increased response amplitudes and decreased latencies as the stimulus is intensified. Consistent with previous reports, the response saturates at relatively dim light levels, corresponding to an operating range of 2–3 log units. However, when light stimulation is increased beyond

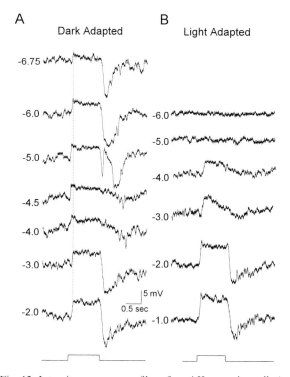

A Dark Adapted   B Light Adapted

-6.75

-6.0   -6.0

-5.0   -5.0

-4.5   -4.0

-4.0   -3.0

-3.0   -2.0

|5 mV
0.5 sec

-2.0   -1.0

Fig. 12. Intensity-response profiles of an AII amacrine cell. **A:** Responses of a dark-adapted AII cell to presentation of a 75 μm diameter spot of light of varying intensity centered over the cell. Values to the left of each trace indicate the log intensity of the stimulus; maximum intensity (log 0.0) = 2.37 mW/cm². Trace at bottom indicates onset and offset of the light stimulus. The ON-center response of the dark-adapted AII cell showed a threshold of about log −6.75. More intense light stimuli, up to about log −4.5, produced an increase in the amplitude of the response and a decreased latency (dashed line). The response saturated at about log −4.5 to −4.0 stimulus intensities. However, presentation of brighter stimuli (log −3.0 and brighter) evoked a robust depolarizing response. Note that the peak latency of these responses to bright lights were longer that those of the saturated responses but similar to those of the responses to the dimmest stimuli. **B:** Responses of the same AII cell to the 75 μm diameter spots of light, but following a 10 minute exposure to a bright background light (log −2.0). The threshold of the light-adapted AII cell was log −4.0, almost 3 log units brighter than that displayed by the cell under dark adapted conditions. Increases in stimulus intensity evoked larger amplitude ON-center responses. These responses showed saturation at between log −1.0 and 0.0. [From Xin and Bloomfield, 1999]

the saturating level, the AII response surprisingly recovers and, in fact, increases in amplitude. Figure 12B shows the responses of another AII cell after a 10-min exposure to a moderately intense

adapting light. This AII cell shows a response threshold of log −3.0, about 3 log units higher than that seen for the dark-adapted cell. Further, the response amplitude increases steadily, showing saturation only to the extremely bright stimuli of log −1.0 and 0.0 intensity. These data indicate that AII amacrine cells are responsive over 6–7 log units of light intensity and thus can convey both rod and cone signals.

As aforementioned, dark-adapted AII cells show ON-center–OFF-surround receptive field organization. In contrast, light-adapted AII cells showed ON-center and OFF-center responses but did not display OFF-surround activity (Xin and Bloomfield, 1999). These results suggested that the receptive fields of AII cells are reorganized following changes in adaptational state. To understand the synaptic pathways circuits involved in this reorganization, we carried out a number of pharmacological studies to dissect the circuits underlying the different response components of light-adapted AII cells. Similar to that seen for dark-adapted retinas, application of APB reversibly blocked the ON-center response of light-adapted AII amacrine cells (Fig. 13). However, this blockade revealed a sustained hyperpolarizing response with waveform and receptive field profile suggesting that it is center-mediated. Athough this OFF-center response was insensitive to the application of APB, it was reduced or abolished by CNQX (Bloomfield and Xin, 2000). The OFF-center response, then, likely reflect the inputs from OFF-center cone bipolar cells to AII amacrine cell dendrites in sublamina *a* of the IPL (Strettoi et al., 1992).

As discussed above for dark-adapted cells, the sensitivity of the ON-center response AII cells to APB indicates that these cone-driven signals may be derived by two possible pathways: (1) cone to rod photoreceptors via gap junctions to rod bipolar cells to AII cells and/or (2) cones to ON-center cone bipolar cells to AII cells via gap junctions. To distinguish between the two pathways we again took advantage of the finding by Mills and Massey (1995) that NO, acting through a cGMP-mediated cascade, uncouples AII amacrine cells from ON-center cone bipolar cells. Application of the NO donors, SNP or SNAP, or the membrane-permeant analog, 8-bromo-cGMP, abolished the ON-center responses of AII cells and revealed a light-evoked, sustained

196

Light-Adapted AII Cell - 50 μM APB

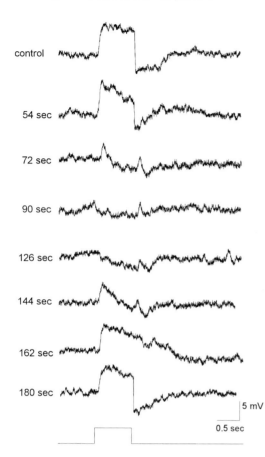

control

54 sec

72 sec

90 sec

126 sec

144 sec

162 sec

180 sec

5 mV

0.5 sec

Fig. 13. Effects of a 40 s application of 50 μm APB on the ON-center responses of a light-adapted AII amacrine cell. Cell was light adapted with a constant background light of log −2.5 intensity. Stimulus was 75 μm diameter spot of light (log −1.5) superimposed on the background light. APB produced a moderate hyperpolarization of the membrane and reversibly blocked the ON-center response. Elimination of the ON-response revealed a small, hyperpolarizing OFF-center response. [From Xin and Bloomfield, 1999]

hyperpolarization corresponding to OFF-center response (Fig. 14); this is in clear contrast to the lack of effect of these drugs on dark-adapted AII cells. These results suggest, then, that the ON-center responses of light-adapted AII cells are derived mainly, if not exclusively, from signals traversing the AII–cone bipolar cell gap junctions. Thus, the ON-center responses of dark- and light-adapted AII cells appear generated by different synaptic circuits.

Light-Adapted AII Cell - 500 μM 8-bromo-cGMP

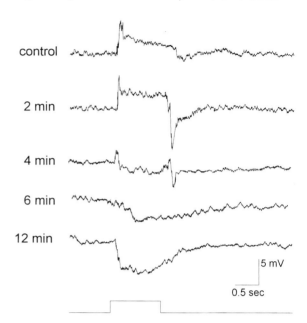

control

2 min

4 min

6 min

12 min

5 mV

0.5 sec

Fig. 14. Effects of a 15 min application of 500 μM 8-bromo-cGMP on the ON-center response of a dark-adapted AII amacrine cell. Cell was adapted with a constant background light (log −3.0) on which a small spot stimulus (75 μm diameter and log −2.0 intensity) was superimposed. The drug produced a small depolarization of the dark membrane potential and blocked the ON-center response, revealing a hyperpolarizing OFF-center response. [From Xin and Bloomfield, 1999]

Conclusions and future directions

Taken together, the results of recent studies indicate that the circuits subserved by AII amacrine cells are highly plastic, being modulated under conditions of changing adaptational state. The light-induced changes in AII–AII cell coupling reflect the need for these vital elements in the rod pathways to be responsive throughout the scotopic/mesopic range. Dark-adapted retinas can be considered analogous to starlight conditions under which rods will only sporadically absorb photons of light. The need, then, is for AII cells to preserve these isolated signals above the background noise. Accordingly, the AII cells are relatively uncoupled under these conditions in that there are few correlated signals to sum and so extensive coupling would serve to dissipate and thereby attenuate the few isolated responses rather than enhance them. Presentation of background lights, analogous to twilight conditions, brings about greater than a 10-fold increase in AII-AII cell coupling. This increased coupling provides for summation of synchronous activity over a wider area, thus preserving the fidelity of these rod-driven, correlated signals at the expense of spatial acuity (cf. Smith and Vardi, 1995). This step-like transition in coupling seen between well dark-adapted retinas and those illuminated with dim background lights suggests two basic operating states for AII cells under scotopic–mesopic light conditions: (1) the ability to respond to single photon events and (2) summing signals over a relatively large area to sum synchronized events above the background noise.

It had been posited that in the transition from rod to cone vision, the AII cells uncouple from the cone bipolar cells to eliminate a large and what was believed to be an inappropriate diversion of cone signals to AII cells (Mills and Massey, 1995; Sterling, 1995). Our recent results indicate quite the opposite. The AII cells have an extensive operating range and clearly remain functional under photopic light conditions. In fact, it appears that the ON-center responses of light-adapted AII cells arise from signals delivered via the gap junctions made with cone bipolar cells indicating that they must remain open under bright ambient light conditions. Interestingly, exogenous application of NO or cGMP effectively modulate the conductance of the AII–cone bipolar cell gap junctions, suggesting an endogenous neuromodulatory mechanism is in place. Understanding the physiological stimuli that set this mechanism in motion is an important direction for future studies. In this regard, it is interesting that in experiments in which AII cells were rapidly light adapted, there was a 1–4 min delay before the ON-center responses reappeared. One notion is that this observation reflects a delay in the opening of AII–cone bipolar cell gap junctions. Clearly, at least some of these junctions must be functional in the dark-adapted state in that they form the sole pathway for ON-center scotopic signals in AII cells to reach the ganglion cells. Is it possible that there are two sets of AII–cone bipolar cell junctions that are rectifying? In this scheme, one set would be active in the dark as signals move from AII to cone bipolar cells, whereas the other set opens during light adaptation to allow transfer of photopic signals in the opposite direction. Interestingly, injection of cone bipolar cells with Neurobiotin fails to label AII cells, indicating rectification of some of these junctions at least in terms of their ability to pass tracers (Mills and Massey, 1995; Vaney, 1994). Recently initiated work on the types of connexins found at the AII-cone bipolar cell junctions (cf. Feigenspan et al., 2001) may provide insights into this provocative idea.

The finding that AII cells continue to operate under photopic light conditions refutes the previous findings of several labs, including our own. In at least our case, the discrepancy stems from the fact that in the past we had carried out amplitude–intensity functions up to the point that we saw saturation of the AII cell responses. Therefore, in a desire to limit light adaptation, we simply never examined AII cell response activity to more intense visual stimuli. Interestingly, both Nelson (1982) and Dacheux and Raviola (1986) described cone-driven signals in AII cells, but these contributed only a small fraction of the amplitude of the rod-driven responses and are thus quite different from the robust cone-driven responses we reported. In any event, as the most abundant amacrine cell type in the retina, AII cells must play a significant role in the processing of photopic signals in the inner retina. The inhibitory feedback synapse made onto axon terminals of OFF-center cone bipolar cells points to one possible function. Understanding the role of AII cells in the processing of cone-driven visual forms another important direction for future research.

One fascinating result concerning the transition of AII cell activity from rod to cone mediation is the reorganization of their receptive fields. Under dark adaptation, AII cells display classic center–surround receptive fields, but under light-adapted conditions the surround activity appears eliminated leaving both ON- and OFF-center responses. Further, the disappearance of AII cell surround activity is opposite to that for brisk ganglion cells whose surrounds are present under light-adapted conditions but are attenuated or completely lost following dark adaptation (Barlow et al., 1957; Rodieck and Stone, 1965; Barlow and Levick, 1976; Muller and Dacheux, 1997). Clearly, then, AII surround receptive fields are not simply imparted to the ganglion cells but instead must dictate how AII

198

cells respond to different stimulus shapes that, in turn, will modify the response activity of post-synaptic ganglion cells. In this regard, the AII cell surround receptive fields appear unique in that they appear exclusively under scotopic light conditions. Synaptic circuitry from horizontal to photoreceptors thought responsible for generating the surrounds of bipolar cells are thought to occur onto cones, but not rods (Baylor et al., 1971, Burkhardt, 1977, but see Linberg and Fisher, 1988). This is consistent with our finding that rod bipolar cells do not generate surround responses. Therefore the appropriate circuitry may not exist in the outer retina to produce surround receptive fields under scotopic conditions and thus this function must be delegated to circuitry in the inner retina. Whether these inner retinal circuits are unique to AII amacrine cells is unclear and only further studies of the surround mechanisms of other amacrine cell types will answer this question. However, Cook and McReynolds (1998) showed recently that amacrine cells play a role in generating surround receptive field of certain ganglion cells in the light-adapted amphibian retina. Thus, inner retinal circuits may play a significant role in generating antagonistic surround receptive fields under a broad range of adaptational conditions.

Finally, we recently proposed that the S1 amacrine cells, acting through inhibitory feedback synapse to rod bipolar cell axon terminals, provide the surround inhibition of AII amacrine cells (Bloomfield and Xin, 2000). Again, the pharmacological data suggest that both $GABA_A$ and $GABA_C$ receptors, both of which have been localized to rod bipolar cell axon terminals (Fletcher et al., 1998), play a role in mediating the AII cell surrounds. Recently, however, Fletcher and Wässle (1999) reported that only $GABA_C$ receptors are localized postsynaptically at the S1-to-rod bipolar cells contacts. These data clearly conflict with the supposition that S1 cells exclusively mediate the surround responds of AII cells. As aforementioned, AII cells also receive direct inhibitory (presumed GABAergic) input from a homogeneous class of amacrine cells that may activate $GABA_A$. Thus, a combination of feed-forward and feedback inhibition may team to provide the surround-mediated activity of AII cells.

Acknowledgments

I thank Drs. Daiyan Xin and Bela Volgyi who carried out many of the experiments described here. This work was supported by NIH grants EY07360, EY06689 and Research to Prevent Blindness, Inc.

References

Akazawa, C., Ohishi, H., Nakajima, Y. Okamoto, N., Shigemoto, R., Nakanishi, S. and Mizuno, M. (1994). Expression of mRNAs of L-AP4-sensitive netabotropic glutamate receptors (mGluR4, mGluR6, mGluR7) in the rat retina. Neurosci. Lett., 171: 52–54.

Barlow, H.B. and Levick, W.R. (1976). Threshold setting by the surround of cat retinal ganglion cells. J. Physiol., 259: 737–757.

Barlow, H.B., Fitzhugh, R. and Kuffler, S.W. (1957). Change of organization of receptive fields of the cat's retina during dark adaptation. J. Physiol., 137: 338–354.

Baylor, D.A., Fuortes, M.G.F. and O'Bryan, P.M. (1971). Receptive field of cones in the retina of the turtle. J. Physiol., 214: 265–294.

Bloomfield, S.A. and Dowling, J.E. (1985a). Roles of aspartate and glutamate in synaptic transmission in rabbit retina. I. Outer plexiform layer. J. Neurophysiol., 53: 699–713.

Bloomfield, S.A. and J.E. Dowling (1985b). Roles of aspartate and glutamate in synaptic transmission in rabbit retina. II. Inner plexiform layer. J. Neurophysiol., 53: 714–725

Bloomfield, S.A. and Miller, R.F. (1986). A functional organization of the ON and OFF pathways in the rabbit retina. J. Neurosci., 6: 1–13.

Bloomfield, S.A. and Xin, D. (2000). Surround inhibition of mammalian AII amacrine cells is generated in the proximal retina. J. Physiol., 523: 771–783.

Bloomfield, S.A., Xin, D. and Persky, S.E. (1995). A comparison of receptive field and tracer coupling size of horizontal cells in the rabbit retina. Vis. Neurosci., 12: 985–999.

Bloomfield, S.A., Xin, D. and Osborne, T. (1997). Light-induced modulation of coupling between AII amacrine cells in the rabbit retina. Vis. Neurosci., 14: 565–576.

Boos, R., Schneider, H. and Wässle, H. (1993). Voltage- and transmitter-gated currents of AII-amacrine cells in a slice preparation of the rat retina. J. Neurosci., 13: 2874–2888.

Brandstätter, J.H., Koulen, P. and Wässle, H. (1997). Selective synaptic distributions of kainate receptor subunits in the two plexiform layers of the rat retina. J. Neurosci., 17: 9298–9307.

Boycott, B.B. and Dowling, J.E. (1969). Organization of the primate retina: light microscopy. Philos. Trans. of the R. Soc. (Lond.) B, 255: 109–184.

Burkhardt, D.A. (1977). Responses and receptive field organization of cones in perch retina. J. Neurophysiol., 40: 53–62.

Cook, P.B. and McReynolds, J.S. (1998). Lateral inhibition in the inner retina is important for spatial tuning of ganglion cells. Nat. Neurosci., 1, 714–719.

Dacheux, R.F. and Raviola, E. (1986). The rod pathway in the rabbit retina: A depolarizing bipolar and amacrine cell. *J. Neurosci.*, 6: 331–345.

Euler, T. and Wässle, H. (1998). Different contributions of GABA$_A$ and GABA$_C$ receptors to rod and cone bipolar cells in a rat retinal slice preparation. *J. Neurophysiol.*, 79: 1384–1395.

Famiglietti, E.V. and Kolb, H. (1975). A bistratified amacrine cell and synaptic circuitry in the inner plexiform layer of the retina. *Brain Res.*, 84: 293–300.

Famiglietti, E.V. and Kolb, H. (1976). Structural basis for ON- and OFF-center responses in retinal ganglion cells. *Science*, 194: 193–195.

Feigenspan, A., Teubner, B., Willecke, K. and Weiler, R. (2001). Expression of neuronal connexin36 in AII amacrine cells of the mammalian retina. *J. Neurosci.*, 21: 230–239.

Fletcher, E.L. and Wässle, H. (1999). Indoleamine-accumulating amacrine cells are presynaptic to rod bipolar cells through GABAC receptors. *J. Comp. Neurol.*, 413: 155–167.

Fletcher, E.L., Koulen, P. and Wässle, H. (1998). GABA$_A$ and GABA$_C$ receptors on mammalian rod bipolar cells. *J. Comp. Neurol.*, 396, 351–365.

Goddard, J.C., Behrens, U.D., Wagner, H.-J. and Djamgoz, M.B.A. (1991). Biocytin: intracellular staining, dye-coupling and immunocytochemistry of the carp retina. *NeuroReport*, 2, 755–758.

Hampson, E.C.G.M., Vaney, D.I. and Weiler, R. (1992). Dopaminergic modulation of gap junction permeability between amacrine cells in mammalian retina. *J. Neurosci.*, 12: 4911–4922.

Hidaka, S., Maehara, M., Umino, O., Lu, Y. and Hashimoto, Y. (1993). Lateral gap junction connections between retinal amacrine cells summating sustained signals. *NeuroReport*, 5: 29–32.

Kaneko, A. (1970). Physiological and morphological identification of horizontal, bipolar and amacrine cells in goldfish retina. *J. Physiol.*, (London) 207: 623–633.

Kolb, H. (1979). The organization of the outer plexiform layer in the retina of the cat: electron microscopic observations. *J. Neurocytol.*, 6:131–153.

Kolb, H. and Famiglietti, E.V. (1974). Rod and cone pathways in the inner plexiform layer of the cat retina. *Science*, 186: 47–49.

Linberg K.A. and Fisher, S.K. (1988). Ultrastructural evidence that horizontal cell axon terminals are presynaptic in the human retina. *J. Comp. Neurol.*, 268: 281–297.

Mangel, S.C. (1991). Analysis of the horizontal cell contribution to the receptive field surround of ganglion cells in the rabbit retina. *J. Physiol.*, 442: 211–234.

Marchiafava, P.L. (1978). Horizontal cells influence membrane potential of bipolar cells in the retina of the turtle. *Nature*, 275: 141–142.

Massey, S.C., Redburn, D.A. and Crawford, M.L.J. (1983). The effects of 2-amino-4-phosphonobutryric acid (APB) on the ERG and ganglion cell discharge of rabbit retina. *Vis. Res.*, 23:1607–1613.

Miller, R.F. and Dacheux, R.F. (1976). Synaptic organization and the ionic basis of ON- and OFF-channels in the mudpuppy retina. I. Intracellular analysis of chloride-sensitive electrogenic properties of receptors, horizontal cells, bipolar cells, and amacrine cells. *J. Gen. Physiol.*, 67: 639–659.

Mills, S.L. and Massey, S.C. (1995). Differential properties of two gap junctional pathways made by AII amacrine cells. *Nature*, 377: 734–737.

Muller, J.F. and Dacheux, R.F. (1997). Alpha ganglion cells of the rabbit retina lose antagonistic surround responses under dark adaptation. *Vis. Neurosci.*, 14: 395–401.

Naka, K.-I. and Nye, P.W. (1971). Role of horizontal cells in the organization of the catfish retinal receptive field. *J. Neurophysiol.*, 34: 785–801.

Naka, K.-I. and Witkovsky, P. (1972). Dogfish ganglion cell discharge resulting from extrinsic polarization of the horizontal cells. *J. Physiol.*, 223: 449–460.

Nakajima, Y., Iwakabe, H., Akazawa, C., Nawa, H., Shigemoto, R., Mizuno, N. and Nakanishi, S. (1993). Molecular characterization of a novel metabotropic glutamate receptor mGLUR6 with a high selectivity for L-2-amino-4-phosphono butyrate. *J. Biol. Chem.*, 268: 11863–11973.

Nelson, R. (1977). Cat cones have rod input: a comparison of response properties of cones and horizontal cell bodies in the retina of the cat. *J. Comp. Neurol.*, 172: 109–136.

Nelson, R. (1982). AII amacrine cells quicken time course of rod signals in the cat retina. *J. Neurophysiol.*, 47: 928–947.

Nomura, A., Shigemoto, R, Nakamura, Y., Okamoto, N., Mizuno, N. and Nakanishi, S. (1994). Developmentally-regulated postsynaptic localization of a metabotropic glutamate-receptor in rat rod bipolar cells. *Cell*, 77: 361–369.

Rodieck, R.W. and Stone, J. (1965). Analysis of receptive fields of cat retinal ganglion cells. *J. Neurophysiol.*, 28: 833–849.

Sandell, J.H., Masland, R.H., Raviola, E. and Dacheux, R.F. (1989). Connections of indoleamine-accumulating cells in the rabbit retina. *J. Comp. Neurol.*, 283: 303–313.

Smith, R.G. and Vardi, N. (1995). Simulation of the AII amacrine cell of mammalian retina: functional consequences of electrical coupling and regenerative membrane properties. *Vis. Neurosci.*, 12: 851–860.

Slaughter, M.M. and Miller, R.F. (1981). 2-Amino-4-phosphonobutyric acid: a new pharmacological tool for retina research. *Science*, 211: 182–185.

Slaughter, M.M. and Miller, R.F. (1985). Characterization of an extended glutamate receptor of the ON bipolar neuron in the vertebrate retina. *J. Neurosci.*, 5: 224–233.

Sterling, P. (1995). Tuning retinal circuits. *Nature*, 377: 676–677.

Strettoi, E., Dacheux, R.F. and Raviola, E. (1990). Synaptic connections of rod bipolar cells in the inner plexiform layer of the rabbit. *J. Comp. Neurol.*, 295: 449–466.

Strettoi, E., Dacheux, R.F. and Raviola, E. (1992). Synaptic connections of the narrow-field, bistratified rod amacrine cell (AII) in the rabbit retina. *J. Comp. Neurol.*, 325: 152–168.

Strettoi, E., Dacheux, R.F. and Raviola, E. (1994). Cone bipolar cells as interneurons in the rod pathway of the rabbit retina. *J. Comp. Neurol.*, 347: 139–149.

Taylor, W.R. (1999). TTX attenuates surround inhibition in rabbit retinal ganglion cells. *Vis. Neurosci.*, 16: 285–290.

Toyoda, J.-I. and Tonosaki, K. (1978). Effect of polarization of horizontal cells on the ON-centre bipolar cell of carp retina. *Nature*, 276: 399–400

Vaney, D.I. (1991). Many diverse types of retinal neurons show tracer coupling when injected with biocytin or neurobiotin. *Neurosci. Lett.*, 125: 187–190.

Vaney, D.I. (1994). Patterns of neuronal coupling in the retina. *Prog. Retin. Eye Res.*, 13: 301–355.

Vardi, N. and Morigiwa, K. (1997). ON cone bipolar cells in rat retina express the metabotropic receptor mGluR6. *Vis. Neurosci.*, 14: 789–794.

Werblin, F.S. and Dowling, J.E. (1969). Organization of the retina of the mudpuppy. *Necturus maculosus.* II. Intracellular recording. *J. Neurophysiol.*, 32: 339–355.

Witkovsky, P. and Dearry, A. (1992). Functional roles of dopamine in the vertebrate retina. *Prog. Retin. Res.*, 10: 247–292.

Xin, D. and Bloomfield, S.A. (1997). Tracer coupling pattern of amacrine and ganglion cells in the rabbit retina. *J. Comp. Neurol.*, 383: 512–528.

Xin, D. and Bloomfield, S.A. (1999). Comparison of the responses of AII amacrine cells in the dark- and light-adapted rabbit retina. *Vis. Neurosci.*, 16: 653–665.

Yamashita, M. and Wässle, H. (1991). Responses of rod bipolar cells isolated from the rat retina to the glutamate agonist 2-amino-4-phosphonobutyric acid (APB). *J. Neurosci.*, 11: 2372–2382.

H. Kolb, H. Ripps and S. Wu (Eds.)
Progress in Brain Research, Vol. 131

CHAPTER 13

Neuromodulation of voltage-dependent K+ channels in bipolar cells: immunocytochemical and electrophysiological studies

Stephen Yazulla[1,*], Keith M. Studholme[1], Shih-fang Fan[1] and Carlos Mora-Ferrer[2]

[1]*Department of Neurobiology and Behavior, SUNY Stony Brook, NY 11794-5230, USA*
[2]*Institut für Zoologie III, J. Gutenberg Universität, 55099 Mainz, Germany*

My major introduction to retinal research was at the Center for Visual Science Meeting in Rochester, NY in 1969. I had just finished my second year in graduate school and a group of us from Allen Granda's lab piled into a van and headed north. It was really quite a show. One of the speakers, Frank Werblin gave a very energetic talk, that literally left the audience breathless. The talk was based on Frank's thesis, in John Dowling's lab, which comprises the classic back-to-back *Journal of Neurophysiology* papers that have set the framework for so much of the retinal electron microscopy and electrophysiology research over the last 30 years. William Rushton then stood up and just laced into Frank, questioning just about everything Frank had said. Frank, as a relatively new PhD, was caught somewhat off guard. John stood up from the audience and calmly said "Why William, I thought you would have understood that" and then he just sat down. William Rushton, in a near rage, roared "**Of course I understood that!**". He then jump up on to the stage and proceeded to answer his own objections on the blackboard. The whole incident made a great impression on me. I do not remember Rushton's objections, but the beauty of those two papers

* Corresponding author: Stephen Yazulla, Tel.: 631-632-9877; Fax: 631-632-6661; E-mail: yazulla@life.bio.sunysb.edu

(Dowling and Werblin, 1969; Werblin and Dowling, 1969) was the predictive value derived from the combined electron microscopy and intracellular recording from the same preparation. For example, the reciprocal synapse between amacrine and bipolar cells was suggested to account for the conversion of the tonic bipolar cell response to a transient amacrine cell response. This hypothesis was tested and supported by Dwight Burkhardt (1972) who showed that amacrine cell responses could be converted from transient to tonic by an antagonist of GABA, a presumed amacrine cell feedback transmitter. The fact that the system is known now to be more complicated is irrelevant to the impetus generated by these early papers. I was fortunate to join John's lab for 2 years as a postdoc (1972–1974) and found an openness with regard to discussion of data and ideas, his ability to get at the most salient feature and an attitude of sharing and interaction towards his work that I have always tried to keep in mind.

From the early 1960s through the mid 1970s, there was an ongoing controversy regarding the retinal locus/loci for the neural component of light and dark adaptation. John, first by himself and then in a series of papers with Harris Ripps and Dan Green, seemed to change their minds with each paper. What struck me and made such an impression was that, given the data, their conclusions were perfectly reasonable and defensible. John, Harris and Dan trusted and listened to their data rather than hang constrained by some hypothesis into which they tried to force the data. The lesson I derived from this was the paramount importance of the data and never to let yourself become so enamoured and personally vested in an hypothesis that you ignore the message of your data. I think that this has served me and my laboratory well.

As I was ending my postdoctoral time in John's lab, he was gearing up to an extensive study of a new type of interneuron, the dopamine interplexiform cell. The results of this initial effort with Berndt Ehinger and graduate student Bill Hedden, were two papers in the *Proceedings of the Royal Society of London* (Dowling and Ehinger, 1978; Hedden and Dowling, 1978). These two papers, continuing the tradition of combining electron microscopy and electrophysiology, have formed the foundation for virtually all subsequent work on the dopamine interplexiform cell; certainly for all of mine. The following overview, I hope, illustrates the broad approach to a problem that has typified John's work and has inspired my laboratory over the years.

Dopamine is the major catecholamine in vertebrate retinae, in which it appears to serve as a signal of light adaptation by reducing photosensitivity (Djamgoz and Wagner, 1992; Witkovsky and Dearry, 1992, for reviews). Behavioral experiments in healthy, dark-adapted humans have demonstrated a decrease in light sensitivity following orally administered levadopa (Gottlob et al., 1994). In addition, depletion of retinal dopamine, whether by reserpine in rats (Malmfors, 1963) or by intraocular injections of 6-hydroxydopamine (6-OHDA) in teleost fish (Lin and Yazulla, 1994a; McCormack and McDonnell, 1994) results in an apparent increase in photosensitivity under photopic conditions. However, Li and Dowling (2000) reported a loss of rod function in zebrafish following dopamine depletion. The intraretinal sites at which effects of dopamine on light sensitivity are mediated are, as yet, unknown but appear likely to occur in the inner retina (Lin and Yazulla, 1994b; Li and Dowling, 2000).

Retinal dopamine in goldfish is contained in a dopaminergic interplexiform cell (DA-IPC) that receives centrifugal input (Zucker and Dowling, 1987) originating from the olfactory bulb

(Stell et al., 1984) and most of its intraretinal input in the inner plexiform layer (IPL) from amacrine cells, while directing most of its output centrifugally to horizontal cell bodies (Dowling and Ehinger, 1978). In addition to horizontal cells, DA-IPCs are in contact with rod- and cone photoreceptor terminals, other DA-IPCs, GABAergic amacrine cells, glycinergic IPCs and bipolar cells (Dowling and Ehinger, 1978; Yazulla and Zucker, 1988; Van Haesendonck et al., 1993; Yazulla and Studholme, 1997). Among the bipolar cells we have focussed on the large ON-type mixed rod–cone (Mb) bipolar cells and their interaction with DA-IPCs.

Mb bipolar cells, comprising at least three subtypes (Stell, 1976; Ishida et al., 1980), receive mixed rod–cone input in the OPL. They have large synaptic terminals in the proximal IPL that receive extensive and near exclusive input from GABAergic amacrine cells (Marc et al., 1978; Yazulla et al., 1987). Contacts with DA-IPCs are relatively rare (Van Haesendonck et al., 1993; Yazulla and Zucker, 1988; Yazulla and Studholme, 1997), perhaps too rare to account for the potent effect of dopamine on voltage-gated calcium currents recorded from the synaptic terminals of Mb bipolar cells (Heidelberger and Matthews, 1994). It appears that the physiological effect of dopamine on Mb bipolar cells greatly exceeds that predicted by the relative sparseness of direct DA-IPC innervation.

Depletion of retinal dopamine by intraocular injections of 6-OHDA in goldfish results in an apparent increase in light sensitivity under photopic backgrounds (Lin and Yazulla, 1994a). This effect occurs by the time DA-IPCs degenerate, i.e., within 10 days, and persists for up to 1 year even though there has been partial reinnervation (10% of control density) of the retina by DA-IPC processes growing in from the marginal zone. The light-activated plasticity of horizontal cell dendritic spinules is inhibited following dopamine depletion with 6-OHDA, but returns to normal with partial reinnervation of the retina with DA-IPC processes (Yazulla and Studholme, 1995; Yazulla et al., 1996). However, DA-IPCs do not reinnervate Mb bipolar cells (Yazulla and Studholme, 1997). This dissociation between the effects of 6-OHDA injection on photopic light sensitivity and light-adaptive spinule formation led us to propose that dopamine acted via two mechanisms in the goldfish retina. First, as a paracrine hormone, the mere presence of dopamine was sufficient to modulate the light-adaptive spinule formation of horizontal cell dendrites in the outer plexiform layer (OPL). The second mechanism required the DA-IPC as an integral part of a circuit for the control of photopic sensitivity (Yazulla et al., 1996), perhaps including the Mb bipolar cell.

Here we will review our efforts over the past several years to elucidate the distribution and function of transmitter receptors and voltage-gated potassium channels on Mb bipolar cells in normal fish as a prelude to studies of fish whose retinas have been depleted of retinal dopamine by intraocular injections of 6-hydroxydopamine. We have used conventional light and electron microscopic immunocytochemistry as well as whole-cell patch-clamp recording techniques. Details of the methodologies can be found in the original publications.

Mb bipolar cells and DA-IPCs

Figure 1 illustrates the distribution of DA-IPC processes in relation to Mb bipolar cells. Double-labeling with tyrosine hydroxylase-immunoreactivity (TH-IR), to identify DA-IPCs and protein kinase C-immunoreactivity (PKC-IR) to identify Mb bipolar cells, shows that there is very little overlap of DA-IPC processes at the levels of the Mb soma, axon and axon terminal (Fig. 1A and B). Despite the extensive DA-IPC arborization in the OPL, ultrastructural analysis has shown that the overwhelming majority

of DA-IPC processes in the OPL are in contact with horizontal cell bodies; less than 4% are onto Mb bipolar cell bodies and dendrites (Van Haesendonck et al., 1993; Yazulla and Studholme, 1997). DA-IPC contacts with the axon terminals are much rarer, and include pre-and postsynaptic morphologies (Yazulla and Zucker, 1988; Yazulla and Studholme, 1997).

Fast transmitter inputs to Mb bipolar cells

Electrophysiological evidence has demonstrated that Mb bipolar cells receive glutamatergic inputs in the OPL from photoreceptors. At least two types of glutamate receptors are involved and appear to depend on whether the input is derived from rods (metabotropic receptors) or cones (glutamate-gated chloride conductance) (Grant and Dowling, 1996). As yet we know of no anatomical probe for the glutamate-gated chloride conductance. However, metabotropic glutamatergic receptors can be visualized with antisera against mGluR6 (unavailable to us) or mGlur1α (Fig. 2B). Double-labeling with mGluR1α and PKC shows that the dendrites of the Mb bipolar cells are strongly immunoreactive for mGluR1α, while the main ascending dendrite and soma are more lightly labeled (Fig. 2B). The axon and axon terminal of Mb bipolar cells are devoid of mGluR1α-IR. It appeared as if the mGluR1αIR was confined to ON-Mb bipolar cells and absent from the ON cone bipolar cells, corroborating the electrophysiological data of Grant and Dowling (1996).

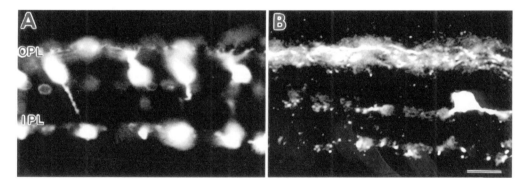

Fig. 1. View of a DA-IPC (**B**) visualized with tyrosine hydroxylase-IR and Mb bipolar cells (**A**), visualized with protein kinase C-IR. DA-IPC have a major projection in the OPL, in which only a small percentage of contacts are with bipolar cells. There are two thinner laminae of DA-IPC processes in the proximal and distal margins of the IPL. Outer plexiform layer (OPL) and inner plexiform layer (IPL). Calibration bar = 25 μm.

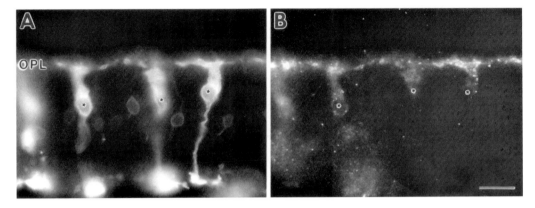

Fig. 2. Distribution of mGluR1α-IR in goldfish retina, visualized with Cy-3. The section was double labeled for PKC-IR (A) and mGluR1α (B) to demonstrate colocalization in Mb bipolar cells. Asterisks (cell bodies) indicate common points in each micrograph. mGluR1α-IR was most prominent on Mb dendrites in the OPL; scattered puncta also were found on the ascending dendrite and soma of the Mb bipolar cells. Calibration bar = 25 μM.

Massive GABAergic input from amacrine cells to the Mb bipolar cell terminals was first indicated by Marc et al. (1978) and has been supported by numerous electrophysiological studies. An electrophysiological study demonstrating bicuculline–benzodiazapine-sensitive GABA$_A$ receptors on Mb terminals (Tachibana and Kaneko, 1987, 1988) was not supported by localization studies of GABA$_A$ receptors by in vitro autoradiography (Yazulla, 1981; Lin and Yazulla, 1994c) or immunocytochemistry of antibodies against GABA$_A$ β2/β3 receptor subunits (Yazulla et al., 1989; Lin and Yazulla, 1994c). A subsequent study (Matthews et al., 1994) showed that GABAergic input to Mb bipolar cells is largely by the so-called GABA$_C$ receptor, an ionotropic GABA receptor that is bicuculline insensitive, and formed by ρ-subunits. Indeed extensive labeling of the Mb synaptic terminals by antibodies against the ρ-subunit has been demonstrated by Koulen et al. (1997).

Modulators of Mb bipolar cells

In addition to the fast transmitter inputs of glutamate in the OPL and GABA in the IPL, Mb bipolar cells are subject to modulation by other neuroactive substances. As mentioned, Mb bipolar cells receive rare contacts from DA-IPCs in the OPL and less so in the IPL. However, antisera against goldfish D1 receptors show a broad distribution all over the Mb bipolar cells (Fig. 3A, B; Mora-Ferrer et al., 1999), suggestive of a dopaminergic influence that greatly exceeds that predicted by the direct DA-IPC innervation that appears restricted to the soma and dendrites in the OPL (Yazulla and Studholme, 1997).

We found that rod bipolar cells of the rat retina were labeled densely by antibodies against cannabinoid CB$_1$ receptors (Yazulla et al., 1999). This was of interest because cannabinoids are reported to increase photosensitivity and thus may serve as a counterpoint to dopamine that, as a light signal, would decrease photosensitivity. We (Yazulla et al., 2000) found that CB$_1$R-IR was found in the OPL, IPL, Müller cells and bipolar cell bodies of goldfish retina. A feature of CB$_1$R-IR in the inner retina of goldfish was labeling in the synaptic terminals of Mb bipolar cells amongst others, as illustrated by colocalization of CB$_1$R-IR with PKC-IR (Fig. 4). In fact, there was a considerable amount of intracellular CB$_1$R-IR in virtually all bipolar-cell terminals. Although CB$_1$R-IR did not entirely fill the Mb bipolar cell terminal, it was rich in areas devoid of mitochondria (Fig. 5A). This restricted distribution accounts for the observation that, at the LM level, CB$_1$R-IR was less extensive in the Mb terminal than indicated by PKC-IR (compare Fig. 4A,B). Membrane-associated CB$_1$R-IR was always opposite an amacrine-cell synapse, but was not necessarily near a bipolar cell synaptic ribbon (Fig. 5B). CB$_1$R-IR was not evenly distributed along the whole plasma membrane; rather it was concentrated at one or two sites, when viewed in single sections. The CB$_1$R-IR extended for

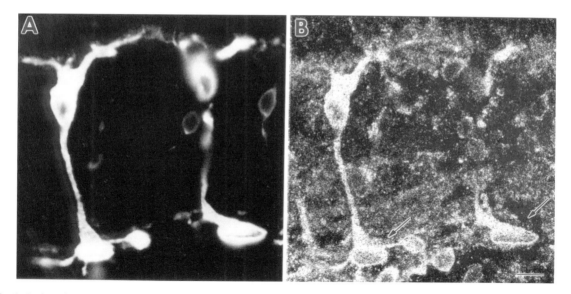

Fig. 3. Red- and green-channel images (presented in black and white) of the same tissue section that was double-labeled with gfD1r-antiserum (Cy3, **B**) and PKC-antiserum (FITC, **A**) in goldfish retina, that were obtained with a Zeiss LSM 510 confocal microscope. Each image is of the same optical section (0.45 μm thick). The large Mb bipolar cells contained numerous overlying puncta, indicative of gfD1r-IR, on the soma, axon, axon terminal in the IPL (arrows), and thick ascending stalk and dendrites in the OPL. Calibration bars = 10 μm. [From Mora-Ferrer et al., 1999]

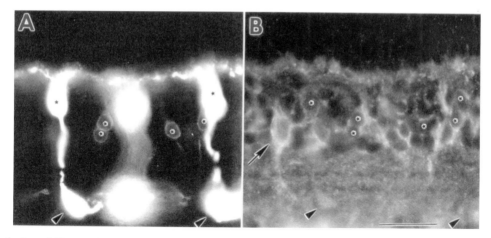

Fig. 4. Distribution of CB_1R-IR in a cryostat section of goldfish retina, visualized with Cy-3. The section was double labeled for PKC-IR **(A)** and CB_1R-IR **(B)** to demonstrate co-localization in ON bipolar cells. Asterisks (cell bodies) and arrowheads (Mb terminals) indicate common points in each micrograph. Faint CB_1R-IR appears to ring each PKC-immunoreactive cell body. Colocalization over the synaptic terminals (arrowheads) is apparent over the terminal at the left side of the micrograph but is not visible at all in the out-of-focus terminals to the right side. The large arrow indicates a CB_1R-immunoreactive Müller Cell. Calibration bar = 25 μm. [Modified from Yazulla et al., 2000]

a short distance into the cytoplasm from the plasma membrane, perhaps due to diffusion of reaction product. This appearance was the case regardless of the bipolar-cell type. However, the relative frequency of membrane-associated CB_1R-IR depended on the bipolar-cell type: 93% ($n = 41$) of the bipolar cell terminals in sublamina b (ON-type), compared to only 33% ($n = 55$) of the terminals in sublamina a (OFF-type). There is thus a marked preference of CB_1R-IR for bipolar cells subserving the ON pathway.

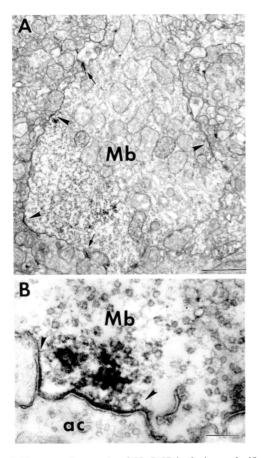

Fig. 5. Electron micrographs of CB$_1$R-IR in the inner plexiform layer of goldfish retina. (**A**) this low power micrograph shows CB$_1$R-IR in an Mb bipolar cell terminal in which there was intracellular labeling mostly on the left side of the terminal as well as membrane-associated labeling (arrowheads). Arrows indicate synaptic ribbons. (**B**). CB$_1$R-IR in the synaptic terminal of an Mb bipolar cell shows extended CB$_1$R-IR along the bipolar cell membrane that was opposed to two amacrine cell processes (ac). Calibration bars = (**A**) 5 µm, (**B**) 0.25 µm. [From Yazulla et al., 2000]

Potassium channel subunits and Mb bipolar cells

Voltage-gated K$^+$ channels comprise a very diverse group of membrane proteins and play an important role in regulating neuronal excitability, including resting membrane potential, action potential firing rate and synaptic transmission (Jan and Jan, 1990; for review). Kv1.1 and Kv1.2, members of the *Shaker* subfamily, and Kv2.1, a member of the *Shab* subfamily of voltage-gated K$^+$ channels, encode a very slowly inactivating "delayed rectifier"- type K$^+$ conductance when expressed as homomultimers in *Xenopus* oocytes; such K$^+$ channels are very sensitive to 4-aminopyridine (4AP) and tetraethylammonium (Stühmer et al., 1989). Calcium-insensitive, delayed rectifiers ($I_{K(V)}$) are a general feature of vertebrate retinae as they have been recorded from a wide variety of retinal neurons (Attwell and Wilson, 1980; Tachibana, 1981; Lipton and Tauck, 1987) including bipolar cells (Attwell et al., 1987; Kaneko et al., 1989; Karschin and Wässle, 1990; Klumpp et al., 1995). Likewise in goldfish, we have recorded $I_{K(V)}$ from Mb bipolar cells (Fan and Yazulla, 1999a, b) and have localized subunits underlying $I_{K(V)}$ to Mb bipolar cells, illustrated for Kv1.2 and Kv2.1 in Fig. 6A and B, respectively. Antibodies against *Shaker*- and *Shab*-like subunits Kv1.1, Kv1.2 (Fig. 6A) and Kv2.1 (Fig. 6B) predominately label the axon of Mb bipolar cells, and lesser label is observed on the axon terminal and cell body; only Kv1.2 labeled dendrites in the OPL (Fig. 6A). Ultrastructural analysis showed that Kv1.2-IR was present at bipolar cell dendrites that contacted cone terminals. In the IPL, Kv-immunoreactivity was present on the plasma membrane but only rarely was it ever associated with a synaptic specialization. Such non-synaptic localization would be expected for voltage-gated rather than chemically gated channels.

Modulation of voltage-dependent K$^+$ currents ($I_{K(V)}$) of Mb bipolar cells

Given the correspondence of immunocytochemical labeling for D1 receptors, CB$_1$ receptors and "Kv" subunits on Mb bipolar cells, we investigated the effects of dopamine D1 ligands and cannabinoid CB$_1$ ligands on $I_{K(V)}$. We used whole-cell patch-clamp techniques on Mb bipolar cells in the goldfish retinal slice.

Dopaminergic effects

Initially we performed control experiments with sodium ascorbate, which has been used routinely to prevent oxidation of dopamine-containing solutions. We found that ascorbate was not neutral but had complex concentration-dependent effects on $I_{K(V)}$

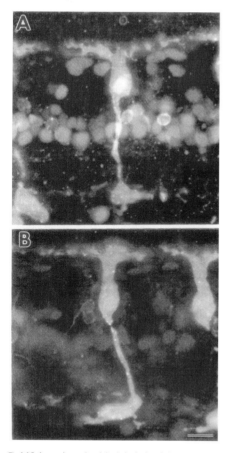

Fig. 6. Goldfish retina double-labeled with anti-PKC (Texas Red) used to identify ON bipolar cells and antibodies against *Shaker*-like Kv1.2 subunit (**A**) and *Shab*-like Kv2.1 subunit (**B**) visualized with FITC. Kv1.2 and Kv2.1 immunoreactivities appear as bright patches that are superimposed on the gray Mb bipolar cells. In general, Kv-IR was sparse but concentrated at the bipolar cell body and proximal portion of the axon. Double-labeling of the ascending dendrite and processes in the OPL was most prominent for anti-Kv1.2 (**A**), although it was present in varying degrees on the other examples. Double-labeling of the axon terminal in the IPL was scattered, and most obvious in the examples illustrated for anti-Kv1.2 (**A**). Note in **A**, the bright oval structure in the soma of the Mb bipolar cell is not the nucleus of that Mb cell, but rather a Kv1.2 immunoreactive cell body lying behind the Mb bipolar cell. This is obvious when the section is viewed in color. calibration bar = 10 μm. [From Yazulla and Studholme, 1998]

(Fig. 7). Increments of 10–20 μM resulted in a long-latency enhancement (Fig. 7A), while large increments (> 40 μM) and decrements of 10–200 μM ascorbate resulted in a rapid suppression of $I_{K(V)}$ (Fig. 7B). These effects were not due to changes in

pH, oxidative stress, lipid peroxidation, any calcium-dependent or sodium dependent action (Fan and Yazulla, 1999a). I–V relations showed that all effects were on the amplitude of $I_{K(V)}$; there was no shift along the x-axis (Fig. 7, bottom). The effects also were prominent between −40 and 0 mV, the approximate operating range of the Mb bipolar cells (Tachibana and Okada, 1991). Amazingly, the effects of ascorbate were blocked by a D1 antagonist SCH 23390 (Fig. 8A) mimicked by dopamine (Fig. 8B) and a D1 agonist SKF 38390 (Fig. 8 C,D). In addition, the effects of ascorbate were blocked completely by the PKA inhibitor Walsh Inhibitor Peptide (Wiptide), but were unaffected by a D2 antagonist, spiperone (Fan and Yazulla, 1999b). We concluded that dopamine and ascorbate acted via D1 receptors and a PKA-dependent mechanism to modulate $I_{K(V)}$ of Mb bipolar cells (Fan and Yazulla, 1999a,b).

The suppressive effect, regardless of whether it was evoked by large increments of ascorbate or decrements of any amount, appeared within the time frame of changing the perfusion media, whereas the enhancement of $I_{K(V)}$ took many minutes to develop. Washout of the effects also took many minutes. In order to study the time course of the effects and whether the bipolar cells had differential spatial sensitivity to D1-mediated modulation, we used puff pipettes to apply the drugs (Fig. 9). The rapid response was the suppression of $I_{K(V)}$, and this was most efficiently induced by a pulsed decrease in the extracellular concentration of ascorbate. This was accomplished by perfusing the slices in saline containing 200 μM ascorbate and recording the responses of $I_{K(V)}$ to puffs of ascorbate-free saline (zero [AA]$_o$). As expected from the perfusion experiments, suppression of $I_{K(V)}$ occurred very quickly, within 80 ms of the applied puff of zero [AA]$_o$ (Fig. 9). Suppression, which reached 50% of control, lasted for several minutes even though the puff was for only 1 s. The puff pipette was positioned upstream of the perfusion flow and orthogonal to different parts of the Mb bipolar cell. $I_{K(V)}$ was suppressed by a puff of zero [AA]$_o$ regardless of whether the puff was aimed at the dendrites in the OPL, the soma or axon terminal (Fig. 9a–d). The null response from the axon (Fig. 9c) is most likely due to the thinness of the axon and its relative inaccessibility within the slice. Mb bipolar

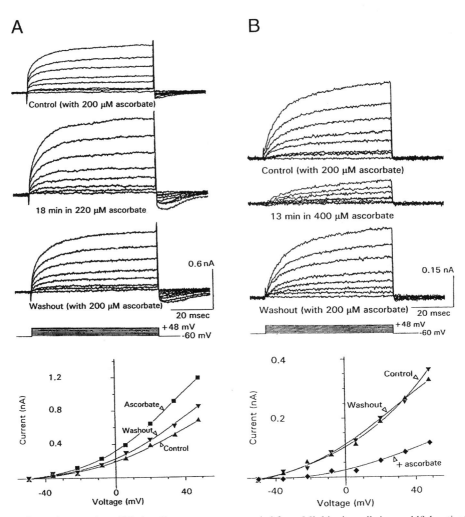

Fig. 7. Modulation of $I_{K(V)}$ by ascorbate. Whole cell currents were recorded from Mb bipolar cells in a goldfish retinal slice. (**A**) $I_{K(V)}$ was reversibly enhanced by an increase of ascorbate concentration from 200 to 220 μM as illustrated in the current records and I–V relation. (**B**) $I_{K(V)}$ was reversibly suppressed by a decrease in ascorbate concentration from 400 to 200 μM as illustrated in the current records and I–V relations. Both effects of ascorbate were on the amplitude of $I_{K(V)}$; there was no shift along the voltage-axis. [From Fan and Yazulla, 1999b]

cells thus appear to be uniformly sensitive to D1 mediated modulation of $I_{K(V)}$. As with the perfusion experiments, the effects of puffed zero ascorbate were blocked by SCH 23390 and Wiptide, but were insensitive to spiperone.

Cannabinergic effects

$I_{K(V)}$, recorded from Mb bipolar cells, was suppressed by the cannabinoid ligands CP 55490 and WIN 151617 (Fig. 10A). The suppression occurred quickly,

reversed rapidly with washout and was suppressed by the CB_1 antagonist SR 141716A (Fig. 10C). The I–V relation also showed a reduction of $I_{K(V)}$ without any shift along the x-axis (Fig. 10B) (Yazulla et al., 2000). Probing the Mb bipolar cell with a puff pipette showed that only the synaptic terminal was sensitive to 1 s puffs of CP 55490; no response was elicited when puffs were directed at the OPL or soma. This finding is consistent with the observation that membrane-associated CB_1R-IR was restricted to the synaptic terminal of Mb bipolar cells (Fig. 5).

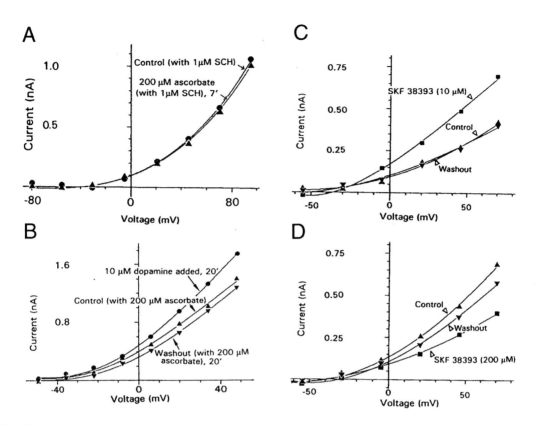

Fig. 8. The effects of ascorbate on $I_{K(V)}$ were mediated by a dopamine D1 receptor mechanism. (**A**) The suppressive effect of a 200 µM increase of ascorbate on $I_{K(V)}$ was blocked by 1 µM SCH 23390, a D1 receptor antagonist. (**B**) 10 µM dopamine still enhanced $I_{K(V)}$ even in the continued presence of 200 µM ascorbate. This is the same effect as obtained with 10–20 µM increments of ascorbate. (**C,D**) SKF 38393 (a D1 agonist) mimicked the effects of ascorbate and dopamine on $I_{K(V)}$. (**C**) The I–V relationships of $I_{K(V)}$ of a cell treated with 5 µM SKF 38393, show a reversible enhancement of $I_{K(V)}$, while in **D**, the I-V curves of $I_{K(V)}$ of a cell treated with 200 µM SKF 38393, show suppression of $I_{K(V)}$. For all data, $I_{K(V)}$ was elicited by a 60 ms, +48 mV depolarizing pulse from a holding potential of -60 mV. [From Fan and Yazulla, 1999b]

Conclusions and future perspectives

Mb bipolar cells receive input from two fast transmitters. Glutamate, from photoreceptors in the OPL, conveys information in the through pathway to ganglion cells, whereas GABA, from amacrine cells in the IPL, potently modulates transmitter release by its action on chloride and calcium currents (Heidelberger and Matthews, 1991; Matthews et al., 1994). In addition, Mb bipolar cells are subject to modulation by other neuroactive agents, as illustrated here, dopamine/ascorbate and cannabinoids. This organization of a glutamatergic neuron, subject to fast GABA inhibition and modulation by dopamine and cannabinoids also is found in the basal

ganglia (Ameri, 1999, for review) and may be a common feature of central nervous system circuits. A well-documented action of both dopamine and cannabinoids is presynaptic modulation of transmitter release by effects on calcium currents (Ameri, 1999, for review). Similarly, in retinal bipolar cells, dopamine potentiates the voltage-dependent influx of calcium by shifting the activation range of calcium current to more negative values (Heidelberger and Matthews, 1994). Cannabinoids simply reduce the amplitude of calcium currents in salamander bipolar cells without altering the activation range (Straiker et al., 1999). Thus, dopamine and cannabinoids can control the amount of transmitter released and hence, the gain of signal transmission from bipolar cells to

210

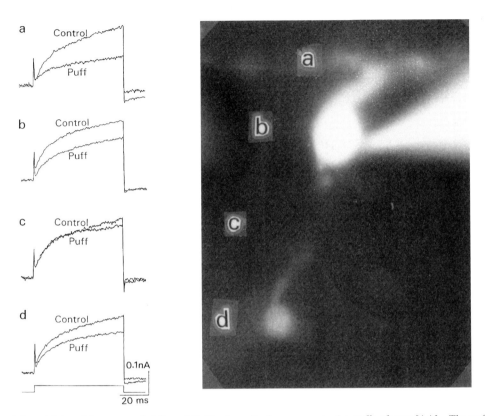

Fig. 9. The spatial sensitivity of $I_{K(V)}$, recorded from Mb bipolar cells, in response to 1 s puffs of zero $[AA]_o$. The puff pipette was placed at various positions along the Mb bipolar cell that was visualized with Lucifer yellow in the recording pipette; $I_{K(V)}$ was elicited first in the absence (Control) and then 80 ms following a 1 s puff of zero $[AA]_o$. The puff of zero $[AA]_o$ caused a reduction of $I_{K(V)}$ when puffed at all parts of the Mb bipolar cell except at the axon. $I_{K(V)}$ was elicited by a 60 ms, +48 mV depolarizing pulse from a holding potential of −60 mV.

ganglion cells. But what about the consequences of modulating $I_{K(V)}$?

$I_{K(V)}$ and the underlying "Kv" subunits are found on goldfish ON bipolar cells but not OFF bipolar cells (Fan and Yazulla, 1999a,b; Yazulla and Studholme, 1998; Yazalla et al., 1999). Activation of $I_{K(V)}$ by depolarizing responses to incremental steps of light will oppose the depolarization, resulting in a relaxation of the ON response. Indeed, virtually all voltage recordings of the large ON bipolar cells of carp and goldfish retina show a pronounced peak and plateau in response to a light flash in contrast to the more tonic response of the large OFF bipolar cells (i.e., Saito and Kujiraoka, 1982; Saito et al., 1984). $I_{K(V)}$ is very insensitive to small increments of either ascorbate or dopamine in that the enhancement takes many minutes to develop. However, small decrements of either dopamine or ascorbate cause a rapid, long

lasting suppression of $I_{K(V)}$, which should delay the relaxation phase of the ON response, that is, make the responses to repetitive flashes more tonic over a period of time. In other glutamatergic regions of the CNS, ascorbate uptake is coupled to glutamate uptake in a heteroexchange process (Rebec and Pierce, 1994). If the same were true for the photo-receptors, extracellular ascorbate would be high in dim light conditions when vesicular glutamate release and transport uptake are high. Incremental flashes would reduce synaptic glutamate release, glutamate transport and consequently extracellular ascorbate. Under these conditions, ascorbate would be a normal and integral component of the photoreceptor-to-bipolar cell synapse. We proposed that the extracellular concentration of dopamine reflects background intensity, whereas extracellular ascorbate reflects local intensity changes. The waveform

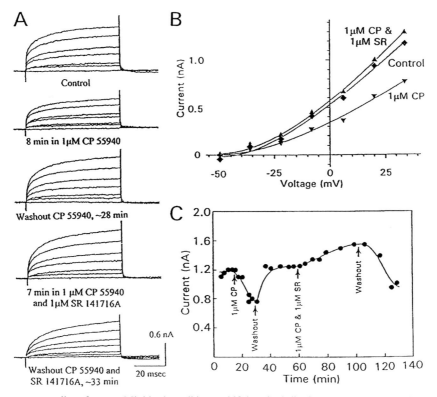

Fig. 10. Whole-cell current recordings from an Mb bipolar cell in a goldfish retinal slice in response to a cannabinoid agonist CP 55940 and antagonist SR 141716A. (**A**) Current recordings to voltage steps from −50 mV to +35 mV in 14 mV steps illustrating the reversible suppression of $I_{K(V)}$ by 1 μM CP 55940 and the blockade of this suppression by 1μM SR 141716A. (**B**) I-V relation illustrating the control, suppression of $I_{K(V)}$ by 1 μM CP 55940 and the blockade of this suppression by 1μM SR 141716A. (**C**) Peak $I_{K(V)}$ elicited by a −50 mV to +35 mV step over a 2 h period. Application of 1 μM CP 55940 produced a 40% decrease in $I_{K(V)}$ that recovered with washout. Subsequent application of 1μM CP 55940 and 1 μM SR 141716A had no initial effect on $I_{K(V)}$. However a slow increase in $I_{K(V)}$ was observed that reversed with washout. (From Yazulla et al., 2000).

(i.e., peak:plateau) of the bipolar cell ON response is determined, in large part, by the amplitude of $I_{K(V)}$. The role of dopamine then, as a signal of background intensity, is to set the boundaries about which changes in ascorbate (local flashes) can modulate the peak:plateau of the ON response of the bipolar cell. This modulation all takes place in the OPL and shapes the response waveform that is presented to the IPL. Signal shaping in the IPL may be even more complicated in that dopamine and a newly described modulator, the cannabinoids, appear to play complementary roles.

Cannabinoids have been reported to increase photosensitivity (i.e., Adams et al., 1978; Kiplinger et al., 1971; West, 1991) and may serve as a dark signal. Their presence on rod bipolar cells of rat and

goldfish retinae is at least consistent with this notion (Yazulla et al., 1999, 2000). Suppression of $I_{K(V)}$ by cannabinoids has a rapid onset as well as offset, in contrast to the long-lasting action of dopamine and ascorbate. As yet, we do not know the source of retinal endocannabinoids nor the speed with which their release and uptake can be modulated by neural activity. Our data show that Mb bipolar cells are more sensitive to short-term modulation by cannabinoids than dopamine/ascorbate. Thus, cannabinoids and dopamine/ascorbate are likely to play different roles in modulating $I_{K(V)}$ under changing conditions of light- and dark-adaptation. Resolution of this issue will require that bipolar cell responses to these drugs be obtained following light stimulation. Still, these studies have provided a framework in which neuroactive substances interact to control a voltage-gated current, the consequence of which may be important in the transition between adaptation states.

There is still disagreement as to the precise role of dopamine in light adaptation. Each of us are listening to our data and taking us where it leads. I suppose that none of us really worries about whose ideas about the role of dopamine turn out to be correct. When I was in John's lab, someone would come up with an idea about an experiment. John would think about it for a bit and his response, etched in memory, has characterized his attitude toward science "That sounds like fun". And so it should be for all of us. Thanks John.

Acknowledgments

This work was supported by NIH Grant EY01682 to SY and GFD Mo 707/1–1 to CMF.

Reference

Adams, A.J., Brown, B., Haegerstrom-Portnoy, G., Flom, M.C. and Jones, R.T. (1978) Marijuana, alcohol, and combined drug effects on the time course of glare recovery. *Psychopharm.*, (Berl) 56: 81–86.

Ameri, A. (1999) The effects of cannabinoids on the brain. *Prog. Neurobiol.*, 58: 315–348.

Attwell, D. and Wilson, M. (1980) Behaviour of the rod network in tiger salamander retina mediated by properties of individual rods. *J. Physiol (Lond.)*, 309: 287–315.

Attwell, D., Mobbs, P., Tessier-Lavinge, M. and Wilson, M. (1987) Neurotransmitter-induced currents in retinal bipolar cells of the axolotl, *Ambystoma mixicanum*. *J. Physiol. (Lond.)*, 387: 125–161.

Burkhardt, D.As. (1972) Picrotoxin, GABA and strychnine: effects upon the proximal negative respons of the frog retina. *Brain Res.*, 43: 246–249.

Djamgoz, M.B.A. and Wagner, H.-J. (1992) Invited review: localization and function of dopamine in the adult vertebrate retina. *Neurochem. Int.*, 20: 139–191.

Dowling, J.E. and Ehinger, B. (1978) The interplexiform cell system-I. Synapses of the dopaminergic neurons of the goldfish retina. *Proc. R. Soc. Lond. [Biol.]*, 201: 7–26.

Dowling, J.E. and Werblin, F.S. (1969) Organization of the mudpuppy retina *Necturus maculosus*. I. Synaptic structure. *J. Neurophysiol.*, 32: 315–338.

Fan, S.F. and Yazulla, S. (1999a) Suppression of voltage-dependent K$^+$ currents in retinal bipolar cells by ascorbate. *Vis. Neurosci.*, 16: 141–148.

Fan, S.F. and Yazulla, S. (1999b) Modulation of voltage-gated K$^+$ currents ($I_{K(v)}$) in retinal bipolar cells by ascorbate is mediated by dopamine D1 receptors. *Vis. Neurosci.*, 16: 928–931.

Gottlob, I., Strenn, K. and Schneider, B.G. (1994) Effect of levadopa on the human dark adaptation threshold. *Graefes Arch. Clin. Exper. Ophthal.*, 232: 584–588.

Grant, G.B. and Dowling, J.E. (1996) On bipolar cell responses in the teleost retina are generated by two distinct mechanisms. *J. Neurophysiol.*, 76: 3842–3849.

Hedden, W.L., Jr. and Dowling, J.E. (1978) The interplexiform system II. Effects of dopamine on goldfish retinal neurones. *Proc. Roy. Soc. Lond. [Biol.]*, 201: 27–55.

Heidelberger, R. and Matthews, G. (1991) Inhibition of calcium influx and calcium current by gamma-aminobutyric acid in single synaptic terminals. *Proc. Nat. Acad. Sci. USA*, 88: 7135–7139.

Heidelberger, R. and Matthews, G. (1994) Dopamine enhances Ca^{2+} responses in synaptic terminals of retinal bipolar neurons. *Neuroreport*, 5: 729–732.

Ishida, A.T., Stell, W.K. and Lightfoot, D.O. (1980) Rod and cone inputs to bipolar cells in goldfish retina. *J. Comp. Neurol.*, 191: 315–335.

Jan, L.Y. and Jan, Y.N. (1990) How might the diversity of potassium channels be generated? *TINS*, 13: 415–418.

Kaneko, A., Pinto, L.H. and Tachibana, M. (1989) Transient calcium current of retinal bipolar cells of the mouse. *J. Physiol. (Lond.)*, 410: 613–629.

Karschin, A. and Wässle, H. (1990) Voltage- and transmitter-gated currents in isolated rod bipolar cells of rat retina. *J. Neurophysiol.*, 63: 860–876.

Kiplinger, G.F., Manno, J.E., Rodda, B.E. and Forney, R.B. (1971) Dose-response analysis of the effects of tetrahydrocannabinol in man. *Clin. Pharm. Therap.*, 12: 650–657.

Klumpp, D.J., Song, E.J., Ito, S., Sheng, M.H., Jan, L.Y. and Pinto, L.H. (1995) The *Shaker*-like potassium channels of the mouse rod bipolar cell and their contributions to the membrane current. *J. Neurosci.* 15: 5004–5013.

Koulen, P., Brandstätter, J.H., Kröger, S., Enz, R., Bormann, J. and Wässle, H. (1997) Immunocytochemical localization of the GABA$_C$ receptor rho subunits in the cat, goldfish, and chicken retina. *J. Comp. Neurol.*, 380: 520–532.

Li, L. and Dowling, J.E. (2000) Effects of dopamine depletion on visual sensitivity of zebrafish. *J. Neurosci.*, 20: 1893–1903.

Lin, Z.S. and Yazulla, S. (1994a) Depletion of retinal dopamine increases brightness perception in goldfish. *Vis. Neurosci.*, 11: 683–693.

Lin, Z.S. and Yazulla, S. (1994b) Depletion of retinal dopamine does not affect the ERG-b wave increment threshold function in goldfish *in vivo*. *Vis. Neurosci.*, 11: 695–702.

Lin, Z.S. and Yazulla, S. (1994c) Heterogeneity of GABA$_A$ receptors in goldfish retina. *J. Comp. Neurol.*, 345: 429–439.

Lipton, S.A. and Tauck, D.L. (1987) Voltage-dependent conductances of solitary ganglion cells dissociated from the rat retina. *J. Physiol. (Lond.)*, 385: 361–391.

Malmfors, T. (1963) Evidence of adrenergic neurons with synaptic terminals in the retina of rats demonstrated with fluorescence and electron microscopy. *Acta Physiol. Scand.*, 58: 99–100.

Marc, R.E., Stell, W.K., Bok, D. and Lam, D.M.K. (1978) GABAergic pathways in the goldfish retina. *J. Comp. Neurol.*, 182: 221–246.

Matthews, G., Ayoub, G.S. and Heidelberger, R. (1994) Presynaptic inhibition by GABA is mediated via two distinct GABA receptors with novel pharmacology. *J. Neurosci.*, 14: 1079–1090.

McCormack, C.A. and McDonnell, M.T. (1994) Abnormal dorsal light response in teleost fish after intraocular injection of 6-hydroxydopamine. *J. Fish Biol.*, 45: 515–525.

Mora-Ferrer, C., Yazulla, S., Studholme, K.M. and Haak-Frendscho, M. (1999) Dopamine D1-receptor immunolocalization in goldfish retina. *J. Comp. Neurol.* 411: 704–714.

Rebec, G.V. and Pierce, R.C. (1994) A vitamin as neuromodulator: Ascorbate release into the extracellular fluid of the brain regulates dopaminergic and glutamatergic transmission. *Prog. Neurobiol.*, 43: 537–565.

Saito, T., Kujiraoka, T. and Toyoda, J. (1984) Electrical and morphological properties of off-center bipolar cells in the carp retina. *J. Comp. Neurol.*, 222: 200–208.

Saito, T. and Kujiraoka, T. (1982) Physiological and morphological identification of two types of On-center bipolar cells in the carp retina. *J. Comp. Neurol.*, 205: 161–170.

Stell, W.K. (1976) Functional polarization of horizontal cell dendrites in goldfish retina. *Invest. Ophthalmol.*, 15: 895–908.

Stell, W.K., Walker, S.E., Chohan, K.S. and Ball, A.K. (1984) The goldfish nervous terminalis: A luteinizing hormone-releasing hormone and molluscan cardioexcitatory peptide immunoreactive olfactoretinal pathway. *Proc. Nat. Acad. Sci. USA*, 81: 940–944.

Straiker, A., Stella, N., Piomelli, D., Mackie, K., Karten, H.J. and Maguire, G. (1999) Cannabinoid CB1 receptors and ligands in vertebrate retina: Localization and function of an endogenous signalling system. *Proc. Natl. Acad. Sci. USA*, 96: 14565–14570.

Stuhmer, W., Ruppersberg, J.P., Schroeter, K.H., Sakmann, B., Stocker, M., Giese, K.P., Perschke, A., Baumann, A. and Pongs, O. (1989) Molecular basis of functional diversity of voltage-gated potassium channels in mammalian brain. *EMBO J.*, 8: 3235–3244.

Tachibana, M. (1981) Membrane properties of solitary horizontal cells isolated from goldfish retina. *J. Physiol. (Lond.)*, 321: 141–161.

Tachibana, M. and Kaneko, A. (1987) γ-Aminobutyric acid exerts a local inhibitory action on the axon terminal of bipolar cells: Evidence for negative feedback from amacrine cells. *Proc. Natl. Acad. Sci. USA*, 84: 3501–3505.

Tachibana, M. and Kaneko, A. (1988) Retinal bipolar cells receive negative feedback input from GABAergic amacrine cells. *Vis. Neurosci.*, 1: 297–305.

Tachibana, M. and Okada, T. (1991) Release of endogenous excitatory amino acids from ON-type bipolar cells isolated from the goldfish retina. *J. Neurosci.*, 11: 2199–2208.

Van Haesendonck, E., Marc, R.E. and Missotten, L. (1993) New aspects of dopaminergic interplexiform cell organization in the goldfish retina. *J. Comp. Neurol.*, 333: 503–518.

Werblin, F.S. and Dowling, J.E. (1969) Organization of the mudpuppy retina *Necturus maculosus.* II. Intracellular recording. *J. Neurophysiol.*, 32: 339–355.

West, M.E. (1991) Cannabis and night vision. *Nature*, 351: 703–704.

Witkovsky, P. and Dearry, A. (1992) Functional roles of dopamine in the vertebrate retina. *Prog. Retinal Res.*, 11: 113–147.

Yazulla, S. (1981) GABAergic synapses in the goldfish retina: an autoradiographic study of ^{3}H-muscimol and ^{3}H-GABA binding. *J. Comp. Neurol.*, 200: 188–195.

Yazulla, S., Lin, Z.S. and Studholme, K.M. (1996) Dopaminergic control of light-adaptive synaptic plasticity and role in goldfish visual behavior. *Vision Res.*, 36: 4045–4057.

Yazulla, S. and Studholme, K.M. (1995) Volume transmission of dopamine may modulate light adaptive plasticity of horizontal cell dendrites in the recovery phase following dopamine depletion in goldfish retina. *Vis. Neurosci.*, 12: 827–836.

Yazulla, S. and Studholme, K.M. (1997) Light adaptation affects synaptic vesicle density but not the distribution of GABA$_A$ receptors in goldfish photoreceptor terminals. *Microsc. Res. Tech.*, 36: 43–56.

Yazulla, S. and Studholme, K.M. (1998) Differential distribution of *Shaker*-like and *Shab*-like K$^+$-channel subunits in goldfish retina and retinal bipolar cells. *J. Comp. Neurol.*, 396: 131–140.

Yazulla, S., Studholme, K.M., McIntosh, H.H. and Deutsch, D.G. (1999) Immunocytochemical localization of cannabinoid CB1 receptor and fatty acid amide hydrolase in rat retina. *J. Comp. Neurol.*, 415: 80–90.

Yazulla, S., Studholme, K.M., McIntosh, H.H. and Fan, S.F. (2000) Cannabinoid receptors on goldfish retinal bipolar cells: Electron-microscope immunocytochemistry and whole-cell recordings. *Vis. Neurosci.*, 17.

Yazulla, S., Studholme, K.M., Vitorica, J. and De Blas, A.L. (1989) Immunocytochemical localization of GABA$_A$ receptors in goldfish and chicken retinas. *J. Comp. Neurol.*, 280: 15–26.

Yazulla, S., Studholme, K. and Wu, J.-Y. (1987) GABAergic input to the synaptic terminals of mb1 bipolar cells in the goldfish retina. *Brain Res.*, 411: 400–405.

Yazulla, S. and Zucker, C.L. (1988) Synaptic organization of dopaminergic interplexiform cells in the goldfish retina. *Vis. Neurosci.*, 1: 13–30.

Zucker, C.L. and Dowling, J.E. (1987) Centrifugal fibres synapse on dopaminergic interplexiform cells in the teleost retina. *Nature*, 330: 166–168.

H. Kolb, H. Ripps and S. Wu (Eds.)
Progress in Brain Research, Vol. 131

CHAPTER 14

Synaptic mechanisms shaping the light-response in retinal ganglion cells

Ethan D. Cohen*

Department of Cellular and Molecular Biology, Harvard University, 16 Divinity Avenue, Cambridge, MA 02138, USA

Introduction

John Dowling has made many fundamental contributions to our understanding of the physiology of the retina. Work in his lab and by his students have strongly influenced my career in the visual neurosciences. John, in a series of classic papers with Frank Werblin (Dowling and Werblin, 1969; Werblin and Dowling, 1969), established the basic cellular pathways of the light-response in the vertebrate retina. Bob Miller worked in John's lab on the B-wave of the electroretinogram, and later with Malcolm Slaughter made many seminal contributions to our understanding of the role of glutamate receptors in retinal function. A collaboration by two of John's students, Ralph Nelson and Helga Kolb helped establish the study of structure-function relationships in the mammalian retina. Finally, I have had the opportunity to work with John. John's ability to think globally, explain complex processes in a simple concise manner, and his enthusiasm towards the work of other young investigators will always be a role model for me to follow.

The ganglion cell forms the final neuron in the retinal pathway of vision. Information about the visual scene is integrated by the retinal ganglion cell, and encoded as a series of action potentials that is sent through the optic nerve to the visual areas of the brain. Retinal ganglion cells are composed of multiple types whose receptive fields form separate arrays that sample the visual scene across the retina. Thus each ganglion cell type sends a different representation of the visual scene to the brain. Recent data garnered from a variety of labs has provided evidence that retinal ganglion cell firing is actively modulated by a variety of new bipolar and amacrine cell pathways and mechanisms. This data has given us new perspectives on how the firing of ganglion cells is modulated by light and also during the process of dark adaptation (see also Bloomfield, this volume). This paper will focus on how bipolar and amacrine cell synaptic mechanisms shape the light response at identified ganglion cell types using new data obtained in mammals and several lower vertebrate species.

Synaptic organization of sustained and transient ganglion cell types in mammals

It has long been recognized that ganglion cells in many vertebrate species display light-evoked firing patterns to stimulation of the receptive field center that can be termed either "transient" or "sustained" (Hartline, 1938). Physiological studies of ganglion cells performed originally in the cat retina by Enroth-Cugell and Robson, 1966 and Cleland et al., 1971; have shown that these response patterns can be associated with distinct types termed "X" and "Y" (see Wassle and Boycott, 1991; Sterling, 1998 for a review). Similar X and Y physiological types are also

* Tel.: 617-495-2559; Fax: 617-496-3321;
E-mail: edcohen@fas.harvard.edu

216

found in the retinas of ferret, rabbit, and mouse, and in the primate retina, are termed "M" and "P" (Dacey, 1999). A key feature to our understanding of these ganglion cells was the discovery that the X and Y physiological types in cat retina correspond to the anatomical types termed "α" and "β". Each type, which can be either ON- or OFF-center, is associated with a unique set of properties.

The receptive fields of Y ganglion cells are large, show transient responses to center spot stimulation, and respond with a strong "non-linear" spatial summation component to drifting gratings. Their axons have the fastest conduction speed of any cat ganglion cell. The morphology of Y or "α" ganglion cells show a wide-field dendritic arbor, and the

largest cell bodies and axons of any cat ganglion cell (Fig. 1A). In addition, Y ganglion cells are coupled homotypically to same-center Y cell neighbors through a series of gap junctions (Vaney, 1991). This coupling can be revealed by recording Y ganglion cells with electrodes containing the tracer neurobiotin (Fig. 1B). Heterotypic coupling is also observed between Y ganglion cells and a series of amacrine cells found in the inner nuclear and ganglion cell layers (Vaney, 1991). Some of these amacrines are wide field axon bearing types.

The receptive fields of X ganglion cells are narrow, show "sustained" light responses to center spot stimulation, display classic center-surround organization, and respond with "linear" spatial

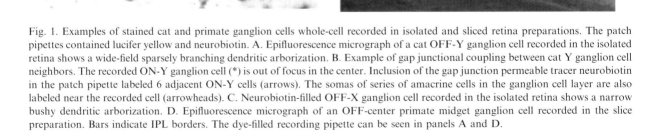

Fig. 1. Examples of stained cat and primate ganglion cells whole-cell recorded in isolated and sliced retina preparations. The patch pipettes contained lucifer yellow and neurobiotin. A. Epifluorescence micrograph of a cat OFF-Y ganglion cell recorded in the isolated retina shows a wide-field sparsely branching dendritic arborization. B. Example of gap junctional coupling between cat Y ganglion cell neighbors. The recorded ON-Y ganglion cell (*) is out of focus in the center. Inclusion of the gap junction permeable tracer neurobiotin in the patch pipette labeled 6 adjacent ON-Y cells (arrows). The somas of series of amacrine cells in the ganglion cell layer are also labeled near the recorded cell (arrowheads). C. Neurobiotin-filled OFF-X ganglion cell recorded in the isolated retina shows a narrow bushy dendritic arborization. D. Epifluorescence micrograph of an OFF-center primate midget ganglion cell recorded in the slice preparation. Bars indicate IPL borders. The dye-filled recording pipette can be seen in panels A and D.

summation to drifting gratings. Their axons have a moderate conduction speed. The morphology of X or "β" ganglion cells show a narrow bush-like dendritic tree and a medium size cell body and axon (Fig. 1C). Unlike Y ganglion cells, X cells are not electrically coupled to their neighbors (Fig. 1C). In primate retina, a corresponding series of narrow and wide field branching ganglion cell types can also be observed (e.g. Fig. 1D). Thus the ability to correlate the anatomy of a known ganglion cell type to its physiology provides a powerful tool for understanding sustained and transient ganglion cell function in the retina.

From the work of Helga Kolb and Ralph Nelson, and the lab of Peter Sterling, we know a great deal about the synaptic inputs to X and Y ganglion cells in the cat retina. Bipolar cells, releasing the excitatory amino acid neurotransmitter glutamate, provide excitatory synaptic input to both X and Y ganglion cell dendrites. ON- and OFF- center X ganglion cells receive bipolar input from 2–3 cone bipolar cell types (McGuire et al., 1984; Cohen and Sterling, 1990). In contrast, the bipolar input to ON- and OFF- Y ganglion cells appears to come largely from a single cone bipolar type (Freed and Sterling, 1988; Kolb and Nelson, 1993). The amount of the bipolar cell input to X and Y ganglion cell types differs substantially. On average, each X ganglion cell receives about 2-5X more bipolar cell input than each Y cell (Kolb 1979; McGuire et al., 1986; Freed and Sterling, 1988; Cohen and Sterling, 1991; Kolb and Nelson, 1993). The remaining synaptic inputs on X and Y cells are from amacrine cells. These inputs are largely inhibitory as both ganglion cell types show strong conductances to the inhibitory neurotransmitters GABA and glycine (Cohen et al., 1994).

While the physiology of these two ganglion cell types have been extensively studied primarily using extracellular recording techniques, little is known about the synaptic currents generating these response patterns. Recently, a series of superfused slice and isolated cat retina preparations have been developed in order to examine the light-evoked synaptic currents shaping X and Y ganglion cells using whole-cell recording techniques (see Cohen et al., 1994; Cohen, 1998 for details). Ganglion cells were recorded in current and voltage clamp mode using patch pipettes that contained physiological levels of chloride in order to separate the reversal potentials of excitatory and inhibitory conductances ($E_{Cl} = \sim -70$ mV). For cellular identification, the dye markers lucifer yellow and neurobiotin were included in the patch pipette (see Fig. 1). This review will focus first on synaptic mechanisms shaping sustained X ganglion cell light-responses.

Light-evoked firing patterns of excitation and corresponding synaptic currents in sustained/X type ganglion cells

The X or "sustained" type ganglion cell comprises about 50% of the cells in the ganglion cell layer of the cat retina (e.g. Stein et al., 1996). Figure 2 shows examples of the light-evoked firing patterns of ON- and OFF-X ganglion cells recorded in current clamp mode to a center spot stimulus (upper panels). The lower panels show the light-evoked currents generating these firing patterns by the same cells in voltage clamp. By holding the ganglion cell near E_{Cl} we can examine the excitatory currents to X ganglion cells in relative isolation. Stimulation of the ON-X ganglion cell with a spot causes excitation and a sustained increase in the cell's firing rate (Fig. 2A). The light-evoked voltage depolarization of the ganglion cell is limited by activation of voltage-dependant sodium and potassium channels during the generation of action potentials. At spot-offset, a short hyperpolarization occurs and the cell's firing rate is reduced. Figure 2B shows the corresponding synaptic current generating this excitatory firing pattern. Spot stimulation evoked a noisy inward current with a large initial transient and smaller sustained component. The inward current declined at spot offset. Figure 2C shows the light-evoked firing pattern of an OFF-X ganglion cell to a dim spot stimulus. Spot stimulation causes a hyperpolarization of the membrane potential and a reduction in firing. Offset of the spot causes excitation and a burst of spikes is seen. Figure 2D shows the corresponding synaptic currents of the same OFF-X cell to spot stimulation. Spot stimulation generates a small net outward current at light-ON that lasts for the duration of the spot. Offset of the spot evokes a rapid inward current. This excitatory current causes the increase in firing seen in OFF-X cells at light-OFF. Thus the firing patterns of X cells are

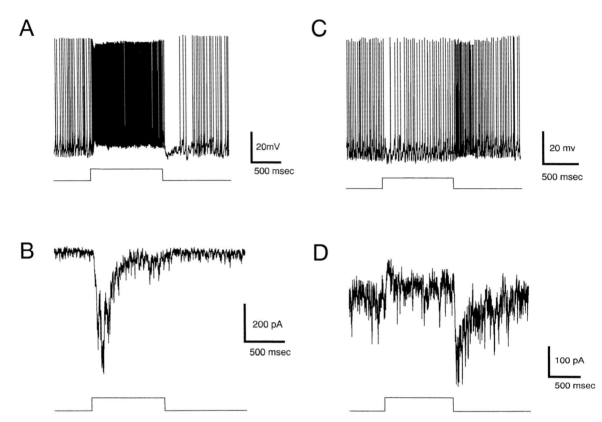

Fig. 2. Comparisons of the light response of cat ON- and OFF-X ganglion cells recorded in current clamp (upper panels) and voltage clamp (lower panels) to center spot stimulation of their receptive field. A. Center spot stimulation of an ON-X ganglion cell in current clamp causes a transient-sustained increase in firing that lasts for the duration of the spot stimulus (lower trace). B. Light-evoked synaptic currents of the same ON-X ganglion cell in voltage clamp. Spot stimulation evoked a transient inward current followed by a smaller sustained component. Holding potential –80 mV. C. Center spot stimulation of an OFF-X cell in current clamp to a dim spot stimulus causes a hyperpolarization and a decrease in firing. At spot offset, a transient increase in firing is observed. D. Light-evoked synaptic current from the same OFF-X cell in voltage clamp. Spot stimulation evokes a small outward current that is sustained and lasts for the spot duration. At light-OFF, a larger inward excitatory current is observed. B, D Holding pot. –80 mV, Potassium-based internal solutions. All cells were recorded in Ames Ringer. (For details, see Cohen, 2000, © American Physiological Society)

shaped by both transient and sustained synaptic current components.

Ganglion cells at rest receive a constant release of glutamate from bipolar cells

When extracellularly recorded, mammalian ganglion cells often show high resting firing rates under light-adapted backgrounds. The nature of these high firing rates appear to be due to a resting release of the excitatory neurotransmitter glutamate from bipolar cells. The upper trace of Fig. 3 shows the raw holding

current record of a cat ON-X ganglion cell in voltage clamp held near the ganglion cell's resting potential. A spot stimulus is applied to the ganglion cell (lower trace). For each presentation, the spot stimulation elicits an inward excitatory current to the ON-X ganglion cell. This excitatory current reflects glutamate release from ON-center bipolar cells. If one blocks ON-bipolar cell input with APB (Slaughter and Miller, 1981; Chen and Linsenmier, 1989) the light-evoked inward current is reduced as expected. However APB also causes a substantial drop in the dark holding current and noise at the ganglion cell (arrow), suggesting it too is glutamate-mediated.

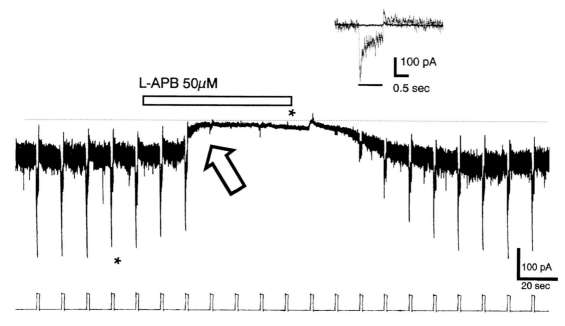

Fig. 3. Bipolar cells provide a resting level of glutamate release onto mammalian ganglion cells. When L-APB, a metabotropic glutamate agonist for ON-bipolar cells is added to the bath, the light-evoked inward currents on this cell are strongly suppressed, and a large decrease in the noise and magnitude of the dark holding current can be seen (arrow) Lower trace: spot stimulus. Inset: shows individual LEC traces (starred) in the control condition (stippled line), and in the presence of APB (solid line). Holding potential, −60 mV (adapted from Cohen, 1998 with permission, © American Physiological Society). Similar reductions in the resting current could also be seen by blocking ionotropic glutamate receptors directly on the ON-X ganglion cell.

The resting glutamatergic synaptic current on cat ganglion cells is substantial, being about 20–25% as large as the light-evoked current. A high resting release rate of glutamate by bipolar cells allows the ganglion cell to encode both positive and negative changes in contrast in the receptive field as respective increases and decreases in their firing rates. What is not clear from these records is what concentration of glutamate (μM) is found at excitatory ganglion cell synapses at rest. This glutamate level may become a significant problem for ganglion cells during retinal insult or disease (see Lipton, this volume).

Inhibitory currents by sustained and transient amacrine cells shape the light-response of X ganglion cells

We can separate the excitatory and inhibitory currents shaping the light-response of X ganglion cells in voltage clamp by holding the ganglion cell at different potentials during the spot stimulus.

Excitatory glutamatergic currents from bipolar cells will open conductances reversing near 0 mV, (e.g. Mittman et al., 1990; Cohen, 1998, 2000), while inhibition from amacrine cells will open chloride-mediated conductances reversing near E_{Cl}, −70 mV. Figure 4A shows an example of this experiment on an ON-X cell. Center spot stimulation of the receptive field center activates a prominent transient-sustained excitatory conductance that reverses positive to −20 mV. At spot-offset a smaller transient inhibitory conductance was activated in many cells. The activation of this inhibitory conductance may correspond to the small hyperpolarization observed on ON-X cells at light-off (e.g. Fig. 2A). Figure 4B shows the results of holding an OFF-X ganglion cell at different potentials during the spot stimulus. Spot stimulation of the receptive field center of an OFF-center X ganglion cell activated a sustained inhibitory conductance at light-ON which was reduced at light-OFF. This conductance reversed near or slightly negative to the calculated E_{Cl} of the internal solution. At light-OFF, an excitatory

220

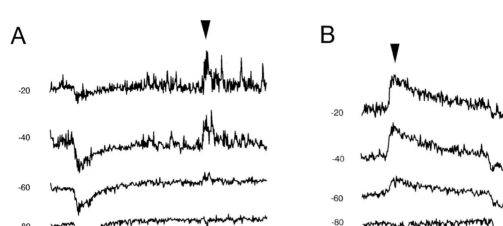

Fig. 4. Light-evoked currents of cat ganglion cells are composed of excitatory and inhibitory conductances arranged in an opposing type of mechanism. A. Light-evoked currents of an ON-center X cell in the cat retinal slice in the presence of TTX (tetrodotoxin) at a series of different holding potentials (indicated at left). During the spot stimulation (bar), light activates an inward current with transient and sustained components that reverses positive to −20 mV. At spot offset a second more transient current is evoked (arrowhead) that reverses at negative potentials. Continued perfusion of the TTX-containing Ringer abolished this current. B. Light-evoked currents of an OFF-X cell in the isolated cat retina held at a series of different holding potentials in the presence of TTX. During the spot stimulus, a sustained inhibitory current (arrowhead) is activated that reverses near the resting potential. At spot offset an inward excitatory current is evoked that reverses positive to −20 mV. Addition of picrotoxin and strychnine blocked the inhibitory currents. (From Cohen, 1998 ©American Physiological Society)

conductance predominated; reversing positive to −20 mV. Thus ON-center X ganglion cells are excited at light-ON by bipolar cells, and transiently inhibited at light-OFF by amacrine cells. In contrast, OFF-center X ganglion cells are actively inhibited at light-ON by amacrine cells, and excited at light-off by bipolar cells. In this fashion, the light-evoked currents of X ganglion cells are shaped by both inhibitory and excitatory currents (see also Belgum et al., 1982).

Sustained AII amacrine cells inhibit OFF-center ganglion cells at light-ON

The AII, or rod amacrine cell provides the main synaptic pathway for rods to modulate the firing of ON-and OFF-center ganglion cells (Famiglietti and Kolb, 1975). In the dark, light stimulation of

rods causes ON-center rod bipolars to release glutamate producing a sustained-ON depolarization in AII amacrine cells (Nelson, 1982; Boos et al., 1993). The AII amacrine cell has a bistratified dendritic tree that spans the ON- and OFF-sublamina of the inner plexiform layer (Nelson, 1982). AII amacrine cells form gap junctions with ON-center cone bipolar cells, which in turn synapse onto ON-center ganglion cells. Thus depolarization of the AII amacrine cell depolarizes electrically coupled ON-center cone bipolar cells which in turn excite ON-center ganglion cells.

However the lobular appendages of AII amacrine cells in the OFF-sublamina also form chemical synapses upon the axon terminals of OFF-center cone bipolar and ganglion cells. These appendages are thought to release the inhibitory neurotransmitter glycine. Application of the inhibitory neurotransmitter glycine to cat OFF-X and Y ganglion cell

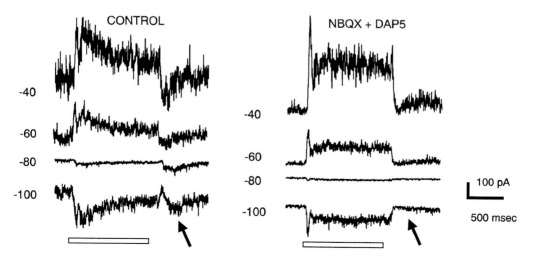

Fig. 5. Evidence for an ON-center cone bipolar cell pathway of inhibition to OFF-center ganglion cells mediated by AII amacrine cells. Whole-cell recording of the light-evoked currents of an OFF-X ganglion cell in voltage clamp at different holding potentials (indicated at left). TTX was added to the Ringer to block sodium currents. Left panel shows the light-evoked currents of the ganglion cell in the control condition. Center spot stimulation (bar), activates a sustained inhibitory conductance that reverses at negative holding potentials near E_{Cl}. At light-OFF, an excitatory current is observed that reverses positive to –40 mV (arrow). The right panel shows the light-evoked currents of the ganglion cell in the presence of the ionotropic glutamate receptor antagonists DAP5 and NBQX. These antagonists block excitatory input to the ganglion cell from OFF-center cone bipolar cells while sparing ON-center cone bipolar function. As expected, the excitatory current at light-OFF is blocked (arrow). However in many cells, the inhibitory current at light-ON prominently remained on the OFF-X ganglion cell. This current appears to be due to glycinergic AII amacrine cell inhibition of OFF-center ganglion cells at light-ON. However under normal conditions it is likely there exist several other pathways of inhibition to OFF-X ganglion cells. (For details, see Cohen, 1998).

dendrites causes opening of chloride channels (Cohen et al., 1994). Consequently, depolarization of the AII amacrine cell at light-ON causes glycine release and a subsequent hyperpolarization of OFF-center cone bipolar and ganglion cells. In this fashion a single ON-center AII amacrine cell can simultaneously excite ON- and inhibit OFF-center pathways to ON- and OFF- center ganglion cells.

Pharmacological evidence for this pathway is often seen in the light-evoked currents of OFF-X ganglion cells (Fig. 5). In the control condition, spot stimulation normally evokes a sustained inhibitory current at light-ON reversing near E_{Cl} (see also Fig. 4). At light-OFF a glutamatergic excitatory current is observed (arrow, left panel). The excitatory current normally comes from OFF-center cone bipolar cells releasing glutamate onto the ionotropic glutamate receptors of OFF-center ganglion cells (Cohen, 1998). If one applies a series of ionotropic glutamate receptor antagonists, OFF-center cone bipolar cell excitation to the OFF-center ganglion cell is blocked, however the inhibition at light-ON curiously remains

unaffected (Fig. 5). This inhibition at light-ON cannot be from ON-center rod bipolars as their ionotropic glutamate receptor synaptic input to the AII amacrine cell will be blocked in the antagonist mixture (Boos et al., 1993). What this experiment reveals is a pathway from cones through ON-center cone bipolars (which use metabotropic glutamate receptors) to the AII amacrine cell. Under these conditions, light can still depolarize ON-center cone bipolar cells which depolarize their electrically coupled AII amacrines, causing them to release glycine onto the OFF-X cell. As a consequence, a direct sustained inhibitory current at light-ON persists on OFF-X ganglion cells (Cohen, 1998; Cohen and Miller, 1999).

Transient spiking amacrine cells also inhibit ganglion cells directly

Recent studies in salamander, rabbit and guinea pig retina have shown that activation of spiking amacrine cells in the receptive field periphery can inhibit the light-evoked response of ganglion cells (Cook et al., 1998; Taylor, 1999; Demb et al., 2000). This synaptic inhibition relies on sodium-dependent action potentials operating in axon-bearing wide field amacrine cells. These experiments have their origin in a classic study by Frank Werblin (1972), who showed that a rotating windmill pattern centered around the receptive field center of a recorded ganglion cell would selectively activate transient type amacrine cell inhibition, but not horizontal cell inhibition. An example of this stimulus paradigm is shown on a current clamp recording of an ON-OFF salamander ganglion cell from a study by Cook et al., (1998) (Fig. 6). The solid trace shows the average voltage response of the ganglion cell (filtered to remove action potentials) to a center spot stimulus. In the control condition, spot stimulion causes the cell to depolarize at spot onset and offset (left panel). Addition of a stationary windmill pattern in the receptive field periphery, has no effect on the ganglion cell's response to the center spot (middle panel). In contrast when the windmill pattern was rotating, the spot-evoked depolarization was inhibited (right panels). When the sodium channel blocker tetrodotoxin was added to the bath, the inhibition of the spot-evoked depolarization by the rotating windmill pattern was now removed. Further experiments showed that the inhibition was direct and mediated by fast glycine receptors (see also Han et al., 1997; Frishman and Linsenmier, 1982). However, it is unclear whether all axon-bearing amacrine cells, such as those electrically coupled to cat Y ganglion cells operate by a similar synaptic mechanism.

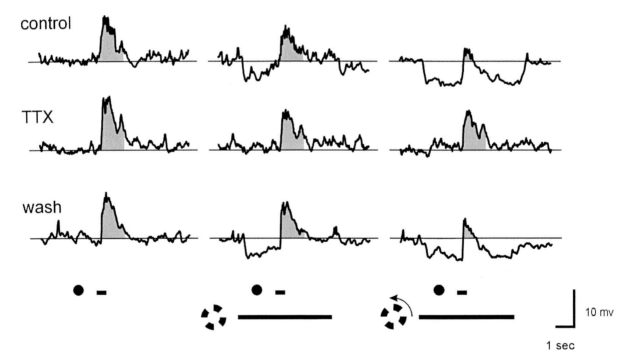

Fig. 6. Tetrodotoxin (TTX) blocks transient amacrine cell inhibition induced by a rotating windmill pattern stimulus on a salamander ON-OFF ganglion cell recorded in current clamp mode. A flashing spot centered over the receptive field, causes a depolarization of the ganglion above its dark resting potential (line). Responses are shown to spot stimulation alone (left traces), the spot response in the presence of a stationary annular windmill pattern (middle traces), and the spot response in the presence of a rotating annular windmill pattern (right traces). Only in the presence of the rotating windmill stimulus, is the spot evoked depolarization of the ganglion cell inhibited. In TTX-containing Ringer, this inhibition was removed. Lower traces show stimulus timing. From Cook et al., 1998. © 1998 Society for Neuroscience.

Light-evoked currents driving X/sustained and Y/transient ganglion cells are similar in form

Figure 7 shows a comparison of the light-evoked currents of X/sustained and Y/transient cat ganglion cells to center spot stimulation. Activation of either ON-center ganglion cell type evokes a transient inward excitatory current at light-ON that declined to a smaller sustained component. Center stimulation of OFF-center ganglion cell types both show a small sustained outward current activated at light-ON and a larger inward excitatory current activated at light-OFF. What is quite remarkable is the about these synaptic currents is that the light-evoked current kinetics of X and Y ganglion cells are remarkably similar in form. This probably reflects the commonality of the main cone bipolar input to both ON-center X and Y ganglion cells from type CBb_1 bipolar cells, and for OFF-center X and Y cells from type CBa_1 (McGuire et al., 1986; Freed and Sterling, 1988; Kolb and Nelson, 1993). A similar kinetic form of light-evoked currents can be seen on a few primate parvocellular ganglion cells recorded in the isolated retina (Fig. 7). Thus the question is raised: what biophysical properties of X and Y ganglion cells makes their light-evoked firing patterns significantly different?

What makes X and Y cells different?

Using the whole-cell recording technique, I have recorded the current-voltage relations and light-evoked currents of ON- and OFF-Y ganglion cells in the slice and isolated retina of the cat ($n = 20$, 15 cells, respectively). What is quite remarkable about both ON- and OFF-Y ganglion cells is that their membrane resistance values are unusually low. This resistance difference can be seen in the light-evoked current records of Fig. 7 as a lower level of noise in the Y ganglion cell records compared to their X ganglion cell counterparts.

One source of this low membrane resistance could be electrical coupling of Y ganglion cells to their like-center neighbors and amacrine cells (see Fig. 1B, and Vaney, 1991). Using neurobiotin-filled patch electrodes, an average of 7.0 ± 1.9 cat Y cells were prominently labeled around a recorded Y cell in the

isolated retina (mean $\pm$ s.d., $n = 7$ cells). In addition, the processes of several wide field amacrines form extensive junctional appositions against neighboring alpha ganglion cell dendrites. This electrical coupling explains why Mastronarde, (1983) found antidromic activation of one Y cell caused 0.7–4% of the spikes recorded in a Y cell neighbor to be synchronized on a sub-millisecond time scale. While Y ganglion cell receptive field centers might be expected to be enlarged by cellular coupling with axon bearing wide field amacrine cells, measurements of Y cell centers obtained under mesopic conditions show they are only ~1.4X larger than their dendritic fields (Peichle and Wassle, 1983). These results suggest that cellular coupling cannot account for the low membrane resistance of Y cells.

Current-voltage relations of Y ganglion cells in the isolated retina show a large linear leak conductance at holding potentials near the resting potential of the ganglion cell. This leak conductance could be reduced by placing cells in the potassium channel blocker barium suggesting the conductance is leakage channel mediated (Cohen, unpublished data, See also Fink et al., 1998). Estimates of the membrane resistance of Y ganglion cells using potassium-based electrodes (taken as the chord conductance near the 0 current holding potential level) were remarkably low in the isolated peripheral retina. Their resistances averaged 30.9 ± 16.2 MΩ in normal Ringer (mean $\pm$ s.d., $n = 12$ cells (7 ON-, 5 OFF-center)). In contrast the membrane resistance of X ganglion cells measured in the same region showed values that were 5 fold higher, averaging 162 ± 73 MΩ (mean $\pm$ s.d., $n = 16$ cells (11 ON-, 5 OFF-center)). In theory, Y ganglion cells could have larger light-evoked excitatory currents to compensate for their lower membrane resistances. However measurements of the light-evoked currents of 27 X and 11 Y cells obtained in the isolated peripheral retina both showed roughly equal excitatory synaptic current magnitudes averaging ~400 pA at –80 mV (Cohen, 1998).

How might a low membrane resistance value explain why Y ganglion cells show fast transient responses to light? Presumably by providing some sort of a leak conductance, the lower values of membrane resistance help reduce the time constant of the larger Y ganglion cell membrane, making its voltage response quicker. A model accounting for X

224

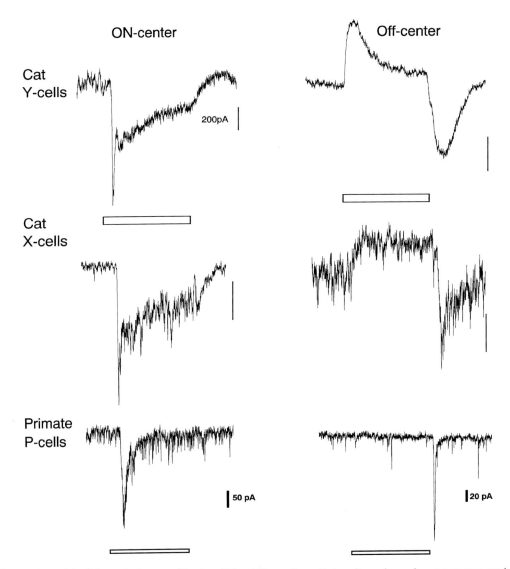

Fig. 7. Comparison of the light-evoked current kinetics of X and Y ganglion cells in voltage clamp show a common mode of excitation between ganglion cell types. A 1 s spot stimulus (indicated by the lower bar) was centered over the receptive field of each ganglion cell. Center spot stimulation of ON-Y ganglion cells shows a transient-sustained pattern of excitatory inward currents similar to that seen on ON-X cells. The light-evoked current kinetics of OFF-X and Y ganglion cells show a similar correspondence. Note the current noise of Y cells is lower than X cells (current bars all denote 200 pA). Ganglion cells were recorded in the presence of TTX Ringer at a holding potential of −80 mV. The light-evoked currents of a few primate midget ganglion cells recorded in the isolated retina are shown for comparison.

and Y ganglion cell firing patterns is shown in Fig. 8. Stimulation of an ON-Y ganglion cell with a spot of light over its receptive field center generates a transient-sustained light-evoked excitatory inward current similar to that observed in the ON-X ganglion cell. However given the Y cell's lower

membrane resistance, only the transient component of the light-evoked excitatory current is able to bring the ganglion cell above spike threshold. This seems plausible given the resting potential of cat ganglion cells average ∼ − 58 mV, close to the sodium channel activation range of –50 mV (Cohen, 1998). In this

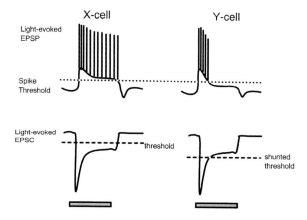

Fig. 8. Model of the transient firing mechanism on Y ganglion cells compared to X cells. Each ganglion cell is stimulated with a spot over its receptive field center (bar). Lower panels: Light-evoked excitatory postsynaptic current (EPSC) from ON-bipolar cells generates an EPSC in X and Y ganglion cells with a transient and sustained component. This current is integrated by the ganglion cell membrane in current clamp mode to form the light-evoked excitatory postsynaptic potential (EPSP, upper panels) which drives the ganglion cell above spike threshold (dotted trace). Further excursions above spike threshold are limited by activation of sodium channels and their subsequent activation of potassium currents to repolarize the membrane. This converts all depolarizing current above spike threshold into an *increase in the rate of firing* (See Diamond and Copenhagen, 1995). Because the light-evoked EPSC of the Y ganglion cell is more strongly shunted, mainly transient component(s) of the light-evoked EPSC are able to drive the ganglion cell membrane above spike threshold. Consequently, more transient firing is produced by the spot stimulus.

fashion, only the larger more transient portion of the Y cell's light-evoked EPSC reaches above spike threshold, resulting in a more transient burst of action potentials. In contrast the higher membrane resistance of X ganglion cells allows both the transient and sustained portion of the light-evoked excitatory postsynaptic current to reach spike threshold, generating a more sustained pattern of firing. Evidence of this shunting mechanism can be seen in a comparison of the current to firing frequency relations (f–I) of an X and Y ganglion cell recorded in current clamp mode (Fig. 9). For X cells, small positive current steps elicit large depolarizations and vigorous sustained firing rates. In contrast, small positive current steps in Y cells generate only small depolarizations. Strong current steps above spike threshold in Y cells cause increased spiking rates that

rapidly adapt probably due to activation of calcium activated potassium currents (Mobbs et al., 1992; Fohlmeister and Miller, 1997). Only extreme currents generate sustained firing patterns.

Several different mechanisms have been proposed to account for the generation of transient signals in the retina such as that found for the light-responses of Y ganglion cells. These include an amacrine circuit truncating the light-response of a bipolar cell (Werblin et al., 1988), V-amacrine cells in mouse retina (Nirenberg and Meister, 1997), potassium currents (Mobbs et al., 1992) and filtering through gap junctions between photoreceptors (Attwell et al., 1983). While the model shown above accounts for the transient light-evoked response properties of Y ganglion cells, it is likely to be an oversimplification of the actual cellular circuitry. Given the low membrane resistance of Y ganglion cells, our ability to maintain adequate space clamp of the dendrites of these ganglion cells is likely to be poor. In addition, recent studies also indicate retinal ganglion cell dendrites can in some cases form action potentials due to sodium channels (Velte and Masland, 1999). Further research will be required to understand the remarkably complex biophysical mechanisms operating in transiently responding neurons.

Effects of neuromodulators on synaptic transmission to ganglion cells

Finally, one area that has remained unexamined in ganglion cell function is how neuromodulatory substances effect synaptic transmission to ganglion cells. Recently, Li and Dowling (2000) have shown that fish vision in the scotopic range is dependant on a dopaminergic mechanism operating in the inner retina. In John Dowling's lab, we are currently examining how dopamine effects neurotransmission from bipolar to ganglion cells in the cyprinid retina. Figure 10 shows the effect of dopamine on the spontaneous miniature excitatory postsynaptic currents (mEPSCs) recorded in a zebrafish retinal ganglion cell. When dopamine is applied to ganglion cells, an increase in the frequency and amplitude of mEPSCs is observed, suggesting synaptic release from bipolar cells is enhanced (Cohen and Dowling, 2000). Such a mechanism could prove

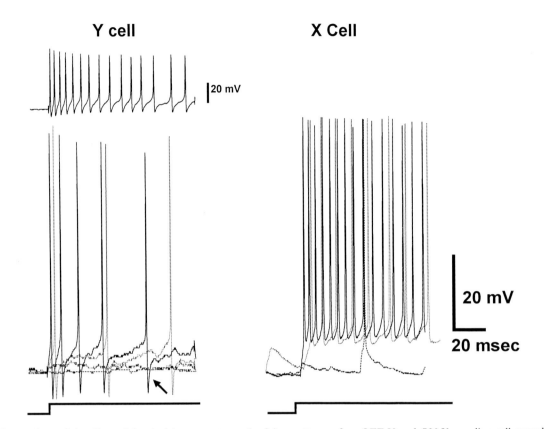

Fig. 9. Comparison of the effect of depolarizing currents on the firing patterns of an OFF-Y and ON-X ganglion cell recorded in current clamp mode from the isolated retina. Cells were held hyperpolarized below spike threshold, and a series of increasing current steps were injected into each cell (starting at 0 pA) to elicit spiking. Lower trace indicates stimulus current timing. Left panel: Firing pattern of a Y cell to four 200 pA current steps from a resting potential of –67 mV. Large currents ($\geq$ 400 pA) elicit spike rate increases that adapt rapidly probably due to hyperpolarizations caused by activation of calcium activated potassium currents (arrow). Only massive currents (1 nA) elicited sustained firing in these cells (inset). Right panel: Firing pattern of an X cell to three 100 pA current steps from a resting potential of –73 mV. Even a single 100 pA step elicits strong sustained firing. There is little firing rate adaptation observed.

advantageous at scotopic light levels where it would raise a small photon signal above the firing/detection threshold of the ganglion cell. It will be interesting to see how other compounds such as melatonin and neuropeptides shape the light-evoked synaptic currents recorded in retinal ganglion cells.

Conclusions and future perspectives:

With the turn of the new millennia, many questions remain unanswered about retinal ganglion cells:

- What are the functions of the many other ganglion cell types besides X and Y?

- How do amacrine and bipolar cells form specific connections with certain ganglion cell types?
- How are do different ganglion cell types become specified during development, and become ON- and OFF-center?
- What are the synaptic mechanisms involved in the modulation of color opponent retinal ganglion cell receptive fields?
- What are the synaptic mechanisms involved in the generation of direction-selective ganglion cell receptive fields? Can we go beyond models of shunting inhibition?
- How do the receptive fields of ganglion cells operate during natural eye behavior?

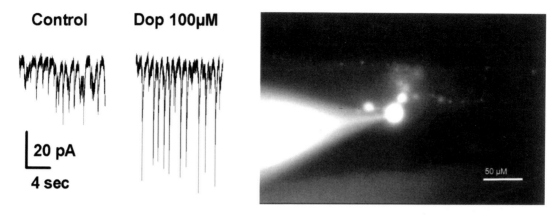

Fig. 10. Dopamine increases the rate of mEPSCs recorded in cyprinid ganglion cells. Left panels show 15 sec segments of the raw current record of an ON-center zebrafish ganglion cell recorded in the retinal slice preparation at holding a potential of −70 mV. The bath Ringer contained tetrodotoxin, picrotoxin, and strychnine to block inhibitory currents. When dopamine (DOP) was added to the Ringer, the amplitude and frequency of the mEPSCs was increased over the control condition. Right panel: Example of a lucifer yellow filled goldfish ON-OFF ganglion cell recorded in the fish retinal slice preparation.

- How are the synaptic currents shaping ganglion cell firing patterns effected by neuromodulators?

With the sequencing of the human genome, an enormous number of new genes have been obtained. However, given the many as yet unknown genes involved in retinal function, it may prove difficult to identify all the genes of interest. A limited fraction of these genes will be studied in the retinae of knockout mice, however many genes will remain unexamined. Suprisingly, this takes us back to a fish (see also Li and Brockerhoff, this volume). The zebrafish is vertebrate model genetic organism that allows one to functionally screen for genes involved in visual behavior, and to study their physiological roles. Thus in tandem with the identified ganglion cell types of mammals, the zebrafish may provide new insights into physiological function in retinal ganglion cells.

Acknowledgments

The author wishes to thank John Troy, Laura Frishman, Robert Miller, Alan Adolph, and John Dowling for helpful discussions. This work was supported by NIH grant EY10617 to E.D.C., Fight for Sight, and a grant from the Zeigler foundation for the Blind.

References

Attwell, D., Werblin, F.S., Wilson, M. and Wu, S.M. (1983) A sign-reversing pathway from rods to double and single cones in the retina of the tiger salamander. *J. Physiol. (Lond.)*, 336: 313–333.

Belgum, J., Dvorak, D. and McReynolds, J. (1982) Sustained synaptic input to ganglion cells of the mudpuppy retina. *J. Physiol.*, 326: 91–108.

Boos R., Schneider, H. and Wassle. H. (1993) Voltage-and transmitter-gated currents of AII amacrine cells in a slice preparation of cat retina. *J. Neurosci.*, 13: 2874–2888.

Chen, E. and Linsenmier, R. (1989) Center components of cone-driven retinal ganglion cells: differential sensitivity to 2-Amino phosphonobutyric acid. *J. Physiol. (Lond.)*, 419: 77–93.

Cohen, E.D. (2000) Role of excitatory amino acid receptors in the light-evoked currents of X-type retinal ganglion cells. *J. Neurophysiol.*, 83: 3217–3229.

Cohen, E.D. (1998) Interactions of excitation and inhibition in the light-evoked currents of X type retinal ganglion cells *J. Neurophysiol.*, 80: 2975–2990.

Cohen, E. and Dowling, J. (2000) Dopamine potentiates synaptic transmission from bipolar cells. *Inv. Ophth. Vis. Sci.*, (Supplement) 41: S936.

Cohen, E.D. and Miller, R.F., (1999) The network-selective actions of quinoxalines on the neurocircuitry of the rabbit retina. *Brain Res.*, 831: 206–228.

Cohen, E. and Sterling, P. (1990) Demonstration of cell types among cone bipolar neurons of cat retina. *Philos. Trans. R. Soc. Lond. B. Biol. Sci.*, 330: 305–321.

Cohen, E. and Sterling, P. (1991) Microcircuitry related to the receptive field center of the on-beta ganglion cell. *J. Neurophysiol.*, 65: 352–359.

Cohen, E.D., Zhou, Z.J. and Fain, G.L. (1994) Ligand-gated currents of alpha and beta ganglion cells in the cat retinal slice. *J. Neurophys.*, 72:1260–1269 .

Cook, P.B., Lukasiewicz, P.D. and McReynolds, J.S. (1998) Action potentials are required for the lateral transmission of glycinergic transient inhibition in the amphibian retina. *J. Neurosci.*, 18: 2301–2308.

Cleland, B.G., Dubin, M.W. and Levick, W.R. (1971) Sustained and transient neurones in the cat's retina and lateral geniculate nucleus, *J. Physiol. (Lond)*, 217: 473–496.

Dacey, D.M. (1999) Primate retina: cell types, circuits and color opponency. *Prog. Retin. Eye Res.*, 18: 737–763.

Demb, J., Haarsma, L., Freed, M. and Sterling, P. (2000) Functional circuitry of the retinal ganglion cell's non-linear surround. *J. Neurosci.*, 19: 9756–9767.

Diamond, J.S. and Copenhagen, D.R. (1995) The relationship between light-evoked synaptic excitation and spiking behaviour of salamander retinal ganglion cells. *J. Physiol. (Lond.)*, 487: 711–725.

Dowling, J.E. and Werblin, F.S. (1969) Organization of retina of the mudpuppy, Necturus maculosus. I. Synaptic structure. *J. Neurophysiol.*, 32: 315–338.

Enroth-Cugell, C. and Robson, J. (1966) The contrast sensitivity of retinal ganglion cells of the cat retina. *J. Physiol. (Lond.)*, 187: 517–552.

Famiglietti, E.V. and Kolb, H. (1975) A bistratified amacrine cell and synaptic ciruicity in the inner plexiform layer of the retina. *Brain Res.*, 84: 293–300.

Fink, M., Lesage, F., Duprat, F., Heurteaux, C., Reyes, R., Fosset, M., and Lazdunski, M. (1998) A neuronal two P domain K^+ channel stimulated by arachidonic acid and polyunsaturated fatty acids. *EMBO J.*, 17(12): 3297–3308.

Fohlmeister, J. and Miller, R. (1997) Impulse encoding mechanisms of ganglion cells in the tiger salamander retina. *J. Neurophysiol.*, 78: 1935–1947.

Freed, M.A. and Sterling, P. (1988) The ON-alpha ganglion cell of the cat retina and its presynaptic cell types. *J. Neurosci.*, 8: 2303–2320.

Frishman, L. and Linsenmier, R. (1982) Effects of picrotoxin and strychnine on non-linear responses of Y type ganglion cells. *J. Physiol. (Lond.)*, 324: 347–363.

Hartline, H.K. (1938). The response of single optic nerve fibers of the vertebrate eye to illumination of the retina. *Am. J. Physiol.*, 121: 400–415.

Han, Y., Zhang, J., and Slaughter, M.M. (1997) Partition of transient and sustained inhibitory glycinergic input to retinal ganglion cells. *J. Neurosci.*, 17: 3392–3400.

Kolb, H. (1979) The inner plexiform layer in the retina of the cat: Electron microscopic observations. *J. Neurocytol.*, 8: 295–329.

Kolb, H. and Nelson, R. (1993) OFF-Alpha and OFF-Beta ganglion cells in cat retina: II. Neural circuitry as revealed by electron microscopy of HRP stains. *J. Comp. Neurol.*, 329: 85–110.

Li, L. and Dowling, J. (2000) Effects of dopamine depletion on visual sensitivity of zebrafish. *J. Neurosci.*, 20: 1893–1903.

Mastronarde D. Interactions between ganglion cells in cat retina. (1983) *J. Neurophysiol.*, 49: 350–365

McGuire, B., Stevens, J. and Sterling, P. (1984) Microcircuitry of bipolar cells in cat retina. *J. Neurosci.*, 4: 2920–2938.

McGuire, B.A. Stevens, J.K. and P. Sterling, (1986) Microcircuitry of beta ganglion cells in cat retina. *J. Neurosci.*, 6: 907–918.

Mittman, S., Taylor, R. and Copenhagen, D. (1990) Concomitant activation of two types of glutamate receptor mediates excitation of salamander retinal ganglion cells. *J. Physiol. Lond.*, 428: 175–197.

Nelson, R., (1982) AII amacrine cells quicken the time course of rod signals in the cat retina. *J. Neurophysiol.*, 47: 928–947.

Mobbs, P., Everett, K. and Cook, A. (1992) A Signal shaping by voltage-gated currents in retinal ganglion cells. *Brain Res.*, 574: 217–223.

Nirenberg, S. and Meister, M. (1997) The light response of retinal ganglion cells is truncated by a displaced amacrine circuit. *Neuron*, 18: 637–650.

Peichle, L. and Wassle, H. (1983) The structural correlate of the receptive field centre of α ganglion cells in the cat retina. *J. Physiol.*, 341: 309–324.

Stein, J.J., Johnson, S.A. and Berson, D.M. (1996) Distribution and coverage of beta cells in the cat retina. *J. Comp. Neurol.*, 372: 597–617.

Sterling, P. (1998) Retina. In: Shepherd G. (Ed.), *The Synaptic Organization of the Brain*. New York: Oxford University Press, pp. 205–233.

Slaughter, M.M. and Miller, R.F. (1981) 2-Amino-4-phosphonobutyric acid: a new pharmacological tool for retina research. *Science Wash. DC*, 211: 182–185.

Taylor, W.R. (1999) TTX attenuates surround inhibition in rabbit retinal ganglion cells. *Vis. Neurosci.*, 16: 285–290.

Vaney D.I. (1991) Many diverse types of retinal neurons show tracer coupling when injected with biocytin or Neurobiotin. *Neurosci. Lett.*, 125: 187–190.

Velte, T.J. and Masland, R.H. (1999) Action potentials in the dendrites of retinal ganglion cells. *J. Neurophysiol.*, 81: 1412–1417.

Wassle, H. and Boycott, B. B. (1991) Functional architecture of the mammalian retina. *Physiol. Rev.*, 71: 447–480.

Werblin, F.S. and Dowling, J.E. (1969) Organization of the retina of the mudpuppy, Necturus maculosus. II. Intracellular recording. *J. Neurophysiol.*, 32: 339–355.

Werblin, F.S. (1972) Lateral interactions at inner plexiform layer of vertebrate retina: antagonistic responses to change. *J. Comp. Physiol. [A]*, 175: 1008–1010.

Werblin, F., Maguire, G., Lukasiewicz, P., Eliasof, S. and Wu, S. (1988) Neural interactions mediating the detection of motion in the retina of the tiger salamander. *Vis. Neurosci.*, 1: 317–329.

H. Kolb, H. Ripps and S. Wu (Eds.)
Progress in Brain Research, Vol. 131

CHAPTER 15

Parallel processing in the mammalian retina: lateral and vertical interactions across stacked representations

Frank Werblin*, Botond Roska and David Balya

Department of Molecular and Cell Biology, Division of Neurobiology, University of California at Berkeley, 145 LSA, Berkeley, CA 94720, USA

Introduction

When Dowling and Boycott (1966; Boycott and Dowling, 1969) outlined the synaptic circuitry of the inner plexiform layer in the mammalian retina, they set in place the key questions of retinal organization that are only beginning to be addressed today. What is the significance of the synaptic "dyad" that they showed so elegantly at which bipolar cell axon terminals make contact with amacrine and ganglion cell processes? What is the role of the amacrine to amacrine synapses, and how do the amacrine to ganglion cell and amacrine to bipolar cell synapses contribute to the organization of the neural message of the retina? Much progress has been made in the last 30 years both confirming and extending the original work of Dowling and Boycott, and the physiological counterparts of their seminal studies are now beginning to fall into place. This paper addresses this physiology and attempts to make some functional inferences about the role of the synapses that Dowling and Boycott first described.

The inner plexiform layer (IPL) of the mammalian retina mediates spatio-temporal integration for a vast array of neurons including 12 types of bipolar cell (Kolb et al., 1981; Euler and Wassle, 1995), 27 types of amacrine cells (Kolb et al., 1981; Masland, 1988; MacNeil et al., 1999) and at least 12 types of ganglion cells (Amthor et al., 1989a,b,c; Kolb et al., 1981; Boycott and Wassle, 1974). The early work of Cajal (1972) showed clearly that the inner plexiform is neatly stratified where the axon terminals of different classes of bipolar cells, as well as the dendrites of different ganglion cells, ramify within very restricted strata at different depths within the IPL (Euler and Wassle, 1995). In terms of function, the work of Nelson et al. (1978) (Nelson and Kolb, 1983; Famiglietti and Kolb, 1976; Famigitti et al., 1977; Kolb and Famiglietti, 1974) showed that there is a major division between ON and OFF activity, splitting the IPL into two main sublamina representing ON and OFF activity. An early prescient paper by Lettvin et al. (1959) and Maturana et al. (1965) suggested that there were "gradients of activity" distributed throughout the IPL, and Famiglietti and Kolb (1976), Wassle and Boycott (1991) and Rodieck (1998) have suggested that the IPL could be further subdivided into regions of more sustained and transient activity. Anatomical evidence suggests that each ganglion cell type "tiles" the retina with a cell density reflecting the dendritic spread of that class (Wassle et al., 1981; Wassle and Boycott, 1991).

*Corresponding author: Frank Werblin, Tel.: 510-642-7236; E-mail: werblin@socrates.berkeley.edu

What is the significance of the stratification within the IPL. What kinds of neural images are carried within these strata, how are the images formed, and how do they interact with each other? To answer these questions we took advantage of a striking anatomical finding: most ganglion cells send their dendrites to just one of the many strata that span the depth of the IPL. This makes it possible to probe individual strata within the IPL by recording from the specific ganglion cells that subserve these strata. We analyzed neural images within each stratum, not by looking at the response properties of individual neurons, but by evaluating the space-time patterns of activity generated by the tiled array of each type of retinal neuron, brought into activity by the presentation of a simple visual stimulus. In particular, we looked at how the representation of a flashed square about 600 μm on a side, about 3 degrees of visual angle, was represented at each stratum. A square is simply a collection of edges in space, and the onset and termination of the square generate "edges" in time. It is the representation of these edges, some sharp, some blurred, some sustained, others transient that characterizes the way each stratum "filters" the original visual input.

Techniques

We describe here only briefly the techniques used to generate the space-time representations of the visual stimuli. Details of recording can be found in the referenced papers. Our goal was to measure excitation, inhibition and spiking as it might exist across an array of retinal neurons. We approached this problem by recording from a single ganglion cell with a patch electrode, then moving the stimulus to many different locations with respect to that cell, similar to the technique pioneered by Ratiff and Hartline (1959) and Baumgartner (1961) and subsequently used by Jacobs and Werblin (1998) and Roska et al. (2000). Each cell served as a representative of many cells of that class at many different positions with respect to the stimulus. Playing back the responses simultaneously, each at its appropriate spatial location, generated a space–time pattern of neural activity representing the responses of excitatory, inhibitory and spiking activity each stratum.

As a further simplification, we "scanned" only across the midline of the square, generating a one dimensional pattern corresponding to the cross section of the representation of the square within the stratum. This decreased the required recording time while allowing us to acquire the most significant aspect of the space-time pattern. The dynamics of this cross section were then displayed as a "space–time surface" as shown in Fig. 1 and some of the subsequent figures. Some interesting variations to the pattern might have been generated at the corners of the square, but we have ignored those for these studies.

Formation of patterns at the Outer Plexiform Layer: horizontal cells and zero crossings

Although we have yet to determine the mechanism by which horizontal cells feed back to cones, the effect of this feedback is the antagonistic interplay between the spatially narrow patterns in the cones and the spatially broad pattern in the horizontal cells (Dowling, 1987). At the peak of this response, typically after about 100 ms, the pattern in response to a square, as measured by a population of OFF bipolar cells, looks like that shown in Fig. 1A. Downward deflection in the space–time surface represents hyperpolarization. At light ON, the surface is hyperpolarized in the region of the stimulus, surrounded by depolarizing peaks outside the region of the stimulus. At light OFF, the cones generate a brief depolarizing response, and at the peak of this response the surface shows a depolarization in the region where the stimulus was, surrounded by hyperpolarizing dimples. Figure 1B shows the responses typical for a depolarizing bipolar cell, the inverse of those in Fig. 1A. Although the details will vary, these patterns will persist over a broad range of horizontal cell space constants and feedback gains. For the OFF bipolars, the peak depolarization of the representation lies *outside* the boundaries of the stimulus at light ON, and inside the boundaries at light OFF. The patterns for the ON bipolars are inverted: here the depolarizing peaks fall inside the boundaries of the stimulus at light ON and outside its boundaries at light OFF. The boundaries themselves lie at the zero crossings of the two bipolar

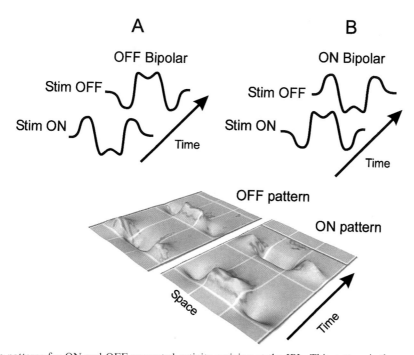

Fig. 1. Space–time patterns for ON and OFF-generated activity arriving at the IPL. This pattern is the result of lateral interactions at the OPL mediated by horizontal cells and expressed at the bipolar terminals. Upper sketches show the cross section of activity at the peak of the ON and OFF responses. Lower sketches show the space time plot of the continuum of activity in space and time of these cross sections. (A) Space–time pattern for the OFF system. Activity appears outside the region of the stimulus at ON and inside the region of the stimulus at OFF. (B) Pattern for the ON system. Activity appears within the region of the stimulus at ON and outside the region of the stimulus at OFF. These patterns form the basis for all subsequent patterns at the inner retina shown in subsequent figures.

cell representations. These patterns are the manifestations of the well known "difference of Gaussians" or "Mexican hat" generated by spot stimuli and historically to classify ganglion cells (Rodieck, 1998). The transformations of the inner retina, shown in this figure for typical ON and OFF dominant activity, will be superimposed upon the surfaces established at the outer retina.

Formation of patterns at the Inner Plexiform Layer

To adequately represent the results, a three dimensional representation in space, time and value, we spread the cross sectional spatial pattern out in time. Thus, by moving from left to right, the reader can follow the development of the spatial activity through the presentation of the stimulus. Two extremes in representation are shown in Fig. 2. Figure 2A illustrates a pattern that would be generated by a population of cells that extract spatial edges, and represent these edges for the full duration of the stimulus. This form of activity is represented by the two horizontal bars in the Fig. 2A. Figure 2B illustrates the pattern that would be generated by a population of cells that represents edges in time, but represents the full extent of the stimulus in space. This activity is represented by the narrow vertical bar appearing just after light ON and lasting for only about 100 ms.

Ordering of the strata in time

Lateral interactions affect response behavior in both space and time. By limiting the stimulus to a small spot we were able to minimize the effects of lateral inhibition and measure the temporal characteristics of the excitatory signals arriving at each stratum. Dark spots were used for the OFF responses; light

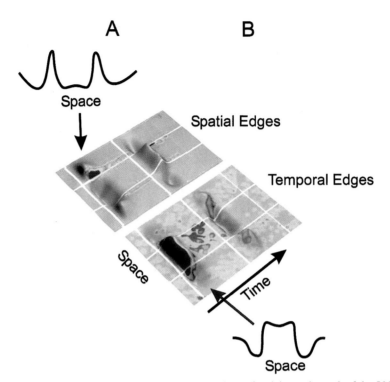

Fig. 2. Patterns for space and time. Individual traces show the cross sections of activity at the peak of the ON response. (A) Space–time pattern generated by a stratum that extracts edges, represented by the two horizontal stripes of activity. The activity appears along the edges of the stimulus, and lasts for the duration of the stimulus. (B) Pattern generated by a stratum that extracts edges in time. Activity appears across the full extent of the stimulus, but appears only briefly when the stimulus is presented.

spots for the ON responses. Figure 3 shows that there is a clear and consistent ordering of temporal response across the strata: For the 8 strata shown here, activity near the midline of the IPL is quite transient, whereas activity closer to the proximal and distal borders of the IPL is more sustained, consistent with the predictions of Wassle and Boycott (1991).

Lateral interactions at the IPL form diversity in spatial profiles

Figure 4 shows a series of spatial profiles derived from 6 ganglion cells that read out the activity of 6 different strata. The representations range from general broad diffuse activity in the traces at the top Fig. 4A to sharp edge extraction in the traces at the bottom. The extraction of these edges appears to be mediated by lateral inhibition via amacrine cell feedback to bipolar cell terminals as illustrated in

the measurements shown in Fig. 4B. The sharp edges remained intact in the presence of glycine and GABA$_A$ blockers, but were completely eliminated with the addition of picrotoxin, a GABA$_C$ receptor blocker, to the bathing solution. Because GABA$_C$ receptors are found exclusively at bipolar cell terminals, this measurement points to feedback at bipolar terminals, presumably from classes of amacrine cells, as the site of this edge-enhancing lateral interaction.

The full spectrum of representations found in the strata

Figure 5 shows an array of patterns found at 7 of the 10 strata of the IPL. The first 4 are from ON cells showing many variations from the typical ON basis response. For example, stratum 1 represents the full extent of the square at light ON, but only very briefly.

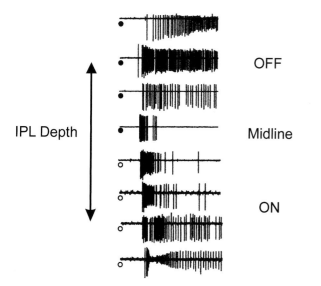

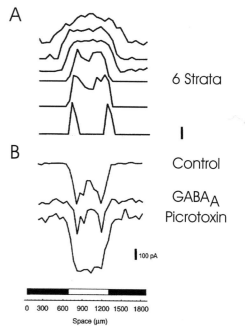

Fig. 3. Strata are ordered in time. Spiking patterns generated by a small stimulus spot to eliminate the effects of lateral interactions on the temporal properties of the response. Under these conditions, the strata near the midline of the IPL at the ON OFF border respond transiently; strata further from the midline respond with more sustained activity. Upper 4 traces from OFF cells in response to a dark spot; lower 4 traces from ON cells in response to a bright spot.

This corresponds to cells of the Y type in cat with brisk, transient activity. The inhibitory component at this stratum shows the typical OFF basis (outside the stimulus at light ON; inside at light OFF), also brief and transient at both light ON and OFF. Stratum 2 represents only the edges of the square at ON, again very briefly, while its inhibitory component is active at light ON throughout the duration of the flash and continues into the OFF time zone. Stratum 3 represents the presence of the square over a longer time period at ON, and shows some edge enhancement. But unlike the other ON strata described above that received inhibition from the OFF system, this stratum receives its inhibitory component from the ON system. Stratum 4 represents the square briefly at ON, its inhibitory component comes from the OFF system.

The three panels on the right show OFF activity. Level 1 is curious because the edges representing the square appear at light ON, but lie in the OFF region of the pattern, outside the stimulus boundaries. This is the only representation the seems to violate the ON OFF rules, suggesting that activity at light ON is

Fig. 4. Spatial profiles for the responses: Traces show the responses for 6 different cell systems at the peak of the response. (A) Different strata show different degrees of edge extraction ranging from those with only a diffuse, blurred pattern (upper) to those with sharp edges (lower). (B) The spatial edges (upper) are completely eliminated by GABA$_C$ blockers (lower) suggesting that lateral inhibition, introduced at the bipolar cell terminals (the site of GABA$_C$ receptors) acts to truncate activity in space.

somehow derived from the OFF system. Inhibition in this stratum is derived from the ON system briefly at light ON and from the OFF system briefly at light OFF. The second excitatory response pattern is typical of the OFF system, and the inhibitory pattern is derived from the ON system. Finally the third OFF stratum shows a typical OFF pattern at light ON and a broad, extended ON-like pattern at light OFF. A most intriguing question is raised by these excitatory and inhibitory patterns: what visual features do these combinations of excitatory and inhibitory patterns extract from the visual environment?

Vertical interactions sharpen the specificity of stratification

The many representations at different strata and the presence of many types of diffuse amacrine cells

234

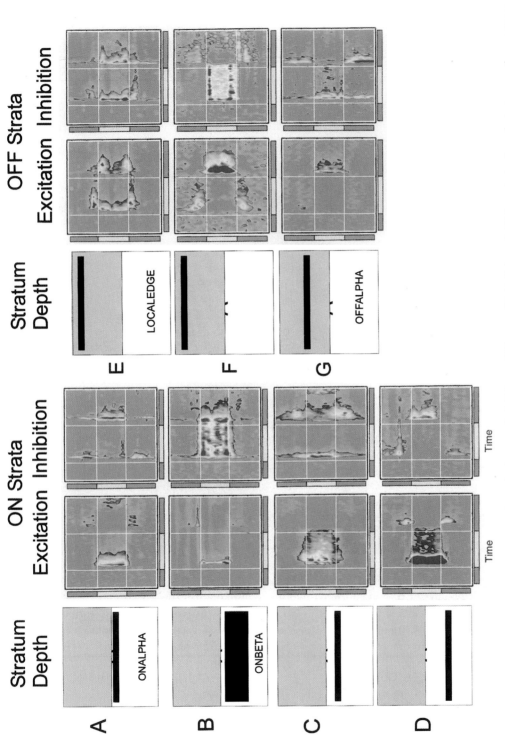

Fig. 5. The spectrum of activities at 7 different strata, shown in the rows: Left Column: ON strata, Right Column Inhibitory strata. In each stratum we show patterns of excitation on the left and patterns of inhibition on the right. Each stratum extracts a unique pair of excitatory and inhibitory patterns from the visual scene. The patterns are described in the text. In many cases the excitatory pattern is derived from the ON system, while the inhibitory pattern is derived from the OFF system. In other cases the excitatory and inhibitory patterns are derived from the same system.

(Masland, 1988; Kolb et al., 1981) suggest that there is *vertical* communication between the strata. Vertical interactions could explain, for example how the ON excitatory activity in a stratum located in the ON sublamina, is combined an inhibitory component that is derived from the OFF sublamina, or how ON-like excitatory activity is combined with OFF-like inhibitory activity as in the first and fourth ON strata and the second OFF strata in Fig. 5. We do not yet understand the underlying "filtering characteristics" for most of these strata, although knowing the forms of excitatory and inhibitory activity should serve as important clues.

Vertical interactions appear to play another role in inter-strata interactions. Figure 6 shows the time courses of activity found in two strata that lie near the ON–OFF boundary, near the midline of the IPL. For these strata, normal is activity is elicited only at light ON, blocking $GABA_C$ activity releases an otherwise invisible OFF component as well. This suggests that there is some diffusion of activity at either the bipolar cell terminals or the ganglion cell dendrites that allows ON and OFF activity to commingle. Vertical interactions, in this case inhibitory inputs from the OFF system, completely eliminate the appearance of OFF activity in these predominantly ON strata. These results suggest that

one role of vertical interactions like that of lateral interactions described above, is image sharpening. But these vertical interactions sharpen in the "feature space" by operating between different strata, rather than in lateral space, acting across strata as shown in Fig. 4.

Representations of natural images

The excitatory and inhibitory patterns shown in Fig. 5 represent a broad spectrum of possible images that are carried by 7 of the 10 strata of the IPL. Excitation and inhibition within each stratum interact to generate a spiking output that is in most cases quite similar to the excitatory patterns under conditions when a flashed square is used as stimulus strata. This suggests that the interactions between excitatory and inhibitory patterns are subtle, and not easily revealed with flashed squares. We could gain a more intuitive notion of the "neural filter" characteristics of the strata by recording the representations of more natural images. The required recording time for such images is prohibitive, so to gain an appreciation for the representations, we created digital "neural filters" for each stratum. The filters utilized the silicon implementation of a retina-like architecture: massively parallel analog array processor (Werblin et al., 1995) that was digitally simulated on a PC as in Jacobs and Werblin (1998). We programmed this processor to generate excitatory and inhibitory patterns at each stratum similar to those shown in Fig. 5, similar to the study described earlier by Werblin (1991). Then we presented each filter with a more natural scene, namely, a face moving back and forth from left to right. The images in Fig. 7 show the snapshots of the representations created in this simulation study. The locations of the patterns correspond to those shown in Fig. 5. Each representation is unique, showing a different quality of edges or combinations of edges and surfaces. Excitation is shown in red, inhibition in green and spiking in white. It is immediately apparent that spiking for all cell classes is quite sparse compared to excitation and inhibition. This was confirmed in some preliminary recordings of natural images using techniques similar to those used

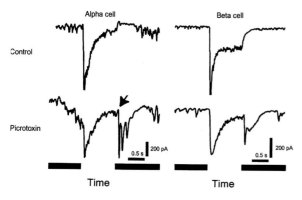

Fig. 6. Vertical Interactions. I. Separating ON and OFF activity in two different cell types. Blocking inhibition reveals OFF activity in this otherwise ON cell type. Upper traces: responses showing purely ON activity measured under normal conditions. Lower traces: responses showing OFF activity that is revealed after $GABA_C$ feedback to bipolar cell terminals is blocked. The blockade of OFF activity is an example of vertical inhibition.

236

On   Off

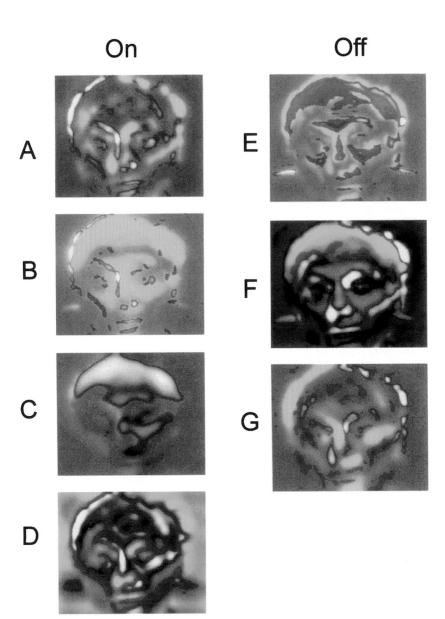

Fig. 7. Responses to natural stimuli. The seven faces shown in this figure were generated by presenting a moving face to seven different "filters" with characteristics similar to those of the seven retinal filters shown in Fig. 5. We tested the filters first with flashed squares to be sure these digital filters generated the same patterns as shown in Fig. 5. The patterns shown here are snapshots taken during the movement of the faces, and correspond to the same retinal filters shown in Fig. 5. Red represents excitation, green inhibition, and white represents spiking. The most striking prediction here is the relative sparseness of spike activity in response to complex patterns. This has been confirmed by some direct physiological measurements from retina in response to this same moving face. It remains to determine what these seven neural filters are designed to specifically detect in the visual environment.

for the flashed squares above. The images represent the expression of a "visual vocabulary" that we do not yet understand, through which the retina represents the visual world to higher centers. The study predicts that complex interactions between excitation and inhibition serve to extract efficient representations of the visual world in the form of spiking output for each ganglion cell class.

Future challenges

These studies uncover a rich set of representations existing in parallel across at least 10 different strata in the IPL. These representations clarify the role of IPL interactions in visual processing. An initial and almost overwhelming center-surround antagonistic pattern is generated at the outer retina via horizontal cell feedback to cones and shown in Fig. 1. This pattern exists at the cone terminals and is "read out" by bipolar cells. Because all retinal cells "view" the world through bipolar cells, this initial form of center surround activity is apparent at every retinal level. The initial center-surround antagonism is further refined, however, via lateral and vertical interactions at the IPL. There, amacrine cells receive input from different strata, then feed back to bipolar cell terminals at $GABA_C$ receptors to extract edges as shown in Fig. 4, to refine the response characteristics as shown in Fig. 6. Amacrine cells receive input at the strata, then feed forward to ganglion cell dendrites at other strata generating inhibitory patterns at each stratum and generating an additional stack of inhibitory representations of the visual world that differ in spatial and temporal dimension as shown in Fig. 5. For flashed squares, the patterns of excitation and spiking are quite similar. But for more complex images interactions between excitation and inhibition at each strata may be more robust and the spiking representations may be more sparse as shown in Fig. 7.

The roles of the dyad, reciprocal, and feedforward synapses, so elegantly revealed in the work of Dowling and Boycott by the early '70s are brought to life in this study. These synapses are the basis and underpinning and represent the fundamental circuit connections upon which the full set of stacked representations of the visual world are built. They represent the basic structure upon which the rich representation of the visual world is created and conveyed to higher visual centers. Our challenge is to understand this vocabulary, to decipher the filter characteristics mediated by excitation and inhibition at each stratum, to follow these representations to higher visual centers, and to understand how this multitude of representations is integrated to generate the full richness of the visual world.

References

Amthor, F.R., Takahashi, E.S. and Oyster, C.W. (1989a) Morphologies of rabbit retinal ganglion cells with concentric receptive fields. *J. Comp. Neurol.*, 280: 72–96.

Amthor, F.R., Takahashi, E.S. and Oyster, C.W. (1989b) Morphologies of rabbit retinal ganglion cells with concentric receptive fields. *J. Comp. Neurol.*, 280: 72–96.

Amthor, F.R., Takahashi, E.S. and Oyster, C.W. (1989c) Morphologies of rabbit retinal ganglion cells with complex receptive fields. *J. Comp. Neurol.*, 280: 97–121.

Baumgartner, G. (1961) Kontrastlichteffekte an retalen Ganglienzellen: Ableitungen vom Tractus opticus der Katze. In: Jung, R. and Kornhuber, H. (Eds.), *Neurophysiologie und Psychophysik des visuellen Systems*. Springer-Verlag, Berlin, pp. 45–53.

Boycott, B.B. and Dowling, J.E. (1969) Organization of the primate retina: Light microscopy. *Phil. Trans. Roy. Soc. Lond. B*, 255: 109–184.

Boycott, B.B. and Wassle, H. (1974) The morphological types of ganglion cells of the domestic cat's retina. *J. Physiol.*, 240: 397–419.

Cajal, S.R. y (1972) *The Structure of the Retina*. Springfield, IL: Charles C. Thomas.

Dowling, J.E. and Boycott, B.B. (1966) Organiztion of the primate retina: Electron microscopy. *Proc. Roy. Soc. Lond. B.*, 166: 80–111.

Dowling, J.E. (1987) *The Retina: An approachable part of the brain*. Cambridge MA: Belknap Press of Harvard University Press.

Euler, T. and Wassle, H. (1995) Immunocytochemical identification of cone bipolar cells in the rat retina. *J. Comp. Neurol.*, 361: 461–478.

Famiglietti, E.V., Jr. and Kolb, H. (1976) Structural basis for ON and OFF-center responses in retinal ganglion cells. *Science Wash DC*, 194: 193–195.

Famiglietti, E.V., Jr., Kaneko, A. and Tachibana, M. (1977) Neuronal architecture of on and off pathways to ganglion cells in carp retina. *Science Wash. DC*, 198: 1267–1269.

Jacobs, A. and Werblin, F.S. (1998) Spatiotemporal patterns at the retinal output. *J. Neurophysiol.*, 80: 447–451

Kolb, H. and Famiglietti, E.V. (1974) Rod and cones pathways in the inner plexiform layer of the cat retina. *Science*, 186: 47–49.

Kolb, H., Nelson, R. and Mariani, A. (1981) Amacrine cells, bipolar cells and ganglion cells of the cat retina a golgi study. *Vis. Res.*, 21: 1081–1114.

Lettvin, J., Maturana, H.R., McCulloch, W.S. and Pitts, W.H. (1959) What the frog's eye tells the frog's brain. *Proc. Inst. Radio Engin.*, 47: 1951–1959.

MacNeil, M.A., Heussy, J.K., Dacheux, R.F., Raviola, E. and Masland, R.H. (1999) The shapes and numbers of amacrine cells: matching of photofilled with golgi-stained cells in the rabbit retina and comparison with other mammalian species. *J. Comp. Neurol.*, 413: 305–326.

Masland, R.H. (1988) Amacrine cells. *TINS*, 11: 405–410.

238

Maturana, H.R., Lettvin, J.Y., McCulloch, W.S. and Pitts, W.H. (1965) Anatomy and Physiology of vision in the frog. *J. Gen. Physiol.*, 129–174.

Nelson, R., Famiglietti, E.V. and Kolb, H. (1978) Intracellular staining reveals different levels of stratification for ON- and OFF-center ganglion cells in the cat retina. *J. Neurophysiol.*, 41: 472–483.

Nelson, R. and Kolb, H. (1983) Synaptic patterns and response properties of bipolar and ganglion cells in the cat retina. *Vis. Res.*, 23: 1183–1195.

Ratiff, F. and Hartline, H.K. (1959) The response of Limulus optic nerve fibers to patterns of illumination on the receptor mosaic. *J. Gen Physiol.*, 42: 1241–1255.

Rodieck, R.W. (1998) *The First Steps in Seeing.* Sunderland, MA: Sinauer Associates.

Roska, B., Nemeth, E., Orzo, L. and Werblin, F.S. (2000) Three levels of Lateral Inhibition in the Tiger Salamander Retina. *J. Neurosci.*, 20: 1941–1951.

Wassle, H., Peichl, L. and Boycott, B.B. (1981) Dendritic territories of cat retinal ganglion cells. *Nature Lond.*, 292: 344–345.

Wassle, H. and Boycott, B.B. (1991) Functional Architecture of the mammalian retina. *Physiol. Rev.*, 71: 447–480.

Werblin, F. (1991) Synaptic connections, receptive fields, and patterns of activity in the tiger salamander retina. *Invest. Ophthalmol. Vis. Sci.*, 32: 459–483.

Werblin, F., Roska, T. and Chua, L.O. (1995) The analogic cellular neural network as a bionic eye. *Int. J. Circuit Theory and Applications*, 23: 541–569.

Neurotransmission and neuromodulation

H. Kolb, H. Ripps and S. Wu (Eds.)
Progress in Brain Research, Vol. 131

CHAPTER 16

Pre- and postsynaptic mechanisms of spontaneous, excitatory postsynaptic currents in the salamander retina

Robert F. Miller[1],*, Jon Gottesman[1], Dori Henderson[1], Mike Sikora[1] and Helga Kolb[2]

[1]*Department of Neuroscience, University of Minnesota, 6-145 Jackson Hall, Minneapolis, MN 55455, USA*
[2]*Department of Ophthalmology, John Moran Eye Center, Salt Lake City, UT 84132, USA*

Introduction

When Dowling first described the ultrastructural details of the inner retina of the primate (Dowling and Boycott, 1966) and later compared it to that of the frog (Dowling, 1968), he advanced a hypothesis about how complexity in retinal neurocircuitry is developed and expressed in ganglion cells. In his comparative analysis, he saw similarities between the primate and frog retinas in the ultrastructural features of synapses in the outer plexiform layer, but found species differences in the inner plexiform layer, in the form of different ratios of amacrine to bipolar synapses. Simple retinas, typified by the primate, had center-surround receptive fields and a comparatively small ratio of amacrine (conventional) to bipolar (ribbon) synapses, while retinas with more complex receptive fields, such as the frog, had a higher ratio of conventional to ribbon synapses. This idea was later evaluated across a number of species by his student Dubin (1970), who carried out an ultrastructural analysis of several different vertebrates and concluded that the ratios of conventional (amacrine) to ribbon (bipolar) synapses in the IPL varied from about 1.7:1 in the human parafovea to

10.8:1 in the pigeon, with the frog at 8.8:1 to 10.9:1. The concept that the retinas of different species process information to different levels of complexity was first advanced by the studies of Lettvin (Maturana et al., 1960) and his colleagues in the frog. This species served as an example of a complex retina in which ganglion cell receptive fields were thought to detect different trigger features of the visible environment. In contrast, earlier studies by Kuffler (1953) in the cat, provided an example of a comparatively simple retina in which ganglion cell receptive fields seemed to be organized as more simple, stereotyped, antagonistic, center-surround units. Thus, Dowling and his colleagues provided an anatomical substrate with which to interpret species differences in the complexity of retinal processing and this hypothesis, developed more than thirty years ago, still influences our thinking about retina processing in different species. Of equal importance, Dowling's pioneering work focused our attention on the microscopic details of retinal synapses and it is the microscopic function of bipolar ribbon synapses to which this article is addressed.

In the intervening decades since Dowling's hypothesis, we have learned a number of additional features about retinal processing and ribbon synapses. We know that ribbon synapses probably package glutamate in their synaptic vesicles and communicate

_____
* Corresponding author: Robert F. Miller, E-mail: rfm@mail.ahc.umn.edu

with postsynaptic cells through an array of glutamate receptors, including ionotropic and metabotropic subtypes (Massey and Maguire, 1995). Furthermore, new insights into ribbon synapses have been revealed by studies of bipolar cell axon terminals, using whole-cell patch recording techniques combined with methods to evaluate changes in membrane capacitance (von Gersdorff et al., 1996). Ribbon synapses of bipolar cells appear to have multiple release zones for a single ribbon and, overall, are capable of large rates of vesicular release for each terminal. Vesicle release is calcium-dependent and the function of the ribbon, a member of a large class of synaptic proteins, appears to be that of tethering vesicles to make them readily available to support the high release rates with which these structures have become synonymous. In conventional synapses, Synapsin I, another synaptic protein is thought to bind vesicles to the cytoskeleton, but this protein is not present in ribbon synapses, presumably because the ribbon assumes that responsibility (Mandell et al., 1992; Mandell et al., 1990; Morgans, 2000).

The "Spillover Hypothesis" of the ribbon synapse

The ribbon synapses of bipolar cells, in the absence of light stimulation, release vesicles spontaneously at a relatively low rate, such that the outcome of single vesicle release can be studied postsynaptically as spontaneous, excitatory postsynaptic currents (sEPSCs). These single vesicle events have been studied with single electrode voltage-clamp (SEVC) techniques in retinal ganglion cells and their pharmacological properties have been analyzed (Taylor et al., 1995; Gao and Wu, 1999). Taylor et al. (1995) reported that the sEPSCs consisted of a single type of event generated by AMPA receptors, while Gao and Wu (1999) reported fast and slow AMPA events and slow NMDA receptor events, the latter observed in On–Off ganglion cells. Because the fast AMPA events appear to be the predominant form of sEPSCs, and light-evoked activity generates some NMDA receptor contribution, the concept of a "spillover" model of the ribbon synapse has been proposed to account for at least some of the postsynaptic ensemble of events.

Figure 1 is a cartoon of a bipolar ribbon synapse with representations of postsynaptic receptors for AMPA, NMDA and KA together with the presynaptic ribbon structure and associated synaptic vesicles. Glutamate transporters are also illustrated, and, while they may be important in affecting the time course of light-evoked, synaptic activity (Tran et al., 1999), blocking their activity does not influence the time course of sEPSCs (Higgs and Lukasiewicz, 1999). The spillover hypothesis suggests that the spontaneous release of synaptic vesicles normally activates AMPA receptors which are located immediately below the active release zones (Fig. 1). When light stimulation induces the release of many vesicles along a single ribbon site, glutamate spillover activates both AMPA and adjacent NMDA receptors. A puff of hyperosmotic sucrose delivered to the IPL through a visually placed pipette is also a means of evoking sufficient release of glutamate to activate NMDA receptors (Yu and Miller, 1995; Velte et al., 1997). The role of KA receptors remains obscure, although immunohistochemical staining of KA receptor subunits has been detected in ganglion cells (Brandstatter et al., 1997).

Spontaneous excitatory postsynaptic currents (sEPSCs)

We have studied sEPSCs in ganglion cells of the neotenous tiger salamander (*Ambystoma tigrinum*) retina using patch-electrode recording techniques in a slice preparation. Figure 2 illustrates a common finding in our pharmacological experiments designed to evaluate the relative contributions of NMDA and AMPA/KA receptors. In this recording, the release rate of sEPSCs was enhanced by using hyperosmotic Ringer (120 mM sucrose added to normal Ringer) as the bathing medium. Under these conditions, both large and small amplitude events are observed (Fig. 2, blue control). The sEPSCs are largely eliminated by NBQX, a highly selective quinoxaline antagonist for AMPA > KA receptors; the loss of synaptic activity by NBQX is associated with a reduction of an inward, background current (or the augmentation of an additional outward current). Note that NBQX did not eliminate all spontaneous events, as small amplitude events persisted; these small events were eliminated when the NMDA antagonist D-AP7 was added to the NBQX bathing medium

(1)

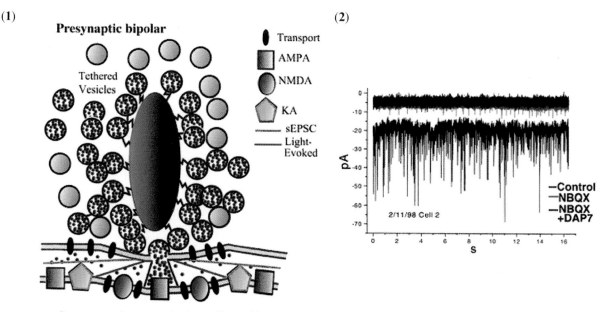

(2)

Fig. 1, 2. In Fig. 1 the spillover concept of a ribbon synapse. A cartoon of the ribbon synapse of a bipolar cell, illustrating the vesicles tethered to the ribbon structure, the extracellular space and the postsynaptic membrane, with representations for AMPA, NMDA and KA glutamate receptors, in addition to glutamate transporters. Active release zones are below the ribbon and fusion of a single vesicle releases glutamate which activates AMPA receptors. When light stimulation or hyperosmotic sucrose stimulation are used to evoke transmitter release, the glutamate is sufficient to spillover and activate the neighboring NMDA receptors. The role of KA receptors is unknown. In Fig. 2 a voltage clamp recording ($V_H = -70$ mV) from a ganglion cell in a retinal slice preparation of the tiger salamander. Under control conditions, the responses consist of rapid, inward currents that are as large as 50 pA and the baseline fluctuates, suggesting that both fast and slow events contribute to the recording. When NBQX was added to the bathing medium, a reduction in inward current was observed associated with a loss of most of the large and small events, was well as the fluctuations in the baseline. However, a small number of low amplitude events persists and these were blocked by adding D-AP7 to the NBQX, which resulted in a further reduction of the inward current.

(Fig 2, black trace). The addition of D-AP7 always further decreased an inward current (or enhanced an outward current), suggesting that tonic NMDA receptors may be active under our recording conditions. This is consistent with our previous studies revealing tonic NMDA receptor activation in ganglion cells of salamander retinal slices (Gottesman and Miller, 1991; Gottesman and Miller, 1992; Gottesman and Miller, 1990). This tonic activation of NMDA receptors serves as a major source of background noise.

Figure 3 shows an expanded view of two traces of sEPSCs observed in a control Ringer environment using hyperosmotic sucrose to enhance the rate of vesicle release. The holding potential for these studies was at −70 mV, near the chloride equilibrium

potential. All of these spontaneous events were blocked by NBQX/D-AP7 and thus presumably depend on AMPA/KA and NMDA receptors. In these records (Fig. 3), numerous, small amplitude events are observed, while larger responses are also apparent. The large amplitude events can be segregated into two classes, one of which appears to be multivesicular, due to the appearance of its jagged rise and decay phase consisting of the summation of many smaller events and an overall, slow time course. In contrast, the single large event in the lower trace does not appear to consist of multiple, smaller events; we believe that these responses reflect the actions of a single vesicle because their decay time is often well described by a single exponential and their rise time is typically smooth.

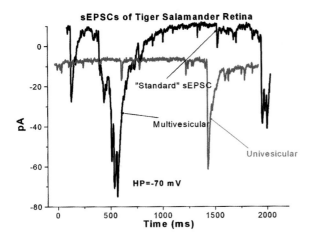

Fig. 3. A waterfall display of two voltage-clamp records from a tiger salamander ganglion cell in a slice preparation. The lower trace indicates the calibrated response plus the resting, inward current level while the upper trace was arbitrarily displaced; it consists of a single, large, multivesicular EPSC comprised of multiple, smaller events. The lower trace shows a single univesicular event which does not consist of multiple, smaller events and a single "average" EPSC is also identified for the purpose of comparison.

Does space clamp failure contribute to EPSC variance?

The sEPSCs were recorded from a retinal slice preparation in which the morphology of the cell and its dendrites were unknown. One can assume that the sEPSCs are generated at different locations along the soma-dendritic tree. Thus one possible source of variance in amplitude and waveform of these spontaneous events relates to the electrotonic distance between the site of generation and the soma-applied SEVC and the possibility of space clamp failure. What contribution to sEPSC variance can be expected from this possible source of error?

Figure 4 illustrates a simulation of a compartmentalized, sustained-On ganglion cell of the mudpuppy retina whose flatmount morphology is illustrated in 4D. For this simulation, we applied a template of a transient change in external glutamate at four different locations from the soma along the dendritic tree (1–4 in the flatmount view), with the most distal input being at a terminal end about 0.70λ from the soma ($R_\mathrm{m} = 70{,}000$ cm^2). To simulate this sEPSC (smEPSC), we applied an exponential function,

$$I_\mathrm{SYN}(t) = G_\mathrm{Max} \cdot \frac{t}{\alpha} \exp\left(1 - \frac{t}{\alpha}\right) \cdot (V_\mathrm{M} - E_\mathrm{SYN}),$$

where $I_\mathrm{SYN}(t) =$ time variant synaptic current, G_Max is the maximum conductance, V_M is the resting or holding potential and E_SYN is the reversal potential for the synaptic current. The parameter α is user defined and determines the peak delay of the exponential function. By adjusting α and G_Max, we simulated a transient change in glutamate, which generated a smEPSC with a peak conductance change of 130 pS and a peak delay of ~1.5 ms which closely matches the average sEPSC first reported by Taylor et al. (1995). The time course of the smESPC was determined by the temporal shape of the change in glutamate and a kinetic scheme for modeling AMPA receptors similar to that of Partin et al., (1996) but modified, based on our own observations with rapid glutamate perfusion using dissociated ganglion cell somas. This kinetic scheme is a two-binding site model with kinetic parameters for activation (bound, open), deactivation (unbound, closed) and desensitization (bound, closed). The kinetic structure is illustrated below with A as the agonist and R as the receptor; the forward and backward rate constants were fit to responses obtained with rapid perfusion experiments.

$$A + R \underset{1'}{\overset{1}{\rightleftharpoons}} AR \underset{2'}{\overset{2}{\rightleftharpoons}} A_2R \underset{3'}{\overset{3}{\rightleftharpoons}} \text{Open}$$

$$4 \Updownarrow 4' \qquad 6 \Updownarrow 6'$$

$$AR_d \underset{5'}{\overset{5}{\rightleftharpoons}} A_2R_d \quad \text{Densensitized}$$

Figure 4C shows the time course of the change in glutamate (lower trace) and the smEPSC (upper trace) recorded from a single compartment postsynaptic structure (soma only). The dark trace shows the temporal course of the smEPSC under normal conditions, whereas the trace in red illustrates the time course of the smEPSC when desensitization is effectively blocked with aniracetam which may operate on the kinetic scheme illustrated above by slowing the closing of the AMPA receptor (step 3′);

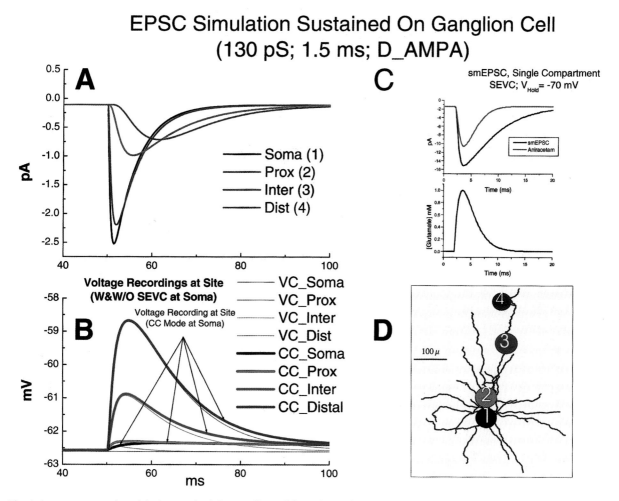

Fig. 4. A compartmental model of a sustained-On ganglion cell from the mudpuppy retina was used to carry out simulations of sEPSCs at different soma-dendritic locations. (D) shows the flatmount morphology of the cell and indicates the four sites of simulated (smEPSC) generation. (C) shows the time course of the glutamate profile (lower trace) which was necessary to generate the smEPSC (upper trace) which had a peak delay of about 1.5 ms and a conductance change of 130 pS ($V_{hold} = -70$ mV). The black trace shows the time course of the smEPSC under normal conditions, while the red trace shows the smEPSC waveform when desensitization was blocked with aniracetam (1 mM) and indicates that desensitization is one element in determining the time course of the AMPA receptor response to single vesicle glutamate release. This recording was generated in a single compartment model, whereas those of (A) and (B) used the model cell of (D). The current records for each site of the smEPSC are illustrated in (A). As the site of injection is moved to more distal locations, the current at the soma is slower and smaller in magnitude; the most distant site of injection was about 0.7λ from the soma. The recordings in (B) show the voltage deflections at the four different sites of smESPC generation and include recordings with (thin lines) and without (thick lines) the voltage clamp applied with an electrode in the soma. In the soma, the voltage response is small due to the low input resistance and the clamp successfully voltage clamps the soma. As the smEPSC injection site is moved distally, the EPSC generates an increasingly larger voltage, due to space clamp failure combined with the increasingly larger input resistance at the distal sites. These simulations suggest that voltage-clamping at the soma can result in significant errors in measuring the time course and amplitude of the synaptic currents which underlie sEPSCs.

this result indicates that the desensitization mechanism is activated by the brief time course of glutamate, consistent with experiments by Taylor et al. (1995) using aniracetum. Figure 4A shows the currents

recorded at the soma using the On-cell multicompartmental model with a single electrode voltage-clamp (SEVC) applied at the soma for each of the four different input locations (1–4). Although

246

the magnitude and time course for the smEPSC are nearly identical at each input location (not illustrated), the responses at the soma show a slower and smaller current as the input site is moved from the soma to the more distal locations. Figure 4B shows voltage responses recorded from each injection site (1–4) under current clamp (CC) and voltage clamp (VC) conditions applied at the soma. For each pair of recordings, the traces with thick lines (arrows) show the voltage under CC conditions, while the thin lines illustrate the recordings at each site for VC conditions applied to the soma electrode. When a smEPSC conductance was applied at the soma, the clamp recorded the input current under good space clamp conditions (no voltage change was detected; VC_Soma). As the site of injection was moved distally, the recording at each site shows that the voltage clamp generated less current to modify the response waveform (thin lines) and the escape voltage at each site was progressively larger. Space clamp failure at progressively distal sites allowed a large escape voltage to occur, which in turn decayed towards the soma with a slower time course and smaller amplitude.

This observation, in which distal smEPSCs generated smaller and slower responses at the soma is an unavoidable consequence of clamping from the soma, which does not see, and therefore cannot compensate, for the conductance change at the site of injection. This is consistent with Rall's concepts about comparisons between the conductance change and the current injected from the conductance change in dendritic tree structures (Rall, 1977). The conductance change does not travel significantly and, as the site of the conductance change becomes more distal, it becomes more difficult to detect it at the soma. In contrast to the difficulty in detecting the conductance change at the soma, the site of the conductance change injects synaptic current that can effectively travel over the cable properties of the dendritic tree and contribute significantly to events recorded at the soma. A very similar analysis has been carried out for dendritic spikes in starburst amacrine cells and for NMDA responses generated in the dendrites of ganglion cells (Velte and Miller, 1998; Velte and Miller, 1996; Velte et al., 1997).

Rall has demonstrated that an EPSP generated at progressively distal locations of the dendritic tree is

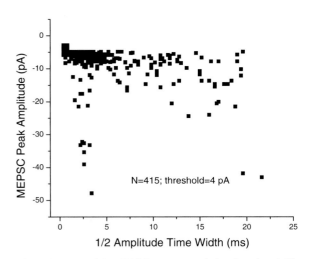

Fig. 5. A group of 415 sEPSCs were recorded and analyzed. The peak amplitude vs half-maximum amplitude time width was plotted and revealed that no simple relationship existed between the two parameters. If cable losses accounted for the data, smaller amplitude responses would have longer half-maximum amplitude time widths; while some large amplitude events did show fast time widths, others were slower. While space-clamp failure may account for some of the data, other factors must contribute to this variance in sEPSC.

seen at the soma as a progressively smaller and slower response. Thus, if spatial displacement is a prominent element which accounts or contributes to the variance in sEPSCs, a plot of sEPSC amplitude vs the half-amplitude time width should provide an inverse relationship, with smaller events associated with longer half times. Figure 5 illustrates a scatter plot of the amplitude vs half-amplitude time width. The scatter of this data does not argue for a simple relationship of any type between the two parameters, and, in general, larger amplitude responses are associated with slower half-amplitude time widths, arguing against clamp failure as the sole determinant of sEPSC variance. Thus, although we cannot dismiss space clamp failure as a contributing factor to sEPSC variance, there appear to be other mechanisms which contribute to the variance we see in sEPSC waveform and amplitude.

Is the ribbon synapse a functional subunit or a source of sEPSC variance?

The anatomy of the ribbon synapse can be viewed as several closely apposed active zones, or release sites,

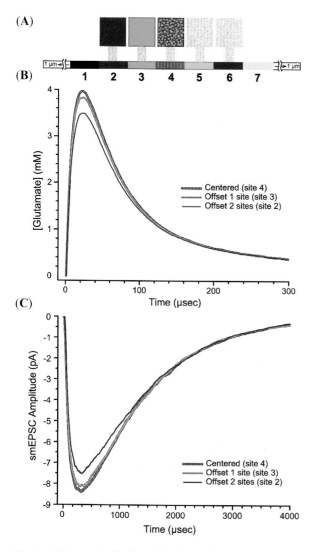

from the center of the ribbon will produce the same postsynaptic response as a vesicle located at one end of the ribbon structure. Intuitively, it would appear that the glutamate transient in the cleft would not be equal for release from central versus distal locations. To gain insight into the extent to which release location could contribute to sEPSC variability, we designed a computer simulated ribbon synapse using MCell software (Stiles et al., 1998). This simulation package implements a random walk of ligand within a user-defined, three-dimensional geometry and includes interactions with ligand-gated receptors.

Figure 6A is a schematic side view of the ribbon structure used in the MCell simulations. The geometry was based on measurements of 9 ribbons from electron microscope images of ultrathin sections of tiger salamander bipolar axon terminals (as in Fig. 7A). The model has 5 possible release sites along the length of the base of the ribbon for vesicles 25 nm in diameter (Fig. 6A, gray boxes). In the simulations, the geometry is restricted to linear volumes and the vesicle representations are cubes with a side length of 25 nm. The vesicles empty their contents through a 10 nm long fusion pore into a synaptic cleft that is 200 Å wide. The pre- and postsynaptic membranes are modeled as "reflective" surfaces to the simulated glutamate. A central region of the postsynaptic surface is an area that is populated with AMPA-type ionotropic receptors modeled after the kinetic scheme of Partin et al. (1996) but based on our own observations using rapid perfusion studies and whole-cell recordings from ganglion cell somas (Fig 4C). The AMPA receptors occupy a surface area of $0.0235 \ \mu m^2$, centered on the ribbon release sites and in the center of a $1 \ \mu m^2$ postsynaptic membrane surface. In the schematic of Fig. 6A, AMPA receptors are located on the bottom of the colored regions (subclefts, Fig. 6A, 1–7). In any given simulation run, the diffusion of 4000 molecules of glutamate (vesicle concentration of 425 mM) was modeled with release from only one site, whose location was varied from the center (site 4, dark vesicle) to the displaced site (site 2 or 3). The movement of molecules, the interaction of the ligand with 126 AMPA receptors and the subsequent behavior of the kinetic model of the receptors is stochastic and simulated with 1 μs time steps.

Fig. 6. **A.** Schematic side view of the base of the modeled ribbon synapse geometry. There are 5 possible release sites, the central vesicle is shown filled with glutamate indicating release will occur for that site alone. **B.** Cleft glutamate concentration for the entire cleft volume (the sum of regions 1–7). Shown are the glutamate stimuli for release from 3 sites: site 2 (red), site 3 (green) and site 4 (blue). **C.** the smEPSCs obtained from the same simulations runs as in **B.** The amplitude was calculated by multiplying the number of open channels by the unitary current of − 0.3 pA.

with vesicles tethered above these sites (Figs. 1 and 6A). Assuming that a cluster of postsynaptic receptors reside adjacent to the synaptic cleft, a natural question arises as to whether the release of a vesicle

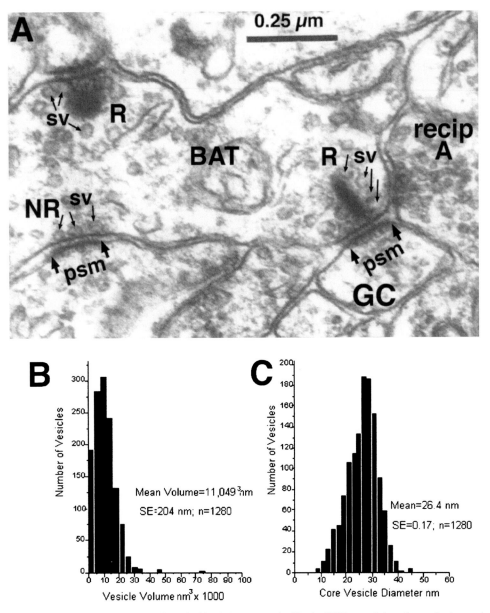

Fig. 7. (A) An electron micrograph shows a portion of a bipolar axon terminal in the ON layer of the salamander inner plexiform layer. These bipolar axon terminals (BAT) are organized into varicosities containing 1–3 ribbons (R). Synaptic vesicles (sv, small arrows) are arranged along the length of the ribbon and are directed at a dyad of postsynaptic structures, one or both of which are amacrine processes (A) and/or a ganglion cell dendrite (GC). The postsynaptic membrane shows some density (psm) and occurs at a slightly widened synaptic cleft containing some striated material (between large arrows). In salamander bipolar terminals it is common to see non ribbon containing synapses directing vesicles at one postsynaptic process (a monad). Most of the postsynaptic amacrine processes make reciprocal synapses to the bipolar terminal (A recip). (B) and (C) show frequency distributions of vesicle diameters and derived values for vesicle volumes, from a sample of 1280 vesicles. While most of the vesicles appear to fall within a unimodal distribution, a significant number are unusually large, having twice the volume of the normal population.

Figure 6B plots the glutamate concentration measured in the cleft for release from sites 2, 3, and 4 in Fig. 6A. The largest glutamate signal is produced by release from the central active zone, site 4. Progressively smaller glutamate signals result from displacing the release site laterally along the ribbon to its end (site 2). Note that the peak delay time in this simulation of glutamate diffusion is much faster than that used to generate the smEPSCs illustrated in Fig. 4. An examination of the physiological data shows that peak delays (10–90% rise times) for the sEPSCs vary from microsecond to millisecond values; averaging many sEPSCs can give an average in the low ms range, but this procedure obscures the physiological variability in this important parameter. At the present time, we do not know whether the variance in peak delay reflects differences in the kinetic behavior of the AMPA receptors, their electrotonic distance from the soma, or whether presynaptic mechanisms, such as variability in the magnitude of the fusion pore can account for the differences we observe in peak delay times for sEPSCs; this issue continues to be a major focus of our simulations and physiological studies.

Figure 6C presents the simulated EPSCs (smEPSC) which arise from the glutamate signals of Fig. 6B. The smEPSC amplitude is calculated assuming a holding potential of − 70 mV, a reversal potential of 0 mV and a single AMPA channel conductance of 10 pS. The data parallel the results seen for glutamate itself, although note the time scale differences between the two graphs. The largest smEPSC is seen for release from the central active zone and the response becomes progressively smaller as the release site is displaced along the ribbon.

While it is true that the location of the release site does make a difference in the amplitude of the smEPSC, these differences are small. In the most extreme case, vesicle release from the most displaced site results in a smEPSC peak amplitude that is only 11% less than that seen for a vesicle released from the center location; this difference cannot account for the observed range of amplitudes in the physiological data. For our symmetrical, five active zone salamander ribbon synapse, if the probability of release is equal for all release sites along the ribbon, then three populations of sEPSCs could be observed; 40% of measured sEPSCs could be attributed to release from the two most lateral sites and represent the smallest amplitude responses; another 40% would be intermediate in amplitude and could be attributed to the two intermediate sites, while a third population would constitute 20% of the pool as the largest event generated by release from the site at the center. However, the amplitude difference in this simulation, between the largest and smallest smEPSC is only 1.1 pA with a single channel conductance of 10 pS. Thus, the smEPSC variance demonstrated by our model would likely fall into one or two amplitude bins (2 pA in width) and would therefore contribute only a small amount to the sEPSC variability we have characterized from physiological data. However, this result is sensitive to the assigned single channel conductance of the model. For example, the difference in peak smEPSC amplitude between central and displaced release sites is 1.8 pA for a single channel conductance of 20 pS vs 0.45 pA for a value of 5 pS. Our main conclusion is that glutamate diffusion within the synaptic cleft of a ribbon synapse is sufficiently fast, that, despite multiple, active release zones, the ribbon synapse operates as a functional unit, with only small variance in the temporal profile of glutamate that can be attributed to positional vesicle release along the dimensions of the ribbon. We conclude that factors such as quantal content, vesicle size or the density of postsynaptic receptors are more likely sources for significant variability to sEPSC amplitudes.

Does vesicle size contribute to the variance in EPSC properties?

We have examined the population of vesicles in presynaptic terminals of bipolar cells in the tiger salamander retina, using electron microscopy and graphical methods (Metamorph, Universal Imaging) for measuring the diameter of vesicles and estimating a derived core vesicle volume. This analysis was very similar to one carried out in fish Mb bipolar terminals (von Gersdorff et al., 1996). While our study is still the subject of ongoing analysis, some preliminary results from this approach bear on the topic of sEPSC variance. Figure 7A shows a single electron micrograph of a ribbon containing synapse of a bipolar terminal. These terminals are organized as varicosities which contain 1–3 ribbons (R, Fig. 7A).

They also contain sites of vesicle accumulation near the membrane that lack a ribbon structure (NR, Fig. 7A), as originally reported by Wong-Riley (1974) for salamander and confirmed in cat and human (Kolb, 1979; Kolb et al., 1992). The two graphs in Fig. 7B and Fig. 7C show the distribution of vesicle diameters and the derived values for vesicle volumes. While most of the vesicles conform to a unimodal distribution around a mean of 26 nm, a small number of vesicles appear to be exceptionally large, around 40 nm. We believe that the large vesicles observed in our material are part of the glutamate, releasable vesicle pool, because we have observed them in the cytosol and within the ribbon structure, close to the presumed sites of vesicle release.

Ordinarily, a finding of two different populations of synaptic vesicles would serve to promote the idea that each vesicle population subserves the packaging and release of two different neurotransmitters, or perhaps the vesicle sizes reflect different states of the endocytotic–exocytotic cycle of a single transmitter system. While we cannot eliminate either of these possibilities, we have observed that members of the large vesicle pool can be observed in different positions of the ribbon-based vesicle release pool cycle, suggesting that they form part of the glutamatergic pool of synaptic vesicles. Figure 8 shows a single electron micrograph from a TS bipolar terminal in which the image was processed to include a visible grid over each large vesicle that had a derived volume of 90,000 nm^3 or more. In this image, seven large vesicles were labeled, four of which seem to be randomly dispersed in the cytosol, while two large vesicles are congregated near a ribbon (arrow), suggesting that these vesicles may have entered into the pool of releasable vesicles associated with the ribbon. For this reason, we are inclined to believe that the large vesicles observed in our material are part of the glutamatergic, releasable vesicle pool; we are presently evaluating how large vs small vesicles could affect the magnitude and time course of the glutamate concentration profile; it is clear that, if the large vesicles contain more glutamate than small vesicles and form part of the releasable vesicle pool, these vesicles will make a substantial contribution to the variance in sEPSCs, assuming that the glutamate released by a small vesicle does not saturate the pool of AMPA receptors, something that appears to be unlikely. However, desensitization of AMPA receptors has been demonstrated in sEPSCs (Taylor et al., 1995), so it remains to be seen whether a larger glutamate release can substantially increase the AMPA receptor response. At the present time, we do not know whether the large, physiological (single vesicle) sEPSCs are generated solely by AMPA receptors, or whether some NMDA receptor contribution to them takes place. Perhaps an additional source of variance in a single synapse is the variance found among synaptic receptors of the same class.

We have wondered whether the vesicles along the ribbon could fuse with each other, before fusing with the cell membrane, to provide a "super vesicle", particularly since the ribbon structure tends to place vesicles into a stack in which vesicle to vesicle opposition is tight. Thus far, no evidence has been observed to support this possibility, in that we have not observed vesicle to vesicle fusion, but functional

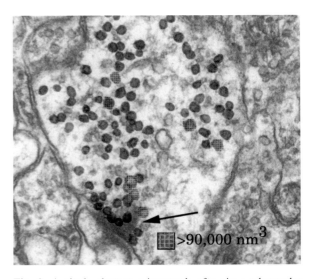

Fig. 8. A single electron micrograph of a tiger salamander bipolar terminal was digitized; each synaptic vesicle was outlined and measured with image processing morphometrics. Those vesicles which had a derived volume (based on an equivalent diameter of the two-dimensional surface area) of 90,000 nm^3 or more, were covered with a visible, square grid. In this image, seven vesicles were identified; four appear to be randomly distributed in the cytosol, but three vesicles are clustered near a synaptic ribbon (arrow), suggesting that they may be part of the ribbon-based, glutamatergic, synaptic vesicle pool.

vesicle fusion could occur with the formation of a fusion pore, without membrane fusion per se; thus we cannot eliminate the possibility of a super vesicle which might contribute to the variance observed in the sEPSC population. However, because some synaptic protein elements, such as syntaxin and SNAP-25 (Morgans, 2000) are necessary to form the fusion pore but are restricted to the presynaptic cell membrane, the likelihood of this type of presynaptic, vesicle fusion is unlikely. Indeed, it seems that this arrangement may be designed expressly to prevent vesicle to vesicle fusion, although the possibility of this type of event cannot be eliminated; perhaps it is made somewhat more likely by the close packing of vesicles around the ribbon structure.

Studies in the electric organ of the electric ray, *Torpedo* have demonstrated that ACh containing vesicles consist of two populations (VP_1 and VP_2) which vary in size and quantal content. The larger VP_1 vesicles, which contain more ACh, undergo exo- and endocytosis and give rise to newly formed, but smaller VP_2 vesicles, which have a higher probability for release under conditions of continuous stimulation (Prior and Tian, 1995). Whether the vesicle size in ribbon synapses is a function of synaptic activity remains to be seen. The animals used in our study were maintained in cold ($4°C$) tanks with a 12 h on / 12 h off light–dark duty cycle (6:00 AM to 6:00 PM) for the flourescent room lights. All animals were sacrificed at about 9:00 AM each day.

How are the large multivesiclular sEPSCs generated?

The large multivesicular events, such as that illustrated in Fig. 2, would not ordinarily be detected in automated peak detection and analysis algorithms. However, we have determined that these events are blocked by D-AP7, suggesting that NMDA receptors play some role in their generation. One possible basis for multivesicular release is through calcium spikes in bipolar terminals (Zenisek and Matthews, 1998) which could give rise to a large, presumably asynchronous release of vesicles. If so, the role of NMDA receptors, which are thought to be primarily

if not exclusively postsynaptic, is, at the moment, completely obscure.

Do postsynaptic receptors contribute to EPSC variance?

AMPA receptors make a substantial contribution to sEPSCs (Taylor et al., 1995; Gao and Wu, 1999), but NMDA receptors also contribute to some responses. Because NMDA receptors have slower offset kinetics than AMPA receptors, sEPSCs with a component from NMDA receptors are likely to show slower offset kinetics compared to those generated exclusively by AMPA receptors. The role of KA receptors, if functional at these synaptic sites, remains to be elucidated.

Conclusions and future directions

More than thirty years after Dowling (1968) proposed that ribbon and conventional synapses interact to generate functional diversity in ganglion cell receptive fields, we are just beginning to understand some of the microscopic details of these synapses. The ribbon synapse seems highly specialized for rapid transmission, through multiple vesicle release zones for each ribbon. In contrast, the more conventional synapses of amacrine cells may be associated with a single release site (Borges et al., 1995). This difference in basic design raises the interesting possibility that, by re-evaluating the idea proposed by Dowling (Dowling, 1968), it might be useful to examine the ratio of active release zones in ribbon vs conventional synapses. If different species have different ribbon sizes and show corresponding differences in the number of active zones per ribbon, then the active zone analysis might also be different for different species.

In the tiger salamander, we estimate that the ribbons are no longer than about 120 nm, whereas in the goldfish, bipolar ribbons are longer and may be up to 400 nm (von Gersdorff et al., 1996); thus, goldfish ribbons could have more release zones for each ribbon. In addition, for these larger structures, the site of release along the ribbon could provide more positional variance than we have estimated for the salamander ribbons. An additional issue which we have not addressed is the possibility that vesicles can be released from non-ribbon sites in bipolar terminals similar perhaps to (Wong-Riley, 1974) non-ribbon release sites in photoreceptors (Ripps and Chappell, 1991). We should also remember that non-ribbon vesicular sites in photoreceptors are typical of the flat cone bipolar contacts which are targeted to the ionotropic glutamate receptors of Off bipolars (Nelson and Kolb, 1983). Could non-ribbon release sites be directed towards different receptor populations in the bipolar axon terminal in the IPL as well? Do non-ribbon release sites have a single or multiple number of active release zones? Are non-ribbon release sites merely ribbon synapses which are undergoing cyclical restructuring of the ribbon? Clearly, there is much to be learned about the microscopic details of ribbon and conventional synapses and, at the present time, we can only speculate on the physiological basis for sEPSC variance.

The variability we and others have observed in the events associated with the release of single vesicles has yet to be accounted for and could include both pre- and postsynaptic mechanisms. The temporal course of glutamate in the synaptic cleft not only relates to the size of the vesicle, but it also to the size of the fusion pore between the vesicle and the cell membrane and the dimensions and properties of the extracellular space. A small component of the variance in the sEPSCs may be attributed to the position of the released vesicle underneath the ribbon, but the larger variance, observed physiologically, is likely to include several other, additional explanations. The possibility that two different sized synaptic vesicles may contribute to the sEPSC variance is a new element; dual vesicle populations were not observed in an analysis of the goldfish (von Gersdorff et al., 1996) bipolar terminal, but they are part of the functional picture of the ACh synapse of the electric organ of *Torpedo*. If two vesicle populations are present, could they be differentially released under different conditions of modulation, such as those associated with light and dark adaptation? If so, then the mean amplitude of sEPSCs could be regulated by neuromodulators. Thus, more than thirty years after Dowling's observations focused our attention onto the microstructure of retinal synapses, we are beginning to understand how these synapses work, the receptor systems which convey their influence and the importance of amacrine vs bipolar inputs into third-order neurons.

Acknowledgment

The authors research has been supported by NIH grants EY03014 and EY12833.

References

Borges, S., Gleason, E., Turelli, M. and Wilson, M. (1995) The kinetics of quantal transmitter release from retinal amacrine cells. *Proc. Natl. Acad. Sci. USA*, 92: 6896–6900.

Brandstatter, J.H., Koulen, P. and Wassle, H. (1997) Selective synaptic distribution of kainate receptor subunits in the two plexiform layers of the rat retina. *J. Neurosci.*, 17: 9298–9307.

Dowling, J.E. (1968) Synaptic organization of the frog retina: an electron microscopic analysis comparing the retinas of frogs and primates. *Proc. R. Soc. Lond. [Biol.]*, 170: 205–228.

Dowling, J.E. and Boycott, B.B. (1966) Organization of the primate retina: electron microscopy. *Proc. R. Soc. Lond. [Biol.]*, 166: 80–111.

Dubin, M.W. (1970) The inner plexiform layer of the vertebrate retina: a quantitative and comparative electron microscopic analysis. *J. Comp. Neurol.*, 140: 479–505.

Gao, F. and Wu, S.M. (1999) Multiple types of spontaneous excitatory synaptic currents in salamander retinal ganglion cells. *Brain Res.*, 821: 487–502.

Gottesman, J. and Miller, R.F. (1990) NMDA-evoked responses in retinal ganglion cells of the larval tiger salamander. *Soc. Neurosci. Abstr.*, 16: 1217.

Gottesman, J. and Miller, R.F. (1991) Do NMDA channels contribute to the resting conductance of retinal ganglion cells? (Abstract) *Soc. Neurosci. Abstr.*, 17(2): 1376.

Gottesman, J. and Miller, R.F. (1992) Pharmacological properties of *N*-methyl-D-aspartate receptors on ganglion cells of an amphibian retina. *J. Neurophysiol.*, 68: 596–604.

Higgs, M.H. and Lukasiewicz, P.D. (1999) Glutamate uptake limits synaptic excitation of retinal ganglion cells. *J. Neurosci.*, 19: 3691–3700.

Kolb, H. (1979) The inner plexiform layer in the retina of the cat: electron microscopic observations. *J. Neurocytol.*, 8: 295–329.

Kolb, H., Li, Z. and Dekorver, L. (1992) Differential staining of neurons in the human retina with protein kinase C Isozymes. *Invest. Ophthalmol. Visual Sci.*, 33: 1173–1173.

Kuffler, S.W. (1953) Discharge patterns and functional organization of mammalian retina. *J. Neurophysiol.*, 16: 37–68.

Mandell, J.W., Czernik, A.J., De Camilli, P., Greengard, P. and Townes-Anderson, E. (1992) Differential expression of synapsins I and II among rat retinal synapses. *J. Neurosci.*, 12: 1736–1749.

Mandell, J.W., Townes-Anderson, E., Czernik, A.J., Cameron, R., Greengard, P. and De Camilli, P. (1990) Synapsins in the vertebrate retina: absence from ribbon synapses and heterogeneous distribution among conventional synapses. *Neuron*, 5: 19–33.

Massey, S.C. and Maguire, G. (1995) *The Role of Glutamate in Retinal Circuitry. Excitatory Amino Acids and Synaptic Transmission*. Academic Press Inc., San Diego, pp. 201–220.

Maturana, H.R., Lettvin, J.Y., McCulloch, W.S. and Pitts, W.H. (1960) Anatomy and physiology of vision in the frog (Rana pipiens). *J. Gen. Physiol.*, 43: 129–175.

Morgans, C.W. (2000) Presynaptic proteins of ribbon synapses in the retina [In Process Citation]. *Microsc. Res. Tech.*, 50: 141–150.

Nelson, R. and Kolb, H. (1983) Synaptic patterns and response properties of bipolar and ganglion cells in the cat retina. *Vision Res.*, 23: 1183–1195.

Partin, K.M., Fleck, M.W. and Mayer, M.L. (1996) AMPA receptor flip/flop mutants affecting deactivation, desensitization, and modulation by cyclothiazide, aniracetam, and thiocyanate. *J. Neurosci.*, 16: 6634–6647.

Prior, C. and Tian, L. (1995) The heterogeneity of vesicular acetylcholine storage in cholinergic nerve terminals. *Pharmacol. Res.*, 32: 345–353.

Rall, W. (1977) Core conductor theory and cable properties of neurons. In: Kandel, E.R. (Ed.), *The Nervous System, Vol. 1*, Williams and Wilkins, Baltimore, pp. 39–97.

Ripps, H. and Chappell, R.L. (1991) Ultrastructural and electrophysiological changes associated with K+-evoked release of neurotransmitter at the synaptic terminals of skate photoreceptors. *Visual Neurosci.*, 7: 597–609.

Stiles, J.R., Bartol, T.M.J., Salpeter, E.E. and Salpeter, M.M. (1998) Monte Carlo simulation of neurotransmitter release using MCell, a general simulator of cellular physiological processes. In: Bower, J.M. (Ed.), *Computational Neuroscience: Trends in Research*, 1998. Plenum Press, New York, pp. 279–284.

Taylor, W.R., Chen, E. and Copenhagen, D.R. (1995) Characterization of spontaneous excitatory synaptic currents in salamander retinal ganglion cells. *J. Physiol-London*, 486: 207–221.

Tran, M.N., Higgs, M.H. and Lukasiewicz, P.D. (1999) AMPA receptor kinetics limit retinal amacrine cell excitatory synaptic responses. *Vis. Neurosci.*, 16: 835–842.

Velte, T.J. and Miller, R.F. (1996) Computer simulations of voltage clamping retinal ganglion cells through whole-cell electrodes in the soma. *J. Neurophysiol.*, 75: 2129–2143.

Velte, T.J. and Miller, R.F. (1998) Spiking and nonspiking models of starburst amacrine cells in the rabbit retina. *Vis. Neurosci.*, 14: 1073–1088.

Velte, T.J., Yu, W. and Miller, R.F. (1997) Estimating the contributions of NMDA and non-NMDA currents to EPSPs in retinal ganglion cells. *Vis. Neurosci.*, 14: 999–1014.

von Gersdorff, H., Vardi, E., Matthews, G. and Sterling, P. (1996) Evidence that vesicles on the synaptic ribbon of retinal bipolar neurons can be rapidly released. *Neuron*, 16: 1221–1227.

Wong-Riley, M.T.T. (1974) Synaptic organization of the inner plexiform layer in the retina of the tiger salamander. *J. Neurocytol.*, 3: 1–33.

Yu, W. and Miller, R.F. (1995) Hyperosmotic activation of transmitter release from presynaptic terminals onto retinal ganglion cells. *J. Neurosci. Methods*, 62: 159–168.

Zenisek, D. and Matthews, G. (1998) Calcium action potentials in retinal bipolar neurons. *Vis. Neurosci.*, 15: 69–75.

H. Kolb, H. Ripps and S. Wu (Eds.)
Progress in Brain Research, Vol. 131

CHAPTER 17

Physiological responses associated with kainate receptor immunoreactivity in dissociated zebrafish retinal neurons: a voltage probe study

Ralph Nelson[1],*, Andrew. T. Janis[1], Toby N. Behar[1] and Victoria P. Connaughton[2]

[1]*Laboratory of Neurophysiology, National Institute of Neurological Disorders and Stroke, NIH, Bethesda, MD 20892, USA*
[2]*Department of Biology, The American University, Washington, DC 20096, USA*

Introduction

A fundamental goal in neurobiology is to understand the relationship between receptor molecules expressed by neurons and the physiological responses of neurons. Armed with such knowledge, a direct interpretation of brain neural circuits might be possible, as the functional role of individual synapses could be ascertained, and the ways in which the nervous system processes information might be inferred. The following chapter examines this idea through studies of the correlation between expression of kainate receptor subunits on retinal neurons and their physiological responses to glutamate. Kainate receptor expression is identified by an antibody against glutamate receptor subunits 5, 6 and 7, (GluR5/6/7) (Huntley et al., 1993), while physiological responses are identified by voltage-probe responses to glutamate or other glutamatergic ligands. Zebrafish has become a significant animal

model for genetic dissection of the vertebrate visual system (Brockerhoff et al., 1995; Fadool et al., 1997). The pattern of visual pathway mutations seen in zebrafish resembles that of humans (Neuhauss et al., 1999). It therefore, appears appropriate to initiate studies of the functional roles of neurotransmitter receptors in this species. On the occasion of this symposium honoring John Dowling's contributions to neuroscience, the topic seems especially appropriate. Studies of the zebrafish visual system are one of John Dowling's recent research initiatives. One of the coauthors of this chapter studied zebrafish retinal cell culture during a Grass Fellowship with John Dowling (Connaughton and Dowling, 1998), while the senior author began a career-long interest in the physiology of ON and OFF bipolar cells while his graduate student (Nelson, 1973).

Retinal glutamate responses

Retina is characterized by a uniquely large diversity of physiological glutamate responses. This includes not only multiple excitatory types, such as AMPA responses seen in retinal horizontal cells (Yang et al., 1998; Blanco and de la Villa, 1999; Shen et al., 1999),

---

* Corresponding author: Ralph F. Nelson, National Institutes of Health, Building 36 Room 2C02, 36 Convent Dr MSC 4066, Bethesda, MD 20892-4066, USA. Tel.: 301-496-8133; Fax: 301-402-1565; E-mail: rnelson@codon.nih.gov

mixed AMPA and NMDA responses seen in retinal ganglion cells (Mittman et al., 1990; Diamond and Copenhagen, 1993; Cohen et al., 1994; Matsui et al., 1998; Gao and Wu, 1999; Cohen, 2000), and kainate responses seen in some OFF-type bipolar cells (DeVries and Schwartz, 1999), but also inhibitory responses seen in ON-type bipolar cells. In particular, ON-type bipolar cells contain multiple inhibitory glutamatergic mechanisms, either metabotropic, in which glutamate suppresses a monovalent cation channel (Nawy and Jahr, 1990; Nawy, 1999), or ionotropic, in which glutamate activates a chloride channel (Grant and Dowling, 1995; Grant and Dowling, 1996; Connaughton and Nelson, 2000). The diversity of glutamate responses in retina provides a good substrate to test the relation between glutamate physiology and molecular markers.

In some cases, the situation would appear to be straightforward. Recently retinal OFF bipolar cells in ground squirrel retina were found to use exclusively kainate receptors in responding to glutamate released by cone photoreceptors (DeVries and Schwartz, 1999). Such exclusive use of kainate receptors at an excitatory synapse is rare in the nervous system being elsewhere found only in dorsal root ganglion cells (Wisden and Seeburg, 1993; Wong and Mayer, 1993). If this arrangement is a general feature of retinal neurocircuitry, then it ought also to be found in zebrafish. In fact, recent electrophysiological evidence suggests, there is a class of zebrafish OFF bipolar cells which are selectively sensitive to kainate (Connaughton and Nelson, 2000). One might expect, then, that a subpopulation of zebrafish retinal bipolar cells would be reactive for a kainate receptor epitope, and that this population should have the physiological response properties of OFF bipolar cells, namely being excited by glutamate.

Connecting receptor subunits to response physiology

In order to test the idea that specific glutamate subunits are associated with unique physiological responses, acutely dissociated retinal neurons were stained by an antibody against kainate receptor subunits to determine which, if any cell types were immunoreactive. Since immunoreactive cells including bipolar cells were in fact found, a double label experiment was performed (Janis et al., 1999). This combined a physiological marker for glutamate responses using oxonol, a distributive voltage-sensitive stain (Waggoner, 1976; Walton et al., 1993; Nelson et al., 1999b), and kainate receptor immunoreactivity. The study identified the physiological properties of retinal neurons which expressed kainate receptors. Results, paradoxically, suggested that the kainate receptor epitope is found in zebrafish ON bipolar cells rather than OFF bipolar cells. In particular labeling was identified in ON types expressing the ionotropic inhibitory mechanism I_{glu}, which is not itself kainate sensitive (Grant and Dowling, 1995).

Receptors in unexpected places

Present results extend anatomical studies in a variety of other vertebrates that suggest that ON bipolar cells express a wider complement of glutamate receptors than physiologically anticipated, including *both* excitatory and inhibitory glutamate receptor subunits (Peng et al., 1995; Vardi et al., 1998; Morigiwa and Vardi, 1999; Vardi et al., 2000). Horizontal cells also label positively for the kainate receptor. While kainate receptor subunits have previously been observed in retinal horizontal cells (Peng et al., 1995; Brandstatter et al., 1997; Morigiwa and Vardi, 1999), excitation by glutamate appears generally to follow an AMPA-like pharmacology, as noted above. In this respect, zebrafish horizontal cells appear similar to most other vertebrate species. The lone exception to this pattern is the NMDA response of catfish horizontal cells (O'Dell and Christensen, 1989). In dissociated zebrafish horizontal cells, the characteristic AMPA-like excitation pattern includes a long-lasting after-hyperpolarization, related to activation of a sodium pump (Nelson et al., 2000).

We also find kainate receptor labeling in zebrafish cones, similar to reports in goldfish retina (Peng et al., 1995). Other ionotropic glutamate subunits (NMDA types) have been observed in mammalian photoreceptors (Goebel et al., 1998; Fletcher et al., 2000). The physiological roles of such subunits in photoreceptors is not yet clear. We have not identified glutamate responses in cones.

The voltage probe recording technique

In retina, where neurotransmitter actions are presumed to last at least as long as the stimuli, the slow kinetics of a distributive voltage probe are appropriate to study at least some facets of neurotransmitter action. Oxonol (Fig. 1A) is a distributive probe with a time constant of several minutes (Nelson et al., 1999b). The fluorophore, though negatively charged, is sufficiently lipophilic to permeate cell membranes, and distributes in Nernstian fashion across them, finding environments particularly favorable to fluorescence (FL) within the cytoplasm (Fig. 1C). Because of the Nernstian relation between cytoplasmic concentration and membrane potential, it is the log of internal concentration (as measured by FL) that measures transmembrane voltage (Walton et al., 1993). Measured sensitivities of 70 mV per log unit

change in FL have been reported (Nelson et al., 1999b). Probe FL increases as cells become depolarized and more of the negatively charged fluorophore is attracted into the cell. FL decreases as cells become hyperpolarized, and the fluorophore is repelled from the cytoplasm. Since the voltage probe technique requires the clean isolation of fluorescent signals from individual cells, it is most appropriate to retinal cell dissociates (Connaughton and Dowling, 1998). A continuous flow chamber used for oxonol recording is shown in Fig 1B.

Single labeling with GluR5/6/7 antibody

When freshly dissociated and fixed cells from zebrafish retina were processed for immunoreactivity (IR) to the Chemicon GluR5/6/7 antibody, cone

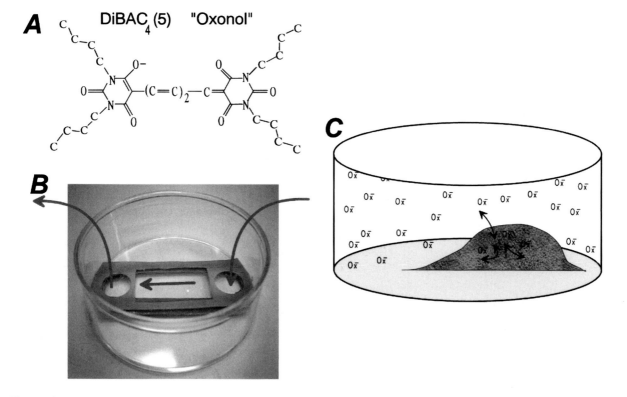

Fig. 1. The oxonol voltage probe is a negatively-charged lipophilic fluorophore (*A*). Oxonol containing perfusate is continuously supplied to, and withdrawn from, the under-cover-glass perfusion chamber. Fluorescence (FL) of dissociated neurons is viewed through the rectangular area (center) as solution flows underneath the gasket-sandwiched cover glass (*B*). Oxonol is attracted into depolarized cells, thereby increasing cellular FL, and repelled from hyperpolarized cells, thereby decreasing FL. Once within the cytoplasm, oxonol becomes concentrated in lipophilic structures, a favorable environment for FL efficiency (*C*).

258

photoreceptors, horizontal cells, and some bipolar cells were positively labeled (Janis et al., 1999). The brightest among these were cones (Fig. 2). Horizontal cells (HC Fig. 3) were moderately immunoreactive, as were some bipolar cells (BC Fig. 3, BC on right Fig. 4). It was clear, however, that bipolar cells were differentially labeled. Large cells with long axons (BC Fig. 3; BC on right, Fig. 4) were as brightly labeled as horizontal cells, while many smaller cells were more faintly labeled. The small bipolar cell with the short axon directed upwards (left BC, Fig. 4) is an example of such an immunonegative bipolar cell.

Immunoreactivity of these three cell types is further summarized in Table 1. We scored 119 total cells (cones, horizontal cells, and bipolar cells), all on the same plate, for relative levels of IR brightness. Horizontal cells, including both morphologically stellate and elongate varieties (Connaughton and Dowling, 1998) consistently showed moderate IR fluorescence. Cones, typically, were brighter than horizontal cells. About 1/4 of bipolar cells were

equally as bright as horizontal cells (Fig. 3B) while the remainder (Fig. 4B, left) were either lightly labeled or immunonegative. Table 1 supports the conclusion that labeling of cones was greater than horizontal cells, labeling of horizontal cells was comparable to some bipolar cells, but that IR among the bipolar cell population was mixed.

The division of bipolar cells into immunoreactive and non-immunoreactive types might be related to classic ON-center and OFF-center physiology. On this theory, OFF-center types might express classic GluR5/6/7 kainate-type receptor subunits. ON-center types would not require any sort of excitatory glutamate mechanism, as they are inhibited by glutamate, and therefore, should not react with the antibody. The morphological evidence (Figs. 3, 4) suggests, however, that, while a relationship between immunoreactivity and physiology might exist, it is

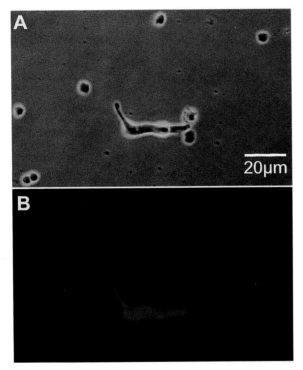

Fig. 2. GluR5/6/7 IR of cone photoreceptor dissociated from zebrafish retina. This example is a long single cone (Connaughton and Dowling, 1998) (**A**) Phase image. (**B**) IR fluorescent image.

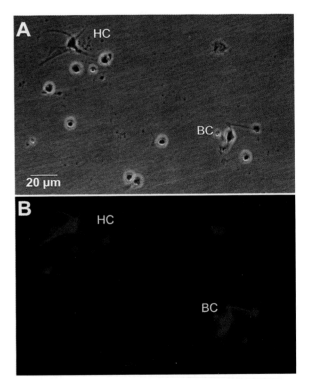

Fig. 3. GluR5/6/7 IR of zebrafish retinal horizontal cell (HC) and bipolar cell (BC). In this example the horizontal cell and the bipolar cell are equally immunoreactive, while other cells in the field are much less reactive. The bipolar cell appears to be a long-axon Mb type (On-center) (**A**) Phase image. (**B**) IR fluorescence image.

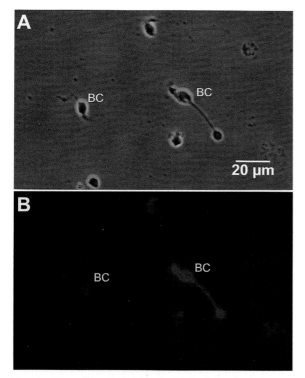

Fig. 4. Not all zebrafish retinal bipolar cells exhibited GluR5/6/7 IR. (A) Phase image; (B) IR fluorescence image. Right, brightly immunoreactive bipolar cell (BC). The morphology, with long axon and large synaptic varicosity, appears similar to Mb types seen in many cyprinids. Left, small bipolar cell with short axon (BC) seen in inverted orientation. The cell is not reactive for the GluR5/6/7 antibody. Based on morphological considerations, the cell on the right is a presumed ON-type, while the cell on the left is a presumed OFF-type.

Table 1. GluR5/6/7 IR of retinal neurons. The data are a subjective scoring of the relative immuno-fluorescence of identified retinal neurons as seen in a single cell-culture field.

Cell Type	No IR	Visible IR	Moderate IR	Bright IR
Cones	0	0	12	21
Horizontal cells	0	6	24	4
Bipolar cells	7	34	11	0

likely to be paradoxical. It is the large bipolar cells with long axons that are immunoreactive. These are most likely ON-center types. The reactive bipolar cell of Fig. 4 (right) resembles the ON-center Mb type identified in cyprinids (Scholes, 1975; Famiglietti

et al., 1977; Ishida et al., 1980; Sherry and Yazulla, 1993). Smaller bipolar cells with short axons, such as the immunonegative bipolar cell in Fig. 4 (left), are likely to be OFF-center types.

Single labeling with the oxonol voltage probe

The more common excitatory responses of zebrafish retinal neurons appear driven primarily by AMPA-type glutamate mechanisms (Fig. 5B–C). Evidence for this was obtained from experiments using (S)-5-Fluorowillardiine, a glutamate agonist selective for AMPA-type receptors (Patneau et al., 1992; Jane et al., 1997), and (2S-4R)-4 Methyl Glutamate, a selective kainate receptor agonist (Jones et al., 1997; Bleakman et al., 1999). Recordings from dendrites, cell body and axon terminal of an ON-center bipolar cell (Fig. 5A) reveal glutamate-evoked inhibition. FL decreases by about 0.2 log units (~15 mV hyperpolarization). These I_{glu}-like inhibitory responses (Grant and Dowling, 1995) were not evoked by kainate, (2S-4R)-4 Methyl Glutamate, or (S)-5-Fluorowillardiine. The metabotropic agonist APB was typically also ineffective (Nelson et al., 1999a). I_{glu} is the most common bipolar-cell glutamate response seen in zebrafish retina (Connaughton and Nelson, 2000).

In Fig. 5B after-hyperpolarizing responses in a horizontal cell (HCell) are observed, while in Fig. 5C depolarizing responses in another retinal neuron (RCell) appear. In both cases, responses are evoked by glutamate, kainate, or (S)-5-Fluorowillardiine, but not (2S-4R)-4 Methyl Glutamate. This pattern suggests that both HCell after hyperpolarization and RCell excitation are activated through an AMPA-like mechanism. After hyperpolarization is an AMPA response of depolarized horizontal cells in which hyperpolarized membrane potential is restored following glutamate application. Other studies suggest that this effect arises as sodium enters through ionotropic glutamate channels and stimulates a sodium pump, which restores membrane potential by hyperpolarizing electrogenic action (Nelson et al., 2000).

The experimental sequence (Fig. 5) finishes with a gramicidin treatment. This permeabilizes all cells to monovalent cations depolarizing them to '0' mV, and

260

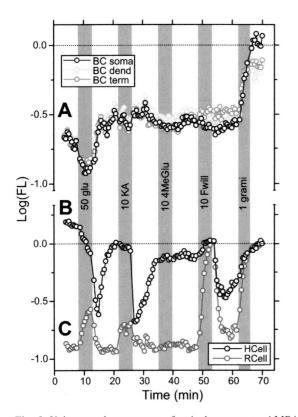

Fig. 5. Voltage-probe responses of retinal neurons to AMPA and kainate selective agonists. (**A**) Simultaneous recordings of oxonol FL from soma, dendrites and axon terminal of ON-center bipolar cell (BC). During glutamate treatment (glu), FL decreased in all cellular regions (hyperpolarizing response). Kainic acid (KA), the kainate-selective agonist (2S-4R)-4 Methyl Glutamic Acid (4MeGlu) and the AMPA selective agonist (S)-5-Fluorowillardiine (Fwill) were ineffective. (**B**) After-hyperpolarizing responses of horizontal cell (Hcell) and (**C**) excitatory responses of another retinal neuron (Rcell). All cells were simultaneously recorded from the same microscope field. The after-hyperpolarizing response, characteristic of horizontal cells (**B**), and the excitatory response of the other retinal neuron (**C**) were evoked by (S)-5-Fluorowillardiine, but not (2S-4R)-4 Methyl Glutamic Acid. This is an AMPA receptor pattern. Here and in Fig. 6, gramicidin permeabilization (grami) determines '0' level of membrane potential (dotted lines), and 1 log unit of FL increase corresponds to ~70 mV of depolarization (Nelson et al., 1999b). Drug concentrations are given in µM.

thereby establishing FL for the '0' level of membrane potential. The increase in FL during gramicidin treatment is a measure of the resting potential. The cell of Fig. 5C exhibits about 1 log unit of membrane potential, corresponding to −70 mV (Nelson et al., 1999b).

Double labeling with oxonol voltage probe and GluR5/6/7 antibody

Voltage-probe protocols were combined with IR staining for kainate receptors to identify possible glutamate subunits involved in observed responses. The GluR5/6/7 IR of 5 major different physiological responses to glutamate are shown in Fig. 6. The top panel (Fig. 6A) illustrates a cell that did not respond to glutamate or kainate. It did, however, maintain a resting potential, as revealed by a large depolarizing response (FL increase) to gramicidin. These findings suggest, there was an appropriate ionic gradient to generate excitatory responses, if any AMPA/kainate activated channels were present. This cell shows virtually no GluR5/6/7 IR, a consistent result. The cell of Fig. 6B was depolarized by both glutamate and kainate (FL increases). This is classic AMPA/kainate physiology. Further, the cell is clearly immunoreactive, which would be consistent with a model in which kainate receptors participated in the excitatory response. The cell of Fig. 6D is a horizontal cell with after-hyperpolarizing responses both to glutamate and kainate. The cell is labeled by the GluR5/6/7 antibody, as previously described (Fig. 3A, HC). Horizontal cells provide a clear example of a correlation between AMPA-like excitatory glutamate responses and GluR5/6/7 IR.

The cells in Fig. 6C and 6E present more paradoxical associations. The cell of 6E is a morphologically identified bipolar cell that was inhibited by glutamate (FL decreases). Based on other experience with such cells, this response is highly likely to be an I_{glu}-type Cl$^-$ response. As anticipated (Fig. 4), it does in fact label with the GluR5/6/7 antibody. The cell of Fig. 6C, on the other hand, is excited by kainate, but much less sensitive to glutamate. This is a pattern seen in OFF-center bipolar cells using patch recording techniques in retinal slice (Connaughton and Nelson, 2000). On this basis, we tentatively identify it as an OFF-type bipolar cell, even though bipolar-cell morphological features were not preserved. This cell, however, does not stain for kainate receptor subunits, even though it displays a kainate preferring, excitatory response physiology.

In total, we were able to correlate physiological glutamate responses with GluR5/6/7 IR for 56 cells in

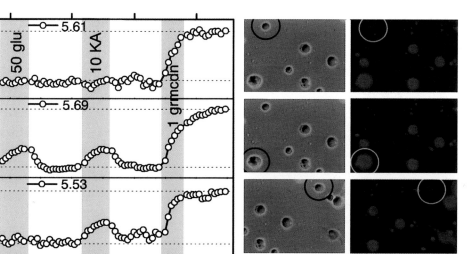

Fig. 6. GluR5/6/7 IR of 5 cells with different glutamate responses. (**A**). (*5.61*): A retinal neuron responded neither to glutamate (glu) nor kainate (KA), but gramicidin treatment revealed a hyperpolarized resting potential. The cell was unreactive for GluR5/6/7. (**B**). (*5.69*): A retinal neuron was depolarized by both glutamate and kainate (FL increases). This cell was reactive for the GluR5/6/7 antibody. (**C**). (*5.53*): A retinal neuron responded to kainate but not glutamate. The cell is poorly reactive for the GluR5/6/7 antibody. (**D**). (*4.49*): After-hyperpolarizing responses for both glutamate and kainate appeared in a horizontal cell. Like other horizontal cells, the cell was brightly reactive for the GluR5/6/7 antibody. (**E**) (*4.24*): This bipolar cell was hyperpolarized by glutamate and is therefore, an ON-center type. It was reactive for the GluR5/6/7 antibody. IR fluorescence is shown in false color.

this microscope field. The histogram (Fig. 7) shows the IR fluorescent pattern for each physiological response category described in Fig. 6. Overall, the correlation between the kainate subunit IR and glutamate responsivity is very high. A contingency table based on the data of Fig. 7 gives a probability of less than 1 in 10,000 that glutamate responses and glutamate receptor expression, as measured by this antibody, are independently distributed. Particularly telling is the persistent lack of IR on cells that do not respond to glutamate.

The table reveals that kainate receptor subunits were found in several unexpected places. First, many cells, such as horizontal cells, which are characteristically excited by a fluorowillardiine-sensitive AMPA-like mechanism, nonetheless appear to express kainate receptor subunits. Second, cells which are inhibited by glutamate are also immunoreactive for kainate subunits. Other studies (Nelson et al., 1999a; Connaughton and Nelson, 2000) indicate that in zebrafish this inhibition is most commonly through I_{glu}-like chloride mechanism (Grant and Dowling,

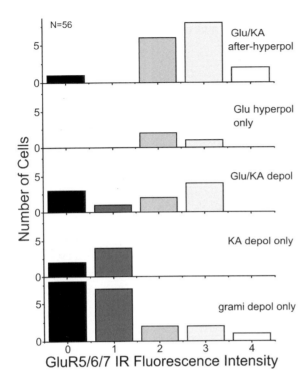

Fig. 7. Intensity of GluR5/6/7 IR among the 5 different physiological types of glutamate response illustrated in Fig. 6. Starting at the top, the brightest and most consistent IR occurred among those cells exhibiting after-hyperpolarizing responses (Glu/KA after-hyperpol). This response was typical of, but not restricted to, excitation of retinal horizontal cells. Next, cells hyperpolarized by glutamate, but not kainate (Glu hyperpol only), typical of ON-center bipolar cells, were found moderately reactive for the GluR5/6/7 antibody. Next, cells depolarized by both glutamate and kainate exhibited a wide range of IR (Glu/KA depol). Next, cells where kainate alone evoked depolarizing responses (KA depol only) were unreactive. This response is characteristic of OFF bipolar cells (Connaughton and Nelson, 2000). Finally, cells where gramicidin revealed membrane potentials, but neither glutamate nor kainate evoked responses, were predominantly unreactive (grami depol only). For scoring GluR5/6/7 IR, fluorescent micrographs were converted to false color scale using NIH image and scored by color. Only cells exhibiting voltage-probe responses for at least 1 of the 3 drug treatments were included.

1995), implying I_{glu} is a type of glutamate response associated with GluR5/6/7 IR. Cells which were excited by glutamate and/or kainate, but were not immunoreactive, also occur (Fig. 7). These are not unexpected, as cells expressing exclusively unreactive AMPA subunits would show such a pattern. In summary, double labeling reveals that the presence of GluR5/6/7 IR on a retinal cell suggests a high probability of a glutamate response on that cell, however, it does not predict the physiological type of glutamate response that may be present.

Conclusions and future perspectives

The Chemicon GluR5/6/7 antibody, selective for kainate receptor subunits, differentially labels zebrafish retinal neurons. Cones and horizontal cells invariably stained. A minority of bipolar cells, often those with large, long-axon, Mb-like morphology (both presumptively and directly identified ON-center cells), stained as brightly as horizontal cells, while other bipolar cells, some with short-axon, OFF-center-like morphology, were very weakly immunoreactive or immunonegative. There was differential staining also among other, unidentified, dissociated cells. In the retina of goldfish, another cyprinid species, an antibody directed against GluR6/7, also selective for kainate receptors, labeled horizontal cells, Mb type (ON-center) bipolar cells, and some cones (Peng et al., 1995). GluR6/7 IR has been found in horizontal cell lateral elements of rat (Brandstatter et al., 1997) and cat retina (Vardi et al., 1998; Morigiwa and Vardi, 1999). Kainate receptor IR appears common to vertebrate horizontal cells. Peng (Peng et al., 1995) noted that GluR6 is phosphorylated by protein kinase-A (PKA), leading to potentiation of synaptic currents. This suggests that enhancement of horizontal-cell glutamate currents by dopamine (Knapp and Dowling, 1987) may be mediated by GluR6 through a PKA mechanism. Cells of the inner retina, amacrine and ganglion cells, also label positively with GluR6/7 antibody (Brandstatter et al., 1997).

Retinal bipolar cells, whether ON-center or OFF-center, appear to express AMPA and/or kainate receptor subunits (Vardi et al., 1998; Morigiwa and Vardi, 1999). OFF-center cells of rat express KA2 type subunits, but not GluR6/7 subunits (Brandstatter et al., 1997), whereas in cat, GluR6/7 subunits are expressed on OFF-center bipolar cells (Morigiwa and Vardi, 1999). AMPA-type subunits are common to ON-center bipolar cells in a range of species (Hughes et al., 1992; Peng et al., 1995;

Hughes, 1997; Morigiwa and Vardi, 1999), while kainate-type subunits, such as reported here, have so far been described only in teleost ON bipolar cells (Peng et al., 1995).

Anatomical inferences relating receptor expression to physiology are extended by combining direct physiological measurement of bipolar-cell responses with antibody staining. The oxonol voltage probe revealed both excitatory and inhibitory glutamate responses in zebrafish retinal neurons. Excitatory responses consisted of either depolarizations or after hyperpolarizations (Nelson et al., 2000). Excitatory responses were AMPA-like in ligand sensitivity, as they were activated by fluorowillardiine. Nonetheless, kainate was also an effective agonist. After-hyperpolarizing responses were particularly characteristic of depolarized horizontal cells. These may arise through activation of an electrogenic Na^+ pump, stimulated by Na^+ entry through AMPA channels (Nelson et al., 2000). Glutamate inhibitory responses, characteristic of ON bipolar cells, were neither AMPA- nor kainate-like in pharmacology. Typically APB, a metabotropic agonist, also failed to evoke such inhibitory responses, even though APB is an effective agonist in a subset of ON-cells in zebrafish retinal slice (Connaughton and Nelson, 2000). Inhibitory responses in dissociated cells appeared to be mainly I_{glu}-type: glutamate-gated Cl^- responses (Connaughton and Nelson, 2000).

Kainate receptor subunit IR was associated with after-hyperpolarizing responses, glutamate-induced hyperpolarizations (I_{glu}), and glutamate/kainate elicited depolarizations. Cells insensitive to glutamate were immunonegative for this antibody. The association of excitatory glutamate receptor subunits with inhibitory glutamate responses confirms inferences from the bipolar-cell immunohistochemical literature cited above. The present work extends this observation to zebrafish retina, where GluR5/6/7 IR, a marker for kainate receptor subunits, appears correlated with an inhibitory I_{glu}-like physiology in ON-center bipolar cells.

Recent evidence in mammalian retina suggests that some OFF-center bipolar cells express kainate receptor physiology (DeVries and Schwartz, 1999). Such neurons are a logical candidate to express a kainate receptor epitope. Zebrafish OFF-bipolar cells often exhibited a kainate-favoring physiology

(Connaughton and Nelson, 2000), but present work suggests they do not express GluR5/6/7 kainate receptor subunits. Possibly such cells utilize either KA1/2 kainate subunits, or even exclusively AMPA subunits (GluR1–4), neither of which should react with the GluR5/6/7 antibody (Huntley et al., 1993). KA2 receptors, but not GluR6/7 receptors, were identified in rat OFF-center bipolar cells, suggesting that KA2 may sometimes form physiologically competent homomeric channels (Brandstatter et al., 1997). On the other hand, AMPA receptors mediate the responses of OFF bipolar cells in salamander retina (Maple et al., 1999).

In brain as in retina, patterns of kainate subunit expression may not invariably overlap with patterns of kainate receptor function (Monaghan and Wenthold, 1997). In retina, horizontal cells express kainate receptor epitopes, but demonstrate AMPA-like patterns of glutamate excitation. Zebrafish bipolar cells reactive for kainate receptor subunits are ON-center types inhibited by glutamate. Neither of these is a classic kainate receptor action. Our findings demonstrate that retinal cells expressing GluR5/6/7 subunit proteins express different functional responses to glutamate, and not necessarily of a kainate type. It appears that, in this sense, the physiological identity of some retinal neurons may be epigenetic. Cells in an environment where glutamate provides a significant source of synaptic signals may express a variety of glutamate-related molecules, but only functionally enable a few of these, while the rest are either supernumary, or utilized in some novel way. Thus, the possibility of defining the physiology of retinal neurons based on selective molecular markers may be limited, even while the overall correlation of glutamate receptor expression with glutamate responsiveness remains strong. The challenge to find molecular markers for patterns of neural integration may be even broader. Neurons such as ON and OFF center ganglion cells can be clearly differentiated based on morphology and physiology (Nelson et al., 1978), but as yet there is no selective molecular tag, nor reason to suspect one. This suggests that progress in understanding the ways in which the nervous system processes visual information will continue to require a broad variety of approaches, including neurophysiological, neuroanatomical, and molecular.

References

Blanco, R. and de la Villa, P. (1999) Ionotropic glutamate receptors in isolated horizontal cells of the rabbit retina. *Eur. J. Neurosci.*, 11: 867–873.

Bleakman, D., Ogden, A.M., Ornstein, P.L. and Hoo, K. (1999) Pharmacological characterization of a GluR6 kainate receptor in cultured hippocampal neurons. *Eur. J. Pharmacol.*, 378: 331–337.

Brandstatter, J.H., Koulen, P. and Wassle, H. (1997) Selective synaptic distribution of kainate receptor subunits in the two plexiform layers of the rat retina. *J. Neurosci.*, 17: 9298–9307.

Brockerhoff, S.E., Hurley, J.B., Janssen-Bienhold, U., Neuhauss, S.C., Driever, W. and Dowling, J.E. (1995) A behavioral screen for isolating zebrafish mutants with visual system defects. *Proc. Natl. Acad. Sci. USA*, 92: 10545–10549.

Cohen, E.D. (2000) Light-evoked excitatory synaptic currents of X-type retinal ganglion cells. *J. Neurophysiol.*, 83: 3217–3229.

Cohen, E.D., Zhou, Z.J. and Fain, G.L. (1994) Ligand-gated currents of alpha and beta ganglion cells in the cat retinal slice. *J. Neurophysiol.*, 72: 1260–1269.

Connaughton, V.P. and Dowling, J.E. (1998) Comparative morphology of distal neurons in larval and adult zebrafish retinas. *Vis. Res.*, 38: 13–18.

Connaughton, V.P. and Nelson, R. (2000) Axonal stratification patterns and glutamate-gated conductance mechanisms in zebrafish retinal bipolar cells. *J. Physiol. (Lond.)*, 524: 135–146.

DeVries, S.H. and Schwartz, E.A. (1999) Kainate receptors mediate synaptic transmission between cones and 'Off' bipolar cells in a mammalian retina. *Nature*, 397: 157–160.

Diamond, J.S. and Copenhagen, D.R. (1993) The contribution of NMDA and non-NMDA receptors to the light-evoked input-output characteristics of retinal ganglion cells. *Neuron*, 11: 725–738.

Fadool, J.M., Brockerhoff, S.E., Hyatt, G.A. and Dowling, J.E. (1997) Mutations affecting eye morphology in the developing zebrafish (Danio rerio). *Dev. Genet.*, 20: 288–295.

Famiglietti, E.V. Jr., Kaneko, A. and Tachibana, M. (1977) Neuronal architecture of on and off pathways to ganglion cells in carp retina. *Science*, 198: 1267–1269.

Fletcher, E.L., Hack, I., Brandstatter, J.H. and Wassle, H. (2000) Synaptic localization of NMDA receptor subunits in the rat retina. *J. Comp. Neurol.*, 420: 98–112.

Gao, F. and Wu, S.M. (1999) Multiple types of spontaneous excitatory synaptic currents in salamander retinal ganglion cells. *Brain Res.*, 821: 487–502.

Goebel, D.J., Aurelia, J.L., Tai, Q., Jojich, L. and Poosch, M.S. (1998) Immunocytochemical localization of the NMDA-R2A receptor subunit in the cat retina. *Brain Res.*, 808: 141–154.

Grant, G.B. and Dowling, J.E. (1995) A glutamate-activated chloride current in cone-driven ON bipolar cells of the white perch retina. *J. Neurosci.*, 15: 3852–3862.

Grant, G.B. and Dowling, J.E. (1996) On bipolar cell responses in the teleost retina are generated by two distinct mechanisms. *J. Neurophysiol.*, 76: 3842–3849.

Hughes, T.E. (1997) Are there ionotropic glutamate receptors on the rod bipolar cell of the mouse retina? *Vis. Neurosci.*, 14: 103–109.

Hughes, T.E., Hermans-Borgmeyer, I. and Heinemann, S. (1992) Differential expression of glutamate receptor genes (GluR1–5) in the rat retina. *Vis. Neurosci.*, 8: 49–55.

Huntley, G.W., Rogers, S.W., Moran, T., Janssen, W., Archin, N., Vickers, J.C., Cauley, K., Heinemann, S.F. and Morrison, J.H. (1993) Selective distribution of kainate receptor subunit immunoreactivity in monkey neocortex revealed by a monoclonal antibody that recognizes glutamate receptor subunits GluR5/6/7. *J. Neurosci.*, 13: 2965–2981.

Ishida, A.T., Stell, W.K. and Lightfoot, D.O. (1980) Rod and cone inputs to bipolar cells in goldfish retina. *J. Comp. Neurol.*, 191: 315–335.

Jane, D.E., Hoo, K., Kamboj, R., Deverill, M., Bleakman, D. and Mandelzys, A. (1997) Synthesis of willardiine and 6-azawillardiine analogs: pharmacological characterization on cloned homomeric human AMPA and kainate receptor subtypes. *J. Med. Chem.*, 40: 3645–3650.

Janis, A.T., Behar, T.N., Connaughton, V.P. and Nelson, R. (1999) Kainate receptors and glutamate responses of zebrafish retinal neurons. *Soc. Neurosci. Abstr.*, 25: 1433.

Jones, K.A., Wilding, T.J., Huettner, J.E. and Costa, A.M. (1997) Desensitization of kainate receptors by kainate, glutamate and diastereomers of 4-methylglutamate. *Neuropharmacol.*, 36: 853–863.

Knapp, A.G. and Dowling, J.E. (1987) Dopamine enhances excitatory amino acid-gated conductances in cultured retinal horizontal cells. *Nature*, 325: 437–439.

Maple, B.R., Gao, F. and Wu, S.M. (1999) Glutamate receptors differ in rod- and cone-dominated off-center bipolar cells. *Neuroreport*, 10: 3605–3610.

Matsui, K., Hosoi, N. and Tachibana, M. (1998) Excitatory synaptic transmission in the inner retina: paired recordings of bipolar cells and neurons of the ganglion cell layer. *J. Neurosci.*, 18: 4500–4510.

Mittman, S., Taylor, W.R. and Copenhagen, D.R. (1990) Concomitant activation of two types of glutamate receptor mediates excitation of salamander retinal ganglion cells. *J. Physiol. (Lond.)*, 428: 175–197.

Monaghan, D.T. and Wenthold, R.J. (1997) *The ionotropic glutamate receptors*, Humana Press, Totowa, NJ.

Morigiwa, K. and Vardi, N. (1999) Differential expression of ionotropic glutamate receptor subunits in the outer retina. *J. Comp. Neurol.*, 405: 173–184.

Nawy, S. (1999) The metabotropic receptor mGluR6 may signal through G(o), but not phosphodiesterase, in retinal bipolar cells. *J. Neurosci.*, 19: 2938–2944.

Nawy, S. and Jahr, C.E. (1990) Suppression by glutamate of cGMP-activated conductance in retinal bipolar cells. *Nature*, 346: 269–271.

Nelson, R. (1973) A comparison of electrical properties of neurons in *Necturus* retina. *J. Neurophysiol.*, 36: 519–535.

Nelson, R., Famiglietti, E.V. Jr. and Kolb H. (1978) Intracellular staining reveals different levels of stratification for on- and off-center ganglion cells in the cat retina. *J. Neurophysiol.*, 41: 472–483.

Nelson, R., Bender, A.M. and Connaughton, V.P. (2000) AMPA excitation restores membrane potential to tonically depolarized retinal horizontal cells. *Soc. Neurosci. Abstr.*, 26: 1327.

Nelson, R., Connaughton, V.P. and Schaffner, A.E. (1999a) Voltage probe measurements of glutamate responses form acutely dissociated zebrafish retinal neurons. *Invest. Ophthalmol. Vis. Sci.*, 40: S242.

Nelson, R., Schaffner, A.E., Li, Y.X. and Walton, M.K. (1999b) Distribution of GABA$_C$-like responses among acutely dissociated rat retinal neurons. *Vis. Neurosci.*, 16: 179–190.

Neuhauss, S.C., Biehlmaier, O., Seeliger, M.W., Das, T., Kohler, K., Harris, W.A. and Baier, H. (1999) Genetic disorders of vision revealed by a behavioral screen of 400 essential loci in zebrafish. *J. Neurosci.*, 19: 8603–8615.

O'Dell, T.J. and Christensen, B.N. (1989) Horizontal cells isolated from catfish retina contain two types of excitatory amino acid receptors. *J. Neurophysiol.*, 61: 1097–1109.

Patneau, D.K., Mayer, M.L., Jane, D.E. and Watkins, J.C. (1992) Activation and desensitization of AMPA/kainate receptors by novel derivatives of willardiine. *J. Neurosci.*, 12: 595–606.

Peng, Y.W., Blackstone, C.D., Huganir, R.L. and Yau, K.W. (1995) Distribution of glutamate receptor subtypes in the vertebrate retina. *Neuroscience*, 66: 483–497.

Scholes, J.H. (1975) Colour receptors, and their synaptic connexions, in the retina of a cyprinid fish. *Philos. Trans. R. Soc. Lond. B Biol. Sci.*, 270: 61–118.

Shen, Y., Lu, T. and Yang, X.L. (1999) Modulation of desensitization at glutamate receptors in isolated crucian carp horizontal cells by concanavalin A, cyclothiazide, aniracetam and PEPA. *Neuroscience*, 89: 979–990.

Sherry, D.M. and Yazulla, S. (1993) Goldfish bipolar cells and axon terminal patterns: a Golgi study. *J. Comp. Neurol.*, 329: 188–200.

Vardi, N., Duvoisin, R., Wu, G. and Sterling, P. (2000) Localization of mGluR6 to dendrites of ON bipolar cells in primate retina. *J. Comp. Neurol.*, 423: 402–412.

Vardi, N., Morigiwa, K., Wang, T.L., Shi, Y.J. and Sterling, P. (1998) Neurochemistry of the mammalian cone 'synaptic complex'. *Vision Res.*, 38: 1359–1369.

Waggoner, A. (1976) Optical probes of membrane potential. *J. Membr. Biol.*, 27: 317–334.

Walton, M.K., Schaffner, A.E. and Barker, J.L. (1993) Sodium channels, GABA$_A$ receptors, and glutamate receptors develop sequentially on embryonic rat spinal cord cells. *J. Neurosci.*, 13: 2068–2084.

Wisden, W. and Seeburg, P.H. (1993) A complex mosaic of high-affinity kainate receptors in rat brain. *J. Neurosci.*, 13: 3582–3598.

Wong, L.A. and Mayer, M.L. (1993) Differential modulation by cyclothiazide and concanavalin A of desensitization at native alpha-amino-3-hydroxy-5-methyl-4-isoxazolepropionic acid- and kainate-preferring glutamate receptors. *Mol. Pharmacol.*, 44: 504–510.

Yang, J.H., Maple, B., Gao, F., Maguire, G. and Wu, S.M. (1998) Postsynaptic responses of horizontal cells in the tiger salamander retina are mediated by AMPA-preferring receptors. *Brain Res.*, 797: 125–134.

H. Kolb, H. Ripps and S. Wu (Eds.)
Progress in Brain Research, Vol. 131

CHAPTER 18

GABA transporter function in the horizontal cells of the skate

Robert Paul Malchow[1,2,*] and Kristen A. Andersen[1,†]

[1]*Department of Biological Sciences, University of Illinois at Chicago, 840 West Taylor Street, Chicago, IL 60607, USA*
[2]*Departments of Ophthalmology and Visual Sciences, University of Illinois at Chicago, 840 West Taylor Street, Chicago, IL 60607, USA*

Introduction

γ-amino butyric acid (GABA) is believed to play a crucial role in the processing of visual information by cells of the vertebrate retina. This inhibitory neurotransmitter has been implicated in functions as diverse as the regulation of the dynamic range of retinal neurons, the establishment of the surround portion of the receptive field of neurons, the establishment of color opponency, mediation of movement detection within the retina, and involvement in the process of visual adaptation (cf. Wu, 1992a,b for review). There is much anatomical evidence that GABA is the neurotransmitter of certain classes of horizontal cells, the retinal neurons thought to be important in establishing lateral inhibitory pathways in the distal retina. Studies supporting this contention include the autoradiographic demonstration of uptake of tritiated GABA into horizontal cells, the detection of high quantities of GABA by immunohistochemical techniques, and immunocytochemical detection of the enzymes necessary for the synthesis of this neurotransmitter (cf. Yazulla, 1986;

Freed, 1992; Marc, 1992). The postsynaptic effects of GABA are mediated by a heterogeneous set of proteins, the GABA receptors, which have been classified into three groups, known as $GABA_A$, $GABA_B$, and $GABA_C$ receptors (Djamgoz, 1995; Qian and Dowling, 1993). The different types of GABA receptors are located in discrete populations of neurons, have distinct pharmacologies and postsynaptic effects, and are believed to play differing roles in the processing of visual information (see Fig. 1).

Specific proteins that mediate the transport of GABA into and out of cells are likely to be key regulators of the effects of GABA within the retina. Uptake of GABA into neurons and surrounding glia is believed to be the primary mechanism for the termination of the postsynaptic effects of GABA (Iversen, 1971; Iversen and Kelly, 1975). Moreover, it has been suggested that these transporters may be involved in the sodium-dependent, but calcium independent, release of GABA into the extracellular space. Much anatomical, biochemical and autoradiographic evidence supporting non-vesicular release of GABA has been accumulated (cf. Schwartz, 1982; Yazulla and Kleinschmidt, 1983; Yazulla, 1983; Ayoub and Lam, 1984; Yazulla et al., 1985), but perhaps the most convincing demonstration of calcium-independent release of GABA has come from the elegant experiments of Schwartz (1987), in which cells possessing GABA receptors were used as

---

*Corresponding author: Robert Paul Malchow, M/C 067, 840 West Taylor Street, Chicago, IL 60607, USA., Tel.: 312-413-1552; Fax: 312-996-2805; E-mail: paulmalc@uic.edu
†Present address: Kristen A. Andersen, Department of Medicine, University of Chicago, 5841 S. Maryland Avenue, MC 6094, Chicago, IL 60637, USA.

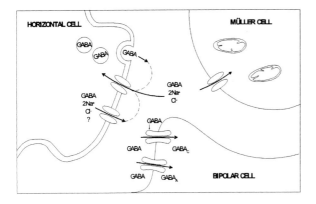

Fig. 1. Schematic representation of GABA pathways in the retina of the skate. Horizontal cells release GABA into the extracellular space, where GABA$_A$ and GABA$_C$ receptors on the dendritic tips of bipolar cells are activated. The extracellular GABA is taken up back into horizontal cells and Muller cells by specific transport proteins. Moreover, the transporter of the horizontal cells may play a key role in the sodium-dependent but calcium-independent release of GABA into the extracellular space.

probes to monitor the release of GABA from isolated retinal horizontal cells. The role that GABA transporters play in processing neuronal information may, therefore, be considerably more complicated than acting simply as sponges to soak up excess GABA in the extracellular space.

Molecular biological studies have made clear that there are several subtypes of GABA transporter that belong to the family of sodium–chloride-coupled transporters. Four distinct GABA transporters (GAT1-4) have been cloned from murine brain (Liu et al., 1993; Schloss, et al., 1994), and three of these transporters have been found to be expressed in ocular tissue. Antibody and in-situ-hybridization studies done in rat retina suggest that a GAT-1 transporter is heavily expressed in amacrine cells, with weaker staining appearing in the Muller cells (Brecha and Weigmann, 1994). A GAT-3 transporter appears to be expressed primarily in rat Muller cells and some amacrine cells, and GAT-2 immunoreactivity was found to be present in the retinal pigment epithelium, the nerve fiber layer, and the ciliary body (Johnson et al., 1996). Location of GABA transporters in tiger salamander retina revealed the presence of a GAT-1 like transporter in selective subtypes of bipolar cells, amacrine cells, interplexiform cells and ganglion cells, while GAT-3 immunoreactivity was detected in certain amacrine cells and cells in the ganglion cell layer (Yang, et al., 1997). Curiously, with one exception (Ekstrom and Anzelius, 1998), these techniques have failed to reveal the presence of GABA transporters in horizontal cells, despite considerable physiological evidence for the presence of such transporters (e.g., Malchow and Ripps, 1990; Cammack and Schwartz, 1993).

Despite the wealth of molecular detail now available regarding the sequence of the various GABA transporters, much remains unknown about the nature and role of the GABA transporter expressed by retinal horizontal cells. Moreover, an understanding of the regulation and modulation of the transport of GABA by horizontal cells remains at a rudimentary level. We have been examining these questions using a model system first introduced by Dowling and Ripps in the 1970s: the retina of the skate (*Raja erinacea/R. ocellata*). These investigators were originally drawn to the retinas of these elasmobranchs because of observations suggesting that these species appeared to possess only rod photoreceptors, thus greatly simplifying studies designed to examine neuronal mechanisms of visual adaptation (Dowling and Ripps, 1970). An additional advantage, of particular relevance to our own work, concerns the fact that the horizontal cells of these species are particularly large, with cell somas having diameters in excess of 100 μm. The large size of the horizontal cells permitted Dowling and Ripps to make stable, long-term electrophysiological recordings, leading to seminal studies not only on the nature of light adaptation but also on the process of synaptic transmission from photoreceptors to second order retinal neurons (Dowling and Ripps, 1970, 1971, 1972, 1973). In our own studies, the large size of the skate horizontal cells greatly facilitates the detection of the transport of GABA using electrophysiological techniques. Transport proteins generate significantly less electrical current than ion channels, with turnover rates estimated to be near 1000 ions per second compared to the millions of ions per second through ionic channels (Hille, 1992). Consequently, GABA transport currents are more easily studied in large cells possessing large numbers of transport proteins. The very large size of the horizontal cells, coupled with the all-rod complement of photoreceptors and the resulting relative simplicity of photoreceptor to second order neuronal connections in these species, continue to make the skate retina a particularly attractive model system to this day.

Characteristics of GABA transport currents from skate horizontal cells

We have examined the GABA transport process in horizontal cells enzymatically isolated from the skate retina using the whole-cell version of the patch clamp technique (Malchow et al., 1990a). To examine GABA transport, cells are typically voltage-clamped at –70 mV, which is the normal resting potential for these cells when isolated. At this voltage, we obtain currents suitable for observing the influx of GABA into the horizontal cells (Malchow and Ripps, 1990). The skate retina possesses two types of horizontal cells that can be readily distinguished based on morphological criteria: the particularly large and thick external horizontal cells, and the more slender internal horizontal cells, whose cell bodies are located just beneath (vitread to) the external horizontal cells (Malchow et al., 1990a). Our electrophysiological

studies support the contention that both types of horizontal cells possess transporters for GABA. The upper trace in Fig. 2A shows the inward current that results when 1 mM GABA is superfused onto a voltage-clamped horizontal cell, and the middle trace shows that the electrical current induced by GABA depends critically on the presence of external sodium. Thus, replacing all the extracellular sodium chloride with lithium chloride completely abolishes the electrical current induced by GABA. The inward current is believed to reflect the transport of GABA in combination with sodium and chloride into the cell. Our own work and electrophysiolgical studies of GABA transporters in a number of other cell types and expression systems indicate that the stoichiometry for transport is 2 sodium ions and 1 chloride ion transported with each (uncharged) GABA molecule. Figure 2B shows that the electrical current elicited by GABA is also abolished by 300 μM of the compound SKF 89976-A, which is known to specifically inhibit GABA transport in a wide variety of preparations (Larsson et al., 1988; Lewin et al., 1994). Based on such experiments, we conclude that both external and internal horizontal cells of the skate possess electrogenic transport systems for GABA. It is worth emphasizing that this result differs from that seen in

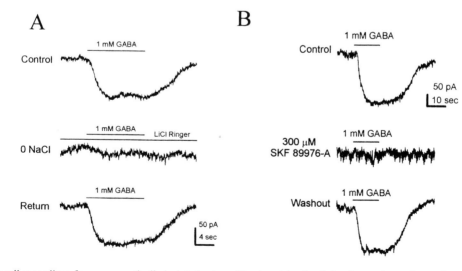

Fig. 2. Whole-cell recordings from enzymatically isolated external horizontal cells of the skate voltage-clamped at –70 mV. **A.** 1 mM GABA evokes an inward current when the cells are superfused in normal skate Ringer's solution. Replacement of the sodium chloride in the Ringer with lithium chloride eliminates the GABA-elicited current. **B.** Recording from another isolated horizontal cell first in normal Ringer, then in Ringer containing 300 μM of the GABA transporter blocking agent SKF 89976-A; this compound completely abolishes the current elicited by GABA, but as shown in the lowest trace, the effect is reversible.

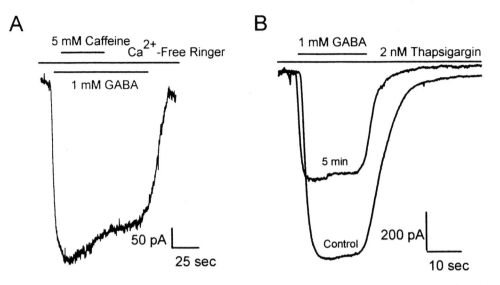

Fig. 5. **A.** Caffeine reduces the GABA transport current. Recordings from a single horizontal cell voltage-clamped at –70 mV. 1 mM GABA induces an inward current, which becomes less when 5 mM caffeine is superfused onto the cell. **B.** Thapsigargin, an agent which prevents reuptake of calcium into internal stores and so induces increases in intracellular calcium, reduces the GABA transport current. Responses from a single cell to 1 mM GABA with the cell voltage-clamped at –70 mV in normal Ringer and 5 min after the addition of 2 nM thapsigargin. The GABA transport current was reduced by one-half the control value.

issue concerns the relative spatial relationship of the GABA transporters with respect to sites for the vesicular release of GABA from retinal horizontal cells. It is conceivable that GABA extruded via calcium-dependent vesicular mechanisms could act at distinct sites and exert a different physiological function from that released by reverse transport.

One conceivable scenario is that down regulation of GABA transport by internal calcium may enhance the postsynaptic effects of the extracellular GABA that has been released through vesicular mechanisms. This could strengthen the lateral inhibitory effects exerted by horizontal cells and increase the effective weight of the visual surround created by the horizontal cells. High levels of internal calcium are expected to be present in horizontal cells in the intact retina in the dark, for several reasons. Photoreceptors are believed to continuously release glutamate in the dark, which would be expected to depolarize horizontal cells and promote the opening of voltage-sensitive L-type calcium channels, thus permitting an influx of calcium. In addition, the glutamate channels present on horizontal cells are themselves permeable to calcium, providing a second pathway for the influx of extracellular calcium into the interior of the

cells (Linn and Christensen, 1992; Malchow and Ramsey, 1999). Finally, the influx of extracellular calcium is likely to lead to calcium-dependent calcium release in the horizontal cells, further elevating intracellular calcium levels. Given our results with caffeine and thapsigargin, we would expect the transport of GABA into horizontal cells to be reduced by these increases in calcium. Our hypothesis would also suggest that direct application of glutamate onto horizontal cells should lead to down-regulation of the GABA transporter, and indeed we have obtained preliminary evidence indicating that the transport of GABA into voltage-clamped horizontal cells is reduced by prior applications of glutamate. It is also important to recall that the transport of GABA into cells is highly voltage-dependent, with depolarization significantly reducing the transport of GABA into cells. Thus, in the intact retina, the depolarization of horizontal cells induced by the glutamate released by photoreceptors by itself should also result in decreased uptake of GABA. Finally, the elevation in intracellular calcium brought about in darkness in the horizontal cells is likely to enhance vesicular-dependent GABA release from the these cells.

We have previously reported that extracellular ATP can also down-regulate the transport of GABA into skate horizontal cells (Malchow and Andersen, 1999; 2000). Interestingly, our current data support the hypothesis that modulation by ATP occurs via a calcium-independent process. In experiments measuring intracellular calcium levels in isolated horizontal cells using the calcium-indicator dye Fura-2, we find that while glutamate and the glutamate analogue kainate both elevate calcium, 1 mM ATP produces no change in intracellular calcium levels in non-voltage clamped external horizontal cells. It appears, therefore, that there are multiple and independent pathways by which the GABA transporter of skate horizontal cells can be modulated (Fig. 6).

Where and when is the ATP released? One likely source would be from the photoreceptor terminals themselves, which are believed to be continuously liberating glutamate in the dark. If this were true, then peak quantities of ATP would likely be released also in the dark, acting to still further depress the transport of GABA into the horizontal cells. We thus envision that the calcium-independent ATP-mediated down regulation of the transport of GABA into horizontal cells might be acting synergistically with the calcium-dependent modulation of the transporter to increase the post-synaptic effects of vesicularly released GABA in the synaptic cleft, again potentially enhancing the contribution of the surround portion of the receptive field. There is little data available with respect to which cells in the retina release ATP and under what lighting conditions, and this will likely be an area receiving much experimental attention in the future.

Conclusion and perspectives

Many questions concerning the regulation of the GABA transporter of horizontal cells remain to be answered. The cellular signal transduction pathways involved in the down-regulation by calcium and ATP

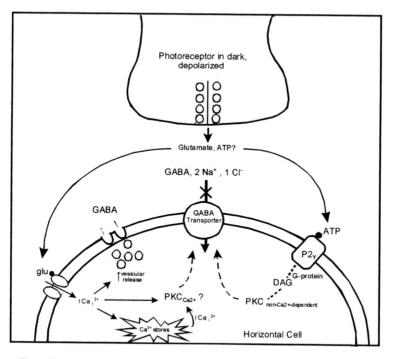

Fig. 6. Schematic diagram illustrating our working hypothesis concerning modulatory pathways of GABA transport in retinal horizontal cells. Two pathways appear to be capable of modulation of the uptake of GABA into horizontal cells: an ATP-activated, calcium independent pathway, and a calcium-dependent pathway involving the activation of internal stores of calcium in the horizontal cell.

remain to be completely established. Our preliminary data suggest that a calcium-independent protein kinase C may play an important role in the ATP-modulation of GABA transport, and experiments are planned to determine if the calcium-dependent modulation relies upon activation of a calcium-sensitive isoform of the enzyme. Also, our present set of experiments have examined only the influx of GABA; we have not yet directly examined the effects of calcium or ATP on carrier-mediated efflux. It is conceivable that efflux through the transporter could be either enhanced or depressed by these agents, and experiments are underway to address these questions. Ultimately, we expect that the model system that Dowling and Ripps originally found so fruitful will continue to yield vital information about the nature of synaptic processing within the outer plexiform layer of the vertebrate retina.

Acknowledgments

This work was supported by grant EYO9411 from the National Eye Institute, a Campus Research Board grant from the University of Illinois at Chicago, and a core grant (EY01792) to the Department of Ophthalmology. We would like to thank Mr. Marek Mori for expert machine shop assistance, Dr. Haohua Qian for his many thoughtful discussions on this manuscript in particular and retinal function in general, and Drs. Ripps and Dowling for their insight, friendship, and past years of fruitful collaborative efforts.

References

Ayoub, G.S. and Lam, D.M. (1984) The release of gamma-aminobutyric acid from horizontal cells of the goldfish (Carassius auratus) retina. J. Physiol. (Lond.), 355: 191–214.

Brecha, N.C. and Weigmann, C. (1994) Expression of GAT-1, a high-affinity gamma-aminobutyric acid plasma membrane transporter in the rat retina. J. Comp. Neurol., 345: 602–611.

Cammack, J.N. and Schwartz E.A. (1993) Ions required for the electrogenic transport of GABA by horizontal cells of the catfish retina. J. Physiol. (Lond.), 472: 81–102.

Djamgoz, M.B.A. (1995) Diversity of GABA receptors in the vertebrate outer retina. Trends Neurosci., 18: 118–120.

Dong, C.J., Picaud, S.A. and Werblin, F.S. (1994) GABA transporters and GABAC-like receptors on catfish cone- but not rod-driven horizontal cells. J. Neurosci., 14: 2648–2658.

Dowling, J.E. and Ripps, H. (1970) Visual adaptation in the retina of the skate. J. Gen. Physiol., 56: 491–520.

Dowling, J.E. and Ripps, H. (1971) S-potentials in the skate retina. Intracellular recordings during light and dark adaptation. J. Gen. Physiol., 58: 163–189.

Dowling, J.E. and Ripps, H. (1972) Adaptation in skate photoreceptors. J. Gen. Physiol., 60: 698–719.

Dowling, J.E. and Ripps, H. (1973) Effect of magnesium on horizontal cell activity in the skate retina. Nature, 242: 101–103.

Ekstrom, P. and Anzelius, M. (1998) GABA and GABA-transporter (GAT-1) immunoreactivities in the retina of the salmon (Salmon salar L.). Brain Res., 812: 179–185.

Freed, M.A. (1992) GABAergic circuits in the mammalian retina. Prog. Brain Res., 90: 107–131.

Haugh-Scheidt, L., Malchow, R.P. and Ripps, H. (1995) GABA transport and calcium dynamics in horizontal cells from the skate retina. J. Physiol. (Lond.), 488: 565–576.

Hille, B. (1992) Ionic channels of excitable membranes. Sutherland, MA: Sinauer Associates.

Iversen, L.L. (1971) Role of transmitter uptake mechanisms in synaptic transmission. Br. J. Pharmacol., 41: 571–591.

Iversen, L.L. and Kelly, J.S. (1975) Uptake and metabolism of gamma-aminobutyric acid by neurons and glial cells. Biochem. Pharmacol. 24: 933–938.

Johnson, J., Chen, T.K., Rickman, D.W., Evans, C. and Brecha, N.C. (1996) Multiple gamma-Aminobutyric acid plasma membrane transporters (GAT-1, GAT-2, GAT-3) in the rat retina. J. Comp. Neurol., 375: 212–224.

Karwoski, C.J. and Proenza, L.M. (1987) Sources and sinks of light-evoked delta [K +]o in the vertebrate retina. Can. J. Physiol. Pharmacol., 65: 1009–1017.

Kline, R.P., Ripps, H. and Dowling, J.E. (1985) Light-induced potassium fluxes in the skate retina. Neuroscience, 14: 225–235.

Larsson, O.M., Falch, E., Krogsgaard-Larsen, P. and Schousboe, A (1988) Kinetic characterization of inhibition of gamma-aminobutyric acid uptake into cultured neurons and astrocytes by 4,4-diphenyl-3-butenyl derivatives of nipecotic acid and guvacine. J. Neurochem. 50: 818–823.

Lewin, L., Mattsson, M.O., Grahn, B. and Sellstrom, A, (1994) Inhibition of SKF 89976-A of the gamma-aminobutyric acid release from primary neuronal chick cultures. Acta Physiol. Scand., 152: 173–179.

Linn, C.P. and Christensen, B.N. (1992) Excitatory amino acid regulation of intracellular Ca2 + in isolated catfish cone horizontal cells measured under voltage- and concentration-clamp conditions. J. Neurosci., 12: 2156–2164.

Liu, Q.R., Lopez-Corcuera, B., Mandiyan, S., Nelson, H. and Nelson, N. (1993) Molecular characterization of four pharmacologically distinct gamma-aminobutyric acid trans-porters in mouse brain [corrected] [published erratum appers in J. Biol. Chem. 1993 Apr 25; 268(12): 9156]. J. Biol. Chem., 268: 2106–2112.

Malchow, R.P., Qian, H.H., Ripps, H. and Dowling, J.E. (1990a) Structural and functional properties of two types of horizontal cell in the skate retina. *J. Gen. Physiol.*, 95: 177–198.

Malchow, R.P. and Ripps, H. (1990) Effects of gamma-aminobutyric acid on skate retinal horizontal cells: evidence for an electrogenic uptake mechanism. *Proc. Natl. Acad. Sci. USA*, 87: 8945–8949.

Malchow, R.P. and Andersen, K.A. (1999) Purinergic modulation of the gamma-aminobutyric acid (GABA) transporter present in horizontal retinal cells. *Soc. Neurosci. Abs.*, 25: 1430

Malchow, R.P. and Andersen, K.A. (2000) Modulation of GABA transport in skate retinal horizontal cells by extra-cellular ATP. *Invest. Ophthalmol. Vis. Sci.*, 40: S113

Malchow, R.P. and Ramsey, D.J. (1999) Responses of retinal Muller cells to neurotransmitter candidates: a comparative survey. *Biol. Bull.* 197: 229–230.

Marc, R.E. (1992) Structural organization of GABAergic circuitry in ectotherm retinas. *Prog. Brain Res.*, 90: 61–92.

Qian, H. and Dowling, J.E. (1993) Novel GABA responses from rod-driven retinal horizontal cells. *Nature*, 361: 162–164.

Sakai, H.M. and Naka, K. (1986) Synaptic organization of the cone horizontal cells in the catfish retina. *J. Comp. Neurol.*, 245: 107–115.

Schloss, P., Puschel, A.W. and Betz, H. (1994) Neurotransmitter transporters: new members of known families. *Curr. Opin. Cell Biol.*, 6: 595–599.

Schwartz, E.A. (1982) Calcium-independent release of GABA from isolated horizontal cells of the toad retina. *J. Physiol. (Lond.)*, 323: 211–227.

Schwartz, E.A. (1987) Depolarization without calcium can release gamma-aminobutyric acid from a retinal neuron. *Science*, 238: 350–355.

Treiman, M., Caspersen, C. and Christensen, S.B. (1998) A tool coming of age: thapsigargin as an inhibitor of sarco-endoplasmic reticulum Ca(2 +)-ATPases. *Trends Pharmacol. Sci.*, 19: 131–135.

Wu, S.M. (1992a) Feedback connections and operation of the outer plexiform layer of the retina. *Curr. Opin. Neurobiol.*, 2: 462–468.

Wu, S.M. (1992b) Functional organization of GABAergic circuitry in ectotherm retinas. *Prog. Brain Res.*, 90: 93–106.

Yang, C.Y., Brecha, N.C. and Tsao, E. (1997) Immunocyto-chemical localization of gamma-aminobutyric acid plasma membrane transporters in the tiger salamander retina. *J. Comp. Neurol.*, 389: 117–126.

Yazulla, S. (1983) Stimulation of GABA release from retinal horizontal cells by potassium and acidic amino acid agonists. *J. Gen. Physiol.*, 275: 61–74.

Yazulla, S. and Kleinschmidt, J. (1983) Carrier-mediated release of GABA from retinal horizontal cells. *Brain Res.*, 263: 63–75.

Yazulla, S., Cunnihgham, J. and Neal, M. (1985) Stimulated release of endogenous GABA and glycine from the goldfish retina. *Brain Res.*, 345: 384–388.

Yazulla, S. (1986) GABAergic mechanisms in the retina. *Prog. Ret. Res.*, 5: 1–52.

H. Kolb, H. Ripps and S. Wu (Eds.)
Progress in Brain Research, Vol. 131
© 2001 Elsevier Science B.V. All rights reserved

CHAPTER 19

Physiological and pharmacological characterization of glutamate and GABA receptors on carp retinal neurons

Xiong-Li Yang*, Ping Li, Tao Lu, Ying Shen and Ming-Hu Han

*Institute of Neurobiology, Fudan University and Shanghai Institute of Physiology,
Chinese Academy of Sciences, 220 Han-Dan Road, Shanghai 200433, China*

Introduction

Glutamate is a major excitatory neurotransmitter in the retina. Photoreceptors and bipolar cells in most vertebrate species release glutamate, which changes the activity of the postsynaptic neurons (horizontal and bipolar cells for photoreceptors in the outer retina; amacrine and ganglion cells for bipolar cells in the inner retina) by directly altering membrane permeability to ions and/or by activating intracellular enzyme systems (for review, see Barnstable, 1993). In the study of photoreceptor transmitters, Dowling and Ripps (1972), in addition to other labs (Cervetto and MacNichol, 1972; Murakami et al., 1972), first showed that L-glutamate depolarized horizontal cells in skate, suggesting that this agent may be a photoreceptor neurotransmitter. Later, Dowling and his colleagues initiated a series of important studies on the pharmacological properties of isolated horizontal cells, further strengthening this supposition and providing insights into the mechanism of action of L-glutamate on horizontal cells (Lasater and Dowling, 1982; Dowling et al., 1983; Lasater et al., 1984).

It is known that there are at least five subtypes of glutamate receptors: kainate, α-amino-3-hydroxy-5-methyl-4-isoxazolepropionic acid (AMPA), N-methyl-D-aspartate (NMDA), L-AP4 and trans-1-aminocyclopentane-1, 3-dicarboxylic acid (ACPD) receptors (Hollmann and Heinemann, 1994). The first three receptors are all ionotropic. The L-AP4 receptor appears to be an autoreceptor which self-regulates the release of neurotransmitter. The ACPD receptor is believed to be involved in activating inositol phosphate (IP) metabolism.

On the other hand, γ-Aminobutyric acid (GABA) is a principal inhibitory neurotransmitter in the retina. It is known to be released by most horizontal and amacrine cells, and it modulates the function of bipolar cells, ganglion cells and even photoreceptors (Yazulla, 1986). GABA receptors are categorized into three subtypes ($GABA_{A/B/C}$ receptors). $GABA_A$ receptors are ionotropic, which means that they are directly coupled to anion channels, and thus cause an increase in chloride permeability of the postsynaptic membranes. $GABA_B$ receptors belong to the family of G-protein coupled receptors and act via intracellular second messengers, resulting in an increased K^+ conductance and the inhibition of voltage-sensitive Ca^{2+} channels (Bormann, 1988). The novel $GABA_C$ receptor, recently added to the above subtypes, like the $GABA_A$ subtype, consists of chloride channels, but is insensitive to the specific $GABA_A$ receptor antagonist bicuculline (BIC) and the $GABA_B$ agonist baclofen (Lukasiewicz, 1996;

* Corresponding author: Xiong-Li Yang, Tel.: (8621)5561-2874; Fax: (8621)5561-2876; E-mail: xlyang@fudan.edu.cn

Cherubini and Strata, 1997). In the retina, Dowling and his colleagues first showed novel $GABA_C$ receptor mediated responses from rod-driven horizontal cells (Qian and Dowling, 1993) and then studied the $GABA_C$ responses from bipolar cells (Qian and Dowling, 1995).

In recent years our laboratory has tried to characterize glutamate receptors of horizontal and amacrine cells, and GABA receptors of bipolar and amacrine cells in carp retina, using patch-clamp techniques. We have also examined the modulation by Zn^{2+}, an endogenous retinal modulator, of the AMPA receptors of horizontal cells and the GABA receptors of bipolar and amacrine cells. We have further found a strong synergistic interaction between the $GABA_A$ receptor and the glycine receptor in the amacrine cells. In this chapter we review some of the results.

Glutamate receptors of horizontal cells

Characterization of receptor subtype and splice variant composition

Glutamate depolarizes horizontal cells, which is associated with a suppression of their light responses. In most cases, L-AP4 and NMDA fail to induce any responses from horizontal cells, whereas the actions of kainate and AMPA on both membrane potential and light responses mimic those of glutamate. These actions persist even after the release of glutamate from the pre-synaptic terminals is blocked by cobalt ions, suggesting that they act on horizontal cells, but not on the presynaptic cells (Yang and Wu, 1991a). Furthermore, kainate- and AMPA-induced depolarization of horizontal cells could be completely blocked by CNQX, a specific antagonist of non-NMDA receptors (Yang and Wu, 1991a). All these results indicate that there are AMPA/KA receptors on horizontal cells.

The current responses to glutamate and AMPA recorded from isolated horizontal cells, using the whole-cell configuration of the patch clamp technique, in combination with a rapid solution changer, are very similar and show significant and rapid desensitization (Fig. 1a and 1b). That is, the currents

rapidly decrease to a steady state level of much lower amplitude (equilibrium state) soon after they reach a peak value. The time constant of desensitization is less than 2 ms. In contrast, the responses induced by kainate are invariably sustained and no desensitization is observed (Fig. 1c). We have determined the values of EC_{50} (the concentration of ligand producing half-maximal response) for glutamate- and AMPA-induced peak currents as about 1 mM, nearly 7-fold higher than that for kainate (Lu et al., 1998). These results are consistent with the pharmacological characteristics of AMPA receptors, suggesting that the glutamate receptor on horizontal cells may be an AMPA preferring subtype.

A selective AMPA receptor antagonist, GYKI 53655, has been recently developed (Lerma et al., 1997). GYKI 53655 completely blocks glutamate-induced currents in horizontal cells at a very low concentration (10 μM) (Fig. 2a and 2b), further strengthening the notion that horizontal cells may exclusively express the AMPA subtype of glutamate receptors (Lu et al., 1998).

Desensitization is a ubiquitous characteristic of ligand-gated channels. Microscopically, desensitization is thought of as a process in which receptors enter a deactivation state from the resting or open state (Jones and Westbrook, 1996). Much evidence has revealed that there exist two alternative splice variants named flip and flop, which are generated by the gene splicing in RNA editing (Sommer et al., 1990). The two splice variants each have different physiological properties (Mosbacher et al., 1994; Partin et al., 1996). In both native and recombinant receptors, it was reported that differences in the proportion of flip/flop variants at AMPA receptors may result in different rates and extents of desensitization (Sommer et al., 1990). In expressed glutamate receptors, some desensitization modulators have been found to differentially modulate flip and flop receptors and thus used to identify splice variants composing glutamate receptors (Partin et al., 1994; Johansen et al., 1995; Sekiguchi et al., 1997). Therefore, we have examined the effects of the desensitization modulators concanavalin A (Con A), cyclothiazide (CTZ), aniracetam and 4-[2-(phenylanl-fonylamino)ethylthio]-2, 6-difluoro-pheynoxy acetamide (PEPA), on AMPA receptors-mediated responses in horizontal cells (Shen et al., 1999a).

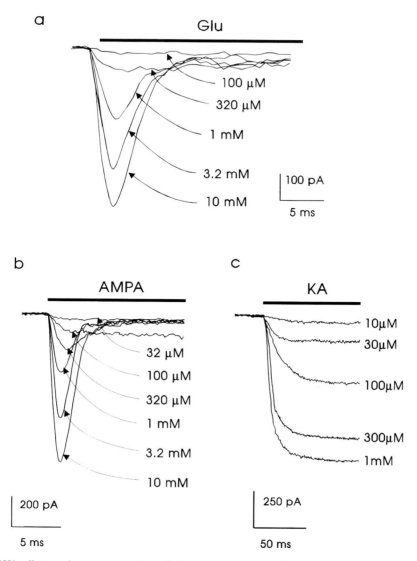

Fig. 1. Responses of H1 cells to various concentrations of glutamate receptor agonists. (a, b, c) responses from three different H1 cells to various concentrations of glutamate (Glu), AMPA and kainate (KA), respectively. Note that the responses to glutamate and AMPA, but not to kainate, usually show striking desensitization. With the application of glutamate and AMPA, peak currents steadily increased with increasing concentrations of these agonists (indicated by arrows), while the equilibrium currents did not. Durations of drug application are indicated by the horizontal bars above each set of responses. Adapted from Lu et al. (1998).

Incubation with Con A suppresses the peak response but weakly potentiates the equilibrium response of horizontal cells to glutamate. CTZ blocks glutamate-induced desensitization in a dose-dependent manner, which results in a steady increase of the equilibrium current and shifts the dose-response relationship of the equilibrium current to the right, but slightly suppresses the kainate-induced sustained current. In

reference to the results obtained in *Xenopus* oocytes, HEK cells and other neurons (Partin et al., 1993; Wong and Mayer, 1993), these effects of Con A and CTZ not only further demonstrate that glutamate receptors expressed in carp horizontal cells may be an AMPA preferring subtype, but also led us to speculate that these receptors may predominantly carry the flop splice variants. This speculation is

280

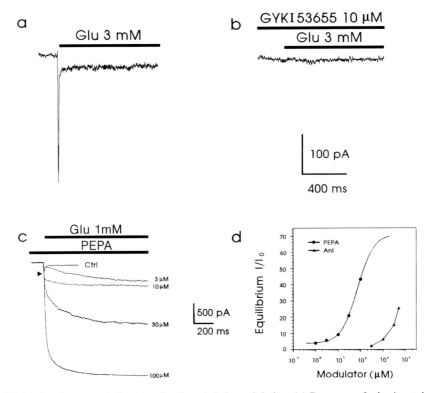

Fig. 2. Glutamate (Glu)-induced currents in horizontal cells and their modulation. (a) Response of a horizontal cell to application of 3 mM glutamate, showing significant desensitization. (b) In the continuous presence of 10 μM GYKI 53655, glutamate fails to induce any response from the same cell. (c) Responses of another horizontal cell to 1 mM glutamate in the presence of PEPA of increasing concentrations. Control (Ctrl) peak response is marked by a triangle. (d) PEPA (circle) and aniracetam (triangle) dose-response relationships for modulation of 1 mM glutamate-induced responses. Ordinate is fold potentiation given as the equilibrium current (I) induced by co-application of PEPA and glutamate/the corresponding response (I_0) recorded without PEPA. Adapted from Lu et al. (1998) and Shen et al. (1999a).

further supported by the actions of aniracetam and PEPA, both flop-preferring modulators of AMPA receptors, on glutamate-induced responses of horizontal cells. These chemicals have been found to considerably block desensitization of glutamate-induced currents in horizontal cells in a dose-dependent manner, but only slightly potentiate kainate-induced currents (Johansen et al., 1995; Sekiguchi et al., 1997), Fig. 2c shows how the response of a horizontal cell to 1 mM glutamate is potentiated by PEPA of increasing concentrations. For comparison, potentiation-dose relationships for aniracetam and PEPA are shown in Fig. 2d. It is evident that PEPA is 1000 fold more potent than aniracetam at these receptors (Shen et al., 1999a). These experiments all suggest that the AMPA

receptor on carp horizontal cells may be predominantly assembled from flop splice variants.

Zn^{2+} modulation of AMPA receptors

Zn^{2+} has been demonstrated to be present in synaptic vesicles of a subset of glutamatergic boutons in certain brain regions. It is believed to function as an endogenous modulator of ligand- and voltage-gated ion channels when co-released with glutamate into the synapse during activity. In the outer retina, Zn^{2+} is localized in the terminals of photoreceptors, providing a possibility that Zn^{2+} may be released from the terminals and thus modulate the activities of retinal second-order neurons (Wu et al., 1993).

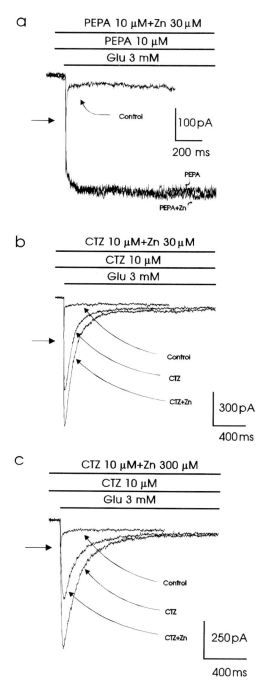

Fig. 3. Zn^{2+} fails to modulate PEPA-potentiated responses, but it has dual effect on cyclothiazide-potentiated glutamate responses of H1 cells. (a) Response of an H1 cell to 3 mM glutamate is greatly potentiated by 10 μM PEPA, and the addition of 30 μM Zn^{2+} hardly changes the response. (b,c) Responses of two isolated H1 cells to 3 mM glutamate (Glu) recorded in normal Ringer's (control), in the presence of 10 μM

Previous work has shown that Zn^{2+} has different effects on NMDA and non-NMDA receptors expressed in *Xenopus* oocytes (Rassendren et al., 1990) and that the action of Zn^{2+} may correlate with receptor structures and/or splice variants (Hollmann et al., 1993). The results described above have demonstrated that glutamate responses of carp horizontal cells consist of a major component mediated by the AMPA receptor flop splice variant, with a minor contribution from the flip splice variant (Shen et al., 1999a).

To investigate whether Zn^{2+} modulation might be relevant to splice variants, PEPA, a flop variant-preferring AMPA receptor potentiator, and cyclothiazide, a flip variant-preferring AMPA receptor potentiator (Johansen et al., 1995), were used to "amplify" the corresponding components of glutamate responses mediated by the flop and flip variants respectively, and then the effects of Zn^{2+} on these "amplified" components were examined (Shen and Yang, 1999). It was found that the PEPA-amplified component of the glutamate (3 mM) response was not changed much by 30 μM Zn^{2+} (Fig. 3a). In contrast, Zn^{2+} had a dual effect on the cyclothiazide-amplified glutamate peak responses: potentiating them at a low concentration (30 μM) (Fig. 3b), but suppressing them at a higher concentration (300 μM) (Fig. 3c). This dual effect is quite similar to results reported for AMPA receptors of superior colliculus neurons and those expressed in *Xenopus* oocytes (Bresink et al., 1996; Rassendren et al., 1990), which consist of flip splice variants. For comparison, we examined the effects of Zn^{2+} on isolated hippocampal neurons which were demonstrated pharmacologically to be flip variant-dominated. For these cells 30 μM Zn^{2+} caused a large potentiation of the glutamate response, which is consistent with the observation that excitatory transmission at the CA3 neuron synapses could be modulated by Zn^{2+} (Hesse, 1979). Taken together, these results suggest that Zn^{2+} modulation of the AMPA receptor may be relevant to splice variants and Zn^{2+} may exert differential effects on glutamatergic transmission

cyclothiazide (CTZ), and under co-application of cyclothiazide and Zn^{2+} (CTZ + Zn). Zn^{2+} concentration is 30 μM (b) and 300 μM (c), respectively. Control response peaks are marked by arrows. Adapted from Shen and Yang (1999).

mediated by receptors consisting of different splice variants.

Glutamate receptors of amacrine cells

Characterization of receptor subtype

In the inner retina amacrine cells receive glutamatergic synaptic input from bipolar cells (Dowling, 1987), and morphological evidence indicates the expression of glutamate receptors in amacrine cells (Brandstäter et al., 1998). In addition, depolarizing responses of amacrine cells to glutamate receptor agonists have been demonstrated electrophysiologically (Dixon and Copenhagen, 1992). Our analysis of glutamate receptors on carp amacrine cells (Shen et al., 1999b) yields results similar to those obtained with horizontal cells.

Whole-cell inward membrane currents induced from carp amacrine cells by glutamate show significant desensitization. In contrast, kainate invariably induces sustained currents from these cells. GYKI 53655 completely blocks the response of amacrine cells to 10 mM glutamate (Fig. 4), suggesting that amacrine cells, like horizontal cells, may predominantly express AMPA receptors.

Single channel conductance of AMPA receptors

Single channel properties of the AMPA receptors of carp amacrine cells have been determined from the fluctuations of kainate-induced non-desensitizing currents. In these experiments, amacrine cells were voltage-clamped at -60 mV and five different concentrations of kainate were applied. As shown in Fig. 5a, the current fluctuations of the equilibrium responses are comparatively small at lower and higher concentrations of kainate, but relatively larger at the intermediate concentration (100 μM), which is close to the EC_{50} of the kainite-induced current (97.5 μM). The current (I) versus variance (σ) relationship could be reasonably well filled with the equation: $\sigma^2 = iI - (i^2/N)$, where the unitary current (i) and the channel number (N) of AMPA receptors were derived to be 0.380 pA and 1202, respectively, for this cell (Fig. 5b). Since the reversal potential of the kainate current is 0 mV and the holding potential

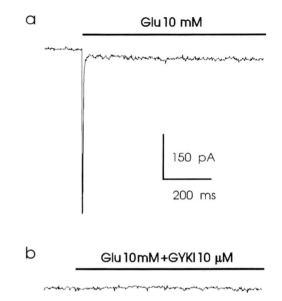

Fig. 4. GYKI 53655 completely blocks glutamate-induced currents from amacrine cells. (a) Response of an amacrine cell to application of 10 mM glutamate (Glu). (b) In the continuous presence of 10 μM GYKI 53655 (GYKI), glutamate fails to induce any response from the cell. Adapted from Shen et al (1999b).

is -60 mV, γ_{noise} (single channel conductance) was calculated to be 6.33 pS for this cell. Based on the same kind of analysis made for 12 other cells, the mean γ_{noise} was 5.70 ± 1.67 pS, close to the values obtained in recombinant receptors (Swanson et al., 1997) and white perch retinal horizontal cells (Schimidt, 1997). The mean number of AMPA was 1643 ± 1063.

Splice variant composition

PEPA and CTZ were used to study the splice variant composition of amacrine cells. CTZ potentiates both the glutamate peak and equilibrium currents and potentiation caused by 100 μM CTZ is nearly a 10-fold increase over control values. 100 μM PEPA, however, produces a nearly a 50-fold increase of the glutamate response. It was recently reported that a comparison of the actions of PEPA versus CTZ (P/C ratio) facilitates the detection of the splice variant heterogeneity (Sekiguchi et al., 1998). The P/C ratio for the glutamate equilibrium current of the amacrine

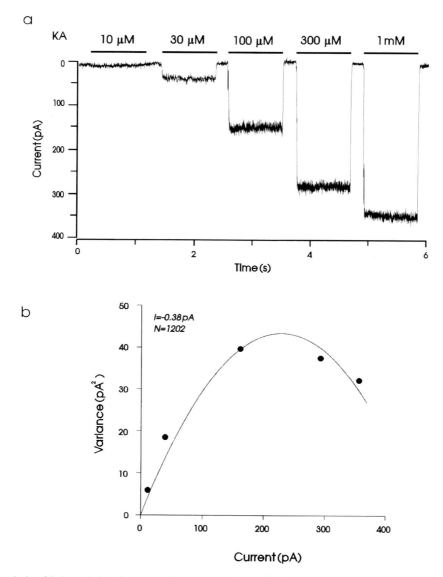

Fig. 5. Fluctuation analysis of kainate-induced currents from an amacrine cell. (a) Responses of an amacrine cell to five different concentrations of kainate (KA). Duration of drug application is indicated by the horizontal bars above the responses. (b) The variance of the current fluctuations (V_{Hold} of -60 mV; V_{Rev} of 0 mV) is plotted against the current amplitude. The curve is the expected variance from the equation: $\sigma^2 = iI - (i^2/N)$, for 2102 channels with a conductance level of 6.33 pS. Abscissa is response amplitude; ordinate is the total variance of all sampling points of whole steady-state currents recorded at different concentrations. Note that the plot of the current variance versus current the amplitude is parabolic. Adapted from Shen et al. (1999b).

cells is high (4.39) (see Fig. 6), suggesting that these cells carry the flop splice variants (Shen et al., 1999b).

Rather fast kinetics of the flop AMPA receptors in amacrine cells may contribute to the conversion of sustained light responses of retinal bipolar cells into transient signals of amacrine cells. Dixon and Copenhagen (1992) found that the light-induced

excitation of amacrine cells is mediated principally through glutamatergic synapses from bipolar cells and these transient responses are not the result of any voltage- or time-dependent conductance in the postsynaptic amacrine cell membrane. However, voltage-dependent calcium current through $GABA_B$ receptors in bipolar cell terminals, possibly truncating

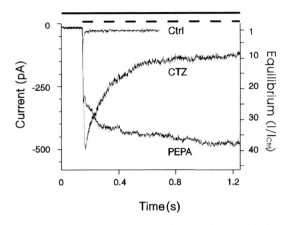

Fig. 6. Comparison of potentiation of 3 mM glutamate-induced currents (Ctrl) by 30 μM cyclothiazide (CTZ) and PEPA from a single amacrine cell. Duration of drug application is indicated by the horizontal bars above the responses; dashed for glutamate and solid for modulators. 1 and 10 are current amplitudes with or without modulators, respectively. Adapted from Shen et al. (1999b).

neurotransmitter release, may be crucial to this conversion (Maguire et al., 1989). Another work, however, suggests that the formation of transient responses of ganglion cells may be due to a different mechanism because baclofen enhances ganglion cell transient responses (Slaughter and Bai, 1989). Desensitization of glutamate receptors is also supposed to participate in shaping light responses of ganglion cells, as cyclothiazide was found to enhance the amplitude and duration of both the on and off light-evoked excitatory postsynaptic currents recorded in ON–OFF ganglion cells (Lukasiewicz et al., 1995), suggesting the involvement of AMPA/ KA receptors. Although no similar work has been conducted in amacrine cells, it could be also the case for these cells.

Gaba receptors of bipolar cells

Characterization of receptor subtypes

Most horizontal and amacrine cells are GABAergic in the retina. Bipolar cells receive feedforward signals from both photoreceptors and horizontal cells in the outer plexiform layer (Yang and Wu, 1991b) and feedback signals from amacrine cells via the reciprocal synapses in the inner plexiform layer (Muller and

Marc, 1990). GABA was recently found to suppress light responses of the color-opponent bipolar cells, which respond to red and green lights with depolarization and hyperpolarization respectively, with the response driven by input from red cones being invariably suppressed to a greater extent. Both $GABA_A$ and $GABA_C$ receptors on bipolar cells may be involved in this suppression (Zhang and Yang, 1997).

We have systematically studied the GABA receptor mediated whole cell responses in carp rod-dominant ON bipolar cells. These cells have an enlarged characteristic axon terminal (Tachibana and Kaneko, 1987), which is easily identified in the light microscope after enzyme digestion and mechanical trituration (Lu and Yang, 1995).

GABA application induces inward currents with significant desensitization in bipolar cells (Fig. 7a). Local application of GABA to the axon and dendrites of bipolar cells could both induce currents, suggesting that GABA released from both horizontal and amacrine cells may influence these cells. This result is consistent with observations made in bullfrog bipolar cells, using retinal slice preparations (Du and Yang, 2000). GABA-induced responses are only partially blocked by 800 μM BIC (Fig. 7b), and the remaining BIC-resistant component is insensitive to baclofen, but dramatically inhibited by the co-application of 14AA, a specific competitive $GABA_C$ receptor antagonist (Fig. 7c) (Han et al., 1997). These results clearly indicate that both $GABA_A$ and $GABA_C$ receptors co-exist in carp bipolar cells.

A number of authors claim that $GABA_C$ receptor-mediated responses show minimal desensitization in contrast to significant desensitization of $GABA_A$ receptor-mediated responses (Feigenspan et al., 1993; Calvo et al., 1994; Qian and Dowling, 1995). It has been suggested that $GABA_A$ receptors mediate transient signals, whereas $GABA_C$ receptors are important for mediating sustained signals (Qian and Dowling, 1995; Djamgoz, 1995). However, we found that the $GABA_C$ response induced from carp bipolar cells shows striking desensitization (see Fig. 7b), even with low concentrations (3 μM) of GABA (Han et al., 1997), suggesting that the $GABA_C$ receptor may play a role in mediating transient signal as well. Actually, it was found in isolated retina that

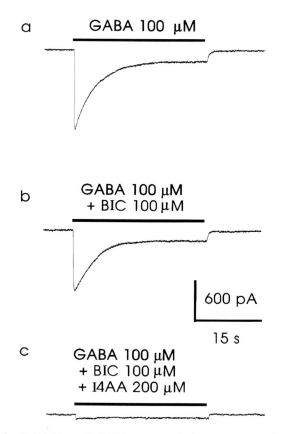

a

GABA 100 μM

b

GABA 100 μM
+ BIC 100 μM

600 pA

15 s

c

GABA 100 μM
+ BIC 100 μM
+ I4AA 200 μM

Fig. 7. GABA_A and GABA_C receptor-induced response of a rod-dominant ON bipolar cell. (a) inward current induced by 100 μM GABA. (b) GABA_C receptor-mediated current separated from the response to 100 μM GABA by application of 100 μM bicuculline (BIC). Note that the GABA_C receptor-mediated current shows striking desensitization. (c) the GABA_C current is potently suppressed by 200 μM I4AA. Adapted from Han et al. (1997).

suppression of transient responses of amacrine cells by GABA could be mediated by GABA_C receptors while suppression of sustained responses could be mediated by GABA_A receptors (Zhang et al., 1999). Existence of the desensitizing GABA_C receptor further suggests that there may exist several subtypes of GABA_C receptors, which may be distinct in intracellular mechanisms and/or subunit composition.

Kinetic characteristics of GABA receptors

Since GABA receptors modulate neuronal spiking, coincidence detection and the output of synchronized neuronal circuitry by affecting the inhibitory

postsynaptic current (IPSC) (McDonald and Olsen, 1994), it is speculated that the neural activity could be modulated at different levels by influencing the decay and duration of the IPSC. Now that we know GABA_A and GABA_C receptors coexist in bipolar cells, it is of interest to explore the differences in kinetics between these two receptors and how the receptor kinetics are modulated. It is essential to address these questions in order to understand the role of GABA in inhibitory synaptic transmission and its underlying mechanism.

Kinetic characteristics of GABA_A and GABA_C receptors studied in our experiments included activation, desensitization and deactivation. In these experiments, 100 μM BIC and 100 μM 14AA were used to suppress the GABA_A and GABA_C response components, respectively, so that the response kinetics of these components could be separately characterized. Step application of GABA allowed us to record the whole course of activation and desensitization of receptors, whereas the recovery of current after pulse application of GABA represented deactivation of receptors (Partin et al., 1996; Han et al., 2000). The top row of Fig. 8 shows a comparison of activation (a), desensitization (b) and deactivation (c) between GABA_C and GABA_A receptors of a bipolar cell.

Activation kinetics of both GABA_A and GABA_C receptors could be well fitted by monoexponential functions, but the time constant (τ) for the GABA_C component is much longer than that for the GABA_A component. Similarly, although both GABA_C and GABA_A receptors desensitize during continued application of GABA, desensitization of the former is much slower. Moreover, the desensitization of the GABA_C response is well fitted by a monoexponential function, while the decay of the GABA_A response is characterized by a fast and a slow component, suggesting that the mechanisms underlying desensitization of the two receptors are different. Furthermore, the sum of two (a fast and a slow) exponentials is required to adequately describe deactivation of both receptors, with the GABA_C being much slower. Overall, the GABA_C receptor has slower kinetics than the GABA_A receptor on the bipolar cells (Han et al., 2000).

It was reported that GABA inhibits the Ca^{2+} influx into bipolar cell terminals, which is mediated

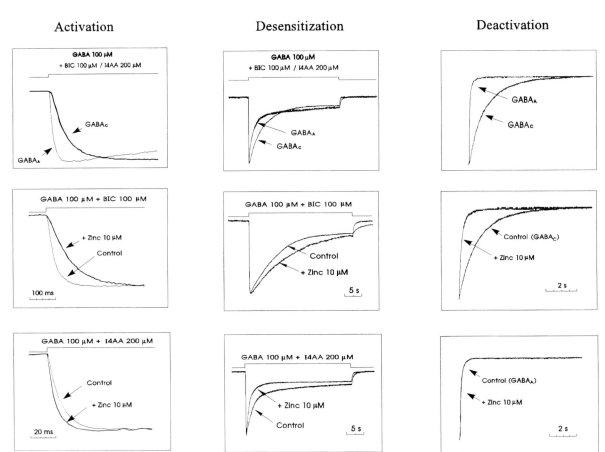

Fig. 8. Comparison of kinetic characteristics of GABA$_C$ and GABA$_A$ receptors on bipolar cells and differential modulation by Zn^{2+} of activation (a), desensitization (b) and deactivation (c) of GABA$_C$ and GABA$_A$ responses. BIC, bicuculline. The kinetics of GABA$_C$ is slower than that of GABA$_A$, and the responses are both normalized in the upper panel. The effects of 10 μM Zn^{2+} on the GABA$_C$ and GABA$_A$ responses recorded from a single bipolar cell are shown in middle and bottom panels, respectively. For comparison, control and Zn^{2+} responses are normalized. Note the differences in time scales for different panels. Adapted from Han and Yang (1999) and Han et al. (2000).

via both GABA$_A$ and GABA$_C$ receptors (Matthews et al., 1994). Activation of GABA$_A$ receptors suppresses the Ca^{2+} influx with fast kinetics and a narrow dynamic range, whereas GABA$_C$ receptors cause inhibition of the Ca^{2+} influx with slow onset and a wider dynamic range (Pan and Lipton, 1995). This difference is apparently due to the distinct kinetics of these two receptors. It is intriguing to speculate that the desensitizing GABA$_C$ receptors may be involved in processing relatively slower signals, whereas the GABA$_A$ receptors may mainly participate in relatively faster signal transmission.

Zn^{2+} modulation of GABA receptor kinetics

In the salamander retina, Zn^{2+} blocks the GABA-induced depolarization of horizontal cells (Wu et al., 1993). In skate bipolar cells, the GABA$_C$-induced responses are invariably down-regulated in amplitude by Zn^{2+} (Qian and Dowling, 1995; Qian et al., 1997). In regard to the modulation of GABA$_A$-induced responses by Zn^{2+}, the results now available are inconsistent. Unlike the significant potentiation of GABA$_A$ responses by low concentrations (0.1–100 μM) of Zn^{2+} in skate bipolar cells (Qian et al., 1997), we consistently observed suppression of the GABA$_A$ responses by Zn^{2+} on carp bipolar cells (Han and Yang, 1999).

Our recent results further show that Zn^{2+} exerts differential effects on the kinetics of the GABA$_A$ and GABA$_C$ responses (middle and bottom rows of Fig. 8): it slows down activation and desensitization of the GABA$_C$ response whereas it accelerates those of the GABA$_A$ response; it accelerates deactivation of the GABA$_C$ response, but has no apparent effect on that of the GABA$_A$ response (Han and Yang, 1999).

Gaba receptors of amacrine cells

Characterization of receptor subtype

In the inner retina, GABA also plays important roles in shaping signal transmission (Yazulla, 1986; Dowling, 1987). Amacrine cells, which are involved in modulating receptive field properties of ganglion cells (Mangel, 1998), receive GABAergic input through serial synapses from neighboring amacrine cells (Dowling, 1987; Muller and Marc, 1990; Zhang et al., 1997). We have previously reported that exogenous GABA application preferentially suppresses the OFF light response of amacrine cells in isolated superfused carp retina (Zhang and Yang, 1997). Also, GABA$_A$ receptors have been demonstrated to be present on amacrine cells immunohistochemically (Grigorenko and Yeh, 1994; Wässle et al., 1998).

Whole-cell recordings were made from carp amacrine cells which are characterized by a small (10–12 μm in diameter) pyriform-shaped soma with one or two principal processes (see Fig. 1, Shen et al., 1999b). GABA could induce inward currents from these cells, which had a reversal potential of 0∼5 mV, close to the chloride equilibrium potential (3.8 mV under our experimental conditions). Fig. 9a shows the response of an amacrine cell to continued application of GABA (100 μM), which showed significant desensitization. The GABA-induced current could be completely abolished by co-application of 100 μM bicuculline (Fig. 9b), but not by I4AA (200 μM) (Fig. 9c), suggesting that the response was exclusively mediated by activation of GABA$_A$ receptors.

Strong synergism between GABA$_A$ and glycine receptors

Analysis of the synaptic organization in the inner retina indicates that GABAergic and glycinergic neurons, which make up the majority of amacrine cells, have extensive interactions between their dendrites (Muller and Marc, 1990; Yazulla and Studholme, 1991). GABA receptors and glycine

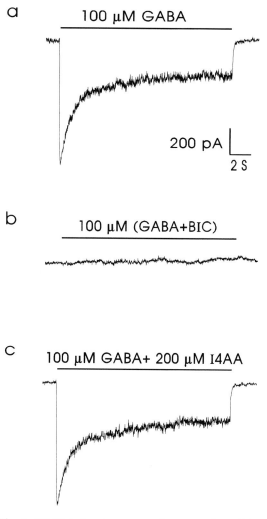

Fig. 9. GABA-induced response of an amacrine cell in carp retina. (a) The response to 100 μM GABA shows pronounced desensitization. (b) The GABA current is completely abolished by co-application of 100 μM bicuculline (BIC) (c) The GABA$_C$ receptor antagonist, I4AA, hardly affects the GABA-induced current. The recordings were made when the cell was clamped at −60 mV. Adapted from Li and Yang (1998).

receptors may also coexist on retinal third-order neurons (Zhou and Fain, 1995). It is generally thought that interactions can take place between receptors for chemical signals at the neuronal membrane level (receptor–receptor interaction) (Zoli et al., 1993). That is, a neurotransmitter, while binding to its receptor, can modulate the characteristics of the receptor for another transmitter. It has been shown that glycine-induced responses of carp amacrine cells are completely blocked by co-application of strychnine, whereas the addition of 5,7-dichlorokynurenic acid (DCKA), has no apparent effect (Li and Yang, 1998). It is likely that there are only strychnine-sensitive glycine receptors on these cells. We have found that there is a strong synergistic interaction between the $GABA_A$ and glycine receptors on isolated carp amacrine cells.

In 58 out of 153 cells (37.9%) tested, GABA and glycine of 10 μM induce no distinguishable (n = 53) or small currents (< 20 pA, n = 5) when applied alone, but co-application of the two chemicals at this concentration caused a substantial response potentiation (403.05 ± 319.98 pA). This phenomenon is illustrated in Fig. 10. The induced response reverses polarity at 5 mV, very close to the chloride equilibrium potential, and it could be completely blocked by the addition of 500 μM picrotoxin (Fig. 10b). The response potentiation induced by the co-application varies from cell to cell. On average, there is at least a 9-fold increase in response size when GABA and glycine are co-applied. Preconditioning a cell with GABA (or glycine) would not alter the potentiation of its response to glycine (or GABA). Furthermore, the induced response could be abolished when bicuculline and strychnine are applied together, but not separately (Li and Yang, 1998). These results indicate that activation of both $GABA_A$ and glycine receptors contributes to the response potentiation.

This interaction is obviously different from the "potentiating" effect induced by co-application of GABA and glycine observed in *Xenopus* oocytes expressing exclusively homomeric $GABA_C$ receptors (Calvo and Miledi 1995). This result is also different from the interaction between GABA and glycine currents previously reported in rat hippocampal neurons, which is due to cross-modulation related to shifts of the chloride reversal potential (Grassi,

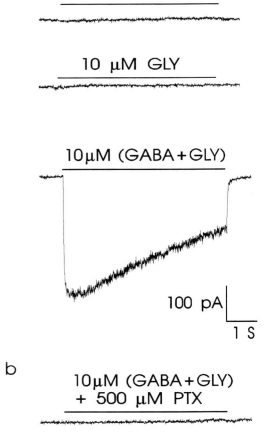

Fig. 10. Strong synergistic interaction between $GABA_A$ and glycine (GLY) receptors. (a) Top and middle traces show that neither 10 μM GABA nor 10 μM GLY induces distinguishable currents from the cell. Bottom trace shows that the response of the cell is markedly potentiated by co-application of 10 μM GABA and 10 μM GLY. (b) The potentiated current is completely abolished by the addition of 500 μM picrotoxin (PTX). All the recordings were made from a single cell when it was clamped at − 60 mV. Adapted from Li and Yang (1998).

1992). The synergistic interaction between $GABA_A$ and glycine receptors observed in amacrine cells may obviously provide a versatility for modulating synaptic transmission in the inner retina.

Zn^{2+} modulation of $GABA_A$ receptor

Zn^{2+} also modulates the $GABA_A$ receptor of carp amacrine cells. As shown in Fig. 11a, the response to 100 μM GABA is reduced in amplitude by 10 μM

Zn^{2+} and completely suppressed by 1 mM Zn^{2+}. This effect of Zn^{2+} is similar to that on carp bipolar cells (see section above). As a comparison, we also investigated modulation by Zn^{2+} of glycine receptors in these cells. The glycine-induced currents are steadily potentiated by Zn^{2+} at lower concentrations (0.1 μM–10 μM), while they are dose-dependently inhibited by Zn^{2+} at higher concentrations (> 100 μM) (Fig. 11b). Both of these effects involve changes in apparent glycine affinity of the glycine receptor (Li and Yang, 1999).

Conclusions and future perspectives

Using electrophysiological and pharmacological approaches, our recent work demonstrates that the glutamate receptors of both horizontal and amacrine cells in carp retina may be the AMPA-preferring subtype, predominantly consisting of the flop splice variant. Since subunits involved in forming native AMPA receptors may have important implications for synaptic transmission at a particular synapse (Mosbacher et al., 1994), the findings reported in this work raise the question as to whether alternative splice variants may be related to specialized functions of AMPA receptors in neurons. While most central neurons use action potentials to transmit information, sensory receptor cells and their postsynaptic interneurons, including horizontal cells, often respond with graded-potentials. Differing from the discontinuous transmitter release caused by presynaptic action potentials in spiking neurons, graded-potential neurons have some distinct morphological features at their synapses, which are probably linked to the high rate of vesicle fusion required for

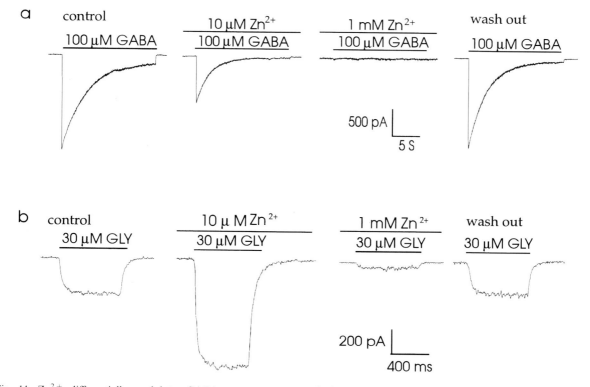

Fig. 11. Zn^{2+} differentially modulates $GABA_A$ receptors versus glycine receptors in isolated carp retinal amacrine cells. (a) Suppression by Zn^{2+} of the $GABA_A$ response observed in an amacrine cell. The response of the cell to 100 μM GABA is partially suppressed by 10 μM Zn^{2+} and completely blocked by 1 mM Zn^{2+}. The Zn^{2+} effect is reversible. (b) Dual effect of Zn^{2+} on 30 μM glycine (Gly) induced currents from an amacrine cell. The glycine response is potentiated by 10 μM Zn^{2+}, while being inhibited by Zn^{2+} of higher concentrations (>100 μM). The Zn^{2+} effects are reversible. Durations of drug application are indicated by the horizontal bars above each response trace. Adapted from Li and Yang (1999).

continuous transmitter release (Juusola et al., 1996). It is also reasonable to predict that there should be receptor characteristics at synapses between graded-potential neurons which match graded and continuous transmitter release. It would be certainly intriguing to explore the physiological implication of rapid desensitization at AMPA receptors, such as those on carp horizontal and amacrine cells, which may be predominantly composed of the flop variants, for synaptic transmission between graded-potential neurons.

It was further found that Zn^{2+}, an endogenous modulator in the retina, modulates flop- and flip-isoform mediated components of the glutamate responses of horizontal cells differentially. Compelling evidence suggests that the flip/flop region of alternative splicing of glutamate receptors located at the end of the L3 loop is extracellular (Hollmann and Heinemann, 1994). In NMDA receptors, Zn^{2+} is found to only potentiate the splice variants lacking a 63-bp insertion near the $5'$ end, indicating that the binding of Zn^{2+} on these subunits is relevant to extracellular structure (Hollmann et al., 1993). As the AMPA receptor shares the same topology with the NMDA receptor, it is reasonable to speculate that this splice variant-related modulation by Zn^{2+} may be due to the difference in extracellular spatial conformation between the flip and flop variants.

$GABA_A$ and $GABA_C$ receptors coexist in carp rod-dominant ON bipolar cells, with the latter showing more significant desensitization. Response kinetics (activation, deactivation and desensitization) of the $GABA_C$ receptors are slower overall than those of the $GABA_A$ receptors. The differences in kinetics between the two receptors may result from distinct subunit composition and/or intracellular mechanisms (Verdoorn et al., 1990; Tia et al., 1996).

GABA receptors may be involved in organizing the center-surround antagonistic receptive fields of both bipolar and ganglion cells. It has been demonstrated that receptor desensitization may play an important role in shaping synaptic transmission and in modulating neuronal excitability (Jones and Westbrook, 1996). Given the continuous release of GABA from horizontal cells in the dark, most GABA receptors on bipolar cells are mainly in the bound-open equilibrium state. When GABA in the synaptic cleft is removed by illumination, the kinetics of the

unbinding steps (deactivation) are the main determinants of functional recovery of GABA receptors, thus directly influencing the following frequency of the synapse. Different deactivation kinetics of the $GABA_C$ and $GABA_A$ receptors suggest that the two receptors may differentially modify synaptic transmission in the frequency domain.

Zn^{2+} exerts differential effects on the kinetics of the $GABA_A$ and $GABA_C$ responses. Although we have not further explored the underlying mechanisms, the differential effects of Zn^{2+} on the kinetics of the $GABA_A$ and $GABA_C$ receptors may result from distinct subunit compositions of these receptors. It was revealed that recombinant receptors lacking γ subunits were more sensitive to Zn^{2+} whereas γ subunit-containing receptors were resistant to Zn^{2+} (Verdoorn et al., 1990; Smart et al., 1994). It was further found that the homomeric $\rho 1$ receptors had two Zn^{2+} binding sites: one competitive and one noncompetitive (Chang et al., 1995). It is thus plausible to speculate that the events occurring at these two binding sites may be somewhat involved in the Zn^{2+} effects reported here. Provided Zn^{2+} is indeed co-released with glutamate from photoreceptor terminals, our data raise the possibility that modulation by Zn^{2+} of $GABA_A$ and $GABA_C$ receptors may be functionally important in regulating signal transmission in the retina.

Carp amacrine cells appear to possess only $GABA_A$ receptors. It is revealed that there is a strong synergistic interaction between the $GABA_A$ receptor and the strychnnine-sensitive glycine receptors on these cells. It has been established that a transmitter may allosterically modulate the ligand-gated receptor activated by another transmitter. It was previously observed in goldfish Mauthner cells that GABA allosterically potentiated glycine binding to glycine receptors (Werman, 1979). Consequently, it may be speculated that GABA and glycine allosterically modulate each other's receptors, which results in the synergistic interaction described in this work. An alternative mechanism may be that the interaction is caused by modifying consensus phosphorylation sites which exist on major intracellular loops of $GABA_A$ and glycine receptors (McDonald and Olsen, 1994).

Our results further demonstrate that Zn^{2+} invariably suppresses the GABA-induced currents, but positively or negatively modulates the glycine-induced currents depending on the concentration of Zn^{2+}. It is obvious that Zn^{2+} at certain levels (1 μM–10 μM) in the inner retina may exert opposite modulation for glycine receptors versus $GABA_A$ receptors: potentiating the glycine response, while inhibiting the $GABA_A$ response, so as to differentially modulate inhibitory synaptic inputs converging on most amacrine cells.

Acknowledgments

The work was supported by grants from the National Programme of Basic Research sponsored by the Ministry of Science and Technology of China (G1999054000), the National Foundation of Natural Science of China (No. 39800041), the Shanghai Metropolitan Fund for Development of Science and Technology (00JC14040) and the Shanghai Institutes of Biological Sciences, the Chinese Academy of Sciences, and the Shanghai–Unilever Research and Development Fund (2004).

References

Barnstable, C.J. (1993) Glutamate and GABA in retinal circuitry. *Curr. Opin. Neurobiol.*, 3: 520–525.

Bormann, J. (1988) Electrophysiology of $GABA_A$ and $GABA_B$ receptor subtypes. *Trends. Neurosci.*, 11: 112–116.

Brandstäter, J.H., Koulen, P. and Wässle, H. (1998) Diversity of glutamate receptors in the mammalian retina. *Vision Res.*, 38: 1385–1397.

Bresink, I., Ebert B., Parsons, C.G. and Mutschler E. (1996) Zinc changes AMPA receptor properties: Results of binding studies and patch clamp recordings. *Neuropharmacology.*, 35: 503–509.

Calvo, D.J. and Miledi, R. (1995) Activation of $GABA_C$ receptors by glycine and alanine. *NeuroReport*, 6: 1118–1120.

Calvo, D.J., Vazquez, A.E. and Miledi, R. (1994) Cationic modulation of ρ1-type γ-aminobutyrate receptors expressed in *Xenopus* oocytes. *Proc. Natl. Acad. Sci. USA*, 91: 12725–12729.

Cervetto, L. and MacNichol, E.F., Jr. (1972) Inactivation of horizontal cells in turtle retina by glutamate and asparate. *Science*, 178: 767–768.

Chang, Y.C., Amin, J.S. and Weiss, D.S. (1995) Zinc is a mixed antagonist of homomeric ρ1 γ-aminobutyric acid-activated channels. *Mol. Pharmacol.*, 47: 595–602.

Cherubini, E. and Strata, F. (1997) $GABA_C$ receptors: a novel receptor family with unusual pharmacology. *News in Physiological Science*, 12: 136–141.

Dixon, D.B. and Copenhagen, D.R. (1992) Two types of glutamate receptors differentially excite amacrine cells in the tiger salamander retina. *J. Physiol. (Lond.)*, 449: 589–606.

Djamgoz, M.B.A. (1995) Diversity of GABA receptors in the vertebrate outer retina. *Trends Neurosci.*, 18: 118–120.

Dowling, J.E. (1987) The Retina: *an Approachable Pad of the Brain.*, The Belknap Press of Harvard University, Cambridge, 1987, pp. 81–123.

Dowling, J.E., Lasater, E.M., Van Buskirk, R. and Watling, K.J. (1983) Pharmacological properties of isolated fish horizontal cells. *Vision Res.*, 23: 421–432.

Dowling, J.E. and Ripps, H. (1972) Adaptation in skate photoreceptors. *J. Gen. Physiol.*, 60: 698–719.

Du, J.L. and Yang, X.L. (2000) Subcellular localization and complements of $GABA_A$ and $GABA_C$ receptors on bullfrog retinal bipolar cells. *J. Neurophysiol.*, 84: 666–676.

Feigenspan, A., Wässle, H. and Bormann, J. (1993) Pharmacology of GABA receptor Cl^- channels in rat retinal bipolar cells. *Nature*, 361: 159–162.

Grassi, F. (1992) Cl^--mediated interaction between GABA and glycine currents in cultured rat hippocampal neurons. *Brain Res.*, 594: 115–123.

Grigorenko, E.V. and Yeh, H.H. (1994) Expression profiling of $GABA_A$ receptor beta-subunits in the rat retina. *Vis. Neurosci.*, 11: 379–387.

Han, M.H., Li, Y. and Yang, X.L. (1997) Desensitizing $GABA_C$ receptors on carp retinal bipolar cells. *NeuroReport*, 8: 1331–1335.

Han, M.H. and Yang, X.L. (1999) Zn^{2+} differentially modulates kinetics of $GABA_C$ versus $GABA_A$ receptors in carp retinal bipolar cells. *NeuroReport*, 10: 2593–2597.

Han, M.H., Shen, Y. and Yang, X.L. (2000) Differences in kinetics between $GABA_C$ and $GABA_A$ receptors on carp retinal bipolar cells. *Sci. China (Ser. C)*, 43: 526–534.

Hesse, G.W. (1979) Chronic Zn^{2+} deficiency alters neuronal function of hippocampal mossy fibers, *Science*, 205: 1005–1007.

Hollmann, M., Boulter, J., Maron, C., et al. (1993) Zinc potentiates agonist-induced currents at certain splice variants of the NMDA receptor, *Neuron*, 10: 943–954.

Hollmann, M. and Heinemann, S. (1994) Cloned glutamate receptors. *Annu. Rev. Neurosci.*, 17: 31–108.

Johansen, T.H., Chaudhary, A. and Verdoorn, TA. (1995) Interactions among GYKI 52446, cyclothiazide, and anir-acetam at recombinant AMPA and kainate receptors. *Mol. Pharmacol.*, 48: 946–955.

Jones, M.V. and Westbrook, G.L. (1996) The impact of receptor desensitization on fast synaptic transmission. *Trends Neurosci.*, 19: 96–101.

Juusola, M., French, A.S., Uusitalo, R.O. and Weckström, M. (1996) Information processing by graded-potential transmission through tonically active synapses. *Trends Neurosci.*, 19: 292–297.

Lasater, E.M. and Dowling, J.E. (1982) Carp horizontal cells in culture respond selectively to L-glutamate and its agonists. *Proc. Natl. Acad. Sci. USA*, 79: 936–940.

Lasater, E.M., Dowling, J.E. and Ripps, H. (1984) Pharmacological properties of isolated horizontal and bipolar cells from the skate retina. *J. Neurosci.*, 4: 1966–1975.

Lerma, J., Morales, M., Vicente, M.A., et al. (1997) Glutamate receptors of the kain ate type and synaptic transmission. *Trends Neurosci.*, 20: 9–15.

Li, P. and Yang, X.L. (1998) Strong synergism between $GABA_A$ and glycine receptors on isolated carp third-order neurons. *NeuroReport*, 9: 2875–2879.

Li, P. and Yang, X.L. (1999) Zn^{2+} differentially modulates glycine receptors versus $GABA_A$ receptors in isolated carp retinal third-order neurons. *Neurosci. Lett.*, 269: 75–78.

Lu, T., Shen, Y. and Yang, X.L. (1998) Desensitization of AMPA receptors on horizontal cells isolated from crucian carp retina. *Neurosci. Res.*, 31: 123–135.

Lu, T. and Yang, X.L. (1995) Dissociation, pharmacology and physiological characteristics of retinal horizontal cells. *Chin. J. Neuroanat.*, 11: 299–306.

Lukasiewicz, P.D. (1996) $GABA_C$ receptors in the vertebrate retina. *Mol. Neurobiol.*, 12: 181–194.

Lukasiewicz, P.D., Lawrence, J.E. and Valentino, T.L. (1995) Desensitizing glutamate receptors shape excitatory synaptic inputs to tiger salamander retinal ganglion cells. *J. Neurosci.*, 15: 6189–6199.

Maguire, G., Lukasiewicz, P. and Werblin, F. (1989) Amacrine cell interactions underlying the response to change in the tiger salamander retina. *J. Neurosci.*, 9: 726–735.

Mangel, S.C. (1998) The generation of directionally selective responses in the retina. *J. Physiol. (Lond.)*, 512: 316–328.

Matthews, G., Ayoub, G.S. and Heidelberger, R. (1994) Presynaptic inhibition by GABA is mediated via two distinct GABA receptors with novel pharmacology. *J. Neurosci.*, 14: 1079–1090.

McDonald, R.L., Olsen, R.W. (1994) $GABA_A$ receptor channels. *Annu. Rev. Neurosci.*, 17: 569–602.

Mosbacher, J., Schoepfer, R., Monyer, H., et al. (1994) A molecular determinant for submillisecond desensitization in glutamate receptors. *Science*, 266: 1059–1062.

Muller, J.F. and Marc, R.E. (1990) GABAergic and glycinergic pathways in the inner plexiform layer of the goldfish retina. *J. Comp. Neurol.*, 291: 281–304.

Murakami, M., Ohtsu, K. and Ohtsuka, T. (1972) Effects of chemicals on receptors and horizontal cells in the retina. *J. Physiol.*, 227: 899–913.

Pan, Z.H. and Lipton, S.A. (1995) Multiple GABA receptor subtypes mediate inhibition of calcium influx at rat retinal bipolar cell terminals. *J. Neurosci.*, 15: 2668–2679.

Partin, K.M., Fleck, M.W. and Mayer, M.L. (1996) AMPA receptor flip/flop mutants affecting deactivation, desensitization, and modulation by cyclothiazide, aniracetam, and thiocyanate. *J. Neurosci.*, 16: 6634–6647.

Partin, K.M., Patneau, D.K. and Mayer, M.L. (1994) Cyclothiazide differentially modulates desensitization of α-amino-3-hydroxy-5-methyl-4-isoxazole propionic acid receptor splice variants. *Mol. Pharmacol.*, 46: 129–138.

Partin, K.M., Patneau, D.K., Winters, C.A., et al. (1993) Selective modulation of desensitization at AMPA versus kainate receptors by cyclothiazide and Concanavalin A. *Neuron*, 11: 1069–1082.

Qian, H. and Dowling, J.E. (1993) Novel GABA responses from rod-driven retinal horizontal cells. *Nature*, 361: 162–164.

Qian, H. and Dowling, J.E. (1995) $GABA_A$ and $GABA_C$ receptors on hybrid bass retinal bipolar cells. *J. Neurophysiol.*, 74: 1920–1928.

Qian, H., Li, L., Chappell, R.L., et al (1997) GABA receptors of bipolar cells from the skate retina: actions of Zn^{2+} on GABA-mediated membrane currents. *J. Neurophysiol.*, 78: 2402–2412.

Rassendren, F.A., Lory, P., Pin, J.P. and Nargeot, J. (1990) Zinc has opposite effects on NMDA and non-NMDA receptors expressed in *Xenopus* oocytes. *Neuron*, 4: 733–740.

Schimidt, K.F. (1997) Properties of glutamate-gated ion channels in horizontal cells of the perch retina. *Vis. Res.*, 37: 2023–2028.

Sekiguchi, M., Fleck, M.W., Mayer, M.L., et al. (1997) A novel allosteric potentiator of AMPA receptors: 4-[2-(Phenylsulfonylamino)ethylthio]-2,6-DifluoroPhenoxy acetamide. *J. Neurosci*, 17: 5760–5771.

Sekiguchi, M., Takeo, J., Harada, T., et al. (1998) Pharmacological detection of AMPA receptor heterogeneity by use of two allosteric potentiators in rat hippocampal cultures. *Br. J. Pharmacol.*, 123: 1294–1303.

Shen, Y. and Yang, X.L. (1999) Zinc modulation of AMPA receptors may be relevant to splice variants in carp retina. *Neurosci. Lett.*, 259: 177–180.

Shen, Y., Lu, T. and Yang, X.L. (1999a) Modulation of desensitization at glutamate receptors in isolated crucian carp horizontal cells by concanavalin A, cyclothiazide, aniracetam and PEPA. *Neuroscience*, 89: 979–990.

Shen, Y., Zhou, Y. and Yang, X.L. (1999b) Characterization of AMPA receptors on isolated amacrine-like cells in carp. *Eur. J. Neurosci.*, 11: 4233–4240.

Slaughter, M.M. and Bai, S.-H. (1989) Differential effects of baclofen on sustained and transient cells in the mudpuppy retina. *J. Neurophysiol.*, 61: 374–381.

Smart, T.G., Xie, X. and Krishek, B.J. (1994) Modulation of inhibitory and excitatory amino acid receptor ion channels by zinc. *Prog. Neurobiol.*, 42: 393–441.

Sommer, B., Keinnen, K., Verdoorn, T.A., et al. (1990) Flip and flop: a cell-specific functional switch in glutamate-operated channels of the CNS. *Science*, 249: 1580–1585.

Swanson, G.T., Kamboj, S.K. and Cull-Candy, S.G. (1997) Single-channel properties of recombinant AMPA receptors depend on RNA editing, splice variation, and subunit composition. *J. Neurosci.*, 17: 58–69.

Tachibana, M. and Kaneko, A. (1987) γ-Aminobutyric acid exerts a local inhibitory action on the axon terminal of bipolar cells: evidence for negative feedback from amacrine cells. *Proc. Natl. Acad. Sci. USA*, 84: 3501–3505.

Tia, S., Wang, J.F., Kotchabhakdi, N. and Vicini, S. (1996) Distinct deactivation and desensitization kinetics of recombinant GABA_A receptors. *Neuropharmacology.*, 35: 1375–1382.

Verdoorn, T.A., Draguhn, A., Ymer, S., et al. (1990) Functional propertied of recombinant rat GABA_A receptors depend upon subunit composition. *Neuron*, 4: 919–928.

Wässle, H., Koulen, P., Brandstätter, J.H., et al. (1998) Glycine and GABA receptors in the mammalian retina. *Vision Res.*, 38: 1411–1430.

Werman, R. (1979) Stiochiometry of GABA-receptor interactions: GABA modulates the glycine-receptor interaction allosterically in a vertebrate neuron. In: Mandel P and DeFeudis F.V. (Eds.), *GABA—Biochemistry and CNS Functions: Advances in Experimental Medicine and Biology.* Plenum Press, New York, pp. 287–301.

Wong, L.A. and Mayer, M.L. (1993) Differential modulation by cyclothiazide and concanavalin A of desensitization at native α-amino-3-hydroxy-5-methyl-4-isoxazolepropionic acid- and kainate-preferring glutamate receptors. *Mol. Pharmacol.*, 44: 504–510.

Wu, S.M., Qiao, X., Yang, X.L., et al. (1993) Localization and modulatory actions of Zn^{2+} in vertebrate retina. *Vision Res.*, 33: 2611–2616.

Yang, X.L. and Wu, S.M. (1991a) Coexistence and functions of multiple types of glutamate receptor in the horizontal cells of the tiger salamander retina. *Vis. Neurosci.*, 7: 377–382.

Yang, X.L. and Wu, S.M. (1991b) Feedforward lateral inhibition: Input-output relation of the horizontal cell to bipolar synapse in the tiger salamander retina. *Proc. Natl. Acad. Sci. USA*, 88: 3310–3313.

Yazulla, S. (1986) GABAergic Mechanisms in the Retina. *Progress in Retinal Research.*, 5: 1–52.

Yazulla, S. and Studholme, K.M. (1991) Glycine-receptor immunoreactivity in retinal bipolar cells is postsynaptic to glycinergic and GABAergic amacrine cell synapses. *J. Comp. Neurol.*, 310: 11–20.

Zhang, D.Q. and Yang, X.L. (1997) OFF pathway is preferentially suppressed by the activation of GABA_A receptors in carp retina. *Brain Res.*, 759: 160–162.

Zhang, D.Q., Yang, R. and Yang, X.L. (1999) Suppression of sustained and transient on signals of amacrine cells by GABA is mediated by different receptor subtypes. *Sci. China (Ser. C)*, 42: 395–400.

Zhang, J., Jung, C.S. and Slaughter, M.M. (1997) Serial inhibitory synapses in retina. *Vis. Neurosci.*, 14: 553–563.

Zhou, Z.J. and Fain, G.L. (1995) Neurotransmitter receptors of starburst amacrine cells in rabbit retinal slices. *J. Neurosci.*, 15: 5334–5345.

Zoli, M., Agnati, L.F., Hedlund, P.B., et al. (1993) Receptor-receptor interactions as an integrative mechanism in nerve cells. *Mol. Neurobiol.*, 7: 293–334.

H. Kolb, H. Ripps and S. Wu (Eds.)
Progress in Brain Research, Vol. 131

CHAPTER 20

The GABA$_C$ receptors of retinal neurons

Haohua Qian* and Harris Ripps

*Department of Ophthalmology and Visual Sciences, University of Illinois at Chicago,
1855 West Taylor Srteet, Chicago, IL 60612, USA*

Introduction

γ-aminobutyric acid (GABA), the main inhibitory neurotransmitter in the central nervous system, exerts its effects by activating GABA receptors (GABARs) on cell membranes. Table 1 summarizes some general properties of the three types of GABAR that have been characterized thus far. GABA$_A$ receptors are a family of ligand-gated chloride channels that mediate rapid inhibitory reactions, inactivate quickly, and have a diverse molecular composition. At least seven subunits and their multiple variants have been identified, providing the potential to form an enormous number of receptors with different response properties (Seeburg et al., 1990; McKernan and Whiting, 1996; Bonnert et al., 1999). The various GABA$_A$Rs are antagonized by bicuculline, and are modulated by a broad range of compounds, many of which serve therapeutically as anaesthetics and sedatives. In contrast, GABA$_B$ receptors belong to the G-protein-coupled receptor superfamily, whose inhibitory actions are mediated indirectly by second messengers that gate potassium and calcium channels (Bowery, 1989). These receptors are insensitive to bicuculline, are activated by baclofen, and are antagonized by phaclofen and saclofen (Bormann, 1988).

GABA$_C$ receptors are the most recently identified members of the GABA receptor family (cf. Drew et al., 1984; Johnston, 1986, 1994, 1996). This class of receptor is bicuculline- and baclofen-insensitive, and although linked to chloride channels, receptor activity is not affected either by benzodiazepines or barbiturates, agents that modulate the responses of GABA$_A$ receptors. Moreover, unlike the fast, transient responses of GABA$_A$Rs, activation of GABA$_C$Rs give rise to sustained responses that desensitize very slowly, and inactivate over a prolonged time course following exposure to GABA. GABA$_C$Rs are distributed throughout the central nervous system (Sivilotti and Nistri, 1991; Albrecht et al., 1997; Boue-Grabot et al., 1998; Wegelius et al., 1998; Enz and Cutting, 1999), and are expressed prominently on neurons of the vertebrate retina. One of the earliest studies revealing the presence of GABA$_C$Rs on retinal neurons was conducted in John Dowling's laboratory on the rod-driven

*Corresponding author: Haohua Qian, Tel.: 312-413-7347; Fax: 312-996-7773; E-mail: hqian@uic.edu

Table 1. Characteristics of GABA receptors

	GABA$_A$ R	GABA$_B$ R	GABA$_C$ R
Category	Ligand-gated chloride channel	G-protein coupled receptor	Ligand-gated chloride channel
Subunits	α, β, γ, δ, ε, π, θ	GBR1, GBR2	ρ
Agonists	Muscimol THIP	Baclofen	
Antagonists	Bicuculline Picrotoxin	Phaclofen	TPMPA Picrotoxin
Desensitization	Yes	No	No
Modulator	Benzodiazepines Barbiturates		Zinc

(H4) horizontal cell of the white perch retina (Qian and Dowling, 1993), and it remains the only cell type in which the GABA response is mediated solely by GABA$_C$Rs.

The properties of the homooligomeric receptors formed in oocytes by expression of GABA ρ subunits suggest strongly that they participate in forming the GABA$_C$Rs on neuronal membranes (cf. Cutting et al., 1991; Wang et al., 1994). However, the exact molecular composition of neuronal GABA$_C$ receptors has yet to be determined. In the following sections we will consider in greater detail the GABA$_C$R-mediated responses of retinal neurons, and the pharmacological, physiological, and molecular properties of GABA$_C$Rs and their subunits.

GABA$_C$ responses of retinal neurons

Figure 1 shows typical current recordings from a morphologically-identifiable perch H4 cell. Note that GABA elicits a sustained response which shows negligible desensitization despite the long exposure to GABA. The slow kinetics of the GABA$_C$-mediated response is best seen at the termination of drug

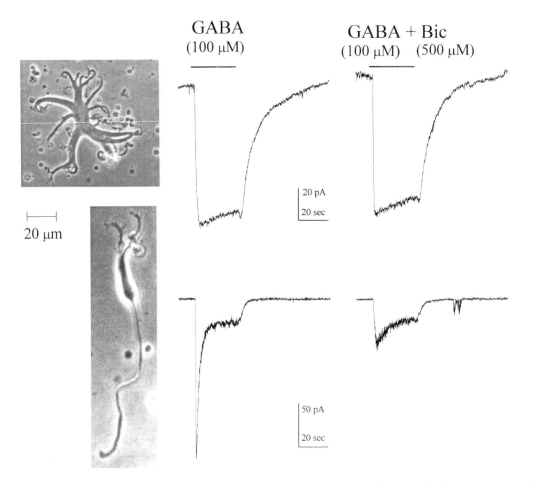

Fig. 1. GABA responses elicited from a rod-driven horizontal cell (top) and a bipolar cell (bottom) of white perch retina. With the membrane potential held at -70 mV, GABA (100 μM) induced inward chloride currents on both types of neuron. Only GABA$_C$ receptors are present on rod-driven horizontal cells, and the GABA induced response is insensitive to 500 μM bicuculline. In contrast, both GABA$_A$ and GABA$_C$ receptors are present on the bipolar cells. The addition of bicuculline (500 μM) blocks most of the current contributed by the GABA$_A$ receptor, leaving a relatively sustained response mediated by GABA$_C$ receptors.

application; at offset, the membrane current gradually returns to baseline with a time constant of ~15 seconds. Both the sustained nature of the response and its slow kinetics are well suited to react to variations in the slow graded potentials generated by neurons of the distal retina.

Although the H4 horizontal cell provides a useful model for examining the response properties of GABA$_C$Rs, immunocytochemical and in situ hybridization studies indicate that GABA$_C$ receptors are present predominantly on bipolar cells (Enz et al., 1995, 1996; Qian et al., 1997a; Koulen et al., 1997), and GABA$_C$R-mediated responses have been recorded from the bipolar cells of every species studied (Feigenspan et al., 1993; Lukasiewicz et al., 1994; Qian and Dowling, 1995; Pan and Lipton, 1995; Qian et al., 1997b; Lukasiewicz and Wong, 1997; Nelson et al., 1999). However, in each instance, the GABA-induced response results from activation of more than one type of GABA receptor and/or transporter. As shown in Fig. 1B, there are transient and sustained components to the GABA response of perch bipolar cells. The former, mediated by GABA$_A$Rs, is suppressed in the presence of bicuculline, thereby isolating the GABA$_C$-mediated component, and both phases of the response are blocked by picrotoxin (not shown). In addition to bipolar cells, responses with similar properties have been obtained from other retinal neurons, including cone-driven horizontal cells (Dong et al., 1994; Kaneda et al., 1997), cone photoreceptors (Picaud et al., 1998), and some types of ganglion cells (Zhang and Slaughter, 1995). Clearly, their presence on so many neuronal cell types suggests that GABA$_C$Rs play an important role in shaping the signals transmitted between neurons of the vertebrate retina.

Pharmacology of GABA$_C$ receptors

In addition to a lack of sensitivity to bicuculline and baclofen, the GABA$_C$Rs on retinal neurons are also insensitive to the competitive antagonists of either GABA$_A$ receptors e.g. SR95531 and hydrastine, or GABA$_B$ receptors e.g. phaclofen and saclofen (Polenzani et al., 1991; Qian and Dowling, 1993). Since competitive antagonists are thought to interact with the receptor's GABA binding sites, these results

suggest that GABA$_C$Rs display a special structural configuration. In agreement with this notion, specific agonists of GABA$_A$ and GABA$_B$ receptors either have no effect (isonipecotic acid, baclofen), serve as partial agonists (isoguvacine, muscimol), or exert an antagonistic effect (THIP, P4S, 3-APA and 3-APMPA) on GABA$_C$ receptors (Woodward et al., 1993; Qian and Dowling, 1994). Interestingly, I4AA, a partial agonist of GABA$_A$ receptors, acts as a potent antagonist on the GABA$_C$Rs of retinal neurons, but is a partial agonist on GABA$_C$Rs expressed in *Xenopus* oocytes (Qian and Dowling, 1994; Qian et al., 1998). Neuroactive steroids, another class of GABA$_A$R modulator, can also have different effects on the responses of GABA$_C$ receptors expressed in *Xenopus* oocytes. Whereas some steroids modulate receptor activity, others do not (Woodward et al., 1992a; Morris et al., 1999); their actions on neuronal GABA$_C$ receptors have yet to be determined.

Although both GABA$_A$ and GABA$_C$ receptors are linked to chloride channels, the GABA$_C$R channel exhibits a significantly lower single channel conductance (Qian and Dowling, 1995; Chang and Weiss, 1999), and TBPS, an agent that blocks GABA$_A$R-gated chloride channels, fails to block the responses mediated by GABA$_C$Rs (Woodward et al., 1992b; Qian and Dowling, 1994). Other properties that distinguish between the two receptor types include their reactions to the chloride channel blocker, picrotoxin, and their relative sensitivities to divalent cations. Unlike its non-competitive blocking action on GABA$_A$R channels, picrotoxin inhibition of GABA$_C$R-mediated activity displays both competitive and non-competitive mechanisms (Qian and Dowling, 1994; Wang et al., 1995a). In rat retina, however, the GABA$_C$ receptors of bipolar cells are surprisingly insensitive to picrotoxin (Feigenspan et al., 1993; Pan and Lipton, 1995), an unusual feature attributable to substitution of a single amino acid residue in the second membrane-spanning domain of the receptor subunit (Zhang et al., 1995). Also noteworthy is the observation that GABA$_C$ receptors are particularly sensitive to modulation by divalent cations (Calvo et al., 1994; Dong and Werblin, 1995; Chang et al., 1995; Kaneda et al., 1997). Their unusually high sensitivity to inhibition by Zn^{2+} has been shown to result from the presence of histidine residues on the extracellular domain of the GABA$_C$R subunits (Wang et al., 1995b).

Much remains to be learned with regard to the pharmacology and functional significance of GABA$_C$Rs, but inroads are being made (Lukasiewicz and Werblin, 1994; Wellis and Werblin, 1995; Dong and Werblin, 1998; Yang et al., 1999), and it is likely that our understanding will be greatly enhanced by the development of specific inhibitors of receptor activity. The availability of a novel compound (TPMPA), thought to be a selective inhibitor of the GABA$_C$R (Murata et al., 1996; Ragozzino et al., 1996), has already proven of value in this regard (Chebib et al., 1998).

Modulation of GABA$_C$ receptor-mediated responses

The action of GABA on the GABA$_C$R-gated current is subject to modulation by a variety of endogenous substances and second messenger systems (Fig. 2). For example, the discharge of glutamate from photoreceptor terminals, which serves as the principal excitatory input to bipolar cells, has been shown to modulate GABA$_C$Rs in rat bipolar cells via activation of protein kinase C (Feigenspan and Bormann, 1994a), and a similar regulatory mechanism has been demonstrated in *Xenopus* oocytes expressing human ρ1 and ρ2 receptors (Kusama et al., 1995, 1998). In fact, both serotonin and glutamate are capable of binding to metabotropic receptors on bipolar cells, resulting presumably in the activation of phospholipase C and the release of diacylglycerol, which, in turn, could induce a protein kinase C-mediated phosphorylation of the GABA$_C$R. Thus, the GABA- mediated inhibitory inputs to bipolar cells from horizontal and amacrine cells may be down regulated by these coupled intracellular mechanisms. In addition, it has been reported that dopamine modulates the GABA$_C$ receptor activity on both catfish cone-driven horizontal cells and tiger salamander bipolar cell terminals (Dong and Werblin, 1994; Wellis and Werblin, 1995). In the salamander, dopamine reduces GABA$_C$R-mediated inhibition through a D1 dopamine receptor linked to a cAMP second messenger pathway.

Although it is questionable whether horizontal cells express a similar metabotropic glutamate receptor (cf. Thoreson and Witkovsky, 1999), the GABA$_C$RS of rod- and cone-driven horizontal cells in fish retina may be autoregulated by the release of

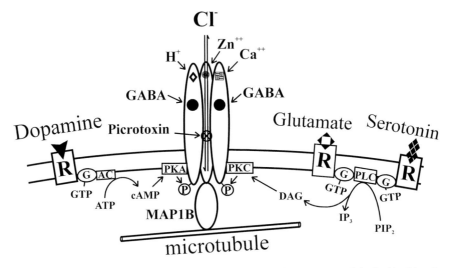

Fig. 2. Modulation of the GABA$_C$ receptor on retinal neurons. Picrotoxin inhibits receptor activity by blocking the chloride channels, whereas protons, Zn^{2+}, Ca^{2+}, and other divalent cations bind to the extracellular domain of the receptor and allosterically modulate the channel current. Metabotropic receptors for neurotransmitters, such as dopamine, serotonin and glutamate, are linked to intracellular second messenger pathways that activate protein kinases (PKA and/or PKC) which lead, in turn, to phosphorylation of the receptor protein and a reduction of the GABA$_C$-mediated current. The GABA$_C$ receptors also interact with the cytoskeleton via a MAP1B protein.

GABA, and modulated by other changes in the composition of the extracellular millieu. Divalent cations such as Ca^{2+} and Zn^{2+} have been shown to exert opposite effects on $GABA_C$-gated currents; calcium augments and zinc inhibits the $GABA_CR$ current in cone-driven horizontal cells of the catfish retina (Dong and Werblin, 1995; Kaneda et al., 1997). Since zinc is presumed to be released (together with glutamate) from dark-adapted receptor terminals, its effect would be to suppress the inhibitory effect of GABA both on bipolar cells and on the horizontal cell itself. In addition, there is evidence that the rat ρ1 receptor, transiently expressed in an HEK293 cell line, is strongly down regulated by protons (Wegelius et al., 1996). Thus, despite the intrinsic buffering capacity of retinal neurons (cf. Haugh-Scheidt and Ripps, 1998), changes in extracellular pH may alter the gating properties of $GABA_CRs$. Surprisingly, these various ionic effects appear to be mediated through distinct binding sites on the extracellular domain of the $GABA_CR$ (see Fig. 2).

Molecular biology of $GABA_C$ receptors

The molecular composition of neuronal $GABA_C$ receptors is another area of importance that is not fully understood despite major breakthroughs in the cloning and expression of $GABA_CR$ subunits (Polenzani et al., 1991; Cutting et al., 1991,1992). $GABA_CRs$ are members of a superfamily of ligand-gated channels which, by analogy with the well studied nicotinic acetylcholine receptors, are presumed to be pentamers, requiring five subunits to constitute a functional receptor (Amin and Weiss, 1996). The topology shown schematically in Fig. 3A indicates that each subunit is composed of four membrane-spanning domains, the second of which lines the receptor channel. The long extracellular N-terminal domain contains two cystine residues that are thought to form a disulfide bond, and the large intracellular loop between the third and fourth transmembrane domains contains consensus sequences representing putative phosphorylation sites. Recent evidence suggests that phosphorylation may be required for internalization of the receptor (Filippova et al., 1999), and that the large intracellular loop is involved in mediating receptor clustering through its interaction with other intracellular proteins (Hanley et al., 1999). Fig. 3B illustrates the organization of the subunits to form the centrally located ionic pore, with ligand binding and modulatory sites on the extracellular side. A conformational change in receptor structure, which occurs when GABA binds to the receptor, opens the channel to gate the transmembrane flux of Cl^-.

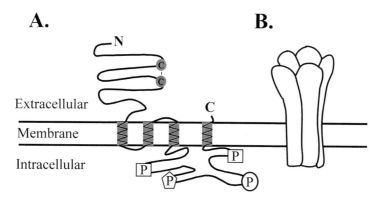

Fig. 3. Schematic diagram of $GABA_C$ receptors. (**A**). Each of the $GABA_C$ receptor subunits has a long extracellular N-terminal region which contains two cystine residues that are thought to form a disufate bond. The extracellular domain forms the GABA binding sites and other modulatory sites. The subunit crosses the cell membrane four times with a short C-terminal region at the outside of the cell. The second transmembrane domain lines the ionic channel of the receptor. There are several putative phosphorylation sites on the large intracellular loop between the third and the fourth transmembrane domain, indicated by the letter P; squares denote PKA sites, a pentagon indicates a PKC site, and the circle is the putative site for a type II Ca-calmodulin-dependent kinase (CaM-KII). (**B**). The functional receptors are formed by five subunits with an ionic channel in the middle of the receptor.

The ρ Subunits of GABA_C Receptors

There is abundant evidence that GABA_C receptors are composed of GABA ρ subunits, which were cloned initially from a human retinal cDNA library (Cutting et al., 1991, 1992). When expressed in *Xenopus* oocytes, GABA ρ subunits form functional homooligomeric GABA-activated chloride channels with pharmacological properties that resemble in many respects those of the GABA_CRs present on retinal neurons (Shimada et al., 1992), as well as those of GABA_CRs expressed in oocytes injected with poly(A)$^+$RNA from mammalian retina (Polenzani et al., 1991). In addition, expression of GABA ρ subunits has been detected in retinal neurons from which GABA_CR-mediated responses were recorded (Enz et al., 1995, 1996; Qian et al., 1997a). Moreover, it is highly likely that heteromeric GABA_CRs also

exist. Rat ρ₁ and ρ₂ subunits coassemble to form a heteromeric receptor in the oocyte expression system (Zhang et al., 1995), and in situ hybridization as well as single cell RT-PCR studies in rat retina show that the two subunits are colocalized in rat retinal bipolar cells (Enz et al., 1995). A similar conclusion was reached based on co-immunoprecipitation results indicating in vitro interaction of human ρ₂ subunits with the N-terminal region of human ρ₁ subunits (Hackam et al., 1997).

To explore further the subunit composition of retinal neurons, and to compare in greater detail the functional properties of GABA_CRs in native cells with the behavior of GABA ρ subunits expressed in *Xenopus* oocytes, we began by cloning the ρ subunits from a white perch retinal cDNA library. Five different GABA ρ subunits were identified (Qian et al., 1997a, 1998), and Fig. 4 shows both their

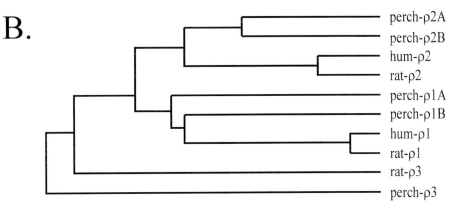

A.

	Perch-ρ1A	Perch-ρ1B	Perch-ρ2A	Perch-ρ2B	Perch-ρ3
Perch-ρ1A	-	84.4 (74.8)	81.0 (68.8)	79.3 (66.2)	70.0 (56.1)
Perch-ρ1B	84.4 (74.8)	-	83.6 (72.4)	81.1 (70.2)	72.2 (60.1)
Perch-ρ2A	81.0 (68.8)	83.6 (72.4)	-	91.7 (84.6)	74.5 (59.4)
Perch-ρ2B	79.3 (66.2)	81.1 (70.2)	91.7 (84.6)	-	77.4 (62.1)
Perch-ρ3	70.0 (56.1)	72.2 (60.1)	74.5 (59.4)	77.4 (62.1)	-

B.

perch-ρ2A
perch-ρ2B
hum-ρ2
rat-ρ2
perch-ρ1A
perch-ρ1B
hum-ρ1
rat-ρ1
rat-ρ3
perch-ρ3

Fig. 4. GABAρ subunits cloned from a white perch retinal cDNA library. (**A**). Homologies between the five GABA ρ subunits from the white perch retina. Entries indicate percent similarities in the amino acid sequences, together with (in parentheses) the percent identity. (**B**). Dendrogram showing the relation of the GABA ρ subunits cloned from the white perch retina to those cloned from human and rat retinas. Note that the divergence between different forms of perch ρ subunits (A and B forms) is greater than between human and rat ρ subunits, suggesting that the various forms of GABA ρ subunits in the white perch retina arise at an early stage of evolution. The ρ3 subunits, on the other hand, show relatively low homology with either the ρ1 or ρ2 subunits. Analysis was performed based on the deduced amino acid sequences of each subunit.

sequence homologies and their relation to the ρ subunits cloned from mammalian retinas. Note that unlike the mammalian retina, where only one form of ρ₁ and ρ₂ subunit has been cloned, there are two isoforms of both the perch ρ₁ and perch ρ₂ subunit. The ρ₃ subunit, which shows less sequence homology to the other perch subunits, is more closely related to the ρ₃ subunit cloned from rat retina (Ogurusu and Shingai, 1996). However, in contrast to the results obtained with the rat ρ₃ subunit (Shingai et al., 1996), no GABA-induced ionic current was recorded when the homomeric perch ρ₃ subunit was expressed in *Xenopus* oocytes. Conversely, all four of the other subunits formed functional homooligomeric receptors in oocytes, and in accordance with their deduced amino acid sequences and the properties of the various receptors, each ρ₁ and ρ₂ family was subdivided into A and B forms (Qian et al., 1998).

In every case, the GABA-activated response from oocytes expressing these receptors was sustained, bicuculline-insensitive, and not modulated either by benzodiazepines or barbiturates, features typical of neuronal GABA_C receptors. Although each of the GABA ρ receptors was shown to gate a chloride channel, and there were many similarities in their functional properties, each displayed a unique pattern of responses that readily distinguished one from the other. For example, each of the subunits was differentially sensitive to activation by GABA, and to inhibition by picrotoxin and zinc. In addition, I4AA behaved as an antagonist on A-type ρ receptors, whereas it acted as a partial agonist on the B-type ρ receptors (Qian et al., 1998).

Another important aspect of a ligand-gated response is its time course. Response kinetics provide insight into the nature of the receptor, and play an important role in shaping the neuronal signal that is transmitted intercellularly. Accordingly, we attempted to analyze more closely the temporal features of the GABA-induced responses from oocytes expressing the various ρ subunits, and to assess the degree to which they mirror the GABA-activated currents recorded from bipolar cells. Interestingly, each of the homooligomeric receptors formed by the individual subunits exhibited different response kinetics. As shown in Fig. 5A, membrane currents recorded from *Xenopus* oocytes expressing

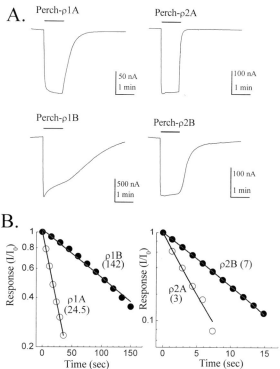

Fig. 5. GABA-induced responses from white perch GABA-ρ subunits expressed in Xenopus oocytes. (**A**). Current responses elicited by 10 μM GABA on oocytes expressing the different forms of GABA-ρ subunit. The duration of GABA application is shown by the bar above each trace. Variations in response amplitude often result from different levels of receptor expression in individual oocytes; response kinetics is a relatively stable parameter independent of amplitude. (**B**). Semilogarithmic plot of membrane currents recorded at various times following GABA offset; the responses have been normalized to their initial amplitudes at the time of offset. The responses are well fit by straight lines, indicating that the relation can be described by single exponential functions. The slope of the line is equal to the time constant of the current decay (τ values are shown in parentheses).

the various white perch GABA-ρ subunits display significantly different waveforms in response to application of 10 μM GABA.

This feature is most evident at response offset, i.e. in the current trace after GABA application is terminated. To quantitate this aspect of the GABA response kinetics, the time course of the offset currents were plotted on a semilogarithmic scale with the amplitudes normalized to their initial values (Fig. 5B). In each case, the data were fit by a straight line, indicating that the off responses are well described by a single exponential function in which the time constant (τ) of decay is obtained from the slope of the line. As indicated by the τ values for each of the ρ subunits, there are consistent differences between the response kinetics of the two receptor families as well as between their subgroups. The GABA-induced responses of ρ_1 receptors are significantly slower than those of ρ_2 receptors, and as we have shown, this difference is determined in large part by a single residue in the second transmembrane domain of the subunits (Qian et al., 1999). Thus, the ρ_1 subunits, which have a proline at amino acid position 320, constitute receptors with slower kinetics, whereas ρ_2 subunits, which contain a serine at that site, form receptors with more rapid response kinetics. This dichotomy is seen also in embryonic kidney cells (HEK-293) transfected with human ρ subunits; the homomeric receptors formed by human ρ_1 subunits show slower response kinetics than receptors formed by human ρ_2 subunits (Enz and Cutting, 1999).

The subunit composition of neuronal GABA$_C$ receptors

Despite the broad range of τ values for the deactivation kinetics of the various perch ρ subunits, none matched the rapid decay phase of the GABA$_C$-mediated response of perch bipolar cells (Fig. 6, inset), nor did expresssion of any of the subunits produce a receptor with faster deactivation kinetics. We mentioned earlier the likelihood that heteromeric receptors can be formed by coassembly of different ρ subunits, but we found that coexpression of different combinations of ρ subunits did not eliminate the disparity. However, it is important to recall that the bipolar cell response to GABA is mediated by both GABA$_A$ and GABA$_C$ receptors. This led us to consider whether the GABA ρ subunits might interact with one of the subunits essential for the formation of a functional GABA$_A$ receptor. To test this possibility we chose the human GABA$_A$ γ_2 subunit (Qian and Ripps, 1999). There were several compelling reasons for choosing the γ subunit from among the many GABA$_A$ subunits. First, the results of earlier studies suggested that human

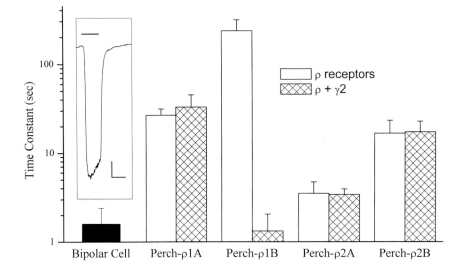

Fig. 6. The kinetics of the GABA responses. Bar graphs illustrate the time constants of GABA offset responses elicited from bipolar cells (solid bar), from homooligomeric perch ρ receptors (clear bars), and from heteromeric receptors composed of ρ and γ_2 subunits (hatched bars). Insert, current traces of GABA$_C$ response recorded from a bipolar cell in the presence of 100 μM bicuculline. Scale bar, 25 pA and 5 s. The time constants obtained from heteromeric γ_2 and ρ_{1B} receptors are significantly different from the values for homomeric ρ_{1B} receptors, but are comparable to the those obtained from retinal bipolar cells.

ρ subunits do not coassemble with either the α or the β subunit of GABA$_A$Rs (Hackam et al., 1998; Koulen et al., 1998); second, perch γ subunits had not yet been cloned; third, and perhaps most important, the γ$_2$ subunit fails to produce a homo-oligomeric GABA-sensitive receptor when expressed in oocytes (Sigel et al., 1990), and was therefore less likely to confound the interpretation of our results.

When coexpressed with each of the perch ρ subunits, the human γ$_2$ subunit was without effect on three of the ρ subunits, but it produced a striking change in the kinetics of the ρ$_{1B}$ receptor (Fig. 6). Note that the perch ρ$_{1B}$ subunit forms a homo-oligomeric receptor in which the time constant of deactivation ($\tau = 234 \pm 76$ s) is more than 180 fold greater than that of the perch bipolar cell ($\tau = 1.6 \pm 0.8$ s). Nevertheless, after coexpression with the GABA$_A$ γ$_2$ subunit, the responses elicited from the resultant receptor were significantly different from those obtained with either of its individual components. Especially noteworthy is the marked increase in the rate of deactivation ($\tau = 1.3 \pm 0.7$ s), which now closely approximates the value obtained from perch bipolar cells.

Despite the change in kinetics, coassembly of the GABA$_A$ γ$_2$ and ρ$_{1B}$ subunits produced a receptor that retained the distinguishing features of a GABA$_C$ receptor, namely, a sustained response to GABA that was insensitive to bicuculline and baclofen, and to the modulatory effects of diazepam. Although there was an enhanced response to pentobarbital, typical of GABA$_A$ receptors, and for which we have no explanation, the formation of this heteromeric ρ$_{1B}$γ$_2$ receptor gave rise to significant changes in receptor pharmacology that brought the results more in line with the pharmacology of native perch bipolar cells. As shown in Fig. 7, there were increases in the receptor's sensitivity to inhibition by picrotoxin and zinc, a reduced sensitivity to activation by GABA, and a reduction in the I4AA-activated current. In each case, the responses of the heteromeric receptors closely approximated those obtained from perch bipolar cells. Clearly, both the kinetic and the pharmacological data suggest that heteromeric receptors consisting of ρ and γ subunits may be involved in the formation of GABA$_C$ receptors on retinal bipolar cells.

A rationale for molecular diversity

The diversity of GABA$_C$Rs, their unique properties, and their prominent expression on different classes of retinal neuron, amply justify the view that these receptors play important roles in retinal signal processing. Although a comprehensive account of how the responses of GABA$_C$Rs affect the functional properties of the retina has yet to emerge, the extreme sensitivity of the receptors to GABA, and the sustained nature of GABA$_C$R-gated currents are well suited to the dynamics of GABA activity in the retina. The two principal sources of GABA are the distally located horizontal cells, and the more proximally placed amacrine cells (Freed et al., 1987; Wässle and Chun, 1989). Processes of both cell types make synaptic contacts with bipolar cells, and each may interact with other neurons in their immediate vicinity, i.e. the photoreceptors and ganglion cells, respectively. Moreover, there is the potential for autoregulation of the GABAergic neurons themselves. Indeed, although species dependent, it appears that every class of retinal neuron may express GABA$_C$ receptors, and the distinctive properties of the different cells suggest the presence of multiple receptor subtypes. It is evident from our earlier discussion that some of this diversity can result from coassembly of subunits representing different classes of GABA receptor (Qian and Ripps, 1999). In addition, it is becoming increasingly apparent that the formation of novel receptors with unique response profiles may occur through promiscuous coassembly of seemingly incompatible receptor subunits (van Hooft et al., 1998). The extent to which this mechanism contributes to the composition of native neuronal receptors is only now being explored.

Comparing the general features of GABA$_C$R-mediated responses of the various cell types suggests that there may be systematic differences in the GABA$_C$Rs of cells located in the outer and inner retina. Thus, the different kinetic properties of GABA$_C$Rs might reflect the receptor's role in responding to the GABA release mediated by the graded potentials of horizontal cells, and the more rapid transient responses of amacrine cells. For example, GABA$_C$Rs in the outer retina, such as found on rod-driven horizontal cells of white perch (Qian and Dowling, 1994), cone-driven horizontal

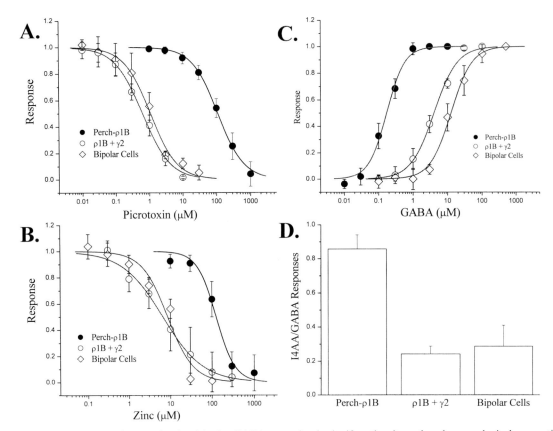

Fig. 7 Co-assembly of the perch-ρ_{1B} subunit with the GABA$_A$-γ_2 subunit significantly alters the pharmacological properties of homomeric ρ_{1B} receptor. (**A**). Dose-response data for the inhibitory action of picrotoxin. At each drug concentration, the response represents the fractional change in the current evoked by GABA when applied at concentrations of 2 μM (for homomeric perch-ρ_{1B} receptors), 10 μM (for heteromeric $\rho_{1B}\gamma_2$ receptors), and 30 μM (for bipolar cells). Data were fit by Hill equations with IC$_{50}$ values of 100 μM, 0.63 μM, and 1.1 μM, and Hill coefficients of 1.1, 1.0 and 1.1 for ρ_{1B} receptors (filled circles), ρ_{1Bg2} receptors (open circles), and the GABA$_C$Rs of bipolar cells (diamonds), respectively. (**B**). Inhibition by zinc. Curves are Hill equations with IC$_{50}$ values of 125 μM, 6.5 μM, and 8.5 μM, and Hill coefficients of 1.9, 0.9 and 1.4 for homo- and hetero-meric GABA ρ receptors and bipolar cells, respectively. (**C**). GABA dose-response curves obtained from homomeric perch-ρ_{1B} receptors and heteromeric perch-ρ_{1B} and γ_2 receptors expressed in *Xenopus* oocytes, and from GABA$_C$Rs on perch bipolar cells. The data for bipolar cells were obtained in the presence of 500 μM bicuculline to block the activity of the GABA$_A$ receptor. The curves are Hill equations with EC$_{50}$ values of 0.17, 4.04 and 12.5 μM and Hill coefficients of 1.6, 1.3 and 1.4 for homomeric (ρ_{1B}), heteromeric ($\rho_{1B}\gamma_2$), and bipolar cell (GABA$_C$) receptors, respectively. (**D**). Normalized amplitude of I4AA-activated response from oocytes expressing perch-ρ_{1B} subunit alone, the ρ_{1B} and γ_2 subunits, and from bipolar cells. For oocytes, responses to 100 μM I4AA were normalized to the responses activated by 10 μM GABA; for bipolar cells, response to 200 μM I4AA were normalized to responses activated by 100 μM GABA. The different GABA concentrations were required to elicit maximal responses under the two conditions.

cells of catfish (Dong and Werblin, 1995) and cone photoreceptors (Picaud et al., 1998), tend to exhibit slower kinetics and are more sensitive to GABA than the GABA$_C$Rs of the inner retina, which are localized primarily on the axon terminals of bipolar cells (Feigenspan and Bormann, 1994b; Qian and Dowling, 1995; Qian et al., 1997b; Lukasiewicz and Wong, 1997). This is apparently well suited to the

properties of GABAergic neurons in these retinal regions. The release of GABA from horizontal cells is mediated primarily by reversal of a voltage- and sodium-dependent GABA transporter, rather than by the calcium-regulated discharge of synaptic vesicles (Schwartz, 1982, 1987). Although the magnitude of the transport current suggests that comparatively fewer molecules of GABA are released, the more than

10-fold greater GABA sensitivity of GABA$_C$Rs (Amin and Weiss, 1994; Qian and Ripps, 1999) makes it likely that they will be more responsive to the transmitter than the GABA$_A$Rs of bipolar cells. Thus, a feedforward signal to the GABA$_C$Rs on bipolar cell dendrites, and/or a feedback signal to the GABARs on cone photoreceptor terminals, probably contributes to the inhibitory surround of the bipolar cell receptive field. In contrast, both GABA$_C$Rs and GABA$_A$Rs are present on horizontal cells of tiger salamander (Kamermans and Werblin, 1992), and it appears that in this instance the two receptor types contribute equally to the autoregulatory effects mediated by the endogenous release of GABA (Yang et al., 1999). In darkness, for example, the GABA-induced chloride conductances of GABA$_C$Rs and GABA$_A$Rs result in a sustained membrane depolarization that extends the operating range of the horizontal cell.

In more proximal regions, the light-evoked release of GABA from amacrine cells occurs both via sodium-dependent action potentials (sensitive to TTX), and an action potential-independent depolarization that is insensitve to TTX (Bieda and Copenhagen, 1999). The two components would tend to promote a rapid transient release of GABA that relaxes and becomes more sustained. Activation of GABA$_A$ and GABA$_C$ receptors clustered on the axon terminals of bipolar cells can then modulate the release of the cell's excitatory transmitter either directly (Lukasiewicz and Werblin, 1994), or indirectly by a dopamine-activated second messenger system that relieves the inhibitory effect mediated by the GABA-induced response of GABA$_C$ receptors (Wellis and Werblin, 1995).

Future directions

It is evident that the GABARs of bipolar cells are in a position to differentially affect the flow of signals from bipolar cells to third order neurons, and the different kinetic properties of GABA$_A$ and GABA$_C$ receptors suggest that they play different roles in mediating the inhibitory effects of GABA at the bipolar cell terminal (Qian et al., 1997b; Lukasiewicz and Shields, 1998), and in shaping the edge enhancement of the ganglion cell receptive field (Jacobs and Werblin, 1998). In this connection, it is noteworthy that there are often different proportions of GABA$_A$ and GABA$_C$ receptors on morphologically different bipolar cells (Qian and Dowling, 1995; Euler and Wässle, 1998; Shields et al., 2000), and the presence of receptors containing various mixtures of their subunits is a distinct possibility. In addition, it is possible that other membrane receptors, unrelated to the GABAR family, can influence via protein–protein interactions the response properties of the GABA receptors (Hanley et al., 1999; Liu et al., 2000). Clearly, further studies are needed to reveal the molecular and functional diversity of the GABA$_C$ receptors on retinal neurons, and to better understand how the various classes of GABA receptor participate in GABA-mediated inhibitory actions within the neuronal circuitry of the retiuna.

Acknowledgments

We are especially indebted to Dr. John Dowling for his important contributions to the studies reported in this paper. The research was supported by grants EY-12028 and EY-06516 from the National Eye Institute.

Abbreviations

GABA (γ-aminobutyric acid), THIP (4,5,6, 7-tetrahydroisoxazolo[5,4-c]pyridin-3-ol], P4S (piperidine-4-sulfonic acid), TBPS (*tert*-burtylbocyclophosphorothionate), 3-APA (3-aminopropyl phosphonic acid), 3-APMPA (3-aminopropyl [methyl]-phosphinic acid), I4AA (imidazol-4-acetic acid), TPMPA ((1,2,5,6-tetrahydropyridin-4-yl)methylphosphinic acid, SR95531 (Gabazine), PKA (protein kinase A), PKC (protein kinase C), PLC (phospholipase C), DAG (diacylglycerol), IP3 (inositol 1,4,5-triphosphate).

References

Albrecht, B.E., Breitenbach. U., Stuhmer, T., Harvey, R.J. and Darlison, M.G. (1997). *In situ* hybridization and reverse transcription–polymerase chain reaction studies on the expression of the GABA$_C$ receptor ρ1- and ρ2-subunit genes in avian and rat brain. *Eur. J. Neurosci.*, 9: 2414–2422.

Amin, J. and Weiss, D.S. (1994). Homomeric ρ1 GABA channels: activation properties and domains. *Recept. Channels*, 2: 227–236.

Amin, J. and Weiss, D.S. (1996). Insights into the activation mechanism of ρ1 GABA receptors obtained by coexpression of wild type and activation-impaired subunits. *Proc. Roy. Soc.* 263: 273–282.

Bieda, M.C. and Copenhagen, D.R. (1999). Sodium action potentials are not required for light-evoked release of GABA or glycine from retinal amacrine cells. *J. Neurophysiol.*, 81: 3092–3095.

Bonnert, T.P., McKernan, R.M., Farrar, S., Le Bourdelles, B., Heavens, R.P., Smith, D.W., Hewson, L., Rigby, M.R., Srinathsinghji, D.J.S., Brown, N., Wafford, K.A. and Whiting, P.J. (1999) θ, a novel γ-aminobutyric acid type A receptor subunit. *Proc. Natl. Acad. Sci. USA*, 96: 9891–9896.

Bormann, J. (1988). Electrophysiology of GABA$_A$ and GABA$_B$ receptor subtypes. *Trends Neurosci.*, 11: 112–116.

Boue-Grabot, E., Roudbaraki, M., Bascles, L., Tramu, G., Bloch, B. and Garret, M. (1998). Expression of GABA receptor ρ subunits in rat brain. *J. Neurochem.*, 70: 899–907.

Bowery, N.G. (1989). GABA$_B$ receptors and their significance in mammalian pharmacology. *Trends Pharmcol. Sci.*, 10: 401–407.

Calvo, D.J., Vazquez, A.E. and Miledi, R. (1994) Cationic modulation of ρ1-type γ-aminobutyrate receptors expressed in *Xenopus* oocytes. *Proc. Natl. Acad. Sci. USA*, 91: 12725–12729.

Chang, Y., Amin, J. and Weiss, D.S. (1995) Zinc is a mixed antagonist of homomeric ρ1 γ-aminobutyric acid-activated channels. *Mol. Pharmacol.*, 47: 595–602.

Chang, Y. and Weiss, D.S. (1999). Channel opening locks agonist onto the GABA$_C$ receptor. *Nature Neurosci.*, 2: 219–225.

Chebib, M., Mewett, K.N. and Johnston, G.A.R. (1998). GABA$_C$ receptor antagonists differentiate between human ρ1 and ρ2 receptors expressed in *Xenopus* oocytes. *Eur. J. Pharmacol.*, 357: 227–234.

Cutting, G.R., Lu, L., Zoghbi, H., O'Hara, B.F., Kasch, L.M., Montrose-Rafizadeh, C., Donovan, D.M., Shimada, S., Antonarakis, S.E., Guggino, W.B., Uhl, G.R. and Kazazian, H.H., Jr. (1991). Cloning of the γ-aminobutyric acid (GABA) ρ1 cDNA: a GABA receptor subunit highly expressed in the retina. *Proc. Natl. Acad. Sci. USA*, 88: 2673–2677.

Cutting, G.R., Curristin, S., Zoghbi, H., O'Hara, B., Selden, M.F. and Uhl, G.R. (1992). Identification of a putative γ-aminobutyric acid (GABA) receptor subunit rho$_2$ cDNA and colocalization of the genes encoding rho$_2$ (GABRR2) and rho$_1$ (GABRR1) to humanf chromosome 6q14–q21 and mouse chromosome 4. *Genomics*, 12: 801–806.

Dong, C.J. and Werblin, F.S. (1994). Dopamine modulation of GABA$_C$ receptor function in an isolated retinal neuron. *J. Neurophysiol.*, 71: 1258–1260.

Dong, C.J. and Werblin, F.S. (1995). Zinc downmodulates the GABA$_c$ receptor current in cone horizontal cells acutely isolated from the catfish retina. *J. Neurophysiol.*, 73: 916–919.

Dong, C.J. and Werblin, F.S. (1998). Temporal contrast enhancement via GABA$_C$ feedback at bipolar terminals in the tiger salamander retina. *J. Neurophysiol.*, 79: 2171–2180.

Dong, C.J., Picaud, S.A. and Werblin, F.S. (1994). GABA transporters and GABA$_C$-like receptors on catfish cone- but not rod-driven horizontal cells. *J. Neurosci.*, 14: 2648–2658.

Drew, C.A., Johnston, G.A.R. and Weatherby, R.P. (1984). Bicuculline-insensitive GABA receptors: studies on the binding of (-)-baclofen to rat cerebellar membranes. *Neurosci. Lett.*, 52: 317–321.

Enz, R. and Cutting, G.R. (1999). GABA$_C$ receptor ρ subunits are heterogeneously expressed in the human CNS and form homo- and heterooligomers with distinct physical properties. *Eur. J. Neurosci.*, 11: 41–50.

Enz, R., Brandstätter, J.H., Hartveit, E., Wässle, H. and Bormann, J. (1995). Expression of GABA receptor ρ1 and ρ2 subunits in the retina and brain of the rat. *Eur. J. Neurosci.*, 7: 1495–1501.

Enz, R., Brandstätter, J.H., Wässle, H. and Bormann, J. (1996). Immunocytochemical localization of the GABA$_C$ receptor ρ subunits in the mammalian retina. *J. Neurosci.*, 16: 4479–4490.

Euler, T. and Wässle, H. (1998). Different contributions of GABA$_A$ and GABA$_C$ receptors to rod and cone bipolar cells in a rat retinal slice preparation. *J. Neurophysiol.*, 79: 1384–1395.

Feigenspan, A. and Bormann, J. (1994a). Modulation of GABA$_C$ receptors in rat retinal bipolar cells by protein kinase C. *J. Physiol.*, 481: 325–330.

Feigenspan, A. and Bormann, J. (1994b). Differential pharmacology of GABA$_A$ and GABA$_C$ receptors on rat retinal bipolar cells. *Eur. J. Pharmacol.*, 288: 97–104.

Feigenspan, A., Wässle, H. and Bormann, J. (1993). Pharmacology of GABA receptor Cl$^-$ channels in rat retinal bipolar cells. *Nature*, 361: 159–163.

Filippova, N., Dudley, R. and Weiss, D.S. (1999). Evidence for phosphorylation-dependent internalization of recombinant human ρ1 GABA$_C$ receptors. *J. Physiol. (Lond.)*, 518: 385–399.

Freed, M.A., Smith, R.G. and Sterling, P. (1987). Rod bipolar array in the cat retina: pattern of inputs from rods and GABA-accumulating amacrine cells. *J. Comp. Neurol.*, 266: 445–455.

Hackam, A.S., Wang, T.-L., Guggino, W.B. and Cutting, G.R. (1997). The N-terminal domain of human GABA receptor ρ1 subunits contains signals for homooligomeric and heterooligomeric interaction. *J. Biol. Chem.*, 272: 13750–13757.

Hackam, A.S., Wang, T.-L., Guggino, W.B. and Cutting, G.R. (1998). Sequences in the amino termini of GABA ρ and GABA$_A$ subunits specify their selective interaction in vitro. *J. Neurochem.*, 70: 40–46.

Hanley, J.G., Koulen, P., Bedford, F., Gordon-Weeks, P.R. and Moss, S.J. (1999).The protein MAP-1B links GABA$_C$ receptors to the cytoskeleton at retinal synapses. *Nature*, 397: 66–69.

Haugh-Scheidt, L. and Ripps, H. (1998). pH regulation in horizontal cells of the skate retina. *Exp. Eye Res.*, 66: 449–464.

Jacobs, A.L. and Werblin, F.S. (1998). Spatiotemporal patterns at the retinal output. *J. Neurophysiol.*, 80: 447–451.

Johnston, G.A.R. (1986). Multiplicity of GABA receptors. In: Olsen, R.W. and Venter, J.C. (Eds.), *Receptor Biochemistry and Methodology*. Vol. 5, Alan R. Liss. Inc., pp. 57–71.

Johnston, G.A.R. (1994). GABA$_C$ receptors. *Progr. Brain Res.*, 100: 61–65.

Johnston, G.A.R. (1996). GABA$_C$ receptors: relatively simple transmitter -gated ion channels? *Trends Pharmacol. Sci.*, 17: 319–323.

Kamermans, M. and Werblin, F. (1992). GABA-mediated positive autofeedback loop controls horizontal cell kinetics in tiger salamander retina. *J. Neurosci.*, 12: 2451–2463.

Kaneda, M., Mochizuki, M. and Kaneko, A. (1997). Modulation of GABA$_C$ response by Ca^{2+} and other divalent cations in horizontal cells of the catfish retina. *J. Gen. Physiol.*, 110: 741–747.

Koulen, P., Brandstätter, J.H., Kröger, S., Enz, R., Bormann, J. and Wässle, H. (1997). Immunocytochemical localization of the GABA$_C$ receptor ρ subunits in the cat, goldfish, and chicken retina. *J. Comp. Neurol.*, 380, 520–532.

Koulen, P., Brandstätter, J.H., Enz, R., Bormann, J. and Wässle, H. (1998). Synaptic clustering of GABA$_C$ receptor ρ subunits in the rat retina. *Eur. J. Neurosci.*, 10: 115–127.

Kusama, T., Sakurai, M., Kizawa, Y., Uhl, G.R. and Murakami, H. (1995). GABA ρ1 receptor: inhibition by protein kinase C activators. *Eur. J. Pharmacol.*, 291: 431–434.

Kusama, T., Hatama, K., Sakurai, M., Kizawa, Y., Uhl, G.R. and Murakami, H. (1998). Consensus phosphorylation sites of human GABA$_C$/GABAρ receptors are not critical for inhibition by protein kinase C activation. *Neurosci. Lett.*, 255: 17–20.

Liu, F., Wan, Q.I., Pristupa, Z.B., Yu, X.-M., Wang, Y.-T. and Niznik, H.B. (2000). Direct protein-protein coupling enables cross-talk between dopamine D5 and gamma-aminobutyric acid A receptors. *Nature*, 403: 274–280.

Lukasiewicz, P.D. and Werblin, F.S. (1994). A novel GABA receptor modulates synaptic transmission from bipolar to ganglion and amacrine cells in the tiger salamander retina. *J. Neurosci.*, 14: 1213–1223.

Lukasiewicz, P.D. and Wong, R.O.L. (1997). GABA$_C$ receptors on ferret retinal bipolar cells: a diversity of subtypes in mammals? *Vis. Neurosci.*, 14: 989–994.

Lukasiewicz, P.D. and Shields, C. R. (1998). Different combinations of GABA$_A$ and GABA$_C$ receptors confer distinct temporal properties to retinal synaptic responses. *J. Neurophysiol.*, 79: 3157–3167.

Lukasiewicz, P.D., Maple, B.R. and Werblin, F.S. (1994). A novel GABA receptor on bipolar cell terminals in the tiger salamander retina. *J. Neurosci.*, 14: 1202–1212.

McKernan, R.M. and Whiting, P.J. (1996). Which GABA$_A$-receptor subtypes really occur in the brain? *Trends Neurosci.*, 19: 139–143.

Morris, K.D., Moorefield, C.N. and Amin, J. (1999). Differential modulation of the γ-aminobutyric acid type C receptor by neuroactive steroids. *Mol. Pharmacol.*, 56: 752–759.

Murata, Y., Woodward, R.M., Miledi, R. and Overman, L.E. (1996). The first selective antagonist for a GABA$_C$ receptor. *Bioorg. Medicinal Chem. Lett.*, 6: 2073–2076.

Nelson, R., Schaffner, A.E., Li, Y.-X. and Walton, M.C. (1999). Distribution of GABA$_C$-like responses among acutely dissociated rat retinal neurons. *Vis. Neurosci.*, 16: 179–190.

Ogurusu, T. and Shingai, R. (1996). Cloning of a putative γ-aminobutyric acid (GABA) receptor subunit ρ3 cDNA. *Biochim. Biophys. Acta*, 1305: 15–18.

Pan, Z.-H. and Lipton, S.A. (1995). Multiple GABA receptor subtypes mediate inhibition of calcium influx at rat retinal bipolar cell terminals. *J. Neurosci.*, 15: 2668–2679.

Picaud, S., Pattnaik, B., Hicks, D., Forster, V., Fontaine, V., Sahel, J. and Dreyfus, H. (1998). GABA$_A$ and GABA$_C$ receptors in adult porcine cones: evidence from a photo-receptor-glia co-culture model. *J. Physiol.*, 513: 33–42.

Polenzani, L., Woodward, R. M. and Miledi R (1991). Expression of mammalian γ-aminobutyric acid receptors with distinct pharmacology in *Xenopus* oocytes. *Proc. Natl. Acad. Sci. USA*, 88: 4318–4322.

Qian, H. and Dowling, J.E. (1993). Novel GABA responses from rod-driven retinal horizontal cells. *Nature*, 361: 162–164.

Qian, H. and Dowling, J.E. (1994). Pharmacology of novel GABA receptors found on rod horizontal cells of the white perch retina. *J. Neurosci.*, 14: 4299–4307.

Qian, H. and Dowling, J.E. (1995). GABA$_A$ and GABA$_C$ receptors on hybrid bass retinal bipolar cells. *J. Neurophysiol.*, 74, 1920–1928.

Qian, H. and Ripps, H. (1999). Response kinetics and pharmacological properties of heteromeric receptors formed by coassembly of GABA ρ- and γ$_2$- subunits. *Proc. Roy. Soc. B*, 266: 2419–2425.

Qian, H., Dowling, J.E. and Ripps, H. (1998) Molecular and pharmacological properties of GABA-rho subunits from white perch retina. *J. Neurobiol.*, 37, 305–320.

Qian, H., Dowling, J.E. and Ripps, H. (1999) A single amino acid in the second transmembrane domain of GABA ρ subunits is a determinant of the response kinetics of GABA$_C$ receptors. *J. Neurobiol.*, 40: 67–76.

Qian, H., Hyatt, G., Schanzer, A., Hazra, R., Hackam, A., Cutting, G. R. and Dowling, J.E. (1997a) A comparison of GABA$_C$ and rho subunit receptors from the white perch retina. *Vis. Neurosci.*, 14: 843–851.

Qian, H., Li, L., Chappell, R.L. and Ripps, H. (1997b) GABA receptors of bipolar cells from the skate retina: actions of zinc on GABA-mediated membrane currents. *J. Neurophysiol.*, 78: 2402–2412.

Ragozzino, D., Woodward, R.M., Murata, Y., Eusebi, F., Overman, L.E. and Miledi, R. (1996). Design and in vitro pharmacology of a selective γ-aminobutyric acid$_C$ receptor antagonist. *Mol. Pharmacol.*, 50: 1024–30.

308

Schwartz, E.A. (1982). Calcium-independent release of GABA from horizontal cells of the toad retina. *J. Physiol.*, 323: 211–227.

Schwartz, E.A. (1987). Depolarization without calcium can release γ-aminobutyric acid from a retinal neuron. *Science*, 238: 350–355.

Seeburg, P.H., Wisden, W., Verdoorn, T.A., Pritchett, D.B., Werner, P., Herb, A., Luddens, H., Sprengel, R. and Sakmann, B. (1990). The GABA$_A$ receptor family: molecular and functional diversity. *Cold Spring Harb. Symp. Quant. Biol.*, 55: 29–40.

Shields, C., Tran, M.N., Wong, R.O.L. and Lukasiewicz, P.D. (2000) Distinct iontropic GABA receptors mediate presynaptic and postsynaptic inhibition in retinal bipolar cells. *J. Neurosci.*, 20: 2673–2682.

Shimada, S., Cutting G. and Uhl, G.R. (1992). γ-aminobutyric acid A or C receptor? γ-aminobutyric acid ρ1 receptor RNA induces bicuculline-, barbiturate-, and benzodiazepine-insensitive γ-aminobutyric acid responses in *Xenopus* oocytes. *Mol. Pharmacol.*, 41: 683–687.

Shingai, R., Yanagi, K., Fukushima, T., Sakata, K. and Ogurusu, T. (1996). Functional expression of GABA ρ3 receptors in *Xenopus* oocytes. *Neurosci. Res.*, 26: 387–390.

Sigel, E., Baur, R., Trube, G., Möhler, H. and Malherbe, P. (1990). The effect of subunit composition of rat brain GABA$_A$ receptors on channel function. *Neuron*, 5: 703–711.

Sivilotti, L. and Nistri, A. (1991). GABA receptor mechanisms in the central nervous system. *Progr. Neurobiol.*, 36: 35–92.

Thoreson, W.B. and Witkovsky, P. (1999) Glutamate receptors and circuits in the vertebrate retina. *Prog. Retinal. Eye Res.*, 18: 765–810.

Van Hooft, J.A., Spier, A.D., Yakel, J.L., Lummis, S.C.R. and Vijverberg, H.P.M. (1998). Promiscuous coassembly of serotonin 5-HT$_3$ and nicotinic α4 receptor subunits into Ca^{2+}-permeable ion channels. *Proc. Natl. Acad. Sci. USA*, 95: 11456–11461.

Wang, T.-L., Hackam, A.S., Guggino, W.B. and Cutting, G.R. (1994) A novel γ-aminobutyric acid receptor subunit (ρ2) cloned from human retina forms bicuculline-insensitive homooligomeric receptors in Xenopus oocytes. *J. Neurosci.*, 14: 6524–6531.

Wang, T.L., Hackam, A., Guggino, W.B. and Cutting, G.R. (1995a). A single amino acid in γ-aminobutyric acid ρ1 receptors affects competitive and noncompetitive components of picrotoxin inhibition. *Proc. Natl. Acad. Sci. USA*, 92: 11751–11755.

Wang, T.L., Hackam, A., Guggino, W.B. and Cutting, G.R. (1995b). A single histidine residue is essential for zinc inhibition of GABA ρ1 receptors. *J. Neurosci.*, 15: 7684–7691.

Wässle, H. and Chun, M.-H.(1989). GABA-like immunoreactivity in the cat retina: light microscopy. *J. Comp. Neurol.*, 279: 43–54.

Wegelius, K., Pasternack, M., Hiltunen, J.O., Rivera, C., Kaila, K., Saarma, M. and Reeben, M. (1998). Distribution of GABA receptor ρ subunit transcripts in the rat brain. *Eur. J. Neurosci.*, 10: 350–357.

Wegelius, K., Reeben, M., Rivera, C., Kaila, K., Saarma, M. and Pasternack, M. (1996) The rho 1 GABA receptor cloned from rat retina is down-modulated by protons. *Neuroreport*, 12: 2005–2009.

Wellis, D.P. and Werblin, F.S. (1995). Dopamine modulates GABAc receptors mediating inhibition of calcium entry into and transmitter release from bipolar cell terminals in tiger salamander retina. *J. Neurosci.*, 15: 4748–4761.

Woodward, R. M., Polenzani, L. and Miledi, R. (1992a). Effects of steroids on γ-aminobutyric acid receptors expressed in *Xenopus* oocytes by poly(A)+ RNA from mammalian brain and retina. *Mol. Pharmacol.*, 41: 89–103.

Woodward, R.M., Polenzani, L. and Miledi, R. (1992b). Characterization of bicuculline/baclofen-insensitive γ-aminobutyric acid receptors expressed in *Xenopus* oocytes. I. effects of Cl- channel inhibitors. *Mol. Pharmacol.*, 42: 165–173.

Woodward, R.M., Polenzani, L. and Miledi, R. (1993). Characterization of bicuculline/baclofen-insensitive (ρ-like) γ-aminobutyric acid receptors expressed in *Xenopus* oocytes. II. pharmacology of γ-aminobutyric acidA and γ-aminobutyric acidB receptor agonists and antagonists. *Mol. Pharmacol.*, 43: 609–625.

Yang, X.-L., Gao, F. and Wu, S.M. (1999). Modulation of horizontal cell function by GABA$_A$ and GABA$_C$ receptors in dark-and light-adapted tiger salamander retina. *Vis. Neurosci.*, 16: 967–979.

Zhang, D., Pan, Z.H., Zhang, X., Brideau, A.D. and Lipton, S.A. (1995). Cloning of a γ-aminobutyric acid type C receptor subunit in rat retina with a methionine residue critical for picrotoxinin channel block. *Proc. Natl. Acad. Sci. USA*, 92: 11756–11760.

Zhang, J. and Slaughter, M. M. (1995) Perferential suppression of the ON pathway by GABA$_C$ receptors in the amphibian retina. *J. Neurophysiol.*, 74: 1583–1592.

H. Kolb, H. Ripps and S. Wu (Eds.)
Progress in Brain Research, Vol. 131
© 2001 Elsevier Science B.V. All rights reserved

CHAPTER 21

Retinoic acid, a neuromodulator in the retina

Reto Weiler*, Mark Pottek, Konrad Schultz and Ulrike Janssen-Bienhold

Neurobiology, University of Oldenburg, D-26111 Oldenburg, Germany

Introduction

In 1960 John Dowling together with George Wald published their seminal paper about the biological function of vitamin A (Dowling and Wald, 1960), opening a new window towards an understanding of the biochemical and biological aspects of retinoids. In the subsequent years the interests of John and his collaborators shifted more towards an understanding of the neuronal mechanisms within the retinal network and in particular to neuromodulation. He pioneered the work on the role of dopamine which eventually resulted in the general recognition of dopamine as a light signal in the retina (Dowling, 1987). It was on this topic that we both collaborated during two summers in Woods Hole (Mangel et al., 1994; Baldridge et al., 1995; Weiler et al., 1997). One of the key findings of this collaboration was the biochemical confirmation of previous electro-physiological findings that although dopamine was a reliable signal for flickering light, it was not a robust signal for the ambient light condition. This finding together with many other observations made by our group, stimulated our search for additional signals that were able to transmit the information about the ambient light conditions to the neuronal retina. And this search incidentally brought us back to that 1960 article about the biological function of vitamin A.

Vitamin A or retinoids are very important biological molecules which serve two very different functions: in the form of retinoic acid they activate a large family of transcription factors which rule important aspects of development and in the form of retinaldehyde they constitute the light-sensitive component of rhodopsin which endows most species with vision. Indeed, the latter function is responsible for their name because for a long period only their photoreceptive role was known (Wald, 1935). Their function as a morphogenetic factor (in the form of retinoic acid) was only discovered recently (Giguère et al., 1987) but has gained widespread interest and led to very deep insight into the molecular events that regulate the axis and pattern formation of the vertebrate body. At the same time these studies have opened a window to an understanding of molecular processes that are at the core of malfunction and potentially linked to tumorgenesis. This research has sparked the interest of the pharmaceutical industry and made retinoic acid an important drug in cancer research and cosmetic applications.

It is the eye where the two biological functions of retinoids still meet (Dräger and McCaffery, 1997). Here, retinoic acid is formed as a consequence of the phototransduction process (McCaffery et al., 1996) and the pattern formation of the retina is determined through retinoic acid activated transcription factors (Wagner et al., 1992). It was therefore proposed that the transcriptional role of retinoic acid which is only found in vertebrates, originated from its phototransductive role. Only in the vertebrates, but not in the

_____

*Corresponding author: Reto Weiler, Tel.: 49-441-798-2581; Fax: 49-441-798-3423

310

invertebrate eye, does light induce the generation of retinoic acid.

Very recently, a third biological role for retinoids in the retina was proposed, that of a neuromodulator (Weiler et al., 1998; Weiler et al., 1999, 2000; Pottek and Weiler, 2000). This proposal is based on the observations that retinoic acid affects many features of the neuronal retina, intimately linked with light adaptation without involving the transcriptional level. This review will concentrate on this newly discovered role of retinoids and will summarize some of the recent findings in support of such a role.

Generation of retinoic acid in the adult retina

When a rhodopsin molecule captures a photon, its light-catching chromophore is converted from the bent form of 11-*cis* retinaldehyde to the straightened form of all-*trans* retinaldehyde. This straightening is followed by a break in the bond between the chromophore and the protein portion of the molecule, opsin. The freed all-*trans* retinaldehyde is now converted to all-*trans* retinol by a membrane bound, NADPH-requiring retinol dehydrogenase. The all-*trans* retinol is then shuttled to the retinal pigment epithelium with the help of the interphotoreceptor retinoid binding protein. In the pigment epithelium it is esterified by an acyltransferase and converted to 11-*cis* retinol by an isomerohydrolase. Another retinol dehydrogenase converts the 11-*cis* retinol into 11-*cis* retinaldehyde, the visual chromophore ready again for incorporation into opsin which is transferred back to the photoreceptor (Saari, 1994) (Fig. 1). All-*trans* retinaldehyde, instead of being subjected to the above metabolism, known as dark regeneration, can also be converted to retinoic acid mediated primarily by the enzyme aldehyde dehydrogenase (Futterman, 1962; McCaffery and Dräger, 1995).

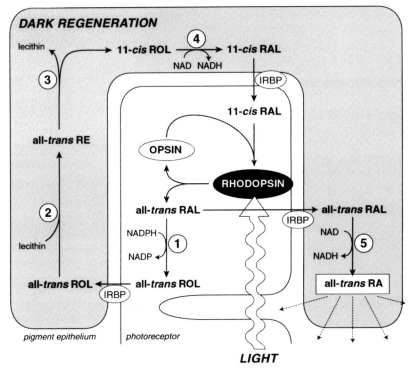

Fig. 1. Retinoid pathway in the outer vertebrate retina. Light stimulation leads to all-*trans* retinaldehyde which is re-converted to the chromophore 11-*cis* retinaldehyde in a sequence of reactions leading to dark regeneration of rhodopsin. Alternatively, it serves as the substrate for the production of retinoic acid. Abbreviations: IRBP, interphotoreceptor retinoid binding protein; RA, retinoic acid; RAL, retinaldehyde; RE, retinyl ester; ROL, retinol; ① membrane-bound retinol dehydrogenase; ② lecithin:retinol acyltransferase; ③ isomerohydrolase; ④ microsomal retinol dehydrogenase; ⑤ aldehyde dehydrogenase.

In a series of papers, Dräger and her collaborators have demonstrated that there is a spatial and temporal expression pattern of different aldehyde dehydrogenases in the developing eye that is responsible for the formation of the dorso-ventral axis, the expression patterns of rods and cones, and the formation of positional cues (reviewed in: Dräger and McCaffery, 1997). Based on the presence of aldehyde dehydrogenase, it appears that during development, most cells of the neuronal retina and the pigment epithelium are capable of synthesizing retinoic acid. The substrate for this synthesis at this stage does not derive from the phototransduction process but from the nutrients, and it has been known for a long time that vitamin A deficiency leads to severe distortions of normal eye development which can be rescued by supplementation of retinoic acid (Dowling and Wald, 1960). Since this review focuses on the role of retinoic acid as a putative neuromodulator in the mature retina, the developmental aspect will not be treated further.

In the mature and functioning retina, the synthesis of retinoic acid becomes light-dependent (McCaffery et al., 1996). The mechanisms accounting for this light-dependency is obvious: all-*trans* retinaldehyde released from bleached rhodopsin will increase with light stimulation and some of it will escape the dark regeneration process and will be converted into retinoic acid by the corresponding dehydrogenase given its presence in the mature retina. Thus, generation of retinoic acid appears to be an unavoidable side effect of the transduction process in particular during bright light stimulation. Since the oxidation step is irreversible, there are good reasons to assume that the amount of retinoic acid depends on the amount of bleached rhodopsin in some nonlinear fashion. The presence of the enzyme aldehyde dehydrogenase has been confirmed in the adult mouse and bovine retina (McCaffery et al., 1996; Saari et al., 1995; Milam et al., 1997) and we could demonstrate its presence also in the adult carp retina (Fig. 2). The strongest label was present in the pigment epithelium and in photoreceptors, in addition Müller cells were also labeled. These data confirm that the enzyme responsible for the conversion of all-*trans* retinaldehyde to retinoic acid is present in the mature retina and found in locations that are very likely to gain access to the substrate.

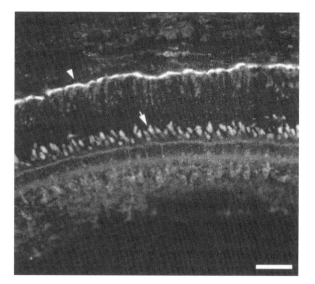

Fig. 2. Micrograph of a cross section of the carp retina labeled with a monoclonal antibody directed against the enzyme aldehyde dehydrogenase. Strong label is present in the retinal pigment epithelium (arrowhead) and in the outer segments of photoreceptors (arrow). Scale bar, 50 µm.

Using very sensitive assays based on retinoic acid reporter cells combined with HPLC techniques, it was possible to directly monitor the light-induced increase of retinoic acid formation in the living mouse eye. A significant increase of retinoic acid was detected already after 10 min of light (McCaffery et al., 1996). We were able to confirm such a light-induced increase also in the carp retina (Fig. 3). The light stimulus in this case was a constant bright white light (50 W halogen bulb) applied for 15 min which significantly increased the amount of retinoic acid.

The data from the mouse and the carp retina confirm the presence of a functional metabolic pathway that converts all-*trans* retinaldehyde to retinoic acid in the mature retina. In addition, the efficacy of this pathway is light-dependent, and retinoic acid, its endproduct, correlates with the ambient light condition. These are excellent prerequisites for a neuromodulator that would signal the ambient light condition to the neuronal retina. In particular since retinoic acid, due to its lipophilic character, can easily cross membranes and, it could affect not only the cell of its origin but also cells in the neighbourhood. We therefore analyzed the potential role of retinoic acid as a neuromodulator by using

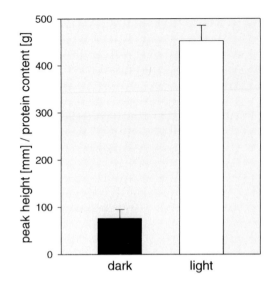

Fig. 3. Endogenous release of RA in the carp eye following dark and light adaptation. Data (mean ± S.D.) were obtained from 15 eyecups. Amount of all-*trans* RA is given as the peak height in the chromatogram relative to the protein content of the sample.

parameters that are known to be affected by light adaptation.

Effects of retinoic acid on the receptive field properties of horizontal cells

The following data were obtained from an inverted eye-cup preparation of the carp retina. Animals were kept under a strict 12-h light–dark cycle and preparation was done in the light phase in order to prevent any detachment of the pigment epithelium. The eye was hemisected and the posterior part was everted on a wooden dome and subsequently dark-adapted. The superfusate was delivered at the apex of the everted retina and drained off by small pieces of tissue paper. Light evoked recordings were made from horizontal cells using sharp electrodes.

(a) Light responsiveness

Light responsiveness was determined using white light, full-field stimuli, which evoke horizontal cell light responses that are independent of the coupling between these cells. After 30–40 min of dark adaptation, a mean maximal light response amplitude

of 30 mV was recorded with a shallow increase over the last 1.2 log units. In contrast, response–intensity relationship of light-adapted cells revealed a steeper increase and peaked at about a mean amplitude of 45 mV (Fig. 4). At low intensities, however, the responsiveness was reduced compared to the dark-adapted retina. Retinoic acid, added during the dark-adapted condition resulted in a response profile that shared many similarities with that of cells after light adaptation.

(b) Spatial properties

Receptive field size is a strongly light-correlated feature of horizontal cells. It is best described by the length constant and the ratio of the response amplitudes resulting from stimulation of its centre and its periphery. Nonsaturating white-light stimuli (spot 0.9 mm diameter; annulus, 1.1 mm inner and 3.2 mm outer diameter) were applied to dark- or light-adapted retinas and to dark-adapted retinas superfused with retinoic acid (Fig. 5A). The ratio of the response amplitudes to annular and spot stimulation (A/S) was plotted against the intensity (Fig. 5B). Ten minutes of light adaptation and 10 min of superfusion with retinoic acid had almost identical effects on the A/S ratio. The observed dependence of the A/S ratio of the stimulus intensity was fully conserved after retinoic acid superfusion. More quantitative data about the receptive field size were obtained by calculating the length constant (λ) of the horizontal cell network, using a series of spot stimuli of increasing size at different intensities. The data were fitted using a root mean square-minimizing routine (Lamb, 1976; Owen and Hare, 1989). In the dark-adapted retina, the majority of length constants were between 400 and 600 µm. Light adaptation decreased the length constant to values between 200 and 400 µm and a similar decrease was obtained with retinoic acid.

(c) Chromatic properties

The above recordings were all made from H1 horizontal cells, which are of the luminosity type and respond to all wavelengths with hyperpolarizations. We also recorded from horizontal cells of the

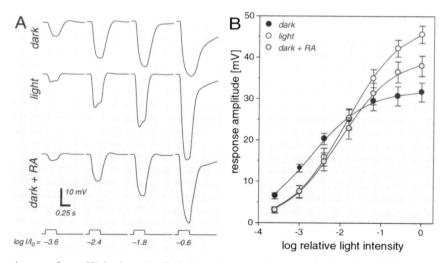

Fig. 4. Light responsiveness of carp H1 horizontal cells is dependent upon the state of adaptation. (A) Response profiles evoked by white light full-field stimulation with different intensities (log I/I_0). Each profile represents the averaged response of 8 cells. (B) Response–intensity diagram for 15 (dark; light) and 10 cells (dark + RA). RA added to the dark-adapted retina led to curve characteristics also obtained after light adaptation. Data representing mean ± S.E.M.

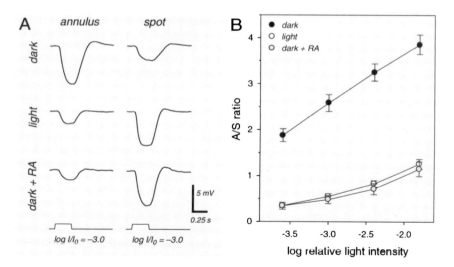

Fig. 5. Spatial properties of carp H1 horizontal cell responses. (A) Responses to white light annular and centered spot stimulation of the same intensity (log I/I_0) averaged from 10 cells. (B) Annulus/spot (A/S) ratio of the response amplitudes for different light intensities. Following light adaptation A/S ratios were substantially reduced compared to the dark-adapted condition. RA given to the dark-adapted retina mimicked the effect of light. Data (mean ± S.E.M.) were obtained from 10 cells under each condition.

chromaticity type H2. In the dark-adapted retina, these cells also respond with hyperpolarization to all wavelengths, whereas in the light-adapted retina their response to stimuli of the longer wavelength range turns into a depolarization (Weiler and Wagner, 1984). The same behavior was seen, when a dark-adapted retina was superfused with retinoic acid (Fig. 6). Again, superfusion with retinoic acid approximated the effects of light adaptation.

Taken together, these data show, that retinoic acid very closely mimics the effects of light adaptation on the receptive field properties of horizontal cells. In all these cases, photically isomerized retinoic acid, used as a control, was without effect.

314

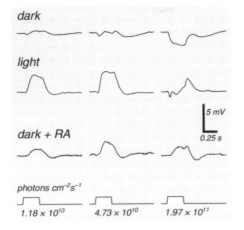

dark

light

dark + RA

5 mV

0.25 s

photons cm⁻²s⁻¹

1.18×10^{10} 4.73×10^{10} 1.97×10^{11}

Fig. 6. Response characteristics of carp H2 horizontal cells with respect to long wavelength stimulation. Full-field responses to 621 nm flashes of different intensity were averaged from 7 (dark; light) and 3 cells (dark + RA). As in the case of light adaptation, RA caused stable depolarizations in the dark-adapted retina.

Effects of retinoic acid on gap junctional coupling

Retinoic acid decreased the length constant of the horizontal cell network as shown above. The length constant is defined as $\lambda = (R_m/R_c)^{0.5}$ and shrinkage of the receptive field may therefore reflect a decrease in the cell's membrane resistance R_m as well as an increase of the coupling resistance R_c. Horizontal cells are extensively coupled with each other and numerous studies have demonstrated that the coupling conductivity is affected by the ambient light conditions and several neuromodulators (reviewed in: Baldridge et al., 1998). Given the potential role of retinoic acid as a light signal and its effect on the receptive field size of the horizontal cell network, we analyzed whether it also affects the coupling conductivity. Conductivity was monitored using either Lucifer Yellow or neurobiotin injection. The spread of the marker injected into a single cell in the living retina is a reliable index of gap junctional conductivity. This set of experiments was not only done with the carp retina but also with the retinas of rabbit and mouse. Lucifer Yellow injection into a H1 cell of a dark-adapted (30 min) carp retina results typically in 6–13 labeled somata. Following application of retinoic acid for 20 min, the spread of the dye was restricted to one or two cells (Fig. 7A). In the rabbit retina the injection of the dye into A-type horizontal

cell results typically in 15–30 min labeled neighboring A-type cells. After about 30 min of superfusion with retinoic acid the coupling was completely abolished (Fig. 7B). The tracer neurobiotin was used to inject horizontal cells in the mouse retina, and typically labeled a network of 150–250 neighboring somata. Again after about 30 min of superfusion with retinoic acid, this coupling was completely abolished (Fig. 7C). In all cases, there was a gradual reduction of the coupling over the superfusion time and in all cases a concentration of 100–150 µM retinoic acid was effective.

Retinoic acid is a highly lipophilic substance which is barely soluble in Ringer. The physiological active concentration around the horizontal cells might therefore be considerably lower. In most of the experiments it was possible to reverse the effect of retinoic acid by extended wash out periods up to 60 min. Again the effect of retinoic acid on gap junctional coupling was stereo-specific since light-isomerised retinoic acid and the 9-*cis* form were without effect (Fig. 8A,B).

Effects of retinoic acid on spinule dynamics

The formation of spinules is a well described phenomenon in the fish retina that is linked to light adaptation. Spinules are spine-like protrusions of the terminal dendrites of horizontal cells invaginating the cone pedicle. They form part of the synaptic ribbon complex within the pedicle, and the number of spinules is directly related to the light-adaptive level of the retina and also correlates with the strength of the negative feedback from horizontal cells onto cones (Weiler and Wagner, 1984; Wagner and Djamgoz, 1993). Several studies have shed light on the cellular and molecular processes that are involved in spinule formation during light adaptation and spinule retraction during dark adaptation (Weiler et al., 1988; Weiler et al., 1991; Weiler and Janssen-Bienhold, 1993; Weiler and Schultz, 1993; Weiler et al., 1995, 1996; Okada et al., 1999). However, despite all these efforts, the signal that transmits the information about the ambient light condition and feeds into the cellular cascades remained elusive. We were therefore analyzing whether retinoic acid could be such a signal.

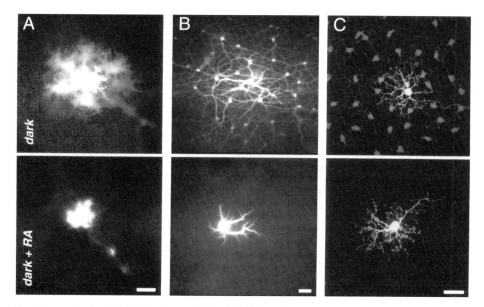

Fig. 7. Dye coupling between horizontal cells in the carp (A), rabbit (B), and mouse retina (C). In the dark-adapted condition, injected dye spread from the recorded cell to several neighboring cells of the same subtype. Following RA treatment, dye spread was absent. Scale bar, 25 µm.

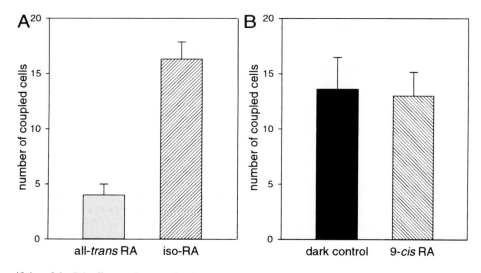

Fig. 8. Stereospecificity of the RA effect on dye coupling between rabbit A-type horizontal cells. (A) Application of light-isomerized all-*trans* RA (iso-RA; $n = 3$) or (B) the 9-*cis* isomer ($n = 5$) revealed no reduction of dye coupling in the dark-adapted retina. Data representing mean ± S.D.

In control experiments, carps were dark-adapted for 3 h and then subsequently light-adapted for 45 min. Cross sections of cone pedicles revealed a synaptic complex typical of light-adapted retinas (Fig. 9A). Numerous spinules were extruded from the horizontal cell dendrites and the quantitative analysis resulted in a spinules per synaptic ribbon (spr) value of 2.51 ± 0.51. In another series of experiments, after 3 h of dark adaptation, the right eyes received an injection of retinoic acid at an estimated intra-ocular concentration of 0.5 µM. The left eye received an injection of the vehicle. Injections were made

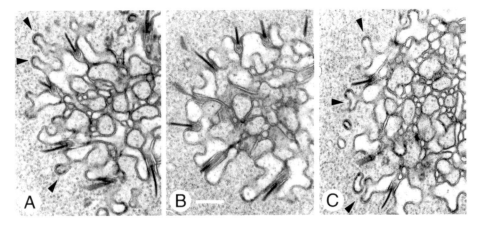

Fig. 9. Effect of RA on spinule dynamics in the carp retina. Electron micrographs of tangential sections at the level of the cone pedicles. (A) Light adaptation gave rise to numerous spinules (arrowheads). Micrographs in (B) and (C) were obtained from the left and right eye of the same dark-adapted animal. Whereas in the dark control (B) no spinules were present, RA treatment (C) led to spinule formation. Scale bar, 0.5 μm.

under dim red light and lasted about 1 min; thereafter the animal was allowed to swim for another 45 min in the dark. Analysis of the cone synaptic complex of the two eyes revealed remarkable differences. Whereas the left eye showed all the features of a dark-adapted retina, the right eye showed all the features of a light-adapted retina (Fig. 9B and C). In the left eye, spinules were almost completely absent and the terminal dendrites showed a rounded shape in the tangential sections. The spr value was 0.72 ± 0.39. In the right eye numerous spinules were present and the spr value was 2.74 ± 0.41, matching that of a light-adapted control.

The effect of retinoic acid was very site-specific. Only the dendrites of horizontal cells invaginating the cone pedicle and laterally flanking the synaptic ribbon produced spinules following retinoic acid injection. These sites are identical to the ones that also produce spinules upon light adaptation. No other dendrites in the cone pedicle—horizontal cell dendrites central to the ribbon or bipolar cell dendrites—produced spinules, nor did the horizontal cell dendrites that are invaginating the rod spherules. These dendrites do not form spinules following light adaptation.

These experiments demonstrated that exogenously administered retinoic acid is a potent signal for the induction of spinules with high specificity for the site. The interesting question now was whether retinoic acid formed in vivo during light adaptation was also

able to induce the formation of spinules. In order to address this question, we used the drug citral, which is known to inhibit the enzyme aldehyde dehydrogenase responsible for the oxidation of retinaldehyde to retinoic acid. Citral at a concentration of 200 μM was injected under dim red light into the right eyes of carps that had been dark-adapted for 3 h. The animal were then allowed to swim for another 25 min in the dark before they were light-adapted for 60 min. Examination of the left eye revealed the presence of numerous spinules and the spr value was 3.12 ± 0.68. The retinae injected with citral, however, showed an overall morphology that closely resembled that of a dark-adapted retina and the number of spinules was significantly lower (spr $= 1.91 \pm 0.53$; Fig. 10). The citral-induced inhibition of spinule formation could be rescued completely by the subsequent injection of 0.5 μM retinoic acid. These experiments strongly support the idea that retinoic acid is a potent in vivo signal for the formation of spinules. The build-up of retinoic acid following light-isomerization of retinaldehyde and its diffusion to horizontal cells is most likely a comparably slow process. Therefore, it is very unlikely that retinoic acid could be a signal for fast changing light conditions. Rather it appears that retinoic acid would be an ideal signal for ambient light conditions, integrating over a certain period of time. It is very tempting to speculate that retinoic acid signals the average, sustained conditions, whereas dopamine is responsible for the signalling of changing

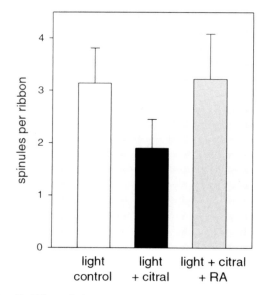

Fig. 10. Effect of the RA-synthesis inhibitor citral on light-induced spinule formation in the carp retina. Citral ($n = 5$) inhibited spinule formation compared to the light-adapted control condition. Spinule formation was restored by subsequent RA treatment ($n = 2$). Data representing mean ± S.D.

events. Indeed, the two signals are independent and the effect of retinoic acid were not blocked by dopaminergic antagonists (Pottek and Weiler, 2000).

At present not much is known about the pathways and the molecular cascades through which retinoic acid exerts its effects in the retina. The well described transcriptional pathway, where retinoic acid activates nuclear receptors, seems not to be involved. Blockade of transcriptional activity using the drug actinomycin did not inhibit the different light-adaptive effect of retinoic acid (Weiler et al., 1998). On the other hand, the observed stereospecificity of its effects suggests the involvement of a receptor. It will therefore be very interesting to unravel the mechanisms that give retinoic acid neuromodulatory power.

Conclusions

The major challenge for all sensory organs is to maintain a wide operating range without loosing high incremental sensitivity. Evolution has developed a plethora of strategies to cope with this dilemma, and we have just begun to recognize and to understand a few of them.

Over the years, many studies have revealed that in the retina such strategies are found at an early stage. Besides the phototransduction process, it appears that the first synaptic transmission between the photoreceptors and the horizontal cells is particularly prone to corresponding mechanisms, which we call neuronal adaptation. The basic principle of neuronal adaptation is the comparison of a local signal with a signal averaged over time and space and the corresponding resetting of the local synaptic transfer.

Such a mechanism involves the transmission of an averaged signal which acts as a neuromodulator. This short report has summarized some of the recent findings that strongly suggest that retinoic acid is such a signal in the retina and consequently can be regarded as a neuromodulator. It is quite fascinating to see that retinoic acid takes over such a function in the retina because it highlights once more that nature often prefers simple solutions for complex tasks. Retinoic acid is an unavoidable byproduct of the phototransduction process and as such directly correlated with the ambient light conditions, and it is highly reactive. It is then very straightforward and economic to combine this molecule with neuromodulatory power.

On a personal side, it is quite rewarding to see that the discovery of retinoic acid as a neuromodulator has bridged two essential lines of research championed by John Dowling during his outstanding career: one being the biological role of retinoids, the other being neuromodulation in the retina. And both lines somehow meet at the horizontal cell, the retinal cell type whose exploration is ultimately linked with the work of John Dowling.

Acknowledgements

Our work on the role of retinoic acid was supported by the Deutsche Forschungsgemeinschaft and the Volkswagen-Stiftung. In 1991, John Dowling and Reto Weiler were the recipients of the Max-Planck-Research Award jointly given by the Max Planck Society and the Alexander von Humboldt Foundation. The award allowed them a collaboration during two summers in Woods Hole, working together with William Baldridge and Stuart Mangel on neuromodulation.

318

References

Baldridge, W.H., Weiler, R. and Dowling, J.E. (1995) Dark-suppression and light-sensitization of horizontal cell responses in the hybrid bass retina. *Vis. Neurosci.*, 12: 611–620.

Baldridge, W.H., Vaney, D.I. and Weiler, R. (1998) The modulation of intercellular coupling in the retina. *Semin. Cell Dev. Biol.*, 9: 311–318.

Dowling, J.E. and Wald, G. (1960) The biological function of vitamin A acid. *Proc. Natl. Acad. Sci. USA*, 46: 587–608.

Dowling, J.E. (1987) *The Retina*. The Belknap Press of Harvard University Press, Cambridge, MA and London, GB.

Dräger, U.C. and McCaffery, P. (1997) Retinoic acid and development of the retina. In: Osborne, N.N. and Chader, G. (Eds.), *Progress in Retinal and Eye Research*, Elsevier Science, pp. 323–351.

Futterman, S. (1962) Enzymatic oxidation of vitamin A aldehyde to vitamin A acid. *J. Biol Chem.*, 237: 677–680.

Giguère, V., Ong, E.S., Segui, P. and Evans, R.M. (1987) Identification of a receptor for the morphogen retinoic acid. *Nature*, 624.

Lamb, T.D. (1976) Spatial properties of horizontal cell responses in the turtle retina. *J. Physiol. (Lond.)*, 263: 239–255.

Mangel, S.C., Baldridge, W.H., Weiler, R. and Dowling, J.E. (1994) Threshold and chromatic sensitivity changes in fish cone horizontal cells following prolonged darkness. *Brain Res.*, 659: 55–61.

McCaffery, J.M. and Dräger, U.C. (1995) Retinoic acid synthesizing enzymes in the embryonic and adult vertebrate. *Adv. Exp. Med. Biol.*, 372: 173–183.

McCaffery, P. and Dräger, U.C. (1994) High levels of a retinoic acid-generating dehydrogenase in the meso-telencephalic dopamine system. *Proc. Natl. Acad. Sci. USA*, 91: 7772–7776.

McCaffery, P., Mey, J. and Dräger, U.C. (1996) Light-mediated retinoic acid production. *Proc. Natl. Acad. Sci. USA*, 93: 12570–12574.

Milam, A.H., Possin, D.E., Huang, J., Fariss, R.N., Flannery, J.G. and Saari, J.C. (1997) Characterization of aldehyde dehydrogenase-positive amacrine cells restricted in distribution to the dorsal retina. *Vis. Neurosci.*, 14: 601–608.

Okada, T., Schultz, K., Geurtz, W., Hatt, H. and Weiler, R. (1999) AMPA-preferring receptors with high Ca^{2+} permeability mediate dendritic plasticity of retinal horizontal cells. *Eur. J. Neurosci.*, 11: 1085–1095.

Owen, W.G. and Hare, W. (1989) Signal transfer from photoreceptors to bipolar cells in the retina of the tiger salamder. *Neurosci. Res. Suppl.*, 10: S77–S88.

Pottek, M. and Weiler, R. (2000) Light-adaptive effects of retinoic acid on receptive field properties of retinal horizontal cells. *Eur. J. Neurosci.*, 12: 437–445.

Saari, J.C. (1994) Retinoids in photosensitive systems. In: Sporn, M.B., Roberts, A.B. and Goodmann, D.S. (Eds.), *The Retinoids: Biology, Chemistry, and Medicine*, Raven Press, New York, pp. 351–385.

Saari, J.C., Champer, R.J., Asson-Batres, M.A., Garwin, G.G., Huang, J., Crabb, J.W. and Milam, A.H. (1995) Characterization and localization of an aldehyde dehydrogenase to amacrine cells of the bovine retina. *Vis. Neurosci.*, 12: 263–272.

Wagner, H.-J. and Djamgoz, M.B.A. (1993) Spinules: a case for retinal synaptic plasticity. *Trends Neurosci.*, 16: 201–206.

Wagner, M., Han, B. and Jessell, T.M. (1992) Regional differences in retinoid release from embryonic neural tissue detected by an in vitro reporter assay. *Development*, 116: 55–66.

Wald, G. (1935) Carotenoids and the visual cycle. *J. Gen. Physiol.*, 19: 351–361.

Weiler, R. and Wagner, H.-J. (1984) Light-dependent change of cone-horizontal cell interactions in carp retina. *Brain Res.*, 298: 1–9.

Weiler, R., Kohler, K., Kirsch, M. and Wagner, H.-J. (1988) Glutamate and dopamine modulate synaptic plasticity in horizontal cell dendrites of fish retina. *Neurosci. Lett.*, 87: 205–209.

Weiler, R., Kohler, K. and Janssen, U. (1991) Protein kinase C mediates transient spinule-type neurite outgrowth in the retina during light adaptation. *Proc. Natl. Acad. Sci. USA*, 88: 3603–3607.

Weiler, R. and Janssen-Bienhold, U. (1993) Spinule-type neurite outgrowth from horizontal cells during light adaptation in the carp retina: An actin-dependent process. *J. Neurocytol.*, 22: 129–139.

Weiler, R. and Schultz, K. (1993) Ionotropic non-*N*-methyl-D-aspartate agonists induce retraction of dendritic spinules from retinal horizontal cells. *Proc. Natl. Acad. Sci. USA*, 90: 6533–6537.

Weiler, R., Schultz, K. and Janssen-Bienhold, U. (1995) Retraction of spinule-type neurites from retinal horizontal cell dendrites during dark adaptation involves the activation of Ca^{2+}/calmodulin-dependent protein kinase II. *Eur. J. Neurosci.*, 7: 1914–1919.

Weiler, R., Schultz, K. and Janssen-Bienhold, U. (1996) Ca^{2+}-dependency of spinule plasticity at dendrites of retinal horizontal cells and its possible implication for the functional role of spinules. *Vision Res.*, 36: 3891–3900.

Weiler, R., Baldridge, W.H., Mangel, S.C. and Dowling, J.E. (1997) Modulation of endogenous dopamine release in the fish retina by light and prolonged darkness. *Vis. Neurosci.*, 14: 351–356.

Weiler, R., Schultz, K., Pottek, M., Tieding, S. and Janssen-Bienhold, U. (1998) Retinoic acid has light-adaptive effects on horizontal cells in the retina. *Proc. Natl. Acad. Sci. USA*, 95: 7139–7144.

Weiler, R., He, S. and Vaney, D.I. (1999) Retinoic acid modulates gap junctional permeability between horizontal cells of the mammalian retina. *Eur. J. Neurosci.*, 11: 3346–3350.

Weiler, R., Pottek, M., He, S. and Vaney, D.I. (2000) Modulation of coupling between retinal horizontal cells by retinoic acid and endogenous dopamine. *Brain Res. Rev.*, 32: 121–129.

H. Kolb, H. Ripps and S. Wu (Eds.)
Progress in Brain Research, Vol. 131
© 2001 Elsevier Science B.V. All rights reserved

CHAPTER 22

Properties of turtle retinal ganglion cell GABA receptors

Eric M. Lasater[1,*] and Yun Liu[1,2]

[1]*Moran Eye Center, University of Utah Health Sciences Center, University of Utah, 50 North Medical Drive,*
Salt Lake City, UT 84132, USA
[2]*Department of Ophthalmology, University of Texas, Health Sciences Center,*
7703 Floyd Curl Drive, San Antonio, TX 78284, USA

Introduction

The synapses between retinal ganglion cells and second order neurons, which comprise the inner plexiform layer, are the last stage of processing of the visual signal before it is conveyed to higher brain centers. Few would argue that γ-aminobutyric-acid (GABA), the principal inhibitory neurotransmitter in the CNS, is an important neurotransmitter in the inner plexiform layer of the vertebrate retina at synapses from amacrine cells onto ganglion cells (Pasantes-Morales et al., 1972; Vaughn et al., 1981; Ariel and Adolph, 1985; Marc et al., 1988; Guiloff and Kolb, 1993; Lukasiewicz and Shields, 1998). In turtle, GABAergic amacrine cells make up nearly 30% of proximal inner nuclear somata (Weiler et al., 1991) and have been shown to have direct input onto ganglion cells (Guiloff and Kolb, 1993) with as much as 90–95% of the inner plexiform layer covered by GABAergic processes. A variety of pharmacologic and physiologic studies have demonstrated that GABA inhibits the responses of ganglion cells to visual stimuli in a wide variety of vertebrate species (see Massey and Redburn, 1987). In addition, it has been shown that GABAergic inhibition participates in the formation of transient and sustained light responses (Maguire et al., 1989; Slaughter et al., 1989). Similarly, GABA may play an important role in directionally selective responses of ganglion cells (Caldwell et al., 1978; Ariel and Adolph, 1985). However, at the cellular level very little is known of the mechanisms which underlie those actions of GABA on retinal ganglion cells. The majority of what we know has been derived from recordings in the intact retina or the retinal slice (for example see Lukasiewicz and Shields, 1998) and so far the data indicates that GABA responses in ganglion cells is predominantly the result of GABA$_A$ receptor activation; we found this not to be the case in turtle.

In a variety of neuronal cell types, GABA has been shown to operate through three classes of GABA receptors (Bormann, 2000). GABA$_A$ receptors are ligand-activated chloride channels while GABA$_B$ receptors modulate voltage-dependent potassium and calcium channels through G-protein activation and an intracellular second messenger pathway. Recent studies have identified in the retina a new subtype of GABA receptor which has been termed the GABA$_C$ receptor (Qian and Dowling, 1993; Feigenspan et al., 1993; Lukasiewicz et al., 1994). These receptors are also coupled to Cl$^-$ channels but unlike GABA$_A$ receptors they are more sensitive to GABA and are insensitive to bicuculline and to channel modulators. While the receptor was

---

*Corresponding author: Eric M. Lasater, Tel.: 801-585-6503;
Fax: 801-581-3357; E-mail: Eric.Lasater@hsc.utah.edu

originally found by Cutting et al. (1991), a great deal of work on it has been carried out in the retina by Dowling and his associates (Qian and Dowling, 1993, 1994, 1995; Qian et al., 1998, 1999). Much of this work has centered on studies of horizontal cells and bipolar cells, since in many species, it appears that the $GABA_C$ receptor resides primarily on these cell types. The bipolar cell in particular seems to have a high concentration at its axon terminal (Feigenspan et al., 1993; Qian and Dowling, 1995; Lukasiewicz and Shields, 1998). In our work, we have found that a large portion of the GABAergic response in turtle ganglion cells can be ascribed to the activation of $GABA_C$ receptors.

In our studies of the inhibitory processes that impinge on retinal ganglion cells, we sought to characterize the properties of GABA evoked responses in turtle ganglion cells. Isolated, cultured ganglion cells were used in an effort to identify the types of GABA receptors involved in GABAergic transmission at the ganglion cell layer in the inner turtle retina and to study the effect on the cell's membrane properties when these receptors were activated. While we describe the results of the activation of all three GABA receptor types, because of the novelty of the finding, we focused on the $GABA_C$ response. From this, we will get a better understanding of how inhibition is carried out at the cellular level in the turtle retina.

Responses of ganglion cells to GABA

Figure 1A shows a response typical of that recorded from an isolated turtle ganglion cell with application of 40 μM GABA for 30 s. The cell was voltage clamped and the membrane potential was held at −70 mV. Two components to the response were observed; one rapidly desensitized and the other was sustained. Similar inward currents with two components were induced in all ganglion cells we tested with GABA ($n > 100$).

The relaxation phase of the transient GABA response, in most cells tested, (in the dosage range of 40–100 μM) was very well fit with a first order exponential equation plus a constant (Fig. 1B). The steady state current calculated from the equation fit on top of the actual sustained current measured at

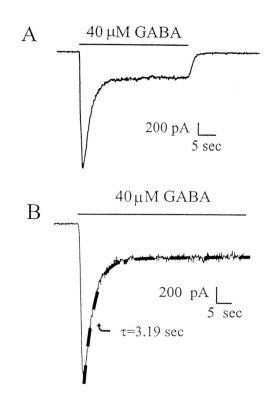

Fig. 1. GABA-induced response in an isolated ganglion cell. (A) GABA current evoked by 40 μM GABA produced a response with an initial transient component which relaxed to a sustained current. (B) First order fit of the relaxation of the GABA current in a second cell. It was fit with a first order exponential equation plus a constant: $I = (I_p^{-t/\tau}) + C$. Where I is the GABA induced current; I_p the GABA induced peak current; τ the time constant of the fast decay; and C was a constant. The value of C was almost equal to the magnitude of the sustained current. The heavy, dashed line represents the fit of the curve with this equation.

the end of a 30 s GABA application. This finding suggested to us that there was probably more than one mechanism mediating the GABA-induced responses.

The time constant for the transient current decay elicited by 40 μM GABA was 4.71 s ($n = 41$), while that for the current evoked by 100 μM GABA was 4.58 s. No significant difference between these two groups was found, even though 100 μM GABA always induced a much larger peak current than 40 μM GABA. The time constant of decay then is independent of the amplitude of the current. These data indicate that the rate of the fast decay was determined by the intrinsic properties of the GABA receptors and did not depend on the magnitude of current flow.

We tested this idea by measuring membrane conductance two seconds before, during and after the application of GABA under various ionic conditions (not shown). We used both symmetric and asymmetric chloride concentrations across the membrane. We found that when the current and conductance were normalized to their maximum values and plotted together as a function of time, the GABA induced currents changed in parallel with the conductance. This suggested that the decay of the current was due to true desensitization of the receptors rather than a change in the chloride reversal potential caused by a very large flow of current which altered equilibrium potentials. Recovery from the desensitization was slow after a 30 s pulse of 100 µM GABA; it was complete after about 1.5–2 min (not shown). Because of this GABA was applied at 2 min intervals, in the experiments described below, to avoid the effect of desensitization of the GABA receptor.

We went on to examine the kinetic properties of the two components of the GABA current. It was found that they were different, consistent with the idea that there could be more than one mechanism underlying the GABA responses in turtle ganglion cells. GABA evoked responses for different concentrations of GABA are shown in Fig. 2. At concentrations lower than 10 µM, GABA elicited only one current component. This current component activated very slowly and showed no desensitization during a 30 s GABA exposure. This slow current component closely resembled the response evoked by the activation of GABA$_C$ receptors seen in other systems (Pan and Lipton, 1995; Qian and Dowling, 1995). At higher concentrations, a the second current component was activated. It had substantially different kinetics than did the first component. It was like the typical currents induced by the activation of CNS GABA$_A$ receptors (Sivilotti and Nistri, 1991). This component activated faster, was transient or rapidly desensitized, and was the larger of the two in magnitude. Interestingly, the concentration at which maximum responses were induced, however, was the same for both currents (~100 µM).

The notion that the two components of the GABA responses were mediated by two different

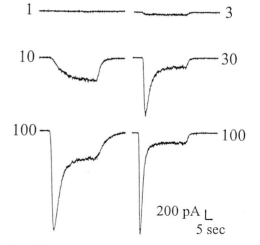

Fig. 2. Different concentrations of GABA evoked different responses. The left column represents current obtained from one cell and those on the right from a second cell. The concentration of GABA applied (µM) is indicated to the left of each trace. At low concentrations the onset of the response was slow and the peak response sustained. Higher concentrations evoked a fast desensitizing response followed by a sustained plateau.

receptor-channel complexes was further supported by fitting the dose response curves for the two GABA currents with the Hill equation as seen in Fig. 3. The sustained currents were measured at the end of a 30 s application of GABA. The transient currents were obtained by subtracting the sustained from the peak currents since the measured sustained current (at 30 s.) is not likely to be contaminated by the transient current. Both currents were normalized to their corresponding maximum responses induced by 100 µM GABA. The GABA concentration-response relation was fit with the following equation:

$$\frac{I}{I_{max}} = \frac{C^n}{(C^n + EC_{50}{}^n)} \qquad (1)$$

In the equation, I is the observed GABA-induced current at a given concentration, I_{max} is the maximum current induced by 100 µM GABA, C is the GABA concentration, n is the Hill coefficient, and EC_{50} is the concentration which evokes a half-maximal response. The EC_{50} for the transient GABA currents was 3.3×10^{-5} M. This is like those found for typical GABA$_A$ receptor channel complexes in other systems (Akaike et al., 1985; Itabashi et al., 1992).

322

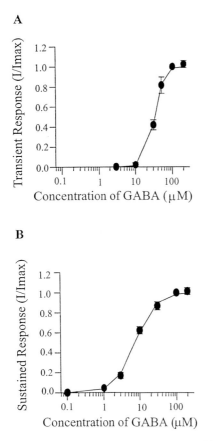

A

B

Fig. 3. Dose response curves were constructed in A for the transient and in B for the sustained GABA currents. To obtain the transient current we subtracted the sustained current measured at the end of a 30 s application from the peak GABA current. The lines going through the points represents the fit with the Hill equation. Error bars are the standard deviations.

While on the contrary, the EC_{50} for the sustained GABA current was 7.6×10^{-6} M. This is considerably lower than that for the $GABA_A$ receptors but is similar to that seen at $GABA_C$ receptors (Woodward et al., 1993; Qian and Dowling, 1994). The Hill coefficient for the transient GABA current was 3.6, suggesting that four molecules of GABA are required to combine with or interact in a cooperative fashion with the GABA receptor for activation. That is the binding of GABA to one receptor facilitates the binding of a second or facilitates the opening of other receptor-channel complexes. The activation of the sustained GABA current, however, requires the binding of probably only two molecules of GABA

as indicated by a Hill coefficient of 1.4. The results of these studies indicated to us that the turtle ganglion cell GABA response is made up of the combined responses resulting from the activation of both $GABA_A$- and $GABA_C$ receptor types.

Unlike what has been observed in other retinas (Lukasiewicz and Shields, 1998), we found that GABA induced both $GABA_A$- and $GABA_C$-like responses in every turtle ganglion cell tested. However, the fraction of the total current produced by these two receptors varied from cell to cell. By dividing the sustained currents by the peak currents we obtained the relative proportion of $GABA_C$-like responses for 80 cells. This is plotted in Fig. 4. The ratio of $GABA_C$-like/total GABA response for individual cells varied from 0.10 to 0.35, with an average value of 0.21 ± 0.05 for 80 cells.

$GABA_C$ immunohistochemistry

In order to confirm the existence of $GABA_C$ receptors on turtle ganglion cells we labeled rho receptors on ganglion cells using antibodies to the rho-1 and rho-2 receptor subunits. The antibodies

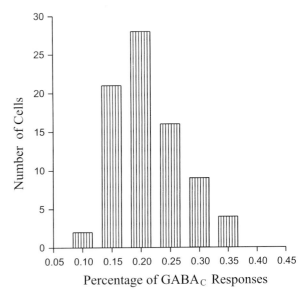

Fig. 4. A histogram illustrating the proportion of $GABA_C$ responses on turtle retinal ganglion cells. The percentages were obtained by dividing the sustained current at the end of a 30 s GABA application (100 μM) by the corresponding peak current. The response of the majority of cells consisted of a high percentage of the $GABA_C$ component; between 20 and 35%.

323

were kindly provided by Drs. Heinz Wässle and
Dongxian Zhang. Isolated, cultured cells were labeled
as well as cells in cryostat sections. An example of a
labeled isolated ganglion cell is shown in Fig. 5A. The
red represents rhodamine labeled antibody. The
antibody labels the membrane of the cell body and
the processes. Note the heavy labeling at the ends
of the processes. In whole retinal sections (Fig. 5B)
there is extensive labeling in the inner plexiform
layer and the ganglion cell layer. Prominent labeling
occurs in layers S1 and S3 and in the ganglion cell
layer; the cell bodies of ganglion cells (arrows) are
heavily labeled.

The results of the labeling study confirm the presence of rho-1 and -2 receptor subunits in the turtle
retina. The subunits are concentrated in the inner
plexiform layer and the ganglion cell layer. The

labeling pattern indicates a significant contribution
of the GABA$_C$ receptor to ganglion cell physiology.

Two GABA-activated receptor-ion channel complexes in turtle ganglion cells

In our studies of turtle ganglion cells, we found that
GABA evoked currents in the cells which consisted of
two components, one transient and the other
sustained. We examined the kinetics of activation
and inactivation of the currents and also investigated
their pharmacological properties. Our results suggest
that the two components are mediated by different
GABA receptor subtypes. Classical GABA$_A$ receptors appear to mediate the transient current while the
sustained current shares some properties with the

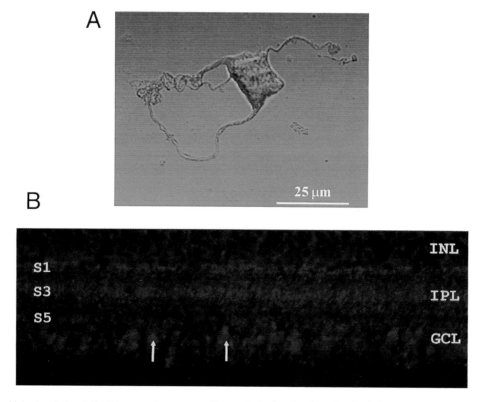

Fig. 5. Immunohistochemisrty of GABA$_C$ receptors on ganglion cells. Isolated cells and retinal slices were labeled with antibodies to rho-1 and -2 receptor subunits. In A is shown a single cell viewed with a combination of transmitted and fluorescence illumination; the red indicates antibody location. The cell plasma membrane and the end of the processes are particularly well labeled. In B is a labeled retinal cross section. Sublamina 1 and 3 are heavily labeled. Likewise the ganglion cell layer is also heavily labeled. The arrows indicate labeled cell bodies. Magnification in B is 400 ×.

current induced by GABA$_C$ receptor activation seen in other systems. The current observed due to GABA$_C$ receptor activation can, in some cells, be a significant portion ($> 25\%$) of the total GABA evoked current. While ganglion cells have been shown to possess GABA$_C$ receptors, such a large contribution of the receptors to ganglion cell activity has not been previously observed in other preparations (Zhang and Slaughter, 1995; Lukasiewicz and Shields, 1998). Several lines of evidence support the idea that GABA$_C$ receptors make a significant contribution to ganglion cell function.

First, the two receptors activate over different ranges and exhibit distinct kinetics. The GABA$_A$ receptors have a narrow activation range while that of the GABA$_C$ receptors is much broader. The kinetics of the GABA$_A$ currents in our cells are transient as in other systems. The fast decay of this current is a true desensitization, similar to that shown by Tauck et al. (1988) in rat. We found that the GABA$_C$ currents activate more slowly, and show little, if any, desensitization (Pan and Lipton, 1995).

In addition, these two receptors show different affinities for GABA. The ganglion cell GABA$_C$ receptors have a greater affinity for GABA than the GABA$_A$ receptors. This was seen in the lower activation threshold and smaller EC_{50} for the sustained GABA current. The high affinity of GABA$_C$ receptors is similar to that seen in other retinal neurons (Qian and Dowling, 1993; Matthews et al., 1994; Pan and Lipton, 1995) and in expressed receptors (Polenzani et al., 1991). Even so, we found that GABA was more efficacious at GABA$_A$ receptor sites. Like Qian and Dowling (1993) and Zhang and Slaughter (1995), we found that the maximum response induce by activation of GABA$_A$ receptors was much greater than that seen with GABA$_C$ receptor stimulation (Zhang and Slaughter, 1995). This could occur if GABA$_A$ receptor-channel complexes are expressed by these cells at a higher relative percentage, or if the single channel conductance of the GABA$_A$-receptor/channel complex is greater. Feigenspan et al. (1993) demonstrated that in rat bipolar cells, consistent with the later, the bicuculline-sensitive GABA receptor had a single channel conductance of 27 pS while that of the bicuculline-resistant GABA receptor was only 7 pS.

Our data indicate that the GABA evoked currents in turtle retinal ganglion cells are carried by the flow of Cl$^-$ ions similar to the GABA currents seen in other retinal ganglion cells (Tauck et al., 1988; Cohen et al., 1989; Lukasiewicz et al., 1994; Zhang and Slaughter, 1995). The observed reversal potential agreed well with that calculated for the Cl$^-$ equilibrium potential as did the amplitude and polarity of the current observed under different conditions. The gating of the GABA-activated Cl$^-$ channels are independent of membrane voltage as indicated by a linear current-voltage relationship for the GABA activated currents (Feigenspan et al., 1993; Tauck et al., 1988; Qian and Dowling, 1993; Ozawa and Yuzaki, 1984; Bormann et al., 1987).

GABA response pharmacology

As mentioned, the above results led us to conclude that the two components of the GABA response in turtle retinal ganglion cells was mediated by two different types of receptor; the GABA$_A$- and GABA$_C$ receptors. We explored this notion in the following experiments. First, we investigated the effect of the specific GABA$_A$ receptor blocker, bicuculline, on the currents. When low concentrations of bicuculline ($1 \sim 10$ μM) were applied, we found it inhibited only the transient GABA current. The sustained current remained intact. The effect recovered completely after bicuculline was washed out of the bath. This is shown in Fig. 6A. Here the cell was exposed to 10 μM bicuculline immediately preceding the application of a mixture of GABA and bicuculline. One can see that the transient current is far more sensitive to the bicuculline than is the sustained current.

If the concentration of bicuculline was increased to as high as 100–250 μM, we saw that the sustained current was reduced but it failed to completely block the current. This is seen in Fig. 6B for a different cell. Application of 100 μM bicuculline reduced the sustained current by about 60%. Interestingly the onset of the current was more rapid than in the first cell but still slower than the transient current. These results seen in Fig. 7 indicate that turtle ganglion cells possess both bicuculline-sensitive and bicuculline-resistant GABA receptors. The transient or rapidly desensitizing GABA current is mediated

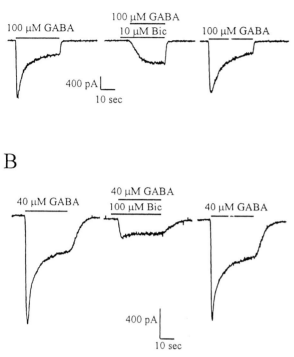

Fig. 6. Separation of the two GABA responses in two cells. In (A) the GABA$_A$ receptor antagonist, bicuculline, was co-applied with GABA. The bicuculline (10 μM) selectively blocked the transient current as seen in the middle trace. Note the slow onset of the response. The cell recovered following drug washout. In (B), a second cell was tested with a higher concentration of bicuculline (100 μM). This reduced but did not completely block the sustained GABA$_C$ response indicating that in turtle bicuculline can have some effect on the GABA$_C$ response. We never saw bicuculline completely block the GABA$_C$ response.

by the bicuculline sensitive receptors, while activation of the bicuculline-resistant receptors generates the sustained component.

The conformationally restricted analogue of GABA, *cis*-4-aminocrotonic acid (*cis*-ACA), has been shown to activate the GABA$_C$ receptor (Qian and Dowling, 1993, 1994). In turtle ganglion cells it evoked an inward current similar to the sustained component of the response to GABA (at concentrations lower than 600 μM). The current induced by higher concentrations of *cis*-ACA, however, often manifest both a transient and a sustained component. The *cis*-ACA however, was considerably (14 times) less potent than GABA. We found that the *cis*-ACA response, like those of GABA, were completely blocked by 100 μM picrotoxin and partially antagonized by 10 μM bicuculline. The GABA receptor-Cl$^-$ channel agonist, muscimol, elicited a current like that evoked by GABA (Fig. 8). However it was about three times more potent than GABA for activation of both the transient and the sustained currents. In this same vein, we tested the ability of the specific GABA$_C$ receptor antagonist, TPMPA (Ragozzino et al., 1996) for its ability to block the sustained current. At 100 μM it reduced the current by 60% (data not shown).

We went on to investigate the effects of known modulators of GABA responses. The results are described below. In studies of CNS neurons, the benzodiazepine, diazepam, has been shown to selectively modulate the activity of GABA$_A$ receptors (Bormann, 2000). We tested it on three ganglion cells and found it to increase the transient GABA current at a concentration of 1 μM. There was no effect on the sustained component. Interestingly, in two other ganglion cells, diazepam had no effect on either current components. These findings suggested to

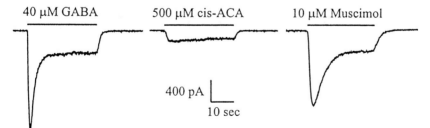

Fig. 7. Responses elicited by different analogs of GABA. The conformationally restricted analogue of GABA, *cis*-ACA, generated a sustained, GABA$_C$ like current (middle trace). Muscimol, a GABA$_A$ receptor agonist, evoked a current like that seen with the application of GABA, i.e. there was both a transient and sustained component.

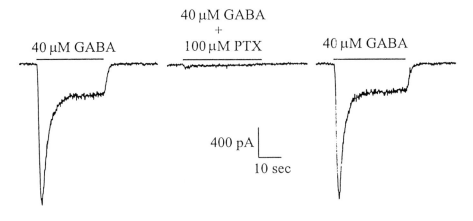

Fig. 8. Picrotoxin inhibits the GABA response. A control response to GABA is shown in the left trace. Picrotoxin applied with GABA almost completely abolishes the GABA response (center trace). Following washout of the drug (right trace) the response returned to control values.

us that a heterogeneous population of $GABA_A$ receptors may exist on these cells. This could come about because of variations in the $GABA_A$ receptor subunit composition from cell to cell.

Zinc is thought to be an indogenous neuromodulator in the vertebrate retina (Wu et al., 1993). In experiments on fish and skate bipolar cells, Dowling and his group (Qian and Dowling, 1995; Qian et al., 1997) showed that zinc specifically inhibited the $GABA_C$ response. We found that in the majority of turtle ganglion cells tested (68%), zinc at a concentration of 20 μM, attenuated or blocked the sustained current but left the transient response intact. Interestingly, the level of inhibition varied from one cell to another. We found that it could inhibit as little as 15% of the response in some cells and completely abolish it in others. In three of the tested cells in which there was only partial block induced by exposure to 20 μM zinc increasing the concentration of zinc to 200 μM did not affect the level of inhibition. These data indicate that the sustained GABA response in turtle retinal ganglion cells may be mediated by different subtypes of $GABA_C$ receptors. In 31% of the cells tested, zinc surprisingly blocked both the transient and the sustained current. At the same concentration (20 μM), zinc always blocked more sustained than transient current. This seems to indicate that the $GABA_C$ receptors are more sensitive to zinc than $GABA_A$ receptors in these cells. These data again raise the possibility of a heterogeneous population of $GABA_A$ receptors and suggest

as well, a heterogeneous population of $GABA_C$ receptors in these cells.

Pharmacology of the GABA evoked currents

The two GABA elicited current components exhibit distinct pharmacological characteristics consistent with the activation of two discrete receptors. The sensitivity to the antagonist, bicuculline, is often used to differentiate $GABA_A$ from $GABA_C$ receptors (Johnston et al., 1986; Shimada et al., 1992; Qian and Dowling, 1995). We found the transient current in turtle ganglion cells to be very sensitive to bicuculline. The sustained current was relatively unaffected by the blocker. In addition, only the transient GABA current was potentiated by the allosteric modulator of $GABA_A$ receptors, diazepam.

Hill coefficients determined from dose response curves suggest that at least three molecules of GABA seem to be required to activate the $GABA_A$ receptors. Only one molecule appears to be needed for $GABA_C$ receptor activation. This indicates that there exists cooperativity among $GABA_A$ receptors or among $GABA_A$ binding sites but not among the $GABA_C$ receptors. Similar cooperativity of $GABA_A$ receptors has been suggested in other systems (Brooks and Werman, 1973; Gallagher et al., 1978; Matthews et al., 1994). It is interesting that the concentration of GABA needed to evoke a maximal response is the same for the two currents, while the slopes of the dose response curves are different. This may be a result of cooperativity.

We found that the GABA receptor agonist muscimol was effective at eliciting both currents. Muscimol has generally been seen to be more potent than GABA at $GABA_A$ receptor sites in a variety of preparations (Mathison and Dreifuss, 1980; Curtis et al., 1980; Nakagawa et al., 1991). But the relative potency of muscimol and GABA at $GABA_C$ receptor sites varies. In retinal horizontal cells, muscimol is less effective than GABA in generating a current (Qian and Dowling, 1993; Dong et al., 1994). In turtle ganglion cells, we found it more potent similar to what has been seen in frog optic tectum (Nistri and Sivilotti, 1985; Sivilotti and Nistri, 1989). The conformationally restricted analogue of GABA, *cis*-ACA, has been seen to be a relatively selective agonist for $GABA_C$ receptors in some preparations (Johnston et al., 1986; Sivilotti and Nistri, 1989). Contrary to this, we found, as did Zhang and Slaughter (1995), that it was a weak agonist for both $GABA_A$ and $GABA_C$ receptors in turtle. Similarly, the antagonist TPMPA blocked the sustained response but to varying degrees. We also found that the effect of imidazole-4-acetic acid, a $GABA_C$ antagonist on white perch horizontal cells, was weak and inconsistent in our cells.

Zinc potently inhibited the $GABA_C$ response similar to that seen in other work (Calvo et al., 1994; Dong and Werblin, 1994; Wang et al., 1994; Qian and Dowling, 1995). The effect of zinc on the $GABA_A$ response was heterogeneous; most responses were not affected but some were. Studies on recombinant $GABA_A$ receptors demonstrated that the γ subunit, which confers diazepam sensitivity to the receptor, confers zinc insensitivity; those $GABA_A$ receptors devoid of γ subunits will be inhibited by zinc (Draguhn et al., 1990; Smart et al., 1991). Evidence exists suggesting that in many systems the $GABA_C$ receptors are a homomeric pentamer of ρ subunits (Cutting et al., 1991; Shimada et al., 1992) but in some tissue they may not be (Qian and Ripps, 1999). Our result with zinc agrees with the first view although we can't rule out a receptor composed of rho and non-rho subunits. The subunit composition of the native $GABA_A$ receptor in turtle is not known. But our results with diazepam and zinc suggest that ganglion cells express at least two subtypes of

$GABA_A$ receptors, one has the γ subunit and the other does not.

Hence, the bicuculline-sensitive GABA receptors in turtle ganglion cells when activated generate a response resembling that of the classical $GABA_A$ evoked response of other preparations. The response resulting from activation of the bicuculline-resistant GABA receptors resembles the $GABA_C$ receptor-activated response seen in other neurons. However, the turtle receptors are somewhat different in that they display pharmacological properties unique to turtle. This unique pharmacological profile for turtle $GABA_C$ receptors is likely the result of subunit composition. The $GABA_C$ receptor is believed to be assembled of ρ subunits (Shimada et al., 1992), of which at least three types have been cloned (Cutting et al., 1991; Albrecht and Darlison, 1995; Enz and Cutting, 1998, 1999; Ogurusu et al., 1999). Although in contrast to this, there is some evidence that certain $GABA_C$ receptors are assembled from rho and non-rho, $GABA_A$ subunits (Qian and Ripps, 1999).

GABA receptor-channel complex ion selectivity

As previously pointed out, GABA induced ionic currents in vertebrate central nervous system neurons are mediated through two types of GABA receptors, $GABA_A$ and $GABA_C$ receptors (Bormann, 2000; Sivilotti and Nistri, 1991; Qian and Dowling, 1993; Feigenspan et al., 1993; Lukasiewicz et al., 1994; Enz and Cutting, 1998). Both receptor types are linked to Cl^- channels. To study the ionic mechanisms of the GABA-evoked currents in turtle ganglion cells, whole cell current-voltage relationships were examined by varying the Cl^- concentration in the recording pipette. We obtained I-V relationships by subtracting the current response recorded in the presence of GABA (100 μM) from that in the absence of GABA (not shown). The relationship was a line with a positive slope ($\sim$7.5) indicating that there was an increase in the membrane conductance during exposure to GABA. The reversal potential was always around 0 mV, very close to the equilibrium potential for Cl^- calculated from the Nernst equation (-0.9 mV). Similar results were obtained when the I-V curve was constructed by measuring the peak GABA current recorded at different holding potentials. Both the peak and the sustained GABA currents always had the same reversal potential. These data indicate that the two components of the GABA activated current were carried by Cl$^-$ ions. Further more, when the intracellular Cl$^-$ ions were partially replaced by equimolar gluconate, the reversal potential was shifted to more negative voltages, very close to the calculated E_{Cl}, for this solution and the amplitude of the current response was smaller, as would be expected for Cl$^-$ channels.

When the selective Cl$^-$ channel antagonist, picrotoxin, was co-applied with GABA at a concentration of 100 μM, we observed complete and reversible blocked of both current components (Fig. 8). The same effect was observed in all cells tested. These results support the notion that the two current components resulting from GABA application are carried through Cl$^-$ channels.

Effect of metabotropic GABA receptor activation

Lastly, as a point of comparison with other ganglion cells, we looked for effects of the activation of the metabotropic GABA$_B$ receptor. As in other ganglion cells we found that GABA$_B$ receptor stimulation affected ganglion cell calcium currents; calcium currents were inhibited. This is illustrated in Fig. 9. In the first left hand panel is shown a control, L-type, calcium current evoked by a voltage ramp under voltage-clamp. Following the application of baclofen

(2nd panel) the current was reduced by about 30%. This effect then recovered after several minutes (middle panel). The effect was largely inhibited by the GABA$_B$ receptor antagonist saclofen applied together with baclofen (fourth panel) indicating specific GABA$_B$ receptor activation lead to the reduction in the calcium current. Although we did not look at this, past studies (Bormann, 2000) suggest that the effect of GABA$_B$ receptor activation in turtle ganglion cells is mediated via a G-protein pathway.

Conclusions and future perspectives

The role of multiple types of GABA receptors in turtle ganglion cell physiology

Our studies of the action of GABA on retinal ganglion cells demonstrate that at least three types of GABA receptors coexist in turtle ganglion cells. The coexistence of GABA$_A$ and GABA$_C$ receptors in a single retinal neuron has been reported in bipolar cells of rat (Pan and Lipton, 1995), and salamander (Lukasiewicz et al., 1994; Lukasiewicz and Shields, 1998) and perch horizontal cells (Qian and Dowling, 1993). Although both GABA$_A$ and GABA$_C$-like receptors are coupled to Cl$^-$ channels, they display distinct physiological and pharmacological properties. As with our findings, calcium channel modulating GABA$_B$ receptors have also been observed in goldfish ganglion cells (Bindokas and Ishida, 1991) and salamander bipolar cells

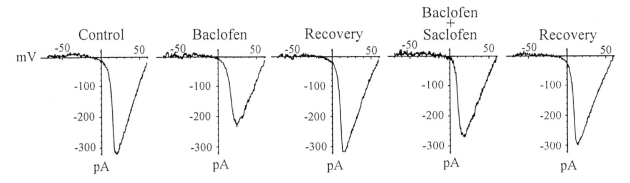

Fig. 9. GABA$_B$ receptor activation modulates a high-voltage activated calcium current in ganglion cells. The Ca^{++} current was elicited by a voltage ramp which changed the membrane potential from a holding potential of -70 mV$-+60$ mV (left trace). Baclofen (200 μM, second trace), a GABA$_B$ receptor agonist, decreased the Ca^{++} current by about 30%. Its voltage-dependence was not affected. Following washout the current recovered to its original amplitude (recovery). The GABA$_B$ receptor antagonist, saclofen, inhibited the response to baclofen (trace second from right). Washout of the drugs resulted in recovery of the response to GABA (right trace).

(Maguire et al., 1989). A unique baclofen-insensitive GABA$_B$-like receptor was identified and shown to coexist with GABA$_A$ receptors in the presynaptic terminal of goldfish bipolar cells. These receptors were sensitive to submicromolar *cis*-ACA and directly modulated Ca^{2+} channels (Heidelberger and Matthews, 1991; Matthews et al., 1994). However, there is very little evidence (Zhang and Slaughter, 1995) of substantial mixing of GABA-A and C receptor types on ganglion cells.

The fact that there is a large percentage of GABA$_C$ receptors on the postsynaptic membranes of turtle ganglion cells will significantly impact the cell's function. Similar to what is seen in bipolar cells, the activation of GABA$_A$ receptors will generate a very large transient inhibition of the ganglion cell response. Subsequent activation of the GABA$_C$ receptors will then result in a low level of long-lasting sustained inhibition. This, of course, will depend on the pattern of GABA release from presynaptic amacrine cells. If release is transient, the GABA$_C$ receptors will probably have little impact on the ganglion cell response. However, if release is sustained, the GABA$_C$ receptor activation will play a big role in the cell's response to bipolar cell input; the cell's activity could be substantially reduced. Overlying this will be the effect of the activation of the GABA$_B$ receptors on these cells. GABA$_B$ receptor activation reduces the calcium current which subsequently results in a decrease in firing rate in these cells. As a result, it will have a generalized inhibitory effect on the cell's response. Thus, the relative combinations of GABA receptors found on a cell are going to largely determine how the cell might respond to excitatory bipolar cell input.

Dowling and his colleagues have contributed significantly to our understanding of the action of GABA on distal neurons in the retina. In particular, they have told us a lot about what occurs through the activation of the GABA$_C$ receptor in these neurons. Our work has taken our understanding of GABA action in the retina a step further by describing its effects on turtle retinal ganglion cells. Surprisingly, like some distal retinal neurons GABA$_C$ receptors make up a large percentage of the cohort of GABA receptors found on these neurons. There is still a great deal to do to further our understanding of the interplay of GABA receptors on ganglion cell response properties. For example, varying the relative ratios of receptors will impact the cells response characteristics. It will be interesting to determine if cells that respond transiently to light input have a larger percentage of GABA$_A$ receptors and those that respond in a more sustained fashion have fewer. We won't put it past John to somehow have a hand in these sorts of studies.

Acknowledgments

This work was supported by NIH grant EY05972 to E.M.L. and an unrestricted grant from Research to Prevent Blindness, Inc. to the Department of Ophthalmology and Visual Sciences.

References

Akaike, N., Hattori, K., Inomata, N. and Oomura, Y. (1985) γ-Aminobutyric acid- and pentobarbitone-gated chloride currents in internally perfused frog sensory neurones. *J. Physiol.*, 360: 367–386.

Albrecht, B.E. and Darlison, M.G. (1995) Localization of the rho 1- and rho 2-subunit messenger RNAs in chick retina by in situ hybridization predicts the existence of gamma-aminobutyric acid type C receptor subtypes. *Neurosci. Lett.*, 189: 155–158.

Ariel, M. and Adolph, A.R. (1985) Neurotransmitter inputs to directionally sensitive turtle retinal ganglion cells. *J. Neurophysiol.*, 54: 1123–1143.

Bindokas, V.P. and Ishida, A.T. (1991) (-)-Baclofen and gamma-aminobutyric acid inhibit calcium currents in isolated retinal ganglion cells. *Proc. Natl. Acad. Sci. USA*, 88: 10759–10763.

Bormann, J. (2000) The 'ABA' of GABA receptors. *Trends Pharmacol. Sci.*, 21: 16–19.

Bormann, J., Hamill, O.P. and Sakmann, B. (1987) Mechanism of anion permeation through channels gated by glycine and γ-aminobutyric acid in mouse cultured spinal neurones. *J. Physiol.* (Cambridge), 385: 243–286.

Brooks, N. and Werman, R. (1973) The cooperativity of γ-aminobutyric acid action on the membrane of locust muscle fibers. *Mol. Pharmacol.*, 9: 571–579.

Caldwell, J.H., Daw, N.W. and Wyatt, H.J. (1978) Effects of picrotoxin and strychnine on rabbit retinal ganglion cells: lateral interactions for cells with more complex receptive fields. *J. Physiol.* (Cambridge), 276: 277–298.

Calvo, D.J., Vazquez, A.E. and Miledi, R. (1994) Cationic modulation of rho$_1$-type gamma-aminobutyrate receptors expressed in *Xenopus* oocytes. *Proc. Natl. Acad. Sci. USA*, 91: 12725–12729.

Cohen, B.N., Fain, G.L. and Fain, M.J. (1989) GABA and glycine channels in isolated ganglion cells from the goldfish retina. *J. Physiol.*, 417: 53–82.

Curtis, D.R., Bornstein, J.C. and Lodge, D. (1980) In vivo analysis of GABA receptors on primary afferent terminations in the cat. *Brain Res.*, 194: 255–258.

Cutting, G.R., Lu, L., O'Hara, B.F., Kasch, L.M., Montrose-Rafizadeh, C., Donovan, D.M., Shimoda, S., Antonarakis, S.E., Guggino, W.B., Uhl, G.R. and Kazazian, H.H., Jr. (1991) Cloning of the gamma-aminobutyric acid (GABA) rho$_1$ cDNA: A GABA receptor subunit highly expressed in the retina. *Proc. Natl. Acad. Sci. USA.*, 88: 2673–2677.

Dong, C-J., Picaud, S.A. and Werblin, F.S. (1994) GABA transporters and GABA$_C$-like receptors on catfish cone- but not rod-driven horizontal cells. *J. Neurosci.*, 14(5): 2648–2658.

Dong, C.-J. and Werblin, F.S. (1994) Dopamine modulation of GABA$_C$ receptor function in an isolated retinal neuron. *J. Neurophysiol.*, 71: 1258–1260.

Draguhn, A., Verdorn, T.A., Ewert, M., Seeburg, P.H. and Sakmann, B. (1990) Functional and molecular distinction between recombinant rat GABAA receptor subtypes by Zn2+. *Neuron*, 5: 781–788.

Enz, R. and Cutting, G.R. (1998) Molecular composition of GABAC receptors. *Vision Res.*, 38: 1431–1441.

Enz, R. and Cutting, G.R. (1999) GABAC receptor rho subunits are heterogeneously expressed in the human CNS and form homo- and heterooligomers with distinct physical properties. *Eur. J. Neurosci.*, 11: 41–50.

Feigenspan, A., Wassle, H. and Bormann, J. (1993) Pharmacology of GABA receptor Cl⁻ channels in rat retinal bipolar cells. *Nature*, 361: 159–161.

Gallagher, J.P., Higashi, H. and Nishi, S. (1978) Characterization and ionic basis of GABA-induced depolarizations recorded *in vitro* from cat primary afferent neurones. *J. Physiol.*, 275: 263–282.

Guiloff, G. and Kolb, H. (1993) Synaptic inputs onto a directional sensitive ganglion cells in turtle retina. *Invest. Ophthalmol. Vis. Sci.*, 34(4): 986.

Heidelberger, R. and Matthews, G. (1991) Inhibition of calcium influx and calcium current by gamma-aminobutyric acid in single synaptic terminals. *Proc. Natl. Acad. Sci. USA*, 88: 7135–7139.

Itabashi, S., Aibara, K., Sasaki, H. and Akaike, N. (1992) γ-Aminobutyric acid-induced response in rat dissociated paratracheal ganglion cells. *J. Neurophysiol.*, 67(4): 1367–1374.

Johnston, D., Rutecki, P.A. and Lebeda, F.J. (1986) Synaptic events underlying spontaneous and evoked paroxysmal discharges in hippocampal neurons. *Adv. Exp. Med. Biol.*, 203: 391–400.

Lasater, E.M. and Witkovsky, P. (1990) Membrane currents of spiking cell isolated from turtle retina. *J. Comp. Physiol. A*, 167: 11–21.

Liu, Y. and Lasater, E.M. (1994a) Calcium currents in turtle retinal ganglion cells II. Dopamine modulation via a cyclic AMP-dependent mechanism. *J. Neurophysiol.*, 71(2): 743–752.

Liu, Y. and Lasater, E.M. (1994b) Multiple GABA receptors of ganglion cells in the turtle retina. *Invest. Ophthalmol. Vis. Sci.*, 35(4): 2154.

Lukasiewicz, P.D., Maple, B.R. and Werblin, F.S. (1994) A novel GABA receptor on bipolar cell terminals in the tiger salamander retina. *J. Neurosci.*, 14: 1213–1223.

Lukasiewicz, P.D. and Shields, C.R. (1998) Different combinations of GABAA and GABAC receptors confer distinct temporal properties to retinal synaptic responses. *J. Neurophysiol.*, 79: 3157–3167.

Maguire, G., Lukasiewicz, P. and Werblin, F. (1989) Amacrine cell interactions underlying the response to change in the tiger salamander retina. *J. Neurosci.*, 9: 726–735.

Marc, R.E., Liu, W-L.S. and Muller, J.F. (1988) Multiple GABA-mediated surround channel in goldfish retina. *Invest. Ophthalmol. Vis. Sci.*, 29: 272.

Massey, S.C. and Redburn, D.A. (1987) Transmitter circuits in the vertebrate retina. *Prog. Neurobiol.*, 28: 55–96.

Mathison, R.D. and Dreifuss, J.J. (1980) Structure-activity relationships of a neurohypophysial GABA receptor. *Brain. Res.*, 187: 476–480.

Matthews, G., Ayoub, G.S. and Heidelberger, R. (1994) Presynaptic inhibition by GABA is mediated via two distinct GABA receptors with novel pharmacology. *J. Neurosci.*, 14: 1079–1090.

Nakagawa, T., Wakamori, M., Shirasaki, T., Nakaye, T. and Akaike, N. (1991) γ-Aminobutyric acid-induced response in acutely isolated nucleus solitarii neurons of the rat. *Am. J. Physiol.*, 260(29): C745–C749.

Nistri, A. and Sivilotti, L. (1985) An unusual effect of gamma-aminobutyric acid on synaptic transmission of frog tectal neurones in vitro. *Br. J. Pharmacol.*, 85: 917–921.

Ogurusu, T., Yanagi, K., Watanabe, M., Fukaya, M. and Shingai, R. (1999) Localization of GABA receptor rho 2 and rho 3 subunits in rat brain and functional expression of homooligomeric rho 3 receptors and heterooligomeric rho 2 rho 3 receptors. *Receptors Channels*, 6: 463–475.

Ozawa, S. and Yuzaki, M. (1984) Patch-clamp studies of chloride channels activated by γ-aminobutyric acid in cultured hippocampal neurons of rat. *Neurosci. Res.*, 1: 275–293.

Pan, Z-H. and Lipton, S.A. (1995) Multiple GABA receptor subtypes mediate inhibition of calcium influx at rat retinal bipolar cell terminals. *J. Neurosci.*, 15(4): 2668–2679.

Pasantes-Morales, H., Klethi, J., Ledig, M. and Mandel, P. (1972) Free amino acids of chicken and rat retina. *Brain Res.*, 41: 494–497.

Polenzani, L., Woodwaard, R.M. and Miledi, R. (1991) Expression of mammalian γ-aminobutyric acid receptors with distinct pharmacology in *Xenopus* oocytes. *Proc. Natl. Acad. Sci. USA*, 88: 4318–4322.

Qian, H. and Dowling, J.E. (1993) Novel GABA Responses from Rod-driven Retinal Horizontal Cells. *Nature*, 361: 162–164.

Qian, H. and Dowling, J.E. (1994) Pharmacology of Novel GABA Receptors Found on Rod Horizontal Cells of the White Perch Retina. *J. Neurosci.*, 14(7): 4299–4307.

Qian, H. and Dowling, J.E. (1995) GABAA and GABAC receptors on hybrid bass retinal bipolar cells. *J. Neurophysiol.*, 74: 1920–1928.

Qian, H., Li, L., Chappell, R.L. and Ripps, H. (1997) GABA receptors of bipolar cells from the skate retina: Actions of Zinc GABA-medicated membrane currents. *J. Neurophysiol.*, 78: 2402–2412.

Qian, H., Dowling, J.E. and Ripps, H. (1998) Molecular and pharmacological properties of GABA-rho subunits from white perch retina. *J. Neurobiol.*, 37: 305–320.

Qian, H., Dowling, J.E. and Ripps, H. (1999) A single amino acid in the second transmembrane domain of GABA rho subunits is a determinant of the response kinetics of GABAC receptors. *J. Neurobiol.*, 40: 67–76.

Qian, H. and Ripps, H. (1999) Response kinetics and pharmacological properties of heteromeric receptors formed by coassembly of GABA rho- and gamma 2-subunits. *Proc. Roy. Soc. Lond. B Biol. Sci.*, 266: 2419–2425.

Ragozzino, D., Woodward, R.M., Murata, Y., Eusebi, F., Overman, L.E. and Miledi, R. (1996) Design and in vitro pharmacology of a selective gamma-aminobutyric acid C receptor antagonist. *Mol. Pharmacol.*, 50: 1024–1030.

Shimada, S., Cutting, G.R. and Uhl, G.R. (1992) Gamma-aminobutyric acid A or C receptor? Gamma-aminobutyric acid rho$_1$ receptor RNA induces bicuculline- barbiturate-, and benzodiazepine-insensitive gamma-aminobutyric acid responses in *Xenopus* oocytes. *Mol. Pharmacol.*, 41: 683–687.

Sivilotti, L. and Nistri, A. (1989) Pharmacology of a novel effect of gamma-aminobutyric acid on the frog optic tectum in vitro. *Eur. J. Pharmacol.*, 164: 205–212.

Sivilotti, L. and Nistri, A. (1991) GABA receptor mechanisms in the central nervous system. *Prog. Neurobiol.*, 36: 35–92.

Slaughter, M.M., Bai, S-H. and Pan, Z.H. (1989) Desegregation: bussing of signals through the retinal network. In: Weiler and Osborne, N.N. (Eds.), *Neurobiology of the Inner Retina*. Springer-Verlag, Berlin, pp. 335–348.

Smart, T.G., Moss, S.J., Xie, X. and Huganir, R.L. (1991) GABAA receptors are differentially sensitive to zinc: dependence on subunit composition. *Br. J. Pharmacol.*, 103: 1837–1839.

Tauck, D.L., Frosch, M.P. and Lipton, S.A. (1988) Characterization of GABA- and glycine-induced currents of solitary rodent retinal ganglion cells in culture. *Neuroscience*, 27(1): 193–203.

Vaughn, J.E., Famiglietti, E.V. Jr., Barber, R.P., Saito, K., Roberts, E. and Ribak, C.E. (1981) Gabaergic amacrine cells in rat retina: immunocytochemical identification and synaptic connectivity. *J. Comp. Neurol.*, 197: 113–127.

Wang, T.-L., Guggino, W.B. and Cutting, G.R. (1994) A novel gamma-aminobutyric acid receptor subunit (rho$_2$) cloned from human retina forms bicuculline-insensitive homooligomeric receptors in *Xenopus* oocytes. *J. Neurosci.*, 14: 6524–6531.

Weiler, R., Ball, A.K. and Ammermuller, J. (1991) Neurotransmitter systems in the turtle retina. *Progress in Retinal Research.*, 10: 1–26.

Woodward, R.M., Polenzani, L. and Milledi, R. (1993) Characterization of bicuculline/baclofen-insensitive (ρ-like) γ-aminobutyric acid receptors expressed in *Xenopus* oocytes. II. Pharmacology of γ-aminobutyric acid$_A$ and γ-aminobutyric acid$_B$ receptor agonists and antagonists. *Mol. Pharmacol.*, 43: 609–625.

Wu, S.M., Qiao, X., Noebels, J.L. and Yang, X.L. (1993) Localization and modulatory actions of zinc in vertebrate retina. *Vision Res.*, 33: 2611–2616.

Zhang, J. and Slaughter, M.M. (1995) Preferential suppression of the ON pathway by GABAC receptors in the amphibian retina. *J. Neurophysiol.*, 74: 1583–1592.

Photoreceptors, visual adaptation and the ERG

H. Kolb, H. Ripps and S. Wu (Eds.)
Progress in Brain Research, Vol. 131
© 2001 Elsevier Science B.V. All rights reserved

CHAPTER 23

The rhodopsin cycle: a twist in the tale

Harris Ripps*

*Department of Ophthalmology and Visual Sciences, University of Illinois College of Medicine,
1855 West Taylor Street, Chicago, IL 60612, USA*

Introduction

It was my good fortune to meet John Dowling when we attended the Cold Spring Harbor Symposium on Sensory Receptors in 1965. Our mutual interest in the mechanisms governing visual adaptation and the problems associated with night-blinding disease, led to our first collaborative research project in 1969 at the Marine Biological Laboratory in Woods Hole. Plans were laid to find a local marine animal having a retina that contained an unusually high rod : cone ratio, in order to minimize the contribution of cones to our electrophysiological and photochemical recordings of visual adaptation. Our success exceeded expectations. We discovered elasmobranchs (*Raja erinacea* and *R. ocellata*) with all-rod retinas swimming the waters of Cape Cod. Although the adaptive range of the skate visual system spans more than 10 logarithmic units, cones have never been seen histologically, and no sign of cone activity has ever been detected electrophysiologically. Over the next 15 years, John and I met each summer at the MBL to explore "photochemical" and "network" adaptation in its various aspects in every cell type of this splendid beast, and we collaborated intermittently thereafter, together with other colleagues, on many related studies. Eventually, John's interest in visual system development led to his enormously fruitful research on zebrafish, and I became enamored of the proteins that mediate intercellular communication and those that are engaged in retinoid transport. Here too, John's pioneering studies of retinal gap junctions, and the transfer of retinoids between photoreceptors and the underlying pigment epithelium, provided the foundation upon which my later work was based. John continues to be a source of inspiration and encouragement, and I am eternally grateful to him for sharing with me his wisdom and insight over these many years. Above all else, I value the close bonds of friendship that developed between John's lovely family and my own. It is a privilege to contribute to a Festschrift honoring Professor John Dowling on the occasion of his 65th birthday; I wish him many happy returns of the day and years of good health.

The rhodopsin cycle[1]

In a landmark paper published more than a century ago, Boll (1876) reported that the retina of a dark-adapted frog has a reddish-purple color, but after exposure to light, it turns pale yellow, and eventually becomes colorless. The significance of this observation did not escape the attention of Willy Kühne (1878), whose superior resources enabled him to

* Tel.: 312-996-2001; Fax: 312-996-7773;
E-mail: harrripp@uic.edu

---

[1]The "rhodopsin cycle" is, with some justification, often referred to as the "visual cycle". However, it is not vision that is being recycled. Indeed, the bleaching and regeneration of rhodopsin proceeds at normal rates in various forms of congenital night blindness (Ripps, 1982), as well as after pressure-induced total blindness (Craik and Vernon, 1941).

336

isolate the substance underlying these chromatic changes, and to provide incontrovertible evidence that the mediator of this phenomenon was the photosensitive pigment subserving rod vision. To the insoluble protein he had extracted with bile salts he gave the name "sehpurpur" (visual purple), which was changed subsequently to "rhodopsin". Moreover, Kühne showed that the original color of the retina could be restored in darkness by simply placing the "bleached" tissue on the surface of the pigment epithelium. Thus, although nothing was known of the chemical reactions involved, or the nature of the exchange that was taking place between the retinal pigment epithelium and the photoreceptors, there was already an indication that the bleaching and regeneration of rhodopsin was a cyclical process.

More than 50 years elapsed before George Wald undertook the formidable task of identifying the substances that were responsible for these chromatic changes (cf. Wald, 1933, 1934). In the course of his research, Wald, together with Ruth Hubbard and a cadre of outstanding co-workers produced a remarkable series of papers elucidating the role of vitamin A in vision, and the physico-chemical processes that propel the rhodopsin cycle. Among their many discoveries, perhaps the most startling was that rhodopsin consists of a bent and twisted form of vitamin A aldehyde (11-*cis* retinaldehyde) bound to the protein opsin, and that the sole action of light in vision is to unbend and untwist the chromophore into the all-*trans* configuration of retinal (Fig. 1). We know now that the *cis–trans* isomerization occurs within a few femtoseconds following the absorption of a single quantum of photic energy (Schoenlein et al., 1991). And as Wald proposed, all subsequent events, including the formation of an active

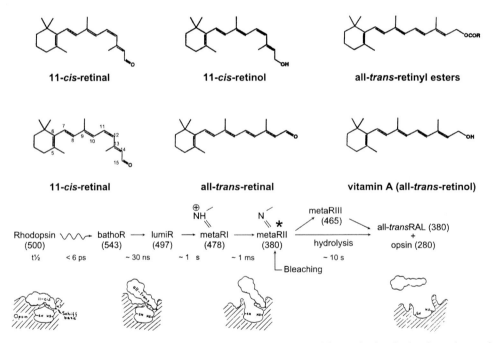

Fig. 1. Structural formulas of retinoids identified by Wald and co-workers as participants in the rhodopsin cycle are shown in the upper section of the figure. The cartoon in the lower section depicts stages in the bleaching of rhodopsin. The rhodopsin chromophore (11-*cis* retinaldehyde) sits within a pocket in opsin. The only action of light is to isomerize retinaldehyde from the 11-*cis* to the all-*trans* configuration (bathorhodopsin, formerly called pre-lumirhodopsin). As opsin unfolds, the molecule degrades thermally through a series of spectrally-distinct intermediates until ultimately the retinaldehyde is hydrolyzed from the apoprotein and reduced to all-*trans* retinol. At an earlier stage (metaRII), the Schiff-base linkage that joins retinaldehyde and opsin becomes deprotonated (*), and the chromoprotein is capable of activating transducin to initiate visual excitation. Transition times give the approximate half-lives of the intermediates at room temperature. Enclosed in parentheses under each intermediate is its absorption maximum. Modified from Wald, 1968, and Rando, 1990.

intermediary that triggers the electrical response of the visual cell, the conformational changes in opsin that free the chromophore from its binding pocket in opsin, and the reduction of all-*trans* retinaldehyde to form vitamin A (all-*trans* retinol), are essentially thermal, no longer requiring the presence of light.

However, it was John Dowling who provided the first quantitative analysis of the exchange of retinoids between the photoreceptors and retinal pigment epithelium (RPE) in the course of light- and dark-adaptation. Soon after he joined the Wald laboratory, John produced the now classic paper that described both the kinetics of the exchange process, as well as the still poorly understood log-linear relation that exists between bleached rhodopsin and visual sensitivity (Dowling, 1960). As illustrated in Fig. 2, the dark-adapted albino rat retina is rich in retinaldehyde (RAL) bound to opsin, but contains only a small amount of vitamin A (all-*trans* ROL), and neither retinoid is detected in the rat RPE. However, the situation changes dramatically during prolonged exposure to bright light. Within the retina, the level of retinaldehyde falls and that of vitamin A rises as the chromophore is liberated from opsin and

is reduced to retinol. But soon thereafter, the level of vitamin A within the retina declines as free retinol is transferred to the RPE. In darkness, the processes are reversed; the vitamin A level within the RPE slowly declines, and the retinaldehyde content of the retina is restored as rhodopsin is regenerated. The inset to Fig. 2 shows that during this period of dark adaptation, the recovery of rhodopsin (expressed on a linear scale) results in a concomitant fall in (log) visual threshold, measured electroretinographically. Thus, even after 50% of the bleached rhodopsin has regenerated, threshold is elevated by about 1.75 log unit (dashed line), far above the 0.3 log unit loss that can be attributed to the reduced probability of quantal absorption.

Although it was now evident that the all-*trans* retinol released on bleaching enters the RPE where it is esterified with long chain fatty acids and stored (Hubbard and Dowling, 1962; Berman et al., 1980), the vitamin A congener returned to the rod outer segment (ROS), and its stereoisomeric configuration remained conjectural. However, these two very elusive issues were resolved when the enzymatic mechanism driving the all-*trans* to 11-*cis*

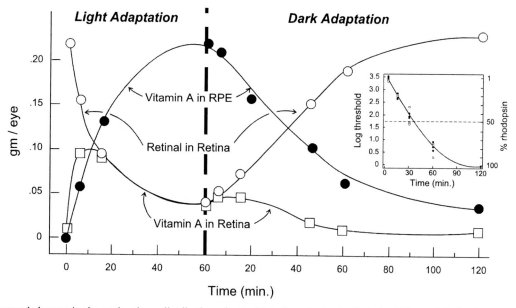

Fig. 2. Temporal changes in the ocular tissue distribution of retinaldehyde and vitamin A during light- and dark-adaptation. See text for details. The values for retinal (open circles) have been increased by 15% to correct for the lower extraction efficacy as compared to vitamin A. Inset: the parallel changes in log threshold (measured electroretinographically) and the rhodopsin content of the retina during dark-adaptation. Note that when 50% of the rhodopsin has been regenerated, threshold remains elevated by more than 1.5 log units. Modified from Dowling, 1960.

338

isomerization, and the site where it occurs, were identified.The elegant and highly innovative studies of Robert Rando and co-workers convincingly demonstrated that the transformation takes place in the RPE under the control of an isomerohydrolase, which processes all-*trans*-retinyl esters (mainly retinyl palmitate) into 11-*cis* retinol (Bernstein et al., 1987; Rando et al., 1991). As a result of their work, and of others, we now have a firmer grasp of the sequence of enzymatic reactions in the biochemical pathway that

leads to the reconstitution of 11-*cis* retinaldehyde (cf. Saari, 1990, 2000).

Figure 3 illustrates schematically some of the key events that comprise the rhodopsin cycle. All-*trans* retinaldehyde is released from opsin after bleaching, and is then rapidly reduced by a retinol dehydrogenase and reduced nicotinamide dinucleotide phosphate in the rod outer segment to all *trans*-retinol. The vitamin A then diffuses or is transported to the RPE where it is esterified by lecithin retinol

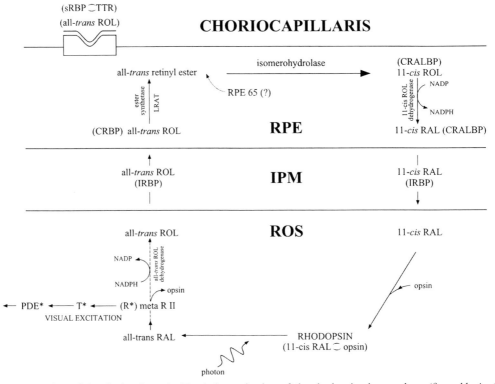

Fig. 3. Schematic overview of the rhodopsin cycle. Photic isomerization of the rhodopsin chromophore (from 11-*cis*- to all-*trans*-retinaldehyde) leads to conformational changes in opsin and the formation within the rod outer segment (ROS) of an active intermediary (metaR II) capable of activating transducin (T*) and thus triggering the enzymatic cascade responsible for generating an electrical signal (the onset of visual excitation). The chromophore ultimately separates from opsin, is enzymatically reduced to all-*trans* retinol, and is transferred through the IPM to the RPE. There it is converted to all-*trans* retinyl ester, the substrate for an isomerohydrolase that yields 11-*cis* retinol, which is then oxidized by 11-*cis* retinol dehydrogenase to 11-*cis* retinaldehyde. In this isomeric form, the retinoid is returned to the outer segments where it binds to opsin for the resynthesis of rhodopsin and completion of the cycle. The functional roles of the various cellular and extracellular retinoid-binding proteins are not fully understood. RPE65 is an essential protein in the isomerization pathway (Redmond et al., 1998), and mutations in the RPE65 gene are associated with severe retinal dysrophies (Gu et al., 1997; Morimura et al., 1998); its mode of action has yet to be elucidated. The supply of all-*trans* retinol is replenished from the blood stream carried by the RBP : TTR complex; a receptor for RBP on the basolateral surface of the RPE mediates the internalization of the retinoid (Bok and Heller, 1976; Pfeffer et al., 1986). Abbreviations: 11-*cis* RAL (11-*cis* retinaldehyde); all-*trans* ROL (vitamin A); RBP (serum retinol-binding protein); TTR (transthyretin); CRALBP (cellular retinaldehyde-binding protein); CRBP (cellular retinol-binding protein); LRAT (lecithin-retinol acyltransferase); NADP (nicotinamide adenine dinucleotide phosphate); NADPH (reduced NADP); R*, T*, PDE* (active forms of rhodopsin, transducin and phosphodiesterase generated sequentially in the transduction cascade).

acyltransferase to long-chain fatty acids for storage, and subsequently isomerized and oxidized to 11-*cis* retinaldehyde. In this form, the retinoid moves to the photoreceptors, where it becomes covalently linked to its active-site lysine in opsin by means of a protonated Schiff base (Bownds, 1967) to reform rhodopsin and complete the cycle.

The intercellular translocation of retinoids

Despite the many significant advances, there are still large gaps in our knowledge of the rhodopsin cycle, notably, the roles played by the various intra- and extra-cellular retinoid-binding proteins (Table 1) as well as other essential proteins, e.g. RPE65 (Redmond et al., 1998). Because free retinol and other retinoids tend to be cytotoxic, poorly soluble, and subject to oxidative degradation in aqueous solutions (cf. Bangham et al., 1964; Crouch et al., 1992), retinoid-binding proteins are generally considered essential for protection, translocation, and the maintenance of functional integrity. However, the manner in which they serve these various functions, particularly in regard to the transport of retinoids, remains unclear. Nevertheless, in some instances it has been shown that retinoid-binding proteins enhance the efficacy of metabolic reactions that are integral to the rhodopsin cycle. Thus, enzymatic esterification of retinol within the RPE is about 3 times more effective when the retinoid is bound to CRBP than when free (Berman et al., 1980), and the

action of the isomerohydrolase, i.e. the rate of 11-*cis* retinol synthesis from all-*trans* retinyl esters, is about 13 times more rapid in the presence of CRALBP (Winston and Rando, 1998).

One of the perplexing issues, and the main subject of this paper, concerns the movement of retinoids between the three principal compartments that participate in the rhodopsin cycle: the photoreceptors (PRs), the retinal pigment epithelium (RPE), and the interphotoreceptor matrix (IPM) that fills the extra-cellular space separating the PRs and the apical surface of the RPE. The properties of interphoto-receptor retinoid-binding protein (IRBP) (cf. Table 2), a soluble glycoprotein synthesized and extruded by the visual cells (Hollyfield et al., 1985; Rodrigues et al., 1986; van Veen et al., 1986), have made it a strong candidate for the carrier that transports retinoids bidirectionally through the IPM (Adler and Martin, 1982; Liou et al., 1982; Lai et al., 1982; Lin et al., 1989).

There are several reasons for holding this view (cf. Pepperberg et al., 1993): (i) IRBP occupies a strategic position in the IPM where it is confined by barriers formed distally by the tight junctions of the RPE (Cohen, 1965) and proximally by the junctional complexes of the external limiting membrane (Tonus and Dickson, 1979; Bunt-Milam et al., 1985); (ii) In most species, IRBP is the major retinoid-binding protein localized within the IPM (Pfeffer et al., 1983; Adler and Martin, 1982); (iii) The isomeric form of retinoid bound to IRBP varies in accordance with the adaptive state of the

Table 1. Retinoid-binding proteins

Protein	M_r	Localization	Ligands
Intracellular			
CRBP	15,500	RPE, Müller cells	all-*trans* retinol*
			all- *trans* retinal
CRALBP	36,400	RPE, Müller cells	11-*cis* retinal*
			11-*cis* retinol*
Extracellular			
RBP complexed to	21,000	Serum, IPM, Neural retina	all-*trans* retinol*
Transthyretin	55,000	Serum, IPM, Neural retina	
Albumin	67,000	Serum, IPM	all-*trans* retinol, 11-cis retinal
IRBP	140,000	IPM	all-*trans* retinol, 11-cis retinal
			other retinoids, vitamin E,
			docosahexaenoic acid and
			other fatty acids

* High affinity binding.

Table 2. Interphotoreceptor retinoid binding protein (IRBP)

- A large glycoprotein (MW 140 kDa)
- Found in all vertebrate species (cartilagenous fish to primates)
- Uniquely localized to subretinal space
- Synthesized in rods and cones and secreted into IPM
- Early expression of mRNA for IRBP (precedes opsin)
- Loosely binds retinoids (e.g., $K_d = 1.3 \times 10^{-6}$ for all-*trans* ROL) tocopherol, cholesterol, fatty acids
- Ligand binding is modulated by light (no change in concentration of IRBP) *In darkness*: IRBP binds ~2 times more 11-*cis* RAL than all-*trans* ROL *On exposure to light*: IRBP binding of all-*trans* ROL increases by a factor of 5, and binding of 11-*cis* RAL decreases by a factor of 4

retina; when the retina is exposed to bright light, the principal endogenous ligand is all-*trans* retinol, whereas in darkness, the predominant ligand is 11-*cis* retinaldehyde (Adler and Spencer, 1991); (iv) IRBP promotes the delivery of all-*trans* retinol to the RPE (Okajima et al., 1989; Flannery et al., 1990), and it serves effectively to extract 11-*cis* retinaldehyde from the RPE (Okajima et al., 1990; Pepperberg et al., 1991; Carlson and Bok, 1992; Edwards and Adler, 2000) and deliver it through an aqueous medium to restore the rhodopsin content of bleached photoreceptors (Jones et al., 1989; Okajima et al., 1990); (v) Studies on the effect of IRBP on rhodopsin regeneration in the experimentally-detached skate retina indicate that the presence of IRBP can significantly enhance the rate of regeneration and the amount of rhodopsin that is regenerated after bleaching (Sun and Ripps, 1992; Duffy et al., 1993). Figure 4 shows that after bleaching almost all of the available rhodopsin, regeneration in the normal eyecup preparation (dashed line) is complete after about 2 hrs in darkness. Detaching the retina from the RPE/eyecup, immersing the entire complement of tissue in Ringer solution to significantly dilute the normal constituents of the IPM, and then replacing the retina on the surface of the RPE, reduces to about 30% the amount of rhodopsin that is regenerated after the bleach (filled circles). However, adding one stage to the protocol, i.e. introducing a 5 μl aliquot of ligand-free IRBP (132 μM) between the neural retina and RPE, results in a more rapid rate of regeneration and a large increase in the fraction of bleached rhodopsin

that is regenerated (open circles). Although both parameters remain below those obtained from the undisturbed eyecup, the addition of IRBP clearly has a beneficial effect on rhodopsin regeneration.

Translocation without transporters

Despite this impressive body of evidence, questions are often raised as to whether IRBP or any other binding protein is required to chaperone retinoids through the short distance (~0.1 μm) that is *presumed* to separate the PR membranes from the apical processes of the RPE. Estimates of the solubility of retinoids range from ~1 nM (Yoshikami and Nöll, 1978) to ~100 nM (Szuts and Harosi, 1991), and although relatively low, they are not incompatible with diffusion through the aqueous phase over subcellular distances. This probably accounts for the findings reported by several investigators in which it was shown that retinoids are readily transferred between membrane-bound vesicles in the absence of retinoid-binding proteins (Rando and Bangerter, 1982; Fex and Johannesson, 1988), and that both the spontaneous transfer of all-*trans* retinol from retinol-binding protein to unilamellar liposomes (Fex and Johannesson, 1987), and from liposomes to rod outer segment membranes (Ho et al., 1989), can occur through an aqueous medium. These observations prompted the suggestion that a transport protein is not an essential component of the rhodopsin cycle. On this view, the likely role of IRBP is to serve as an extracellular buffer to prevent the aqueous degradation of retinoids, and to suppress the potentially cytotoxic effect of retinol when large amounts are released into the IPM.

The exchange of lipophilic molecules across adjacent phospholipid membranes is hardly surprising. However, it is noteworthy that in each of the foregoing studies the separation between donors and acceptors is minuscule. This is not the case for the distance between membranes of the apical processes of the RPE and the plasma membrane enclosing proximal regions of the ROS. The mammalian rod outer segment is on the order of 25–35 μm in length (Fig. 5A), and contains approximately 1000 rhodopsin-bearing bimembraneous discs. At the distal end, the RPE extends processes that envelop, at most, only a third of the ROS (Spitznas and Hogan, 1970; Zinn and Benjamin-Henkind, 1979), and serve primarily to engulf packets of shed disc membranes and incorporate them into phagosomes during the disc renewal process (Young, 1971; Steinberg and Wood, 1979). Thus, the basal end of the rod outer segment, where the discs first encounter the incident light, is far removed from the apical

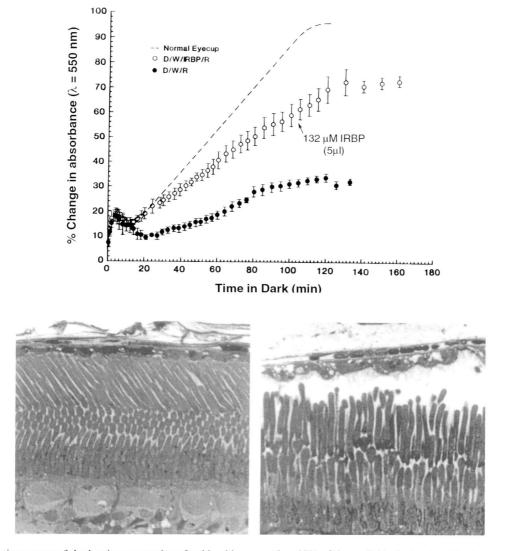

Fig. 4. The time course of rhodopsin regeneration after bleaching more than 97% of the available rhodopsin in the dark-adapted skate retina. The data are derived from absorbance changes measured at 550 nm, and expressed as a percentage of the density change resulting from the bleaching exposure. The results are averages of five experimental runs under each of the following conditions: (i) a normal eyecup preparation (dashed line) in which the retina remained adherent to the RPE (microgaph at lower left); (ii) the retina is experimentally detached, and the separated tissues are immersed in a large volume of Ringer solution before replacing the retina on the RPE (filled circles); and (iii) following the same protocol as in (ii) except that a 5 μl aliquot of 132 μM IRBP is deposited on the RPE before replacing the retina (open circles). During the first 10 min of dark adaptation, the changes associated with rhodopsin regeneration are masked by the formation and decay of a late intermediate, metarhodopsin III. At later times, the normal rate of regeneration and the amount of rhodopsin regenerated are markedly attenuated by the retinal detachment and dilution of the subretinal space. Although the retina remains detached (micrograph at lower right), the introduction of IRBP enhances both the fraction of rhodopsin regenerated and the rate at which it occurs. Modified from Duffy et al., 1993.

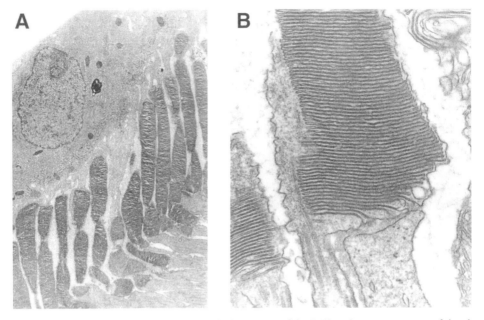

Fig. 5. Electron micrographs illustrating the relation of the apical processes of the RPE to the outer segments of the photoreceptors. **A**. This low-power view shows that the processes extend only a short distance along the rod photoreceptor outer segments, and probably serve primarily to engulf packets of disc membranes for incorporation into phagosomes in the disc-shedding/renewal process. Note the long apical processes extending down to reach a cone outer segment. **B**. The apical processes are not seen at the basal portion of the outer segment near its junction with the inner segment.

processes of the RPE (Fig. 5B). Nevertheless, the retinoid released from each of its bleached rhodopsin molecules must make the journey to the RPE for processing, and ultimately return to the ROS to reconstitute the photopigment. It seems highly unlikely that free retinoids can diffuse over distances of 20 μm or more without undergoing degradation or inducing cytotoxic reactions.

The IRBP 'Knockout' mouse

Although the available evidence clearly favors an essential role for IRBP in the rhodopsin cycle, the controversy surrounding this issue prompted us to undertake the study of an animal model in which the IRBP gene was inactivated through homologous recombination (Liou et al., 1998). A gene targeting protocol was designed to disrupt mouse IRBP by replacing the promoter region and the first exon of the IRBP gene with a neomycin resistant gene driven by a phosphoglycerate-kinase promoter (Fig. 6A), thereby effectively eliminating the production of IRBP. RT-PCR performed on total RNA isolated

from whole mouse eyes, Western blot analysis, and immunocytochemistry on retinal sections (Fig. 6B) confirmed the absence of the protein in IRBP$-/-$ mice (Liou et al., 1998).

Histological examination of IRBP$-/-$ mice and normal littermates (IRBP$+/+$) showed that the retinas of mice lacking IRBP have far fewer photoreceptor nuclei, and abnormally short outer segments containing distorted, poorly organized disc membranes (Figs. 6C, D). As expected from the appearance of the retina of these young (P30) mice, both the photopic (not shown) and scotopic electroretinogram (ERG) were significantly reduced in amplitude (Fig. 7A). However, it was surprising to find that both the ultrastructural appearance of the photoreceptors (Fig. 6D) and the ERG potentials (Fig. 7B) showed far less deterioration than we had anticipated over a period of six months (Ripps et al., 2000).

The twist in the tale

But the real surprise came when we recorded, by electroretinography and by spectrophotometry,

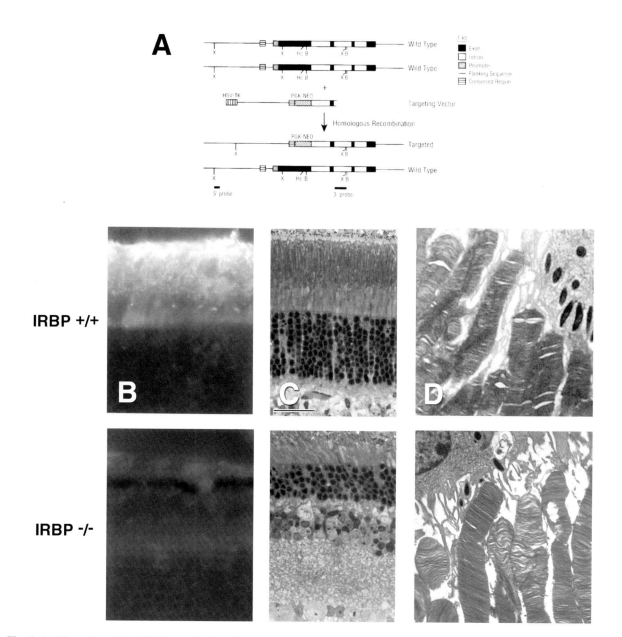

Fig. 6. **A**. Disruption of the IRBP gene by homologous recombination; see text and Liou et al., 1998 for details. **B**. IRBP was not detected in the retina of IRBP−/− mice by immunocytochemistry using monoclonal or polyclonal antibodies against various epitopes on the protein. In normal (IRBP+/+) mice, IRBP is localized to the IPM and extends from the apical margin of the RPE to the outer limiting membrane. Here the antigen is visualized with a rabbit anti-monkey polyclonal antibody and FITC-labeled goat anti-rabbit IgG. **C**. Light micrographs of the mid-peripheral retina from one-month-old IRBP−/− and normal (IRBP+/+) mice. More than half of the photoreceptors have been lost in the IRBP−/− mouse, and their receptor outer segments are shorter than normal, poorly aligned, and clearly disorganized. **D**. Electron micrograph of the IRBP+/+ retina (upper panel) shows the normal appearance of the disc membranes at the interface between the photoreceptors and RPE. In contrast, the apical processes of the RPE of six-month old IRBP−/− mice appear shredded, and there is vacuolization and gross disorganizaton of the outer segment disc membranes. However, some photoreceptors throughout the retina appear to be relatively unaffected, and are able to retain their seemingly normal structure. Retinal ultrastructure of younger (P30) IRBP−/− mice (not shown) were indistinguishable from that seen at six months of age.

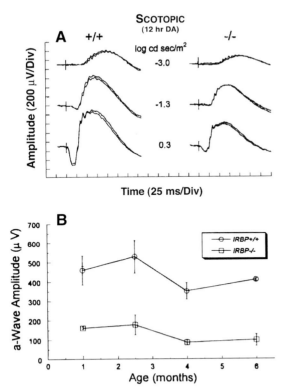

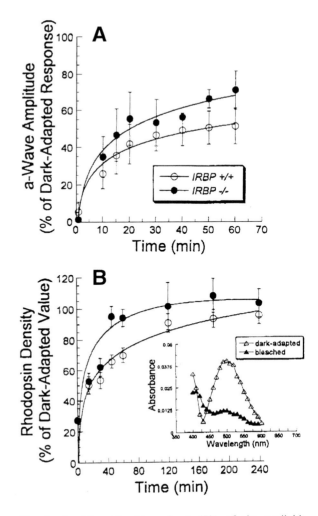

Fig. 7. **A.** ERG recordings from wild type (IRBP+/+) and IRBP−/− littermates to flash stimuli spanning an intensity range of 3.3 log units, i.e., from below cone threshold (−3.0 log cd s/m^2) to one capable of eliciting a response of near maximal amplitude (0.3 log cd s/m^2). The amplitudes of both the a- and b-waves of IRBP−/− mice are reduced by more than 50% compared to wild-type animals. **B.** The photoreceptor potential (a-wave) of the ERG in IRBP−/− mice shows relatively little deterioration in response amplitude over a period of six months.

the recovery of visual sensitivity and rhodopsin after exposure to an intense bleaching light. ERG recordings from the eyes of anesthetized animals obtained at various times after exposure to an intense illumination that bleached about 70% of the available rhodopsin showed that the recovery of the electroretinographic response during dark-adaptation occurred in IRBP−/− mice with seemingly faster kinetics than normal (Fig. 8A). This was confirmed by spectrophotometric analysis of rhodopsin in extracts from retinal homogenates obtained under similar experimental conditions. The results illustrated in Fig. 8B show that the resynthesis of rhodopsin during dark-adaptation also proceeded at a more rapid rate in the IRBP−/− mouse than in the

Fig. 8. **A.** After bleaching about 67% of the available rhodopsin, the a-wave amplitude of IRBP−/− mice recovers at a faster rate than normal, and as shown in **B**, a similar result is obtained from spectrophotometric determinations of rhodopsin density on retinal homogenates collected at various times following the bleaching exposure. Modified from Ripps et al., 2000.

normal. Thus, despite the significant loss of photoreceptors, the reduced rhodopsin content of the retina, and the pronounced loss of visual (ERG) sensitivity, the rhodopsin cycle is not seriously impaired in the IRBP−/− mouse (Palczewski et al., 1999; Ripps et al., 2000). Clearly the abnormalities we observed in structure and function could not be attributed, as first thought, to a deficiency in the vitamin A content of the affected retina resulting from a failure of the rhodopsin cycle (Liou et al., 1998).

Alternative pathways

The importance of retinoids in development, in the maintenance of tissue integrity, and in the visual process, may dictate the need for redundancy in the preservation of the many vital functions in which retinoid-binding proteins participate. Although we had not expected the rhodopsin cycle to be intact in IRBP−/−mice, there have been numerous studies in which deletion of proteins considered vital to the functional integrity of various tissues revealed little or no phenotypic abnormalities (cf. Rudnicki et al., 1992; Weintraub, 1993). Indeed, the findings are consistent with those of related studies on animal models and humans lacking other retinoid-binding proteins or enzymes considered essential for normal development or the rhodopsin cycle. For example, an earlier study by Gorry et al. (1994) showed that mice carrying a null mutation in cellular retinoic acid-binding protein I (CRABPI) were phenotypically indistinguishable from wild type mice at early stages of development as well as in adult life. Comparable results were obtained under conditions that produced deficiencies in serum retinol-binding protein (RBP). RBP is synthesized primarily in the liver, and after binding retinol, is secreted to the circulation where it forms a 1:1 molar complex with transthyretin (prealbumin) for the transport of retinol to target tissues throughout the body (Blaner, 1989). Considering that this is the major route by which the tissue demands of vitamin A are met, it seems remarkable that neither widespread systemic disease nor severe visual deficits are seen in individuals carrying mutations in the gene for retinol-binding protein (Biesalski et al., 1999), or in mice with targeted disruption of the RBP gene (Quadro et al., 1999). At birth, RBP "knockout" mice have lowered blood levels of retinol, and a reduction in ERG amplitude suggestive of a visual defect. However, the animals are viable and fertile, and when kept on a conventional animal diet, normal visual function (determined electroretinographically) is restored within a few months despite the persistantly low levels of blood retinol. Since liver stores of retinol cannot be mobilized, the cellular supply of vitamin A must have been maintained by alternative means, possibly from circulating retinyl esters, β-carotene, chylomicrons, or retinoic acid.

Further evidence for the presence of alternative routes in sustaining the rhodopsin cycle was demonstrated recently in a study of patients with fundus albipunctatus, an unusual disease that results from mutations in RDH5, the gene encoding 11-cis retinol dehydrogenase (Yamamoto et al., 1999; Gonzalez-Fernandez et al., 1999; Cideciyan et al., 2000). In the latter study, it was shown that the Arg157Trp mutation resulted in inactivation of RDH, which would be expected to prevent the oxidation of 11-cis retinol and thereby interrupt the rhodopsin cycle (Fig. 3). Nevertheless, patients with this and other forms of the disorder are able to regenerate rod and cone pigments and recover visual sensitivity after extensive photopigment bleaching, albeit over an extremely prolonged time course (Carr et al., 1974; Ripps, 1982; Yamamoto et al., 1999; Gonzalez-Fernandez et al., 1999; Cideciyan et al., 2000). Moreover, studies on microsomal preparations from bovine RPE using competition assays to analyze the cofactors involved in the activation of RDH, provided evidence strongly suggestive of the presence of alternative oxidative pathways for the production of 11-cis retinaldehyde (Cideciyan et al., 2000).

Because of its profound impact on vision, a similar situation probably applies to the exchange of retinoids between the RPE and photoreceptors. Several retinoid-binding proteins are present within the IPM (Table 1), and each may take part to some extent in the exchange process, particularly in the absence of IRBP. Both RBP and transthyretin are expressed early in development, are synthesized within the RPE (Martone et al., 1988a,b; Cavallaro et al., 1990; Herbert et al., 1991; Ong et al., 1994), and are secreted across the apical membrane into the IPM (Ong et al., 1994). Also found within the IPM is serum albumin (Adler and Edwards, 2000), another protein that is capable of binding retinoids of the rhodopsin cycle (Horwitz and Heller, 1973). RBP and/or albumin could serve as carriers for the bi-directional exchange of retinoids, although whether either protein is capable of mediating the rapid regeneration kinetics displayed by IRBP−/− mice is a question that needs to be addressed. RBP, for example, binds retinoids more tightly than does IRBP (Cogan et al., 1976; Adler et al., 1985), but it is present in the IPM in extremely low concentration, i.e. the molar ratio of RBP to IRBP is only about 0.015 (Adler and Edwards, 2000). The relatively tight binding, which would tend to retard retinoid release to its target tissues, the apparent absence of receptors for RBP on the apical surface of the RPE (Bok and Heller, 1976; Pfeffer et al., 1986), and the paucity of RBP in the IPM, suggest that RBP may not be a significant player in the transport process.

In contrast, the concentration of albumin in human IPM is about two-fold greater than IRBP, and it is present in even greater abundance relative to IRBP in the rodent retina (Adler and Edwards, 2000). However, the efficiency with which albumin binds retinol is only about 3% that of IRBP (Okajima et al., 1989), and its ability to remove 11-*cis*-retinaldehyde from RPE in situ or from isolated RPE membranes is significantly less than IRBP (Okajima et al., 1990; Edwards and Adler, 2000). Nevertheless, in their studies on the uptake and processing of retinoids by primary cultures of human RPE, Das et al. (1990) observed that the RPE is able to incorporate ^{3}H-retinol, convert it to 11-*cis* retinaldehyde and release the retinoid into the culture medium for transfer to rod outer segments. Moreover, these authors found that the amount of 11-*cis* retinaldehyde transferred to the ROS was in direct proportion to the amount of albumin present in the culture medium. Clearly, the role of serum albumin, and of RBP, in the intercellular exchange of retinoids warrant further study. The creation of mouse models in which the genes coding for these proteins are disrupted, as well as studies on "double knockouts" lacking IRBP and albumin, or IRBP and RBP, would go a long way toward resolving this issue (cf. Rudnicki et al., 1993).

The IRBP−/− phenotype

Evidence that the directed flow of all-*trans* retinol and 11-*cis* retinaldehyde is not adversely affected in IRBP−/− mice (Fig. 8) is a good indication that the early loss of photoreceptors and the outer segment abnormalities seen in these animals (Fig. 6) cannot be attributed to a localized vitamin A deficiency. However, it is important to recall that in addition to its ability to bind retinoids, IRBP binds other hydrophobic ligands such as cholesterol and vitamin E (Alvarez et al., 1987), and it binds fatty acids with a single high-affinity (covalent) binding site as well as several low-affinity binding sites (Bazan et al., 1985). These compounds are essential membrane constituents, and the binding properties of IRBP suggest that it is well suited to facilitate the movement of fatty acids and other lipids through the IPM (Fliesler and Schroepfer, 1986; Putilina et al., 1993). It is particularly noteworthy that docosahexanoic acid (DHA), the major fatty-acid constituent of the disc membranes (Fliesler and Anderson, 1983), does not undergo de novo synthesis in the retina, and must be derived from the choroidal circulation (Anderson et al., 1974; Fliesler and Anderson, 1983). IRBP binds DHA in preference to other fatty acids (Chen et al., 1993), and thus the transport of DHA to the photoreceptors, and its recycling during the disc renewal process, may be critically dependent upon the availability of IRBP. Interestingly, significantly reduced levels of DHA have been reported in IRBP−/− mice and in transgenic animals with other forms of retinal degeneration (Anderson et al., 1999).

Considering that IRBP gene expression occurs early in photoreceptor differentiation (Gonzalez-Fernandez and Healy, 1990; Hauswirth et al., 1992; Liou et al., 1994), it is quite possible that the structural defects in IRBP−/− mice reflect a failure in the transport of lipids and other essential fatty acids that are required for normal photoreceptor development. Our histological studies of P11 mice lacking IRBP tend to support this view (Liou et al., 1998); abnormalities resulting from lipid depletion could induce early changes in disc membrane composition, and ultimately, the disruption and loss of photoreceptors. A defect of this sort may account for the observation that a reduction in IRBP in rd/rd, rds/rds mutant mice significantly precedes the loss of visual cells (van Veen et al., 1988). Similarly, a reduction in the level of IRBP gene expression occurs well before the onset of photoreceptor cell death in Abyssinian cats homozygous for hereditary rod–cone degeneration (Narfström et al., 1989; Wiggert et al., 1994). And as was shown for the IRBP "knockout" mice (Palczewski et al., 1999; Ripps et al., 2000), the reduced levels of IRBP in the affected Abyssinian cats appear to have no deleterious effect on rhodopsin kinetics or the time course of visual adaptation (Narfström et al., 1993).

Conclusions and future directions

This brief review included some key events in the history of the rhodopsin cycle, a summary of experiments aimed at defining the mechanisms by which retinoids are transferred betweeen the photoreceptors and retinal pigment epithelium, and the results of studies showing the functional consequences of selectively inactivating binding proteins that are considered essential for the solubilization, protection, and translocation of retinoids. The observation that disruption of the genes coding for several of these proteins does not produce the adverse effects one might expect is a good indication that the mechanism by which retinoids move between cellular compartments is still unclear. However, the fact that the rhodopsin cycle continues unabated in the absence of IRBP does not rule out the possibility that IRBP subserves the intercellular exchange of retinoids under normal physiological conditions. In its absence, another retinoid-binding protein of the interphotoreceptor matrix, or one derived from cells that border the IPM, may fulfill the need for a retinoid transporter.

Although I have stressed the possibility that back-up systems may be in play when there is a deficiency in one or another retinoid-binding protein, the view that a vehicle is required for the intercellular movement of retinoids between the RPE and photoreceptors is based largely on indirect evidence. Functional studies of double-knockout mice, in which the genes for IRBP and one or another retinoid-binding protein of the IPM are inactivated, warrant further study, and may help to resolve this issue.

The late 19th century ushered in the modern era of visual photochemistry. Not too surprisingly, we arrive at the dawn of the 21st century, and have yet to understand fully the workings of the rhodopsin cycle.

Acknowledgments

I gratefully acknowledge the important contributions of Drs. Gerald Chader, Mark Duffy, Gregory Liou, Ting-Ing Okajima, Neal Peachey, David Pepperberg, Barbara Wiggert, and Jane Zakevicius to the studies described here. Research in the author's laboratory was supported by grant EY-06516 and core grant (EY-01792) from the National Eye Institute, and an unrestricted award to the Department of Ophthalmology and Visual Sciences from Research to Prevent Blindness Inc., New York.

References

Adler, A.J. and Edwards, R.B. (2000) Human interphotoreceptor matrix contains serum albumin and retinol-binding protein. *Exp. Eye Res.*, 70: 227–234.

Adler, A.J., Evans, C.D. and Stafford, W.F. (1985) Molecular properties of bovine interphotoreceptor retinoid-binding protein. *J. Biol. Chem.*, 260: 4850–4855.

Adler, A.J. and Martin, K.J. (1982) Retinol-binding proteins in bovine interphotoreceptor matrix. *Biochem. Biophys. Res. Commun.*, 108: 1601–1608.

Adler, A.J. and Spencer, S.A. (1991) Effect of light on endogenous ligands carried by interphotoreceptor retinoid-binding protein. *Exp. Eye Res.*, 53: 337–346.

Alvarez, R.A., Liou, G.I., Fong, S.-L. and Bridges, C.D.B. (1987) Levels of α- and γ- tocopherol in human eyes: evaluation of the possible role of IRBP in intraocular α-tocopherol transport. *Amer. J. Clin. Nutr.*, 46: 481–487.

Anderson, R.E., Benolken, R.M., Dudley, P.A., Landis, D.J. and Wheeler, T.G. (1974) Polyunsaturated fatty acids of photoreceptor membranes. *Exp. Eye Res.*, 18: 205–213.

Anderson, R.E., Maude, M.B., Chen, H., Wong, F., Petters, R.M., Liou, G.I., Bok, D., Acland, G.M. and Aguirre, G.D. (1999) Lower ROS docosahexaenoic acid phenotype in animals with inherited retinal degenerations. *Invest. Ophthalmol. Vis. Sci. (Abst.)*, 40: S473.

Bangham, A.D., Dingle, J.T. and Lucy, J.A. (1964) Studies on the mode of action of excess of vitamin A. 9. Penetration of lipid monolayers by compounds in the vitamin A series. *Biochem. J.*, 90: 133–140.

Bazan, N.G., Reddy, T.S., Redmond, T.M., Wiggert, B. and Chader, G.J. (1985) Endogenous fatty acids are covalently and noncovalently bound to interphotoreceptor retinoid-binding protein in the monkey retina. *J. Biol. Chem.*, 260: 13677–13680.

Berman, E.R., Horowitz, J., Segal, N., Fisher, S. and Feeney-Burns, L. (1980) Enzymatic esterification of vitamin A in the pigment epithelium of bovine retina. *Biochim. Biophys. Acta*, 630: 36–46.

Bernstein, P.S., Law, W.C. and Rando, R.R. (1987) Isomerization of *all-trans* retinoids to *11-cis retinoids in vitro*. *Proc. Natl. Acad. Sci. USA*, 84: 1849–1853.

Biesalski, H.K., Frank, J., Beck, S.C., Heinrich, F., Illek, B., Reifen, R., Gollnick, H., Seeliger, M.W., Wissinger, B. and Zrenner, E. (1999) Biochemical but not clinical deficiency results from mutation in the gene for retinol binding protein. *Amer. J. Clin. Nutr.*, 69: 931–936.

348

Blaner, W.S. (1989) Retinol-binding protein: the serum transport protein for vitamin A. *Endocr. Rev.*, 10: 308–316.

Bok, D. and Heller, J. (1976) Transport of retinol from the blood to the retina: an autoradiographic study of the pigment epithelial cell surface receptor for plasma retinol-binding protein. *Exp. Eye Res.*, 22: 395–402.

Boll, F. (1876) Zur Anatomie und Physiologie der Retina. *Monatsberichte der Berliner Acadamie.*, 12 November: 783–787.

Bownds, D. (1967) Site of attachment of retinal in rhodopsin. *Nature*, 216: 1178–1181.

Bunt-Milam, A.H. and Saari, J.C. (1983) Immunocytochemical localization of two retinoid-binding proteins in vertebrate retina. *J. Cell Biol.*, 97: 703–712.

Bunt-Milam, A.H., Saari, J.C., Klock, I.B. and Garwin, G.G. (1985) Zonulae adherents pore size in the external limiting membrane of the rabbit retina. *Invest. Ophthalmol. Vis. Sci.*, 26: 1377–1380.

Carlson, A. and Bok, D. (1992) Promotion of the release of 11-cis retinal from cultured retinal pigment epithelium by interphotoreceptor retinoid-binding protein. *Biochemistry*, 31: 9056–9062.

Carr, R.E., Ripps, H. and Siegel, I.M. (1974) Visual pigment kinetics and adaptation in fundus albipunctatus. *Doc. Ophthalmologica Proc. Series*, 9: 193–204.

Cavallaro, T., Martone, R.L., Dwork, A.J., Schon, E.A. and Herbert, J. (1990) The retinal pigment epithelium is the unique site of transthyretin synthesis in the rat eye. *Invest. Ophthalmol. Vis. Sci.*, 31: 497–501.

Chen, Y., Saari, J.C. and Noy, N. (1993) Interactions of all-*trans*-retinol and long-chain fatty acids with interphotoreceptor retinoid-binding protein. *Biochem.*, 32: 11311–11318.

Cideciyan, A.V., Haeseleer, F., Fariss, R.N., Aleman, T.S., Jang, G.-F., Verlinde, C.L.M.J., Marmor, M.F., Jacobson, S.G. and Palczewski, K. (2000) Rod and cone visual cycle consequences of a null mutation in the 11-*cis*-retinol dehydrogenase gene in man. *Visual Neurosci.*, 17: 667–678.

Cohen, A.I. (1965) A possible cytological basis for the "R" membrane in the vertebrate eye. *Nature (Lond.)*, 205: 1222–1223.

Cogan, U., Kopelman, M., Mokady, S. and Shinitzky, M. (1976) Binding affinities of retinol and related compounds to retinol-binding proteins. *Eur. J. Biochem.*, 65: 71–78.

Craik, K.J.W. and Vernon, M.D. (1941) The nature of dark adaptation. *Brit. J. Psychol.*, 32: 62–81.

Crouch, R.K., Hazard, E.S., Lind, T., Wiggert, B., Chader, G. and Corson, D.W. (1992) *Photochem. Photobiol.*, 56: 251–255.

Das, S.R., Bhardwaj, N. and Gouras, P. (1990) Synthesis of retinoids by human retinal epithelium and transfer to rod outer segments. *Biochem. J.*, 268: 201–206.

Dowling, J.E. (1960) Chemistry of visual adaptation in the rat. *Nature (Lond.)*, 188: 114–118.

Duffy, M., Sun, Y., Wiggert, B., Duncan, T., Chader, G.J. and Ripps, H. (1993) Interphotoreceptor retinoid binding protein (IRBP) enhances rhodopsin regeneration in the experimentally detached retina. *Exp. Eye Res.*, 57: 771–782.

Edwards, R.B. and Adler, A.J. (2000) IRBP enhances removal of 11-*cis*-retinaldehyde from isolated RPE membranes. *Exp. Eye Res.*, 70: 235–245.

Fex, G. and Johannesson, G. (1987) Studies of the spontaneous transfer of retinol from the retinol : retinol-binding complex to unilamellar liposomes. *Biochim. Biophys. Acta.*, 901: 255–264.

Fex, G. and Johannesson, G. (1988) Retinol transfer across and between phospholipid bilayer membranes. *Biochim. Biophys. Acta.*, 944: 249–255.

Fliesler, S.J. and Anderson, R.E. (1983) Chemistry and metabolism of lipids in the vertebrate retina. *Progr. Lipid Res.*, 22: 79–131.

Fliesler, S.J. and Schroepfer, G.J.Jr. (1986) *In vitro* metabolism of mevalonic acid in the bovine retina. *J. Neurochem.*, 46: 448–460.

Flannery, J.G., O'Day, W., Pfeffer, B.A., Horwitz, J. and Bok, D. (1990) Uptake, processing and release of retinoids by cultured human retinal pigment epithelium. *Exp. Eye Res.*, 51: 717–728.

Gonzalez-Fernandez, F. and Healy, J.I. (1990) Early expression of the gene for interphotoreceptor retinol-binding protein during photoreceptor differentiation suggests a critical role for the interphotoreceptor matrix in retinal development. *J. Cell Biol.*, 111: 2775–2784.

Gonzalez-Fernandez, F., Kurz, D., Bao, Y., Newman, S., Conway, B.P., Young, J.E., Han, D.P. and Khani, S.C. (1999) 11-*cis* retinol dehydrogenase mutations as a major cause of the congenital night-blindness disorder known as fundus albipunctatus. *Mol. Vision*, 5: 41–46.

Gorry, P., Lufkin, T., Dierich, A., Rochette-Egly, C., Decimo, D., Dolle, P., Mark, M., Durand, B. and Chambon, P. (1994) The cellular retinoic acid binding protein I is dispensable. *Proc. Natl. Acad. Sci. USA*, 91: 9032–9036.

Gu, S.-M., Thompson, D.A., Srikumari, C.R.S., Lorenz, B., Finckh, U., Nicoletti, A., Murthy, K.R., Rathmann, M., Kumaramanickavel, G., Denton, M.J. and Gal, A. (1997) Mutations in RPE65 cause autosomal recessive childhood-onset severe retinal dystrophy. *Nat. Genet.*, 17: 194–197.

Hauswirth, W.W., Langerijt, A.V.D., Timmers, A.M., Adamus, G. and Ulshafer, R.J. (1992) Early expression and localization of rhodopsin and IRBP in the developing fetal bovine retina. *Exp. Eye Res.*, 54: 661–670.

Herbert, J., Cavallaro, T. and Martone, R. (1991) The distribution of retinol-binding protein and its mRNA in the rat eye. *Invest. Ophthalmol. Vis. Sci.*, 32: 302–309.

Ho, M.-T.P., Massey, J.B., Pownall, H.J., Anderson, R.E. and Hollyfield, J.G. (1989) Mechanism of vitamin A movement between rod outer segments, inter-photoreceptor retinoid-binding protein and liposomes *J. Biol. Chem.*, 264: 928–935.

Hollyfield, J.G., Fliesler, S.J., Rayborn, M.E., Fong, S.-L., Landers, R.A. and Bridges, C.D. (1985) Synthesis and secretion of interstitial retinol-binding protein by the human retina. *Invest. Ophthalmol. Vis. Sci.*, 26: 58–67.

Horwitz, J. and Heller, J. (1973) Interactions of all-*trans*-, 9-, 11, and 13-*cis* retinal, all-*trans*-retinyl acetate, and retinoic acid with human retinol-binding protein and prealbumin. *J. Biol. Chem.*, 248: 6317–6324.

Hubbard, R. and Dowling, J.E. (1962) Formation and utilization of 11-*cis* vitaminA by the eye tssue during light and dark adaptation. *Nature (Lond.)*, 193: 341–343.

Jones, G.J., Crouch, R.K., Wiggert, B., Cornwall, M.C. and Chader, G.J. (1989) Retinoid requirements for recovery of sensitivity after visual-pigment bleaching in isolated photoreceptors. *Proc. Natl. Acad. Sci. USA*, 86: 9606–9610.

Kühne, W. (1878) *On the Photochemistry of the Retina and on Visual Purple.* (Translated from the German and edited by M. Foster), Macmillan, London, UK.

Lai, Y.-L., Wiggert, B., Liu, Y.P. and Chader, G.J. (1982) Interphotoreceptor retinol-binding proteins : possible transport vehicles between compartments of the retina. *Nature* 298: 848–849.

Lin, Z.-S., Fong, S.-L. and Bridges, C.D.B. (1989) Retinoids bound to interstitial retinol-binding protein during light and dark-adaptation. *Vision Res.*, 29: 1699–1709.

Liou, G.I., Bridges, C.D.B., Fong, S.-L., Alvarez, R.A. and Gonzalez-Fernandez, F. (1982) Vitamin A transport between retina and pigment epithelium-an interstitial protein carrying endogenous retinol (interstitial retinol-binding protein) *Vision Res.*, 22: 1457–1468.

Liou, G.I., Fei, Y., Peachey, N.S., Matragoon, S., Wei, S., Blaner, W.S., Wang, Y., Liu, C., Gottesman, M.E. and Ripps, H. (1998) Early onset photoreceptor abnormalities induced by targeted disruption of the interphotoreceptor retinoid-binding protein gene. *J. Neurosci.*, 18: 4511–4520.

Liou, G.I., Wang, M. and Matragoon, S. (1994) Timing of interphotoreceptor retinoid-binding protein (IRBP) gene expression and hypomethylation in developing mouse retina. *Dev. Biol.*, 161: 345–356.

Martone, R.L., Herbert, J., Dwork, A. and Schon, E.A. (1988a) Transthyretin is synthesized in the mammalian eye. *Biochem. Biophys. Res. Commun.*, 151: 905–912.

Martone, R.L., Schon, E.A., Goodman, D.S., Soprano, D.R. and Herbert, J. (1988b) Retinol-binding protein is synthesized in the mammalian eye. *Biochem. Biophys. Res. Commun.*, 157: 1078–1084.

Morimura, H., Fishman, G.A., Grover, S.A., Fulton, A.B., Berson, E.L. and Dryja, T.P. (1998) Mutations in the RPE65 gene in patients with autosomal retinitis pigmentosa or Leber congenital amaurosis. *Proc. Natl. Acad. Sci. USA*, 95: 3088–3093.

Narfström, K., Ivert, L., Yamamoto, S. and Gouras, P. (1993) Adaptation of rod and cone electroretinograms in the Abyssinian cat hereditary rod–cone degeneration. *Clin. Vision Sci.*, 8: 177–185.

Narfström, K., Nilsson, S.E., Wiggert, B., Lee, L., Chader, G.J. and vanVeen, T. (1989) Reduced level of interphotoreceptor retinoid-binding protein (IRBP), a possible cause for retinal degeneration in the Abyssinian cat. *Cell Tissue Res.*, 25: 631–639.

Okajima, T.-I., Pepperberg, D.R., Ripps, H., Wiggert, B. and Chader, G.J. (1989) Interphotoreceptor retinoid-binding protein: role in delivery of retinol to the pigment epithelium. *Exp. Eye Res.*, 49: 629–644.

Okajima, T.-I., Pepperberg, D.R., Ripps, H., Wiggert, B. and Chader, G.J. (1990) Interphotoreceptor retinoid-binding proteinpromotes rhodopsin regeneration in toad photoreceptors. *Proc. Natl. Acad. Sci. USA*, 87: 6907–6911.

Ong, D.E., Davis, J.T., O'Day, W.T. and Bok, D. (1994) Synthesis and secretion of retinol-binding protein and transthyretin by cultured retinal pigment epithelium. *Biochemistry*, 33: 1835–1842.

Palczewski, K., van Hooser, J.P., Garwin, G.G., Chen, J., Liou, G.I. and Saari, J.C. (1999) Kinetics of visual pigment regeneration in excised mouse eyes and in mice with a targeted disruption of the gene encoding interphotoreceptor retinoid-binding protein or arrestin. *Biochem.*, 38: 12012–12019.

Pepperberg, D.R., Okajima, T.-I., Ripps, H., Chader, G.J. and Wiggert, B. (1991) Functional properties of interphotoreceptor retinoid-binding protein. *Photochem. Photobiol.*, 54: 1057–1060.

Pepperberg, D.R., Okajima, T.-I., Wiggert, B., Ripps, H., Crouch, R.K. and Chader, G.J. (1993) Interphotoreceptor retinoid-binding protein (IRBP): molecular biology and physiological role in the visual cycle of rhodopsin. *Molecular Neurobiol.*, 7: 61–85.

Pfeffer, B.A., Clark, V.M., Flannery, J.G. and Bok, D. (1986) Membrane receptors for retinol-binding protein in cultured human retinal pigment epithelium. *Invest. Ophthalmol. Vis. Sci.*, 27: 1031–1040.

Pfeffer, B., Wiggert, B., Lee, L., Zonnenberg, B., Newsome, D. and Chader, G. (1983) The presence of a soluble interphotoreceptor retinol-binding protein (IRBP) in the retinal interphotoreceptor space. *J. Cellular Physiol.*, 117: 333–341.

Putilina, T., Sittenfeld, D., Chader, G.J. and Wiggert, B. (1993) Study of a fatty acid binding site of interphotoreceptor retinoid-binding protein using fluorescent fatty acids. *Biochemistry*, 32: 3797–3803.

Quadro, L., Blaner, W.S., Salchow, D.J., Vogel, S., Piantedosi, R. Gouras, P., Freeman, S., Cosma, M.P., Colantuoni, V. and Gottesman, M.E. (1999) Impaired retinal function and vitamin A availability in mice lacking retinol-binding protein. *EMBO J.*, 18: 4633–4644.

Rando, R.R. (1990) The chemistry of vitamin A and vision. *Angew. Chem. Int. Ed. Engl.*, 29: 461–480.

Rando, R.R. and Bangerter, F.W. (1982) The rapid intermembraneous transfer of retinoids. *Biochem. Biophys. Res. Commun.*, 104: 430–436.

Rando, R.R., Bernstein, P.S. and Barry, R.J. (1991) New insights into the visual cycle. *Progr. Ret. Res.*, 10: 161–178.

Redmond, T.M., Yu, S., Lee, E., Bok, D., Hamaasaki, D., Chen, N., Goletz, P., Ma, J.-X., Crouch, R.K. and Pfeiffer, K. (1998) *Rpe65* is necessary for production of 11-*cis*-vitamin A in the retinal visual cycle. *Nature Genetics*, 20: 344–350.

Ripps, H. (1982) Night blindness revisited: from man to molecules. The Proctor Lecture. *Invest. Ophthalmol. Vis. Sci.*, 23: 588–609.

Ripps, H., Peachey, N.S., Xu, X., Nozell, S.E., Smith, S.B. and Liou, G.I. (2000) The rhodopsin cycle is preserved in IRBP "knockout" mice despite abnormalities in retinal structure and function. *Visual Neurosci.*, 17: 97–105.

Rodrigues, M.M., Hackett, J., Gaskins, R., Wiggert, B., Lee,L., Redmond, M. and Chader, G.J. (1986) Interphotoreceptor retinoid–binding protein in retinal rod cells and pineal gland. *Invest. Ophthalmol. Vis. Sci.*, 27: 844–850.

Rudnicki, M.A., Braun, T., Hinuma, S. and Janeisch, R. (1992) Inactivation of *myoD* in mice leads to up-regulation of the myogenic HLH gene *myf-5* and results in apparently normal muscle development. *Cell*, 71: 383–390.

Rudnicki, M.A., Schnegelsberg, P.N.J., Stead, R.H., Braun, T., Arnold, H.H. and Janeisch, R. (1993) *MyoD* or *myf5* is required for the formation of skeletal muscle. *Cell*, 75: 1351–1359.

Saari, J.C. (1990) Enzymes and proteins of the mammalian visual cycle. *Progr. Ret. Res.*, 9: 363–381.

Saari, J.C. (2000) Biochemistry of visual pigment regeneration. The Friedenwald Lecture. *Invest. Ophthalmol. Vis. Sci.*, 41: 337–348.

Spitznas, M. and Hogan, M.J. (1970) Outer segments of photoreceptors and the retinal pigment epithelium. *Arch. Ophthalmol.*, 84: 810–819.

Steinberg, R.H. and Wood, I. (1979) The relationship of the retinal pigment epithelium to photoreceptor outer segments in human retina. In: Zinn, K.M. and Marmour, M.F. (Eds.), *The Retinal Pigment Epithelium*, Chapter 2, Harvard University Press, Cambridge, MA, pp. 32–44.

Sun, Y. and Ripps, H. (1992) Rhodosin regeneration in the normal and in the detached/replaced retina of the skate. *Exp. Eye Res.*, 55: 679–689.

Szuts, E.Z. and Harosi, F.I. (1991) Solubility of retinoids in water. *Arch. Biochem. Biophys.*, 287: 297–304.

Tonus, J.G. and Dickson, D.H. (1979) Neuro-glial relationships at the external limiting membrane of the newt retina. *Exp. Eye Res.*, 28: 93–110.

van Veen, T., Ekstrom, P., Wiggert, B., Lee, L., Hirose, Y., Sanyal, S. and Chader, G.J. (1988) A developmental study of interphotoreceptor retinoid-binding protein (IRBP) in single and double homozygous rd and rds mutant mouse retinae. *Exp. Eye Res.*, 47: 291–305.

van Veen, T., Katial, A., Shinohara, T., Barrett, D.J., Wiggert, B., Chader, G.J. and Nickerson, J.M. (1986) Retinal photoreceptor neurons and pinealocytes accumulate mRNA for interphotoreceptor retinoid-binding protein (IRBP) *FEBS Lett.*, 208: 133–137.

Wald, G. (1933) Vitamin A in the retina. *Nature*, 132: 316–317.

Wald, G. (1934) Carotenoids and the vitamin A cycle in vision. *Nature*, 134: 65.

Wald, G. (1968) Molecular basis of visual excitation. *Science*, 162: 230–239.

Weintraub, H. (1993) The myoD family and myogenesis: redundancy, networks, and thresholds. *Cell*, 75: 1241–1244.

Wiggert, B., van Veen, T., Kutty, G., Lee, L., Nickerson, J., Si, J.-S., Nilsson, S.E.G., Chader, G.J. and Narfström, K. (1994) An early decrease in interphotoreceptor retinoid-binding protein gene expression in Abyssinian cats homozygous for hereditary rod–cone degeneration. *Cell Tissue Res.*, 278: 291–298.

Yamamoto, H., Simon, A., Eriksson, U., Harris, E., Berson, E.L. and Dryja, T.P. (1999) Mutations in the gene encoding 11-*cis* retinol dehydrogenase cause delayed dark adaptation and fundus albipunctatus. *Nature Gen.*, 22: 188–191.

Yoshikami, S. and Nöll, G.N. (1978) Isolated retinas synthesize visual pigments from retinol congeners delivered by liposomes. *Science*, 200: 1393–1395.

Young, R.W. (1971) Shedding of discs from rod outer segments in the Rhesus monkey. *J. Ultrastruct. Res.*, 34: 190–203.

Zinn, K.M. and Benjamin-Henkind, J.V. (1979) Anatomy of the human retinal pigment epithelium. In Zinn, K.M. and Marmour, M.F. (Eds.), *The Retinal Pigment Epithelium*, Chapter 1, Harvard University Press, Cambridge, MA, pp. 3–31.

H. Kolb, H. Ripps and S. Wu (Eds.)
Progress in Brain Research, Vol. 131
© 2001 Elsevier Science B.V. All rights reserved

CHAPTER 24

Insights into the rod rhodopsin regeneration process using the excised mouse eye

Sanford E. Ostroy*

Department of Biological Sciences, Purdue University, Lilly Hall of Life Sciences, West Lafayette, IN 47907-1392, USA

Introduction

The Dowling (1960) study of the bleaching and regeneration of the rhodopsin in the rod photoreceptors of the rat was such a major landmark that most of our present view of this process is still based on that work (for examples see Chader et al., 1998; Saari, 2000). A particularly unique feature of that study was that it maintained the physiological viability of the system by bleaching in live animals and permitting the rhodopsin regeneration to occur under those same conditions. In developing an excised albino mouse eye preparation, Ostroy et al., (1992) sought to incorporate a major aspect of that study—maintaining the integrity of the structural components of the eye during the bleaching and regeneration cycles. The preparation was also developed in order to test various perfusion factors, to monitor the rhodopsin concentration changes directly, to follow the rhodopsin regeneration at low bleaching levels, to obtain data in a mammal, and to take advantage of the powerful array of genetic tools available for the mouse. Two of those studies are presented: (1) rhodopsin regeneration in diabetic mice and (2) the rhodopsin regeneration process at low bleaching levels.

General properties of rhodopsin regeneration in the excised albino mouse eye

Representative experiments are presented in Figs. 1 and 2. Fig. 1 illustrates the rates and amounts of rhodopsin regeneration after multiple bleaches. Following the first two bleaches, complete regenerations occur. Thus a two-bleach protocol could be used to reversibly test the effect of various conditions. To show such an experiment and illustrate original data, a glucose experiment is presented in Fig. 2. With no glucose in the extracellular perfusate only minimal rhodopsin regeneration follows the first bleach (spectra 2 and 3). After restoration of normal extracellular glucose concentration (5.1 mM) a second bleach is followed by a high level of rhodopsin regeneration (spectra 3–5; see figure caption for additional details).

The two-bleach protocol was used to test the effects of extracellular glucose concentration (Ostroy et al., 1992) and hypoxia (Ostroy et al., 1993). Because of the characteristics of diffusion of gases one can be certain that modified levels of oxygen concentration will diffuse throughout the whole eye. However, the hypoxic and extracellular glucose concentration results were comparable—reducing the available metabolic energy reduced or eliminated rhodopsin regeneration—and the effects were reversible. Under hypoxic conditions no rhodopsin regeneration was observed but after oxygen was re-introduced, bleaches were followed by complete

* Tel.: 765-494-4942; Fax: 765-494-0876;
E-mail: sostroy@bilbo.bio.purdue.edu

352

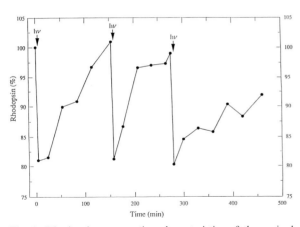

Fig. 1. Rhodopsin regeneration characteristics of the excised mouse eye preparation. Thirty second fluorescent light bleaches of 19%, 20% and 19% followed by regenerations of 105%, 90% and 62%, respectively. From Ostroy et al. (1992); Fig. 1 (modified). Originally published in *Experimental Eye Research* 55: 419–423. Reproduced with permission. Copyright © 1992 by Academic Press.

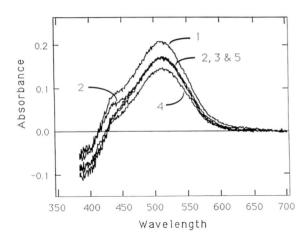

Fig. 2. Rhodopsin absorption spectra of the albino excised mouse eye preparation and the effect of extracellular glucose concentration. Shows the inhibitory effect of 0 mM extracellular glucose on rhodopsin regeneration. Spectrum no. 1, original rhodopsin spectrum after subtraction of the final spectrum. Spectrum no. 2 following an illumination (with 0 mM extracellular glucose in the perfusate) that bleached 19% and spectrum no. 3, $3\frac{1}{3}$ h later showing the lack of major rhodopsin regeneration (17%). Spectrum 4 following a second illumination (in the presence of 5.1 mM glucose) that bleached 16% followed by a regeneration of 93% (spectrum 5, after 3 h). From Ostroy et al. (1992); Fig. 3 (modified). Originally published in *Experimental Eye Research* 55: 419–423. Reproduced with permission. Copyright © 1992 by Academic Press.

regeneration (Ostroy et al., 1993). For extracellular glucose concentration the lowest amounts of rhodopsin regeneration occurred at 1 mM extracellular glucose, with low regeneration at 0 mM glucose (8% and 20%, respectively). As the extracellular glucose concentration was raised above 1 mM the rhodopsin regeneration improved until normal levels of regeneration were observed from 4 mM to 10 mM glucose (normal is 5.1 mM). High concentrations of extracellular glucose of 20 mM (Ostroy et al., 1994) and 30 mM (Knapp, 1997) decreased the levels of rhodopsin regeneration, possibly mimicking the effect of diabetes (see next section).

Mechanistically, these studies showed that the rhodopsin regeneration process is reversibly dependent on aerobic glycolysis and presumably the ATP that is derived from this pathway. In the prevailing view of the rhodopsin regeneration process, the only step known to have such a dependence was the recycling of NADPH and its role in the reduction of all-trans retinal to all-trans retinol (Schnetkamp and Daemen, 1981, Ostroy et al., 1992). However, we did not observe any major changes in the amount or rate of change of retinal concentration under conditions of hypoxia or low glucose (Knapp, 1997). A more recent study that showed the importance of rim protein as an ATP dependent ABC transporter of all-trans retinal from within the rod disk may provide a mechanistic explanation for these and other results (Illing et al., 1997; Sun et al., 1999; Weng et al., 1999; see below "Rim protein or acidification: A potential role in diabetes and other disorders"). It should be noted that while the ability to obtain data at low bleaches has the advantage of providing data in the physiologically functional range of the rod photoreceptors, unless the effect is very obvious, it is limited in its ability to obtain mechanistic information. Concentration differences of 15% or less are almost impossible to detect.

Following from the data on the effects of extracellular glucose, one focus of further studies was to determine if diabetes would adversely affect the process of rhodopsin regeneration. Another focus was to utilize lower bleaching levels that would both require less metabolic energy and more closely approach the bleaching levels encountered in the normal functioning of rod photoreceptors.

Rhodopsin regeneration in diabetic mice

Diabetes is responsible for physiological problems in a number of systems, including the visual system (Pickup and Williams, 1994). Although our studies focused on the specific issue of rod rhodopsin regeneration, the responsible mechanism, acidity within the rod photoreceptors, could potentially be responsible for a number of the abnormalities caused by diabetes.

The initial data clearly showed that diabetic mice had some abnormalities in their rod rhodopsin regeneration. The initial study used bleaching levels of 15–20% and streptozotocin-induced diabetic mice, mimicking Type I diabetes (Ostroy et al., 1994). The diabetic mice exhibited reductions in the regeneration following a bleach with the amount of reduction dependent on the severity of the diabetes. At normal extracellular glucose, severely diabetic mice exhibited regeneration levels of 64% and more moderately diabetic mice exhibited regeneration levels of 74%. To enhance the information on the rhodopsin regeneration of diabetics a genetic line of albino diabetic mice was developed mimicking Type II diabetes. In addition, it became possible to further reduce the bleaching levels. Under these conditions, both the genetic and streptozotocin-induced diabetic mice showed similar effects—a slowing in the rate of rhodopsin regeneration accompanied by the formation of a rhodopsin intermediate that is only observed under acid conditions. The data for the genetic diabetic mouse and comparable data for the non-diabetic mouse are presented in Figs. 3 and 4. N-Retinylidene-Opsin (NRO440), the acid form of the Schiff's base between retinal and opsin, is quite evident in the diabetic mouse eye but absent in the non-diabetic mouse eye. This is most easily observed in the difference spectra which show a distinct peak at 440 nm in the diabetic (Fig. 3B) but not in the non-diabetic (Fig. 4B). The time course of the formation of NRO440 in the diabetic as well as the decay of retinal380 over that same time period in the non-diabetic are presented in Figs. 3A and 4A. In the diabetic approximately 30% of the photoproducts proceeded to NRO440.

Extracellular glucose concentration affected the rhodopsin in diabetic mice and non-diabetic mice in expected ways. In non-diabetic mice high

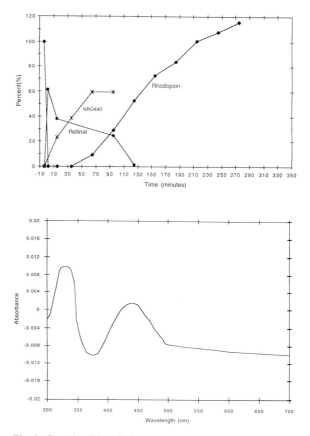

Fig. 3. Genetic albino diabetic mouse. Showing the time course of retinal380, rhodopsin and N-Retinylidene-Opsin (NRO440) concentrations (A) and the difference spectrum that shows the spectral changes soon after the illumination (B). Difference spectrum (B) is the 15 min spectrum subtracted from the 2 min spectrum (timed from the end of the illumination). Bleach of 10.8%. From Ostroy (1998; Fig. 2). Originally published in *Current Eye Research* 17: 979–985.

extracellular glucose concentrations slowed the rate (20 mM and 30 mM; Knapp, 1997) and reduced the amount (20 mM; Ostroy et al., 1994) of rhodopsin regeneration. In diabetic mice the amount of rhodopsin regeneration was increased by high extracellular glucose concentration (20 mM; Ostroy et al., 1994).

Acidity, caused by the presence of excess glucose proceeding to lactic acid because it cannot be metabolized through the TCA cycle, is a well known biochemical pathway. However, its potentially detrimental cellular effects have not been particularly recognized. One possible reason for this is the experimental difficulty of attributing any modifications

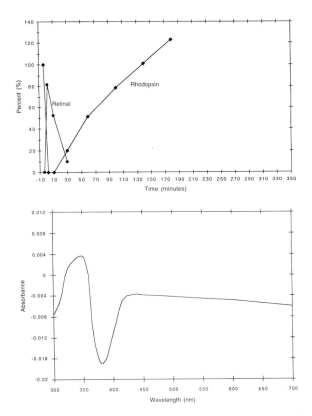

Fig. 4. Non-diabetic albino mouse. Showing the time course of retinal380 and rhodopsin concentrations (A) and the difference spectrum that shows the spectral changes soon after the illumination (B). Difference spectrum (B) is the 15 min spectrum subtracted from the 2 min spectrum (timed from the end of the illumination). Bleach of 14.6%. From Ostroy (1998; Fig. 3). Originally published in *Current Eye Research* 17: 979–985.

of cellular processes to acidity. These data may assist in focusing on such a mechanism. In the visual system, the observation that good glucose control can reduce some of the detrimental effects of diabetes is consistent with such a mechanism.

Rim protein or acidification: a potential role in diabetes and other disorders

A report by Weng et al. (1999) on the characteristics of an ABCR knockout mouse would appear to have direct relevance to our diabetic studies. The mouse lacks rim protein, a rod photoreceptor localized protein that had been shown to be an

ABC transporter (Illing et al., 1997). Weng et al. (1999) indicate that this protein transports an all-*trans* retinal/phosphatidylethanolamine covalently bound complex (N-retinylidene-PE) from the inside to outside of the disk membrane. Moreover, mice lacking this transporter exhibited high concentrations of the acid form of the N-retinylidene-PE, with an absorbance peak at 450 nm. This result appears to coincide with our own observation of NRO440 in diabetic mice (Fig. 3). In a reinterpretation of our own data it may be that we observed the acid form of N-retinylidene-PE rather than NRO440 (N-retinylidene-opsin). Alternatively, it may be that the rod photoreceptors of both the diabetic mice and the ABCR knockout mice experienced an increased acidity—causing the formation of both acidic forms. In normal rod photoreceptor cell functioning only the alkaline form of N-retinylidene-PE is observed (Weng et al., 1999) and neither form of N-retinylidene-opsin is observed (Abrahamson and Ostroy, 1967). In addition, one of the characteristics of individuals lacking rim protein in Stargardt's Disease includes a slowing of rod dark adaptation (Fishman et al., 1991). This appears to correspond with our observation of a slowed rhodopsin regeneration in the diabetic mice (Fig. 3A). Thus it seems possible that the rhodopsin regeneration abnormalities that are observed in diabetic mice may be related to the abnormalities that occur when rim protein is defective. In addition to Stargardt's Disease, the other rim protein defective disorders include fundus flavimaculatus, recessive retinitis pigmentosa, recessive cone–rod dystrophy, and possibly age-related macular degeneration (see Weng et al., 1999).

Complexities of rhodopsin regeneration and some new ideas

Our data also begin to address a more fundamental issue—the present view of rhodopsin recovery in rod photoreceptors. In particular, the view that each 11-*cis* chromophore is utilized only once and must return to the retinal pigment epithelium before being re-isomerized. Human rod photoreceptors function at bleaching levels of 0.00004% (Hecht et al., 1942) to 5% (Campbell and Rushton, 1955), with steady light at rod saturation associated with a 5% level of bleaching (Campbell and Rushton, 1955; Rodieck, 1973). At a static level this means that from 4 opsins to 500,000 opsins need new 11-*cis* chromophore in each of 120 million rod photoreceptors. To illustrate the difficulties, Fig. 5 presents a dimensionally proportional retinal pigment epithelium and human rod photoreceptor with 5% of the opsins in a bleached state. Most striking is the distance of some of the opsins from the retinal pigment epithelium and their extensive distribution among the many disks of the rod photoreceptor. A major question is how new 11-*cis* retinals (that are reactive aldehydes) being supplied from outside of the photoreceptors could find and react with the opsins that require new chromophore.

Some of our studies have been directed at this issue with the assumption that, particularly at low bleaches, the opsins are able to re-utilize their retinal. To date we have been unable to obtain direct data showing such a mechanism. We have, however, been able to show that light stimulates the process of rhodopsin regeneration beyond the amount needed to replace only the bleached rhodopsins, particularly at low bleaching levels. Directly derived from these data is the notion that not all of the bleached opsins are immediately supplied with new 11-*cis* chromophore and that some opsins remain without 11-*cis* chromophore—to be replaced when light activates the regeneration process (Ostroy, 2001).

The rhodopsin regeneration process at low bleaching levels

On the assumption that bleaching levels above 5% already exceed rod saturation and that some mechanisms may operate only at the lower bleaching levels, we have focused some of our studies at those lower levels. The results for animals dark adapted for 24 h are presented in Fig. 6. As the bleaching levels were lowered below 5%, increasing amounts of rhodopsin regeneration, up to 400%, were observed. Thus the data directly show that light stimulates the process of rhodopsin regeneration. In other words, light does not simply begin the regeneration process for the rhodopsins it has just bleached but initiates a more extensive process. With regards to 11-*cis* retinal, our results show that light has stimulated either the

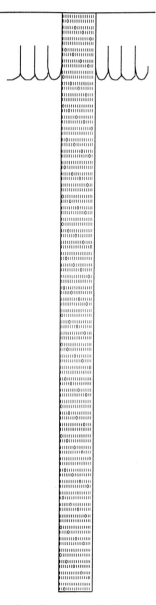

Fig. 5. Representation of a uniform 5% bleach in a human rod photoreceptor. The illustration shows the relative positions and dimensions of a rod photoreceptor outer segment, the individual disks, bleached(0) and unbleached (|) rhodopsins, and the retinal pigment epithelium. Representing 110–150 million rod photoreceptors (Osterberg, 1935) with each photoreceptor containing approximately 1,000 disks (Dowling, 1967) and each disk containing approximately 10,000 rhodopsin molecules. Shows the relationship of the dark or light adapted human rod photoreceptor with 12% in possible contact with the retinal pigment epithelium (Burnside and Laties, 1979); illustrates 1570 unbleached rhodopsins (of 9.5 million) and 82 bleached rhodopsins (of 0.5 million) in 51 disks (of 1,000).

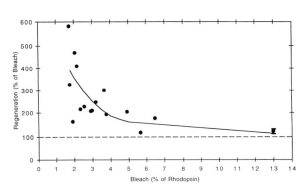

Fig. 6. Rhodopsin regeneration as a function of bleach level in albino mice dark adapted for 24 h. Line is a best fit polynomial. (Presented by Ostroy, 2001.)

production or transport of 11-*cis* retinal. Moreover, the amounts of 11-*cis* retinal that are now available exceeds the amount needed to simply replace the bleached chromophores by at least 300%. It may even be much higher since our lowest bleach is 1.7%—a comparatively high bleach when compared to the range of rod photoreceptor function. Since the regeneration of rhodopsin requires both 11-*cis* retinal and available opsins these data provide information about both of these components. With regard to the opsins, it shows that some opsins are without native chromophore even after 24 h of dark adaptation. At 24 h of dark adaptation 4.7% of the opsins of the rod photoreceptor were without native chromophore (Ostroy, 2001).

Conclusions and future perspective

Some aspects of our studies of rod rhodopsin regeneration in the excised mouse eye have served to confirm previous studies or ideas. In particular, our determination that the metabolic energy (presumably ATP) supplied by glucose or oxygen were important to the rhodopsin regeneration process, confirms other studies that came to similar conclusions (Rando et al., 1990). We obtained additional information by determining the concentration profile of extracellular glucose. This led directly to the studies of diabetic mice and the new findings of reduced or altered rhodopsin regeneration in mouse models of Type I and Type II diabetes. That acidity within the rod photoreceptors may cause the altered rhodopsin regeneration in diabetic mice is of

potential importance. The common features of modified rhodopsin regeneration in diabetic mice and both mice and humans lacking in rim protein are intriguing. Finally, we have begun to more directly address the current model of rhodopsin regeneration. At lower bleaching levels, both a light stimulated mechanism and opsins that remain for some time without 11-*cis* chromophore, have been revealed. Will it be found that the rhodopsins within rod photoreceptors are able to re-utilize their chromophore following a bleach?

Future scientists would do well to mimic the high quality of science and high principles exemplified by John E. Dowling. In my own areas of pursuit I look forward to a better understanding of the mechanisms behind the physiological problems caused by diabetes while molecular biological advances eliminate the genetic forms of this disease. In the rhodopsin regeneration process much is yet to be found— many steps and factors yet to be discovered—with many surprises along the way. It has been a privilege to be a part of this era of vision research.

References

Abrahamson, E.W. and Ostroy, S.E. (1967) The photochemical and macromolecular aspects of vision. *Prog. Biophys. Mol. Biol.*, 17: 179–215.

Burnside, B. and Laties, A.M. (1979) Pigment movement and cellular contractility in the retinal pigment epithelium. In: Marmor, M.F. and Zinn, K.M. (Eds.), *The Retinal Pigment Epithelium*, Harvard University Press, Cambridge, MA.

Campbell, F.W. and Rushton, W.A.H. (1955) Measurement of the scotopic pigment in the living human eye. *J. Physiol.*, 130: 131–147.

Chader, G., Pepperberg, R., Crouch, B. and Wiggert, B. (1998) Retinoids and the pigment epithelium. In: Marmor, M.F. and Wolfensberger, T.J. (Eds.), *The Retinal Pigment Epithelium, Function and Disease*, Oxford University Press, New York.

Dowling, J.E. (1960) Chemistry of visual adaptation in the rat. *Nature*, 188: 114–118.

Dowling, J.E. (1967) The organization of vertebrate visual receptors. In: Allen, J.M. (Ed.), *Molecular Organization and Biological Function*, Harper & Row, New York, pp. 186–210.

Fishman, G.A., Farbman, J.S. and Alexander, K.R. (1991) Delayed rod dark adaptation in patients with Stargardt's disease. *Ophthalmology*, 98: 957–962.

Hecht, S., Shlaer, S. and Pirenne, M.H. (1942) Energy, quanta, and vision. *J. Gen. Physiol.*, 25: 819–840.

Illing, M., Molday, L.L. and Molday, R.S. (1997) The 220-kDa rim protein of retinal rod outer segments is a member of the ABC transporter superfamily. *J. Biol. Chem.*, 272: 10303–10310.

Knapp, J.D. (1997) The effect of glucose concentration on rhodopsin regeneration and the all-trans retinal to retinol reaction in the eyes of diabetic and non-diabetic mice. Honors Research Thesis, Purdue University, Department of Biological Sciences, West Lafayette, IN 47907.

Osterberg, G. (1935) Topography of the layer of rods and cones in the human retina. *Acta. Ophthal.*, (Suppl. 6): 1–103.

Ostroy, S.E., Friedmann, A.L. and Gaitatzes, C.G. (1992) Extracellular glucose dependence of rhodopsin regeneration in the excised mouse eye. *Exp. Eye Res.*, 55: 419–423.

Ostroy, S.E., Gaitatzes, C.G. and Friedmann, A.L. (1993) Hypoxia inhibits rhodopsin regeneration in the excised mouse eye. *Invest. Ophthalmol. Vis. Sci.*, 34: 447–452.

Ostroy, S.E., Frede, S.M., Wagner, E.F., Gaitatzes, C.G. and Janle, E.M. (1994) Decreased rhodopsin regeneration in diabetic mouse eyes. *Invest. Ophthalmol. Vis. Sci.*, 35: 3905–3909.

Ostroy, S.E. (1998) Altered rhodopsin regeneration in diabetic mice caused by acid conditions within the rod photoreceptors. *Curr. Eye Res.*, 17: 979–985.

Ostroy, S.E. (2001) Light stimulation of the rhodopsin regeneration process. *Biophys. J.*, 80: 605a.

Pickup, J.C. and Williams, G. (Eds.) (1994) *Chronic Complications of Diabetes*, Blackwell Science, Inc.

Rando, R.R., Bernstein, P.S. and Barry, R.J. (1990) New insights into the visual cycle. In: Osborne, N. and Chader, G. (Eds.), *Progress in Retinal Research*, Pergamon Press, New York, pp 114–118.

Rodieck, R.W. (1973) In: Kennedy, D. and Park, R.B. (Eds.), *The Vertebrate Retina: Principles of Structure and Function*, Freeman and Company, San Francisco.

Saari, J.C. (2000) Biochemistry of visual pigment regeneration. The Friedenwald Lecture. *Invest. Ophthalmol. Vis. Sci.*, 41: 337–348.

Schnetkamp, P.P.M. and Daemen, F.J.M. (1981) Transfer of high-energy phosphate in bovine rod outer segments: a nucleotide buffer system. *Biochim. Biophys. Acta.*, 672: 307–312.

Sun, H., Molday, R.S. and Nathans, J. (1999) Retinal stimulates ATP hydrolysis by purified and reconstituted ABCR, the photoreceptor-specific ATP-binding cassette transporter responsible for Stargardt disease. *J. Biol. Chem.*, 274: 8269–8281.

Weng, J., Mata, N.L., Azarian, S.M., Tzekov, R.T., Birch, D.G. and Travis, G.H. (1999) Insights into the function of rim protein in photoreceptors and etiology of Stargardt's disease from the phenotype in *abcr* knockout mice. *Cell*, 98: 13–23.

H. Kolb, H. Ripps and S. Wu (Eds.)
Progress in Brain Research, Vol. 131

CHAPTER 25

The response gradient along the rod outer segment: cGMP, age and calcium

K.N. Leibovic*

SUNY at Buffalo, Buffalo, NY 14214, USA and MCV/VCU, Richmond, VA, USA

Introduction

Between 1979 and 1980 I spent an extended sabbatical in John Dowling's laboratory at Harvard. I had been more interested in theoretical problems before then. The time with John marked a turning point. I not only learned some essential techniques, but got a first hand, down to earth appreciation of the mentality of a superb experimentalist, who could express his thoughts in clear and simple language.

At Harvard we worked on photoreceptor adaptation using intracellular recordings from Bufo rods. I had long maintained that the major part of light and dark adaptation takes place in the photoreceptors and our results confirmed this. Threshold changes at light ON and OFF in rods mirror psychophysical measurements. We derived the Weber law for light backgrounds, quantified threshold elevation with bleaching from 0% to over 90% and we showed that, similarly to the psychophysical findings there was an equivalence between bleaching and backgrounds in terms of threshold elevation and response compression. But a critical difference between bleaching and background adaptation lies in the response kinetics (Leibovic et al., 1987).

On my return to Buffalo I continued the work on photoreceptors, but got more interested in transduction. One finding which intrigued me was that of the response gradient along the rod outer segment (ROS): the light responses at the tip are smaller and slower than at the base (Lamb et al., 1981; Baylor and Lamb, 1982; Schnapf, 1983). I should like to summarize our work in relation to this phenomenon.

Disc renewal and aging

The ROS and its contents are constantly renewed by forming new membrane at the base and discarding it at the tip where it is phagocytosed in the pigment epithelium (PE). Differences between the base and tip have been reported with regard to membrane composition (Beosze-Battaglia et al., 1990), rhodopsin phosphorylation (Shichi and Williams, 1979) and recovery from bleaching (Pepperberg et al., 1992). These observations, including the response gradient, have been proposed to be due to the aging of the outer segment as it grows out towards the tip. This raises a number of questions:

1. While it is true that the tip is older than the base, could the response gradient be due to some other cause, such as interactions between the rod inner segment (RIS) and its outer segment, rather than aging?
2. What would happen if one could manipulate the age of the tip relative to the base? Would it have an effect on the response gradient?

* 105 High Park Blvd., Buffalo, NY 14226, USA.
E-mail: bphknl@acsu.buffalo.edu

3. It has been suggested that the response gradient is due to a [Na] gradient with [Na] being higher at the tip. But does Ca, which is pivotal in transduction, play a role?

We have carried out a series of experiments to answer these questions.

The experiments

The animals used in these studies were *Bufo marinus* and *Xenopus laevis*. The eye was dissected, and pieces of eye-cup were placed in the media we developed for maintenance and dissociation of photoreceptors (Leibovic, 1986). Responses were obtained from individual rods either in isolation or in clumps of cells with the suction electrode (Baylor et al., 1979) using optical and data acquisition systems described previously (Leibovic et al., 1987; Leibovic and Pan, 1994).

Light intensities, presented in arbitrary N.D. units throughout, can be converted to photons absorbed per rod in accordance with the following calibration: a 100 ms flash attenuated by a 6.6 N.D. filter delivered on average 1 photon to a 45 μm long ROS with a collecting area (Baylor et al., 1979) of 15.7 μm^2. Similarly, a steady background attenuated by a 6.5 N.D. filter delivered 12.4 photons/s to a ROS of equivalent length.

To assess the gradient along the ROS, we used the saturated responses to strong light flashes of varying lengths L of ROS drawn into the suction electrode. As this length increases, the saturation time T decreases and the response amplitude A increases. Fig. 1 shows that these changes are linear and that T and A are linearly related. Therefore, by recording T for different lengths L of ROS one obtains $|\Delta T/\Delta L|$ as a measure of the response gradient. It turns out that $|\Delta L/\Delta T|$ is numerically more convenient, and it is therefore used in what follows instead of $|\Delta T/\Delta L|$.

The saturation time T was measured as shown in Fig. 5, from the end of the initial upstroke to the end of the flat horizontal part of the current response. We compared this method with two others: in the first we extrapolated the linear upstroke (i.e. the rapid current shutoff) and the exponential recovery after saturation, respectively, to the flat horizontal trace where the response is saturated and then measured

T between the corresponding points of intersection; in the second method we measured T between the points at 10% below the maximum, saturated response at upstroke and decay. There was no difference in either the consistency or the variability of the results between the three methods.

cGMP: is the response gradient due to RIS-ROS interactions?

In a general way the response waveform tells us something about the underlying mechanisms. Specifically, the duration of the saturated response T marks the time when all the cGMP sensitive channels are closed, i.e. from the moment that all the free cGMP is hydrolyzed to when new cGMP becomes available.

From Fig. 1 it is evident that the tip takes longer to recover from saturation than the base. There could be several possibilities for this. One is that cGMP

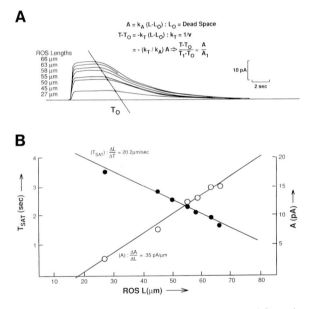

Fig. 1. A. A series of superimposed responses, traced from the original responses of a dark adapted rod, to a 100 ms flash $I_F = 3.5$ which isomerized an estimated 1260 rhodopsin molecules in a collecting area of 15.7 μm^2. Different lengths of the ROS, as indicated on the left, were sucked into the electrode. The response amplitude varies linearly with ROS length, as does the saturation time T. T_0 is the limit of T when $L = L_0$, the electrode dead space. The curves are aligned on the left, at the beginning of the response. B. Plots of A and T from panel A (Leibovic and Pan, 1994).

is regenerated in the RIS and takes longer to reach the tip. G-cyclase which is required for the production of cGMP is present in the OS but has been reported to be heavily concentrated around the axonemes at the RIS–ROS junction (Fleishman and Danisevich, 1979). Thus, cGMP could be generated there as well as inside the ROS. Moreover, it must be recalled that most of the cGMP is in bound form (Kilbride and Ebrey, 1979; Woodruff and Fain, 1982; Cohen and Blazinski, 1988; Yamazaki et al., 1988; Cote et al., 1989), so that free cGMP to terminate saturation could also come from bound stores.

To decide between the various alternatives we made use of the fact that light adapted responses are faster than dark adapted ones, as we had shown in John's laboratory. One can quantify this further by finding the values of $|\Delta L/\Delta T|$ under dark adapted and light adapted conditions. Table 1 gives such values at two flash intensities (I_F) for 5 cells in the dark (DA) and in the presence of two backgrounds (I_{BX}, I_{BY}). For I_{BX}, a weak background, the full background beam was attenuated by a 6.5 ND and I_{BY}, a moderate background, by a 5.5 ND filter.

$|\Delta L/\Delta T|$ has the dimensions of speed. If fresh cGMP was generated in the region of the axonemes and moved from there through the ROS, then $|\Delta L/\Delta T|$ would be the speed of movement, which could be due to diffusion or to some form of active transport. When recording from shorter lengths of ROS it would take longer for the cGMP to get there and hence T would be longer. Although the data points lie close to a straight line, which is not what one would expect with diffusion, it might be only an approximation due to the short length of the ROS. However, we can dismiss the possibility of diffusion on several counts. First, it would be difficult to account for faster diffusion in the presence of a light background, as demonstrated in Table 1. Second, the diffusion coefficient in a rod has been measured to be between 3 and 10 $\mu m/s^2$ (Cameron and Pugh, 1990).

As a rough estimate of the diffusional displacement Δ of a particle in time t one can use the equation:

$$\Delta = (2Dt)^{1/2} = (2 \times \{3 - 10\} \times 1)^{1/2}$$
$$= 2.4 - 4.5 \ \mu m \text{ in } 1 \text{ s}.$$

where D = diffusion coefficient. For longer times Δ/t decreases. This is much smaller than the observed values of $|\Delta L/\Delta T|$, even in dark adapted cells. Finally, it can be shown from calculations based on the diffusional concentration profile that T should not be linear with L even over the length of the ROS.

There remains the possibility of active transport of cGMP from the RIS. But there is also the possibility that cGMP is not produced in the RIS–ROS region, but locally in the RIS and that T gets longer due to the slowing kinetics from base to tip. To decide between these possibilities, i.e. transport from the RIS vs. slowing of local kinetics, we devised the following experiment.

About half the ROS was sucked into the electrode. An opaque, blackened shield could be placed over the other half of the ROS (and RIS) outside the electrode. A background light, either I_{BX} or I_{BY}, was projected over the preparation. Without the shield the whole cell was light adapted and T was recorded for a given light flash I_F. This was then repeated with the shield covering the part of the rod outside the electrode. The configuration is sketched in Fig. 2, and shows that the presence of the shield did not affect the recorded responses. Fig. 3A shows that the shield was effective in excluding light (from light scattering and diffraction) up to 1 log unit. This was sufficient to shield the rod outside the electrode from both I_{BX} and I_{BY} which displaced the response operating curve of the rod by at most 1 log unit as shown in Fig. 3B.

Now if there is transport of cGMP along the ROS after a saturating flash, then since a background would speed this up, T should be shorter without than with the shield. This is because the part of the ROS proximal to the RIS is light adapted without and dark adapted with the shield. On the other hand, if cGMP is supplied locally, there should be no difference with or without the shield.

Fig. 4 shows the results of such an experiment which has been repeated with unvarying reproducibility on other cells. As before, the slopes of the lines in Fig. 4 differ between different cells, but there is no

Table 1. Values of $|\Delta L/\Delta T|$ in $\mu m/s$ (Leibovic and Pan, 1994)

Cell ID	280592	290592	300592	070193	090193
I_F (ND)	3	3	3	3.5	3.5
DA	18	25	15	11	14
I_{BX}	–	29	17	12	36
I_{BY}	52	35	–	35	60

362

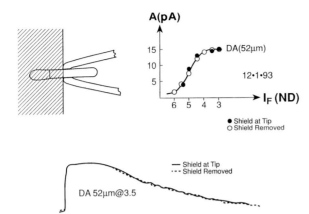

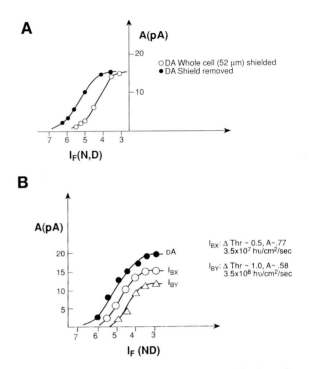

Fig. 2. A (top left). Sketch of a rod, half sucked into the electrode, with an opaque shield covering the part outside the electrode. Top right: Plot of response amplitude A vs. flash intensity I_F (in units of N.D. attenuation) shows that the shield, when it does not cover the OS inside the electrode, has no effect on the responses. Bottom: Superimposed response waveforms with and without the shield as in B are identical (Leibovic and Pan, 1994).

difference with or without the shield in any of the cells. We therefore conclude that new free cGMP is generated locally, but the kinetics for its supply are slowed as we go from base to tip of the ROS.

At a flash intensity $I_F = 3$, as in Fig. 4, we estimate that 4×10^3 rhodopsin molecules have been activated. This is about 5–10 times the intensity which first saturates the response and from the data of Cohen and Blazinski (1988) the amount of cGMP hydrolyzed is then well in excess of the free cGMP present. In principle, the lengthening of T along the OS could be due to the slowing release of cGMP from bound states or to its slower regeneration involving G-cyclase; but one cannot exclude the possibility that any of the steps preceding the hydrolysis of cGMP may be controlling (Pepperberg et al., 1992) and may inactivate more slowly near the tip than the base, or that we are dealing with a combination of factors. In any event, it remains true that response saturation does not end until new, free cGMP becomes available, and our results show that this occurs locally and is progressively delayed as one goes from base to tip of the ROS. In addition, the independence of different parts of the ROS, as in the experiment of Fig. 4, reinforces the notion that the ROS can be considered as a stack of modules (Leibovic, 1990; Leibovic and Moreno-Diaz Jr., 1992) with each

Fig. 3. A. Response vs. flash intensity for a rod fully drawn into the electrode and wholly shielded (open circles) and with the shield removed (filled circles), showing that the shield effectively attenuates the light by 1 log unit. B. The backgrounds I_{BX} and I_{BY} raise the flash intensity for a threshold response by 0.5 and 1.0 log units respectively and reduce the maximum A to 0.77 and 0.58 of the dark adapted (DA) value (Leibovic and Pan, 1994).

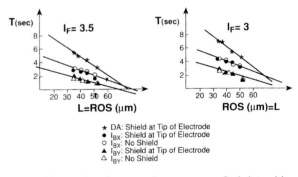

Fig. 4. The results of an experiments at two flash intensities, $I_F = 3.5$ and 3.0 and two backgrounds I_{BX} and I_{BY}. There is no difference in the saturation time T for different lengths L, with or without the shield in the configuration of Fig. 2A (Leibovic and Pan, 1994).

containing within it all the machinery necessary for transduction and adding its contribution linearly to the response of the whole ROS.

Age of tip vs. base: effects of light and temperature on response gradient

If the response gradient is due to the age gradient between base and tip, then there should also be differences in the response gradients between outer segments with different age gradients. In fact, it is possible to control the rates of ROS regeneration, and thus the age gradients, by varying the temperature. It has been shown that lowering the temperature slows ROS regeneration and raising the temperature accelerates it (Hollyfield, 1979; Hollyfield et al., 1977; Young, 1967). In the following experiments we used Xenopus laevis.

The animals were divided into three groups: Tc, Tn and Tw. The Tc group was kept at 14.5°C, the Tn group at 20 to 21°C and the Tw group at 29.5°C. All were exposed to normal diurnal lighting near the window in our laboratory. Allowing time for complete ROS renewal, the animals were sacrificed after about two months exposure to their respective temperatures and the rod responses to a saturating flash were recorded as described above. There was the usual variability between the responses of different cells with regard to amplitude and kinetics and there was overlap in these characteristics between the Tc, Tn and Tw groups. However, statistically there were significant differences as shown in Table 2.

According to the t-test, the hypothesis that the means are equal in Table 2 is rejected with a probability greater than 99.9% for the Tc vs. the Tn and the Tn vs. the Tw groups. n = number of samples in a group.

The values of $|\Delta L/\Delta T|$ increase monotonically from Tc through Tn to Tw, showing that the gradient from base to tip is greatest in the cold reared and least in the warm reared animals. This is as expected if the response gradient is due to aging of the membrane in temperature dependent ROS renewal.

Table 2. Mean values. ± S.D. at $I_F = 3$, for $|\Delta L/\Delta T|$ for the groups Tc, Tn and Tw (Leibovic and Bandarchi, 1997a)

Group	Tc	Tn	Tw
$\|\Delta L/\Delta T\|$	4.45± 1.26	9.29± 2.50	13.71± 3.26
N	13	15	12

Moreover, having demonstrated earlier that the recovery from response saturation at any point along the ROS is driven by local processes and is not dependent on the transport of metabolites from the RIS, the implication is that the age gradient is correlated with local changes in the transduction cycle which generates the light response.

Ionic correlates of the response gradient: the role of Ca

Since Ca plays such an important part in cellular regulation in general and in phototransduction and light adaptation in particular, we examined the Ca exchange across the ROS membrane in order to determine if there are any differences between base and tip. In these experiments we used Bufo marinus and Xenopus laevis. The results for both species are quite similar.

Data analysis

When one examines in some detail the waveform of the saturated response, one first sees a rapid reduction of the inward current, followed by a secondary decrease to a plateau of zero current (Fig. 5). It has been shown that the secondary decrease is due to the relaxation of the Ca exchange current (Yau and Nakatani, 1985; Nakatani and Yau, 1988) which exchanges 1 Ca + 1 K going out with 4 Na coming into the cell (Cervetto et al., 1989). The exchange current is therefore proportional to the Ca extruded from the ROS. It has also been shown (Nakatani and Yau, 1988) and confirmed by us that this exchange current is essentially independent of flash intensity and that it decays exponentially with time. A single exponential is generally adequate, although a better fit is sometimes achieved with two exponentials (Gray-Keller and Detwiler, 1994).

As a rule the exchange current j depends on time t as well as the length x of ROS from which it is recorded. The exponential decay parameter τ also depends on length: τ increases as the length of ROS inside the suction electrode decreases. Therefore

$$j(x, t) = j(x, 0) \exp \{-t/\tau(x)\} \quad (1)$$

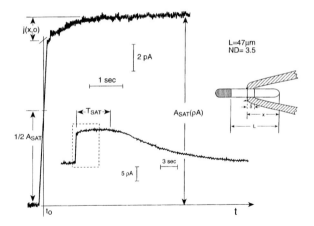

Fig. 5. The inset on the right shows a rod of ROS length L μm with x μm drawn into the recording electrode. The mouth of the electrode of thickness is a dead space from which no current is collected. The smaller tracing shows the saturated response of a rod. T_{SAT} is the saturation time. The dashed rectangle is enlarged and shown as the larger tracing. A_{SAT} is the saturated response amplitude, $j(0,0)$ is the Ca exchange current extrapolated back to t_0, the time at half maximum amplitude (Leibovic and Bandarchi, 1997b).

After a saturating flash, the charge transfer over the length x is

$$q(x) = \int_0^\infty j(x,t)dt \qquad (2)$$
$$= j(x,0)\tau(x)$$

Let $i(x,t)$ be the current density along the ROS. Then

$$j(x,0) = \int_\delta^x i(z,0)dz$$

where δ is the dead space at the tip of the electrode (see Fig. 5).

We consider three cases:

(a) $i = i_0 =$ constant.

Then $j(x,0) = i_0 x - i_0 \delta \qquad (3a)$

(b) $i = i_0 \pm i_1 x$.

Then $j(x,0) = \pm \left(\frac{1}{2}\right) i_1 x^2$
$$+ i_0 x \pm \left(-\frac{1}{2}\right) i_1 \delta^2 - i_0 \delta \quad (3b)$$

(c) $i = i_0 \exp(i_1 x)$.

Then $j(x,0) = (i_0/i_1) \times \{\exp(i_1 x) - \exp(i_1 \delta)\}$
$$(3c)$$

i_0 and i_1 are constants which can be positive or negative.

The original records were enlarged for ease of measurement as illustrated in Fig. 5 and the exchange current was read as a function of time. In all cases the current could be represented by Eq. (1). In order to deal with the variability between different cells, the values of j and τ were normalized by fitting a least squares regression line to the data for each cell and setting to 1 the fitted value for a standard length x of 50 μm.

Calcium extrusion along the ROS

The t-test applied to the mean values of $j(50,0)$ and $\tau(50)$ to Bufo and Xenopus before normalization showed no significant differences between the two species. The means for the combined data sets before normalization were

$$j(50,0) = 1.7 \text{ pA} \quad \text{and} \quad \tau(50) = 0.55 \text{ s}.$$

The normalized values of $j(x,0)$ and $\tau(x)$ are plotted in Fig. 6. It is apparent that the values for Bufo and Xenopus fall within the same ranges. The values of $q(x)$ from Eq. (2) are plotted in Fig. 7. Least squares fitting of the data to linear, quadratic and exponential functions was performed to distinguish between the alternatives in Eq. (3) for j and to find the best fit for τ. The quadratic fit did not conform to Eq. (3b). The exponential fit was statistically better than the linear fit (multiple correlation $R^2 = 0.95$ vs. 0.78), but gave an unrealistic value for δ. The best linear fit was

$$j(x,0) = 0.038x - 0.871 \qquad (4)$$

Accordingly, based on our analysis, the normalized exchange current density is constant. Then using Eq. (3a), $i_0 = 0.038$ pA/μm and $\delta = 23$ μm approximately.

The best fit for τ was

$$\tau(x) = 0.73 + 2.98 \ \exp(-0.049x); \ (R^2 = 0.99)$$
$$(5)$$

From Eqs. (2), (4) and (5) we can calculate the charge transfer after a saturating flash near the base, near the tip and for a fixed length of ROS. After correcting for the normalizations we get:

$$q(50) = 0.92\,\text{pC}$$
$$q(50) - q(49) = 0.023\,\text{pC} \qquad (6)$$
$$q(\delta + 1) - q(\delta) = 0.064\,\text{pC}$$

These figures correspond to an extrusion of 3.87×10^5 Ca ions near the tip (23–24 μm from the tip of the ROS), 1.37×10^5 near the base (49–50 μm

from the tip of the ROS) an 5.93×10^6 over the length of a 50 μm OS. By contrast, a ROS with a free internal Ca concentration of, say, 400 nM (Korenbrot and Miller, 1989; Lagnado, et. al., 1992, McCarthy et al., 1994), a length of 50 μm, a diameter of 5.5 μm and half the ROS space occupied by discs, contains 1.43×10^5 Ca ions. Since there is no influx of Ca while the response remains saturated, these figures imply that most of the extruded Ca comes from internally buffered stores and once more points to the important role of Ca in transduction.

Calcium exchange and concentration

To explore the effects of external Ca concentration on Ca exchange, the IS was sucked into the recording electrode and the OS was perfused with a Ringer solution in which Ca was reduced to 0.1 of its normal value (0.1 CaR). The dark current was larger and the saturation time shorter in 0.1 Ca. Table 3 gives the mean values of the Ca exchange current $j(x,0)$ and peak dark current A for four different recordings from four cells.

It can be seen that although A is larger, j is smaller in 0.1 CaR. In the steady state the Ca influx is equal to the efflux. Therefore, since the dark current carries primarily Na and Ca, it follows that the ratio of Ca:Na entering the ROS is also reduced. Moreover

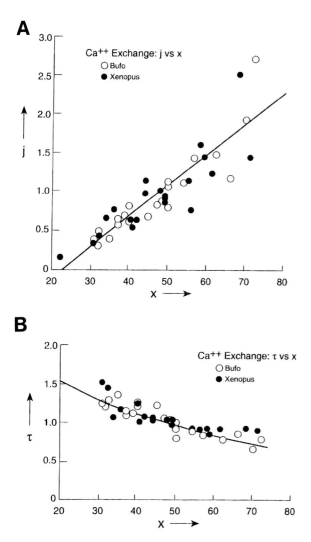

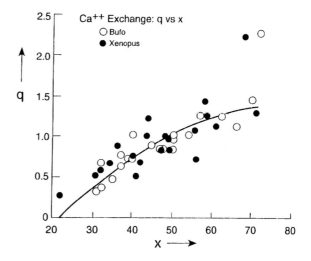

Fig. 6. **A.** The normalized exchange current $j(0,0)$ is plotted vs. ROS length x. The least squares regression line is $j = 0.038x - 0.871$; ($R^2 = 0.78$). (Leibovic and Bandarchi, 1997b). **B.** Plot of normalized time constant τ vs. x with least squares exponential fit; $\tau = 0.73 + 2.98\exp(-0.049x)$; ($R^2 = 0.99$) (Leibovic and Bandarchi, 1997b).

Fig. 7. Plot of charge transfer $q = j\tau$ vs. x. The current through the experimental points is the product of the fitted equations for j and τ. (Leibovic and Bandarchi, 1997b).

Table 3. Comparison of steady state Ca exchange in RR and 0.1 CaR (mean ± s.d.) (Leibovic and Bandarchi, 1997b)

	x	j(RR)	A(RR)	j/A(RR)	j(0.1 CaR)	A(0.1 CaR)	j/A(0.1 CaR)
mean ± s.d.	3.8 ± 5.5	1.49 ± 0.28	25.9 ± 5.1	0.058 ± 0.008	0.89 ± 0.14	42 ± 7.4	0.021 ± 0.002

the Ca exchange current has been shown to obey the equation

$$\frac{j}{j_{sat}} = \frac{[Ca]_i}{([Ca]_i + K)} \qquad (7)$$

over a wide range of conditions (Lagnado et al., 1992; Nakatani and Yau, 1988). j_{sat} is the maximum exchange current reached at a saturating concentration of internal free Ca and K is a Michaelis constant which is several times larger than the internal free Ca. Consequently, as a rough estimate from Eq. (7) and Table 3 , the reduction of j in 0.1 CaR implies the reduction of the internal free Ca to approximately 0.5–0.6 of its value in regular Ringer (RR).

Calcium exchange and saturation time

We next looked at the relationship between T and τ along the ROS for a given flash intensity. It has been shown before in experiments using Ca loading and substitution of Li for Na (Hodgkin et al., 1987) that the light sensitive current recovers as soon as internal Ca has dropped sufficiently. Although that situation is somewhat different from the one considered here, it points to a possible connection between internal Ca and response saturation.

Fig. 8 is a plot of the raw values of T_{sat} vs. τ for different lengths x of ROS in the same cells as in Figs. 6–8 for Bufo marinus. The linear regression line is

$$T = 7.06\tau + 1.19; \quad (R^2 = 0.89) \qquad (8)$$

Thus the kinetics of Ca exchange are correlated with those of response recovery at the given flash intensity. However, T outlasts Ca extrusion (see Fig. 5). The end of T signals the availability of new cGMP, which depends on the activity of G-cyclase as well as the preceding steps in the transduction cycle. The correlation of T with τ suggests that the kinetics of these steps are coordinated with those of Ca exchange. This is not surprising, since Ca also exerts its control on rhodopsin phosphorylation and the resulting inactivation of phosphodiesterase.

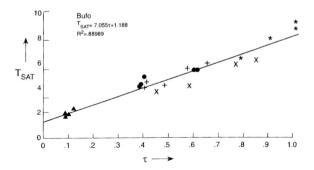

Fig. 8. Plot of T_{sat} vs. τ from the Bufo records at N.D.3. The least squares regression line is $T_{sat} = 7.005 + 1.188$. ($R = 0.89$). The different symbols correspond to different cells. (Leibovic and Bandarchi, 1997b).

Calcium and response gradient

In summary, we have shown that after a saturating flash more Ca is extruded at the tip than at the base; that τ, like T, is longer at the tip than the base and that it is correlated with T; and that lowering external Ca, which also lowers internal Ca, speeds up the responses and increases their amplitude. We now have to ask whether our results can explain the response gradient from base to tip.

It has been known for some time that higher external [Ca] slows the response and decreases its amplitude (Yoshikami and Hagins, 1973). Since there is a correlation between internal and external Ca according to Eq. (7) and the results from Table 3, it may be tempting to assume that internal [Ca] is higher at the tip than the base. But this is not borne out by our results according to Eq. 4. There is, however an alternative explanation which has to do with Ca buffering.

We have already alluded to the importance of Ca buffering in transduction. If the amount of buffer increases from base to tip, then the total internal Ca will rise, while the free Ca can stay essentially constant. This will prolong the extrusion of Ca after a saturating flash and explains why T and τ are longer at the tip and it is also consistent with the greater charge transfer at the tip (see Eq. (6)). Effectively, the internal Ca is higher during the light response and this can account for the smaller response amplitude and slower kinetics.

In principle an internal Na concentration increasing towards the tip could also give rise to a response gradient (Schnapf, 1983). But there is no direct evidence for such a Na gradient.

Ca and OS shedding

As the newly formed ROS membrane migrates from base to tip, the process of renewal at the RIS–ROS junction is balanced by shedding at the tip. Small packets of plasma membrane containing a few disks are pinched off at the tip and phagocytosed in the PE. The shedding is stimulated by light (LaVail, 1976). Now it is well known that Ca is also involved in membrane fusion, which is part of the process in pinching off the tip from the ROS. It is therefore reasonable to hypothesize that there is a link between ROS shedding and the high concentration of Ca near the tip.

Conclusion

It has long been thought that the response gradient along the ROS has something to do with aging as the membrane is regenerated near the base and moves towards the tip of the ROS. But there was no experimental evidence for this. Moreover, it would have been difficult to explain if the light response was generated by the ROS acting as a unit, rather than through local processes inside it.

Our work in relation to cGMP has confirmed that responses are generated locally. By manipulating the age gradient through the control of the rate of ROS regeneration, we have demonstrated that age and response gradients are, indeed, correlated. Finally we have shown that there is a gradient of bound Ca inside the ROS and that this can explain the observed response gradient through the actions of Ca on transduction. In addition, the higher Ca levels near the tip may play a role in disk shedding.

Obviously there are a number of things which can go wrong with the normal processes underlying the response gradient and it will be interesting to find their correlations with photoreceptor disease. As in so many areas of retinal research, John was the first to correlate a disease, viz. retinal dystrophy, with physiological, biochemical and morphological measures (Dowling and Sidman, 1962). It remains to be seen how the response gradient along the ROS may be affected by disease.

In conclusion, I am grateful to have been able to do this work, which was carried out with the help of my students K.-Y. Pan, J. Bandarchi and M. Panaro. It all began with the start I got in John's laboratory.

References:

Baylor, D.A., Lamb, T.D. and Yau, K-W. (1979) The membrane current of single rod outer segments. *J. Physiol.*, 288: 589–611.

Baylor, D.A. and Lamb, T.D. (1982) Local effects of bleaching in retinal rods of the toad. *J. Physiol.*, 328: 49–71.

Boesze-Battaglia, K., Fiesler, S.J. and Albert, A.D. (1990) Relationship of cholesterol content to age of disc membranes of retinal rod outer segments. *J. Biol. Chem.*, 265: 18867–18870.

Cameron, D.A. and Pugh, E.N. Jr. (1990) The magnitude, time course and spatial distribution of current induced in salamander rods by cyclic guanisine nucleotides. *J. Physiol.*, 430: 419–439.

Cervetto, L., Lagnado, L., Perry, R.J., Robinson, D.W. and McNaughton, P.A. (1989) Extrusion of calcium from rod outer segments is driven by sodium and potassium gradients. *Nature*, 337: 740–743.

Cohen, A.I. and Blazinski, C. (1988) Light induced losses and dark recovery rates of cGMP of rod outer segments of intact amphybian photoreceptors. *J. Gen. Physiol.*, 92: 731–746.

Cote, R.H., Nicol, G.D., Burke, S.A. and Bownds, M.D. (1989) cGMP levels and membrane current during onset recovery and light adaptation of the photoresponse of detached frog photoreceptors. *J. Biol. Chem.*, 264: 15384–15391.

Dowling, J.E. and Sidman, R.L. (1962) Inherited retinal dystrophy in the rat. *J. Cell Biol.*, 14: 73–109.

Fleishman, D. and Danisevich, M., (1979) Guanylate cyclase of isolated bovine retinal rod axonemes. *Biochemistry*, 18: 5060–5066.

Gray-Keller, M.P. and Detwiler, P.B. (1994) The calcium feedback signal in thew phototransduction cascade of vertebrate rods. *Neuron*, 13: 849–861.

Hodgkin, A.L., McNaughton, P.A. and Nunn, B.J. (1987) Measurement of sodium-calcium exchange in salamander rods. *J. Physiol.*, 391: 347–370.

Hollyfield, J.G. (1979) Membrane addition to photoreceptor outer segments. *Invest. Ophthalm. & Visual Sci.*, 18: 977–981.

Hollyfield, J.G., Besharse, J.C. and Rayborn, M.E. (1977) Turnover of rod photoreceptor outer segments I: membrane addition and loss in relation to temperature. *J. Cell Biol.*, 75: 490–506.

368

Kilbride, P. and Ebrey, T.G. (1979) Light initiated changes of cGMP levels in the frog retina measures with quick freezing techniques. *J. Gen. Physiol.*, 74: 415–426.

Korenbrot, J.I. and Miller, D.L. (1989) Cytoplasmic free calcium concentration indark adapted retinal rod outer segments. *Vis. Res.*, 29: 939–948.

Lagnado, L., Cervetto, L. and McNaughton, P.A. (1992) Calcium homeostasis in the outer segments of retinal rods from the tiger salamander. *J. Physiol.*, 455: 111–142.

Lamb, T.D., McNaughton, P.A. and Yau K-W. (1981) Spatial spread of activation and background desensitization in toad rod outer segments. *J. Physiol.*, 319: 463–496.

La Vail, M.M. (1976) Rod outer segment disc shedding in rat retina: relation to cyclic lighting. *Science*, 194: 1071–1074.

Leibovic, K.N. (1986) A new method of nonenzymatic dissociation of the Bufo retina. *J. Neurosci. Methods.*, 15: 301–306.

Leibovic, K.N. (1990) Vertebrate Photoreceptors. In: Leibovic, K.N. (Ed.), *Science of Vision*, pp. 16–52. Springer Verlag, N.Y.

Leibovic, K.N. and Moreno-Diaz, R. Jr. (1992) Rod outer segments are designed for optimum photon detection. *Biol. Cybern.*, 66: 301–306.

Leibovic, K.N. and Bandarchi, J. (1997a) Effects of light and temperature on the response gradient of retinal rod outer segments. *Brain Res.*, 750: 321–324.

Leibovic, K.N. and Bandarchi, J. (1997b) Phototransduction and calcium exchange along the retinal rod outer segment. *NeuroReport* 8: 1295–1300.

Leibovic, K.N., Dowling, J.E. and Kim, Y.Y. (1987) Background and bleaching equivalence in steady state bleaching of vertebrate rods. *J. Neurosci.*, 7: 1056–1063.

Leibovic, K.N. and Pan, K-Y. (1994) The saturated response of vertebrate rods and its relation to cGMP metabolism. *Brain Res.*, 653: 325–329.

McCarthy, S.T., Younger, J.P. and Owen, W.G. (1994) Free calcium concentration in bullfrog rods determined in the presence of multiple forms of Fura-2. *Biophys. J.*, 67: 2076–2089.

Nakatani, K. and Yau, K-W. (1988) Calcium and magnesium fluxes across the toad rod outer segment. *J. Physiol.*, 395: 695–729.

Pepperberg, D.R., Cornwall, M.C., Kahlert, M., Hoffman, K.P., Jin, J., Jones, J.G. and Ripps, H. (1992) Light dependent delay in the falling phase of the retinal rod photoresponse. *Vis. Neurosci.*, 8: 9–18.

Schnapf, J.L. (1983) Dependence of the single photon response on longitudinal position of absorption in toad photo-receptors. *J. Physiol.*, 343: 147–159.

Shichi, H. and Williams, T.C. (1979) Rhodopsin phosphorylation suggests biochemical heterogeneities of retinal rod discs. *J. Supramolecular Struct.*, 12: 419–424.

Woodruff, M.L. and Fain, G.L. (1982) Ca dependent changes in cGMP levels are not correlated with the opening and closing of the light dependent permeability of toad photo-receptors. *J. Gen. Physiol.*, 80: 537–555.

Yamazaki, A., Sen, I., Bitenski, M.W., Casnelli, J.E. and Greengard, P. (1988) Cyclic GMP specific, high affinity noncatalytic binding sites on light activated phosphodiesterase. *J. Biol. Chem.*, 255: 11619–11624.

Yau, K-W. and Nakatani, K. (1985) Light induced reduction of cytoplasmic free calcium in retinal rod outer segments. *Nature*, 313: 579–582.

Yoshikami, S. and Hagins, W.A. (1973) Control of the dark current in vertebrate rods and cones. In: Langer, H. (Ed.), *Biochemistry and Physiology of Visual Pigments*, pp. 245–255. Springer Verlag, N.Y.

Young, R.W. (1967) The renewal of photoreceptor cell outer segments. *J. Cell. Biol.*, 33: 61–72.

H. Kolb, H. Ripps and S. Wu (Eds.)
Progress in Brain Research, Vol. 131

CHAPTER 26

The flash response of rods in vivo

David R. Pepperberg*

Lions of Illinois Eye Research Institute, Department of Ophthalmology and Visual Sciences, University of Illinois at Chicago, College of Medicine, 1855 West Taylor Street, Chicago, IL 60612, USA

Introduction

Electrophysiological studies of rod photoreceptors in vitro have, over the past three decades, provided a wealth of information on the phototransduction process in these remarkable cells of the retina. These studies, in concert with the large and still rapidly growing body of information on the biochemistry of phototransduction, have led to a good overall understanding of the mechanisms underlying the sensitivity, kinetics and adaptation properties of the electrical response of rods to light, though many important issues as yet remain unsolved. My own introduction to this exciting area was as a postdoc in the Dowling laboratory in the 1970s, a period of intensive focus within the lab on rod phototransduction and adaptation mechanisms (Dowling and Ripps, 1972; Fain and Dowling, 1973; Green et al., 1975; Kleinschmidt and Dowling, 1975; Fain, 1976; Pepperberg et al., 1976, 1978; Lipton et al., 1977a,b; Gold, 1979). As it has in so many areas of visual neuroscience, John's work over the years has had enormous impact on the field of photoreceptor electrophysiology, and it continues to inspire and guide new studies in this important area.

Knowledge gained from in vitro electrophysiological studies of rods naturally stimulates interest in better understanding the properties of rod phototransduction in the living eye. Such "in vivo" information clearly is of importance for determining,

for example, the sensitivity and time course of the flash response in the native microenvironment of the rods; the dependence of rod light and dark adaptation on the rods' association with the retinal pigment epithelium; and the properties of visual signal transmission from rods to bipolar and horizontal cells of the retina.

A window into the operation of visual processes in the intact eye is provided by the electroretinogram (ERG), a multicomponent electrical signal that can be recorded at the cornea upon flash stimulation (Granit, 1933). For more than a century the technique of electroretinography has been used in both clinical and fundamental studies to investigate response properties of retinal neurons. Work within the past several decades (Penn and Hagins, 1969; Sillman et al., 1969; Dowling and Ripps, 1970, 1972; Heynen and van Norren, 1985; Hood and Birch, 1990; Robson and Frishman, 1996) has established, in particular, that the leading edge of the rod-mediated ERG a-wave is an approximate monitor of the massed response of the rods themselves. Recent studies have further shown that analysis of the ERG a-wave in relation to quantitative models of rod transduction can yield information on specific properties of the activating reactions in the transduction cascade (Hood and Birch, 1990, 1993; Lamb and Pugh, 1992; Breton et al., 1994; Cideciyan and Jacobson, 1996; Robson and Frishman, 1996).

Electrical signaling in the retina is, of course, more than a matter of response generation by the photoreceptors (!), and contributions to the ERG from post-receptor processes severely limit the window on

---
* Tel.: 312-996-4262; Fax: 312-996-7773;
E-mail: davipepp@uic.edu

photoreceptor activity provided by the conventional ERG. The constraint, recognized for many years, is that post-receptor components such as the b-wave and oscillatory potentials begin to dominate the ERG and thus mask the a-wave response early in development of the overall ERG waveform. In mammals, for example, masking of the a-wave by b-wave intrusion begins at post-flash times of about 25 ms or earlier, depending on flash strength. As in vitro photoreceptor data indicate the rod flash response to last several hundred milliseconds or more (Baylor et al., 1984; Nakatani et al., 1991; Kraft et al., 1993), rod activity monitored by the a-wave represents merely a tiny initial portion of the response. A number of questions regarding phototransduction in the intact eye could in principle be addressed if there were a means to determine the full course of the rod response. Approaches involving treatment of the retina with agents that abolish or suppress post-receptor responses have provided substantial information (e.g. Sieving et al., 1994; Robson and Frishman, 1995) but are obviously invasive in nature.

The aim of this chapter is to describe a recently developed electroretinographic technique, here termed the "paired-flash" ERG method, that makes possible the approximate determination of the full time course of the rod flash response in vivo. I first describe the method and then review specific findings obtained in paired-flash studies on mice and on human subjects. The main points emphasized are determinations of the amplitude–intensity function, the kinetics of the response to a flash of fixed strength, and the adapting effect of steady background light. The experiments to be highlighted have been conducted in close collaboration with Dr. David G. Birch (Retina Foundation of the Southwest), Dr. Donald C. Hood (Columbia University) and Dr. John R. Hetling (University of Illinois at Chicago), and I am grateful to these colleagues for their major contributions to this work.

Description of the method

The paired-flash ERG method is based on a rod response property described in numerous in vitro studies, that of *photocurrent saturation*. Saturation of the response, i.e. a decrease in rod circulating current to essentially zero value, develops as a result of the transiently high level of activated cGMP phosphodiesterase (PDE*) produced by a bright flash. This burst of PDE* activity causes the intracellular level of free cGMP to drop to near-zero, and the near-zero concentration of free cGMP leads in turn to closure of essentially all of the cGMP-gated channels in the plasma membrane of the rod outer segment.

The *rapid development* of the ERG a-wave response to a bright test flash (see above), and the nature of saturation as a *fixed reference condition* (complete channel closure) presumably independent of simultaneously occurring, post-receptor ERG potentials, underlie the concept of the paired-flash technique. As shown schematically in Fig. 1, the method involves presentation of a test flash of fixed intensity, and of a probe flash of fixed high intensity, in each of a series of trials. The interflash interval, termed t_{probe} below (see legends of Figs. 2 and 6), is varied among trials, and the family of rod-mediated a-wave responses to the probe flash is analyzed for amplitude. The idea is that the bright probe flash, delivered at a defined time after the test flash, rapidly drives the rods to their saturating limit and thus titrates the prevailing level of rod circulating current. The a-wave of the probe response is analyzed for amplitude at a near-peak time, and the measured amplitude is referenced to that obtained with presentation of the probe flash delivered alone ("probe-alone" response), i.e. in the absence of recent presentation of the test stimulus. These measurements of probe response amplitude yield determinations of $A(t)$, the derived response to the test flash, through the relation

$$A(t) = A_{mo} - A_m(t) \qquad (1)$$

where A_{mo} is the amplitude of the probe-alone response, and $A_m(t)$ is the probe response amplitude determined in a paired-flash trial. By fixing the interflash interval and varying the test flash strength, one can similarly obtain the amplitude–intensity function at a fixed chosen time after presentation of the test flash. The essence of the procedure in both cases is the recording of the ERG a-wave response to the *probe* flash, and analysis of the probe response to derive the rod response to the *test* flash.

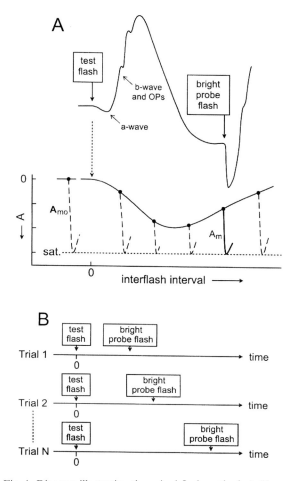

Fig. 1. Diagram illustrating the paired-flash method. **A.** Hypothetical ERG response to a test flash and a subsequently presented, bright probe flash. The lower part of the panel shows hypothetical responses to a group of probe flashes presented at differing times. Peaks of these responses are aligned to reflect the presumed fixed state of the rods that corresponds with photocurrent saturation. The diagram ignores the contribution of cones to the probe response. **B.** Protocol for paired-flash trials to determine time course of the derived response to a fixed test flash. Adapted from Pepperberg et al., (2000) with permission of Academic Press.

The photostimulator used for paired-flash ERG experiments employs full-field (i.e. ganzfeld) flashes generated by two flash lamps. The short duration of the stimuli produced by these flash lamps ($\sim$2 ms or less) satisfies the requirement, in these experiments, for delivery of the test or probe flash within an interval that is small by comparison with that of a-wave development. In mouse the a-wave peak time obtained with our standard probe flash,

$\sim$300–400 scotopic candela second per m^2 (sc cd s m^{-2}), is typically $\approx$7–8 ms. In human subjects, where the probe flash strength typically is about 1.6×10^4 scotopic troland seconds (sc td s), the time-to-peak of the probe response is about 8–9 ms. Additional aspects of the methodology will be noted below; full details of procedures for recording and data analysis have been described in detail (Pepperberg et al., 1997, 2000; Hetling and Pepperberg, 1999).

Derived responses

Amplitude–intensity relation

Varying the test flash strength and keeping the interval between the test and probe flashes constant allows determination of the amplitude–intensity function at a given post-test-flash time. This is illustrated by Fig. 2, which presents amplitude–intensity results for the mouse derived response at a post-test flash time $t = 86$ ms, a time near the observed time-to-peak for the weak-flash response (see below). Panel A shows probe responses obtained a representative experiment and illustrates the rapid development of the probe-flash-generated a-wave. These responses were obtained with an interflash interval (t_{probe}) of 80 ms and were analyzed for amplitude at a fixed time, 6 ms, after probe flash presentation (see figure legend). Light traces illustrate probe responses obtained in paired-flash trials; the heavy trace marked PA is the probe-alone response; and the vertical arrow identifies the 6-ms time of amplitude determination of each response. With increasing test flash intensity, the peak amplitude of the probe response becomes smaller, reflecting an increasing amplitude of the response to the test flash (cf. Eq. 1). Furthermore, at all but the highest test flash strengths, the probe responses exhibit an approximate kinetic similarity, i.e. rising phases of the amplitude-scaled probe responses are similar. This latter point is illustrated by Fig. 2B, which shows selected panel A responses that have been rescaled to provide a match of amplitudes at 6 ms after probe flash presentation (labels accompanying these rescaled waveforms indicate test flash strengths in sc cd s m^{-2}). With Eq. (1), the amplitudes $A_{\text{m}}(86)$ and A_{mo} determined in a given experiment yield

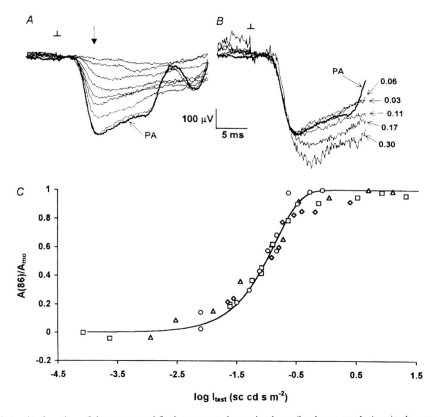

Fig. 2. Amplitude–intensity function of the mouse rod flash response determined at a fixed near-peak time in the response (86 ms). Here and in Figs. 3–5, the quoted post-test-flash time t represents the sum of the interflash interval t_{probe} (interval between the test and probe flash) and the "determination time" t_{det} of the probe flash response; t_{det}, which was 6 ms unless otherwise stated, represents the period between probe flash presentation and the time of determination of the probe response amplitude. **A.** Light traces are probe responses obtained paired-flash trials; test flash strengths were (top to bottom) 11.0, 0.98, 0.30, 0.17, 0.11, 0.06, 0.03 and 0.0003 sc cd s m^{-2}. **B.** Rescaled probe responses, illustrating kinetics of the leading edge of the a-wave. Accompanying labels indicate the test flash strength in sc cd s m^{-2}. **C.** Amplitude of the derived response, plotted as a function of log test flash strength (I_{test}). Data collected in four experiments. Results from a given experiment are shown by identical symbols. The curve plots Eq. (2) with $k = 7.0$ (sc cd s m^{-2})$^{-1}$. Data from a given experiment have been shifted horizontally by a fixed small amount (< 0.15 log sc cd s m^{-2}) to bring the Eq. (2) fitted curve for each data set into alignment. Adapted from Hetling and Pepperberg (1999) with permission of The Physiological Society.

$A(86)/A_{mo}$, the normalized derived response at 86 ms after the test flash. Fig. 2C shows the results collected in four experiments of the type just described. Here the normalized derived response $A(86)/A_{mo}$ is plotted against the logarithm of the test flash strength, with data from a given experiment shifted horizontally by a fixed small amount (<0.15 log sc cd s m^{-2}; see figure legend). The data are well described by the exponential function (curve in Fig. 2)

$$A(86)/A_{mo} = 1 - \exp(-k\,I_{test}) \qquad (2)$$

where k, a sensitivity parameter, has the value 7.0 (sc cd s m^{-2})$^{-1}$. The exponential behavior of

the amplitude–intensity relation at this near-peak time is in agreement with previous studies of both mammalian and amphibian rods in vitro, for which the amplitude–intensity relation for the photocurrent response shows a similar dependence on test flash strength (Lamb et al., 1981; Baylor et al., 1984; Nakatani et al., 1991; Kraft et al., 1993; Xu et al., 1997).

Response kinetics

Keeping the test flash strength constant and varying the interval between the test and probe flashes allows determination of the full time course of the response. Shown in Fig. 3 is the course of the rod response to a weak test flash, obtained in a group of experiments on mice. The derived response exhibits a peak near 90 ms and a falling phase that extends over several hundred milliseconds, properties generally similar to those of photocurrent recordings from mouse rods in vitro (Sung et al., 1994; Xu et al., 1997).

With increasing test flash strength, the derived response reaches saturation and exhibits a progressively longer period of near-saturation before beginning the recovery to baseline. Using the paired-flash technique, one can investigate the falling phase of the response to a relatively bright flash, as shown in Fig. 4. This figure shows probe responses obtained in an experiment that employed a saturating test flash of 4.37 sc cd s m^{-2}. Panel A of the figure shows probe responses obtained with interflash intervals in the range of 10–60 ms. Here the evident rapid decline of the probe response with increasing interflash interval describes the rapid climb of the derived response toward saturation. Panel B shows probe responses obtained with interflash intervals spanning the range of 40–1200 ms, and describes the return of the probe response toward its nominal, probe-alone (PA) form. As shown in Fig. 4B, a small extent of

recovery abruptly develops at ~70 ms after presentation of the test flash (note differences among probe responses obtained with t_{probe} values over the range of 40–400 ms). We interpret this rapidly developing, small change as due to recovery of the *cone* photoreceptor response to the test flash. This early recovery is followed by a slower process, attributable to recovery of the rod response to the test flash, that leads to near-complete return of the probe response on a time scale of about one second (Fig. 4B–C).

A topic of intense current interest in phototransduction is the nature of processes that govern the recovery kinetics of the flash response. Information on this issue comes from the experiment of Fig. 5, which examined the responsiveness of the rods during the slow recovery from a bright conditioning flash. Each trial in this experiment involved the presentation of three flashes: a fixed *conditioning* flash at time zero; a fixed *test* flash presented at defined time during the recovery (here, 10 s or 12 s); and a *probe* flash presented at varying times after the test stimulus. The experiment was designed to obtain the derived response to a test flash presented during the long recovery phase of the conditioning flash response.

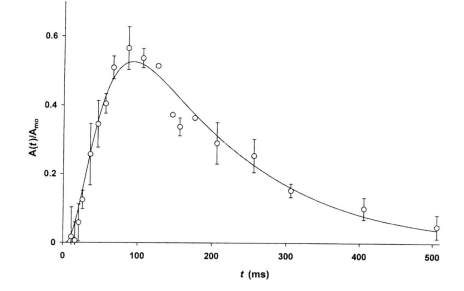

Fig. 3. Full time course of the derived response of mouse rods to a weak test flash. Results collected from five experiments. The derived normalized response A/A_{mo} is plotted as a function of time after a weak test flash ($I_{test} = 0.12 \pm 0.02$ sc cd s m^{-2}). Adapted from Hetling and Pepperberg (1999) with permission of The Physiological Society.

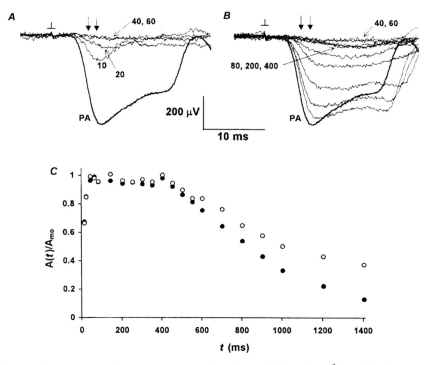

Fig. 4. Recovery of the probe flash response after a saturating test flash ($I_{test} = 4.37$ sc cd s m^{-2}). *A–B.* Probe responses. Labels indicate time t_{probe}, in ms. Values of t_{probe} for the five unlabeled responses in *B* were (top to bottom): 500, 600, 800, 1000 and 1200 ms. Note the small extent of recovery that occurs at post-flash times near ~70 ms, interpreted as recovery of the cone photoreceptors. The slower, more extensive phase of growth of the probe response is interpreted as rod recovery. *C.* Normalized amplitudes plotted as a function of post-test-flash time. Open and filled circles indicate results obtained with determination times t_{det} of 6 and 7.5 ms, respectively (vertical arrows in panels *A* and *B*). Adapted from Hetling and Pepperberg (1999) with permission of The Physiological Society.

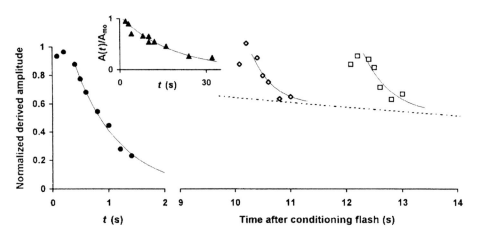

Fig. 5. Derived response of mouse rods to a fixed test flash (2.57 sc cd s m^{-2}) presented during the slow recovery after a bright conditioning flash. Open diamonds and open squares: results obtained with test flash presentation at 10 s and 12 s, respectively, after conditioning flash presentation. Filled circles at the left indicate the derived response to the test flash in the absence of recent presentation of the conditioning flash. *Inset*: Filled triangles show recovery from the conditioning flash presented alone. The dotted curve in the main part of the figure is a segment of the smooth curve fitted to the data of the inset. Adapted from Hetling and Pepperberg (1999) with permission of The Physiological Society.

We first consider the data of the Fig. 5 inset (filled triangles), which show the slow recovery from the conditioning flash itself, i.e. a recovery proceeding over a period of about 30 s. The data in the left part of the figure (filled circles) serve as a further reference; they describe the derived response to the fixed test flash (2.57 sc cd s m^{-2}) presented under dark-adapted conditions, i.e., in the absence of conditioning flash stimulation. As shown by the filled circles, this nominal derived response to the test flash exhibited a duration of ~1 s. The same 2.57 sc cd s m^{-2} flash was then used as the test stimulus presented at 10 s (open diamonds) or 12 s (open squares) during the slow recovery from the conditioning flash (right-hand part of Fig. 5). Together, these results address the basis of the process that rate-limits recovery of the rods from the conditioning flash. If this rate-limiting process were the resynthesis of cGMP and resulting opening of the cGMP-gated channels in the rod plasma membrane, excitation in the transduction cascade produced by the test flash should "set back" the progress of this cGMP replenishment, and the falling phase of the response to the test flash should show the same slow kinetics as that of the baseline recovery from the conditioning flash (dotted curve in the figure). This is clearly not the case. Rather, the response recovery after test flash presentation is comparable to that of the response obtained in the absence of the conditioning flash. This result indicates that recovery of the baseline is being governed by a slow decay of one or more excitatory inter-mediates of the cascade, rather than by the formation of cGMP.

In the mouse, the contribution of cones to the overall excursion of the response to the bright probe flash is small (see, e.g., Fig. 4) (Hetling and Pepperberg, 1999; Lyubarsky et al., 1999). However, in human subjects, the cone response can be substantial relative to the overall excursion of the rod-mediated response. This necessitates subtraction of the cone-mediated component of the raw probe response obtained in a paired-flash trial. The putative cone response to the probe flash is determined by measuring the response to a long-wavelength ("red") probe flash that is photopically matched to the short-wavelength ("blue") probe stimulus nominally used in the paired-flash trials. This cone contribu-tion is then computationally subtracted from the raw response to the short-wavelength probe flash to yield the putative "rod-only" response to the short-wavelength probe.

Figure 6 shows paired-flash ERG data obtained from a human subject, and illustrates the use of this cone-subtraction method to determine the rod response to a test flash of 11 sc td s. Waveforms at the upper left are raw probe responses to the fixed probe flash delivered at varying times after the test in a series of paired-flash trials. Also shown (response "C") is the response to the photopically matched probe flash delivered alone. Shown at the upper right (panel B) are the probe responses after subtraction of response C. These presumed rod-only probe responses were analyzed for amplitude at the peak time in the probe response. Panel C of the figure illustrates determination of the derived response to the test flash. Here the probe responses are positioned with their negative peaks aligned at a fixed ordinate value, representing the presumed fixed condition of photocurrent saturation (cf. Fig. 1). The resulting family of probe responses, positioned along the time axis according to the time of probe flash presentation, defines a family of pre-probe baselines (filled circles in Fig. 6C) that collectively represent the derived response to the 11 sc td s test flash. The response to this relatively weak test flash, as well as responses to test flashes nearer saturation (44 sc td s; filled circles in Fig. 7), exhibit a peak at post-test-flash times near 170 ms, and a falling phase that extends over several hundred milliseconds.

As in the mouse, and consistent with in vitro photocurrent data, paired-flash ERG analysis of human rod recovery after a bright flash shows evidence of a saturation period followed by a gradual fall to pre-flash baseline. The example shown in Fig. 8A–B describes the recovery of the probe a-wave after a flash of 2×10^3 sc td s. Note here the period of apparent rod saturation, about 1200 ms, during which the rod-mediated portion of the a-wave is essentially zero. Figure 8C summarizes results obtained over a range of saturating test flash strengths that correspond with rhodopsin bleaches of up to about 12%. As analyzed with an exponential recovery function to yield the apparent period of rod saturation (see Fig. 8B and legend), the Fig. 8C data show a progressive increase in apparent saturation period with increasing flash strength.

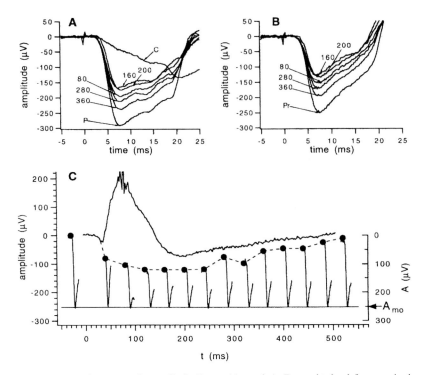

Fig. 6. Derived response of human rods to a weak test flash ($I_{test} = 11$ sc td s). Data obtained from a single subject. Here and in Figs. 7–9 (results describing the human rod derived response), quoted values of the post-test-flash time t represent the interflash interval t_{probe}. **A.** Raw probe flash responses obtained at differing times after the test flash (labels accompanying waveforms). Response C: obtained with photopically matched long-wavelength probe flash. **B.** Cone-corrected probe responses. **C.** Derived response. Cone-corrected probe responses are positioned according to the time of probe flash presentation, and vertically shifted so that the negative peaks are aligned (presumed saturation condition). Filled circles, which represent the pre-probe baseline, describe the derived rod-mediated response. Reproduced from Pepperberg et al., (1997) with permission of Cambridge University Press.

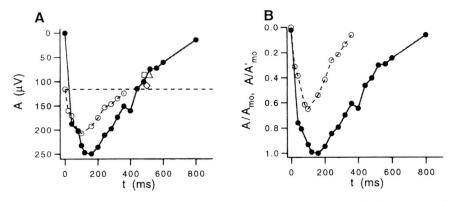

Fig. 7. Derived response of human rods to a 44 sc td s test flash, in darkness (filled circles) and in the presence of steady background light (32 sc td) (open circles). Data obtained from a single subject. **A.** The data indicate derived amplitudes, A, in μV. The dashed line represents the derived rod response maintained by the steady background. The nominal probe flash strength was 1.2×10^4 sc td s; the open diamond, open triangle and open square show, respectively, results obtained in darkness with probe flash strengths of 2.5×10^3, 5.0×10^3, and 2.4×10^4 sc td s. **B.** Filled circles replot the panel A dark-adapted response normalized to A_{mo}, the maximal amplitude of the dark-adapted flash response. Open circles replot the panel A light-adapted response normalized to A'_{mo}, the maximal amplitude of the response to a flash superimposed on the background. Adapted from Pepperberg et al., (1997) with permission of Cambridge University Press.

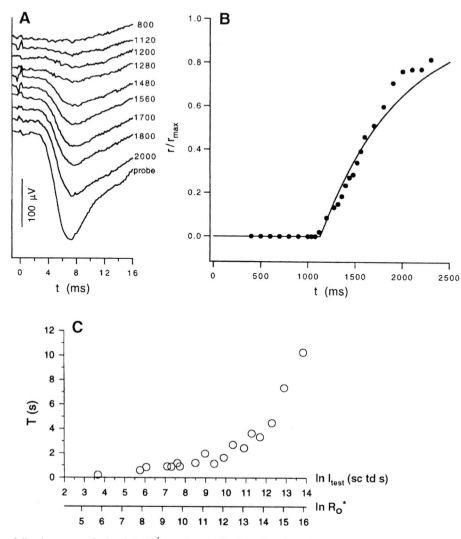

Fig. 8. Recovery following a test flash of 2×10^3 sc td s. **A.** Rod-mediated portion of the probe response, after computational subtraction of the cone-mediated component. **B.** Recovery time course. Solid curve plots the function $r/r_{max} = 1 - \exp[-(t - T)/\tau_r]$, with T, the apparent period of saturation, equal to 1.2 s; and with τ_r, a recovery time constant, equal to 0.82 s. **C.** Flash-dependence of the period T of apparent rod saturation. Data obtained from a single subject. Values of T were obtained by fitting an exponential decay function to the recovery data, as in panel B. Adapted from Pepperberg et al., (1996) with permission of The Optical Society of America.

Light adaptation

The rods of both mammals and lower vertebrates exhibit light adaptation, a regulatory process that is critical for maintaining responsiveness over a wide range of illumination conditions (Dowling and Ripps, 1970, 1972; Kleinschmidt and Dowling, 1975; Fain et al., 1989; Tamura et al., 1989; Nakatani et al., 1991; Matthews, 1991; Kraft et al.,

1993). Figs. 7 and 9 provide in vivo evidence for light adaptation in human rods. In Fig. 7A, the time course of the derived rod response to a 44 sc td s test flash was determined in the absence and presence of a steady background light (filled and open circles, respectively). In background light the same test flash yielded a derived response that recovered more quickly to the prevailing baseline, despite the fact that the total combined amount of light incident on the rods (background plus test flash) exceeded that incident under the dark-adapted condition. This accelerated recovery to baseline is apparent also when the responses are plotted as normalized to the prevailing excursion of the rod response (Fig. 7B; see figure legend).

Fig. 9 describes the effects of background light on properties of the amplitude–intensity relation. Panel A shows the amplitude–intensity function obtained from a single subject in darkness and in background light, using a 170-ms interflash interval. The signature of background desensitization is the shift in the normalized amplitude–intensity function, i.e., a displacement, to higher value, of the flash strength required to produce half-saturation of the prevailing function. Panel B shows the action of backgrounds of different intensity. With increasing background strength there occurs a progressively greater shift in the flash intensity needed to produce a criterion fractional saturation of the response (see figure legend). Note that much of the overall shift exhibited over the range of backgrounds investigated is already evident with the background that maintained a steady (baseline) response of only about 34% of the overall excursion.

Conclusions and future perspective

The in vivo response of rods to a test flash can to good approximation be determined through paired-flash ERG measurements, as now demonstrated in a number of studies (Birch et al., 1995; Lyubarsky and Pugh, 1996; Pepperberg et al., 1997, 2000; Cideciyan et al., 1998; Hetling and Pepperberg, 1999; Robson and Frishman, 1999). The technique naturally complements in vitro methods of studying photoreceptor responses, and should be useful in future studies of both fundamental transduction processes and mechanisms of photoreceptor disease.

An important question in need of further investigation by both in vivo and in vitro measures of rod activity is the nature of shut-off and recovery mechanisms in phototransduction. The present Fig. 5 has shown an example of how in vivo data can provide information constraining the possible mechanisms at work at a given flash strength. An obvious advantage of the in vivo approach to studies of this type is the capacity for full recovery of the rods after illumination. A flash stimulation condition of particular interest is that which produces on the order of one to several photoactivated rhodopsins (R*) per disk

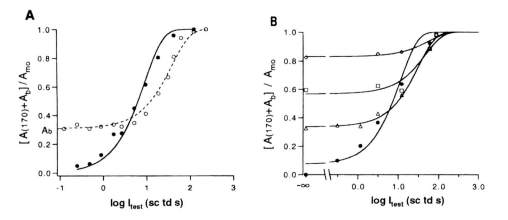

Fig. 9. Effect of background light on amplitude–intensity relation for the human rod flash response. **A.** Amplitude–intensity function for the rod response in darkness (filled symbols) and in background light (32 sc td; open symbols), with an interflash interval of 170 ms. Curves show the fit of saturating exponential functions to the data. The fitted functions are of the form, $A(170)/A_{mo}$ [or $A(170)/A'_{mo}$] $= 1 - \exp(-k\, I_{test})$, where $A(170)$ is the derived rod amplitude obtained with an interflash interval of 170 ms; where A_{mo} and A'_{mo} are, respectively, dark- and light-adapted maximal amplitudes of the derived flash response; and where k is a sensitivity parameter. Data obtained from a single subject. **B.** Effect of differing background intensities. Data were obtained from a single subject, with background intensities of 0, 50, 200 and 630 sc td (filled circles, open triangles, open squares, and open diamonds, respectively). Sensitivity values k for these functions are, respectively, 0.089, 0.032, 0.022 and 0.017 (sc td s)$^{-1}$. Adapted from Pepperberg et al., (1997) with permission of Cambridge University Press.

surface in the outer segment, i.e., one thousand to several thousand R*s per rod. Biochemical and biophysical data suggest that this flash strength is sufficient to produce near-complete transient activation of the transducin-PDE stages in the transduction cascade (Liebman and Pugh, 1982; Pepperberg et al., 1988) and to transiently overwhelm the action of the RGS-9, an outer segment protein that accelerates the hydrolysis of activated transducin's GTP ligand and thereby deactivates transducin (Chen et al., 2000). It will be of interest to determine how this overwhelming of RGS-9 activity contributes to the progressive slowing of rod recovery seen in vivo with increasing strength of very bright test flashes and to investigate further the dependence of this slowed recovery on the active lifetime of R* (cf. Birch et al., 1995; Pepperberg, et al., 1996)

A further topic of substantial interest, one tied closely to John Dowling's classic studies on rhodopsin and visual adaptation (Dowling, 1960, 1963), is to understand the in vivo behavior of rods during recovery from rhodopsin bleaching illumination. As emphasized in several talks at this meeting, a lot is known but much remains to be learned as to the dependence of rod dark adaptation on rhodopsin regeneration, and on the support of regeneration by retinoid processing in the retina and retinal pigment epithelium. Data from several studies [e.g. Pepperberg et al., 1996 (present Fig. 8C); Thomas and Lamb, 1999], provide a foundation for further examining rod recovery from bleaching illumination by paired-flash ERGs. One question in need of resolution is whether recovery processes of differing kinetic order govern the progress of rhodopsin regeneration and the associated process of dark adaptation at different bleach levels. For example, the reduction of all-*trans* retinal has been hypothesized to be rate-limiting for clearing of the chromophore site of illuminated rhodopsin (Hofmann et al., 1992; Saari et al., 1998) and, as hypothesized by Laitko and Hofmann (1998), the accelerating nature of the relation between bleach extent and rod saturation period (cf., e.g., present Fig. 8C) may signify onset of a zero-order reaction dependent on the removal of all-*trans* retinal from opsin. The availability of techniques to determine levels of visual cycle retinoids in mouse eye tissues (Saari et al., 1998; Qtaishat et al., 1999; Saari, 2000) suggests

the feasibility of investigating, in parallel biochemical and paired-flash ERG experiments, how flash response properties of the rods correlate with the progress of all-*trans* retinal removal from opsin, as well as the course of 11-*cis* retinal formation in the RPE and its delivery to the rods.

An exciting goal of paired-flash ERG work on human subjects is to develop this technique further as a diagnostic tool in studies of retinal diseases. Such clinical application of the method may, in particular, help to identify abnormalities in the recovery reactions of phototransduction. For example, in patients with retinitis pigmentosa and the pro-23-his mutation of rhodopsin, paired-flash ERG data reported by Birch et al. (1995) reveal an abnormally long course of rod recovery following a bright test flash. Similar ERG methods can be used to determine in vivo response properties of human cone photoreceptors. To date, several investigations have provided information on cone response kinetics in normal subjects and in patients (Hood et al., 1996; Cideciyan et al., 1998; Friedburg and Lamb, 2000).

Finally, it will be important to combine results from investigations of the photoreceptor response with emerging new insights coming from ERG analysis of post-receptor processing in the retina. Studies in experimental animals, employing pharmacological treatments that differentially inhibit specific components of the rod- and cone-mediated ERG response, have provided important information on post-receptor processes in the retina (e.g. Sieving et al., 1994; Robson and Frishman, 1995, 1999; Dong and Hare, 2000). A future goal of importance to both fundamental and clinical understanding of visual function will be further study of in vivo rod and cone responses in combination with these techniques for examining post-receptor events.

Acknowledgments

I acknowledge with many thanks the major contributions of my collaborators, Drs. David G. Birch, Donald C. Hood and John R. Hetling, to the studies highlighted in this review. I also thank Dr. Hetling, Dr. Dwight A. Burkhardt, Dr. Jennifer Kang Derwent and Mr. Gabriel A. Silva for helpful comments on the manuscript. Research in my

380

laboratory is supported by NIH grants EY-05494 and EY-01792, by The Foundation Fighting Blindness (Baltimore, MD), and by a departmental award from Research to Prevent Blindness (New York, NY).

References

Baylor, D.A., Nunn, B.J. and Schnapf, J.L. (1984) The photocurrent, noise and spectral sensitivity of rods of the monkey *Macaca fascicularis*. *J. Physiol.*, 357: 575–607.

Birch, D.G., Hood, D.C., Nusinowitz, S. and Pepperberg, D.R. (1995) Abnormal activation and inactivation mechanisms of rod transduction in patients with autosomal dominant retinitis pigmentosa and the pro-23-his mutation. *Invest. Ophthalmol. Vis. Sci.*, 36: 1603–1614.

Breton, M.E., Schueller, A.W., Lamb, T.D. and Pugh, E.N., Jr. (1994) Analysis of ERG *a*- wave amplification and kinetics in terms of the G-protein cascade of phototransduction. *Invest. Ophthalmol. Vis. Sci.*, 35: 295–309.

Chen, C.-K., Burns, M.E., He, W., Wensel, T.G., Baylor, D.A. and Simon, M.I. (2000) Slowed recovery of rod photo-response in mice lacking the GTPase accelerating protein RGS-9. *Nature*, 403: 557–560.

Cideciyan, A.V. and Jacobson, S.G. (1996) An alternative phototransduction model for human rod and cone ERG *a*-waves: Normal parameters and variation with age. *Vision Res.*, 36: 2609–2621.

Cideciyan, A.V., Zhao, X., Nielsen, L., Khani, S.C., Jacobson, S.G. and Palczewski, K. (1998) Null mutation in the rhodopsin kinase gene slows recovery kinetics of rod and cone phototransduction in man. *Proc. Natl. Acad. Sci. USA*, 95: 328–333.

Dong, C.-J. and Hare, W.A. (2000) Contribution to the kinetics and amplitude of the electroretinogram b-wave by third-order retinal neurons in the rabbit retina. *Vision Res.*, 40: 579–589.

Dowling, J.E. (1960) Chemistry of visual adaptation in the rat. *Nature*, 188: 114–118.

Dowling, J.E. (1963) Neural and photochemical mechanisms of visual adaptation in the rat. *J. Gen. Physiol.*, 46: 1287–1301.

Dowling, J.E. and Ripps, H. (1970) Visual adaptation in the retina of the skate. *J. Gen. Physiol.*, 56: 491–520.

Dowling, J.E. and Ripps, H. (1972) Adaptation in skate photoreceptors. *J. Gen. Physiol.*, 60: 698–719.

Fain, G.L. (1976) Sensitivity of toad rods: dependence on wavelength and background illumination. *J. Physiol.*, 261: 71–101.

Fain, G.L. and Dowling, J.E. (1973) Intracellular recordings from single rods and cones in the mudpuppy retina. *Science*, 180: 1178–1181.

Fain, G.L., Lamb, T.D., Matthews, H.R. and Murphy, R.L.W. (1989) Cytoplasmic calcium as the messenger for light adaptation in salamander rods. *J. Physiol.*, 416: 215–243.

Friedburg, C. and Lamb, T.D. (2000) Deriving the complete time course of the human cone photoreceptor response in vivo using the ERG and the paired-flash technique. *Invest. Ophthalmol. Vis. Sci.*, 41: S493 (abstr.).

Gold, G.H. (1979) Photoreceptor coupling in retina of the toad, *Bufo marinus*. II. Physiology. *J. Neurophysiol.*, 42: 311–328.

Granit, R. (1933) The components of the retinal action potential in mammals and their relation to the discharge in the optic nerve. *J. Physiol.*, 77: 207–239.

Green, D.G., Dowling, J.E., Siegel, I.M. and Ripps, H. (1975) Retinal mechanisms of visual adaptation in the skate. *J. Gen. Physiol.*, 65: 483–502.

Hetling, J.R. and Pepperberg, D.R. (1999) Sensitivity and kinetics of mouse rod flash responses determined *in vivo* from paired-flash electroretinograms. *J. Physiol.*, 516: 593–609.

Heynen, H. and van Norren, D. (1985) Origin of the electroretinogram in the intact macaque eye. I. Principal component analysis. *Vision Res.*, 25: 697–707.

Hofmann, K.P., Pulvermüller, A., Buczyłko, J., Van Hooser. P. and Palczewski, K. (1992) The role of arrestin and retinoids in the regeneration pathway of rhodopsin. *J. Biol. Chem.*, 267: 15701–15706.

Hood, D.C. and Birch, D.G. (1990) A quantitative measure of the electrical activity of human rod photoreceptors using electroretinography. *Vision Res.*, 33: 1605–1618.

Hood, D.C. and Birch, D.G. (1993) Light adaptation of human rod receptors: The leading edge of the human a-wave and models of rod receptor activity. *Vision Res.*, 33: 1605–1618.

Hood, D.C., Pepperberg, D.R. and Birch, D.G. (1996) The trailing edge of the photoresponse from human cones derived using a two-flash ERG paradigm. *Opt. Soc. Amer., 1996 Tech. Digest Series*, 1: 64–67.

Kleinschmidt, J. and Dowling, J.E. (1975) Intracellular record-ings from gecko photoreceptors during light and dark adaptation. *J. Gen. Physiol.*, 66: 617–648.

Kraft, T.W., Schneeweis, D.M. and Schnapf, J.L. (1993) Visual transduction in human rod photoreceptors. *J. Physiol.*, 464: 747–765.

Laitko, U. and Hofmann, K.P. (1998) A model for the recovery kinetics of rod phototransduction, based on the enzymatic deactivation of rhodopsin. *Biophys. J.*, 74: 803–815.

Lamb, T.D., McNaughton, P.A. and Yau, K.-W. (1981) Spatial spread of activation and background desensitization in toad rod outer segments. *J. Physiol.*, 319: 463–496.

Lamb, T.D. and Pugh, E.N., Jr. (1992) A quantitative account of the activating steps involved in phototransduction in amphibian photoreceptors. *J. Physiol.*, 449: 719–758.

Liebman, P.A. and Pugh, E.N., Jr. (1982) Gain, speed and sensitivity of GTP binding vs PDE activation in visual excitation. *Vision Res.*, 22: 1475–1480.

Lipton, S.A., Ostroy, S.E. and Dowling, J.E. (1977a) Electrical and adaptive properties of rod photoreceptors in *Bufo marinus*. I. Effects of altered extracellular Ca^{2+} levels. *J. Gen. Physiol.*, 70: 747–770.

Lipton, S.A., Rasmussen, H. and Dowling, J.E. (1977b) Electrical and adaptive properties of rod photoreceptors in *Bufo marinus*. II. Effects of cyclic nucleotides and prosta-glandins. *J. Gen. Physiol.*, 70: 771–791.

Lyubarsky, A.L. and Pugh, E.N., Jr. (1996) Recovery phase of the murine rod photoresponse reconstructed from electroretinographic recordings. *J. Neurosci.*, 16: 563–571.

Lyubarsky, A.L., Falsini, B., Pennesi, M.E., Valentini, P. and Pugh, E.N., Jr. (1999) UV-and midwave-sensitive cone-driven retinal responses of the mouse: a possible phenotype for coexpression of cone photopigments. *J. Neurosci.*, 19: 442–455.

Matthews, H.R. (1991) Incorporation of chelator into guinea-pig rods shows that calcium mediates mammalian photoreceptor light adaptation. *J. Physiol.*, 436: 93–105.

Nakatani, K., Tamura, T. and Yau, K.-W. (1991) Light adaptation in retinal rods of the rabbit and two other nonprimate mammals. *J. Gen. Physiol.*, 97: 413–435.

Penn, R.D. and Hagins, W.A. (1969) Signal transmission along retinal rods and the origin of the electroretinographic *a*-wave. *Nature*, 223: 201–205.

Pepperberg, D.R., Birch, D.G., Hofmann, K.P. and Hood, D.C. (1996) Recovery kinetics of human rod phototransduction inferred from the two-branched *a*-wave saturation function. *J. Opt. Soc. Amer. A*, 13: 586–600.

Pepperberg, D.R., Birch, D.G. and Hood, D.C. (1997) Photoresponses of human rods *in vivo* derived from paired-flash electroretinograms. *Vis. Neurosci.*, 14: 73–82.

Pepperberg, D.R., Birch, D.G. and Hood, D.C. (2000) Electroretinographic determination of human rod flash response *in vivo*. In: Palczewski, K. (Ed.), *Methods in Enzymology*, Vertebrate Phototransduction and the Visual Cycle, Part B, Vol. 316, Academic Press, San Diego, pp. 202–223.

Pepperberg, D.R., Brown, P.K., Lurie, M. and Dowling, J.E. (1978) Visual pigment and photoreceptor sensitivity in the isolated skate retina. *J. Gen. Physiol.*, 71: 369–396.

Pepperberg, D.R., Kahlert, M., Krause, A. and Hofmann, K.P. (1988) Photic modulation of a highly sensitive, near-infrared light-scattering signal recorded from intact retinal photoreceptors. *Proc. Natl. Acad. Sci. USA*, 85: 5531–5535.

Pepperberg, D.R., Lurie, M., Brown, P.K. and Dowling, J.E. (1976) Visual adaptation: effects of externally applied retinal on the light-adapted, isolated skate retina. *Science*, 191: 394–396.

Qtaishat, N.M., Okajima, T.-I.L., Li, S., Naash, M.I. and Pepperberg, D.R. (1999) Retinoid kinetics in eye tissues of VPP transgenic mice and their normal littermates. *Invest. Ophthalmol. Vis. Sci.*, 40: 1040–1049.

Robson, J.G. and Frishman, L.J. (1995) Response linearity and kinetics of the cat retina: The bipolar cell component of the dark-adapted electroretinogram. *Vis. Neurosci.*, 12: 837–850.

Robson, J.G. and Frishman, L.J. (1996) Photoreceptor and bipolar-cell contributions to the cat electroretinogram: A kinetic model for the early part of the flash response. *J. Opt. Soc. Amer. A*, 13: 613–622.

Robson, J.G. and Frishman, L.J. (1999) Dissecting the dark-adapted electroretinogram. *Doc. Ophthalmologica*, 95: 187–215.

Saari, J.C. (2000) Biochemistry of visual pigment regeneration. The Friedenwald Lecture. *Invest. Ophthalmol. Vis. Sci.*, 41: 337–348.

Saari, J.C., Garwin, G.G., Van Hooser, J.P. and Palczewski, K. (1998) Reduction of all-*trans*-retinal limits regeneration of visual pigment in mice. *Vision Res.*, 38: 1325–1333.

Sieving, P.A., Murayama, K. and Naarendorp, F. (1994) Push-pull model of the primate photopic electroretinogram: a role for hyperpolarizing neurons in shaping the b-wave. *Vis. Neurosci.*, 11: 519–532.

Sillman, A.J., Ito, H. and Tomita, T. (1969) Studies on the mass receptor potential of the isolated frog retina. I. General properties of the response. *Vision Res.*, 9: 1435–1442.

Sung, C.-H., Makino, C., Baylor, D. and Nathans, J. (1994) A rhodopsin gene mutation responsible for autosomal dominant retinitis pigmentosa results in a protein that is defective in localization to the photoreceptor outer segment. *J. Neurosci.*, 14: 5818–5833.

Tamura, T., Nakatani, K. and Yau, K.-W. (1989) Light adaptation in cat retinal rods. *Science*, 245: 755–758.

Thomas, M.M. and Lamb, T.D. (1999) Light adaptation and dark adaptation of human rod photoreceptors measured from the *a*-wave of the electroretinogram. *J. Physiol.*, 518: 479–496.

Xu, J., Dodd, R.L., Makino, C.L., Simon, M.I., Baylor, D.A. and Chen, J. (1997) Prolonged photoresponses in transgenic mouse rods lacking arrestin. *Nature*, 389: 505–509.

H. Kolb, H. Ripps and S. Wu (Eds.)
Progress in Brain Research, Vol. 131

CHAPTER 27

Dark adaptation

Gordon L. Fain*

*Departments of Physiological Science and Ophthalmology, University of California, Los Angeles,
Los Angeles, CA 90095-1527, USA*

Introduction

When I first joined the Dowling laboratory as a graduate student in the late sixties, one of John's principal interests was the mechanism of adaptation in the retina. Psychophysical measurements of visual threshold in humans had shown that bright bleaching light produces a large decrease in the sensitivity of the eye (see Barlow, 1964; Hecht, 1937), too large to be produced merely by the decrease in the concentration of the visual pigment (i.e. the decrease in quantum catch). If the decrease in sensitivity is not solely the result of the decrease in the concentration of pigment, some other process must make an important contribution to this decrease. Since bleaching desensitization closely resembles in many respects the desensitization produced by steady background light, Stiles and Crawford (1932) suggested that the bleaching of photopigment may produce an "equivalent background", but the nature of this equivalent background was for a long time entirely unclear.

For his thesis with George Wald, John had worked principally on vitamin A deprivation. By feeding rats a diet deprived of vitamin A, he showed that the visual threshold of the rats decreases as the concentration of rhodopsin in the eye decreases, with the logarithm of the threshold for the electroretinogram (ERG) approximately linear and inversely proportional to the concentration of rhodopsin (Dowling and Wald, 1958; Dowling and Wald, 1960). These

observations led him to inquire whether a similar relationship exists during dark adaptation.

Log-linear relationship between threshold and pigment concentration

To answer this question, John exposed several rats to a bright bleaching light and then measured the change in threshold of the ERG with time after the illumination (Dowling, 1960). He then exposed rats to the same light in parallel experiments and measured the rhodopsin concentration in the photoreceptors as a function of time during recovery from the bleach. The results of these experiments are shown in Fig. 1. The closed symbols give the $\log_{10}$ of the threshold relative to the threshold in the dark-adapted animal, and the open symbols give the decline in rhodopsin concentration. When the data are plotted in this way, there is a clear relationship between sensitivity and visual pigment concentration. This relationship is shown even more clearly in Fig. 2, in which the log threshold and rhodopsin concentration are directly compared. A similar proportionality was found by Rushton (1961) for human rod vision.

In addition to these observations, John also showed that, after bleaching, the chromophore of the visual pigment leaves the photoreceptors presumably in its all-*trans* configuration and travels to the pigment epithelium; and during dark adaptation, the chromophore comes back, presumably as 11-*cis* (Dowling, 1960; Hubbard and Dowling, 1962). This surprising result has created a whole new field of

* Tel.: 310-206-4281; E-mail: gfain@ucla.edu

384

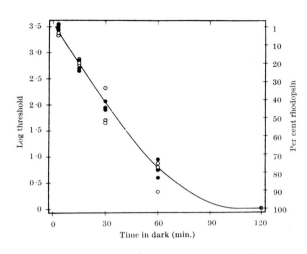

Fig. 1. Dark adaptation and rhodopsin concentration in the rat retina. Ordinate gives (left) the log of the threshold of the electroretinogram (ERG), normalized to the threshold in darkness (set at 1.0 or $\log_{10} = 0$); and (right) rhodopsin concentration as a per cent of the concentration in darkness. Abscissa gives time after exposure to a bright light bleaching approximately 100% of the rhodopsin. Filled circles are measurements of threshold from anaesthetized rats, and open circles parallel measurements of rhodopsin concentration from pigment extracted from isolated retinas. Reprinted with permission from Dowling (1960).

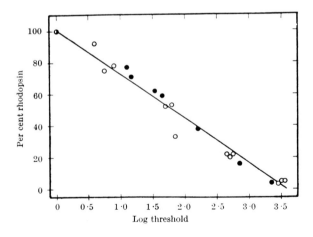

Fig. 2. Relationship between rhodopsin concentration and log threshold. Measurements were made as in Fig. 1 from rat retina. Ordinate gives rhodopsin content as a per cent of the rhodopsin in the dark-adapted eye, and abscissa gives the log of the threshold of the ERG Open circles are taken from experiments like those in Fig. 1 for recovery of sensitivity after a strong bleach, and closed circles are for the desensitization produced by vitamin A deprivation (Dowling and Wald, 1958). Reprinted with permission from Dowling (1960).

research into the mechanism of chromophore transport and regeneration, which has been the subject of many detailed investigations (for reviews, see Crouch et al., 1996; Saari, 2000a).

Bleaching adaptation in photoreceptors

When I began my graduate work, the log-linear relationship between threshold and pigment concentration was firmly established, but the reason for this relationship was poorly understood. As John himself recognized, there were evident problems. The data in Fig. 2 are for recovery from large bleaches, but small bleaches produce disproportionately large increases in threshold; furthermore, threshold does not appear to rise more steeply as the rhodopsin concentration goes to zero, as might be expected from a strictly log-linear relationship (see Pepperberg, 1984; Wald, 1961). There is in addition, the more fundamental difficulty of explaining why, even for bleaches between 10 and 90%, the log-linear relationship in Fig. 2 gives such a good fit. If, as Stiles and Crawford suggested, bleaching produces an "equivalent background", one might expect this background to excite the photoreceptors and produce a signal like that produced by real light (Barlow, 1964). But excitation by real light in a photoreceptor is linearly proportional to intensity, at least for dim illuminations (see for example, Baylor et al., 1979). If bleaching adaptation were originating from a signal in the photoreceptors, would it not seem more likely that the relationship between bleached pigment and equivalent excitation would be linear rather than log-linear (Lamb, 1981; Pepperberg, 1984)?

The role of the photoreceptors in bleaching desensitization and the effect of bleached pigment on receptor sensitivity began to be investigated in more detail, as recordings began to be made from single rods and cones. Measurements from the rods themselves (Grabowski and Pak, 1975), including those made within the Dowling laboratory (Kleinschmidt and Dowling, 1975), showed that most of the decrease in sensitivity produced by bright bleaching light occurs within the photoreceptors. Furthermore, the photoreceptors behave as if they were excited by an equivalent bleaching light (Leibovic et al., 1987). John and his collaborators also showed that, for weak bleaches, the log-linear relationship appears not to hold, and the decrease in sensitivity in the rod seems in fact to be linearly related to the decrease in pigment concentration (Leibovic et al., 1987).

Bleached pigment excites the visual cascade

One particularly helpful approach to investigate the nature of bleaching desensitization has been to expose isolated photoreceptors to bright light and to record the effect of bleaching on the response of the cell with suction electrode recording (see for example Lamb, 1980; Cornwall et al., 1983; Cornwall et al., 1989; Cornwall et al., 1990; Leibrock et al., 1994; Leibrock and Lamb, 1997). Since isolated photoreceptors have little capacity to regenerate pigment, large bleaches produce a stable concentration of bleached pigment in the outer segment. Furthermore, as David Pepperberg and coworkers in the Dowling laboratory first showed (Pepperberg et al., 1976), the bleached rhodopsin can be regenerated by exposing the rod outer segment to exogenous 11-*cis* retinal, either in ethanolic solution or in liposomes (Yoshikami and Noll, 1982). This makes it possible effectively to produce variable amounts of

bleached pigment in the outer segment and then to study reversibly the effect of bleached pigment on the physiology of the photoreceptor.

Recordings with the suction electrode technique show that bleached rods have many of the attributes of rods exposed to steady background light (see also Leibovic et al., 1987): the circulating current is smaller, the sensitivity of the rod is depressed, and light responses to dim flashes have a more rapid time course of current decay (see Fain and Cornwall, 1993). This can be seen for a salamander rod in Fig. 3. The responses in this figure were all recorded from the same isolated salamander rod, first in darkness, then over a period of about an hour after presentation of a light bleaching 90% of the photopigment, and finally after addition of exogenous 11-*cis* retinal. The bleaching exposure caused a large desensitization, which was only partially reversible. Even an hour after the bleach, the rod remained desensitized, and the wave form of the light response had a more rapid time course of decay (Fig. 3, Insert). Other experiments have shown that in an isolated rod for which little regeneration of photopigment can occur, this steady-state desensitization is stable even for many days (Corson et al., 1996). If, however, the rod is exposed to liposomes containing 11-*cis* retinal, the

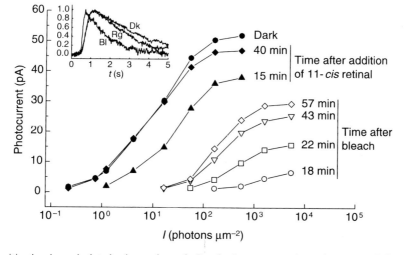

Fig. 3. Bleaching desensitization in an isolated salamander rod. Graph gives response-intensity curves all for the same rod for peak amplitude of the photocurrent measured with a suction electrode, as a function of the intensity of 520 nm flashes under the following conditions: in darkness (filled circles), after exposure to a light that bleached approximately 90% of the visual pigment (open symbols), and after addition to the bleached rod of exogenous 11-*cis* retinal in phospholipid vesicles (filled triangles and diamonds). *Inset* gives normalized small amplitude responses for this same rod when dark-adapted (*Dk*), at steady state after the bleach (*Bl*), and after recovery of sensitivity following exposure to exogenous 11-*cis* retinal (*Rg*). Reprinted with permission from Fain et al. (1996).

sensitivity and wave form of response can both recover nearly to those recorded at the beginning of the experiment from the dark-adapted receptor.

The evident similarity of desensitization of photoreceptors after bleaching and in the presence of background light reinforces the notion that bleached photopigment may produce an equivalent background excitation by stimulating the transduction cascade. Carter Cornwall and I reasoned that if bleached pigment stimulated transduction, we ought to be able to detect a stable increase in the enzymes of phototransduction after bleaching. We therefore used a method developed by Alan Hodgkin and Brian Nunn (1988) to estimate the rate of the phosphodiesterase from isolated rods. We rapidly exposed an isolated cell to a solution for which all of the Na^+ was replaced with Li^+. Since Li^+ cannot replace Na^+ in Na^+/K^+-Ca^{2+} exchange, the Ca^{2+} concentration in the outer segment increases rapidly in this solution and rapidly inhibits the guanylyl cyclase (Koch and Stryer, 1988). The photocurrent then declines nearly exponentially as the phosphodiesterase (PDE) in the outer segment hydrolyzes cyclic guanosine monophosphate (cGMP), and the time constant of current decline can be used as a measure of the rate of the PDE.

Typical results from our experiments are shown in Fig. 4 (from Cornwall and Fain, 1994). The records in the column on the left show the change in photocurrent during the change from Na^+ solution to Li^+ solution, and these same responses are shown on the right, but with the negative of the current plotted on a log_{10} scale. In the dark, the current of the rod in Li^+ solution declines slowly, with a time constant of about 1 s. In this same rod, 22% of the rhodopsin was bleached, and 40 min later, after the responses of the cell had come to steady state, the cell was again exposed to Li^+ solution. The decline of current is more rapid, indicating that the rate of the PDE after a bleach in an isolated rod is continuously accelerated, even in darkness. A further light exposure producing a total bleach of 52% of the rhodopsin produced an even greater stable acceleration in the PDE of this rod, which could be completely reversed to the rate characteristic of the dark-adapted cell by exposing the rod to exogenous 11-*cis* retinal.

In addition to stimulating the PDE, bleached pigment also accelerates the rate of the guanylate

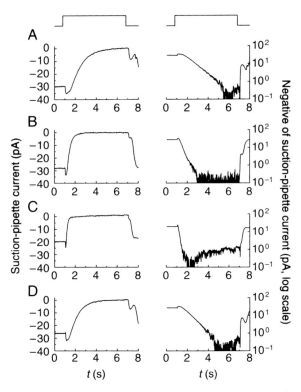

Fig. 4. Bleached pigment activates the transduction cascade. Salamander rods were rapidly stepped into a solution for which the Na^+ was replaced with Li^+. Since Li^+ does not substitute for Na^+ in Na^+/Ca^{2+}-K^+ exchange, the free Ca^{2+} concentration in the rod increased rapidly, blocking the guanylyl cyclase. The photocurrent declined as the phosphodiesterase (PDE) hydrolyzed cGMP, and the rate of decline of current is therefore a measure of PDE velocity (see text and Hodgkin and Nunn, 1988). Records to the right show the effect of Li^+ substitution on the photocurrent in darkness (A), at steady state after bleaching 22% of the pigment (B), at steady state after bleaching a total of 52% of the pigment (C), and after pigment regeneration with exogenous 11-*cis* retinal (D). Bleaching produces an increase in the rate of decline of current after Li^+ substitution, reflecting an increase in PDE velocity, which is reversed upon addition of 11-*cis* retinal. Curves to right give the negative of the suction pipette current plotted on a log scale and indicate that the log of current declines nearly linearly with time, with a time constant that becomes shorter with bleaching and is restored to its original value upon addition of 11-*cis* retinal. Reprinted with permission from Fain et al. (1996).

cyclase. Cornwall and I showed this by rapidly exposing outer segments to isobutylmethyl xanthine (IBMX), which blocks the photoreceptor PDE. When the PDE is blocked, the rod circulating current *increases*, as the cyclase synthesizes additional cGMP. From the initial rate of the current increase, it is possible to estimate the rate of the guanylyl cyclase, which also increases after bleaching and can be reversed by exposure to exogenous 11-*cis* retinal. Similar effects were subsequently also see in bleached cones (Cornwall et al., 1995).

One of the most interesting observations Cornwall and I made was that the increases in the rates of both the PDE and the cyclase after bleaching vary linearly with the increase in the concentration of bleached pigment. This can be seen in Fig. 5 (from Cornwall and Fain, 1994). The increase in the PDE velocity relative to that in darkness (β/β^D) is shown as the filled circles, and the relative increase in cyclase velocity (α'/α'^D) as the open circles. The open squares give the expected increase in the cyclase velocity, calculated from the increase in the PDE and the change in circulating current. This was always larger than the measured increase, but a more recent analysis taking into account the effect of Ca^{2+} on the cyclic-nucleotide-gated channels gives measured increases for the cyclase much closer to those expected (Kefalov et al., 1999).

The linear increase in PDE and cyclase rates with increasing percent bleach has an important implication. The excitation of transduction is linear with the amount of bleached pigment, probably because each bleached pigment molecule has an equal probability of exciting the visual cascade. Since increases in the PDE and cyclase rates are stable for long periods after the bleach, it is likely that the form of bleached pigment responsible for the stable excitation is simply opsin, that is pigment without chromophore, and additional experiments from the Cornwall laboratory strongly support this conclusion, at least for cones (Jin et al., 1993). Furthermore, the excitation is produced via activation of the G protein transducin, apparently in a manner similar to that produced by real light (Matthews et al., 1996).

Comparison of the magnitude of PDE and cyclase rates after bleaching with those produced by steady backgrounds suggests that rod opsin is only about 10^{-6}–10^{-7} as effective as metarhodopsin II or Rh*, the active form of the pigment produced by light (see also Leibovic et al., 1987). A similar estimate has been obtained from biochemical measurements of transducin activation in photoreceptor membranes by rod metarhodopsin II on the one hand, and rod opsin on the other (Melia et al., 1997). The low gain

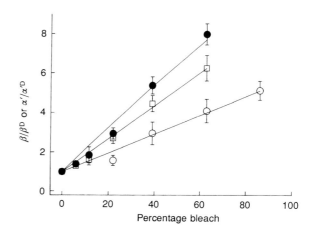

Fig. 5. Increase in the velocities of PDE and cyclase are linear with the concentration of bleached pigment. Filled circles give for salamander rods the mean increase in PDE velocity relative to that in darkness (β/β^D), measured as in Fig. 4, as a function of per cent rhodopsin bleached. Open circles give mean increase in cyclase velocity relative to that in darkness (α'/α'^D), determined from the initial rate of current increase after stepping photoreceptors into a solution containing the PDE blocker isobutylmethyl xanthine (IBMX). Open squares give values for α'/α'^D calculated from β/β^D and the values of the circulating current at steady state after the bleach and in darkness (see Cornwall and Fain, 1994). Bars give S.E.M.s. Straight lines are best-fitting linear regressions constrained to pass through $\beta/\beta^D = 1$ and $\alpha'/\alpha'^D = 1$ at zero bleach (i.e. in darkness). Reprinted with permission from Cornwall and Fain (1994).

of transduction activation by bleached pigment probably reflects a low probability of excitation of transducin. The gain of activation of transducin by opsin is probably also low, since stably bleached photoreceptors show little current noise (Jones, 1998), in marked contrast to rods exposed to steady background light.

In summary, bleached pigment probably as opsin produces an excitation of the transduction cascade that is linear with the concentration of opsin in the outer segment. This excitation seems to occur by a reaction between opsin and transducin in a manner similar to that between meta II and transducin as produced by real light. However, the probability of a successful collision between opsin and transducin appears to be rather low, and the gain of this first stage of activation is also low, probably because opsin does not exist in a special conformation like metarhodopsin II, capable of repeated and multiple activation of transducin molecules over a relatively long duration. One must imagine instead a rare event for which an opsin molecule assumes by chance and with low probability a conformation that can activate transducin. Thus the activation of transduction by bleached photopigment has a gain much smaller than that of Rh*, and opsin activation has little effect on the physiology of the photoreceptor unless large amounts of pigment are bleached. After large bleaches, the persistent excitation of the transduction cascade by the bleached pigment produces an equivalent background light and adapts the photoreceptor, much like a steady background light.

A simple model for bleaching desensitization

Photoreceptors are adapted by steady light according to the well-known Weber-Fechner relation (Fain et al., 2000),

$$\frac{S_F}{S_F^D} = \frac{I_0}{I_0 + I_B} \tag{1}$$

where S_F is the flash sensitivity of the photoreceptor, S_F^D is the flash sensitivity in the background, I_B is the background light intensity, and I_0 is a constant called the dark light. Eq. (1) can be re-arranged to an equation linear in background intensity (Baylor and Hodgkin, 1974):

$$\frac{S_F^D}{S_F} - 1 = \frac{I_B}{I_0} \tag{2}$$

This equation has been used to plot the data in Fig. 6A for the sensitivity of salamander rods in steady backgrounds (Jones et al., 1996).

Now suppose that bleached pigment produces an equivalent background light by exciting transduction linearly, with each bleached pigment molecule activating transducin and phosphodiesterase with the same probability and gain (see Fig. 5). It should be possible to replace I_B/I_0 in Eq. (2) with a term proportional to the fraction of pigment bleached, provided the flash sensitivity is first corrected for the decrease in the concentration of rhodopsin in the outer segment. The flash sensitivity after a bleach will be the result of the desensitization produced by the activation of the transduction

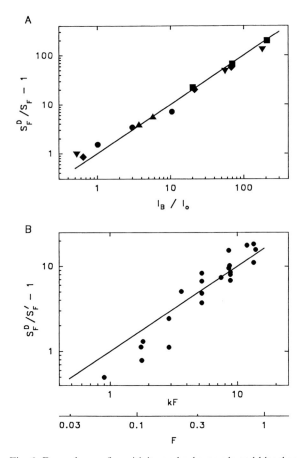

Fig. 6. Dependence of sensitivity on backgrounds and bleaches for salamander rods. **A.** Sensitivity in steady background light (S_F), normalized to sensitivity in darkness (S_F^D), linearized as in Eq. (2) and plotted as a function of background intensity. Each symbol represents data from a different cell, normalized to the value of the constant I_0 measured in that cell. **B.** Sensitivity at steady state after bleaching, corrected for the decrease in quantum catch with Eq. (3), normalized to sensitivity in darkness (S_F^D), and linearized as in Eq. (4). Each data point is from a single bleach in a single cell. Reprinted with permission from Jones et al. (1996).

cascade as well as by the decrease in quantum catch, that is

$$\frac{S_F}{S_F^D} = (1 - F)\frac{S_F'}{S_F^D} \tag{3}$$

where F is the fraction of pigment bleached and S_F'/S_F^D is the sensitivity decrease due to the activation of the cascade by the bleached pigment. The value of S_F'/S_F^D can therefore be obtained from the measured values of S_F/S_F^D after bleaching by dividing by $(1-F)$, estimated from the photosensitivity of the pigment and the intensity of the bleaching beam (Jones et al., 1996). The value of S_F'/S_F^D should be proportional to the fraction bleached, that is

$$\frac{S_F^D}{S_F'} - 1 = kF \qquad (4)$$

where k is a constant (Jones et al., 1996).

The stable decrease in sensitivity after bleaching in a number of salamander rods has been fitted with this equation in Fig. 6B. Although for small bleaches there is a tendency for S_F' to be larger (that is, for the desensitization to be smaller) than this equation would predict, for small bleaches, it is likely that some of the rhodopsin will have been regenerated, even in an isolated rod (Azuma et al., 1977; Cocozza and Ostroy, 1987; Donner and Hemila, 1975). This may have accounted for the anomalously large sensitivity after dim bleaches.

If we combine Eqs. (3) and (4), we can calculate the total decrease in sensitivity in a bleached photoreceptor due both to the decrease in quantum catch and the excitation of the visual cascade by the bleached pigment,

$$\frac{S_F}{S_F^D} = \frac{(1-F)}{(1+kF)} \qquad (5)$$

This equation has been plotted as the solid line in Fig. 7. The data points give the total decrease in sensitivity for a number of different salamander rods as a function of the fraction of photopigment bleached and are similar to previously published measurements (see for example Leibovic et al., 1987; Pepperberg, 1984). The dashed line gives the decrease in sensitivity predicted from the decrease in quantum catch alone. The satisfactory fit of Eq. (5) to the data in Fig. 7 indicates that, for rods at steady state after illumination bleaching a significant fraction of the visual pigment, a simple linear relationship between bleached pigment and sensitivity is adequate to explain bleaching desensitization in an isolated photoreceptor (Jones et al., 1996). A similar relationship also satisfactorily accounts for the decrease in sensitivity at steady state after bleaching in an isolated cone (Jones et al., 1993).

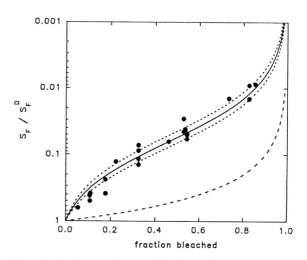

Fig. 7. The decrease in sensitivity in a photoreceptor after bleaching is produced by an equivalent background light whose intensity increases linearly with the fraction of rhodopsin bleached. Data points give for salamander rods the total change in sensitivity (S_F/S_F^D), uncorrected for the decrease in quantum catch, measured at steady state after bleaching from salamander rods. Each point is for a single bleach from a single cell. The solid line is the curve predicted by Eq. (5) for $k = 16.2$, and the short dashed lines are those for $k = 13.0$ or 20.7, corresponding to increases or decreases in the estimated photosensitivity $\pm15\%$. The line of longer dashes gives the decrease in normalized sensitivity predicted only from the decrease in quantum catch. Reprinted with permission from Jones et al. (1996).

Role of Ca^{2+} in bleaching desensitization

In background light, there is considerable evidence that Ca^{2+} is the primary second messenger responsible for producing the changes in sensitivity (see Fain et al., 2000). Changes in the concentration of Ca^{2+} produce changes in the rate of the guanylyl cyclase, transduction gain, and channel cGMP affinity that, together with the change in the rate of turn over of cGMP by the PDE and cyclase, seem to be mostly responsible for the changes in the sensitivity and wave form of the receptor response (Koutalos et al., 1995).

Since the effects of backgrounds and bleaches on rods are so similar (Fain and Cornwall, 1993; Jones et al., 1996; Leibovic et al., 1987; Leibrock et al., 1994), it would be reasonable to suppose that Ca^{2+} also plays an important role in bleaching desensitization. A role for Ca^{2+} is indicated by experiments for which the change in outer segment Ca^{2+} concentration was impeded by perfusion with low $Ca^{2+}/0$ Na^+ solution. This treatment prevents the changes in wave form and sensitivity normally produced by the bleach (Matthews et al., 1996).

Additional evidence for a role of Ca^{2+} in bleaching desensitization has been obtained from actual measurements in the free Ca^{2+} concentration with a fluorometric dye (Sampath et al., 1998). A typical result from a salamander rod is given in Fig. 8, which compares circulating current, sensitivity, and fluorescence from the Ca^{2+}-sensitive dye fluo3, previously incorporated into the photoreceptor outer segments. The first illumination with the laser was used to estimate the dark resting Ca^{2+} concentration, which other measurements suggest to be in the neighborhood of 650–700 nM in salamander and Gekko rods (Gray-Keller and Detwiler, 1994; Sampath et al., 1998). This first laser exposure was sufficiently bright to have bleached a large fraction of the photopigment in the rod. During time in darkness after this exposure, the sensitivity and circulating current slowly recover to stable values lower than those in the dark-adapted cell. The cell was again exposed to the laser to measure the free Ca^{2+} in the bleached receptor, and the fluo3 fluorescence was clearly smaller than in the dark-adapted cell. When the rod was subsequently presented with 11-*cis* retinal in lipid vesicles, circulating current and sensitivity both recovered as in Fig. 3, and the fluorescence of fluo3 (and hence the concentration of free Ca^{2+}) returned to near the dark-adapted value. Similar measurements with similar results have been made from salamander cones (Sampath et al., 1999).

Mechanism of dark adaptation

The experiments I have described have given us some notion of how desensitization occurs in an isolated rod after the bleaching of a significant percentage of the photopigment. The bleached pigment probably as opsin produces a linear excitation of the transduction cascade that activates the PDE and cyclase, reduces the intracellular free Ca^{2+} concentration, and desensitizes the photoreceptor much as steady background light. It is now appropriate to ask how far this

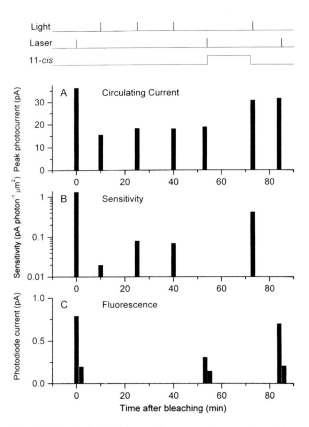

Fig. 8. Effect of bleaching and regeneration on circulating current, sensitivity, and fluo-3 fluorescence for salamander rod. All measurements from the same experiment on same cell. **A.** Circulating current was estimated from amplitude of light response to saturating flash intensity. **B.** Sensitivity is plotted as the ratio of the current response (in pA) to the light intensity (in photon μm^{-2}). Currents for A. and B. were recorded with a suction pipette. **C.** Rods were incubated in fluo-3AM at the beginning of the experiment, and fluo-3 fluorescence was elicited with an argon laser. Values plotted are the maximum and minimum fluorescence values for laser flashes given in darkness and after complete suppression of the circulating current. The first set of laser exposures bleached a significant fraction of the pigment in the photoreceptor. During the succeeding 50–60 min, the circulating current and sensitivity reached steady state. A second set of laser exposures were given to estimate the free-Ca^{2+} concentration in the bleached rod. The cell was then exposed to liposomes containing 11-*cis* retinal, and a final set of laser exposures were given after sensitivity and circulating current had recovered to near to their dark-adapted levels. Reprinted with permission from Sampath et al. (1998).

description of bleaching desensitization in an isolated rod or cone helps us understand how the visual system in a behaving organism loses and then slowly recovers sensitivity during dark adaptation.

One useful way of answering this question is to examine carefully the time course of recovery after bright bleaching light. Fig. 9 summarizes measurements of the e.r.g. of the rat retina during and after exposure to bright light (Dowling, 1963). The open circles show the decrease in threshold during a 5 min exposure to steady background light, and the x's, the recovery of sensitivity after the background light was extinguished. The filled circles and dashed line give the concentration of rhodopsin measured in parallel experiments after the 5 min exposure to the background.

These experiments provided two interesting insights into the mechanism of dark adaptation. First, the rate of recovery varies considerably with the amount of previous light exposure (see also Dowling and Ripps, 1972), becoming increasingly slower the greater the amount of rhodopsin bleached. Second, there are two phases of dark adaptation, a rapid and a slow, which John called "neural" and "photochemical". Although in this study on rat it was possible that some contribution to adaptation was made from cones as well as rods (Gouras, 1967), thus accounting in part for the two phases of recovery, similar rapid and slow phases were subsequently observed in skate (Dowling and Ripps, 1970), for which the retina most probably contains only a single receptor type (Cornwall et al., 1989; Ripps and Dowling, 1991).

We still do not understand what is responsible for determining the rate of recovery of sensitivity after a strong bleach, either in single photoreceptors or in the visual system as a whole. The bleaching of a significant fraction of rhodopsin will initially produce a large concentration of metarhodopsin II, which will be phosphorylated, capped by arrestin, and, then, slowly converted to metarhodopsin III and/or opsin. It seems possible that all of these intermediates activate the visual cascade, with the greatest activation produced by unphosphorylated meta II and the least by opsin; but at present nothing is known about activation by phosphorylated meta II or meta III. Several attempts have been made to measure the time course of the conversion of intermediates of bleaching after bright light exposure and to correlate these events with the time course of change in sensitivity (summarized in Fain et al., 2001), but studies of this sort have invariably used isolated photoreceptors

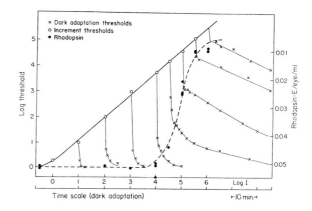

Fig. 9. Time course of dark adaptation in the rat retina. The electroretinogram (ERG) was measured from anaesthetized, albino rats with a cotton wick electrode, and rhodopsin measurements were made in parallel experiments by extracting the pigment from the retinas. The retina was exposed to a steady background light for 5 min, and the threshold of the ERG in the presence of the background is shown as the open circles. The light was then extinguished, and the time course of dark adaptation of the ERG threshold is shown as the x's. Closed circles and dashed line give the rhodopsin concentration, measured as extinction $(eye)^{-1}$ $(ml\ extract)^{-1}$ as rapidly as possible after the end of the 5 min light exposure. Reprinted with permission from Dowling (1963).

or retina, so that, changes in pigment absorbance can be measured conveniently with a spectrophotometer. Unfortunately, little pigment regenerates under these conditions, and we do not yet know how to mimic the time course of normal regeneration by adding exogenous chromophore. One interesting approach has been to use small bleaches for which regeneration can occur even in the isolated receptor, and experiments of this kind have argued for a role of phosphorylated metarhodopsin II (Leibrock and Lamb, 1997). Other experiments suggest that the conversion of all-*trans* retinal to all-*trans* retinol by retinol dehydrogenase is rate-limiting in the regeneration of pigment (Hofmann et al., 1992; Saari, 2000b; Saari et al., 1998), and that accumulation of all-*trans* retinal in the outer segment may desensitize the photoreceptor (Buczylko et al., 1996).

It has long been realized that desensitization in the visual system is produced not only by events occurring in the photoreceptors but also by mechanisms that exist in the retina and perhaps elsewhere in the visual pathway (for reviews, see Dowling, 1987; Rushton, 1965). One of the clearest demonstrations of this phenomenon is shown in Fig. 10

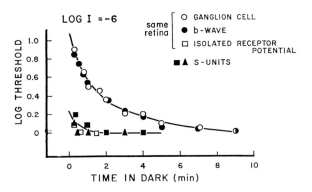

Fig. 10. Field adaptation in the skate retina. Graph compares time course of dark adaptation for horizontal cells (S-units), ganglion cells, the b-wave of the ERG, and the aspartate-isolated a-wave (receptor potential) of the ERG after the same 1 min light exposure. Note difference in rate of recovery for distal cells (a-wave and horizontal cells) and for proximal cells (b-wave and ganglion cells). Reprinted with permission from Green et al. (1975).

(from Green et al., 1975). The squares show measurements of the recovery of sensitivity after a bright light exposure in the skate retina for photo-receptors and horizontal cells, and the circles similar measurements for ganglion cells and the b-wave of the ERG. The recovery of sensitivity is slower in more proximal cells. Fig. 10 gives data for a rather dim bleaching exposure, but a similar (though quantitatively smaller) difference between distal and proximal cells is seen when a significant fraction of the visual pigment is bleached (Green et al., 1975). It would therefore appear that the time course of dark adaptation at the level of the ganglion cells and the visual system as a whole, though mostly the result of desensitization in the photoreceptors, can also be influenced by events in other cells in the retina. It is possible that these differences in rates of recovery in the photoreceptors and in the proximal retina may be responsible at least in part for the fast and slow ("neural" and "photochemical") phases of sensitivity recovery in the ERG like those shown in Fig. 9.

The contribution to the time course of recovery of sensitivity during dark adaptation produced by proximal cells in the retina, called "field adaptation", is probably the result of the summation of signals somewhere in the retina. John first suggested that at least one location where signals may be summed and sensitivity altered is the bipolar cell (Dowling, 1967). This remains an eminently reasonable proposal.

Bipolar cells receive direct input from photoreceptors and are perfectly positioned to sum their signals, and recent experiments indicate that depolarizing bipolar cells have special mechanisms of Ca^{2+}-dependent adaptation perhaps similar to those present in the photoreceptors (Shiells and Falk, 1999). Photoreceptors after small bleaches produce spontaneous, photon-like responses (Lamb, 1980) that are poorly correlated with the desensitization occurring in the photoreceptor itself (Leibrock et al., 1994) but could sum to produce additional desensitization somewhere else in the visual pathway (Leibrock and Lamb, 1997). Techniques presently available are probably adequate to resolve these issues, but the experiments still remain to be done.

Summary and future perspectives

From the time of the first description of the relation between bleached pigment and sensitivity, we have made considerable progress understanding how bleaching desensitization occurs. In single photoreceptors, desensitization is largely produced by a change in the rate of turnover of the PDE, and by the modulation of the rates of enzymes (such as guanylyl cyclase and rhodopsin kinase) and the opening probability of the cyclic-nucleotide-gated channels by the change in Ca^{2+} concentration, produced largely by the change in circulating current (see Fain et al., 2000). The equivalent background is produced by activation of the visual cascade by bleached pigment, and this activation (at least for opsin) is linear with the fraction bleached. We still do not know which bleaching intermediates are actually responsible for desensitization during dark adaptation in the behaving organism, for which pigment regeneration occurs normally. It now seems clear that most of the desensitization and recovery of sensitivity after exposure to bright light occurs in the photoreceptors. There is also some contribution from field adaptation in other cell types in the retina and perhaps elsewhere in the visual pathway, and one of these "summation pools" may very well occur at the level of the bipolar cells.

One of our greatest priorities for the future is a greater understanding of the role of various bleaching intermediates, including all-*trans* retinal, in the time course of sensitivity recovery during adaptation. Many of the genetic forms of diseases of retinal degeneration, including retinitis pigmentosa, produce abnormalities in the rate of recovery of sensitivity after bleaching (see for example Goto et al., 1995; Jacobson et al., 1994). If we had more information about the role of different forms of the visual pigment in determining the time course of dark adaption, we might be able to understand how these abnormalities occur.

Acknowledgments

Many of the ideas in the paper grew out of a long and very productive association with Carter Cornwall and Gregor Jones of the Boston University School of Medicine, and Hugh Matthews of Cambridge University. I am grateful to Carter for reading an earlier version of the manuscript. Work in my laboratory is supported by EY01844 of the National Eye Institute.

References

Azuma, K., Azuma, M. and Sickel, W. (1977) Regeneration of rhodopsin in frog rod outer segments. *J. Physiol. (Lond.)*, 271: 747–759.

Barlow, H.B. (1964) Dark-adaptation: a new hypothesis. *Vision Res.*, 4: 47–57.

Baylor, D.A. and Hodgkin, A.L. (1974) Changes in time scale and sensitivity in turtle photoreceptors. *J. Physiol. (Lond.)*, 242: 729–758.

Baylor, D.A., Lamb, T.D. and Yau, K.W. (1979) The membrane current of single rod outer segments. *J. Physiol. (Lond.)*, 288: 589–611.

Buczylko, J., Saari, J.C., Crouch, R.K. and Palczewski, K. (1996) Mechanisms of opsin activation. *J. Biol. Chem.*, 271: 20621–20630.

Cocozza, J.D. and Ostroy, S.E. (1987) Factors affecting the regeneration of rhodopsin in the isolated amphibian retina. *Vision Res.*, 27: 1085–1091.

Cornwall, M.C. and Fain, G.L. (1994) Bleached pigment activates transduction in isolated rods of the salamander retina. *J. Physiol. (Lond.)*, 480: 261–279.

Cornwall, M.C., Fein, A. and MacNichol, E.F., Jr. (1983) Spatial localization of bleaching adaptation in isolated vertebrate rod photoreceptors. *Proc. Natl. Acad. Sci. USA.*, 80: 2785–2788.

Cornwall, M.C., Fein, A. and MacNichol, E.F., Jr. (1990) Cellular mechanisms that underlie bleaching and background adaptation. *J. Gen. Physiol.*, 96: 345–372.

Cornwall, M.C., Matthews, H.R., Crouch, R.K. and Fain, G.L. (1995) Bleached pigment activates transduction in salamander cones. *J. Gen. Physiol.*, 106: 543–557.

Cornwall, M.C., Ripps, H., Chappell, R.L. and Jones, G.J. (1989) Membrane current responses of skate photoreceptors. *J. Gen. Physiol.*, 94: 633–647.

Corson, D.W., Gunasinghe, S. and Fleury, T.W. (1996) Persistence of opsin desensitization. *Invest. Ophthalmol. Vis. Sci.*, 37: S239.

Crouch, R.K., Chader, G.J., Wiggert, B. and Pepperberg, D.R. (1996) Retinoids and the visual process. *Photochem. Photobiol.*, 64: 613–621.

Donner, K.O. and Hemila, S. (1975) Kinetics of long-lived rhodopsin photoproducts in the frog retina as a function of the amount bleached. *Vision Res.*, 15: 985–995.

Dowling, J.E. (1960) Chemistry of visual adaptation in the rat. *Nature*, 188: 114–118.

Dowling, J.E. (1963) Neural and photochemical mechanisms of visual adaptation in the rat. *J. Gen. Physiol.*, 46: 1287–1301.

Dowling, J.E. (1967) The site of visual adaptation. *Science*, 155: 273–279.

Dowling, J.E. (1987) *The Retina: An Approachable Part of the Brain*. Harvard University Press, Cambridge.

Dowling, J.E. and Ripps, H. (1970) Visual adaptation in the retina of the skate. *J. Gen. Physiol.*, 56: 491–520.

Dowling, J.E. and Ripps, H. (1972) Adaptation in skate photoreceptors. *J. Gen. Physiol.*, 60: 698–719.

Dowling, J.E. and Wald, G. (1958) Vitamin A deficiency and night blindness. *Proc. Natl. Acad. Sci.*, 44: 648–661.

Dowling, J.E. and Wald, G. (1960) The biological function of vitamin A acid. *Proc. Natl. Acad. Sci.*, 46: 587–608.

Fain, G.L. and Cornwall, M.C. (1993) Light and dark adaptation in vertebrate photoreceptors. In: Shapley R. and Lam, D.M.-K. (Eds.), *Contrast Sensitivity. Proceedings of the Retina Research Foundation Symposia*, MIT Press, Cambridge, MA, pp. 3–32.

Fain, G.L., Matthews, H.R., et al. (1996) Dark adaptation in vertebrate photoreceptors. *Trends Neurosci.*, 19: 502–507.

Fain, G.L., Matthews, H.R., Cornwall, M.C. and Koutalos, Y. (2001) Adaptation in vertebrate photoreceptors. *Physiol. Rev.*, 81: 117–151.

Goto, Y., Peachey, N.S., Ripps, H. and Naash, M.I. (1995) Functional abnormalities in transgenic mice expressing a mutant rhodopsin gene. *Invest. Ophthalmol. Vis. Sci.*, 36: 62–71.

Gouras, P. (1967) Visual adaptation: its mechanism. *Science*, 157: 583–584.

Grabowski, S.R. and Pak, W.L. (1975) Intracellular recordings of rod responses during dark-adaptation. *J. Physiol. (Lond.)*, 247: 363–391.

Gray-Keller, M.P. and Detwiler, P.B. (1994) The calcium feedback signal in the phototransduction cascade of vertebrate rods. *Neuron*, 13: 849–861.

Green, D.G., Dowling, J.E., Siegel, I.M. and Ripps, H. (1975) Retinal mechanisms of visual adaptation in the skate. *J. Gen. Physiol.*, 65: 483–502.

Hecht, S. (1937) Rods, cones, and the chemical basis of vision. *Physiol. Rev.*, 17: 239–290.

Hodgkin, A.L. and Nunn, B.J. (1988) Control of light-sensitive current in salamander rods. *J. Physiol. (Lond.)*, 403: 439–471.

Hofmann, K.P., Pulvermuller, A., Buczylko, J., Van Hooser, P. and Palczewski, K. (1992) The role of arrestin and retinoids in the regeneration pathway of rhodopsin. *J. Biol. Chem.*, 267: 15701–15706.

Hubbard, R. and Dowling, J.E. (1962) Formation and utilization of 11-*cis* vitamin A by the eye tissues during light and dark adaptation. *Nature*, 193: 341–343.

Jacobson, S.G., Kemp, C.M., Cideciyan, A.V., Macke, J.P., Sung, C.-H. and Nathans, J. (1994) Phenotypes of stop codon and splice site rhodopsin mutations causing retinitis pigmentosa. *Invest. Ophthalmol. Vis. Sci.*, 35: 2521–2534.

Jin, J., Crouch, R.K., Corson, D.W., Katz, B.M., MacNichol, E.F. and Cornwall, M.C. (1993) Noncovalent occupancy of the retinal-binding pocket of opsin diminishes bleaching adaptation of retinal cones. *Neuron*, 11: 513–522.

Jones, G.J. (1998) Membrane current noise in dark-adapted and light-adapted isolated retinal rods of the larval tiger salamander. *J. Physiol. (Lond.)*, 511: 903–913.

Jones, G.J., Cornwall, M.C. and Fain, G.L. (1996) Equivalence of background and bleaching desensitization in isolated rod photoreceptors of the larval tiger salamander. *J. Gen. Physiol.*, 108: 333–340.

Jones, G.J., Fein, A., MacNichol, E.F., Jr. and Cornwall, M.C. (1993) Visual pigment bleaching in isolated salamander retinal cones. Microspectrophotometry and light adaptation. *J. Gen. Physiol.*, 102: 483–502.

Kefalov, V.J., Cornwall, M.C. and Crouch, R.K. (1999) Occupancy of the chromophore binding site of opsin activates visual transduction in rod photoreceptors. *J. Gen. Physiol.*, 113: 491–503.

Kleinschmidt, J. and Dowling, J.E. (1975) Intracellular recordings from gecko photoreceptors during light and dark adaptation. *J. Gen. Physiol.*, 66: 617–648.

Koch, K.W. and Stryer, L. (1988) Highly cooperative feedback control of retinal rod guanylate cyclase by calcium ions. *Nature*, 334: 64–66.

Koutalos, Y., Nakatani, K. and Yau, K.W. (1995) The cGMP-phosphodiesterase and its contribution to sensitivity regulation in retinal rods. *J. Gen. Physiol.*, 106: 891–921.

Lamb, T.D. (1980) Spontaneous quantal events induced in toad rods by pigment bleaching. *Nature*, 287: 349–351.

Lamb, T.D. (1981) The involvement of rod photoreceptors in dark adaptation. *Vision Res.*, 21: 1773–1782.

Leibovic, K.N., Dowling, J.E. and Kim, Y.Y. (1987) Background and bleaching equivalence in steady-state adaptation of vertebrate rods. *J. Neurosci.*, 7: 1056–1063.

Leibrock, C.S. and Lamb, T.D. (1997) Effect of hydroxylamine on photon-like events during dark adaptation in toad rod photoreceptors. *J. Physiol. (Lond.)*, 501: 97–109.

Leibrock, C.S., Reuter, T. and Lamb, T.D. (1994) Dark adaptation of toad rod photoreceptors following small bleaches. *Vision Res.*, 34: 2787–2800.

Matthews, H.R., Cornwall, M.C. and Fain, G.L. (1996) Persistent activation of transducin by bleached rhodopsin in salamander rods. *J. Gen. Physiol.*, 108: 557–563.

Matthews, H.R., Fain, G.L. and Cornwall, M.C. (1996) Role of cytoplasmic calcium concentration in the bleaching adaptation of salamander cone photoreceptors. *J. Physiol. (Lond.)*, 490: 293–303.

Melia, T.J., Jr., Cowan, C.W., Angleson, J.K. and Wensel, T.G. (1997) A comparison of the efficiency of G protein activation by ligand-free and light-activated forms of rhodopsin. *Biophys. J.*, 73: 3182–3191.

Pepperberg, D.R. (1984) Rhodopsin and visual adaptation: analysis of photoreceptor thresholds in the isolated skate retina. *Vision Res.*, 24: 357–366.

Pepperberg, D.R., Lurie, M., Brown, P.K. and Dowling, J.E. (1976) Visual adaptation: effects of externally applied retinal on the light-adapted, isolated skate retina. *Science*, 191: 394–396.

Ripps, H. and Dowling, J.E. (1991) Structural features and adaptive properties of photoreceptors in the skate retina. *J. Exp. Zool. Suppl.*, 5.

Rushton, W.A.H. (1961) Rhodopsin measurement and dark-adaptation in a subject deficient in cone vision. *J. Physiol.*, 156: 193–205.

Rushton, W.A.H. The Ferrier Lecture. (1965) *Proc. R. Soc. Lond.*, B162: 20–46.

Saari, J. (2000a) Biochemistry of visual pigment regeneration: the Friedenwald lecture. *Invest. Ophthalmol. Vis. Sci.*, 41: 337–348.

Saari, J.C. (2000b) Biochemistry of visual pigment regeneration. *Invest. Ophthalmol. Vis. Sci.*, 41: 337–348.

Saari, J.C., Garwin, G.G., Van Hooser, J.P. and Palczewski, K. (1998) Reduction of all-trans-retinal limits regeneration of visual pigment in mice. *Vision Res.*, 38: 1325–1333.

Sampath, A.P., Matthews, H.R., Cornwall, M.C., Bandarchi, J. and Fain, G.L. (1999) Light-dependent changes in outer segment free Ca^{2+} concentration in salamander cone photoreceptors. *J. Gen. Physiol.*, 113: 267–277.

Sampath, A.P., Matthews, H.R., Cornwall, M.C. and Fain, G.L. (1998) Bleached pigment produces a maintained decrease in outer segment Ca^{2+} in salamander rods. *J. Gen. Physiol.*, 111: 53–64.

Shiells, R.A. and Falk, G. (1999) A rise in intracellular Ca^{2+} underlies light adaptation in dogfish retinal 'on' bipolar cells. *J. Physiol.*, 514.

Stiles, W.S. and Crawford, B.H. (1932) Equivalent adaptation levels in localized retinal areas. In: *Report of a Joint Discussion on Vision, June 3, 1932, Imperial College of Science*. Physical Society, London pp. 194–211.

Wald, G. (1961) The molecular organization of visual systems. In: McElroy, W.D. and Glass, B. (Eds.), *A Symposium on Light and Life*. The Johns Hopkins Press, Baltimore, pp. 724–753.

Yoshikami, S. and Noll, G.N. (1982) Technique for introducing retinol analogs into the isolated retina. *Methods Enzymol.*, 81: 447–451.

H. Kolb, H. Ripps and S. Wu (Eds.)
Progress in Brain Research, Vol. 131
© 2001 Elsevier Science B.V. All rights reserved

CHAPTER 28

Evaluation of the contributions of recoverin and GCAPs to rod photoreceptor light adaptation and recovery to the dark state

James B. Hurley[1],* and Jeannie Chen[2]

[1]*Department of Biochemistry, 357350, University of Washington, Seattle, WA 98195, USA*
[2]*Doheny Eye Institute, BMT-401, University of Southern California, Los Angeles, CA 90033, USA*

Introduction

Among the many important aspects of the retina that John Dowling has studied is the ability to adapt to illumination conditions. His studies showed that adaptation occurs both at the receptor level and also at the network level. During the past thirteen years since Dowling summarized this aspect of vision in his book, "The Retina, an approachable part of the brain" the molecular basis for photoreceptor light and dark adaptation has become more clear. Important biochemical reactions and the enzymes that catalyze them have been identified. In this report we will describe some studies that provide evidence for physiological functions of these biochemical reactions.

Phototransduction is initiated when light stimulates visual pigments in rod and cone photoreceptors. In rods, light isomerises 11-*cis* retinal on rhodopsin to an all-*trans* configuration. That induces changes in the rhodopsin structure that transform it into an activator of a G-protein, transducin. Transducin is structurally and functionally related to other heterotrimeric G-proteins, such as Gs, Go and others

(Hurley et al., 1984; Hurley, 1990). Its α subunit binds GTP upon activation (Fung et al., 1981) and relieves constraints caused by an inhibitory subunit of a cGMP phosphodiesterase (Hurley, 1980; Hurley et al., 1981; Hurley and Stryer, 1982). The ensuing hydrolysis of cGMP causes closure of cGMP-gated cation channels in the photoreceptor plasma membrane (Fesenko et al., 1985). Components of the phototransduction cascades in rods and cones are similar but in many cases they are derived from different genes (e.g. Lerea et al., 1986; Hamilton and Hurley, 1990).

Continuous illumination of photoreceptors presents two problems to the phototransduction apparatus. First, if the illumination is bright enough to drive a photoreceptor into saturation, then significant biochemical adjustments must occur in order for the photoreceptor to respond to further increments in light intensity. This requires re-opening a fraction of the channels that were closed by the saturating light. A reduction in photosensitivity may also occur, although the evidence for this aspect of light adaptation is controversial (Pugh et al., 1999). The second problem is that a photoreceptor must also undergo a change in identity from being just a detector of increments of light to being a detector of both increments and decrements of light. With few exceptions (Normann and Perlman, 1979;

*Corresponding author: James B. Hurley, Tel.: 206-543-2871; Fax: 206-685-2320; E-mail: jbhhh@u.washington.edu

Burkhardt, 1994), this important aspect of photo-receptor function has been neglected in most physiological studies of phototransduction (Baylor, 1998). But the need for it is obvious when one considers how survival can depend on rapid detection of the shadow of a predator, for example. Adjustments to the biochemical state of a photoreceptor that allow darkness to cause rapid opening of cation channels are required.

A consequence of phototransduction is that closure of cGMP-gated cation channels blocks entry of Ca^{2+}. Since Ca^{2+} continues to leave photoreceptors via a Na^+/Ca^{2+}, K^+ exchanger the concentration of free cytoplasmic Ca^{2+} falls from $\sim$500 to $\sim$50 nM (Gray-Keller and Detwiler, 1994). This lowering of free $[Ca^{2+}]$ is required for cation channels to re-open upon exposure of photoreceptors to continuous illumination (Nakatani and Yau, 1988; Matthews et al., 1988).

Three biochemical reactions linked to phototransduction are known to be sensitive to Ca^{2+}. Guanylyl cyclase activity is stimulated by low $[Ca^{2+}]$ (Koch and Stryer, 1988), rhodopsin phosphorylation is inhibited by high $[Ca^{2+}]$ (Kawamura, 1993) and the affinity of cGMP-gated channels for cGMP is reduced by high $[Ca^{2+}]$ (Hsu and Molday, 1993). The Ca^{2+}-dependencies of these reactions measured in vitro vary, but they are close enough to the physiological range of $[Ca^{2+}]$ in photoreceptors that roles for each of these reactions in light adaptation or flash response recovery have been rationalized (Gray Keller et al., 1993; Gorczyca et al., 1994; Erickson et al., 1998).

Inhibition of rhodopsin kinase and activation of guanylyl cyclase have been studied extensively using in vitro biochemical methodology. These reactions are catalyzed by rhodopsin kinase and photoreceptor membrane guanylyl cyclase, respectively and each of these enzymes is regulated by a different Ca^{2+}-binding protein. Rhodopsin kinase is regulated by the Ca^{2+}-binding protein, recoverin (Kawamura, 1993; Chen et al., 1995) and guanylyl cyclase is regulated by other Ca^{2+}-binding proteins known as guanylyl cyclase activator proteins, or GCAPs (Dizhoor and Hurley, 1999). Two GCAP-sensitive guanylyl cyclases (Dizhoor et al., 1994; Lowe et al., 1995) and two types of GCAPs (Dizhoor et al., 1995; Gorczyca et al., 1995) have been identified that

are expressed and functional in vertebrate retinas. A third type of GCAP has also been cloned but the only reported evidence for its expression in photoreceptors is not convincing (Haeseleer et al., 1999). Recoverin and GCAPs are members of a sub-family of EF-hand Ca^{2+} binding proteins that also include hippocalcins, neurocalcins and frequenins.

Recoverin and rhodopsin phosphorylation

Recoverin was first purified (Dizhoor et al., 1989) from bovine rod outer segments. Its amino acid sequence was determined (Dizhoor et al., 1991), cDNA encoding it was isolated (Ray et al., 1992) and an effective method for expressing it was developed. The amino-terminus of recoverin is heterogenously acylated (Dizhoor et al., 1992) as are several other photoreceptor proteins that have a myristoylation consensus sequence (Johnson et al., 1994). Recoverin binds Ca^{2+} (Dizhoor et al., 1991) at two sites (Flaherty et al., 1993) that bear resemblance to the EF-hand structures in calmodulin. When recoverin binds Ca^{2+} it undergoes a substantial conformational change (Ames et al., 1997) that pulls the N-terminal fatty acyl moiety from a hydrophobic pocket within recoverin (Zozulya and Stryer, 1992; Dizhoor et al., 1993; Hughes et al., 1995). This increases the affinity of recoverin for membranes by allowing the fatty acyl moiety to function as a membrane anchor (Zozulya and Stryer, 1992; Dizhoor et al., 1993).

Kawamura and Murakami showed that Ca^{2+} and S-modulin, a homologue of recoverin in frogs, prolong cGMP phosphodiesterase activation following a flash of light in vitro (Kawamura and Murakami, 1991). Kawamura subsequently showed that Ca^{2+} together with S-modulin or recoverin also slows light-stimulated rhodopsin phosphorylation in vitro (Kawamura, 1993). This effect of S-modulin/recoverin on phosphorylation is probably responsible for prolongation of phosphodiesterase activity. Recoverin inhibits rhodopsin phosphorylation in vitro by a direct interaction with rhodopsin kinase (Chen et al., 1995). However, a troublesome feature of the effect of recoverin on rhodopsin phosphorylation is that the concentration of Ca^{2+} required for half-maximal effect is higher than the estimated physiological range of free Ca^{2+} in intact rod outer segments. In fact, the Ca^{2+}-dependence of this reaction in vitro is even quite different from the other Ca^{2+}-dependent process to be discussed in this chapter, regulation of guanylyl cyclase by GCAPs. A comparison of the Ca^{2+}-dependence of regulation of these two reactions is shown in Fig. 1.

No hereditary disease of humans has yet been linked to the recoverin gene.

GCAPs and guanylyl cyclase

Guanylyl cyclase was shown to be sensitive to sub-micromolar concentrations of $[Ca^{2+}]$ (Koch and Stryer, 1988). In 1992, a membrane form of guanylyl cyclase, RetGC-1, specifically expressed in photoreceptors was cloned but it was not clear

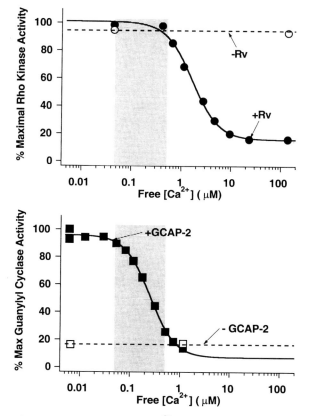

Fig. 1. Comparison of the Ca^{2+} sensitivities of rhodopsin phosphorylation in the presence of recoverin vs guanylyl cyclase in the presence of GCAP-2. Data are replotted from Chen et al. (1995) and from Dizhoor et al. (1994). The shaded area represents an estimate of the range of bulk intracellular free Ca^{2+} in rods (Gray-Keller and Detwiler, 1994).

whether or not this enzyme was the one responsible for Ca^{2+}-sensitive cGMP synthesis in rods (Shyjan et al., 1992). Dizhoor et al. (1994) resolved this issue by showing that RetGC-1 can be stimulated by a purified protein only at low free $[Ca^{2+}]$. The protein was subsequently sequenced and cloned (Dizhoor et al., 1995). A similar protein was independently identified (Gorczyca et al., 1994), cloned (Gorczyca et al., 1995) and christened "Guanylyl Cyclase Activator Protein-1" or "GCAP-1". The name is unfortunately a misnomer because these proteins have the abilities to both activate and inhibit guanylyl cyclase (Dizhoor and Hurley, 1996). However, to be consistent with this nomenclature the protein identified by Dizhoor et al. (1995) was dubbed "GCAP-2". Subsequent studies showed that GCAP-2 is generally expressed in rods whereas GCAP-1 has been detected in both rods and cones (Kachi et al., 1999). A second form of GCAP-sensitive guanylyl cyclase was also identified and named "RetGC-2" (Lowe et al., 1995). RetGC-1 is enriched in cones but also present in rods. RetGC-2 mRNA was localized specifically to photo-receptors (Lowe et al., 1995) but detailed localization of RetGC-2 protein has not yet been reported.

Structural and functional features of RetGCs and GCAPs have been explored by mutagenesis and modeling. RetGCs are composed of dimers of single polypeptide chains that each span the membrane once. On the intracellular side most proximal to the membrane is a domain with homology to protein kinases, followed by a coiled-coil dimerization domain and then a catalytic domain. The extracel-lular domain is not required for regulation by GCAPs (Laura et al., 1996) and evidence suggests that the kinase-like domain is a docking site for GCAPs (Laura and Hurley, 1998). The dimerization domain is not optimized for maximal strength of dimeriza-tion, but instead for the ability to be regulated by the physiologically most appropriate concentration of Ca^{2+} (Tucker et al., 1999). The structure of the RetGC catalytic domain has not yet been determined directly but it has been modeled based on known structures of adenylyl cyclases (Liu et al., 1997). The two amino acids that determine nucleotide specificity have been identified in the catalytic domain (Tucker et al., 1998).

Mutations in RetGC-1 and GCAP-1 have been linked to diseases that cause human retinal degeneration including Leber's Congenital Amaurosis, Autosomal Dominant Cone Dystrophy and Autosomal Dominant Cone–Rod Dystrophy. (Perrault et al., 1996; Kelsell et al., 1998; Payne et al., 1998).

Applications of transgenic mouse methodology to phototransduction

Homologous recombination using embryonic stem cells has become an effective method to inactivate specific genes in mice. Although mouse retinas are heavily enriched with rods, the availability of inbred lines, cell lines and genetic information has made mouse the species of choice for most types of targeted gene disruption experiments. A concerted effort by several investigators has produced mouse strains in which important genes including arrestin (Xu et al., 1997), rhodopsin kinase (Chen et al., 1999), rhodopsin (Lem et al., 1999), and the phosphodiesterase inhibitor subunit (Tsang et al., 1996) have been disrupted. In the studies described in this report we analyzed mice in which the recoverin gene was inactivated and mice in which the two GCAP genes (Howes et al., 1997) were inactivated. Detailed descriptions of the genetic manipulations used to produce these mice will be reported elsewhere.

Recent advances in electroretinography

The a-wave of the rodent electroretinogram appears within milliseconds following an intense flash of light. Recent detailed analyses of electroretinography have shown that the rising phase of the a-wave from mouse retinas is related to phototransduction in rods by the following equation (Lyubarsky and Pugh, 1996; Hetling and Pepperberg, 1999)

$$a = a_{max}(1 - \exp(-0.5\Phi A(t - t_0)^2)) \qquad (1)$$

where a is the a-wave amplitude, a_{max} is the maximal a-wave amplitude that would occur in the absence of b-wave interference, Φ is the number of isomerisations per rod, A is an amplification factor related to the gain of phototransduction, t is the time after the flash and t_0 is a delay time.

The direct relationship between early a-wave kinetics and phototransduction kinetics also formed

the basis for an ERG-based method to monitor recovery kinetics of rod photoreceptors following a light flash (Lyubarsky and Pugh, 1996; Pepperberg et al., 1997). In this method a test flash is first given to elicit a photoresponse that closes some or all of the rod plasma membrane channels. A defined interval passes during which some channels re-open as a consequence of the biochemical reactions that govern recovery to the dark state. Then a second, nearly saturating, probe flash is given to elicit a response whose amplitude is proportional to the fraction of channels that had re-opened by the time of the probe flash. Data from a series of probe flashes at various delay times then defines the time course of recovery to the dark state. These types of analyses agree remarkably well with time courses of recovery based on isolated rod photoreceptor recordings (Lyubarsky and Pugh, 1996).

A similar approach can be used to monitor the closure of channels during light adaptation (Thomas and Lamb, 1999). First a nearly saturating probe flash is given to record the a-wave of the animal in its dark adapted state. Background illumination is applied and the probe flash is given again. By monitoring the a-wave response at a specified time (9 ms in the experiments described here) the fraction of channels closed by the background illumination can be estimated.

ERG analyses of recoverin knock-out mice

ERG flash responses over 8 log units of intensity for normal and recoverin−/− mice are shown in Fig. 2A. A peculiar characteristic of the recoverin−/− response is a second positive potential that appears after the b-wave in response to intermediate flash intensities. This unusual type of response suggests disruption of some sort of feedback mechanism within the retina. The maximal amplitude of the a-wave is also diminished in the recoverin−/− ERGs. Based only on this analysis we cannot determine whether this reflects a difference in the number of open channels in the dark-adapted state or if it reflects a difference in electrical resistance of the retina. The sensitivities and maximal responses of normal and Rv−/− mice are determined in Fig. 2B by fitting the a-wave responses to Eq. 1.

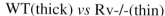

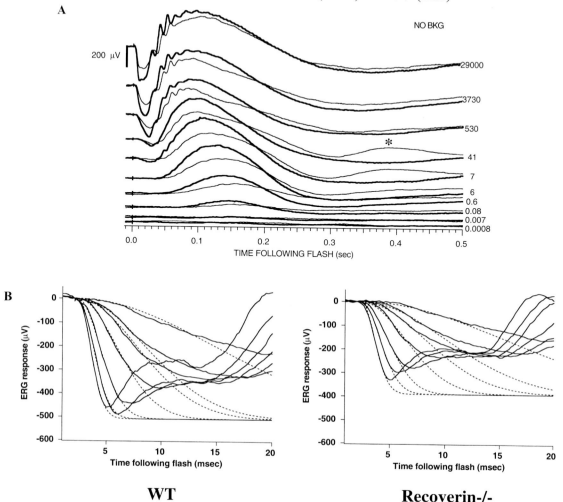

WT

Recoverin-/-

Fig. 2 **A.** ERG responses to white light flashes delivered to normal (heavy traces) and recoverin$-/-$ (thin traces) eyes. Each trace is an average of responses from 6 normal and 6 recoverin$-/-$ mice. The numbers to the right are estimates of the number of photoisomerisations per rod caused by the flashes. The calibration to determine these numbers was done by comparing the wild-type data with the kinetics and sensitivity of the mouse ERGs reported by Lyubarsky and Pugh (1996). Light from a photographic flash unit was filtered and focused onto one end of a bifurcated fiber optic bundle. The other end of the bundle was connected to a constant light source and shutter system. The light emitting from the end of the bifurcated fiber optic bundle was focused onto the cornea of the anaesthetized mouse. ERGs were recorded using a gold ring electrode attached to a translucent plastic disk (Bayer et al., 2000). Electrical potentials measured from the cornea were compared with a ground electrode in the mouse's mouth and were filtered electronically between 1 Hz and 3,000 Hz. The data were digitized and acquired at 5,000 Hz. Data were collected in Igor Pro (Wavemetrics) with an Instrutech ITC-16 analog to digital interface using a library of custom acquisition routines written by Fred Rieke (University of Washington). **B.** Comparison of the flash sensitivities of normal and recoverin$-/-$ mice. a-wave responses of normal (left panel) and recoverin$-/-$ mice (right panel) are shown. The traces are the averages of recordings from 14 wild-type mice and 6 Rv$-/-$ mice. For the second brightest flash the means and standard deviations for the a-wave at 5 ms were 421 ± 105 µV for wild-type and 271 ± 31 µV for Rv$-/-$. Responses to flashes estimated to cause 1,700; 2,200; 3,950; 12,450; 51,900; 164,000 and 519,000 photoisomerisations per rod in normal retinas are shown. The data were fit to Eq. 1 using a Global Fit analysis using Igor Pro analysis software (Wavemetrics). The dotted curves are the fits. The relative a_{max} values calculated from the data fits for Rv$-/-$ compared to normal mice were 309 and 508 µV respectively, and the ratio of amplification factors (A_{Rv}/A_{WT}) averaged over all flash intensities was 0.84 ± 0.11.

The results show that the absence of recoverin does not significantly affect dark-adapted photosensitivity of rods.

Using the paired flash protocol outlined in the previous section we also compared recovery kinetics of normal and recoverin−/− mice (Fig. 3). Recoverin−/− mice returned to the dark state approximately three times faster than normal mice.

Figure 2B shows that this is most likely not caused by a decrease in sensitivity to the test flash. This result appears to be consistent with the expected function of recoverin. In the absence of recoverin the initial rate of rhodopsin phosphorylation would be faster so one would expect recovery to the dark state to be faster. We also measured rates of recovery following flashes that bleached up to 10,000 times

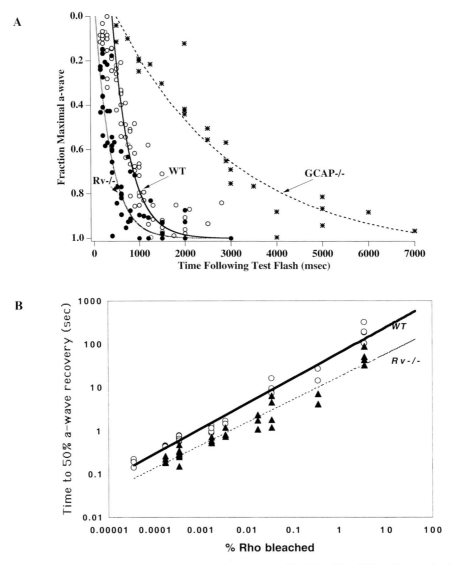

Fig. 3. **A.** Recovery time course following a test flash (100 ms pulse of white light (1.2 μW)) and determined by measuring a-wave responses using a white light probe flash from a photographic flash unit (4.4 μJ or ∼30,000 photoisomerisations per rod). Analyses of normal, recoverin−/− and GCAP−/− mice are shown. Each data set is a compilation of data from 4–7 mice. **B.** Summary of recovery time courses for normal and recoverin−/− mice over a range of test flash intensities. All test flashes were 100 ms long except for the experiments with the highest % rhodopsin bleached. In those experiments 1 s test flash was used.

more rhodopsin than the test flash used in Fig. 3A. Under these conditions recovery to the dark state takes as long as minutes. Recoverin−/− mice continue to return to the dark state about three times faster than normal mice throughout the range of intensities tested in the experiments shown in Fig. 3B.

ERG analyses of GCAP−/− mice

Figure 4 shows flash responses of normal mice and mice in which both GCAP-1 and GCAP-2 genes are inactivated (GCAP−/−). The time course of the b-wave response is extended in GCAP−/− mice and the a-wave amplitudes are reduced. Otherwise, the responses appear normal under dark-adapted conditions. Interpretation of the reduced a-wave amplitude is ambiguous for the same reasons described in the discussion of recoverin−/− responses. Although a detailed analysis of the sensitivity has not been completed, our preliminary results suggest

that the GCAP−/− mutation does not dramatically affect the dark-adapted sensitivity.

Figure 3A shows paired flash analyses of GCAP−/− mice in comparison with normal and recoverin−/− mice. GCAP−/− mice take about three times longer than normal to return to the dark state under these conditions. This result is consistent with a requirement for GCAPs to stimulate guanylyl cyclase to synthesize cGMP and re-open channels following flashes of light.

Effects of steady background illumination on normal and GCAP−/− mice were analyzed by measuring probe flash responses on top of various levels of background illumination as shown in Fig. 5A. In normal mice the background illumination initially closes channels but the molecular mechanisms of light-adaptation then re-open a fraction of the channels to restore sensitivity. Normal, recoverin−/− and GCAP−/− light-adaptation are compared in Fig. 5B. There is perhaps a small effect of the recoverin mutation on light adaptation. But the absence of GCAPs causes rods to shut down

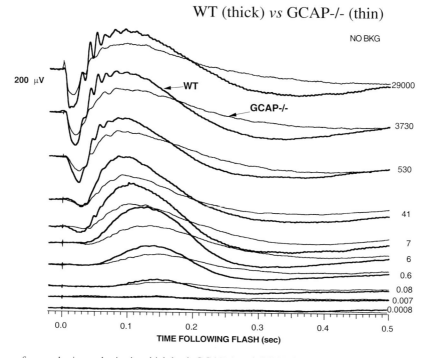

Fig. 4. Flash responses of normal mice and mice in which both GCAP-1 and GCAP-2 genes are inactivated (GCAP−/−). Each trace is an average of responses from 6 normal (heavy traces) and 6 GCAP−/− (thin traces) mice. The numbers to the right are estimates of the number of photoisomerisations per rod caused by the flashes in normal mice.

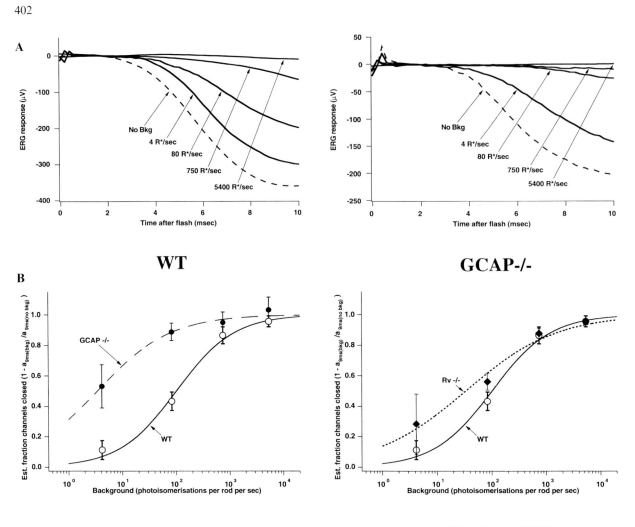

Fig. 5. **A.** Comparisons of light-adaptation in normal, recoverin–/– and GCAP–/– mice. Responses to flashes of white light that cause ~30,000 photoisomerisations per rod were recorded in the absence (dashed line) or presence (solid lines) of white background illumination. The numbers next to each trace represent the estimated rate of bleaching rhodopsin caused by the background illumination. This was based on comparison of the power of the light source measured at the position of the cornea compared with the energy of the flash unit measured in the same way. A photometric filter was used for all measurements. The number of photoisomerisations caused by the flash unit configuration was calibrated as described in Fig. 2. **B.** Comparison of light-adaptation in normal, recoverin–/– and GCAP–/– retinas. The fraction of dark current remaining at each level of background illumination was estimated (Thomas and Lamb, 1999) by calculating a_{bkg}/a_{DA} measured at 9 ms following the probe flash (~30,000 photoisomerisations per rod).

nearly all of their channels and go into saturation at significantly lower background intensities than in normal retinas. This result is also consistent with a requirement for GCAPs to stimulate cGMP synthesis to keep up with the accelerated cGMP hydrolysis caused by steady illumination.

Conclusions and future perspective

The findings reported here are consistent with a central role for GCAPs in light-adaptation. GCAPs repress cGMP synthesis under dark-adapted conditions. But when Ca^{2+} levels are lowered by light GCAPs stimulate cGMP synthesis in order to re-open some of the channels that were initially closed by light.

The recoverin−/− findings reported here are consistent with the expected function of recoverin. As expected, the absence of recoverin shortened the response to dim and moderate intensity flashes presumably because rhodopsin phosphorylation proceeds faster in the absence of recoverin. Other studies are underway in our laboratories to confirm this explanation by direct biochemical analysis.

An important caveat with all experiments such as these is that changes may have occurred in the retinas of these mutant mice to compensate for the absence of recoverin or GCAPs. Preliminary studies from our lab and from other labs analyzing these mice (to be published elsewhere) have so far not revealed any such changes.

These physiological studies highlight the need for a biochemical counterpart, i.e. quantitative biochemical analysis of factors that determine the adaptation-state of photoreceptors. Ideally such biochemical analyses could be performed under conditions identical to those used for the physiological studies. We are currently developing methods to measure rhodopsin phosphorylation, regeneration and the physiological states of photoreceptors under such conditions. This should enhance our ability to experimentally define the specific contributions of these biochemical reactions to light- and dark-adaptation.

Acknowledgments

We wish to thank David Pepperberg and Ed Pugh for many useful discussions about the theory and practice of electroretinography. We thank Fred Rieke for providing his data acquisition software and for advice. These studies were supported by funds from the National Eye Institute (EY06641 to JBH).

Reference

Ames, J.B., Ishima, R., Tanaka, T., Gordon, J.I., Stryer, L. and Ikura, M. (1997) Molecular mechanics of calcium-myristoyl switches. *Nature*, 389: 198–202.

Bayer, A.U., Mittag, T., Cook, P., Brodie, S.E., Podos, S.M. and Maag, K.-P. (2000) Comparisons of the amplitude size and the reproducibility of three different electrodes to record the corneal flash electroretinogram in rodents. *Doc. Ophthalmol.*, 98: 233–246.

Baylor, D. (1998) How photons start vision. *Proc. Natl. Acad. Sci. USA*, 93: 560–565.

Burkhardt, D.A. (1994) Light adaptation and photopigment bleaching in cone photoreceptors in situ in the retina of the turtle. *J. Neurosci.*, 14: 1091–1105.

Chen, C.-K., Inglese, J., Lefkowitz, R.J. and Hurley, J.B. (1995) Ca2+-dependent interaction of recoverin with rhodopsin kinase. *J. Biol. Chem.*, 270: 18060–18066.

Chen, C.K., Burns, M.E., Spencer, M., Niemi, G.A., Chen, J., Hurley, J.B., Baylor, D.A. and Simon, M.I. (1999) Abnormal photoresponses and light-induced apoptosis in rods lacking rhodopsin kinase. *Proc. Natl. Acad. Sci. USA*, 96: 3718–3722.

Chen, C.K., Inglese, J., Lefkowitz, R.J. and Hurley, J.B. (1995) Ca(2+)-dependent interaction of recoverin with rhodopsin kinase. *J. Biol. Chem.*, 270: 18060–18066.

Dizhoor, A.M., Chen, C.-K., Olshevskaya, E., Sinelnikova, V.V., Phillipov, P. and Hurley, J.B. (1993) Role of the acylated amino terminus of recoverin in Ca^{2+}-dependent membrane interaction. *Science*, 259: 829–832.

Dizhoor, A.M., Ericsson, L.H., Johnson, R.S., Kumar, S., Olshevskaya, E., Zozulya, S., Neubert, T.A., Stryer, L., Hurley, J.B. and Walsh, K.A. (1992) The NH_2 terminus of retinal recoverin is acylated by a small family of fatty acids. *J. Biol. Chem.*, 267: 16033–16036.

Dizhoor, A.M. and Hurley, J.B. (1996) Inactivation of EF-hands Makes GCAP-2 (p24) a Constitutive Activator of Photoreceptor Guanylyl Cyclase by Preventing a Ca^{2+}-induced "Activator-to-Inhibitor" Transition. *J. Biol. Chem.*, 271: 19346–19350.

Dizhoor, A.M. and Hurley, J.B. (1999) Regulation of photoreceptor membrane guanylyl cyclases by guanylyl cyclase activator proteins. *Methods*, 19: 521–531.

Dizhoor, A.M., Lowe, D.G., Olshevskaya, E.V., Laura, R.P. and Hurley, J.B. (1994) The human photoreceptor membrane guanylyl cyclase, RetGC, is present in outer segments and is regulated by calcium and a soluble activator. *Neuron*, 12: 1345–1352.

Dizhoor, A.M., Nekrasova, E.R. and Philippov, P.P. (1989) The binding of G proteins to immobilized delipidated rhodopsin. *Biochem. Biophys. Res. Commun.*, 162: 544–549.

Dizhoor, A.M., Olshevskaya, E.V., Henzel, W.J., Wong, S.C., Stults, J.T., Ankoudinova, I. and Hurley, J.B. (1995) Cloning, sequencing and expression of a 24 kDa Ca^{2+} binding protein activating photoreceptor guanylyl cyclase. *J. Biol. Chem.*, 270: 25200–25206.

Dizhoor, A.M., Ray, S., Kumar, S., Niemi, G., Spencer, M., Brolley, D., Walsh, K.A., Philipov, P.P., Hurley, J.B. and Stryer, L. (1991) Recoverin: A calcium sensitive activator of retina rod guanylate cyclase. *Science*, 251: 915–918.

Erickson, M.A., Lagnado, L., Zozulya, S., Neubert, T.A., Stryer, L. and Baylor, D.A. (1998) The effect of recombinant recoverin on the photoresponse of truncated rod photoreceptors. *Proc. Natl. Acad. Sci. USA*, 95: 6474–6479.

404

Fesenko, E.E., Kolesnikov, S.S. and Lyubarsky, A.L. (1985) Induction by cyclic GMP of cationic conductance in plasma membrane of retinal rod outer segment. *Nature*, 313: 310–313.

Flaherty, K.M., Zozulya, S., Stryer, L. and McKay, D.B. (1993) Three-dimensional structure of recoverin, a calcium sensor in vision. *Cell*, 75: 709–716.

Fung, B.K., Hurley, J.B. and Stryer, L. (1981) Flow of information in the light-triggered cyclic nucleotide cascade of vision. *Proc. Natl. Acad. Sci. USA*, 78: 152–156.

Gorczyca, W.A., Gray Keller, M.P., Detwiler, P.B. and Palczewski, K. (1994) Purification and physiological evaluation of a guanylate cyclase activating protein from retinal rods. *Proc. Natl. Acad. Sci. USA*, 91: 4014–4018.

Gorczyca, W.A., Polans, A.S., Surgucheva, I.G., Subbaraya, I., Baehr, W. and Palczewski, K. (1995) Guanylyl cyclase activating protein: a calcium-sensitive regulator of phototransduction. *J. Biol. Chem.*, 270: 22029–22036.

Gray-Keller, M.P., Polans, A.S., Palczewski, K., Detwiler, P.B. and Marshall, C.J. (1993) The effect of recoverin-like calcium-binding proteins on the photoresponse of retinal rods Protein prenylation: a mediator of protein-protein interactions. *Neuron*, 259: 1865–1866.

Gray-Keller, M.P. and Detwiler, P.B. (1994) The calcium feedback signal in the phototransduction cascade of vertebrate rods. *Neuron*, 13: 849–861.

Haeseleer, F., Sokal, I., Li, N., Pettenati, M., Rao, N., Bronson, D., Wechter, R., Baehr, W. and Palczewski, K. (1999) Molecular characterization of a third member of the guanylyl cyclase-activating protein subfamily. *J. Biol. Chem.*, 274: 6526–6535.

Hamilton, S.E. and Hurley, J.B. (1990) A phosphodiesterase inhibitor specific to a subset of bovine retinal cones. *J. Biol. Chem.*, 265: 11259–11264.

Hetling, J.R. and Pepperberg, D.R. (1999) Sensitivity and kinetics of mouse rod flash responses determined in vivo from paired-flash electroretinograms. *J. Physiol. (Lond.)*, 516: 593–609.

Howes, K., Bronson, J.D., Li, N., Zhang, K., Lee, M., Subbaraya, I., Frederick, J., Surguchov, A., Kolb, H., Palczewski, K. and Baehr, W. (1997) Molecular characterization of the mouse GCAP1/GCAP2 gene array and expression of GCAPs in the mouse retina. *Invest. Ophthalmol. Vis. Sci.*, 38: A93.

Hsu, Y.-T. and Molday, R.S. (1993) Modulation of the cGMP-gated channel of rod photoreceptor cells by calmodulin. *Nature*, 361: 76–79.

Hughes, R.E., Brzovic, P.S., Klevit, R.E. and Hurley, J.B. (1995) Calcium-dependent solvation of the myristoyl group of recoverin. *Biochemistry*, 34: 11410–11416.

Hurley, J.B. (1980) Isolation and recombination of bovine rod outer segment cGMP phosphodiesterase and its regulators. *Biochem. Biophys. Res. Commun.*, 92: 505–510.

Hurley, J.B. (1990) A likely history of G-protein genes. *Biochem. Soc. Symp.*, 56: 81–84.

Hurley, J.B., Barry, B. and Ebrey, T.G. (1981) Isolation of an inhibitory protein for the cyclic guanosine $3'5'$-mono-phosphate phosphodiesterase of bovine rod outer segments. *Biochim. Biophys. Acta*, 675: 359–365.

Hurley, J.B., Simon, M.I., Teplow, D.B., Robishaw, J.D. and Gilman, A.G. (1984) Homologies between signal transducing G proteins and ras gene products. *Science*, 226: 860–862.

Hurley, J.B. and Stryer, L. (1982) Purification and characterization of the g regulatory subunit of the cyclic GMP phosphodiesterase from retinal rod outer segments. *J. Biol. Chem.*, 257: 11094–11099.

Johnson, R.S., Ohguro, H., Palczewski, K., Hurley, J.B., Walsh, K.A. and Neubert, T.A. (1994) Heterogeneous N-acylation is a tissue- and species-specific posttranslational modification. *J. Biol. Chem.*, 269: 21067–21071.

Kachi, S., Nishizawa, Y., Olshevskaya, E., Yamazaki, A., Miyake, Y., Wakabayashi, T., Dizhoor, A. and Usukura, J. (1999) Detailed localization of photoreceptor guanylate cyclase activating protein-1 and -2 in mammalian retinas using light and electron microscopy. *Exp. Eye Res.*, 68: 465–473.

Kawamura, S. (1993) Rhodopsin phosphorylation as a mechanism of cyclic GMP phosphodiesterase regulation by S-modulin. *Nature*, 362: 855–857.

Kawamura, S. and Murakami, M. (1991) Calcium-dependent regulation of cyclic GMP phosphodiesterase by a protein from frog retinal rods. *Nature*, 349: 420–423.

Kelsell, R.E., Gregory-Evans, K., Payne, A.M., Perrault, I., Kaplan, J., Yang, R.B., Garbers, D.L., Bird, A.C., Moore, A.T. and Hunt, D.M. (1998) Mutations in the retinal guanylate cyclase (RETGC-1) gene in dominant cone-rod dystrophy. *Hum. Mol. Genet.*, 7: 1179–1184.

Koch, K.-W. and Stryer, L. (1988) Highly cooperative feedback control of retinal rod guanylate cyclase by calcium ions. *Nature*, 334: 64–71.

Laura, R.P., Dizhoor, A.M. and Hurley, J.B. (1996) The Membrane Guanylyl Cyclase, Retinal Guanylyl Cyclase-1, Is Activated through Its Intracellular Domain. *J. Biol. Chem.*, 271: 11646–11651.

Laura, R.P. and Hurley, J.B. (1998) The kinase homology domain of retinal guanylyl cyclases 1 and 2 specifies the affinity and cooperativity of interaction with guanylyl cyclase activating protein-2. *Biochemistry*, 37: 11264–11271.

Lem, J., Krasnoperova, N.V., Calvert, P.D., Kosaras, B., Cameron, D.A., Nicolo, M., Makino, C.L. and Sidman, R.L. (1999) Morphological, physiological, and biochemical changes in rhodopsin knockout mice. *Proc. Natl. Acad. Sci. USA*, 96: 736–741.

Lerea, C.L., Somers, D.E., Hurley, J.B., Klock, I.B. and Bunt-Milam, A.H. (1986) Identification of specific transducin α subunits in retinal rod and cone photoreceptors. *Science*, 234: 77–80.

Liu, Y., Ruoho, A.E., Rao, V.D. and Hurley, J.H. (1997) Catalytic Mechanism of the Adenylyl and Guanylyl Cyclases: Modeling and Mutational Analysis. *Proc. Natl. Acad. Sci. USA*, 94(25): 13414–13419.

Lowe, D.G., Dizhoor, A.M., Liu, K., Gu, Q., Spencer, M., Laura, R., Lu, L. and Hurley, J.B. (1995) Cloning and expression of a second photoreceptor-specific membrane retina guanylyl cyclase (RetGC), RetGC-2. *Proc. Natl. Acad. Sci. USA*, 92: 5535–5539.

Lyubarsky, A.L. and Pugh, E.N., Jr. (1996) Recovery phase of the murine rod photoresponse reconstructed from electroretinographic recordings. *J. Neurosci.*, 16: 563–571.

Matthews, H.R., Murphy, R.L.W., Fain, G.L. and Lamb, T.D. (1988) Photoreceptor light adaptation is mediated by cytoplasmic calcium concentration. *Nature*, 334: 67–69.

Nakatani, K. and Yau, K.-W. (1988) Calcium and light adaptation in retinal rods and cones. *Nature*, 334: 69–71.

Normann, R.A. and Perlman, I. (1979) Signal transmission from red cones to horizontal cells in the turtle retina. *J. Physiol. (Lond.)*, 286: 509–524.

Payne, A.M., Downes, S.M., Bessant, D.A., Taylor, R., Holder, G.E., Warren, M.J., Bird, A.C. and Bhattacharya, S.S. (1998) A mutation in guanylate cyclase activator 1A (GUCA1A) in an autosomal dominant cone dystrophy pedigree mapping to a new locus on chromosome 6p21.1. *Hum. Mol. Genet.*, 7: 273–277.

Pepperberg, D.R., Birch, D.G. and Hood, D.C. (1997) Photoresponses of human rods in vivo derived from paired-flash electroretinograms. *Vis. Neurosci.*, 14: 73–82.

Perrault, I., Rozet, J.-M., Calvas, P., Gerber, S., Camuzat, A., Dollfus, H., Chatelin, S., Souied, E., Ghazi, I., Leowski, C., Bonnemaison, M., Le Paslier, D., Frezal, J., Dufier, J.-L., Pittler, S., Minnich, A. and Kaplan, J. (1996) Retinal-specific guanylate cyclase gene mutations in Leber's congenital amaurosis. *Nat. Genet.*, 14: 461–464.

Pugh, E.N., Jr., Nikonov, S. and Lamb, T.D. (1999) Molecular mechanisms of vertebrate photoreceptor light adaptation. *Curr. Opin. Neurobiol.*, 9: 410–418.

Ray, S., Zozulya, S., Niemi, G.A., Flaherty, K.M., Brolley, D., Dizhoor, A.M., McKay, D.B., Hurley, J.B. and Stryer, L. (1992) Cloning, expression and crystallization of recoverin, a calcium sensor in vision. *Proc. Natl. Acad. Sci. USA*, 89: 5705–5709.

Shyjan, A.W., de Sauvage, F.J., Gillett, N.A., Goeddel, D.V. and Lowe, D.G. (1992) Molecular cloning of a retina-specific membrane guanylyl cyclase. *Neuron*, 9: 727–737.

Thomas, M.M. and Lamb, T.D. (1999) Light adaptation and dark adaptation of human rod photoreceptors measured from the a-wave of the electroretinogram. *J. Physiol. (Lond.)*, 518: 479–496.

Tsang, S.H., Gouras, P., Yamashita, C.K., Kjeldbye, H., Fisher, J., Farber, D.B. and Goff, S.P. (1996) Retinal degeneration in mice lacking the gamma subunit of the rod cGMP phosphodiesterase. *Science*, 272: 1026–1029.

Tucker, C.L., Hurley, J.H., Miller, T.R. and Hurley, J.B. (1998) Two amino acid substitutions convert a guanylyl cyclase, RetGC-1, into an adenylyl cyclase. *Proc. Natl. Acad. Sci. USA*, 95: 5993–5997.

Tucker, C.L., Woodcock, S.C., Kelsell, R.E., Ramamurthy, V., Hunt, D.M. and Hurley, J.B. (1999) Biochemical analysis of a dimerization domain mutation in RetGC-1 associated with dominant cone-rod dystrophy. *Proc. Natl. Acad. Sci. USA*, 96: 9039–9044.

Xu, J., Dodd, R.L., Makino, C.L., Simon, M.I., Baylor, D.A. and Chen, J. (1997) Prolonged photoresponses in transgenic mouse rods lacking arrestin. *Nature*, 389: 505–509.

Zozulya, S. and Stryer, L. (1992) Calcium-myristoyl protein switch. *Proc. Natl. Acad. Sci. USA*, 89: 11569–11573.

H. Kolb, H. Ripps and S. Wu (Eds.)
Progress in Brain Research, Vol. 131

CHAPTER 29

Light adaptation and contrast in the outer retina

Dwight A. Burkhardt*

*Departments of Psychology and Physiology and Graduate Program of Neuroscience, University of Minnesota,
75 E. River Road, Minneapolis, MN 55455, USA*

Introduction

My first glimpse into the world of visual physiology came when I was an optometry student and read Adler's *Physiology of the Eye* (Adler, 1953) in a course in physiological optics at Indiana University. It then seemed clear that there were two giants in the field of visual adaptation: Selig Hecht and George Wald. Only later would I find out that as I was reading Adler's book, a brilliant graduate student of Wald's, by the name of John E. Dowling, was already adding new chapters to the story on visual adaptation (Dowling and Wald, 1958; Dowling, 1960). By the time I had the good fortune to work under John as a postdoctoral fellow at Johns Hopkins, he was widely recognized for his studies on the relation between bleached rhodopsin and visual sensitivity in the normal and vitamin-A deprived retina. In subsequent years, John and his co-workers would go on to make many contributions to our understanding of visual adaptation (Dowling, 1987). For the present purposes, three are of special interest: (1) light adaptation, as revealed by large changes in incremental sensitivity and Weber's Law behavior, can come about without significant bleaching of the visual pigment, rhodopsin; (2) a large component of the sensitivity changes associated with visual adaptation may be ascribed to the photoreceptors themselves; and (3) in addition to the primary mechanisms in

photoreceptors, significant contributions are made by post-receptor or "network" mechanisms.

These three themes have provided the context for research on visual adaptation by many investigators for several decades. In this chapter, we review some of our own research that bears on these themes. It complements and extends some of John's earlier work since we focus on cone photoreceptors and cone photopigment, rather than on rods and rhodopsin, and our research on post-receptor mechanisms is based on intracellular recordings from bipolar cells. In the first part of this chapter, we take up the issue of the relation between photopigment bleaching and mechanisms of light adaptation in cones. In the second part, we examine the nature of contrast processing in bipolar cells and how it is modulated by light adaptation.

Light adaptation and Weber's Law in cones in the turtle retina

Intracellular recordings in response to light from a helium–neon laser were made from cones in the superfused eyecup of the turtle (*Pseudemys scripta elegans*) as previously described in detail (Burkhardt, 1994). In Fig. 1A, the column labeled "Dark", shows superimposed responses of a red-sensitive cone evoked by 632.8 nm flashes of variable intensity presented as 400 ms steps to the dark-adapted retina. These graded responses are typical for vertebrate cones and the resulting amplitude–intensity relation (not shown) was well-described by an equation of the

* Tel.: 612-625-6375, 612-625-0755; Fax: 612-626-2079;
E-mail: burkh001@maroon.tc.umn.edu

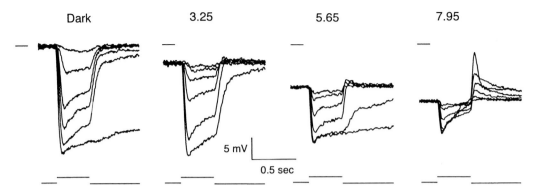

Fig. 1. Superimposed responses of a red-sensitive cone in the turtle retina evoked by 632.8 nm flashes of variable intensity presented as 400 ms steps in the dark-adapted retina (left column, labeled "Dark") and by a series of incremental flashes presented on steady background fields of 3.25, 5.65 and 7.95 log photons s^{-1} μm^{-2}. The incremental responses were evoked by flashes that were 0.09, 0.18, 0.47, 0.90 and 3.0 log units more intense than the background field.

Michaelis-Menten type (Perlman and Normann, 1998). In the column marked 3.25, the cone was exposed to a steady background field of 3.25 log photons s^{-1} μm^{-2}. The superimposed traces show responses evoked by incremental flashes of variable intensity. For the other two sets of responses, the retina was exposed to steady background fields of 5.65 and 7.95 log photons s^{-1} μm^{-2}, respectively, and responses were again evoked by a series of incremental flashes. From these records, it is evident that increasing the background illumination, and hence the state of light adaptation, leads to appreciable changes in the response waveforms along with an increase in the steady, "DC", hyperpolarization of the membrane potential.

Recordings like those of Fig. 1 were obtained from a sample of 15 cones and measurements of response amplitude were plotted against the stimulus intensity to find the flash intensities required to evoke a small criterion response (equivalent to 5% of the cone's maximum response in the dark). The reciprocal of these values, which specifies the step flash sensitivity, is plotted against the background intensity in Fig. 2. The smooth curve, which provides a satisfactory fit to the full range of the data, is given by the equation,

$$S_L/S_D = (1 + I/I_o)^{-1} \qquad (1)$$

where S_L and S_D are the sensitivity to a step (400 ms) in the presence of background light and in the dark, respectively, I is the intensity of the background

light, and I_o is the background intensity that reduces the step sensitivity by one half (Baylor and Hodgkin, 1974a; Matthews et al., 1990; Schnapf et al., 1990). The value for I_o in Fig. 2 is 500 photons s^{-1} μm^{-2}. It follows from Eq. (1) that when the background intensity, I, is very high relative to I_o, sensitivity will be inversely proportional to I. This is the relation classically known as Weber's Law, $\Delta I/I = k$ (where I is the background intensity, ΔI is the increment in light required to evoke a fixed criterion response, and k is a constant). The data in Fig. 2 conform closely to Weber's Law over the upper 7 decades of background illumination. This greatly exceeds the largest range of about 3.5 decades reported previously for Weber's Law behavior in vertebrate cones (Normann and Anderton, 1983). Thus, thanks to the very high intensities available from the helium–neon laser, we have been able to show that light adaptation in the red-sensitive cones holds over an exceedingly large range. The most intense background in Fig. 2 is about 1000 times greater than that of white paper illuminated by sunlight at noon.

Photopigment bleaching and light adaptation in cones

To analyze photopigment bleaching in turtle cones, a method was devised in which a measuring laser beam (632.8 nm) was incident on the back of the eyecup and was subsequently transmitted through the sclera and retina, and then to a

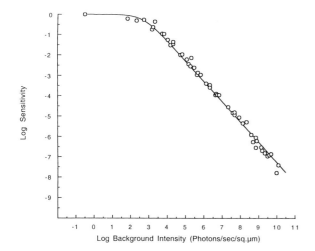

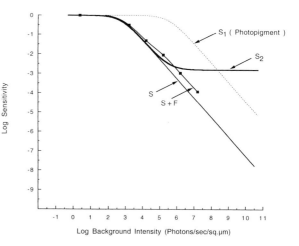

Fig. 2. Incremental step sensitivity measurements for a sample of 15 red-sensitive turtle cones. The equation for the smooth curve is given in the text, with I_o set at 2.70 log photons $s^{-1} \mu m^{-2}$. The open circle at the far left gives the sensitivity in the dark-adapted retina. Reprinted from Burkhardt (1994) with permission from the *Journal of Neuroscience*.

Fig. 3. Factors in light adaptation that influence the incremental sensitivity of cones: S, the intrinsic cone sensitivity (thin smooth curve, from Fig. 2); S_1, the sensitivity expected due to photopigment bleaching; S_2, the sensitivity due to all intrinsic mechanisms except photopigment bleaching; $S + F$, sensitivity due to all intrinsic mechanisms plus feedback from horizontal cells to cones.

measuring photodiode. Spectral measurements confirmed that the measured changes in transmission were restricted to the red-sensitive cones (Burkhardt, 1994). The success in achieving such good isolation with this method seems critically dependent on the facts that the red-sensitive cones are by far the most numerous of all receptor types (including rods) and that the wavelength (632.8 nm) and spectral purity of the measuring laser beam are optimal for selective absorption by the red-sensitive cones. The results were well-fit by the steady-state bleaching equation (Rushton and Henry, 1968; Hollins and Alpern, 1973):

$$P = I_h/(I_h + I) \qquad (2)$$

where I is the intensity of the steady background illumination in photons $s^{-1} \mu m^{-2}$, P is the fraction of pigment present, and I_h is the intensity which reduces P to 0.5, i.e. the half-bleaching constant. As realized at least since the time of Hecht (1937), by reducing the proportion of photons absorbed, photopigment bleaching will lead to a proportional loss of visual sensitivity. Thus, the dashed curve in Fig. 3, labeled S_1, shows the loss of sensitivity predicted by Eq. (1) above. The thin, solid curve labeled S, is the curve previously used to fit the sensitivity data in Fig. 2.

The heavy curve marked S_2 and the curve labeled $S + F$ will be considered later.

The effect of feedback from horizontal cells on the sensitivity of cones

It has been known for a long time that turtle cones receive an antagonistic feedback signal from horizontal cells (Baylor et al., 1971; reviewed in Burkhardt, 1993) and from time to time, it has been suggested that feedback might provide a mechanism for light adaptation in vertebrates. This was investigated in experiments in which the sensitivity for a centered, 150 μm spot was measured on a large and a small background field, 2200 μm and 250 μm in diameter, respectively. Previous work has shown that the influence of feedback should be maximal in the case of the large background field and negligible with the small field. (By the same token, the influence of feedback will be negligible in Fig. 2 since in those experiments, the background was only 100 μm in diameter.) It was found that the sensitivity of the cone was clearly enhanced on the large vs. small background (Burkhardt, 1995). This finding is illustrated by the squares in Fig. 3. At the higher backgrounds intensities, the squares lie above the smooth curve, i.e. the cone sensitivity in the absence of feedback. Thus, these results show that as the background intensity increases, the effect of feedback increases and can then enhance cone sensitivity by as much as ~ 0.5 log unit, i.e. some 3 fold.

Three mechanisms for light adaptation in turtle cones: an overview

Figure 3 leads to several conclusions about mechanisms for light adaptation in cones. The dotted curve, labeled S_1, shows the changes in sensitivity expected from the effects of bleaching, as given by the equation, $S_1 = kP$, where S_1 is the expected sensitivity, P is the fraction of photopigment present (see Eq. (1) above), and the constant k is set to 1.0. Fig. 3 thus shows that bleaching is insignificant at weak to moderate background intensities and can not be responsible for shaping cone sensitivity and Weber's Law behavior over this range. However, at higher intensities, bleaching becomes significant and since it decreases the available photopigment in proportion to the background intensity, it becomes an essential mechanism for preserving Weber's Law behavior at backgrounds of about 6.0–6.5 log photons s^{-1} μm^{-2} and higher. In short, the ability of turtle cones to maintain Weber's Law behavior over the exceedingly intense backgrounds covering the upper 3.5 decades of Fig. 3 is due to bleaching. Bleaching plays no such role in vertebrate rods since the Weber's Law range is limited and rods saturate, becoming totally unresponsive at intensities that bleach negligible amounts of rhodopsin (Pugh et al., 1999).

Since photopigment bleaching acts at the very first stage of the system as a simple scalar to reduce the cone sensitivity, it is possible to assess the contribution of mechanisms that act at later stages from the simple relation: $S = S_1 \times S_2$, where S is the measured cone sensitivity; S_1 is the effect of photopigment on sensitivity as described above; and S_2 is the total contribution of the mechanisms that act at later stages of the light adaptation processes. The heavy solid curve in Fig. 3 shows how S_2 varies with the background intensity. Thus, S_2 is wholly responsible for the change in sensitivity up to a background intensity of about 5 log photons s^{-1} μm^{-2} and by itself, is capable of impressing Weber's Law behavior

over a range of about 1.0–1.5 log units. Thereafter, over backgrounds from 5.0 to 6.5 log photons s^{-1} μm^{-2}, its contribution tends to level off as it acts in concert with bleaching to effectively maintain Weber's Law behavior. At higher backgrounds, all further *changes* in sensitivity are due to bleaching alone. It is tempting to think that the S_2 curve might represent the calcium-mediated control of cyclic GMP, which is generally viewed as the primary biochemical mechanism for photoreceptor light adaptation (Fain and Matthews, 1990; Koutalos and Yau, 1996). However, there appear to be several other nonbleaching mechanisms in rods (Pugh et al., 1999) and so the S_2 curve is probably best viewed as the lumped action of all intrinsic, non-bleaching mechanisms of cone light adaptation. Whatever their identity, Fig. 3 suggests that, in toto, these nonbleaching mechanisms are only designed to regulate sensitivity over about 2.5 decades and to directly accommodate incident light intensities of no more than 6.5 log photons s^{-1} μm^{-2}. Above this intensity, these mechanisms are effectively protected from overload, since their effective input depends on the photoisomerization rate and this is clamped by bleaching to a constant level of about 5×10^6 photoisomerizations s^{-1} (Burkhardt, 1994).

Feedback is an extrinsic mechanism of cone light adaptation since it is mediated by horizontal cells and thus, in Dowling's scheme (Dowling, 1987), qualifies as a network mechanism of light adaptation. It modifies the cone's amplitude–intensity curve (not shown) in a subtractive manner analogous to subtractive mechanisms inferred from human psychophysics (Burkhardt, 1995). In Fig. 3, the effect of feedback is illustrated as an increase in sensitivity from the level of the smooth curve, S, to the level of the squares. This effect appears very modest when viewed on the very large scale (eight orders of magnitude) of Fig. 3. The measurements, however, show that the effect increases with background intensity and can increase sensitivity by as much as $3\times$—a functionally significant change for modulating the detectability and salience of objects in natural environments. Thus, feedback from horizontal cells provides an additional mechanism of light adaptation in which the incremental sensitivity, initially set by intrinsic mechanisms in the outer segment, can be modulated some three-fold at the cone pedicle.

Contrast responses of bipolar cells and cones in the tiger salamander retina

In natural environments, most objects are defined by virtue of their contrast with respect to the ambient background. Hence, the mechanisms for contrast processing are of the utmost importance for retinal function. Although, it is widely appreciated that Weber's Law implies that very low contrasts will generate approximately invariant responses independent of the level of ambient illumination, this is, but a small facet of contrast processing. In natural environments, contrasts range from very low to very high and appear in two polarities: objects may be either brighter (positive contrast) or darker (negative contrast) than their backgrounds.

Pat Fahey and I have analyzed the response of bipolar cells in the retina of the tiger salamander (*Ambystoma tigrinum*) over a large domain of contrast by using a liquid crystal display to stimulate the center of the receptive field with contrast steps of variable magnitude and both polarities (Burkhardt and Fahey, 1998). Figure 4 shows some representative responses for a depolarizing (Bd) and a hyperpolarizing bipolar cell (Bh) while the retina was light-adapted to a steady background of 20 cd m^{-2}. Contrast is specified as the logarithm of the flash/background intensity ratio: Contrast $= \log_{10} (F/B)$, where B is the steady background intensity and F is the light intensity prevailing during the flash. It may be seen that the cells generate remarkably large responses to very small contrast steps (± 0.03),

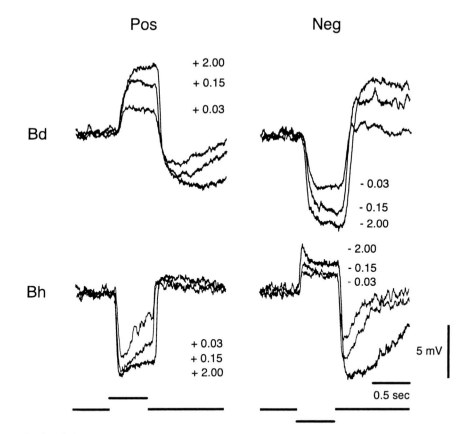

Fig. 4. Responses of a depolarizing bipolar cell (Bd) and a hyperpolarizing bipolar cell (Bh) in the tiger salamander retina to 500 ms steps of positive and negative contrast. The contrast is given to the right of each trace. Background illumination is 20 cd m^{-2}. The contrast gain (see text) for positive and negative contrast is, respectively, 8.1% and 16.2% for the Bd cell and 27% and 8.2% for the Bh cell. Reprinted from Burkhardt and Fahey (1998) with permission from the *Journal of Neurophysiology*.

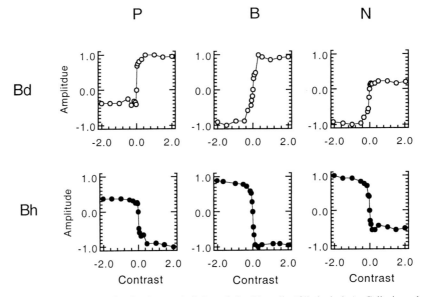

Fig. 5. Contrast–response curves for 3 Bd cells (open circles) and 3 Bh cells (filled circles). Cells in column P are positive-contrast dominant, cells in column N are negative contrast dominant, and cells in column B are balanced. Background illumination is 20 cd m^{-2}.

suggesting that the contrast gain (contrast sensitivity) is very high and that the contrast–response curve might be very steep and saturate at relatively low contrasts. These suggestions are fully borne out by the normalized contrast–response curves shown in Fig. 5 for 3 Bd cells (open circles) and 3 Bh cells (closed circles). These curves underscore the finding that the relative strength of responses to contrasts of opposite polarity varies markedly across both classes of bipolar cells. Thus, the cells in column P give their largest response to positive contrast, while those in column B give relatively balanced responses, and those in column N give their maximum response to negative contrast. Recordings from over 150 bipolar cells (Burkhardt and Fahey, 1998; Fahey and Burkhardt, unpublished) provide strong support for these and other substantial differences across the bipolar cell population. It is thus apparent that bipolar cells play a critical role in expanding the range and complexity of contrast coding.

The overall contrast–response curve of bipolar cells appears very nonlinear, regardless of whether the stimulus is scaled in log contrast, Michelson contrast, or the size of the light step (ΔL). When analyzed with respect to ΔL, the linear range was

found to be very narrow, limited to contrasts of $\sim \pm 0.03$. This result appears at odds with the generalization reached from white-noise analysis in the light-adapted catfish retina, that the bipolar cell response is predominantly linear (Sakai and Naka, 1987; Sakai et al., 1995). At least part of the apparent disagreement might be due to differences in species, the stimulus (steps vs. white noise), criteria for linearity, or the dynamic state of light adaptation. For brief flashes in the dark, the responses of rod-driven bipolar cells in the isolated retina of the tiger salamander are highly nonlinear overall, but show linearity for very small responses (Capovilla et al., 1987).

The contrast responses of cones were investigated under the same conditions as those used for bipolar cells. On the basis of spectral screening tests, all cones were identified as red-sensitive (610 nm) cones. Figure 6 shows the average contrast–response curve for a sample of 8 cones. The results were very similar from cell to cell as is evident by the relatively small error bars in Fig. 6. The dotted curve shows the result expected, if the response were linearly related to the magnitude of the light step, ΔL. The fit is satisfactory for small contrasts ($\sim \pm 0.20$), suggesting that linearity holds for small contrast steps, in

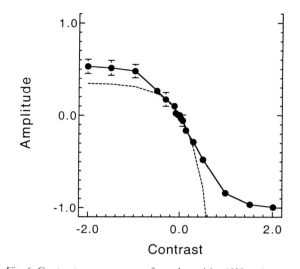

Fig. 6. Contrast–response curve for red-sensitive (610 nm) cones of the tiger salamander retina. Mean and standard deviations (error bars) for a sample of 8 cones. When not shown, error bars are smaller than the data points. Dotted curve shows the relation expected for linearity, i.e. if the amplitude were proportional to the size of the light step, ΔL (see text). Background illumination is 20 cd m^{-2}. Reprinted from Burkhardt and Fahey (1998) with permission from the *Journal of Neurophysiology*.

agreement with past evidence for small-signal linearity in cones. At the other extreme of the response continuum, Fig. 6 shows that the maximum responses of cones are about twice as large for positive than for negative contrast. Thus, unlike bipolar cells (see B and N, Fig. 5), cones are invariably positive-contrast dominant.

Contrast gain and signal transfer from cones to bipolar cells

Measurements of contrast gain, expressed as % of the maximum response/% contrast, were obtained from responses evoked by the smallest contrast (typically, $\pm 3\%$). Contrast is expressed here as % Michelson contrast since this metric has been commonly used in past work on contrast gain. (For low to moderate contrasts, % Michelson contrast is approximately equivalent to log contrast $\times$ 100). Under our standard conditions, the average contrast gain of cones was about 1%, i.e. a contrast of 1% evokes about 1% of the cone's maximum response. The average contrast gain of bipolar cells was much higher, about 10%.

Moreover, many bipolar cells, including the pair in Fig. 4, showed gains as high as 15–25% (see Fig. 4 legend). Thus, an almost imperceptible contrast of 1% was capable of evoking a response of some 15–25% of maximum from the more sensitive bipolar cells. Taken together, our results provide strong evidence for contrast gain amplification in the signal transfer from cones to bipolar cells.

Because the contrast–response curves of the 610 nm cones were very similar from cone to cone and additional tests showed that the bipolar cells in our sample received an overwhelming input from the 610 cones, further aspects of the signal transfer from cones to bipolar cells can be evaluated by plotting the response of individual cone-driven bipolar cells against the corresponding cone responses of Fig. 6.

Figure 7 shows a sample of such cone–bipolar plots for three Bd and three Bh cells. In all these plots, the measurements in the left and right quadrants correspond to responses to positive and negative contrast, respectively. For all cells, the slope for very small contrasts is very steep, implying high gain from cones to bipolar cells, and the response saturates rather quickly with stronger cone input. Normalized amplitude data from 44 cells were analyzed to determine the relative bipolar–cone slope gain by projecting the first point of the cone vs. bipolar plot to the origin and computing the resulting slope in dimensionless units. For positive and negative contrasts, respectively, the mean values were about -9 and -10 for Bd cells and $+12$ and $+7$ for Bh cells. Of the four possible comparisons, only the difference between the gain for positive vs. negative contrast for Bh cells reached statistical significance ($p = 0.006$).

When estimated as voltage gain, our values ranged from 5–9$\times$, and are thus comparable with past findings of voltage gains between 2.5 and 10 for small signals transmitted across the rod $\rightarrow$ bipolar synapse in the isolated retina of the tiger salamander (Capovilla et al., 1987; Yang and Wu, 1993; Wu, 1994). However, contrary to past findings for rod-driven bipolar cells, we did not find a significant difference between the mean gains for Bh vs. Bd cells for the cone-driven cells studied here. Moreover, although Bh cells showed a tendency to generate a somewhat larger total response than Bd cells, the difference in the means (13.1 vs. 10 mV) was not statistically significant. Indeed, over all the results

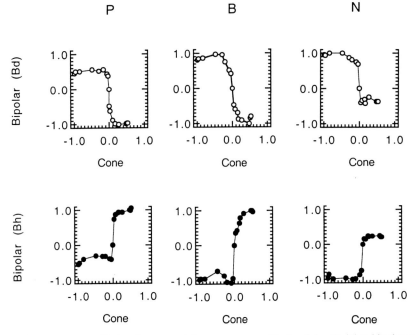

Fig. 7. Relation between the response amplitude of cones and the response amplitude of depolarizing bipolar cells (open circles) and hyperpolarizing bipolar cells (filled circles). Response amplitude is normalized for all cells. Data for the cones are based on the mean results shown in Fig. 6. Background illumination is 20 cd m^{-2}.

of our contrast experiments, the similarities between Bd and Bh cells were, rather surprisingly, more impressive than any differences.

Although the plots in Fig. 7 are compressed, they suggest that the cone–bipolar relation might be linear for a small range of signals. An analysis of this question showed that the range was very small, amounting to only $\sim \pm 5\%$ of the cone response, equivalent to a contrast range of less than ± 0.03. In the large signal domain, the remarkable steepness of the cone–bipolar curves is apparent from the finding that a half-maximal bipolar response is typically evoked by a cone response of some 15% of maximum and in a number of cases, the effective cone response was considerably smaller, falling in the 2–10% range. In absolute terms, on average, cone responses in the 1–2 mV range evoked a half-maximal bipolar response.

Modulation of contrast gain by light adaptation

To pursue the question of how light adaptation might modify contrast gain in bipolar cells and cones,

measurements were obtained on background fields ranging over nearly 4 decades from 0.2 to 1000 cd m^{-2}. Figure 8 gives mean results for a sample of 10 cones (circles), 30 Bh (triangles) and 25 Bd cells (squares). The results show that contrast gain is dependent on the level of light adaptation. As the background is increased from 0.2 to 1000 cd m^{-2}, the contrast gain of cones increases by about $3\times$ while that of bipolars cells increases by about $7\times$. This difference can not be ascribed to a fixed scaling operation since the curves of Fig. 8 clearly differ in shape when plotted in logarithmic co-ordinates. Thus, Fig. 8 suggests that there are at least two adaptation-dependent mechanisms regulating contrast gain. One is manifest in the cone voltage. The other arises between the voltage response of the cones and bipolar cells. It might be presynaptic (modulation of cone transmitter release) and/or postsynaptic, i.e. intrinsic to the bipolar cell.

As a possible mechanism, feedback from horizontal cells to cones has some appeal since: (1) By serving as a common presynaptic mechanism, it could provide a simple explanation for the rather surprising finding that the contrast gain of Bh and Bd cells show very similar variation with background

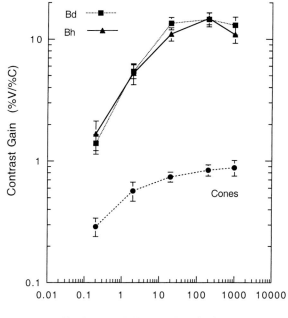

Fig. 8. Contrast gain for depolarizing bipolar cells (Bd, squares), hyperpolarizing bipolar cells (Bh, triangles) and cones (filled circles) as a function of background illumination. Error bars are ±S.E.M.

illumination (Fig. 8); (2) As shown in Fig. 3, feedback increases the incremental sensitivity (contrast gain) with increasing light adaptation in turtle cones (Burkhardt, 1995). However, it has not been possible to test the feedback hypothesis in the salamander retina since, to date, we have been unable to detect feedback in tiger salamander cones, in essential agreement with others (Hare and Owen, 1996; Roska et al., 2000). It remains possible that feedback might modulate synaptic transmission without inducing detectable changes in membrane potential, as has been suggested for goldfish cones (Kammermans and Spekreijse, 1999). On the other hand, quite apart from feedback, there appear to be several other possible mechanisms (Wu et al., 1993; Hare and Owen, 1995; Akopian et al., 2000; Brecha and Witkovsky, 2000; Thoreson et al., 2000) that might modulate transmitter release and contrast gain without affecting the cone membrane potential.

Figure 8 shows that at least part of the increase in contrast gain with light adaptation arises at or before

the generation of the cone response. We have some preliminary evidence that contrast gain and the steady DC potential of cones grow in parallel with background illumination. Given the multiple biochemical pathways implicated in transduction and light adaptation in photoreceptors (Fain and Matthews, 1990; Koutalos and Yau, 1996; Pugh et al., 1999), it seems probable that a common precursor(s) may lie at the root of a relation between contrast gain and DC potential in cones. For example, the decline in calcium that occurs with light adaptation and is believed to modulate the DC potential, might also modulate mechanisms that regulate contrast gain.

Different views of light adaptation: contrast gain vs. incremental sensitivity plots

It is instructive to analyze the present measurements of contrast gain in the context of the incremental sensitivity format that has been widely used in past studies of light adaptation. Because the contrast gain for cones in Fig. 8 is virtually constant over the background range of 20–1000 cd m^{-2} it follows that Weber's Law holds closely over this range. However, at weaker backgrounds (< 20 cd m^{-2}), the contrast gain varies with the background intensity and thus Weber's Law no longer holds.

To illustrate the above results in the context of the conventional incremental sensitivity format, we have converted our cone contrast gain data to incremental sensitivity. The results are shown in Fig. 9 by the filled circles. For comparison, the open circles give, over a sensitivity range of 5 log units, the incremental sensitivity data for turtle cones previously shown in Fig. 2. It is apparent that, the results for salamander and turtle cones are very similar. Both are reasonably well-described by the dashed smooth curve. It represents the general equation previously used in Fig. 2, $S_L/S_D = (1 + I/I_o)^{-1}$. Thus, when I is large relative to I_o, S_L/S_D is inversely proportional to I (Weber's Law) but when the background intensity is much lower and I is very small, the proportionality, and thus Weber's Law, no longer holds. Changes in flash sensitivity in the low-intensity background range of incremental sensitivity plots have often been ignored in the past and indeed, in the conventional,

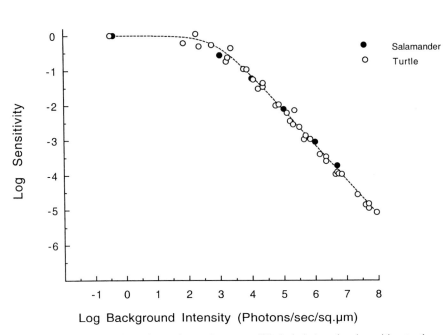

Fig. 9. Incremental sensitivity for red-sensitive tiger salamander cones (filled circles) and red-sensitive turtle cones (open circles). The smooth curve is based on Eq. (1) in the text with I_o set at 800 photons s^{-1} μm^{-2} to fit the salamander data. The data for the turtle cones are taken from Fig. 2. The two symbols at the far left show the sensitivity in the dark-adapted state.

low-resolution plots covering many orders of magnitude (e.g. Figs. 2 and 9), it is tempting to dismiss these changes as an insignificant prelude to the emergence of Weber's Law at higher intensities. To the contrary, our analysis of contrast gain in Fig. 8 displays these changes at higher resolution and thus underscores the fact that light adaptation exerts sizable and functionally important changes in cones and bipolar cells prior to the emergence of Weber's Law.

Conclusions and future perspective

Three stages of light adaptation can be identified from our experiments on turtle cones. The first stage is due to photopigment bleaching. It is negligible at low light levels, but becomes critical for maintaining Weber's Law behavior over moderate to extremely intense levels of background light. The second stage is responsible for light adaptation over the lowest 3 decades of background light, and over the upper 1.0–1.5 decades, is capable of mediating Weber's Law behavior. It acts in concert with photopigment bleaching at more intense backgrounds

and may be largely due to calcium-dependent regulation of cyclic GMP. The third stage is due to feedback from horizontal cells to cones. It provides an additional mechanism of light adaptation by which the incremental sensitivity, initially set by intrinsic mechanisms in the outer and inner segment, can be modulated by some three fold at the cone pedicle. It remains a challenging task for the future to conclusively establish the identity and mode of action of the cellular mechanisms responsible for the second and third stages of light adaptation in cones.

Intracellular recordings show that light adaptation modulates the contrast gain of bipolar cells in the tiger salamander retina. Contrast gain increases with increasing background intensity and then stabilizes at higher intensities, exhibiting Weber's Law behavior and reaching very high values in the 20–30 × range. The Weber's Law behavior arises in cones whereas the high contrast gain is due to amplification arising between the generation of the cone and bipolar voltage responses. The amplification of the bipolar contrast gain varies with the background illumination and is not a fixed multiple of the cone contrast gain. Thus, there appear to be at least two adaptation-dependent mechanisms regulating contrast gain. One is manifest at the level of the cone voltage. The other arises between the voltage response of the cones and bipolar cells. It remains a challenging task for the future to identify the nature of the mechanisms acting at each level. The second mechanism might be postsynaptic, i.e. intrinsic to the bipolar cell and/or presynaptic, e.g. modulation of cone transmitter release by feedback or other mechanisms.

Acknowledgments

This chapter is dedicated to John E. Dowling with deep appreciation for his support, intellectual stimulation, and friendship during my postdoctoral training and for more than 30 years thereafter. I would also like to express my appreciation to the National Eye Institute for supporting my research for many years. The research described here was supported by N.I.H. grant EY00406.

References

Adler, F.H. (1953) *Physiology of the Eye*. C. V. Mosby Co. St. Louis, Mo.

Akopian, A., Johnson, J., Gabriel, R., Brecha, N. and Witkovsky, P. (2000) Somatostatin modulates voltage-gated K^+ and Ca^{2+} currents in rod and cone photoreceptors of the salamander retina. *J. Neurosci.*, 20: 929–936.

Baylor, D.A., Fuortes, M.G.F. and O'Bryan, P.M. (1971) Receptive fields of cones in the retina of the turtle. *J. Physiol.*, 214: 265–294.

Baylor, D.A. and Hodgkin, A.L. (1974) Changes in time scale and sensitivity in turtle photoreceptors. *J. Physiol.*, 242: 729–753.

Burkhardt, D.A. (1995) The influence of center-surround antagonism on light adaptation in cones in the retina of the turtle. *Vis. Neurosci.*, 12: 877–885.

Burkhardt, D.A. (1994) Light adaptation and photopigment bleaching in cone photoreceptors *in situ* in the retina of the turtle. *J. Neurosci.*, 14: 1091–1105.

Burkhardt, D.A. (1993) Synaptic feedback, depolarization, and color opponency in cone photoreceptors. *Vis. Neurosci.*, 10: 981–989.

Burkhardt, D.A. and Fahey, P.K. (1998) Contrast enhancement and distributed encoding by bipolar cells in the retina. *J. Neurophysiol.*, 80: 1070–1081.

Capovilla, M., Hare, W.A. and Owen, W.G. (1987) Voltage gain of signal transfer from retinal rods to bipolar cells in the tiger salamander retina. *J. Physiol.*, 391: 125–140.

Dowling, J.E. and Wald, G. (1958) Vitamin A deficiency and night blindness. *Proc. Natl. Acad. Sci. USA*, 44: 648–641.

Dowling, J.E. (1960) The chemistry of visual adaptation in the rat. *Nature*, 188: 114–118.

Dowling, J.E. (1987) *The Retina: An Approachable Part of the Brain*. Cambridge, Mass: Belknap Press.

Fain, G.L. and Matthews, H.R. (1990) Calcium and the mechanism of light adaptation in vertebrate photoreceptors. *Trends Neurosci.*, 13: 378–384.

Hare, W.A. and Owen, W.G. (1996) Receptive field of the retinal bipolar cell: a pharmacological study in the tiger salamander. *J. Neurophysiol.*, 76: 2005–2019.

Hare, W.A. and Owen, W.G. (1995) Similar effects of carbochol and dopamine on neurons in the distal retina of the tiger salamander. *Vis. Neurosci.*, 12: 443–455.

Hecht, S. (1937) Rods, cones and the chemical basis of vision. *Physiol. Rev.*, 17: 239–290.

Hollins, M. and Alpern, M. (1973) Dark adaptation and visual pigment regeneration in human cones. *J. Gen. Physiol.*, 62: 430–447.

Kammermans, M. and Spekreijse, H. (1999) The feedback pathway from horizontal cells to cones: a mini-review with a look ahead. *Vision Res.*, 39: 2449–2468.

Koutalos, Y. and Yau, K.-W. (1996) Regulation of sensitivity in vertebrate rod photoreceptors by calcium. *Trends Neurosci.*, 19: 73–81.

Matthews, H.R., Fain, G.L., Murphy, R.L.W. and Lamb, T.D. (1990) Light adaptation in cone photoreceptors of the salamander: a role for cytoplasmic calcium. *J. Physiol.*, 420: 447–469.

Normann, R.A. and Anderton, P.J. (1983) The incremental sensitivity curve of turtle cone photoreceptors. *Vision Res.*, 23: 1731–1733.

Perlman, I. and Normann, R.A. (1998) Light adaptation and sensitivity controlling mechanisms in vertebrate photoreceptors. *Progress in Retinal Research*, 17: 523–563.

Pugh, E.N., Nikonov, S. and Lamb, T.D. (1999) Molecular mechanisms of vertebrate photoreceptor adaptation. *Curr. Opin. Neurobiol.*, 9: 410–418.

Roska, B., Nemeth, E., Orzo, L. and Werblin, F.S. (2000) Three levels of lateral inhibition: a space-time study of the retina of the tiger salamander. *J. Neurosci.*, 20: 1941–1951.

Rushton, W.A. and Henry, G.H. (1968) Bleaching and regeneration of cone pigments in man. *Vision Res.*, 8: 617–631.

Sakai, H.M. and Naka, K.-I. (1987) Signal transmission in the catfish retina. V. Sensitivity and circuit. *J. Neurophysiol.*, 58: 1329–1350.

Sakai, H.M., Wang, J.L. and Naka, K.I. (1995) Contrast gain control in the lower vertebrate retinas. *J. Gen. Physiol.*, 105: 815–835.

418

Schnapf, J.L., Nunn, B.J., Meister, M. and Baylor, D.A. (1990) Visual transduction in cones of the monkey, *macaca fascicularis*. *J. Physiol.*, 427: 681–713.

Thoreson, W.B., Nitzan, R. and Miller, R.F. (2000) Chloride efflux inhibits single calcium channel open probability in vertebrate photoreceptors: chloride imaging and cell-attached patch-clamp recordings. *Vis. Neurosci.*, 17: 197–206.

Thoreson, W.B. and Witkovsky, P. (1999) Glutamate receptors and circuits in the vertebrate retina. *Prog. Retin. Eye Res.*, 18: 765–810.

Wu, S., Qiaoxi, X., Noebels, J.L. and Yang, X.L. (1993) Localization and modulatory actions of zinc in vertebrate retina. *Vision Res.*, 33: 2611–2616.

Wu, S.M. (1994) Synaptic transmission in the outer retina. *Annu. Rev. Physiol.*, 56: 141–168.

Yang, X.-L. and Wu, S.M. (1993) Synaptic transmission from rods to rod-dominated bipolar cells in the tiger salamander retina. *Brain Res.*, 613: 275–280.

H. Kolb, H. Ripps and S. Wu (Eds.)
Progress in Brain Research, Vol. 131
© 2001 Elsevier Science B.V. All rights reserved

CHAPTER 30

Synaptic mechanisms of network adaptation in horizontal cells

Douglas G. McMahon*, Dao-Qi Zhang, Larissa Ponomareva and Tracy Wagner

Department of Physiology, University of Kentucky, Lexington, KY 40536-0084, USA

Introduction

In the retina, as in other areas of the brain, neural function emerges from an interplay between the intrinsic properties of neurons and the pattern, strength and functional characteristics of synaptic communication. A primary function of the neural retina, the transformation of photoreceptor signals into spatially and temporally dynamic neural output to the brain, is accomplished by synaptic interactions in the retinal plexiform layers. A fundamental tenet which has emerged from the study of synaptic mechanisms throughout the central nervous system is that synaptic ion channels and receptors are critical sites for the regulation of cell-to-cell signaling and thus are control points for the modulation of neural function. The mechanisms of synaptic plasticity are critical processes by which the nervous system adapts to changes in stimuli, reflects previous experience and shapes neural connections during development. John Dowling and his laboratory made seminal contributions to the study of neuromodulation in the retina, where modulation of transmission at glutamatergic and electrical synapses apparently underlies adaptational changes in the function of retinal neural networks to different levels of illumination (Lasater and Dowling, 1985; Knapp and Dowling, 1987).

The teleost fish retina has long served as a model preparation for studies of retinal neurophysiology and has been of particular importance with regard to understanding retinal neuromodulation. It was in this type of preparation that Dowling and his colleagues began their investigations of retinal neuromodulation (Dowling and Ehinger, 1978; Hedden and Dowling, 1978). The horizontal cell network of teleost fish retinas is both a critical locus for neuromodulation and a highly accessible experimental system which continues to yield insights into mechanisms of retinal synaptic plasticity. My own work, in JED's lab and after, has focused specifically on the ion channels mediating transmission at electrical and glutamatergic synapses because they are principal forms of excitatory communication in retinal networks, and on the modulatory effects of dopamine and nitric oxide on these synaptic conductances because these substances are also widely distributed in vertebrate retinas. In teleost retinas, dopamine is released from dopaminergic interplexiform cells which form an intraretinal feedback system, receiving their input from the inner plexiform layer and making their output in the outer plexiform layer, primarily onto horizontal cells (Dowling and Ehinger, 1978). Nitric oxide synthase, the enzyme which generates nitric oxide, is found in a wide variety of neurons in both the inner and outer teleost retina, including photoreceptors, horizontal cells, bipolar cells, amacrine cells and Muller cells so that there are local sources for this rapidly decaying transmitter substance in all retinal layers (Weiler and Kewitz, 1993; Liepe et al., 1994; Ponomareva et al., 1998). Recent results also suggest that zinc and retinoic acid may play

*Corresponding author: Douglas G. McMahon, Tel.: 859-257-2345; Fax: 859-323-1070; E-mail: dgmcma1@pop.uky.edu

important physiological roles in regulating retinal synaptic transmission at glutamate receptors and gap junctions (Weiler et al., 1998; McMahon et al., 1999; Pottek and Weiler, 2000; Zhang and McMahon, 2000).

Retinal horizontal cells are critical sites of convergence of these modulatory systems. The electrically coupled horizontal cell network is a post-synaptic element of the first visual synapse. It receives glutamatergic input from, and provides negative feedback to, the photoreceptors, influencing the dynamic range, spatial properties and color opponency of visual signals in bipolar cells, and subsequently, in neurons of the inner retina (for review see Dowling, 1987). In teleost fish retinas, horizontal cells also receive input from both major modulatory transmitter systems, through conventional synaptic input from dopaminergic interplexiform cells (Dowling and Ehinger, 1978), and through the NO/cGMP system (Weiler and Kewitz, 1993; Liepe et al., 1994; Ponomareva et al., 1998). These pathways are thought to play critical roles in shaping the functional characteristics of the horizontal cell network through their impact on horizontal cell synaptic communication. Similar mechanisms apparently shape the function of inner retinal circuits in mammals (Hampson et al., 1992; Mills and Massey, 1995).

Two principle synaptic conductances present in horizontal cells, gap junctions and glutamate receptors, are also primary routes for excitatory (sign conserving) signal transmission throughout the retina—glutamatergic transmission primarily mediates radial communication, whereas gap junctional transmission contributes primarily to lateral communication, but also to radial transmission in mammalian rod circuits. In the retina, more than any other region of the brain, it is clear that gap junctions play a critical role in neural function. Gap junctions are widely distributed in all synaptic layers of the retina and are of fundamental importance in transmitting and shaping visual signals (Vaney, 1991; Cook and Becker, 1995). For example, lateral inhibition in retinal receptive fields is directly attributable to electrical synaptic transmission between horizontal cells (Werblin and Dowling, 1969), while transmission of rod signals in the mammalian retina occurs through the AII-cone bipolar electrical synapse (Kolb and Famiglietti, 1974; Strettoi et al., 1992). In many other instances the function of extensive

gap junctional coupling in retinal neural networks remains incompletely understood. Cell-to-cell transmission at electrical synapses is mediated by ion channels composed of proteins called connexins. Molecular cloning has revealed that the connexins form a large gene family of structurally homologous ion channel proteins expressed in gap junctions (Bennett et al., 1994).

Ionotropic glutamate receptors mediate excitatory chemical synaptic transmission in the central nervous system and are widely distributed in all post-receptoral layers of the retina (Hughes et al., 1992; Muller et al., 1992; Hamassaki-Britto et al., 1993). As with gap junctions, horizontal cell glutamate receptors play a critical role in transmitting and shaping visual signals in the outer retina and they have provided a unique preparation for the study of glutamate receptor modulation. The physiological modulation of glutamate receptors was first reported in fish retinal horizontal cells by JED's laboratory, as were the mechanisms of this modulation at the single channel level (Knapp and Dowling, 1987; Knapp et al., 1990). This mechanism is a general one which is thought to be present in amphibian retinas (Witkovsky et al., 1989; Hare and Owen, 1995) and other regions of the vertebrate brain as well (Kalivas and Duffy, 1995). Our laboratory has recently reported novel mechanisms by which NO/cGMP/PKG acts to alter the responsiveness of horizontal cell glutamate receptors (McMahon and Ponomareva, 1996; McMahon and Schmidt, 1999). This is also likely to be of general significance for retinal function given the widespread distribution of both AMPA-type glutamate receptors and the NO transmitter system. The underlying mechanisms of glutamate receptor modulation are important for understanding network adaptation in the retina.

In summary, our research has focused on mechanisms of gap junction and glutamate receptor modulation in the retinal horizontal cell neural network. Through this approach, using fish horizontal cells as a well studied neurobiological system, we can elucidate critical neural mechanisms of visual signal transmission in retinal circuits and of network adaptation. The available evidence suggests that the mechanisms we are studying, while most experimentally accessible in horizontal cells, also operate at many other synapses in the vertebrate retina and brain.

Gap junctions and their modulation

The Dowling Lab and its disciples made primary observations establishing the modulation of neural gap junctions. Eric Lasater, working with JED, and then in his own lab, applied the newly described dual whole cell recording technique to isolated horizontal cell pairs and first established that horizontal cell gap junctional electrical coupling was modulated by dopamine through cAMP and PKA (Lasater and Dowling, 1985; Lasater, 1987). This demonstration of electrical synaptic modulation by a neurotransmitter spawned a high level of interest in the mechanisms by which vertebrate electrical synapses could be regulated and sparked my own work (with JED and then in my own lab) on how horizontal cell gap junctions are affected by neuromodulatory substances. Because a certain percentage of teleost retinal horizontal cells dissociate into primary cell culture as cell pairs, with their gap junction intact, they are a uniquely useful preparation for studying electrical synaptic modulation. One focus has been on elucidating how modulators act at the level of individual gap junction channels.

Gap junctional modulation by dopamine

Whereas Negishi had shown that dopamine modulated coupling between horizontal cells (Negishi and Drujan, 1979) and Lasater and Dowling (1985) had demonstrated that this effect was direct on the horizontal cells and caused their electrical uncoupling, the question still remained—how were the individual cell-to-cell channels which mediate cellular coupling being affected by dopamine? On the single channel level there were essentially three possible mechanisms to reduce the overall junctional conductance. Dopamine could: (i) reduce the conductance of individual gap junction channels through an effect on the ion-conducting pore, or it could; (ii) reduce the number of channels in the junction by removing or inactivating them, or it could; (iii) reduce the average current flowing through individual channels by altering the kinetics of their spontaneous opening and closing. In order to address this, we sought to analyze the currents flowing through individual horizontal cell gap junction channels in the presence or absence of dopamine and determine if any of the above three parameters were altered. The approach we took was to refine the dual whole cell recording technique. At the time we still used white perch horizontal cells in JEDs lab and although they were large and sturdy to facilitate electrophysiology, their strong coupling meant that individual gap junction channel currents could not usually be distinguished directly. At first, we used ensemble variance analysis of current noise from multichannel coupling currents (Fig. 1), and a few recordings in which we could distinguish individual channel openings, to establish that dopamine primarily affected the open probability of horizontal cell gap junction channels and did not appear to significantly affect either unitary conductance or channel number (McMahon et al., 1989). Later, in my own laboratory we extended this work to zebrafish horizontal cells (McMahon, 1994). These cells are quite a bit smaller than those of the perch, and although they are a challenge from which to record, they offer the benefit of true single channel gap junction recordings and a higher bandwidth due to reduced total membrane capacitance. With these advantages, we could better resolve the unitary conductance (50–60 pS for most channels) and distinguish that the reduction in open probability was due to both a reduction in mean open time (ca. 30%) and a decrease in the frequency of channel openings (ca. 50%, McMahon and Brown, 1994, Fig. 2). Thus the main effect of dopamine was to alter the spontaneous gating kinetics of gap junction channels so on average they spent less time in the open state and therefore conducted less current as a population.

What functional consequences does this kinetic form of channel modulation have for the horizontal cell network? One implication is that modulation of metabolic coupling of horizontal cells should scale in agreement with electrical coupling. If dopamine acted by changing pore size (unitary conductance), then it might selectively block the sharing of second messenger molecules which occurs through gap junction channels along with ionic flow. By altering channel kinetics, rather than pore geometry, the relative permeability of the junctions will remain

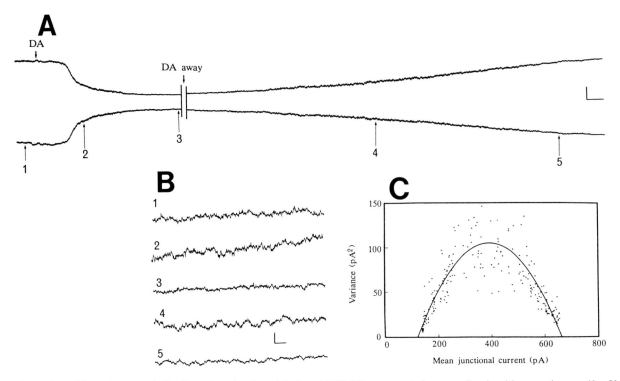

Fig. 1. Ensemble variance analysis of gap junctional modulation. (**A**) Holding currents from a cell pair with a continuous 40 mV transjunctional potential, uncoupling by dopamine is represented as the traces moving together, recovery by them moving apart (calibrations = 500 pA, 8 s). (**B**) Changes in current noise induced by dopamine. One second segments of the recording in (a) shown on an expanded time scale (calibrations = 50 pA, 100 ms). (**C**) Variance analysis of current noise modulation. Points are mean and variance of junctional current binned at one second intervals, line is parabolic fit of the data which gives an estimated change in open probability from 0.83 to 0.18 during dopamine modulation.

similar in the modulated and unmodulated states so that metabolic coupling would "scale" with alterations in electrical coupling.

Gap junctional modulation by nitric oxide

The gaseous neurotransmitter NO had also been identified as a neuroactive substance that uncoupled retinal horizontal cells through a second messenger pathway, in this case cGMP (DeVries and Schwartz, 1989; Miyachi et al., 1990). We sought to elucidate its mechanisms and compare its action with dopamine, given that the two modulatory pathways converged on the same electrical synaptic channels. On the level of second messenger mechanisms there is a strict parallelism with dopamine—that is NO acts on horizontal cell gap junctions through production of cGMP and activation of PKG (Lu and McMahon, 1997). Surprisingly, we found that whereas NO has similar effects to dopamine at the macroscopic level (i.e. electrical uncoupling) its action at the single channel level is distinct. NO achieves its uncoupling effect by altering gap junction channel gating kinetics, but is sole effect is to reduce opening frequency (Lu and McMahon, 1997, Fig. 3). This implies that DA/cAMP and NO/cGMP target different sites in the horizontal cell gap junction channel molecules.

While the above results demonstrate the modulation of electrical coupling by exogenous NO, they did not address the action of endogenously generated NO on horizontal cell coupling. Unlike dopamine, which is known to be secreted from interplexiform cells, the source of modulatory NO for horizontal cell coupling is not completely clear. In several species of fish,

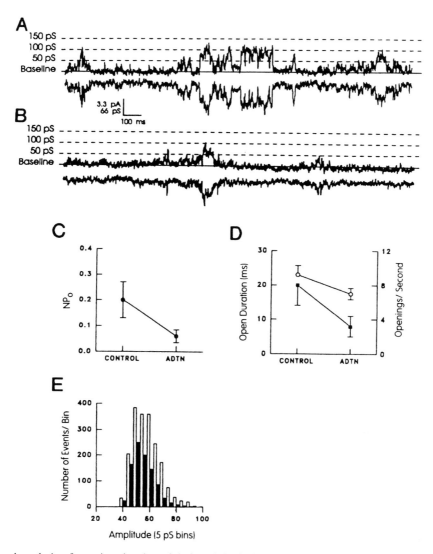

Fig. 2. Single channel analysis of gap junctional modulation. (A) Single channel junctional currents in the control condition, Vj = 50 mV. (B) Single channel junctional current from the same cell pair during application of 100 µM ADTN, a dopamine agonist. Note reduction in channel activity. (C) Reduction in overall open probability by ADTN. (D) Reductions in channel open duration (circles) and opening frequency (squares) by ADTN. (E) Lack of effect on unitary conductance by ADTN. For C–E, N = 5 cell pairs.

including the hybrid striped bass (Fig. 4), the enzyme nitric oxide synthase (NOS), or its markers, are present in a subset of horizontal cells (Weiler and Kewitz, 1993; Liepe et al., 1994), raising the possibility that horizontal cells may be NO sources for each other (by diffusion), or that horizontal cells may be sensitive to their own NO (i.e. self-modulation). NO is generally thought to act by diffusion because the Ca^{++} dependencies of NOS and its target, soluble guanylate cyclase, can fall into different concentration ranges. However, we have recently shown that stimulation of endogenous NOS in horizontal cell pairs in low-density cell culture leads to uncoupling (Ponomareva et al., 1998). In addition, similar treatment of isolated single cells modulates their glutamate responses (McMahon and Ponomareva, 1996). Taken together, these results suggest that horizontal cells are indeed sensitive to their own NO and therefore may self-modulate in situ.

424

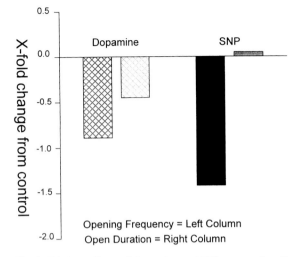

X-fold change from control

Opening Frequency = Left Column
Open Duration = Right Column

Fig. 3. Distinct effects of dopamine and NO on gap junction channel kinetics. Bar graph shows data from dopaminergic modulation of horizontal cell junctions (McMahon and Brown, 1994) compared with NO modulation (Lu and McMahon, 1997).

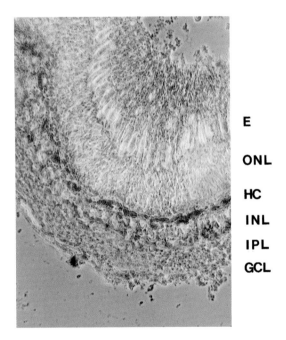

E

ONL

HC

INL

IPL

GCL

Fig. 4. NOS-like immunoreactivity in hybrid bass retina. Binding of anti-nNOS antibody (Transduction Laboratories, 2 µg/ml) visualized with DAB/peroxidase system (VECTOR) in the horizontal cell layers of a frozen section of hybrid bass retina. Abbreviations: E, photoreceptor ellipsoids; ONL, outer nuclear layer; HC, horizontal cell layer; INL, inner nuclear layer; IPL, inner plexiform layer; GCL, ganglion cell layer.

Gap junctional modulation by retinoic acid

Retinoic acid (RA), a retinoid metabolite, is widely distributed in retina and brain. It is conventionally known as a gene regulator via ligand-activated transcription factors, retinoic acid receptors (RARs) and retinoid X receptors (RXRs). As shown in JEDs lab and others, in the vertebrate eye, the RA signaling pathway is involved in early eye and photoreceptor development, through the activation of gene transcription mediated by nuclear receptors (Hyatt et al., 1992; Kelly et al., 1994; Marsh-Armstrong et al., 1994; Hyatt et al., 1996; Hyatt and Dowling, 1997). In the mature retina, however, RA biosynthesis has been shown to be regulated by light (McCaffery et al., 1996), and RA has also recently been reported to affect the structure and physiological coupling of retinal horizontal cells through a mechanism independent of its transcriptional effects (Weiler et al., 1998; Pottek and Weiler, 2000; see chapter by Weiler this volume).

Recently, our laboratory has investigated the mechanisms by which RA affects horizontal cell gap junction channels and several novel findings have emerged (Zhang and McMahon, 2000). All-*trans* RA (at-RA) uncouples cultured hybrid bass horizontal cells with an IC50 in the low micromolar range for horizontal cell pairs (Fig. 5) and in the sub-micromolar range for gap junction hemichannels. The acid moiety is critical because all-*trans* retinaldehyde and all-*trans* retinol are 50–100 times less effective at modulating gap junction channels, but at-RA does not act by altering physiological pH. RA modulates gap junction channels by reducing their open probability (Fig. 6). The effect on the channels is direct—neither second messengers, nor G-proteins are involved. Most surprisingly, the site of action is not on the cytoplasmic face, where most gap junctional modulators act, but is extracellular, both for hemichannels and coupled cell pairs. Dialysis of cells or pairs with RA in the recording pipette has no effect, whereas superfusion of RA closes hemichannels and uncouples pairs. In hemichannel preparations, at-RA acts to competitively inhibit the action of extracellular Ca^{++} on channel activity. Thus, our working hypothesis is that RA acts to close gap junction channels in horizontal cells by interacting with a site on the channels which can also bind

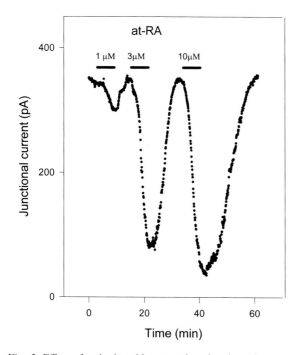

Fig. 5. Effect of retinoic acid on gap junctional conductance. Currents were acquired by stimulating one cell (driver cell) with a transjunctional voltage of 20 mV, 1 s pulses, and by holding another cell (follower cell) at 0 mV, then vice versa. The amplitude of junctional current was reduced by three different concentrations of at-RA.

extracellular Ca^{++} in the hemichannel state. The 5–10 fold increase in IC50 concentration for uncoupling of cell pairs vs hemichannels suggests that the access to or the binding affinity of this site for RA is changed by assembly of the hemichannels into gap junction channels.

Novel connexin physiologies

Most gap junction channels exhibit some form of voltage-dependent closure when voltage differences across the junction are elevated and horizontal cell junctional channels are no exception (McMahon, 1994; Lu and McMahon, 1996a). This channel characteristic may not play a prominent role in physiological modulation of coupling in the intact horizontal cell network as it is hard to imagine the circumstances in which transjunctional potentials sufficient to produce significant uncoupling

(ca. 40 mV) could be sustained between such well coupled cells. However, the degree of voltage-dependence (or lack thereof) has proven to be a useful parameter to distinguish different molecular isoforms of gap junction channels. While doing a careful survey of voltage-dependence in H2-type horizontal cells from the hybrid striped bass, Cheng-biao Lu, in my lab found that even within the population of H2 cell pairs there was an interesting distribution of voltage sensitivity. About on quarter of cell pairs exhibited strong voltage-dependent junctional closure, one half were voltage-dependent to lesser degrees, and one quarter had coupling which was insensitive to transjunctional voltage (Lu et al., 1999, Fig. 7). This voltage-insensitive coupling was indeed due to cell-to-cell channels, rather than cytoplasmic bridges or cellular damage, because these junctions were shown to limit or exclude the passage of Lucifer Yellow dye (Lu et al., 1999). Further characterization of this kind of coupling revealed that in addition to being insensitive to voltage, it was also comparatively insensitive to the physiological uncouplers dopamine and NO, with doses of these modulators near the IC50 for voltage-dependent coupling producing only 5–10% change in voltage independent junctions. Interestingly, coapplication of NO and of dopamine produced synergistic strong uncoupling of the voltage-insensitive junctions. Voltage insensitive junctions were also distinct at the single channel level. Single channels in these junctions exhibited a unitary conductance of 150 pS, rather than the 50–60 pS conductance associated with the previously described voltage-dependent channels in cell pairs of this type and species (Lu and McMahon, 1996a; Lu et al., 1999). Thus we concluded that we had distinguished a second type of horizontal cell coupling which was insensitive to high transjunctional voltages and relatively unresponsive to physiological modulators.

Since we had performed all our experiments with morphologically identified H2-type cell pairs, the clear implication was that there are two types of coupling exhibited by this cell type. One possible explanation for these observations is that the voltage-dependent and voltage-independent types of coupling are representative of two distinct connexin channel isoforms expressed in H2 horizontal cells. In this scenario, most cell pairs show intermediate

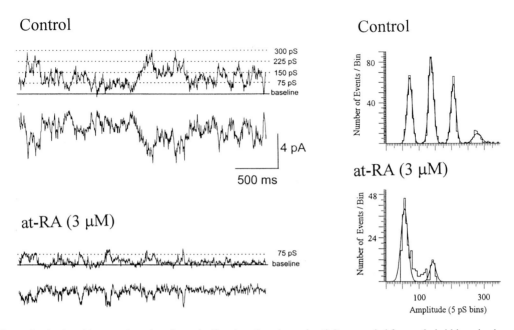

Fig. 6. Effects of retinoic acid on gap junction channels. Gap junction channel activity recorded from a hybrid bass horizontal cell pair using dual whole cell patch clamp. The control traces show multiple levels of conductance from the gating of several active channels. Following application of at-RA (lower traces) the channel activity was reduced, but the unitary conductance was unaffected.

voltage-dependence due to a mixture of junction types, but at the extremes of the distribution are cells in the voltage-dependent or voltage-independent channels dominate. Further molecular analysis will reveal if this speculation is supported, but regardless of the molecular basis, it is interesting to note the presence of two distinct functional forms of gap junctional coupling in a morphologically homogenous cell population.

Although we clearly must be cautious in interpreting the results of these in vitro studies, before similar in vivo work is performed, it is interesting to speculate on the potential functional implications of this distinct form of coupling on the horizontal cell network. Key in this regard is the lack of sensitivity of these junctions to dopamine and NO modulation. The presence of these junctions could act to limit the responsiveness of the network to dopamine and NO. In principle, regulation of their expression could offer a mechanism of tuning the responsiveness of the network to modulators. Alternately, if the modulator-insensitive junctions are expressed only in a subpopulation of H2 cells in situ, then they could form dopamine and NO insensitive subnetworks.

Molecular cloning of retinal connexins

Understanding the molecular basis of electrical synaptic transmission in the retina requires identification and physiological characterization of the gap junction channel isoforms which mediate cellular coupling. Tracy Wagner in my lab cloned, characterized, and functionally expressed a cDNA for a gap junction channel derived from the retina of the teleost fish (*Danio aquipinnatus* cx43, DACX43). The cDNA for DACX43, obtained by screening a danio retinal cDNA library, contains an open reading frame of 1146 nucleotides encoding a connexin protein with a predicted molecular mass of 43.3 kDa. In comparison with previously cloned connexin channel genes, it shares the greatest sequence homology with *Rattus norvegicus* Cx43 (78%). The predicted amino acid sequence (Fig. 8) shows regions of prominent sequence divergence from mammalian cx43 including the third transmembrane segment and the cytoplasmic loop, which have been proposed to mediate channel conductance and its regulation (Bennett et al., 1994; Becker et al., 1995; Wang and Peracchia, 1996). The predicted DACX43 sequence contains several consensus phosphorylation

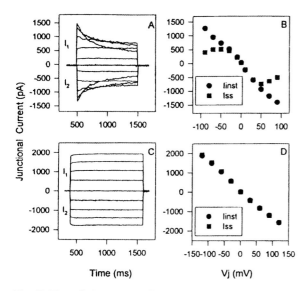

Fig. 7. Two distinct types of electrical coupling in H2-type hybrid bass horizontal cells. Traces show junctional currents recorded in follower cells in response to voltage steps into driver cells of 1 s in duration. Current traces were obtained by stepping driver cell voltage from −120 to +120 mV in 30 mV increments while holding the follower cell at 0 mV. (**A**). Voltage-dependent coupling currents. (**B**). Instantaneous junctional current (Iinst, circles) and steady state junctional current (Iss, squares) for the recording in A plotted as a function of Vj. The current–voltage relationships are linear for Iinst (a slope of 15 nS) and non-linear for Iss. Iss demonstrates voltage-dependent inactivation compared to Iinst beginning at Vj of ±40 mV. (**C**). Voltage-independent coupling current within a voltage range of −90 to +90 mV. (**D**). The current–voltage relations are linear for both instantaneous (Iinst, circles) and steady-state (Iss, squares) currents with a slope of 18 nS.

sequences in the c-terminal region, for PKA/PKG (T347), PKC (T261, S295, S369, S373) and PKC/CAKII (T256), some of which are conserved in mammalian Cx43. Northern blot hybridization revealed that DACX43 is expressed in the brain as well as in the retina. In addition, Southern analysis suggested that there are multiple copies of DACX43, or other closely related sequences, in the *Danio aquipinnatus* genome.

Using gap junction deficient mouse N2A neuroblastoma cells, we successfully established cell lines which stably express DACX43 and make functional gap junctions. Dual whole cell electrophysiology revealed that cell pairs expressing DACX43 mRNA exhibited bidirectional electrical coupling, whereas untransfected cell pairs were not coupled (Wagner

et al., 1998). Thus DACX43 forms functional gap junction channels.

Further characterization of DACX43 junctions in N2A cells has showed that they are not uncoupled by application of heptanol, a nearly universal gap junctional uncoupler, and that they do not exhibit voltage-dependent inactivation at elevated transjunctional voltages (up to ±100 mV). In addition, preliminary experiments stimulating PKA and PKG suggest that DACX43 junctions may be insensitive to these kinases. These unusual physiological and pharmacological properties are similar to those we have recently reported for novel voltage-independent HC gap junctions (Lu et al., 1999) and also to the previously cloned gap junction channel cx56 (Rup et al., 1993).

These results indicate that DACX43, a connexin channel gene expressed in both retina and brain, contains sequence differences from its rat homolog in the pore conducting and regulating region and potential phosphorylation sites for modulation by dopamine/PKA and NO/PKG. Preliminary characterization indicates that junctions composed of DACX43 exhibit similarities to the characteristics of voltage-independent horizontal cell junctions. There is biochemical and immunocytochemical evidence indicating the expression of cx43 in fish retinal horizontal cells (McMahon et al., 1994; Lu and McMahon, 1996b). In addition, recent immunocytochemical reports using antisera to rat cx43 have emphasized the expression of cx43 homologs in Muller cells of the fish retina (Giblin and Christensen, 1997; Ball and McReynolds, 1998; Janssen-Beinhold et al., 1998), but have also indicated the presence of lower levels of immunoreactivity in the OPL (Giblin and Christensen, 1997; Janssen-Beinhold et al., 1998). Taken together, these results suggest that fish homologs of cx43 may be primary component of Muller cell gap junctions, and may constitute a portion of the connexin channels in fish horizontal cell junctions.

Modulators of glutamate receptors

The 1987 paper by Knapp and Dowling, in which they demonstrated that dopamine and cAMP increased glutamate receptor responses in horizontal

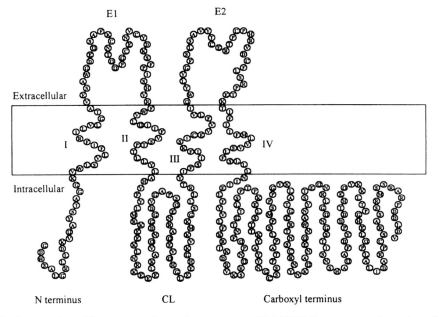

Fig. 8. Predicted primary amino acid sequence and secondary structure of DACX43. Roman numerals mark predicted transmembrane alpha helices, CL marks the cytoplasmic loop, E1 and E2 mark the extracellular channel interaction domains.

cells, represents the primary description of glutamate receptor modulation in the vertebrate central nervous system. This, of course, has become an area of widespread interest because of its potential impact on so many fundamental questions of neural function and disease. My own laboratory has examined the action on horizontal cell glutamate receptors of two other modulators present in the outer plexiform layer, NO and zinc.

Glutamate receptor modulation by nitric oxide

With a role established for NO in modulating horizontal cell electrical coupling, we next sought to examine if it also affected transfer of signal from the photoreceptors by modulation of horizontal cell glutamate-gated currents. Larissa Ponomareva in my lab began to examine this question. Her initial findings were that NO modulation decreased the amplitude of horizontal cell responses to both kainate and glutamate—the opposite of dopamine's action (McMahon and Ponomareva, 1996). This effect could not be blocked with cyclothiazide, suggesting that it was not due to increased receptor desensitization. As

with NO's effect on gap junctions, glutamate receptor modulation was mimicked by application of cGMP and blocked by cellular dialysis with a peptide inhibitor of PKG (McMahon and Ponomareva, 1996). This scheme turned out to be too simplistic as further investigation using a full range of agonist concentrations in the "concentration-ramp" technique developed by K.F. Schmidt, at Justus-Liebig University in Giessen, revealed a dual action of NO on glutamate currents (McMahon and Schmidt, 1999). NO both *decreased* the apparent affinity of receptors for glutamate (i.e. increased the EC50 concentration) and *increased* the maximal current (Fig. 9). The overall dose-response relation resulting from these competing changes exhibited decreased amplitude responses below EC50 and increased amplitude responses at high agonist concentrations. Application of cGMP only produced the rightward shift in EC50, suggesting that the increase in I_{max} was perhaps a direct effect of NO on the receptors.

How might glutamate receptor modulation by NO affect the function of the photoreceptor-horizontal cell synapse? Experiments applying NO to intact retinas revealed that NO had two seemingly contradictory effects on horizontal cell glutamate

A.

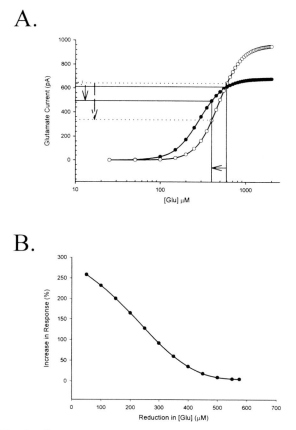

B.

Fig. 9. Effects of SNP on horizontal cell glutamate responses and modeling of predicted effects on resting potential and photoresponses. (**A**) Combined dose-response curves for glutamate and glutamate in the presence of SNP illustrating the increase in I_{max} and rightward shift in affinity. Values for glutamate alone (filled symbols) are an EC_{50} of 287 μM, I_{max} of 681 pA and Hill coefficient of 2.95. The values for glutamate plus SNP (open symbols) are 484 μM, 960 pA and 3.29 respectively. Upper set of horizontal lines show the predicted currents evoked by 600 μM glutamate alone (solid line) and in the presence of SNP (dotted line). Lower set of horizontal lines show the predicted currents evoked by 400 μM glutamate alone (solid line) and in the presence of SNP (dotted line). SNP produces a net increase in inward glutamate current evoked by glutamate concentrations greater than 550 μM but a net decrease in inward current evoked by glutamate concentrations less than this amount. Length of the vertical arrows indicate the size of the response (change in current) evoked by a decrease in glutamate concentration from 600 to 400 μM in the absence of SNP (solid arrow) and the presence of SNP (dotted arrow). (**B**) Changes in horizontal cell photocurrents (i.e. the reduction in inward current due to reduction in glutamate concentration) induced by SNP plotted vs the decrease in glutamate concentration, starting from 600 μM. The predicted increase in photocurrent is proportionally greater for small reductions in glutamate concentration.

transmission—it depolarized the dark resting potential while also increasing the amplitude of the hyperpolarizing light responses (Pottek et al., 1997). While NO is likely to have presynaptic effects as well as those on the post-synaptic horizontal cell receptors (Rieke and Schwartz, 1994; Kurenny et al., 1994; Noll et al., 1994; Savchenko et al., 1997), the specific dual changes in the glutamate receptor dose-response relation induced by NO can qualitatively account for both the effects of NO on horizontal cell membrane potential and on response amplitude (McMahon and Schmidt, 1999). As shown in Fig. 9, if the concentration of glutamate at the receptors in the dark is above the crossover point of the NO and control dose-response relations, then the dark membrane potential will be depolarized due to the increase in I_{max} and the amplitude of responses evoked by decreases in glutamate (light responses) will be increased due to the increase in EC50. Thus, one possible explanation for NO's actions in situ is embodied in the NO-glutamate receptor interactions we have described.

NO, like dopamine, is proposed to act as an adapting retinal neuromodulator. Although the measurements of NO release conditions in retinas are limited, a recent report indicates that overall NO production in the rabbit retina is increased by both flickering and steady background light (Neal et al., 1998). The increased synaptic transfer predicted by the above scheme of NO modulation of glutamate receptors could, in combination with photoreceptor adaptational mechanisms, act to preserve the amplitude of horizontal cell light responses in the presence of background light.

Glutamate receptor modulation by zinc

Zinc is a trace metal which is most strikingly co-localized with glutamate-containing synaptic terminals in the retinal photoreceptor layer and present in presynaptic terminals throughout the retina (Wu et al., 1993). Zinc is taken up and sequestered in glutamate-containing synaptic vesicles by a specific zinc transporter (Palmiter et al., 1996; Wenzel et al., 1997) providing the possibility that zinc may be also co-released with glutamate from synaptic terminals (Wu et al., 1993). Indeed, with intense activity, zinc concentrations as high as 200–300 μM may be obtained in synaptic clefts of the hippocampus (Assaf and Chung, 1984). Therefore, zinc may play an important physiological role in modulating postsynaptic responses to different levels of glutamatergic input to retinal neurons.

In our laboratory, Dao-Qi Zhang has been assaying for Zn effects on horizontal cell glutamate receptors and has found that it produces a unique monotonic decrease in AMPA-type glutamate receptor responses. Whole-cell currents and single channel activity gated by glutamate agonists were recorded from hybrid striped bass retinal neurons dissociated in cell culture. Coapplication of 300 μM zinc decreased the steady state horizontal cell kainate induced currents by ca. 60% and kainate currents recorded from putative amacrine and ganglion cells by ca. 30%. Additional characterization of this effect was performed on horizontal cell AMPA-type glutamate receptor currents which were gated by

AMPA and blocked by GYKI 52446. The dose-inhibition relationship for glutamate and AMPA responses by zinc concentrations from 0.5 to 2000 μM showed inhibition at all concentrations and yielded a half maximal inhibitory concentration of 100–175 μM and a maximal fractional inhibition of ca. 80% (Fig. 10). The inhibitory effects of zinc on glutamate responses persisted in the presence of the desensitization inhibitor cyclothiazide, indicating that it does not act by increasing rapid desensitization. At the single channel level, zinc did not affect single channel conductance, but did significantly reduce channel open probability.

This study in bass retinal neurons demonstrated monotonic inhibition by zinc of currents mediated by AMPA-type glutamate receptors in both desensitized and non-desensitized states. This is clearly distinct from the dual modulation by zinc of AMPA-receptors in superior colliculus neurons

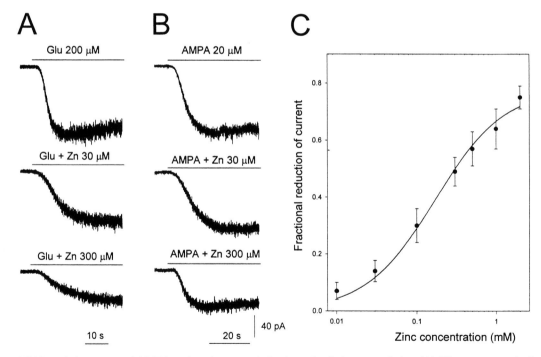

Fig. 10. Inhibition of glutamate and AMPA-activated currents in horizontal cells by external zinc. (**A**). The upper trace is the inward current evoked in a cell by 200 μM glutamate ($V_H = -60$ mV). After washout, the inward current elicited by glutamate slightly decreased in the presence of 30 μM zinc as shown in the middle trace. The lower trace shows the current was decreased with co-application of glutamate and 300 μM zinc. (**B**). Similar results were obtained with AMPA as the agonist. Inward currents induced by 20 μM AMPA were inhibited by 30 μM (middle trace) and 300 μM zinc (lower trace). (**C**). Dose-response curve for the fractional reduction of current produced by different doses of zinc (0.5–2000 μM). Each point shows the means ± S.E.M. of data from 5 cells. Smooth curve is a best-fit by Michaelis-Menten equation with a K_m of 168 μM and R_{max} of 0.78.

(Bresink et al., 1996) and on recombinant non-NMDA receptors expressed in Xenopus oocytes (Rassendren et al., 1990). In those preparations, zinc less than 500–1000 µM potentiated the response mediated by non-NMDA receptors, whereas zinc at higher concentrations inhibited glutamate receptor responses. In our studies, we found only inhibition, even at zinc concentrations in the low micromolar range. Our findings are also unique with respect to retinal neurons. Modulation by zinc of non-NMDA receptors was not found in salamander, carp and perch retinal horizontal cells under physiological conditions (Wu et al., 1993; Schmidt, 1999; Shen and Yang, 1999).

The inhibition of AMPA receptor mediated glutamate responses which we have described in dissociated retinal neurons could significantly modulate glutamatergic transmission in the retina, and by implication, other regions of the CNS. Although retinal zinc is most strikingly localized in photoreceptor terminals, areas of concentration exist in the inner retinal layers as well (Wu et al., 1993). The majority of our studies focused on zinc inhibition of glutamate response in horizontal cells, which are post-synaptic to photoreceptors, but we did find that kainate responses were also reduced in inner retinal neurons putatively identified as amacrine or ganglion cells by morphology. Thus, this mechanism is potentially widespread within the retina. In our cultured cell preparations, 50% inhibition of glutamate currents was achieved at zinc concentrations of 100–200 µM. At present, it is unclear what is the physiological range of zinc concentrations in retinal synaptic clefts (Wu et al., 1993; Spiridon et al., 1998) although concentrations as high as 200–300 µM may occur in the hippocampus during stimulation of glutamatergic synapses (Assaf and Chung, 1984), indicating that our findings are of potential physiological relevance.

Glutamate release from photoreceptors onto horizontal cells is high in the dark, thus presumably zinc, which is thought to be co-released with glutamate, would also obtain its highest synaptic levels under these conditions. The inhibitory mechanism we have described could serve to reduce horizontal cell responses to the continuously released glutamate in the dark adapted retina. However, since multiple sites of action for zinc action have already been identified

in the outer retina, the overall effect of zinc on outer retinal function is likely to be more complex. Zinc released from the photoreceptors may inhibit GABA responses and glutamate transporters of cone photoreceptors in the outer retina (Dong and Werblin, 1995; Spiridon et al., 1998) which could lead to inhibition of horizontal cell GABA feedback to cones and less uptake of glutamate from the synaptic cleft. In addition, exogenously applied zinc blocks glutamate release from photoreceptors, presumably by blocking voltage-dependent calcium channels in photoreceptor terminals (Wu et al., 1993) a mechanism which could come into play if there is spillover of zinc from the synaptic cleft.

The strong suppression of zinc on I_{max} is opposite of the actions of NO and dopamine, two endogenous modulators of glutamate receptors in the retina, which have been shown to enhance the I_{max} (Kruse and Schmidt, 1993; McMahon and Schmidt, 1999). All three modulators are likely participate in modulation of glutamate receptor function in retinal horizontal cells in situ. Additional experiments with intact retinal preparations are needed to further clarify the role of zinc in retinal function.

Dopamine/NO interactions

The fact that the dopamine and NO transmitter systems converge onto cone-driven horizontal cells of fish retinas provokes the question—Do these neuromodulators interact in their regulation of glutamatergic and electrical synapses of horizontal cells? Although NO and dopamine could interact at many levels—from release to second messengers—our previous work demonstrating partial overlap in their influence on gating kinetics of gap junction channels suggested to us that interactions may also take place at the level of their target molecules, the synaptic ion channels of HCs. We therefore tested for positive or negative interactions in the modulation of coupling or glutamate currents during coapplication of dopamine and the NO donor SNP.

We have examined this issue as part of other studies of coupling and GluR modulation. In terms of interactions with gap junctions—we determined dose ranges of SNP and dopamine which each typically decreased coupling (voltage-dependent) in

H2 HCs by approximately 50% (100–300 µM for each modulator, Fig. 11). We then applied both modulators simultaneously which resulted in a 92% reduction in junctional conductance on average. Thus, NO and dopamine act in an additive way to strongly uncouple HCs, as would be expected from their individual actions.

In contrast, dopamine and NO have opposing effects on the amplitude of HC glutamate currents elicited by puffs of agonist (McMahon and Ponomareva, 1996), so that we initially expected that simultaneous application would lead to negative interactions. To examine this, we performed glutamate dose-response curves in the presence of a saturating dose of SNP alone (2 mM) and 2 mM SNP plus a saturating dose of 200 µM dopamine (Fig. 12). Surprisingly, even in the presence of SNP,

dopamine produced a substantial (3-fold) increase in I_{max}, similar to its effects when applied in isolation (Kruse and Schmidt, 1993). Dopamine in the presence of NO also produced a further decrease in receptor affinity (increased EC50 from ca. 400 µM to ca. 700 µM). Thus, when applied together, dopamine and NO do not block each others action, but in fact act synergistically to strongly modulate HC glutamate receptors (McMahon and Schmidt, 1999).

For both horizontal cell glutamate receptors and gap junction channels NO/PKG and DA/PKA produce potent and additive effects upon coapplication. Thus it may be that these transmitters act as comodulators of horizontal cell synaptic physiology in the intact retina. At present, little is known regarding any correlated release or higher order interactions of these modulators which may occur in situ.

Conclusions and future perspectives

When I came to John Dowling's lab in 1986 the concept of neuromodulation in retinal neural networks revolved around dopamine acting as a

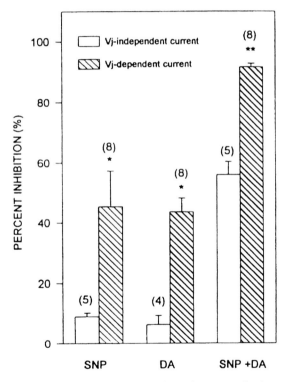

Fig. 11. Effects of SNP and dopamine co-application on voltage-dependent and voltage-independent coupling. Each bar represents mean ± SD. Statistical comparisons were made between Vj-dependent and Vj-independent couplings by Student *t*-test (unpaired). *$p < 0.05$, **$p < 0.01$. The effect of coapplication was additive for voltage-dependent coupling and synergistic (i.e. more than additive) for voltage-independent coupling.

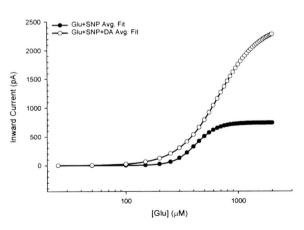

Fig. 12. Synergistic effects of dopamine and NO on glutamate responses. Dose-response curves to glutamate in the presence of 2 mM SNP or in the presence of 2 mM SNP plus 200 µM dopamine. Figure shows average responses for six neurons. An increase in EC50 and in I_{max} were evident in the responses recorded in the presence of both modulators when compared to SNP alone. On average, in the presence of SNP, dopamine further enhanced the increase in EC50 from 422 µM ± 91 to 682 µM ± 200 and tripled I_{max} from 740 pA ± 334 to 2455 pA ± 1485 ($p < 0.05$, paired *t*-tests).

modulator of ion channels at retinal synapses to affect circuit dynamics. The analysis of dopamine as the prototype retinal neuromodulator by JED and his lab—including anatomy, intact retina physiology, biochemistry, cellular and finally molecular physiology by patch clamp—provided the blueprint for defining the roles and actions of additional modulatory neuroactive substances in the retina. Interestingly, the physiological role of dopamine is still a matter of intense research with recent evidence from a mutagenesis approach, reiterating the view that dopamine mediates dark-adapting processes (Li and Dowling, 2000a, 2000b), whereas physiological approaches have favored its release by flickering background light (Weiler et al., 1997).

Our own research has been concentrated at the cellular and molecular levels and has been highly successful at identifying novel mechanisms of synaptic modulation in horizontal cells. As summarized in Fig. 13, these include the effects of NO on gap junction and glutamate receptor ion channel function, synergistic interactions of dopamine and NO in targeting these synaptic conductances (McMahon and Schmidt, 1999; Lu et al., 1999), retinoic acid acting as an external modulator of gap junctional coupling and zinc suppression of the activity of AMPA-type glutamate receptors (McMahon et al., 1999; Zhang and McMahon, 2000). Of note is the

fact that whereas dopamine and NO exert their modulatory effects through second messengers and kinases, retinoic acid and zinc may act directly on the external faces of gap junction and glutamate receptor channels. NO may use both direct and second messenger modes because its effects are only partially mimicked by its second messenger cGMP. These results obtained with patch-clamp recording from isolated cells can precisely describe cellular and subcellular mechanisms of synaptic plasticity and suggest the possibility that these mechanisms could regulate horizontal network function in situ, but cannot resolve their actual contribution to the intact system.

Critical questions raised by the cellular research remain unaddressed in the intact retina. For example—What is the effect of endogenously generated NO in the fish retina and under what conditions is it released? How do dopamine and NO affect one another's regulation of horizontal cell receptive fields and light responses? How does of glutamate receptor modulation contribute to overall regulation of HC network light responses? Do retinoic acid and zinc fulfill their potential roles as synaptic modulators in situ? The ultimate goal of our research is understanding critical retinal mechanisms and not only the workings of retinally expressed ion channels and receptors. Thus, in the future we expect combine our

Synaptic Modulation in Horizontal Cells

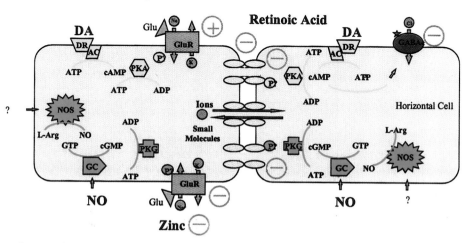

Fig. 13. Summary diagram of synaptic modulation mechanisms in teleost horizontal cells.

434

cellular and molecular studies with electrophysiology in the intact isolated retina. We hope to reveal new and significant information on the molecular basis of network adaptation in the retina, a fundamental visual mechanism.

References

Assaf, S.Y. and Chung, S.H. (1984) Release of endogenous zinc from brain tissue during activity. *Nature (Lond.)*, 308: 734–736.

Ball, A.K. and McReynolds, J.S. (1998) Localization of gap junctions and tracer coupling in retinal Muller cells. *J. Comp. Neurol.*, 393: 48–57.

Becker, D.L., Evans, W.H., Green, C.R. and Warner, A. (1995) Functional analysis of amino acid sequences in connexin43 involved in intercellular communication through gap junctions. *J. Cell. Sci.*, 108: 1455–1467.

Bennett, M.V., Zheng, X. and Sogin, M.L. (1994) The connexins and their family tree. *Soc. Gen. Physiol. Ser.*, 49: 223–233.

Bresink, I., Ebert, B., Parsons, C.G. and Mutschler, E. (1996) Zinc changes AMPA receptor properties: results of binding studies and patch clamp recordings. *Neuropharmacology*, 35: 503–509.

Cook, J.E. and Becker, D.L. (1995) Gap junctions in the vertebrate retina. *Microsc. Res. Tech.*, 31: 408–419.

DeVries, S.H. and Schwartz, E.A. (1989) Modulation of an electrical synapse between solitary pairs of catfish horizontal cells by dopamine and second messengers. *J. Physiol (Lond.)*, 414: 351–375.

Dong, C.-J. and Werblin, F.S. (1995) Zinc downmodulates the GABAC receptor current in cone horizontal cells acutely isolated from the catfish retina. *J. Neurophysiol.*, 73: 916–919.

Dowling, J.E. (1987) *The retina: an approachable part of the brain*. Cambridge, MA: Belknap Press of Harvard University Press.

Dowling, J.E. and Ehinger, B. (1978) The interplexiform cell system. I. Synapses of the dopaminergic neurons of the goldfish retina. *Proc. R. Soc. Lond. B*, 201: 7–26.

Giblin, L.J. and Christensen, B.N. (1997) Connexin43 immunoreactivity in the catfish retina. *Brain Res.*, 755: 146–150.

Hamassaki-Britto, D.E., Hermans-Borgmeyer, I., Heinemann, S. and Hughes, T.E. (1993) Expression of glutamate receptor genes in the mammalian retina: the localization of GluR1 through GluR7 mRNAs. *J. Neurosci.*, 13: 1888–1898.

Hampson, E., Vaney, D.I. and Weiler, R. (1992) Dopaminergic modulation of gap junction permeability between amacrine cells in the mammalian retina. *J. Neurosci.*, 12: 4911–4922.

Hare, W.A. and Owen, W.G. (1995) Similar effects of carbachol and dopamine on neurons in the distal retina of the tiger salamander. *Vis. Neurosci.*, 12: 443–455.

Hedden, W.L. Jr. and Dowling, J.E. (1978) The interplexiform cell system. II. Effects of dopamine on goldfish retinal neurones. *Proc. R. Soc. Lond. B Biol. Sci.*, 201: 27–55.

Hughes, T.E., Hermans-Borgmeyer, I. and Heinemann, S. (1992) Differential expression of glutamate receptor genes (GluR1-5) in the rat retina. *Vis. Neurosci.*, 8: 49–55.

Hyatt, G.A., Schmitt, E.A., Marsh-Armstrong, N.R. and Dowling, J.E. (1992) Retinoic acid-induced duplication of the zebrafish retina. *Proc. Natl. Acad. Sci. USA*, 89: 8293–8297.

Hyatt, G.A., Schmitt, E.A., Fadool, J.M. and Dowling, J.E. (1996) Retinoic acid alters photoreceptor development in vivo. *Proc. Natl. Acad. Sci. USA*, 93: 13298–13303.

Hyatt, G.A. and Dowling, J.E. (1997) Retinoic acid. A key molecule for eye and photoreceptor development. *Invest. Ophthalmol. Vis. Sci.*, 38: 1471–1475.

Janssen-Bienhold, U., Dermietzel, R. and Weiler, R. (1998) Distribution of connexin43 immunoreactivity in the retinas of different vertebrates. *J. Comp. Neurol.*, 396: 310–321.

Kalivas, P.W. and Duffy, P. (1995) D1 receptors modulate glutamate transmission in the ventral tegmental area. *J. Neurosci.*, 15: 5379–5388.

Kelly, M.W., Turner, J.K. and Reh, T.A. (1994) *Development*, 120: 2091–2102.

Knapp, A.G. and Dowling, J.E. (1987) Dopamine enhances excitatory amino acid-gated conductances in retinal horizontal cells. *Nature*, 325: 437–439.

Knapp, A.G., Schmidt, K.F. and Dowling, J.E. (1990) Dopamine modulates the kinetics of ion channels gated by excitatory amino acids in retinal horizontal cells. *Proc. Natl. Acad. Sci. USA*, 87: 767–771.

Kolb, H. and Famiglietti, E.V. (1974) Rod and cone pathways in the inner plexiform layer of cat retina. *Science*, 186: 47–49.

Kruse, M. and Schmidt, K.-F. (1993) Studies on the dopamine-dependent modulation of amino acid-gated currents in cone horizontal cells of the perch (Perca fluviatilis). *Vision Res.*, 33: 2031–2042.

Kurenny, D.E., Moroz, L.L., Turner, R.W., Sharkey, K.A. and Barnes, S. (1994) Modulation of ion channels in rod photoreceptors by nitric oxide. *Neuron*, 13: 315–324.

Lasater, E.M. (1987) Retinal horizontal cell gap junctional conductance is modulated by dopamine through a cyclic AMP-dependent protein kinase. *Proc. Natl. Acad. Sci. USA*, 84: 7319–7323.

Lasater, E.M. and Dowling, J.E. (1985) Dopamine decreases conductance of the electrical junctions between cultured retinal horizontal cells. *Proc. Nat. Acad. Sci.*, 82: 3025–3029.

Li, L. and Dowling, J.E. (2000a) Disruption of the olfactoretinal centrifugal pathway may relate to the visual system defect in *night blindness b* mutant zebrafish. *J. Neurosci.*, 20: 1883–1892.

Li, L. and Dowling, J.E. (2000b) Effects of dopamine depletion on visual sensitivity of zebrafish. *J. Neurosci.*, 20: 1893–1903.

Liepe, B.A., Stone, C., Koistinaho, J. and Copenhagen, D.R. (1994) Nitric oxide synthase in Mueller cells and neurons of salamander and fish retina. *J. Neurosci.*, 14: 7641–7654.

Lu, C. and McMahon, D.G. (1996a) Gap junction channel gating at bass retinal electrical synapses. *Vis. Neurosci.*, 13: 1049–1057.

Lu, C. and McMahon, D.G. (1996b) Partial sequence of a gap junction channel from the hybrid striped bass retina. *Soc. Neurosci. Abs.*, 22: 883.

Lu, C. and McMahon, D.G. (1997) Modulation of hybrid bass retinal gap junctional channel gating by nitric oxide. *J. Physiol.*, 499: 689–699.

Lu, C., Zhang, D.-Q. and McMahon, D.G. (1999) Electrical coupling in retinal horizontal cells mediated by distinct voltage-independent gap junctions. *Vis. Neurosci.*, 16: 811–818.

Marsh-Armstrong, N., McCaffery, P., Gilbert, W., Dowling, J.E. and Drager, U.C. (1994) Retinoic acid is necessary for development of the ventral retina in zebrafish. *Proc. Natl. Acad. Sci. USA*, 91: 7286–7290.

McCaffery, P., Mey, J. and Drager, U.C. (1996) Light-mediated retinoic acid production. *Proc. Natl. Acad. Sci. USA*, 93: 12570–12574.

McMahon, D.G. (1994) Modulation of electrical synaptic transmission in zebrafish retinal horizontal cells. *J. Neurosci.*, 14: 1722–1734.

McMahon, D.G. and Brown, D.R. (1994) Modulation of gap-junction channel gating at zebrafish retinal electrical synapses. *J. Neurophysiol.*, 72: 2257–2268.

McMahon, D.G. and Ponomareva, L.V. (1996) Nitric oxide and cGMP modulate retinal glutamate receptors. *J. Neurophysiol.*, 76: 2307–2315.

McMahon, D.G. and Schmidt, K.F. (1999) Horizontal cell glutamate receptor modulation by NO: mechanisms and implications for the first visual synapse. *Vis. Neurosci.*, 16: 425–433.

McMahon, D.G., Knapp, A.G. and Dowling, J.E. (1989) Horizontal cell gap junctions: single channel conductance and modulation by dopamine. *Proc. Natl. Acad. Sci. USA*, 86: 7639–7643.

McMahon, D.G., Rischert, J.C. and Dowling, J.E. (1994) Protein content and cAMP-dependent phosphorylation of fractionated white perch retina. *Brain Res.*, 659: 110–116.

McMahon, D.G., Zhang, D.Q. and Lu, C. (1999) Zinc modulation of glutamate receptors on retinal horizontal cells. *Invest. Ophthalmol. Vis. Sci.*, 40: S1275.

Mills, S.L. and Massey, S.C. (1995) Differential properties of two gap junctional pathways made by AII amacrine cells. *Nature*, 377: 734–737.

Miyachi, E., Murakami, M. and Nakaki, T. (1990) Arginine blocks gap junctions between retinal horizontal cells. *Neuroreport*, 1: 107–110.

Muller, F., Greferath, U., Wassle, H., Wisden, W. and Seeburg, P. (1992) Glutamate receptor expression in the retina. *Neurosci. Lett.*, 138: 179–182.

Neal, M., Cunningham, J. and Matthews, K. (1998) Selective release of nitric oxide from retinal amacrine and bipolar cells. *Invest. Opthalmol. Vis. Sci.*, 39: 850–853.

Negishi, K. and Drujan, B.D. (1979) Reciprocal changes in center and surrounding S potentials of fish retina in response to dopamine. *Neurochem. Res.*, 4: 313–318.

Noll, G.N., Billek, M., Pietruck, C. and Schmidt, K.F. (1994) Inhibition of nitric oxide synthase alters light responses and dark voltage of amphibian photoreceptors. *Neuropharmacology*, 33: 1407–1412.

Palmiter, R.D., Cole, T.B., Quaife, C.J. and Findley, S.D. (1996) ZnT-3, a putative transporter of zinc into synaptic vesicles. *Proc. Natl. Acad. Sci. USA*, 93: 14934–14939.

Ponomareva, L., Lu, C., Stone, J., deVente, J. and McMahon, D.G. (1998) Effects of nitric oxide on intracellular cGMP in horizontal cells of the hybrid striped bass retina. *Soc. Neurosci. Abstr.*, 24: 642.

Pottek, M., Schultz, K. and Weiler, R. (1997) Effects of nitric oxide on the horizontal cell network and dopamine release in the carp retina. *Vision Res.*, 37: 1091–1102.

Pottek, M. and Weiler, R. (2000) Light-adaptive effects of retinoic acid on receptive field properties of retinal horizontal cells. *Eur. J. Neurosci.* 12: 437–445.

Rassendren, F.A., Lory, P., Pin, J.P. and Nargeot, J. (1990) Zinc has opposite effects on NMDA and non-NMDA receptors expressed in Xenopus Oocytes. *Neuron*, 4: 733–740.

Rieke, F. and Schwartz, E.A. (1994) A cGMP gated current can control exocytosis at cone synapses. *Neuron*, 13: 863–873.

Rup, D.M., Veenstra, R.D., Wang, H.Z., Brink, P.R. and Beyer, E.C. (1993) Chick connexin-56, a novel lens gap junction protein. Molecular cloning and functional expression. *J. Biol. Chem.*, 268: 706–712.

Savchenko, A., Barnes, S. and Kramer, R.H. (1997) Cyclic-nucleotide-gated channels mediate synaptic feedback by nitric oxide. *Nature*, 390: 694–698.

Shen, Y. and Yang, X.L. (1999) Zinc modulation of AMPA receptors may be relevant to splice variants in carp retina. *Neurosci. Lett.*, 259: 177–180.

Schmidt, K.F. (1999) Divalent cations modulate glutamate receptors in retinal horizontal cells of the perch (Perca fluviatilis). *Neurosci. Lett.*, 262: 109–112.

Spiridon, M., Kamm, D., Billups, B., Mobbs, P. and Attwell, D. (1998) Modulation by zinc of the glutamate transportes in glial cells and cones isolated from the tiger salamander retina. *J. Physiol.*, 506: 363–376.

Strettoi, E., Raviola, E. and Dacheux, R.F. (1992) Synaptic connections of the narrow-field, bistratified rod amacrine cell (AII) in the rabbit retina. *J. Comp. Neurol.*, 325: 152–168.

Vaney, D.I. (1991) Many diverse types of retinal neurons show tracer coupling when injected with biocytin or neurobiotin. *Neurosci. Lett.*, 125: 187–190.

Wagner, T.L.E., Beyer, E.C. and McMahon, D.G. (1998) Cloning and functional expression of a novel gap junction channel from the retina of Danio aquipinnatus. *Vis. Neurosci.*, 15: 1137–1144.

Wang, X.G. and Peracchia, C. (1996) Connexin 32/38 chimeras suggest a role for the second half of inner loop in gap junction gating by low pH. *Am. J. Physiol.*, 271: C1743–C1749.

Weiler, R. and Kewitz, B. (1993) The marker for nitric oxide synthase, NADPH-diaphorase, co-localizes with GABA in horizontal cells and cells of the inner retina in the carp retina. *Neurosci. Lett.*, 158: 151–154.

Weiler, R., Baldridge, W.H., Mangel, S.C. and Dowling, J.E. (1997) Modulation of endogenous dopamine release in the

436

fish retina by light and prolonged darkness. *Vis. Neurosci.*, 14: 351–356.

Weiler, R., Schultz, K., Pottek, M., Tieding, S. and Janssen-Beinhold, U. (1998) Retinoic acid has light-adaptive effects on horizontal cells in the retina. *Proc. Natl. Acad. Sci. USA*, 95: 7139–7144.

Wenzel, H.J., Cole, T.B., Born, D.E., Schwartzkroin, P.A. and Palmiter, R.D. (1997) Ultrastructural location of zinc transporter-3 (ZnT-3) to synaptic vesicle membranes within mossy fiber boutons in the hippocampus of mouse and monkey. *Proc. Natl. Acad. Sci. USA*, 94: 12679–12681.

Werblin, F.S. and Dowling, J.E. (1969) Organization of the retina of the mudpuppy, Necturus maculosus, II: Intracellular recording. *J. Neurophysiol.*, 32: 339–355.

Witkovsky, P., Stone, S. and Tranchina, D. (1989) Photoreceptor to horizontal cell synaptic transfer in the Xenopus retina: modulation by dopamine ligands and a circuit model for interactions of rod and cone inputs. *J. Neurophysiol.*, 62: 864–881.

Wu, S.M., Qiao, X., Noebels, J.L. and Yang, X.L. (1993) Localization and modulatory actions of zinc in vertebrate retina. *Vision Res.*, 33: 2611–2616.

Zhang, D.Q. and McMahon, D.G. (2000) Direct gating by retinoic acid of retinal electrical synapses. *Proc. Natl. Acad. Sci. USA*, 97: 14754–14759.

H. Kolb, H. Ripps and S. Wu (Eds.)
Progress in Brain Research, Vol. 131

CHAPTER 31

Triphasic adaptation of teleost horizontal cells

William H. Baldridge*

Retina and Optic Nerve Laboratory, Departments of Anatomy and Neurobiology and Ophthalmology, Dalhousie University, Halifax, NS, Canada B3H 4H7

Introduction

The first intracellular recordings from any vertebrate retina were made from horizontal cells of a teleost (Svaetichin, 1953). Although a great deal was subsequently learned about the response properties, connectivity and functional role of retinal horizontal cells it was not until more than 30 years later that work from the laboratory of John E. Dowling at Harvard University clearly indicated that the response properties of teleost horizontal cells were not static but depended on the adaptation state of the retina. That is, the responses and receptive-field properties of these cells changed dramatically depending on the level of ambient illumination or on the prior light history of the retina. This work profoundly influenced a number of retinal neuroscientists, myself included. For me, the work started by Dowling has culminated in a hypothesis that the effect of ambient illumination on horizontal cell activity is not described by the classical two states of adaptation, dark- and light-adaptation, but is most parsimoniously explained by positing three states of adaptation. In this chapter I will review, more or less historically, the work that ultimately led to the development of the hypothesis of triphasic adaptation of horizontal cells. The focus will be evidence from the teleost retina but the situation in other vertebrate retinas will be briefly considered as will the

functional significance of horizontal cell triphasic adaptation. Although data from many different laboratories shall be considered, the influence of John Dowling on this area of study will be clearly evident.

Horizontal cells in the teleost retina

Horizontal cells are one of two classes of retinal neuron that receive direct synaptic input from photoreceptors, the other being bipolar cells. In teleosts the pattern of synaptic input is usually generalized from the description of goldfish (*Carassius auratus*) horizontal cells (Stell, 1967; Stell and Lightfoot, 1975), with three types of cone-driven horizontal cells and one type of rod-driven horizontal cell. Depending on the species (e.g. Hassin, 1979), one or two of the cone-driven horizontal cell types hyperpolarize regardless of the wavelength of light and hence, are termed luminosity-type horizontal cells (LHCs). The response polarity of the other cone-driven horizontal cell(s) depends on wavelength and, therefore, are termed chromaticity-type horizontal cells (CHCs). Rod horizontal cells receive input exclusively from rods.

The size of the receptive field of horizontal cells is much greater than their dendritic field size due to extensive gap junction coupling between horizontal cells of the same type (Yamada and Ishikawa, 1965; Naka and Rushton, 1967). There is now extensive evidence (for review see Baldridge et al., 1998) that the receptive-field size of horizontal cells is not fixed

---

* Tel.: 902-494-6305; Fax: 902-494-6309;
E-mail: wbaldrid@is.dal.ca

438

but can be reduced by a number of neuromodulators. In most cases these neuromodulators reduce receptive-field size, at least in part, by increasing gap junction resistance (Lasater and Dowling, 1985; McMahon et al., 1989; Lu and McMahon, 1997) but some may also reduce receptive-field size by decreasing membrane resistance (Piccolino et al., 1984). Many of these modulators also reduce the responsiveness of horizontal cells, acting post-synaptically by modulating the synaptic input from photoreceptors (Knapp and Dowling, 1987; McMahon and Ponomareva, 1996). The responsiveness and receptive-field size of teleost horizontal cell is also affected by the adaptation state of the retina and this will be the main focus of the following sections in this chapter.

Prolonged darkness decreases horizontal cell responsiveness and receptive-field size

In 1985 Stuart Mangel and John Dowling were the first[1] to describe changes in the response properties of horizontal cells in the teleost retina as a function of adaptation state. In retinas from goldfish, maintained in complete darkness for a prolonged period (>2 h) prior to isolation, the responsiveness and receptive-field size of LHCs were decreased compared to the situation when the fish were kept in the dark for only a short period (30 min) prior to study (see Fig. 1). The key changes were: (1) that the response amplitude of LHCs to relatively small spot stimuli (for example, 0.4 mm diameter) were greater in retinas subject to prolonged darkness than brief darkness whereas; (2) the response amplitude to large (>6.0 mm diameter) or full-field stimuli were decreased following prolonged darkness. The relative increase of the response to small spot stimuli is consistent with an increase in gap junction resistance and decreased receptive-field size (Piccolino et al., 1984). The response to a large-diameter spot or a full field should not be affected by changes in gap junction coupling (Mangel and Dowling, 1987) and, therefore, the reduced responsiveness is due to a

---

[1] It should be noted that Yang, Tauchi and Kaneko reported evidence of horizontal cell dark-suppression in abstract form in 1982.

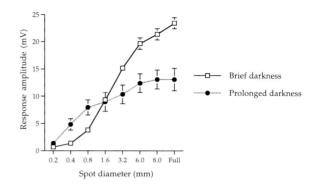

Fig. 1. Effect of brief and prolonged darkness on the responses of goldfish LHCs to spot and full-field stimuli. Horizontal cell responses to small spot stimuli are relatively increased after prolonged darkness ($n = 8$) compared to brief darkness ($n = 16$). Responses to large spot or full-field stimuli are decreased following prolonged darkness. These data indicate that prolonged darkness decreases the receptive-field size and responsiveness of horizontal cells. Error bars are SEM. Data re-plotted from Mangel and Dowling (1985).

mechanism other than one affecting gap junctions. One possible mechanism is modulation of horizontal cell glutamate receptors (Knapp and Dowling, 1987; McMahon and Ponomareva, 1996).

Illumination increases horizontal cell responsiveness and receptive-field size

The observations made by Mangel and Dowling (1985) were followed up by a trio of papers from the Dowling lab (Tornqvist et al., 1988; Yang et al., 1988a, 1988b). These papers described additional features of dark- and light-dependent changes of horizontal cell responsiveness and receptive-field size but in a different teleost, the white perch (*Roccus americanus*). In the first of these papers (Yang et al., 1988a) it was again shown that prolonged darkness decreased the amplitude of LHC responses to a full-field stimulus. In addition, it was shown that exposure to steady or periodic illumination of the isolated retina increased the responsiveness of LHCs previously "suppressed" by maintaining the animal in prolonged darkness. Most of the recordings in this study were made from LHCs but additional data were collected from CHCs. Like the LHCs, the responses of CHCs were suppressed by prolonged darkness and subsequently increased by illumination. The responses of rod-driven horizontal cells, however, were not suppressed by darkness.

Yang, Tornqvist and Dowling (1988a) also noted a change in the dark resting membrane potential of LHCs from prolonged dark-adapted retinas compared to the potential in LHCs following illumination. Following darkness, LHC dark resting membrane potential was relatively depolarized (e.g. −17 mV) but after illumination the potential hyperpolarized (to −24 mV). Yang, Tornqvist and Dowling (1988a) also pointed out that the response kinetics of LHCs subject to prolonged darkness were relatively slow but were gradually increased following illumination.

In the third of the trio of papers (Tornqvist et al., 1988) it was shown that the receptive-field size of LHCs from white perch, like goldfish, were decreased in retinas taken from animals subject to prolonged darkness. Receptive-field size was assessed using the same approach Mangel and Dowling (1985) had used: comparison of small versus large spot or full-field stimuli. Tornqvist, Yang and Dowling (1988) went even further by showing that subsequent illumination of the isolated retina (from an animal subject to prolonged dark-adaptation) increased the receptive-field size. This study also demonstrated that the spread of the fluorescent dye Lucifer yellow was restricted (limited to about 4 cells on average) when injected into horizontal cells from retinas isolated from prolonged dark-adapted fish. Following illumination, the spread of Lucifer yellow was extensive, labeling on average 31 cells. These results again indicated that at least part of the mechanism leading to the decreased receptive-field size of horizontal cells subject to prolonged darkness was a decrease in horizontal cell to horizontal cell gap junction permeability. Conversely, the increased receptive-field size of horizontal cells from retinas subject to illumination (or only brief darkness) could be explained, at least in part, by increased gap junction permeability.

It was in this series of three papers that two new terms were first introduced to describe the effects of dark and light on horizontal cell responses. The term "dark-suppression" was used to describe the decreased responsiveness and receptive-field size of horizontal cells recorded from retinas taken from animals maintained in the dark for a prolonged period. "Light-sensitization" was the term used to describe the light-induced increase of horizontal cell responsiveness and receptive-field size. Retinas subject to only a brief period of darkness were also considered to be "light-sensitized."

Further studies of horizontal cell dark-suppression

I had the opportunity to work with Stuart Mangel, Reto Weiler and John Dowling at the Marine Biological Laboratory at Woods Hole, Massachusetts the summers of 1992 and 1993 and as a result of this work, additional features of horizontal cell dark-suppression were revealed. The first of these was the fact that suppression of horizontal cell responses could be observed by maintaining isolated retina (not just the animal) in darkness (Mangel et al., 1994). To achieve this it was necessary to use a protocol that limited the exposure of the retina to illumination. Horizontal cells were impaled without, or only the limited use of, light flashes. Using this approach it was possible, in several cases, to record an intensity-response series in a cell that had been maintained in complete darkness for 2 h and then exposed to only a single, brief (150 ms), dim test flash. The responses of LHCs to full-field illumination recorded this way were suppressed, with, on average, a response amplitude less than 10 mV for the brightest stimulus used. Responses recorded following a period of steady illumination increased dramatically with, on average, a response amplitude of 28 mV to the brightest stimulus used. In addition, the dark resting membrane potential of the LHCs hyperpolarized by more than 14 mV during the transition from dark-suppressed to light-sensitized.

In addition to response suppression and relative depolarization of the dark resting membrane potential, prolonged darkness also decreased the response threshold of LHCs by at least −2 log units when compared to the same cell following illumination. The response waveform also changed with the response duration exceeding stimulus duration after prolonged darkness but matching stimulus duration after illumination. In addition, the chromatic responses of these cells were changed; after prolonged darkness the responses to short wavelength stimuli (450 nm, 500 nm) were enhanced but the responses to longer wavelength stimuli (650 nm) were decreased,

440

when compared to the responses following illumination. These changes imply that, after prolonged darkness, rod-like signals can be observed in the LHC response (Mangel et al., 1994). If the anatomy of white perch retina conforms to what is known from the retina of the goldfish, such a rod signal cannot be due to direct synaptic input from rods to LHCs (Stell, 1967; Stell and Lightfoot, 1975). However, gap junction coupling between rods and cones (Witkovsky et al., 1974; Scholes, 1975) represents a possible mechanism whereby rod signals could reach cone-driven horizontal cells.

Another study that resulted from the collaborative effort at the Marine Biological Laboratory (Baldridge et al., 1995) described in greater detail how LHCs can be dark-suppressed by maintaining isolated hybrid bass (*Morone chrysops/Morone saxatilis*) retina in the dark and how periods of steady illumination increase the responsiveness or "light-sensitize" LHCs (see Fig. 2). This study also showed that the extent of LHC dark-suppression was influenced by the time of day; although dark-suppression was clearly observed during the day, dark-suppression was greater at night. Stuart Mangel's laboratory at the University of Alabama has investigated this issue in greater detail and revealed a distinct circadian influence on horizontal cell dark-suppression and on the appearance of the rod signal in the LHC response (Wang and Mangel, 1996).

Another interesting and important result that emerged from Baldridge, Weiler and Dowling (1995) was that dark-suppression does not necessarily require prolonged darkness. Starting with light-sensitized LHCs, it was found that as little as 2 min of complete darkness could significantly reduce (by 40%) the response amplitude to a full-field stimulus of fixed intensity. Subsequent exposure to steady illumination for 1 min completely restored the responsiveness to the initial light-sensitized level.

Although several different species of teleosts were used, all the studies of horizontal cell dark-suppression described above employed the isolated retina preparation. Might this preparation be responsible for the suppression of horizontal cell responses in the dark? For example, studies of retinomotor movements in teleosts suggested that millimolar levels of extracellular taurine may be important for normal dark-adaptation (Dearry and Burnside, 1986).

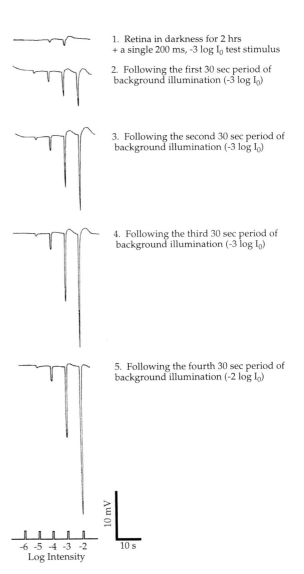

1. Retina in darkness for 2 hrs + a single 200 ms, -3 log I_0 test stimulus

2. Following the first 30 sec period of background illumination (-3 log I_0)

3. Following the second 30 sec period of background illumination (-3 log I_0)

4. Following the third 30 sec period of background illumination (-3 log I_0)

5. Following the fourth 30 sec period of background illumination (-2 log I_0)

10 mV

-6 -5 -4 -3 -2   10 s
Log Intensity

Fig. 2. Dark-suppression and light-sensitization of an LHC from the hybrid bass retina. The upper-most record (1) was obtained from an isolated retina preparation maintained for 2 h in the dark and the cell impaled using only a single 200 ms test flash. The responsiveness of the cell was then characterized using full-field stimuli over a range of intensities (500 ms duration). The next records (2–5) show the responses of the same cell to the same intensity series but after four periods of steady background illumination. Horizontal cell responses are clearly suppressed after darkness but show increased responsiveness following illumination. Adapted from Baldridge, et al. (1995).

My laboratory recently tested the hypothesis that the absence of taurine in the physiological solutions used for isolated retina electrophysiology might be the cause of horizontal cell dark-suppression. We were able to demonstrate that addition of 5 mM taurine to the extracellular solution did not abolish horizontal cell dark-suppression in isolated goldfish retina (Baldridge et al., 2000). Therefore, horizontal cell dark-suppression is not an artifact produced by the absence of extracellular taurine. The strongest evidence that dark-suppression is not an artifact of the isolated retina preparation comes from a technically impressive study where white perch horizontal cells were recorded in vivo (Yang et al., 1994). Horizontal cell dark-suppression was clearly observed in vivo making it unlikely that suppression is simply an artifact of the isolated retina preparation.

There is more than just light and dark: triphasic adaptation

At about the same time that the trio of papers from the Dowling lab describing dark-suppression and light-sensitization were published I had begun studies, as part of my graduate work in the lab of Alexander K. Ball at McMaster University, on the effects of illumination on horizontal cells in the goldfish retina. We soon generated data that seemed at odds with the evidence indicating that teleost horizontal cells are uncoupled in darkness and coupled in the light. We assessed the receptive-field size of goldfish horizontal cells by examining the responses to several sizes of annulus stimuli and comparing them to the responses generated by spot stimuli of similar illuminated area. The ratio of the annulus response/spot response is positively correlated with the receptive-field size; when the receptive-field size is large, and horizontal cells are well-coupled, changes of current originating at peripheral cells (due to stimulation by an annulus) will reach the central, recorded cell. As the receptive-field size decreases, less current will pass to or from the central cell and the response to the annulus will, therefore, decrease. Using this approach, we found that the annulus response/spot response ratio (and therefore the receptive-field size) of all types of cone-driven horizontal cells were relatively increased in retinas obtained from 2 h dark-adapted fish (Fig. 3, Baldridge and Ball, 1991). After exposing the isolated retina to a period of steady bright background illumination the response to both spot and annulus

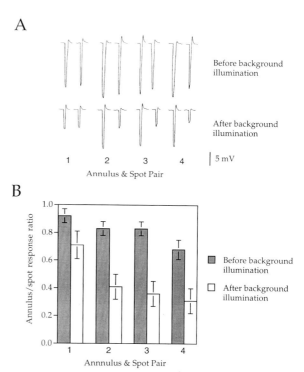

Fig. 3. Effect of background illumination on goldfish horizontal cell receptive-field size. (A) Response of a horizontal cell to 4 pairs of spot and annulus stimuli of similar illuminated area. The annulus/spot response ratio for this cell was decreased by background illumination in the case of the three largest spots and annuli (pairs 2–4). (B) Mean data from all horizontal cells studied ($n = 14$) showing that the annulus/spot ratio decreased following background illumination. The decrease in the annulus/spot ratio is consistent with decreased receptive-field size. Spot diameters (in mm) were 1.25, 2.75, 4.50 and 8.00 for pairs 1–4, respectively. Annulus inner/outer diameters (in mm) were 0.75/1.50, 2.50/3.75, 2.50/5.25, 3.00/8.00 for pairs 1–4, respectively. Error bars are S.E.M. Adapted from Baldridge and Ball (1991).

stimuli decreased. However, the decrease of the response to annulus stimulation was much greater than the response to the corresponding spot of similar illuminated area. In other words, the annulus response/spot response ratio decreased following bright background illumination. We also found extensive spread of Lucifer yellow in the horizontal cell network of "dark-adapted" retina and that such spread was significantly restricted following exposure to a bright adapting light. This suggested that at least part of the mechanism leading to the reduced receptive-field size was a decrease of gap junction coupling.

Taken at face value, our result could not have been more opposite to the conclusions derived from the previous work from the Dowling lab. An explanation that would unify these disparate observations started with the realization that the responses of horizontal cells we recorded from in "dark-adapted" retina were not suppressed and, therefore, the "dark" starting points of our experiments and those of the dark-suppression studies were not the same. Indeed, the robust amplitude of the responses of our "dark-adapted" retinas suggested that they corresponded to what the Dowling laboratory had termed "light-sensitized." In retrospect this is probably because we did not dark-adapt our fish as extensively as in the Dowling lab (where fish were sometimes maintained in the dark overnight) and our fish were always dark-adapted during the day, when dark-suppression is weaker. But if our "dark-adapted" retinas were, in fact, light-sensitized then an important conclusion that can be drawn is that the functional states of teleost horizontal cells cannot be classified simply as "dark" or "light" and that at least three functional states are required to explain the data. The effect of illumination has two different effects depending on the prior light history of the retina. Moderate illumination applied after prolonged darkness increases horizontal cell responsiveness and receptive-field size. Bright illumination applied to an already light-sensitized retina decreases horizontal cell responsiveness and receptive-field size. Consequently, we proposed (Baldridge and Ball, 1991) that horizontal cells in the teleost retina can be described in terms of one of three adaptation states (see Table 1).

Although not well recognized at the time it was published, another laboratory had previously reported that the receptive-field size of carp (*Cyprinus carpio*) LHCs were decreased during and after background illumination (Shigematsu and Yamada, 1988). These investigators mapped the receptive field of horizontal cells using a narrow slit of light. As in Baldridge and Ball (1991) horizontal cell responses from "dark-adapted" retinas seem, in fact, to be light-sensitized. At around the same time as our experiments, studies in the Dowling laboratory, using white perch, also revealed a decrease of LHC receptive-field size (assessed by comparing the responses to a small spot versus a full-field) and Lucifer yellow dye coupling when light-sensitized horizontal cells were exposed to steady bright illumination or following flickering illumination (Umino et al., 1991). These authors also proposed triphasic adaptation as a way to differentiate light-sensitization and light-adaptation.

Using the term "triphasic" to describe the dark- and light-dependent changes of horizontal cell responsiveness and receptive-field size does not mean to imply that the cells are rigidly restricted to one of these three states. Indeed, there is a continuum of changes that can, at least conceptually, be thought of as a bell-shaped relation between horizontal cell responsiveness and receptive-field size as a function of the temporally integrated extent of light exposure. What the term "triphasic" is intended to signal is that the adaptation of teleost horizontal cells cannot be regarded in the traditional "biphasic" sense of dark- or light-adaptation.

Direct evidence for triphasic adaptation

The suggestion of triphasic adaptation is a parsimonious explanation of how different adaptation states produce reductions of teleost horizontal cell receptive-field size and dye coupling. However, since the original proposal of this idea in 1991 there hasn't been much direct evidence to support this hypothesis. Recently, my laboratory has returned to this question and we now have additional evidence that supports the hypothesis of triphasic adaptation.

Table 1. Triphasic adaptation of teleost horizontal cells

Level of illumination	Adaptation state	Responsiveness	Receptive-field size
Dark	Dark-Suppressed	Decreased	Decreased
Moderate	Light-Sensitized	Increased	Increased
Extensive	Light-Adapted	Decreased	Decreased

The most complete evidence at this time comes from studies done by Andrew Wear, a graduate student in my laboratory, who has used Lucifer yellow dye coupling to investigate the hypothesis that there are at least three functional states of teleost horizontal cell adaptation as a function of illumination. We have found, in all types of goldfish cone-driven horizontal cells, that Lucifer yellow injected into horizontal cells is restricted to one (Fig. 4A) or only a few (on average 2) cells (Fig. 5) when the

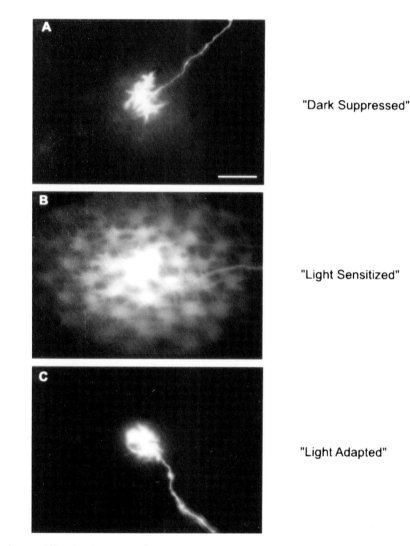

"Dark Suppressed"

"Light Sensitized"

"Light Adapted"

Fig. 4. Effect of background illumination on Lucifer yellow dye coupling between H1 (LHC) goldfish horizontal cells. (**A**) This cell was injected with Lucifer yellow in a retina exposed only to a single test flash after being maintained in complete darkness for 2 h. Dye did not spread beyond the injected cell indicating that the horizontal cell network was relatively uncoupled. (**B**) In this case the retina, after 2 h darkness, was then exposed to background illumination of moderate intensity before a horizontal cell was impaled and injected with Lucifer yellow. The dye passed from the central injected cell into numerous adjacent cells indicating increased coupling between the horizontal cells. (**C**) This cell was injected in a retina that had been exposed (following 2 h complete darkness) to bright background illumination. Dye did not pass to adjacent cells indicating that the horizontal cell network was relatively uncoupled. It is proposed that the three different coupling states observed correspond to the two adaptation states "dark-suppressed" and "light-sensitized" described by Yang, Tornqvist and Dowling (1988a) and the "light-adapted" state described by Baldridge and Ball (1991) and Umino, Lee and Dowling (1991). Scale bar = 40 μm. Data provided by Andrew Wear.

444

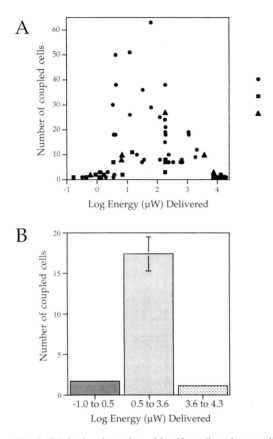

Fig. 5. Triphasic adaptation of Lucifer yellow dye-coupling in goldfish horizontal cells. (A) In retinas maintained in complete darkness for 2 h and then subject to limited light exposure, Lucifer yellow dye coupling is restricted. At moderate levels of light exposure coupling increases. At the brightest levels of light exposure Lucifer yellow dye coupling is decreased. Although the most dramatic increase in dye coupling took place in the case of H1 (LHC) horizontal cells, all three cone horizontal cell types showed increased dye coupling after moderate illumination. (B) Mean number of Lucifer yellow coupled cells as a function of increasing light exposure of retinas maintained in the dark for 2 h. After limited light exposure (−1.0–0.5 log energy delivered) dye spread is restricted to one or only a few cells. Over a range of moderate intensities (0.5–3.6 log energy delivered) dye spread increases but after the brightest illumination (3.6–4.3 log energy delivered) Lucifer yellow dye coupling is decreased. Error bars are SEM. Data provided by Andrew Wear.

isolated retinas are subject to little or no light exposure (Wear and Baldridge, 2000). Moderate levels of illumination increased the spread of dye (Fig. 4B) to include, on average 17 cells (Fig. 5), but exposure to prolonged or bright illumination restricted the spread of dye from the injected cell

(Fig. 4C) to neighboring cells, on average limiting dye solely to the injected cell (Fig. 5). This data is consistent with the proposal that horizontal cell receptive-field size is: (1) decreased in retinas maintained in the dark for a prolonged period; (2) increased following exposure to moderate illumination and (3) decreased again following exposure to bright illumination.

Mechanisms of triphasic adaptation in the teleost retina

The original work from the Dowling laboratory describing horizontal cell dark-suppression (Mangel and Dowling, 1985, 1987; Tornqvist et al., 1988; Yang et al., 1988b) also presented evidence indicating that dopamine was the intra-retinal signal of darkness. Application of dopamine mimicked the effect of prolonged darkness by reducing receptive-field size, decreasing responsiveness, depolarizing the dark resting membrane potential and slowing the response kinetics of horizontal cells. Even more convincing were studies showing that dark-suppression was reversed by application of the D1 dopamine-receptor antagonist SCH-23390 and was abolished in retinas where the endogenous source of dopamine was eliminated by lesioning dopaminergic interplexiform cells with 6-hydroxydopamine (Yang et al., 1988b).

The suggestion that dopamine is a signal of darkness in the retina generated a controversy that, to this day, has not been completely resolved. A number of studies, using a variety of techniques, have questioned the suggestion that dopamine is released during prolonged darkness (for review see Djamgoz and Wagner, 1992; Witkovsky and Dearry, 1992). Indeed, most of these studies reach the opposite conclusion, namely that dopamine release increases with illumination or, under circadian control, during the subjective day (Lei and Dowling, 2000; Mangel and Wang, 2000 but see also Weiler, 1997 #58). It is beyond the scope of this chapter to reconcile the disagreement concerning dopamine release in the teleost retina. Additional studies of the mechanism of horizontal cell dark-suppression seem inevitable and ideas for alternate mechanisms that might explain horizontal cell dark-suppression have already been proposed (Kamermans et al., 1991; Kamermans and Werblin, 1992).

What is the mechanism of light-adaptation?

As part of our study of the effect of illumination on horizontal cell receptive-field size and dye coupling (Baldridge and Ball, 1991) we demonstrated that dopamine was not the signal of horizontal cell light-adaptation. The D1 dopamine receptor antagonist SCH-23390 did not block light-adaptation nor did prior 6-OHDA lesioning. Similar results were obtained by Umino, Lee and Dowling (1991) who showed that the D1 > D2 dopamine receptor antagonist haloperidol did not block horizontal cell light-adaptation. Several other mechanisms of light-adaptation can be imagined (see Baldridge et al., 1998) but few have been tested. The most recent candidate molecule to emerge as a signal for light-adaptation is retinoic acid: application of all-*trans*-retinoic acid uncouples carp horizontal cells and induces spinule formation in horizontal cell dendrites (Weiler et al., 1998). This study also showed that citral, an inhibitor of aldehyde dehydrogenase, an enzyme necessary for the synthesis of retinoic acid, blocked the light-dependent formation of horizontal cell spinules and this may suggest that retinoic acid is also the signal that mediates light-adaptation. If retinoic acid is the mediator of horizontal cell light-adaptation then inhibitors of retinoic acid synthesis should also block the light-adaptive reduction of horizontal cell receptive-field size and dye coupling but this remains to be determined.

Light-adaptation produced by periods of steady illumination does not appear to be mediated by a mechanism that is dependent of dopamine. However, in the case of flickering light-adaptation dopamine does seem to be involved. Umino, Lee and Dowling (1991) showed that the reduction of horizontal cell receptive-field size induced by a 2 Hz flickering light could be blocked by the dopamine receptor antagonist haloperidol. Recently, Mangel and Wang (2000) also demonstrated that the effect of flickering illumination (but not sustained illumination) on horizontal cell receptive-field was blocked by the D1-selective dopamine receptor antagonist SCH-23390. Interestingly, the effect of flickering

light-adaptation was also blocked by tetrodotoxin (TTX), which blocks voltage-gated Na^+ channels, suggesting that the retinal dopamine release induced by flickering light depends on the generation of action potentials.

Triphasic adaptation in other species

Teleosts are not the only group of animals where triphasic adaptation has been demonstrated. Indeed, the first complete demonstration of triphasic adaptation came from the laboratory of Stewart Bloomfield at New York University. Using Neurobiotin tracer-coupling and receptive-field mapping (by translating narrow slits of light) the Bloomfield laboratory showed a triphasic relationship between tracer spread and receptive-field size as a function of background light intensity in A- (see Fig. 6) and B-type horizontal cells and AII amacrine cells of rabbit retina (Bloomfield et al., 1997; Xin and Bloomfield, 1999). The extent of tracer coupling and receptive-field size were restricted following dark-adaptation or in the presence of very dim backgrounds. In the presence of moderate levels of illumination tracer coupling and receptive-field size increased. When background illumination was bright, tracer spread

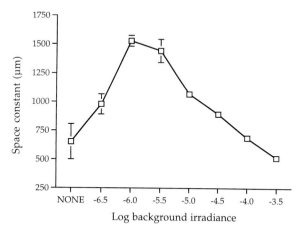

Fig. 6. Triphasic adaptation of A-type horizontal cells in the rabbit retina. Horizontal cell receptive-field size (space constant) is relatively decreased in the absence of background illumination. As the level of background illumination increases so does the receptive-field size. At higher levels of background illumination (> -5.5 log I_0) the receptive-field size decreases. Error bars are S.E.M. Data replotted from Xin and Bloomfield (1999).

and receptive-field size decreased. In teleosts, dark-suppression is mostly descriptive of the reduced responsiveness of horizontal cells after darkness (although we and others have used this term to also include the reduced receptive-field size as well). Is there any evidence for suppression of horizontal cells responses in animals other than teleosts? Given the results from the Bloomfield laboratory, it is perhaps not surprising that there is evidence that rabbit horizontal cell responses are suppressed following periods of darkness and that responses are increased by periods of illumination (Mangel and Wang, 1997; Hanitzsch and Bligh, 1999). Therefore, the data from rabbit retina, taken as a whole, indicates that the triphasic nature of horizontal cell receptive-field size is not a feature limited to teleosts and may well exist in a variety of animals, including mammals.

Despite the demonstration of triphasic adaptation in a mammalian retina, it is not clear how widespread this phenomenon is among vertebrates. In many vertebrate retinas, horizontal cell receptive-field size is expanded under dark or dim light conditions and is reduced only after moderate to bright background illumination (Witkovsky and Shi, 1990; Dong and McReynolds, 1991; Weiler and Akopian, 1992; Hankins, 1995). In addition, the effects of both steady and flickering background illumination are blocked by dopamine receptor antagonists suggesting that, unlike the situation in teleosts, dopamine is the signal of horizontal cell light-adaptation in these animals. It may even be that triphasic adaptation is not a feature of all teleosts or that there are different levels of expression depending on species. For example, Hankins and Jenkins (2001) reported that they were unable to observe horizontal dark-suppression in the retina of roach (*Rutilus rutilus*). An alternate explanation to the absence of dark-suppression in this species would be that the level of dark-suppression varies among teleosts, being weak in roach. There is some precedent for this in that there is a general consensus that the strength of dark-suppression varies from teleost to teleost, being greater in perch-like fishes (Order Perciformes; hybrid bass, white perch) and weaker in carps (Order Cypriniformes; including goldfish and roach). Such a difference might correspond to the different demands on the visual system of perch-like fishes compared to carps.

Significance of triphasic adaptation

As codified in textbooks (e.g. Dowling, 1987, 1992), it is generally believed that an important functional role of horizontal cells is to contribute to the receptive-field surround of bipolar cells which, by extension, means that horizontal cells contribute to the receptive-field surround of ganglion cells. There is pretty good evidence that this is the case: in a variety of vertebrates it has been shown that current injection into horizontal cells, leading to hyperpolarization, produced surround-like responses in bipolar cells (Marchiafava, 1978; Toyoda and Tonosaki, 1978; Toyoda and Kujiraoka, 1982; Sakuranaga and Naka, 1985) and ganglion cells (Naka and Nye, 1971; Naka and Witkovsky, 1972; Sakuranaga and Naka, 1985; Mangel and Miller, 1987; Mangel, 1991). If horizontal cells contribute to the receptive-field surround of bipolar and ganglion cells, it follows that changes in the size and strength of horizontal cell responses might be reflected as changes in the size or strength of the receptive-field surround of bipolar and ganglion cells. What one would predict is that the receptive-field surround should be weak and small under the conditions that lead to horizontal cell dark-suppression, that the surround should grow in size and strength with light-sensitization and, with light-adaptation, that the size of the surround should decrease.

There is evidence that some of these changes may, in fact, occur. In cat (Barlow et al., 1957; Rodieck and Stone, 1965; Maffei et al., 1971; Yoon, 1972; Enroth-Cugell and Lennie, 1975; Barlow and Levick, 1976; Peichl and Wässle, 1983; but see also Troy et al., 1999), frog (Donner and Reuter, 1965) and rabbit (Masland and Ames, 1976; Jensen, 1991; Muller and Dacheux, 1997), the strength of the inhibitory receptive-field surround appears to weaken when ganglion cells are recorded after periods of dark-adaptation and, in goldfish, prolonged darkness abolishes the color-opponent responses of double color-opponent ganglion cells (Raynauld and Laviolette, 1979). Such a reduction of the receptive-field surround during darkness may be a way to increase the sensitivity of the cone system at the expense of contrast sensitivity generated by the antagonistic center-surround receptive fields of bipolar and ganglion cells. It is possible that reduction of the lateral inhibition generated by horizontal cells under such conditions allows the cone system to operate at the lower end of cone sensitivity but above or near rod saturation.

In the context of horizontal cells as a source of the receptive-field surround of ganglion cells, what might be the significance the reduction of horizontal cell receptive-field size following light-adaptation? One would predict that the receptive-field surround would narrow. This would mean that the size of the visual field being sampled by the surround would be smaller and, therefore, permit spatial contrast analysis to be done more locally. It is also worth considering the fact that teleost horizontal cell light-adaptation can be accomplished either by steady illumination or flickering illumination, although the mechanisms appear to be different. It is not completely clear why these two different processes exist, but perhaps it allows horizontal cell receptive-field size to be decreased as ambient illumination level rises in either spatial contrast-rich (equivalent to flickering illumination) or spatial contrast-poor (equivalent to steady illumination) natural scenes.

A more sophisticated analysis of the utility of triphasic adaptation was recently reported by Balboa and Grzywacz (2000a, 2000b). Many models propose that horizontal cells should be coupled under dim light conditions as a way of decreasing photon-absorption noise by averaging thereby increasing the signal-to-noise ratio. However, Balboa and Grzywacz (2000b) suggest that "such an increase at low luminance levels may smooth out basic visual information of natural images." Consequently, they proposed a "minimal-local asperity" hypothesis and suggest that triphasic adaptation would optimize the extraction of certain features in natural images, specifically edge detection, contrast and intensity.

Conclusions and future perspectives

The original description of horizontal cell dark-suppression by Mangel and Dowling in 1985, and subsequent work from the Dowling laboratory and by Dowling's collaborators, have added much to our understanding of how horizontal cell function is modulated by the level of ambient illumination. Without this, the model of horizontal cell triphasic

adaptation would not have emerged. However, many interesting questions remain to be answered. Most important is to understand the mechanisms that mediate dark-suppression and light-adaptation. Equally important is the need for a better understanding of the effect of horizontal cell activity on retinal processing and a clear demonstration of the impact of triphasic adaptation on the generation of the receptive-field surrounds of bipolar and ganglion cells. It is clear that such questions will continue to fascinate retinal neuroscientists well into the new century, building on the legacy established by John E. Dowling.

Acknowledgments

Many agencies have supported my studies of horizontal cells over the years including the Medical Research Council (MRC) of Canada, the Grass Foundation, Sigma Xi and the National Academy of Science. Current horizontal cell research in my laboratory is supported by the Natural Science and Engineering Research Council (NSERC) of Canada and I am, at present, a Canadian Institutes of Health Research (CIHR) RPP Investigator.

References

Balboa, R.M. and Grzywacz, N.M. (2000a) The minimal local-asperity theory of retinal lateral inhibition. *Neural Comp.*, 12: 1485–1517.
Balboa, R.M. and Grzywacz, N.M. (2000b) The role of early lateral inhibition: more than maximizing luminance information. *Vis. Neurosci.*, 17: 77–90.
Baldridge, W.H. and Ball, A.K. (1991) Background illumination reduces horizontal cell receptive-field size in both normal and 6-hydroxydopamine-lesioned goldfish retina. *Vis. Neurosci.*, 7: 441–450.
Baldridge, W.H., McLure, P. and Pow, D.V. (2000) Taurine blocks spontaneous cone contraction but not horizontal cell dark suppression in isolated goldfish retina. *J. Neurochem.*, 74: 2614–2621.
Baldridge, W.H., Vaney, D.I. and Weiler, R. (1998) The modulation of intercellular coupling in the retina. *Cell Develop Biol.*, 9: 311–318.
Baldridge, W.H., Weiler, R. and Dowling, J.E. (1995) Dark-suppression and light-sensitization of horizontal cell responses in the hybrid bass retina. *Vis. Neurosci.*, 12: 611–620.

448

Barlow, H.B., Fitzhugh, R. and Kuffler, S.W. (1957) Change of organization in the receptive fields of the cat's retina during dark adaptation. *J. Physiol.*, 137: 338–354.

Barlow, H.B. and Levick, W.R. (1976) Threshold setting by the surround of cat retinal ganglion cells. *J. Physiol.*, 259: 737–757.

Bloomfield, S.A., Xin, D. and Osborne, T. (1997) Light-induced modulation of coupling between AII amacrine cells in the rabbit retina. *Vis. Neurosci.*, 14: 565–576.

Dearry, A. and Burnside, B. (1986) Dopaminergic regulation of cone retinomotor movement in isolated teleost retinas: I. Induction of cone contraction is mediated by D2 receptors. *J. Neurochem.*, 46: 1006–1021.

Djamgoz, M.B.A. and Wagner, H.-J. (1992) Localization and function of dopamine in the adult vertebrate retina. *Neurochem Int.*, 20: 139–191.

Dong, C.J. and McReynolds, J.S. (1991) The relationship between light, dopamine release and horizontal cell coupling in the mudpuppy retina. *J. Physiol.*, 440: 291–309.

Donner, K.O. and Reuter, T. (1965) The dark-adaptation of single units in the frog's retina and its relation to the regeneration of rhodopsin. *Vision Res.*, 5: 615–632.

Dowling, J.E. (1987) *The retina, an approachable part of the brain.* Belknap Press, Cambridge, MA.

Dowling, J.E. (1992) *Neurons and networks, an introduction to neuroscience.* Belknap Press, Cambridge, MA.

Enroth-Cugell, C. and Lennie, P. (1975) The control of retinal ganglion cell discharge by receptive field surrounds. *J. Physiol.*, 247: 551–578.

Hanitzsch, R. and Bligh, J. (1999) Light potentiation of horizontal cells in the isolated rabbit retina. *Doc. Ophthalmol.*, 97: 41–55.

Hankins, M.W. (1995) Horizontal cell coupling and its regulation. In: Djamgoz, M., Archer, S. and Vallerga S. (Eds.), *Neurobiology and Clincial Aspects of the Outer Retina.* Chapman and Hall, London, pp. 195–220.

Hankins, M.W. and Jenkins, A. (2001) Long-term light history modulates the light response kinetics of luminosity (L)-type horizontal cells in the roach retina. *Brain Res.*, 887: 230–237.

Hassin, G. (1979) Pikeperch horizontal cells identified by intracellular staining. *J. Comp. Neurol.*, 186: 529–540.

Jensen, R.J. (1991) Involvement of glycinergic neurons in the diminished surround activity of ganglion cells in the dark-adapted rabbit retina. *Vis. Neurosci.*, 6: 43–53.

Kamermans, M., Van Dijk, B.W., Spekreijse, H. and Werblin, F. (1991) A model for the changes in coupling and kinetics of cone driven retinal horizontal cells during light/dark adaptation. In: Beckman, F. (Eds.), *Analysis and modeling of neural systems.* Kluwer Academic, Boston, pp. 223–230.

Kamermans, M. and Werblin, F. (1992) GABA-mediated positive autofeedback loop controls horizontal cell kinetics in tiger salamander retina. *J. Neurosci.*, 12: 2451–2463.

Knapp, A.G. and Dowling, J.E. (1987) Dopamine enhances excitatory amino acid-gated conductances in cultured retinal horizontal cells. *Nature*, 325: 437–439.

Lasater, E.M. and Dowling, J.E. (1985) Dopamine decreases conductance of the electrical junctions between cultured retinal horizontal cells. *Proc. Natl. Acad. Sci.*, 82: 3025–3029.

Lei, L. and Dowling, J.E. (2000) Effects of dopamine depletion on visual sensitivity in zebrafish. *J. Neurosci.*, 20: 1893–1903.

Lu, C. and McMahon, D.G. (1997) Modulation of hybrid bass retinal gap junctional channel gating by nitric oxide. *J. Physiol. (Lond.)*, 499: 689–699.

Maffei, L., Fiorentini, A. and Cervetto, L. (1971) Homeostasis in retinal receptive fields. *J. Neurophysiol.*, 34: 579–587.

Mangel, S.C. (1991) Analysis of the horizontal celll contribution to the receptive field surround of ganglion cells in the rabbit retina. *J. Physiol.*, 442: 211–234.

Mangel, S.C., Baldridge, W.H., Weiler, R. and Dowling, J.E. (1994) Threshold and chromatic sensitivity changes in fish cone horizontal cells following prolonged darkness. *Brain Res.*, 659: 55–61.

Mangel, S.C. and Dowling, J.E. (1985) Responsiveness and receptive field size of carp horizontal cells are reduced by prolonged darkness and dopamine. *Science*, 229: 1107–1109.

Mangel, S.C. and Dowling, J.E. (1987) The interplexiform-horizontal cell system of the fish retina: effects of dopamine, light stimulation and time in the dark. *Proc. Roy. Soc. Lond. Ser. B*, 231: 91–121.

Mangel, S.C. and Miller, R.F. (1987) Horizontal cells contribute to the receptive field surround of ganglion cells in the rabbit retina. *Brain Res.*, 414: 182–186.

Mangel, S.C. and Wang, Y. (1997) Light responses of rabbit cone-connected horizontal cells exhibit a diurnal rhythm. *Invest. Ophthalmol. Vis. Sci. (ARVO Suppl.)*, 38: 616.

Mangel, S.C. and Wang, Y. (2000) Two dopamine systems in the fish retina. *Invest. Ophthalmol. Vis. Sci. (ARVO Suppl.)*, 41: S112.

Marchiafava, P.L. (1978) Horizontal cells influence membrane potential of bipolar cells in the retina of the turtle. *Nature*, 275: 141–142.

Masland, R.H. and Ames, A. (1976) Responses to acetylcholine of ganglion cells in an isolated mammalian retina. *J. Neurophysiol.*, 39.

McMahon, D.G., Knapp, A.G. and Dowling, J.E. (1989) Horizontal cell gap junctions: Single-channel conductance and modulation by dopamine. *Proc. Natl. Acad. Sci. USA*, 86: 7639–7643.

McMahon, D.G. and Ponomareva, L.V. (1996) Nitric oxide and cGMP modulate retinal glutamate receptors. *J. Neurophysiol.*, 76: 2307–2315.

Muller, J.F. and Dacheux, R.F. (1997) Alpha ganglion cells of the rabbit retina lose antagonistic surround responses under dark adaptation. *Vis. Neurosci.*, 14: 395–401.

Naka, K.-I. and Nye, P.W. (1971) Role of horizontal cells in organization of the catfish retinal receptive field. *J. Neurophysiol.*, 34: 785–801.

Naka, K.-I. and Witkovsky, P. (1972) Dogfish ganglion cell discharge resulting from extrinsic polarization of the horizontal cells. *J. Physiol.*, 223: 449–460.

Naka, K.I. and Rushton, W.A.H. (1967) The generation and spread of S-potentials in fish (cyprinidae). *J. Physiol.*, 192: 437–461.

Peichl, L. and Wässle, H. (1983) The structural correlate of the receptive field centre of α ganglion cells in the cat retina. *J. Physiol.*, 341: 309–324.

Piccolino, M., Neyton, G. and Gerschenfeld, H.M. (1984) Decrease of gap junction permeability induced by dopamine and cyclic adenosine 3′:5′-monophosphate in horizontal cells of turtle retina. *J. Neurosci.*, 4: 1271–1280.

Raynauld, J.P. and Laviolette, J.R. (1979) Goldfish retina: a correlate between cone activity and morphology of the horizontal cell in cone pedicules. *Science*, 204: 1436–1438.

Rodieck, R.W. and Stone, J. (1965) Analysis of the receptive fields of cat retinal ganglion cells. *J. Neurophysiol.*, 28: 833–849.

Sakuranaga, M. and Naka, K.-I. (1985) Signal transmission in the catfish retina. I. Transmission in the outer retina. *J. Neurophysiol.*, 53: 373–389.

Scholes, J.H. (1975) Colour receptors and their synaptic connexions in the retina of cyprinid fish. *Phil. Transact. R. Soc. Lond. Ser. B*, 270: 61–118.

Shigematsu, Y. and Yamada, M. (1988) Effects of dopamine on spatial poperties of horizontal cell responses in the carp retina. *Neurosci. Res.*, (Suppl. 8): S69–S80.

Stell, W.K. (1967) The structure and relationships of horizontal cells and photoreceptor-bipolar synaptic complexes in goldfish retina. *Am. J. Anat.*, 121: 401–424.

Stell, W.K. and Lightfoot, D.O. (1975) Color-specific interconnections of cones and horizontal cells in the retina of the goldfish. *J. Comp. Neurol.*, 159: 473–502.

Svaetichin, G. (1953) The cone action potential. *Acta. Physiol. Scand.*, 29: 565–600.

Tornqvist, K., Yang, X.-L. and Dowling, J.E. (1988) Modulation of cone horizontal cell activity in the teleost fish retina, III. Effects of prolonged darkness and dopamine on electrical coupling between horizontal cells. *J. Neurosci.*, 8: 2279–2288.

Toyoda, J. and Kujiraoka, T. (1982) Analyses of bipolar cell responses elicited by polarization of horizontal cells. *J. Gen. Physiol.*, 79: 131–145.

Toyoda, J.-I. and Tonosaki, K. (1978) Effect of polarization of horizontal cells on the on-centre bipolar cell of the carp retina. *Nature*, 276: 399–400.

Troy, J.B., Bohnsack, D.L. and Diller, L.C. (1999) Spatial properties of the cat X-cell receptive field as a function of mean light level. *Vis. Neurosci.*, 16: 1089–1104.

Umino, O., Lee, Y. and Dowling, J.E. (1991) Effects of light stimuli on the release of dopamine from interplexiform cells in the white perch retina. *Vis. Neurosci.*, 7: 451–458.

Wang, Y. and Mangel, S.C. (1996) A circadian clock regulates rod and cone input to fish retinal cone horizontal cells. *Proc. Natl. Acad. Sci. USA*, 93: 4655–4660.

Wear, A. and Baldridge, W.H. (2000) Triphasic adaptation of horizontal cells in goldfish retina: A Lucifer yellow dye coupling study. *Invest. Ophthalmol. Vis. Sci. (ARVO Suppl.)*, 41: S942.

Weiler, R. and Akopian, A. (1992) Effects of background illuminations on the receptive field size of horizontal cells in the turtle retina are mediated by dopamine. *Neurosci. Lett.*, 140: 121–124.

Weiler, R., Schultz, K., Pottek, M., Tieding, S. and Janssen-Bienhold, U. (1998) Retinoic acid has light-adaptive effects on horizontal cells in the retina. *Proc. Natl. Acad. Sci. USA*, 95: 7139–7144.

Witkovsky, P. and Dearry, A. (1992) Functional roles of dopamine in the vertebrate retina. *Prog. Retinal. Res.*, 11: 247–292.

Witkovsky, P., Shakib, M. and Ripps, H. (1974) Interreceptoral junctions in the teleost retina. *Invest. Ophthalmol. Vis. Sci.*, 13: 996–1009.

Witkovsky, P. and Shi, X.P. (1990) Slow light and dark adaptation of horizontal cells in the xenopus retina: A role for endogenous dopamine. *Vis. Neurosci.*, 5: 405–413.

Xin, D. and Bloomfield, S.A. (1999) Dark- and light-induced changes in coupling between horizontal cells in mammalian retina. *J. Comp. Neurol.*, 405: 75–87.

Yamada, E. and Ishikawa, T. (1965) The fine structure of the horizontal cells in some vertebrate retinae. *Cold Spring Harbor Symp. Quant. Biol.*, 30: 383–392.

Yang, X.-L., Fan, T.-X. and Shen, W. (1994) Effects of prolonged darkness on light responsiveness and spectral sensitivity of cone horizontal cells in carp retina in vivo. *J. Neurosci.*, 14: 326–334.

Yang, X.-L., Tauchi, M. and Kaneko, A. (1982) Effects of prolonged dark-adaptation on the sensitivity of L-type external horizontal cells. *J. Physiol. Soc. Jpn.*, 44: 421.

Yang, X.-L., Tornqvist, K. and Dowling, J.E. (1988a) Modulation of cone horizontal cell activity in the teleost fish retina, I. Effects of prolonged darkness and background illumination on light responsiveness. *J. Neurosci.*, 8: 2259–2268.

Yang, X.-L., Tornqvist, K. and Dowling, J.E. (1988b) Modulation of cone horizontal cell activity in the teleost fish retina, II. Role of interplexiform cells and dopamine in regulating light responsiveness. *J. Neurosci.*, 8: 2269–2278.

Yoon, M. (1972) Influence of adaptation level on response pattern and sensitivity of ganglion cells in the cat's retina. *J. Physiol.*, 221: 93–104.

H. Kolb, H. Ripps and S. Wu (Eds.)
Progress in Brain Research, Vol. 131
© 2001 Elsevier Science B.V. All rights reserved

CHAPTER 32

Potassium conductances and the glutamate transporter in Müller cells of the turtle retina and their role in potassium siphoning

Ido Perlman[1,*], Eduardo Solessio[2] and Eric M. Lasater[3]

[1]*Bruce Rappaport Faculty of Medicine, Technion-Israel Institute of Technology, Haifa, Israel*
[2]*SUNY Upstate Medical University, Syracuse, NY, USA*
[3]*John Moran Eye Center, University of Utah, Salt Lake City, UT, USA*

Introduction

The Müller cells were paid little attention by retinal researchers until two independent studies suggested that they were the source of the b-wave of the electroretinogram (ERG). One study based its conclusion on a sink-source analysis of the electrical currents underlying the genesis of the ERG b-wave (Faber, 1969). In the second study, intracellular recordings of light-induced potential changes from mudpuppy Müller cells were found to have similar characteristics to those of the ERG b-wave (Miller and Dowling, 1970). These studies constituted a breakthrough in retinal research since they provided the first information on the cellular origin of the ERG that is being widely used as an objective measure of retinal function in human and laboratory animals. Despite the non-neuronal origin of the ERG b-wave, comparison of the ERG b-wave to light-induced electrical activity in retinal neurons showed that the b-wave could be used as a measure of post-receptoral retinal function (Dowling and Ripps, 1970; Green et al., 1975).

The next step in Müller cell research was aimed at revealing the biophysical mechanisms underlying the genesis of their light-induced responses. Miller and Dowling (1970) first suggested that increases in extracellular potassium ions in the outer plexiform layer (OPL) induced the Müller cell photoresponses. Subsequent studies using potassium-sensitive microelectrodes showed that the situation was more complex (Karwoski and Proenza, 1977, 1978; Dick and Miller, 1978; Kline et al., 1978, 1985). As a result of these pioneering studies and subsequent research, it is now widely accepted that the retinal Müller cells play an important role in maintaining potassium homeostasis in the retina (Newman et al., 1984; Karwoski et al., 1989) and in the clearance of neurotransmitters from the retinal extracellular space (Brew and Attwell, 1987; Schwartz and Tachibana, 1990; Biedermann et al., 1994).

Siphoning of potassium ions from the inner retina to large sinks (e.g. blood vessels and vitreous humor) during light-induced increases in extracellular potassium levels becomes possible by the high density of potassium channels that are unevenly distributed along the Müller cells (Brew et al., 1986; Newman, 1987, 1988). Thus, when potassium conductance is reduced with barium ions, the increase in the vitreal potassium level during light stimulation is eliminated

---

* Corresponding author: Ido Perlman, Tel.: (4) 829-5279/5346; Fax: (4) 853-5969; E-mail: Iperlman@tx.technion.ac.il

while intra-retinal changes in potassium ions are unaffected (Karwoski et al., 1989). The type of potassium channels and their exact location vary between species. Müller cells in some species (e.g. axolotl and tiger salamander) were reported to contain only one type of potassium channels, the inward rectifier (Brew et al., 1986; Newman, 1993) while in others (e.g. rabbit, guinea pig) a variety of potassium channels were demonstrated (Nilius and Reichenbach, 1988; Reichelt and Pannicke, 1993; Chao et al., 1994).

Müller cells in the turtle retina, like those in other species, are highly permeable to potassium ions and inward or outward potassium fluxes can be induced depending upon the driving force (Conner et al., 1985; Le Dain et al., 1994; Linn et al., 1998; Solessio et al., 2000). The outward and inward potassium currents in turtle Müller cells can be mediated either by inwardly rectifying potassium channels that are characterized by a significant non-adapting component or by two types of channels; a strong inward rectifier and an ohmic voltage-independent channel (Solessio et al., 2001). The spatial distribution of potassium channels along turtle Müller cells and their role in potassium siphoning remain unclear. Furthermore, the Müller cells in turtle, as in other retinas, have a rather unique morphology. They have one, relatively thick distal process and several long thin processes extending proximally from the cell body and ending in a small, spherical endfoot at the inner limiting membrane (Conner et al., 1985; Linn et al., 1998). In turtle Müller cells 6–8 proximal processes can be seen, while in pigeon up to 25 processes have been observed (Cajal, 1972). This morphology raises concerns about the extent of space clamp in these cells during experiments utilizing voltage-clamp recordings (Newman, 1993; Solessio et al., 2000) as well as their capacity to efficiently siphon potassium ions in the intact retina from the inner retinal layers to the vitreous.

Müller cells are also essential for efficient signal transmission within the retina. Dowling and his co-workers were among the first to suggest that an excitatory neurotransmitter is being continuously released in darkness from the photoreceptors terminals and that the rate of release is reduced during light stimulation (Dowling and Ripps, 1973; Cervetto and Piccolino, 1974). The identity of this neurotransmitter has been the focus of extensive research in a variety of retinal preparations from different species but it was only firmly established as L-glutamate by the study of Lasater and Dowling (1982) who compared the effects of L-glutamate and L-aspartate on horizontal cells that had been isolated from the retina of the white perch. In order to expedite signal transmission from cones to horizontal cells it is not sufficient to reduce the rate of transmitter release, but the transmitter also has to be removed from the vicinity of the horizontal cells (Perlman et al., 1989). Different subtypes of glutamate transporters have been demonstrated in all retinal neurons as well as in Müller cells and astrocytes (Schultz and Stell, 1996; Rauen et al., 1996; Eliasof et al., 1998). These uptake systems are essential for fast synaptic transmission in the outer and inner plexiform layers (Gaal et al., 1998; Matsui et al., 1999; Barnett and Pow, 2000). An additional role for the glutamate transporters is to reduce the basal level of glutamate and thus, to protect retinal neurons from glutamate toxicity (Izumi et al., 1999). Since the glutamate transporters are electrogenic (Brew and Attwell, 1987; Schwartz and Tachibana, 1990; Barbour et al., 1991), they contribute to the membrane potential of Müller cells and may indirectly affect potassium siphoning.

We undertook an investigation on turtle Müller cells in order to evaluate their role in potassium siphoning. We studied the properties of the potassium channels and their distribution along the cells. From the morphological characteristics of the Müller cells and their electrical properties we analyzed their cable properties in order to assess the electrotonic conduction of voltage along the cells. The properties of the glutamate transporter were investigated in order to assess its possible contribution to potassium siphoning. To achieve these goals, Müller cells were isolated from the retina of the turtle *Pseudemys scripta elegans* and studied using the whole-cell patch-clamp technique (Solessio et al., 2000). Current responses to depolarizing and hyperpolarizing voltage pulses were recorded in order to construct the I-V relationship under different conditions.

Distribution of potassium channels

The current responses of one Müller cell to voltage steps of long (1.6 s) duration using whole-cell recording configuration at the cell body are shown in Fig. 1A. The cell was held at −80 mV. A pre-pulse to −100 mV was applied for 200 ms followed by a 1.6 s pulse to different voltage levels ranging from −120 to +40 mV. At the termination of these pulses the cell was stepped back to −100 mV and then to −80 mV. To construct the I-V relationships shown in Fig. 1B, currents were measured 25 ms after onset of voltage pulses and just prior to their termination (vertical dashed lines marked by T and S respectively). It is clear that the inward currents remained relatively constant and did not change with time. However, the outward currents progressively decreased with time until a steady state level had been reached. This is a manifestation of the block of the potassium channels by intracellular magnesium ions and polyamines (Solessio et al., 2001). It is evident from Fig. 1 that even with maximal block, substantial potassium efflux can be induced at depolarizing voltages. These outward currents do not flow through a delayed rectifier or calcium-dependent potassium channels (Linn et al., 1998) but probably through an ohmic, voltage-independent potassium channel or through a non-inactivating component of the inward rectifier (Solessio et al., 2001).

To assess the distribution of potassium channels along the Müller cells, we obtained whole-cell recordings from somas of complete cells (soma and processes), from cells in which we sheared off the processes using a sharp micropipette and from isolated processes (Fig. 2A). The I-V curves were derived from depolarizing and hyperpolarizing voltage pulses (200 ms in duration) that were applied from a holding potential of −70 mV. The I-V curve recorded from the soma before and after cutting away its 4 processes are compared in Fig. 2B (filled and open circles respectively). As expected, the magnitude of the current is considerably larger when recording from the cell with its processes intact and the shape of the I-V curve shows less rectification. In Fig. 2C, the average I-V curve of single, isolated processes ($N = 3$) is compared to that of isolated soma ($N = 5$). The currents were normalized relative to the capacitance of the corresponding cellular parts (151 ± 45 pF for the soma alone, and 35 ± 8 pF for the process alone) and are expressed in the figure as current density (pA/pF). Assuming that the specific capacitance of the membrane in the cell soma is similar to that in the process and endfoot, the curves in Fig. 2C indicate that the density of potassium channels in the process and endfoot is

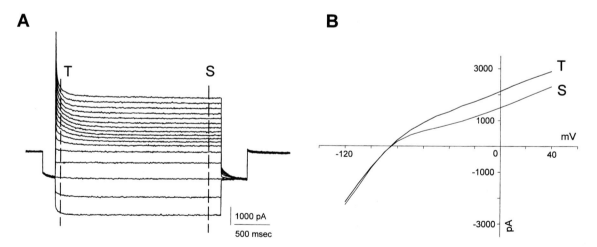

Fig. 1. Ionic currents in a turtle Müller cell that were measured using whole-cell recordings in an isolated cell. (**A**) The cell was held at −80 mV and voltage pulses of long duration (1.6 s) were applied to levels ranging from −120 to +40 mV at 10 mV increments. Each voltage pulse was preceded by a pre-pulse to −100 mV. Currents were measured 25 ms after onset of voltage pulses (vertical line marked by T) and just prior to termination of the voltage pulses (vertical line marked by S). (**B**) I-V relationship for short (T) and long (S) time intervals after onset of voltage pulses.

higher than in the soma. Thus, turtle Müller cells are similar to those in other cold-blooded vertebrates having the highest density of potassium channels in the endfoot region (Brew et al., 1986; Newman, 1987, 1988). Furthermore, the I-V curves of the soma and process have very similar voltage dependency as is evident from Fig. 2D where each of the I-V curves from Fig. 2C was replotted and scaled relative to the current measured at +40 mV. This observation indicates that similar type of potassium channels reside in each structure of the turtle Müller cell and therefore, the decreased rectification observed in

recordings from cells with all their processes intact (Fig. 2B) is a consequence of inadequate space clamping of the cell under voltage-clamp (Newman, 1993).

The cable properties of turtle müller cells

Turtle Müller cells have their cell bodies located in the INL and 6–10 thin processes extend proximally and terminate in an endfoot in the vitreo-retinal border (Conner et al., 1985; Linn et al., 1998).

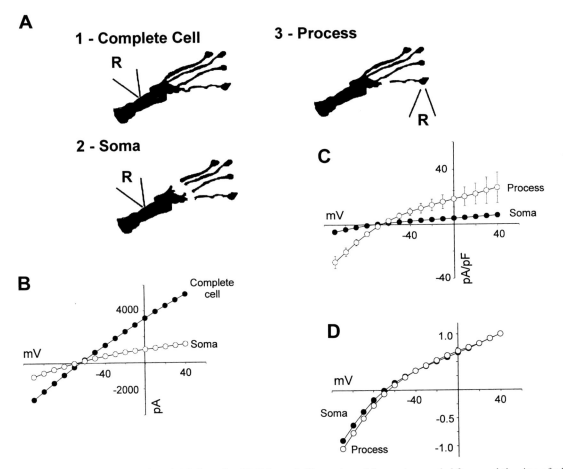

Fig. 2. I-V curves of different parts of turtle Müller cells. (A) Schematic illustration of the parts recorded from and the sites of whole-cell configuration; complete cell with processes intact, isolated soma, cell process with endfoot. (B) I-V curves from a complete cell with its processes and an isolated soma (filled and open circles respectively). In both cases, whole-cell recording was done in the cell soma. (C) Average I-V curves of isolated cell somas ($N = 5$) and of single cell processes with endfoot intact ($N = 3$). Currents densities were derived by dividing the measured currents by the capacitance of each cell part. (D) The I-V curves in Fig. 2C were normalized to the current values measured at $+40$ mV.

As shown in Fig. 2, this structure prevents adequate space clamping when whole-cell voltage-clamp is established in the cell soma of a cell with its processes intact and thus, distorts the I-V curve (Newman, 1993). Furthermore, such structure may prevent electrotonic spread of voltage along the cells during light-induced neuronal activity in the retina and, thus compromises the cell's capacity to efficiently siphon potassium ions. In order to investigate these possibilities, we constructed a compartmental model of turtle Müller cells. Dimensions of the cells were measured from cells in isolation and from lucifer yellow filled cells in the turtle retinal slice (Linn et al., 1998) and are listed in Table 1.

The electrical properties of the soma and the processes of Müller cells were derived as follows using experimental results and several assumptions. The membrane resistivity of the soma, R_m given in $\Omega \, cm^2$, was derived from the equation

$$\tau_m = R_m C_m \qquad (1)$$

where τ_m is the time constant of the exponential function used to fit the voltage response to a depolarizing current pulse and C_m is the membrane capacitance assumed to be 1 $\mu F/cm^2$. The membrane resistivity of the cell soma and the processes were also derived from measurements of the input resistance, computed from the current response to a voltage step of +20 mV that was applied from a holding potential of −70 mV. The axial resistivity, R_i, was given the value 70 Ω cm (Segev et al., 1989).

The remaining electrical properties of the cell soma and processes were derived from the following cable equations (Rall, 1989). The space constant, λ was calculated from

$$\lambda = [(R_m/R_i)/(d/4)]^{1/2} \qquad (2)$$

where d is the diameter of the cellular compartment. The specific resistance, R_s, from

$$R_s = [(4R_m R_i)/(\pi^2 d^3)]^{1/2} \qquad (3)$$

The input resistance, R_{in}, was obtained from

$$R_{in} = R_s/\tanh(L) \qquad (4)$$

And the voltage drop along the cable was derived from

$$V(x)/V_0 = \cosh(L-X)/\cosh(L) \qquad (5)$$

where $V(x)$ is the voltage at distance x from the site where a voltage pulse of V_0 is given. The values of X and L are, respectively, the distance from the site of the applied voltage pulse and the length of the compartment normalized to the space constant λ.

The electrical parameters of the model for turtle Müller cells in isolation are listed in Table 1. We determined the specific membrane resistance of the cell soma at 1700 $\Omega \, cm^2$ while that of each process was 6.8 times smaller (250 $\Omega \, cm^2$). The space constant of the isolated soma is several times its length resulting in a minimal voltage drop (<1%) along the cell body, as required for adequate space clamping. The clamping conditions are not nearly as ideal in the case of the isolated processes for which our estimation predicted a voltage drop of about 13% given their reduced specific membrane resistance and smaller diameter. Because the process is not

Table 1. Measured and computed electrical and spatial parameters of turtle Müller cells

	Parameter	Units	Soma	Process
R_{in}	input resistance (measured) ($n = 3$)	MΩ	87±23	56±10
τ_m	time constant ($n = 3$)	ms	1.76±0.6	–
R_m	membrane resistivity	Ωcm^2	1700	250
R_i	axonal resistivity	Ωcm	70	70
l	length	μm	70	70
d	diameter	μm	10	2
λ	space constant	μm	779	133
R_e	specific resistance	MΩ	6.9	29.8
R_{in}	input resistance (computed)	MΩ	77	62
V/V$_o$	voltage	%	99	87

456

isopotential as we initially assumed, we may have introduced a small error in our computations. However, the close match between the measured and computed input resistance (Table 1) implies that the error is minimal. It should be noted however, that the processes in Müller cells that have been isolated from the retina, tend to swell with time in culture to attain a diameter of about 2 μm compared to 0.5 μm that was measured in the retinal slice. These morphological changes have an impact on the electrotonic properties of the Müller cells as shown below.

In order to compute the voltage drop in a Müller cell with all processes intact, we used a compartmental model that allowed us to estimate the voltage drop in the processes when clamping the cell soma, and conversely, the voltage drop in the soma when clamping the endfoot. For our calculations, we assumed a typical cell being a cylinder of 10 μm diameter and 70 μm length and connected to six processes each of 70 μm length and 0.5 μm diameter. The cell soma and each of the processes were divided into seven equal compartments, each of 10 μm length. Thus, 50 simultaneous equations were derived, one for each node and were solved using the program *Mathematica*. The results of this computation are shown in Fig. 3.

When whole-cell configuration is established in the cell soma and a voltage pulse is applied (Fig. 3A), the entire cell soma is equipotential. However, voltage drop along the thin proximal processes is substantial and the endfoot of each of the 6 processes of the hypothetical cell undergoes a voltage change that is only 60% of that applied in the soma. When whole-cell is established in one of the endfeet (Fig. 3B), a very sharp voltage drop is seen along the process, and the potential change in the cell soma is only 10% of that applied to the endfoot. The remaining five endfeet are very poorly clamped under these conditions.

The data illustrated in Fig. 3 support the notion that interpretations of whole-cell experiments of Müller cells should be done with caution since space clamping is inadequate (Newman, 1993). This is especially true for Müller cells of complex structure such as that of the turtle retina. Our computations show that isolated somas lacking processes are essentially isopotential and since they posses the same potassium channels as the processes and endfeet (Fig. 2), they are well suited for voltage-clamp studies of the ionic currents participating in potassium siphoning by turtle Müller cells (Solessio et al., 2000; Solessio et al., 2001).

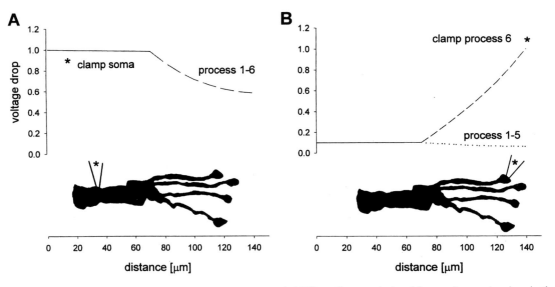

Fig. 3. Using the compartmental model, the voltage drop across turtle Müller cells was calculated for a voltage pulse given in the soma (**A**) and in one endfoot (**B**). If a voltage change is applied in the soma, each of the 6 endfeet will experience about 60% of this change. When the voltage pulse is given to one endfoot, the change in the soma will be about 10% of that applied in the endfoot while none of the other 5 endfeet will experience any voltage change.

Efficiency of potassium siphoning by turtle Müller cells

Measurements of potassium fluxes in response to a sudden increase in potassium concentration near the soma of isolated Müller cell from the tiger salamander retina indicated that the potassium efflux from the endfoot was driven by electromotive and not diffusional forces (Newman et al., 1984). Therefore, the voltage drop along the Müller cells and the relationship between their different parts are of utmost importance when potassium siphoning is analyzed. Potassium influx or efflux depends upon the difference between the membrane potential and the potassium equilibrium potential. If this difference is negative, potassium efflux will occur, whereas a positive difference will cause potassium influx. Thus, for a large potassium influx into the Müller cells to occur in the outer and inner plexiform layers (OPL and IPL), the membrane potential has to remain relatively constant despite local increases in the concentration of extracellular potassium ions. For this situation to occur, the parts of the Müller cell that are exposed to a normal potassium level have to "clamp" the cell to a fixed potential despite local changes in the concentration of extracellular potassium ions. But we have shown in Fig. 3B that the voltage drops by almost 90% from the endfoot to the soma, and thus a thin process cannot prevent the membrane potential from changing when potassium concentration changes around the soma. However, turtle Müller cells contain at least six thin processes each ending with an endfoot at the vitreo-retinal border. Assuming that all these endfeet are exposed to the same environment, and thus have the same potential, the question now becomes how well can these processes clamp the cell soma and prevent its membrane potential from changing in response to light-induced changes in the concentration of extracellular potassium ions.

We calculated the voltage "seen" by the cell soma of a hypothetical Müller cell when one or more processes are clamped at a fixed potential level. As shown in Fig. 4A, when only one process is clamped, the potential at the soma is only 10% of that in the endfoot. However, the quality of the clamp increases as the number of identical endfeet increases, such that with six endfeet the potential in the soma follows

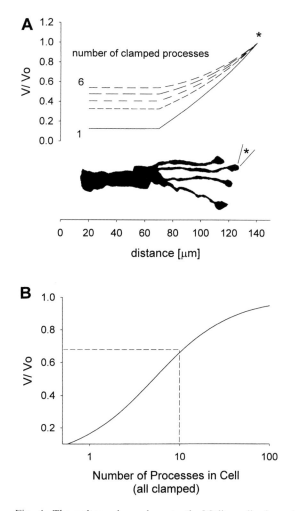

Fig. 4. The voltage drop along turtle Müller cells depends upon the number of process and the voltage at each endfoot. (A) Voltage drop from the endfoot region to the soma as has been calculated for different number of endfeet clamped to the same potential level. The more endfeet are clamped the shallower the voltage drop. When the potential is changed similarly in all six endfeet, the soma will experience close to 50% of this change. (B) The ratio of voltage in soma to voltage in endfeet has been calculated as a function of the number of endfeet being clamped together. For 10 endfeet, the soma will experience close to 70% of the change.

that of the endfeet at more than 50% efficiency. We calculated the voltage experienced by the soma as a function of the number of processes in the cell assuming that all were clamped at the same reference voltage. These results are shown in Fig. 4B. The quality of the clamp rises asymptotically with the number of processes. For a cell with 10 identical processes, the soma potential is more than 70% of that in the endfeet. Thus, numerous thin processes can clamp the membrane potential of the Müller cell despite local changes in potassium equilibrium potential. Under these conditions, when the concentration of extracellular potassium ions increases in a restricted retinal region during neuronal activity, potassium equilibrium increases locally but the membrane potential of the Müller cells hardly changes. Therefore, a large inward potassium current will occur.

In this regard, it appears that a trade-off has evolved in the Müller cells of retinas in certain species like turtle. In the Müller cells of these retinas, reduction in the diameter of the proximal processes seems to be compensated for by increased numbers of processes per cell, thereby maintaining (in theory) a relatively efficient capacity to siphon potassium away from the inner retina. In contrast, Müller cells that posses a single long proximal process of small diameter, like those in the central retina of rabbit and frog, have been shown to act poorly as potassium siphoning devices (Eberhardt and Reichenbach, 1987; Skatchkov et al., 1999).

The glutamate transporter and potassium siphoning

Müller cells also play an important role in synaptic transmission within the retina by actively removing glutamate from the extracellular space. Figure 5 illustrates the effects of glutamate on turtle Müller cells. Depolarizing and hyperpolarizing voltage pulses (100 ms in duration) were applied from a holding potential of −70 mV before and during application of L-glutamate in saturating concentration (200 μM). The I-V curves, constructed from currents that were measured just before the termination of the voltage pulses, are shown in Fig. 5A. In order to derive the glutamate-induced current, the two curves were substracted and the resulting difference I-V curve is shown in Fig. 5B (filled circles). Glutamate induces an inward current that increases as the cell is hyperpolarized.

In order to determine whether the glutamate-induced current flowed through glutamate-gated channels or was carried by an uptake system, we tested the effects of known glutamate agonists and antagonists. Kainic acid, AMPA and NMDA did not induce any measurable current while, D-aspartate did (not shown here). These observations support the notion that the measured glutamate-induced current in turtle Müller cells reflects the activation of an electrogenic uptake system and not the opening of specific glutamate-gated ionic channels. This conclusion is strengthened by the failure of known antagonists to glutamate-gated channels (CNQX and kynurenic acid) to reduce the glutamate-induced current as shown in Fig. 5C. In contrast, in the presence of 50 μM of the transporter blocker L-trans-pyrrolidine-2,4-dicarboxylate (PDC), the magnitude of the glutamate current was considerably reduced (curve marked DIFF in Fig. 5D) relative to the control (curve marked GLU in Fig. 5D). Detailed analysis showed that PDC elicited a standing inward current (marked PDC in Fig. 5D) that had voltage dependency similar to that of glutamate. Raising the concentration of PDC did not alter this current. The effects of PDC and glutamate were not additive, the current elicited by a mixture of glutamate and PDC was similar to that elicited by glutamate alone. Thus, PDC acts as a competitive inhibitor for the glutamate transporter in turtle Müller cells as it does for glutamate transporters in cerebellar granule cells (Griffiths et al., 1994). Consistent with the known stoichiometry of glutamate uptake systems (Schwartz and Tachibana, 1990), replacement of sodium in the extracellular solution with choline ions eliminated the glutamate current (Fig. 5B).

The data in Fig. 5 indicate that the glutamate transporter in turtle Müller cells is an electrogenic one and therefore, exposure to glutamate is expected to induce an inward current associated with depolarization. The magnitude of the glutamate-induced current depends upon the glutamate concentration and the driving force; the more hyperpolarized is the cell the larger the current (Fig. 5). The magnitude of the depolarization depends upon the amplitude of the current and the input resistance of the cell. We have previously shown that blocking potassium conductance with barium ions does not alter the magnitude of the glutamate-induced current but causes a substantial augmentation of the glutamate-induced depolarization (Linn et al., 1998). Since glutamate can modulate the electrical properties of Müller cells,

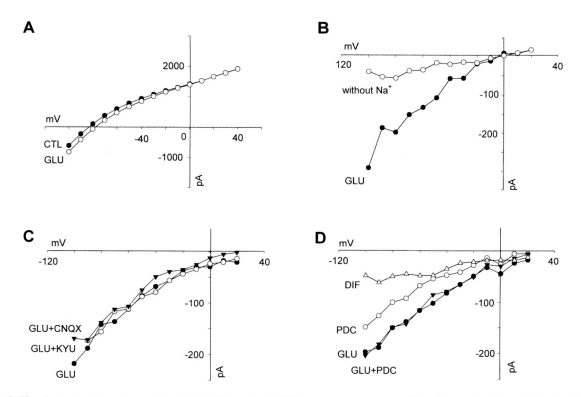

Fig. 5. The glutamate-induced current in turtle Müller cells. (**A**) I-V curves were constructed from hyperpolarizing and depolarizing voltage pulses (100 ms in duration) that were applied from a holding potential of −70 mV. Recordings were done in normal turtle Ringer solution and during application of a glutamate (200 μM) solution (filled and open circles respectively). (**B**) The glutamate-current (filled circles) was derived by substracting the I-V curves shown in (**A**). Replacing sodium ions with choline ions in the extracellular solution eliminated the glutamate current (open circles). (**C**) Antagonists of gluamate-gated channels; CNQX and Kynurenic acid, did not affect the glutamate-induced current in turtle Müller cells. (**D**) PDC (50 μM) elicited current that was smaller than that of glutamate (open and filled circles respectively) but of similar voltage dependency. A mixture of PDC + glutamate (filled inverted triangles) exerted similar effect to glutamate alone. The I-V curve of the glutamate current elicited in the presence of PDC is similar to the difference (DIFF) between the I-V curve obtained with the mixture and that obtained with PDC alone.

it probably contributes to potassium fluxes. It should be noted that the following analysis is concerned only with the contribution of the glutamate transporter to potassium siphoning through its effects on the electrical properties of the Müller cells. We ignore the direct effect of activating the transporter that is associated with counter-transport of potassium ions (Amato et al., 1994).

Possible contribution of the glutamate transporter to potassium siphoning is illustrated schematically in Fig. 6 where the effects of a local increase in potassium alone (A) and exposure to glutamate (B and C) are described. When the concentration of extracellular potassium ions is raised from 2.5 to 5.0 mM and the membrane potential of the cell is allowed to change freely, a new I-V curve will be established with the

membrane potential changing by about 20 mV (pathway a in Fig. 6A) as predicted by the Nernst potential. Being in equilibrium under these conditions, no inward potassium current will be observed. However, if the cell soma is clamped to its original potential, a large inward current will be seen (pathway b in Fig. 6A). This current is countered by an outward current through the clamping micropipette. Since the potential of the soma is clamped by the numerous endfeet (Fig. 4), the outward current will be induced there. Since the endfeet are highly permeable to potassium ions, the outward current will be carried by potassium ions. Thus, the influx of potassium ions in the inner retina where light-induced potassium increases occur is balanced by efflux of potassium into the vitreous.

460

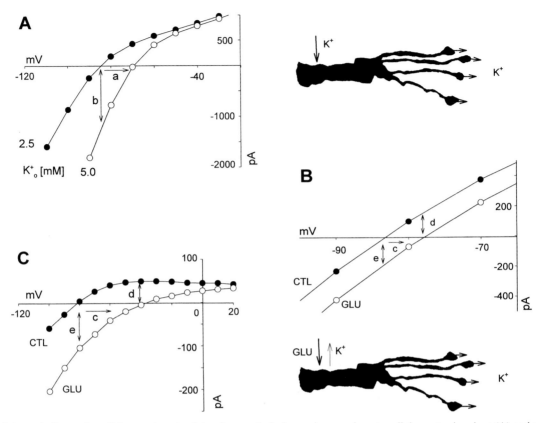

Fig. 6. Schematic illustration of changes in potential and currents during an increase in extracellular potassium ions (A) and a sudden exposure to L-glutamate (B and C). (**A**) When the cell is allowed to change its potential, it will depolarize (a mV) to a new resting potential when extracellular potassium is raised from 2.5 mM to 5.0 mM and no current will be induced. If the membrane potential is clamped by the endfeet to its original level, then a large inward current (b pA) will be induced in the soma and outward potassium currents in the endfeet. (**B**) Exposure to glutamate shifts the I-V curve of a current-clamped cell to the right by c mV and a small outward potassium current (d pA) will be induced in the soma. If the cell soma is clamped by the endfeet, the inward glutamate current (e pA) will be balanced by an outward potassium current of similar magnitude in the endfeet. (**C**) The electrical changes induced by glutamate become relatively larger when the potassium permeability of the Müller cell is reduced with barium ions.

The electrical changes in a Müller cell upon a sudden exposure to glutamate are illustrated in Fig. 6B. Because the effects are rather small relative to the total currents through the cell's membrane, we "zoomed in" on the relevant part of the I-V curves shown in Fig. 5A. If the potential of the Müller cell is allowed to change freely, then the glutamate current will induce a new steady state in which the cell depolarizes by a few millivolts (c in Fig. 6B) and the inward glutamate current is balanced by a small outward potassium current (d in Fig. 6B) mainly in the cell soma since the degree of depolarization in the endfeet will be considerably smaller. However, if the potential of the soma is clamped, the glutamate current will be larger (e in Fig. 6B). This current will

be countered by an outward current through the clamping electrode or the endfeet of the Müller cell. In the latter situation, the outward current will be carried by potassium ions.

The above analysis supports the notion that activation of the glutamate uptake system in Müller cells contributes to potassium siphoning by inducing the extrusion of potassium ions from the intracellular compartment to the vitreous in the region of the endfeet. However, this effect is relatively small in the conditions shown in Fig. 6B; the glutamate currents are of the order of 100 pA and the induced depolarization is on the order of a couple of millivolts (Linn et al., 1998). The relative effect of the glutamate transporter can be augmented in conditions where the potassium conductance is reduced as shown in Fig. 6C. Here, the potassium conductance was reduced with barium ions and the I-V curve shows decreased potassium currents though the reversal potential remains the same. Application of glutamate induces an inward current of similar magnitude to that recorded in the control conditions but the induced depolarization is tens of mVs (Linn et al., 1998) as is also evident from the change in the reversal potential in Fig. 6C. In this situation, the currents induced by glutamate and by changes in potassium are of comparable magnitude and thus, the role of the glutamate transporter in potassium siphoning becomes relevant. In the in vivo situation, the conductance of potassium channels can be modulated by a variety of intracellular and extracellular components. These include polyamines (Solessio et al., 2001), glutamate (Schwartz, 1993; Puro et al., 1996), GABA (Zhang and Yang, 1999), dopamine (Biedermann et al., 1995) and ATP (Kusaka and Puro, 1997).

Conclusions and future perspectives

Giant advances have been made in Müller cell research since the pioneering studies of John Dowling and his colleagues. Thanks to these studies, we learned that these cells were highly and almost exclusively permeable to potassium ions and that light stimuli changed the concentrations of extracellular potassium ions in the different retinal layers. These observations formed the foundations of the concept that the Müller cells were crucial for siphoning the excess potassium from the retina to the vitreous or blood vessels. Maintaining potassium homeostasis is a pre-requisite for normal function of all nervous tissues including the retina. Potassium concentration in the extracellular space is relatively low (about 2.5 mM) and therefore, even small changes in concentration will be reflected in large changes in potassium equilibrium potential across cell membranes, thereby disrupting neuronal activity. In the retina, light-induced increases in the concentration of extracellular potassium (Steinberg et al., 1980; Karwoski et al., 1985; Reichenbach et al., 1992) need to be countered by removal of potassium. Some is

taken up by the Na/K exchanger that exists in all retinal cells but additional mechanisms are needed especially during prolonged photic activation (day vision). Potassium ions can diffuse from sites of high concentration to sites of low concentration but this is a slow process (Newman et al., 1984; Reichenbach et al., 1992). Thus, the role of Müller cells in siphoning potassium from sites of high concentration to large sinks is essential.

In order to contribute to potassium homeostasis, the Müller cells are highly and almost exclusively permeable to potassium ions. Müller cells from every vertebrate retina studied contain inwardly rectifying potassium conductance but other types of channels including delayed rectifier and calcium-dependent potassium channels have been demonstrated (Nilius and Reichenbach, 1988; Reichelt and Pannicke, 1993; Chao et al., 1994). Regardless of the exact type of potassium channels present, the electrical properties of the Müller cells have to be accurately controlled for potassium to be taken up from sites of high potassium and extruded to large sinks. We have shown here that Müller cells with multiple thin processes can support potassium siphoning like Müller cells having one thick proximal process. Since the potential of the soma is efficiently clamped to the resting potential by the numerous endfeet, an inward flow of potassium through the inward rectifying channels is induced when light-induced increases in extracellular potassium ions occur. In analogy to voltage-clamp experiments where the inward current is balanced by an outward current through the clamping electrode, in turtle Müller cells the inward potassium current in the cell soma is balanced by an outward current through the multiple processes and their endfeet. Since the endfeet are mainly permeable to potassium ions, these ions carry the outward current into the vitreous. Thus, the type of potassium channels, their distribution along the Müller cells and the passive electrical properties of the cells that depend upon their structure are essential factors to be considered when potassium siphoning is discussed. Furthermore, the conductance of the potassium channels in retinal Müller cells can be modulated by intracellular and extracellular components (Schwartz, 1993; Biedermann et al., 1995; Puro et al., 1996; Kusaka and Puro, 1997; Zhang and Yang, 1999; Solessio et al., 2001), thus adding a degree of control on the efficacy of potassium siphoning to metabolic pathways in the Müller cells themselves and in the retinal neurons.

However, additional cellular mechanisms may provide further support to potassium siphoning. One of these is the glutamate transporter that is primarily responsible for removal of excess glutamate from the extracellular space. This is an electrogenic transporter that induces a net inward current in the cell soma. The magnitude of the glutamate-induced depolarization depends on how much the cell soma is clamped by the endfeet. As shown here, the multiple processes and their endfeet act as a clamping pipette and therefore, the glutamate-induced inward current is balanced by an outward current in the clamping area (the endfeet). Since the endfeet are almost exclusively permeable to potassium ions, this outward current is carried by potassium ions.

Although the contribution of the glutamate transporter to the siphoning of potassium ions appears to be small in the case of the turtle Müller cells (Fig. 6), the above analysis indicates that cellular mechanisms such as the electrogenic Na/K exchanger (Reichenbach et al., 1992), the GABA transporter (Biedermann et al., 1994; Ehinger, 1977), the nitric oxide system (Kusaka et al., 1996) and probably others need to be considered in the context of Müller cell morphology, the type of potassium channels, and their dependence upon ligands (e.g. polyamines, glutamate, GABA, cGMP, ATP) whenever potassium siphoning is discussed. The relative contribution of these mechanisms to potassium siphoning will vary among species given that their Müller cells vary in their morphology and the expression of the above cellular mechanisms.

References

Amato, A., Barbour, B., Szatkowski, M. and Attwell, D. (1994) Counter-transport of potassium by the glutamate uptake carrier in glial cells isolated from the tiger salamander retina. *J. Physiol. (Lond.)*, 479: 371–380.

Barbour, B., Brew, H. and Attwell, D. (1991) Electrogenic uptake of glutamate and aspartate into glial cells isolated from the salamander (*Ambystoma*) retina. *J. Physiol. (Lond.)*, 436: 169–193.

Barnett, N.L. and Pow, D.V. (2000) Antisense knockdown of GLAST, a glial glutamate transporter, compromises retinal function. *Invest. Ophthalmol. Vis. Sci.*, 41: 585–591.

Biedermann, B., Eberhardt, W. and Reichelt, W. (1994) GABA uptake into isolated retinal Müller glial cells of the guinea-pig detected electrophysiologically. *Neuroreport*, 12: 438–440.

Biedermann, B., Fröhlich, E., Grosche, J., Wagner, H.-J. and Reichenbach, A. (1995) Mammalian Müller (glial) cells express functional D_2 dopamine receptors. *Neuroreport*, 6: 609–612.

Brew, H. and Attwell, D. (1987) Electrogenic glutamate uptake is a major current carrier in the membrane of axolotl retinal glial cells. *Nature*, 327: 707–709.

Brew, H., Gray, P.T.A., Mobbs, P. and Attwell, D. (1986) Endfeet of retinal glial cells have higher densities of ion channels that mediate K^+ buffering. *Nature*, 324: 466–468.

Cajal, S.R.y. (1972) In: Thorpe, S.A. and Glickstein, M. (Eds.), *The Structure of the Retina*, Springfield, ILL, Thomas.

Cervetto, L. and Piccolino, M. (1974) Synaptic transmission between photoreceptors and horizontal cells in the turtle retina. *Science*, 183: 417–419.

Chao, T.I., Henke, A., Reichelt, W., Eberhardt, W., Reinhardt-Maelicke, S. and Reichenbach, A. (1994) Three distinct types of voltage-dependent K^+ channels are expressed by Müller (glial) cells of the rabbit retina. *Pflüg. Arch. Eur. J. Physiol.*, 426: 51–60.

Conner, J.D., Detwiler, P.B. and Sarthy, P.V. (1985) Ionic and electrophysiological properties of retinal Müller (glial) cells of the turtle. *J. Physiol. (Lond.)*, 362: 79–92.

Dick, E. and Miller, R.F. (1978) Light-evoked potassium activity in mudpuppy retina: its relationship to the b-wave of the electroretinogram. *Brain Res.*, 154: 388–394.

Dowling, J.E. and Ripps, H. (1970) Visual adaptation in the retina of the skate. *J. Gen. Physiol.*, 56: 491–520.

Dowling, J.E. and Ripps, H. (1973) Neurotransmission in the distal retina: the effects of magnesium on horizontal cell activity. *Nature*, 242: 101–103.

Eberhardt, W. and Reichenbach, A. (1987) Spatial buffering of potassium by retinal Müller (glial) cells of various morphologies calculated by a model. *Neuroscience*, 22: 687–696.

Ehinger, B. (1977) Glial and neuronal uptake of GABA, glutamic acid, glutamine and glutathione in the rabbit retina. *Exp. Eye Res.*, 25: 221–234.

Eliasof, S., Arriza, J.L., Leighton, B.H., Amara, S.G. and Kavanaugh, M.P. (1998) Localization and function of five glutamate transporters cloned from the salamander retina. *Vision Res.*, 38: 1443–1454.

Faber, D.S. (1969) Analysis of the slow transretinal potential in response to light. Ph.D. dissertation, University of New York, Buffalo, New York, USA.

Gaal, L., Roska, B., Picaud, S.A., Wu, S.M., Marc, R. and Werblin, F.S. (1998) Postsynaptic response kinetics are controlled by a glutamate transporter at cone photoreceptors. *J. Neurophysiol.*, 79: 190–196.

Green, D.G., Dowling, J.E., Siegal, I.M. and Ripps, H. (1975) Retinal mechanisms of visual adaptation in the skate. *J. Gen. Physiol.*, 65: 483–502.

Griffiths, R., Dunlop, J., Gorman, A., Senior, J. and Grieve, A. (1994) L-trans-pyrrolidine-2,4-dicarboxylate and cis-1-aminocyclobutane-1,3-dicarboxylate behave as transportable, competitive inhibitors of the high-affinity glutamate transporter. *Biochem. Pharmacol.*, 47: 267–274.

Izumi, Y., Kirby, C.O., Benz, A.M., Olney, J.W. and Zorumski, C.F. (1999) Müller cell swelling, glutamate uptake and excitotoxic neurodegeneration in the isolated rat retina. *Glia*, 25: 379–389.

Karwoski, C.J., Lu, H.-K. and Newman, E.A. (1989) Spatial buffering of light-evoked potassium increases by retinal Müller (glial) cells. *Science*, 217: 953–955.

Karwoski, C.J., Newman, E.A., Shimazaki, H. and Proenza, L.M. (1985) Light-evoked increases in extracellular K$^+$ in the plexiform layers of amphibian retinas. *J. Gen. Physiol.*, 86: 189–213.

Karwoski, C.J. and Proenza, L.M. (1977) Relationship between Müller cell responses, a local transretinal potential and potassium flux. *J. Neurophysiol.*, 40: 244–259.

Karwoski, C.J. and Proenza, L.M. (1978) Light-evoked changes in extracellular potassium concentration in mudpuppy retina. *Brain Res.*, 142: 515–530.

Kline, R.P., Ripps, H. and Dowling, J.E. (1978) Generation of b-wave currents in the skate retina. *Proc. Natl. Acad. Sci. USA*, 75: 5727–5731.

Kline, R.P., Ripps, H. and Dowling, J.E. (1985) Light-induced potassium fluxes in the skate retina. *Neuroscience*, 14: 225–235.

Kusaka, S., Dabin, I., Barnstable, C.J. and Puro, D.G. (1996) cGMP-mediated effects on the physiology of bovine and human retinal Müller (glial) cells. *J. Physiol. (Lond.)*, 497: 813–824.

Kusaka, S. and Puro, D.G. (1997) Intracellular ATP activates inwardly rectifying K$^+$ channels in human and monkey retinal Müller (glial) cells. *J. Physiol. (Lond.)*, 500: 593–604.

Lasater, E.M. and Dowling, J.E. (1982) Carp horizontal cells in culture respond selectively to L-glutamate and its agonists. *Proc. Natl. Acad. Sci. USA*, 79: 936–940.

Le Dain, A.C., Anderton, P.J., Martin, D.K. and Millar, T.J. (1994) Tetraethyammonium-insensitive inward rectifier K$^+$ channel in Müller cells of the turtle (*Pseudemys scripta elegans*) retina. *J. Memb. Biol.*, 141: 239–245.

Linn, D.M., Solessio, E., Perlman, I. and Lasater, E.M. (1998) The role of potassium conductance in the generation of light responses in Müller cells of the turtle retina. *Vis. Neurosci.*, 15: 449–458.

Matsui, K., Hosoi, N. and Tachibana, M. (1999) Active role of glutamate uptake in the synaptic transmission from retinal nonspiking neurons. *J. Neurosci.*, 19: 6755–6766.

Miller, R.F. and Dowling, J.E. (1970) Intracellular responses of the Müller (glial) cells of mudpuppy retina: their relation to b-wave of the electroretinogram. *J. Neurophysiol.*, 33: 323–341.

Newman, E.A. (1987) Distribution of potassium conductance in mammalian Müller (glial) cell: A comparative study. *J. Neurosci.*, 7: 2423–2432.

Newman, E.A. (1988) Electrophysiology of retinal glial cells. In: Osborne, N.N. and Chader, G.J. (Eds.), *Progress in Retinal Research*. Elsevier Science Ltd., Oxford, pp. 153–171.

Newman, E.A. (1993) Inward-rectifying potassium channels in retinal glial (Müller) cells. *J. Neurosci.*, 13: 3333–3345.

Newman, E.A., Frambach, D.A. and Odette, L.L. (1984) Control of extracellular potassium levels by retinal glial cell K$^+$ siphoning. *Science*, 255: 1174–1175.

Nilius, B. and Reichenbach, A. (1988) Efficient K$^+$ buffering by mammalian retinal glial cells die to cooperation of specialized ion channels. *Pflüg. Arch. Eur. J. Physiol.*, 411: 654–660.

Perlman, I., Knapp, A.G. and Dowling, J.E. (1989) Responses of isolated white perch horizontal cells to changes in the concentration of photoreceptor transmitter agonists. *Brain Res.*, 487: 16–25.

Puro, D.G., Yuan, J.P. and Sucher, N.J. (1996) Activation of NMDA receptor-channels in human retinal Müller glial cells inhibits inwardly-rectifying potassium currents. *Vis. Neurosci.*, 13: 319–326.

Rall, W. (1989) *Cable Theory for Dendritic Neurons*. MIT Press, Cambridge.

Rauen, T., Rothstein, J.D. and Wassle, H. (1996) Differential expression of three glutamate transporter subtypes in the rat retina. *Cell Tissue Res.*, 286: 325–336.

Reichelt, W. and Pannicke, T. (1993) Voltage-dependent K$^+$ currents in guinea pig Müller (glial) cells show different sensitivities to blockade by Ba^{2+}. *Neurosci. Lett.*, 155: 15–18.

Reichenbach, A., Henke, A., Eberhardt, W., Reichelt, W. and Dettmer, D. (1992) K$^+$ ion regulation in retina. *Can. J. Physiol. Pharmacol.*, 70: S239–S247.

Schultz, K. and Stell, W.K. (1996) Immunocytochemical localization of the high-affinity glutamate transporter, EAAC1, in the retina of representative vertebrate species. *Neurosci. Lett.*, 211: 191–194.

Schwartz, E.A. and Tachibana, M. (1990) Electrophysiology of glutamate and sodium co-transport in a glial cell of the salamander retina. *J. Physiol. (Lond.)*, 426: 43–80.

Schwartz, E.A. (1993) L-glutamate conditionally modulates the K$^+$ current of glial cells. *Neuron*, 10: 1141–1149.

Segev, I., Fleshman, J.W. and Burke, R.E. (1989) *Compartmental Models of Complex Neurons*. MIT Press, Cambridge.

Skatchkov, S.N., Krusek, J., Reichenbach, A. and Orkand, R.K. (1999) Potassium buffering by Müller cells isolated from the center and periphery of the frog retina. *Glia*, 27: 171–180.

Solessio, E., Linn, D.M., Perlman, I. and Lasater, E.L. (2000) Charaerization with barium of potassium currents in turtle Müller cells. *J. Neurophysiol.*, 83: 418–430.

Solessio, E., Rapp, K., Perlman, I. and Lasater, E.M. (2001) Spermine mediates inward rectification in potassium channels of turtle Müller cells. *J. Neurophysiol.*, in press.

Steinberg, R.H., Oakley, B.I. and Niemeyer, G. (1980) Light evoked changes in [K$^+$]$_o$ in retina of intact cat eye. *J. Neurophysiol.*, 44: 897–921.

Zhang, J. and Yang, X.L. (1999) GABA(B) receptors in Müller cells of the bullfrog retina. *Neuroreport*, 23: 1833–1836.

H. Kolb, H. Ripps and S. Wu (Eds.)
Progress in Brain Research, Vol. 131
© 2001 Elsevier Science B.V. All rights reserved

CHAPTER 33

Some aspects of the oscillatory response of the retina

Lillemor Wachtmeister*

Department of Clinical Sciences/Ophthalmology, Umeå University, SE-901 85 Umeå, Sweden

Introduction

In 1865 the light-evoked field potentials of the retina, collectively termed the electroretinogram (ERG), were first described by the Swedish physiologist Fritjof Holmgren (1865). The initial component of the corneally recorded ERG is the a-wave, a cornea-negative potential whose leading edge largely reflects the response of the photoreceptors (reviewed by Marmor and Lurie, 1979; Hood and Birch, 1997; Robson and Frishman, 1999). The a-wave is followed by the b-wave, a cornea-positive component that to a large extent indirectly reflects bipolar cell activity (Xu and Karwoski, 1994a,b). Fig. 1A describes the a-wave, b-wave, and subsequent ERG components associated with prolonged photic exposure.

Among the components of the ERG there are several that are oscillatory in nature. After a prolonged light stimulus is switched off there is a negative fast oscillation (FO) that peaks at 45–60 s in humans (Skoog, 1975; Nilsson and Skoog, 1975). After a steady light has been turned on a slow positive oscillation (SO) appears, having its maximum at 10–12 min, which can also be recorded as the light peak of the electrooculogram (EOG) (Arden et al., 1962).

There are also rapid small wavelets superimposed on the ascending b-wave of the ERG (Fig. 1A,B).

These wavelets, termed oscillatory potentials (OPs), were first noticed in the frog ERG by Granit and Münsterhjelm (1937). The OPs have been recorded in all species hitherto tried, from humans to mud-puppies. This rapid oscillatory response has a much higher frequency (90–160 Hz) than that of the a- and b-wave (25 Hz) which has been demonstrated by Fourier analysis in humans (Algvere and Wachtmeister, 1972; Algvere et al., 1972). The OPs are most easily elicited when the retina is stimulated by light with a fast rise time, brief duration and strong intensity, which bleaches negligible amount of rhodopsin (Ronchi and Grazi, 1956; Bornschein and Goodman, 1957; Wachtmeister, 1973).

The present chapter will only deal with the rapid oscillatory response of the retina, the oscillatory potentials (OPs). In the search for knowledge of the origin of the OPs and understanding of the functional role of the OPs John Dowling has contributed in several ways. His vast experience in the field of neurobiology, morphologically as well as physiologically, and brilliant intellect in interpretation of the findings during our collaboration at Harvard Biological Laboratory did indeed initiate and open up new perspectives for all of us working in this field of research. Some experimental and clinical aspects of the OPs will be presented. The paper will focus on the relation of the OPs to neuronal adaptation but it will also point out the clinical use of the OPs in diagnosis of retinal disease and in the description of the phenotype in hereditary retinal dystrophies.

* Tel.: +46-90-785 2470; Fax: +46-90-145997;
 E-mail: Lillemor.Wachtmeister@ophthal.umu.se

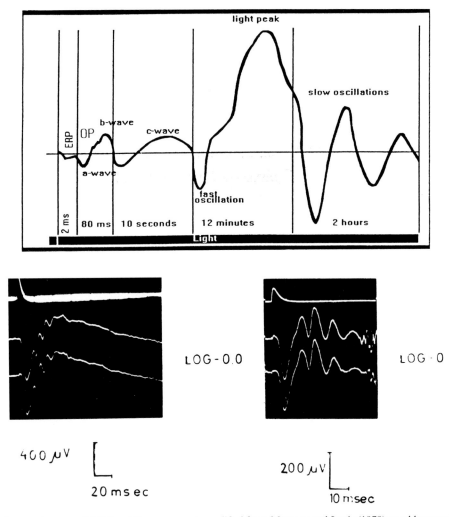

Fig. 1. (A). The electroretinogram (ERG) and its components modified from Marmor and Lurie (1979), used by permission. (B). ERG-recordings in a healthy human subject performed with a long time constant and in response to light of high intensity and a rapid rise time at an interstimulus interval of 30 s (left). The responses to the second and third flashes are shown. On the right are the oscillatory potentials (OPs) of the ERG recorded with a short time constant (T = 15 ms), selectively attenuating the a- and b-waves during the same stimulus conditions. From Wachtmeister (1973), used by permission.

Results and discussion

Experimental aspects – origin

What do the OPs represent? There have been several suggestions. The OPs have been considered to contribute to the b-wave (Granit and Münsterhjelm, 1937), to be a partly derivative version of the ERG (Lachapelle and Benoit, 1994), to be an electrical manifestation of an oscillating retinal membrane (Levitt and Mc Avinn, 1979) and to be an expression of optic nerve activity (Doty and Kimura, 1963; Steinberg, 1966). However, the OPs have been shown to have characteristics and origins distinct from those of the a- and b-waves and thus to be separate to the major, slow components of the ERG (Wachtmeister 1972, Wachtmeister and Dowling, 1978; Heynen et al., 1985).

Data from several experimental studies will illustrate these conclusions. Some of this work (on the mudpuppy) was performed during my post doctoral year with John Dowling at Harvard University.

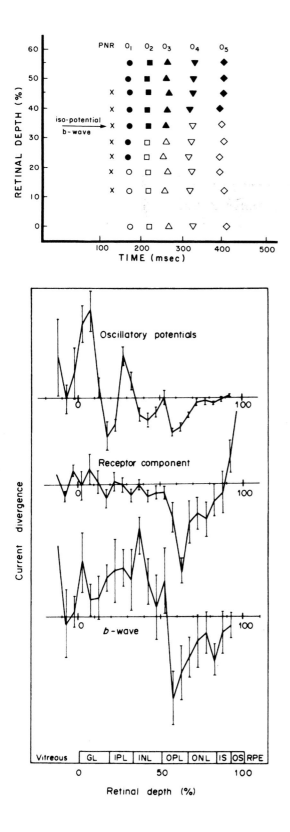

He made his very well equipped laboratory in basic electrophysiology, available for me to learn and work in. This was a prerequisite for the advanced methods which had to be used to collect data, and to investigate the origin of the OPs. Laminar profile of voltages of the mudpuppy retina (Fig. 2A) and in vivo current-source density studies of the monkey ERG (Fig. 2B) demonstrated that the site(s) of origin of the OPs were separate from the b-wave and the receptor components (Wachtmeister and Dowling, 1978; Heynen et al., 1985), and also different from the proximal negative response (PNR), an extracellular response of the amacrine cells (Wachtmeister and Dowling, 1978). In the mudpuppy as well as in the monkey the OPs were found to reflect radial flows of currents in the retina. There was a more proximal distribution of the OP generator(s) than that of the a- and b-waves. In the mudpuppy retina the OPs reversed polarity as a function of depth, unlike the PNR (Fig. 2A). The reversal points were located at different retinal strata, suggesting individual origins in the inner part of the retina. They seem to represent a series of radial current loops moving from the inner to the outer retina, a feedback system, which had been originally suggested by Brown (1968). However, the precise intraretinal site(s) of origin

Fig. 2. (**A**). Peak times of the individual oscillatory peaks of the mudpuppy ERG in relation to retinal depth. Depth is expressed in percent. Open symbols represent peak times of non-reversed positive OPs. Closed symbols represent peak times of reversed negative OPs. Crosses represent the peak of the proximal negative response (PNR). Full-field stimulus of 200 ms duration delivered at an interval of 30 s was used. As the microelectrode penetrates the retina from the vitreous side the b-wave reverses its polarity at about 35% of depth. The PNR remains negative over the entire depth and it can be recorded from about 10 to 50%. The individual oscillatory peaks reverse their polarities at different levels. O_1 at about 20%, O_2 and O_3 at about 30% and O_4 and O_5 at about 40% retinal depth. From Wachtmeister and Dowling (1978), used by permission. (**B**). Current source density profiles of the OPs, the receptor component and the b-wave of the monkey ERG, recorded in one experiment (mean of 9 series). The OP profile represents the mean of all components from the bandpass filtered signals. Error bars denote ±SEM. The intraretinal high pass digitally filtered local ERG and the local resistance were recorded in steps of 20 μm with a bipolar coaxial microelectrode in the intact macaque eye in response, to a 10° stimulus of 10 ms duration, ISI:1.25 s. From Heynen et al. (1985), used by permission.

remains unknown. The OPs are most probably generated by the bipolar cells—but the interplexiform cell cannot be excluded as a generator (Heynen et al., 1985). Pharmacological studies have shown that the OPs seem to primarily reflect neuronal activity in inhibitory neuronal pathways in the inner retina, initiated by the amacrines and most likely the dopaminergic ones (Wachtmeister and Dowling, 1978; Wachtmeister, 1980, 1981; Wachtmeister, 1998). The OPs may be the only post-synaptic neuronal component that can be recorded in the ERG except when structured stimuli are being used (Dawson et al., 1982).

Relation to neuronal adaptation and the importance of the oscillatory response (OPs)

There are two fundamental adaptive processes in the retina—one determined by the concentration of photopigment ("photochemical" adaptation) and the other rapid one depending on non-receptoral neuronal mechanisms ("network" or neural adaptation) and this term was coined by John Dowling in 1963 (Dowling, 1963; Green et al., 1975). Very dim illumination which does not affect receptor or horizontal cell sensitivity was shown to decrease the thresholds of the amacrine cells (PNR) and the ganglion cells in the skate retina in experiments performed by Dowling and Ripps in Woods Hole (Dowling, 1967; Dowling and Ripps, 1977). Therefore, we know that the neuronal adaptive mechanisms of non-receptoral origin are located more proximally in the retina.

After complete dark adaptation, no definite OPs can be recorded. An oscillatory response of optimal energy (and of low frequency) is recorded during mesopic conditions in humans which can be induced by conditioning flashes (Fig. 3A,B), light adaptation to a steady background illumination, or during succeeding dark adaptation after a bright preillumination (Algvere and Wachtmeister, 1972; Wachtmeister, 1973). The OPs were found to be linked to fast adaptational changes unrelated to concentration of photopigments (see also review Wachtmeister, 1998).

An imperative for neuronal adaptation is a system, which quickly reacts to changes of illumination and communicates back to distal retina (Dowling, 1963, 1967). The OPs reflect fast adaptational changes—and represent post-synaptic neuronal activity in feedback circuits from the proximal retina (Ogden, 1973; Wachtmeister and Dowling, 1978; Heynen et al., 1985). The oscillatory response has therefore been used to sensitively assess the neuronal adaptive function of the retina.

The postnatal development of the neuronal adaptive qualities of the retina by monitoring the OPs was investigated by us in a rat model (el Azazi and Wachtmeister, 1990, 1991a,b, 1992). We found that the neuronal adaptive mechanisms appeared later and matured slower than the photochemical one (which was adult-like at the age of 18 days in the rat) (Fulton and Graves, 1980; Fulton and Baker, 1984). The photopically elicited OPs appeared comparatively later postnatally than the scotopically induced ones (Fig. 4A,B). This delay of development of neuronal activity indicated by the retarded maturation of the oscillatory response most probably reflects a functional immaturity of the dopaminergic neuronal system. Moreover the timetable of development of the individual oscillatory peaks is most likely related to the plan of maturation of the different neurotransmitter systems of the retina, and most probably the inhibitory ones.

Recent experimental studies by our group have shown that the neuronal adaptive system, as indicated by the OPs, is a comparatively robust one and may play a vision—preserving role in the rat (Wang et al., 2000). When the rats were exposed to two levels of dim (scotopic) background illuminations there was an increase of the oscillatory response, even though the slow components, the a- and b-waves, were not affected (in the weakest background light) or were decreased (in the somewhat stronger scotopic background light) (Fig. 5). In relatively more intense (low mesopic level) illumination the oscillatory response maximized and the major components further decreased. In the strongest background light (high mesopic level) the OPs diminished about 50% and the a- and b-waves were almost abolished. Thus, the neuronal adaptive system may serve to signal the introduction of dim illumination, and in addition signal the occurrence of an increase in ambient light level over a large range.

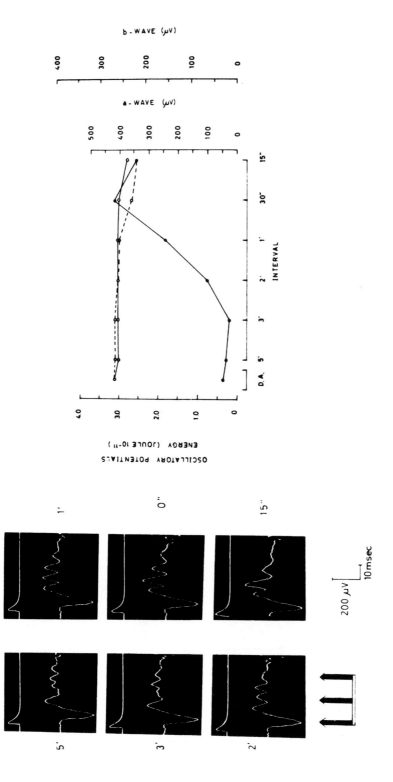

Fig. 3. (A). OPs of the human ERG recorded with a short time constant (T = 15 ms) during dark adaptation in response to flashes of high intensity delivered at different intervals, as indicated. From Wachtmeister (1973), used by permission. (B). Calculated energy of the OPs of the human ERG shown in (A) and the amplitudes of the a- and b-waves in relation to the interval between stimulus flashes of high intensity. Black circles indicate energy of the OPs, open circles and continuous line designate amplitude of the a-wave, and open circles and dashed line indicate the amplitude of the b-wave. The ERGs were recorded in dark adaptation in response to flashes of high intensity delivered at different interstimulus intervals (ISI), varying from 5 min to 15 s. Most prominent OPs were recorded at an interval of 30 s. From Wachtmeister (1973), used by permission.

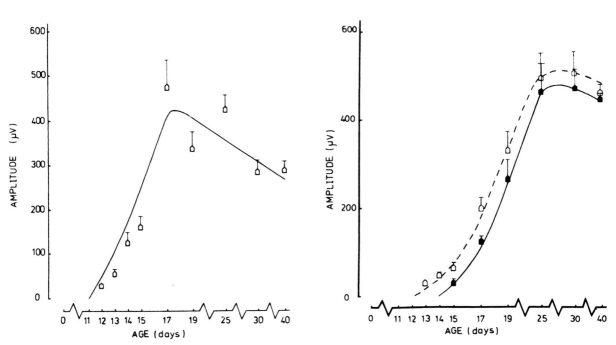

Fig. 4. (**A**). Summed amplitude of the OPs of the rat ERG recorded during relatively extreme scotopic conditions (ISI = 5 min) in relation to postnatal age. Means ± SEM of six experiments at each age. Very small SEMs are not shown graphically. From el Azazi and Wachtmeister (1991b), used by permission. (**B**). Summed amplitudes of the OPs of the rat ERG recorded during relatively extreme (ISI: 10 s) and extreme (ISI:5 s) photopic conditions in relation to postnatal age. Unfilled symbols = ISI:10 s. Filled symbols = ISI:5 s. Very small SEMs are not shown graphically. From el Azazi and Wachtmeister (1991a), used by permission.

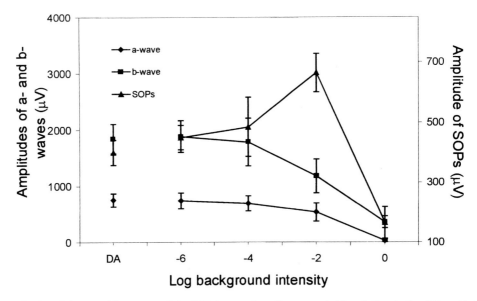

Fig. 5. Mean amplitudes of the a- and b-waves and the SOP (summed oscillatory peaks) in relation to the different intensities of BG (background) -illumination, and measured in dark adaptation and 6 min after the BG light was turned on. Bar indicates 95% confidence interval for the mean ($n = 5$).

Clinical aspects

Clinically, and in medical ophthalmological practice, the oscillatory response is best known to be a good indicator of the functional integrity of the micro-circulation of the inner retina in patients with diabetic retinopathy, retinal vascular occlusions, systemic hypertension, retinopathy of prematurity etc. (see overview Wachtmeister, 1998). Several investigators have analyzed the individual oscillatory peaks in various hereditary degenerative and dystrophic reti-nopathies (Heckenlively et al., 1983; Lachapelle et al., 1983; Miyake and Kawasi, 1984; Miyake et al., 1986; Lachapelle and Little, 1992; Cideciyan and Jacobson, 1993; Lachapelle, 1994).

In congenital stationary night blindness (CSNB) of the Schubert-Bornschein type the oscillatory response has been shown to be a valuable instrument for early detection of neuronal abnormality and defective transmission (Hill et al., 1974; Heckenlively et al., 1983; Lachapelle et al., 1983; Miyake and Kawase, 1984; Miyake et al., 1986). The pathological oscilla-tory response not only reveals an affected rod system but also very sensitively denotes an impaired inter-action between the scotopic and photopic systems. A detailed evaluation discloses a differential absence of the earlier OPs (O_2 O_3) indicating a dysfunction of the rod mediated on-pathways of the inner retina. Moreover, female carriers of CSNB without clinical signs of ocular pathology show a selective reduction of the summed amplitudes of the OPs (with intact timing), probably implying loss of function to patches of retinal area in this X-linked recessive disease (Miyake and Kawase, 1984).

As retinal neurobiology has progressed so also has our molecular understanding of the genetic hetero-geneity of patients with hereditary degenerative and dystrophic retinopathies including retinitis pigmen-tosa (RP). Around 55 different proteins are known to cause various kinds of hereditary retinal dystrophies, if patients carry certain mutations in many different genes (Ehinger, 2000). There may be more than 60 gene loci involved and an updated list is available on Ret Net web (Daiger et al., 2000). Also in RP-patients in which basically the outer retina (photoreceptors and retinal pigment epithe-lium) is affected, the OP-response has been found to be abnormal (Cideciyan and Jacobson, 1993;

Lachapelle, 1994). Diminished or delayed OPs or no measurable OPs have been described (Cideciyan and Jacobson, 1993). Moreover, a disproportionately reduced second, second and third or only fourth oscillatory peak(s) have been observed indicating a disturbed function of primarily the rod mediated on-pathways or mainly the cone-related off-pathways in the inner retina (Lachapelle, 1994). Thus, the OP findings clearly signal a disrupted function in the inner retinal layers already at a comparatively early stage of the RP disease. Hypothetically—these distur-bances of inner retinal function, as indicated by loss or reduction of individual oscillatory peak(s), may reflect abnormal wiring of surviving rods (neurite sprouting) and/or pathological changes of the cone axons which have been observed in RP patients (Li et al., 1995; Fariss et al., 2000). During the degen-erative process of human photoreceptors rod neurites, bypassing the rod bipolar and horizontal cells, that are normally post-synaptic to rod axons, as well as elongated and branched cones, appear in regions of photoreceptor death (Li et al., 1995). These changes of the rods are termed neurite sprouting and some types of amacrine cells and horizontal cells also undergo neurite sprouting. Furthermore, the rod neurites project into the inner retina and make contacts direct to amacrine cells (Fariss et al., 2000).

A variety of clinical phenotypes, including Stargardt's dystrophy (STGD)—Fundus flavimacu-latus (FFM), has been reported in patients with mutations in the retina-specific ABCR-gene (Klevering et al., 1999). A defective peripherin/RDS gene has also been described in patients with a STGD/FFM clinical phenotype, but also other phenotypes, in the same family (Weleber et al., 1993). STGD/FFM-patients exhibit a progressive atrophy of the deeper retinal layers (pigment epithe-lium and choriocapillaris) in combination with degeneration of the photoreceptors. Even though STGD/FFM is an outer retina disease, the patients show relatively early OP abnormalities (Lachapelle et al., 1990; Weleber et al., 1993). A closer analysis revealed a comparatively more decreased third oscillatory peak in STGD and only a slightly delayed second OP in FFM (Lachapelle et al., 1990). In more severe cases (with the peripherin/RDS mutation) there was a general reduction of all the individual OP peaks (Weleber et al., 1993). It is therefore tempting to suggest that the severity of the disease may vary with type of mutation, which also may be expressed as different pattern of OP-morphology and varying degree of disturbed inner retinal function. Such an interpretation is also in accordance with a suggestion that ABCR-mutations may be grouped in different classes of severity (van Driel et al., 1998).

Conclusions and future perspectives

Conclusions

Thus, in summary we conclude that:

1. The oscillatory potentials (OPs) of the retina are separate components of the ERG with different origins compared to the slow dominant components, a- and b-waves.
2. The individual oscillatory peaks most likely represent synaptic activity in feedback neuronal pathways in the inner retina, probably inhibitory ones and initiated by the amacrine cells.
3. The oscillatory response of the ERG may be used as an instrument to monitor the function of the neuronal adaptive system in the proximal retina.
4. The postnatal development of the fast adaptive neuronal process as indicated by the OPs, is slower than that of the photochemical adaptive system.
5. The neuronal adaptive process seem to represent a robust retinal structure and may play a vision preserving role to alert against unwarranted attenuation of the slowly regenerating visual pigment.
6. The OPs of the ERG can be of use in clinical ophthalmology to identify early compromise of retinal neuronal function and microcirculation of the inner retina. The oscillatory response is also a sensitive tool to discover disturbed neuronal function in patients with retinitis pigmentosa, Stargardt's disease, congenital stationary night blindness and other hereditary retinal degenerations and dystrophies.

Future perspectives

Increased knowledge about the relation between phenotype and genotype (i.e. mapped chromosomal location, genomic sequence of the mutation, probable protein involved etc) will eventually enable us to define several different subtypes of RP, retinitis punctata albescens, STGD/FFM etc. Consequently novel entities will evolve. This transformation has already started and for example, recently a new autosomal recessive retinal degenerative disease, Bothnia dystrophy, was characterized to its genotype (Burstedt et al., 1999) and phenotype (Burstedt et al., 2001). Also the oscillatory response will play a role in this process, being a useful clinical instrument to detect and classify early neuronal abnormalities—and hopefully help to link defect gene/protein to retinal function. Furthermore, as clinical gene correction therapy now is becoming available (McNally et al., 1999) and DNA-analysis may be used for development of new treatment strategies in the future, monitoring the oscillatory response will also be of importance to evaluate therapeutic effects and demonstrate functional rescue.

Acknowledgments

The support of NIH, US Health Science Postdoctoral Research Fellowship (F05-TW-2250), the Swedish Medical Research Council (No 05411), the Swedish Medical Society, the Karolinska Institute and Umeå University are greatly acknowledged. I thank Dr. David Pepperberg for helpful comments on the manuscript and Mrs. Birgit Johansson for excellent secretarial work.

References

Algvere, P. and Wachtmeister, L. (1972) On the oscillatory potentials of the human electroretinogram in light and dark adaptation. II. Effect of adaptation to background light and subsequent recovery in the dark. A Fourier analysis. *Acta. Ophthalmol. (Copenh.)*, 50: 837–862.

Algvere, P., Wachtmeister, L. and Westbeck, S. (1972) On the oscillatory potentials of the human electroretinogram in light and dark adaptation. I. Thresholds and relation to stimulus intensity on adaptation to short flashes of light. A Fourier analysis. *Acta. Ophthalmol. (Copenh.)*, 50: 737–759.

Arden, G.B., Barrada, A. and Kelsey, J.H. (1962) New clinical test of retinal function based upon the standing potential of the eye. *Br. J. Ophthalmol.*, 46: 449–467.

Bornschein, H. and Goodman, G. (1957) Studies of the a-wave in the human electroretinogram. *Arch. Ophthalmol.*, 58: 431–437.

Brown, K.T. (1968) The electroretinogram. Its components and their origins. *Vision Res.*, 8: 633–677.

Burstedt, M., Sandgren, O., Holmgren, G. and Forsman-Semb, K. (1999) Bothnia Dystrophia Caused by Mutations in the Cellular Retinaldehyde-Binding Protein Gene (RLBP1) on Chromosome 15q26. *Invest. Ophthalmol. Vis. Sci.*, 40: 995–1000.

Burstedt, M., Forsman-Semb, K., Golovleva, I., Janunger, T., Wachtmeister, L. and Sandgren, O. (2001) Ocular phenotype of Bothnia dystrophy, an autosomal recessive retinitis pigmentosa associated with a R234W mutation in the RLBP1 gene. *Arch. Ophthalmol.*, 119: 260–267.

Cideciyan, A. and Jacobson, S. (1993) Negative Electroretinograms in Retinitis Pigmentosa. *Invest. Ophthalmol. Vis. Sci.*, 34: 3253–3263.

Daiger, S.P., Sullivan, L.S. and Rossiter, B.J. (2000) Web URL: http//www.sph.uth.tmc.edu/Retnet/. Laboratory for Molecular Diagnosis of Inherited Eye Diseases.

Dawson, W.W., Maida, T.M. and Rubin, M.L. (1982) Human pattern-evoked retinal responses are altered by optic atrophy. *Invest. Ophthalmol. Vis. Sci.*, 22: 796–803.

Doty, R.W. and Kimura, D.S. (1963) Oscillatory potentials in the visual system of cats and monkeys. *J. Physiol.*, 168: 205–218.

Dowling, J.E. (1963) Neural and photochemical mechanisms of visual adaptation in the rat. *J. Gen. Physiol.*, 46: 1287–1301.

Dowling, J.E. (1967) The site of visual adaptation. *Science*, 155: 273–279.

Dowling, J.E. and Ripps, H. (1977) The proximal negative response and visual adaptation in the skate retina. *J. Gen. Physiol.*, 57: 57–74.

Ehinger, B. (2000) Tapetoretinal degenerations: Experiences, experiments and expectations. *Acta. Ophthalmol. Scand.*, 78: 244–255.

el Azazi, M. and Wachtmeister, L. (1990) The postnatal development of the oscillatory potentials of the electroretinogram. I. Basic characteristics. *Acta. Ophthalmol. (Copenh.)*, 68: 401–409.

el Azazi, M. and Wachtmeister, L. (1991a) The postnatal development of the oscillatory potentials of the electroretinogram. II. Photopic characteristics. *Acta. Ophthalmol. (Copenh.)*, 69: 6–10.

el Azazi, M. and Wachtmeister, L. (1991b) The postnatal development of the oscillatory potentials of the electroretinogram. III. Scotopic characteristics. *Acta. Ophthalmol. (Copenh.)*, 69: 505–510.

el Azazi, M. and Wachtmeister, L. (1992) The postnatal development of the oscillatory potentials of the electroretinogram. IV. Mesopic characteristics. *Acta. Ophthalmol. (Copenh.)*, 70: 194–200.

Fariss, R.N., Li, Z.-Y. and Milam, A.H. (2000) Abnormalities in rod photoreceptors, amacrine cells, and horizontal cells in human retinas with retinitis pigmentosa. *Am. J. Ophthalmol.*, 129: 215–223.

Fulton, A. and Graves, A. (1980) Background adaptation in the developing rat retina: an electroretinographic study. *Vision Res.*, 20: 819–826.

Fulton, A. and Baker, B. (1984) The relation of retinal sensitivity and rhodopsin in developing rat retina. *Invest. Ophthalmol. Vis. Sci.*, 25: 647–651.

Granit, R.L. and Münsterhjelm, A. (1937) The electrical response of dark adapted frog's eye to monochromatic stimuli. *J. Physiol.*, 88: 436–458.

Green, D.G., Dowling, J.E., Siegel, I.M. and Ripps, H. (1975) Retinal mechanisms of visual adaptation in the skate. *J. Gen. Physiol.*, 65: 483–502.

Heckenlively, J.R., Martin, D.A. and Rosenbaum, A.L. (1983) Loss of electroretinographic oscillatory potentials, optic atrophy and dysplasia in congenital stationary night blindness. *Am. J. Ophthalmol.*, 96: 526–534.

Heynen, H., Wachtmeister, L. and van Norren, D. (1985) Origin of the oscillatory potentials in the primate retina. *Vision Res.*, 10: 1365–1373.

Hill, D.A., Arbel, K.F. and Berson, E.L. (1974) Cone electroretinogram in congenital nyctalopia with myopia. *Am. J. Ophthalmol.*, 78: 127–136.

Holmgren, F. (1865) Metod att objektivera effekten av ljusintryck på retina. *Upsala läkaref. Förhandl.*, 1: 177–191.

Hood, D.C. and Birch, D.G. (1997) Assessing abnormal rod photoreceptor activity with the a-wave of the electroretinogram: applications and methods. *Doc. Ophthalmol.*, 92: 253–267.

Klevering, B.J., van Driel, M., van de Pol, D.J.R., Pinkers, A.J.L., Cremers, F.M. and Hoyng, C.B. (1999) Phenotypic variations in a family with retinal dystrophy as result of different mutations in the ABCR gene. *Br. J. Ophthalmol.*, 83: 914–918.

Lachapelle, P. (1994) The human suprathreshold photopic oscillatory potential in the human electroretinogram. *Doc. Ophthalmol.*, 88: 1–25.

Lachapelle, P. and Little, J. (1992) Abnormal light adaptation of the electroretinogram in some carriers of choroideremia. *Clin. Vision Sci.*, 7: 403–411.

Lachapelle, P. and Benoit, J. (1994) Interpretation of the filtered 100 to 1000 Hz electroretinogram. *Doc. Ophthalmol.*, 86: 33–46.

Lachapelle, P., Little, J. and Polomeno, R. (1983) The Photopic Electroretinogram in Congenital Stationary Night Blindness with Myopia. *Invest. Ophthalmol. Vis. Sci.*, 24: 442–450.

Lachapelle, P., Little, J. and Roy, M.S. (1990) The electroretinogram in Stargardt's disease and fundus flavimaculatus. *Doc. Ophthalmol.*, 73: 395–404.

Levitt, J. and McAvinn, J.D. (1979) Oscillatory potentials in the electroretinogram. *Tower International Technomedical Journal of Life Sciences*, 9: 19–22.

Li, Z.-Y., Kljavin, I. and Milam, A.H. (1995) Rod Photoreceptor Neurite Sprouting in Retinitis Pigmentosa. *J. Neurosci.*, 15: 5429–5438.

Marmor, M.F. and Lurie, M. (1979) In: Zinn, K.M. and Marmor, M.F. (Eds.), *The Retinal Pigment Epithelium*. Harvard University Press, Cambridge, pp. 226.

McNally, N., Kenna, P., Humphries, M.M., Hoch, W., Khan, N.W., Bush, K.A., Sieving, P.A., Humphries, P. and Farrar, G.J. (1999) Structural and functional rescue of murine rod

474

photoreceptors by human rhodopsin transgene. *Hum. Mol. Genet.*, 8: 1309–1312.

Miyake, Y. and Kawase, Y. (1984) Reduced amplitude of oscillatory potentials in female carriers of x-linked recessive congenital stationary night blindness. *Am. J. Ophthalmol.*, 98: 208–215.

Miyake, Y., Yagasaki, K., Horiguchi, M., Kawase, Y. and Kanada, T. (1986) Congenital Stationary Night Blindness with a Negative Electroretinogram. *Arch. Ophthalmol.*, 104: 1013–1020.

Nilsson, S.E.G. and Skoog, K.O. (1975) Covariation of the simultaneously recorded c-wave and standing potential of the human eye. *Acta. Ophthalmol.*, 53: 721–730.

Ogden, T.E. (1973) The oscillatory waves of the primate electroretinogram. *Vision Res.*, 13: 1059–1074.

Robson, J.G. and Frishman, L.J. (1999) Dissecting the dark-adapted electroretinogram. *Doc. Ophthalmol.*, 95: 187–215.

Ronchi, L.A. and Grazi, S. (1956) The dependence of human electroretinogram on the shape of the stimulus as a function of time. *Optica. Acta.*, 3: 188–195.

Skoog, K.G. (1975) The directly recorded standing potential of the human eye. *Acta. Ophthalmol.(Copenh.)*, 53: 120–132.

Steinberg, R. (1966) Oscillatory activity in the optic tract of cat and light adaptation. *J. Neurophysiol.*, 29: 139–156.

van Driel, M.A., Mangeri, A., Klevering, B.J., Hoyng, C.B. and Cremers, F.P. (1998) ABCR unites what ophthalmologists divide(s). *Ophthalmic Genet.*, 19: 117–122.

Wachtmeister, L. (1972) On the oscillatory potentials of the human electroretinogram in light and dark adaptation. *Acta. Ophthalmol. (Copenh.)*, Suppl. 116.

Wachtmeister, L. (1973) On the oscillatory potentials of the human electroretinogram in light and dark adaptation. IV. Effect of adaptation to short flashes of light. Time interval and intensity of conditioning flashes. A Fourier analysis. *Acta. Ophthalmol. (Copenh.)*, 51: 250–273.

Wachtmeister, L. (1980) Further studies of the chemical sensitivity of the oscillatory potentials of the electroretinogram (ERG). I. GABA- and glycine antagonists. *Acta. Ophthalmol. (Copenh.)*, 58: 712–725.

Wachtmeister, L. (1981) Further studies of the chemical sensitivity of the oscillatory potentials of the electroretinogram (ERG). II. Glutamate- aspartate- and dopamine antagonists. *Acta. Ophthalmol. (Copenh.)*, 59: 247–258.

Wachtmeister, L. (1998) Oscillatory Potentials in the Retina: what do they reveal. In: Osborne, N. and Chader, G. (Eds.), *Progress in Retinal and Eye Research*. Vol. 17, No. 4, Elsevier Science Ltd, UK, pp. 485–521.

Wachtmeister, L. and Dowling, J. (1978) The oscillatory potentials of the mudpuppy retina. *Invest. Ophthalmol. Vis. Sci.* 17: 1176–1188.

Wang, L., el Azazi, M., Eklund, A. and Wachtmeister, L. (2000) Background light adaptation of the retinal neuronal adaptive system. I. Effect of background light intensity. (Submitted for publication.)

Weleber, R.G., Carr, R.E., Murphey, W.H., Sheffield, V.C. and Stone, E.M. (1993) Phenotypic Variation Including Retinitis Pigmentosa, Pattern Dystrophy, and Fundus Flavimaculatus in a Single Family With a Deletion of Codon 153 or 154 of the Peripherin/RDS Gene. *Arch. Ophthalmol.*, 111: 1531–1542.

Xu, X.J. and Karwoski, C.J. (1994a) Current source density (CSD) analysis of retinal field potentials. I. Methodological considerations and depth profiles. *J. Neurophysiol.*, 72: 84–95.

Xu, X.J. and Karwoski, C.J. (1994b) Current source density analysis of retinal field potentials. II. Pharmacological analysis of the b-wave and M-wave. *J. Neurophysiol.*, 72: 96–105.

Circadian rhythms

H. Kolb, H. Ripps and S. Wu (Eds.)
Progress in Brain Research, Vol. 131

CHAPTER 34

Light and circadian regulation of retinomotor movement

Beth Burnside*

Department of Molecular and Cell Biology, University of California, Berkeley, 335LSA #3200, Berkeley, CA 94720-3200, USA

Introduction

In fish, amphibians, and birds photoreceptors and RPE pigment granules undergo morphological rearrangements in response to light and circadian signals (Fig. 1). These retinomotor movements reposition rod and cone photoreceptor outer segments and the shielding pigment of the RPE for optimal light capture by appropriate photoreceptors under photopic or scotopic conditions (cf. Burnside and Nagle, 1983; Wagner et al., 1993). Light induces cones to contract, rods to elongate and pigment granules to disperse into the long apical projections of the RPE cells. These movements position cone outer segments first in line for light reception and bury rod outer segments in the shielding RPE pigment, thereby protecting the rod visual pigment from overstimulation (Douglas, 1982). Darkness reverses these movements, thereby denuding the rod outer segments and positioning them first in line for light reception. First described more than a century ago (Mueller, 1856), retinomotor movements have since been the subject of an astonishing number of publications, variously describing their phylogenetic distribution and attempting to understand their regulation (see reviews by Garten, 1907; Arey, 1915, 1916; Parker, 1932; Walls, 1942; Detweiler, 1943; Ali, 1975;

Burnside and Nagle, 1983; Wagner et al., 1993; Cahill and Besharse, 1995).

Welsh and Osborne (1937) first recognized that retinomotor movements were regulated not only by light but also by circadian signals. They observed that in catfish maintained in constant darkness, cones elongated at subjective dusk and contracted at subjective dawn. Circadian retinomotor movements have subsequently been shown to be widespread in fish and amphibian species (see reviews by Burnside and Nagle, 1983; Wagner et al., 1993; Cahill and Besharse, 1995). All species so far studied exhibit circadian regulation of cone movements; rod and/or RPE movements are much less common.

For several years my lab has sought to identify the cytoskeletal elements responsible for retinomotor movements in teleost rods, cones, and RPE cells and to characterize the regulatory pathways by which light and circadian signals control these movements. Since retinomotor movements are robust and easily quantified, they provide a useful model for understanding diurnal or circadian regulation of widespread but more complex cyclic photoreceptor processes, such as outer segment disk assembly and shedding.

I happened upon retinomotor movements in 1973 when I gave a seminar in Philadelphia about amphibian neurulation. After my talk, Paul Liebman pointed out with only mild impatience that photoreceptor retinomotor movements were much better models for investigating regulated cell shape change than amphibian neural plate cells. I looked into the

* Tel.: 510-642-3200; Fax: 510-643-6791;
E-mail: burnside@socrates.berkeley.edu

DARK ADAPTED   LIGHT ADAPTED

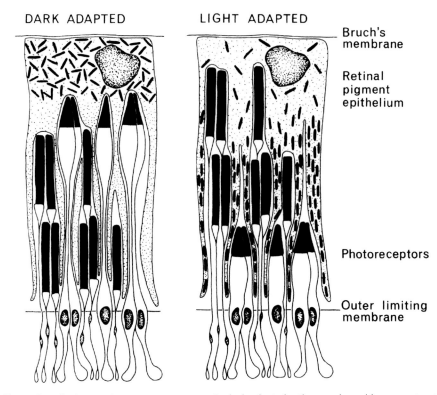

Bruch's membrane

Retinal pigment epithelium

Photoreceptors

Outer limiting membrane

Fig. 1. Schematic illustration of teleost retinomotor movements. In dark adapted retinas, rod myoids are contracted, cone myoids are elongated, and melanin pigment granules are aggregated to the base of the retinal pigment epithelial (RPE) cells. In light adapted retinas, rods elongate, cones contract, and pigment granules disperse into the RPE apical projections.

literature, decided he was right, and appreciated the tip. Since the most dramatic retinomotor movements are found in fishes, I began to work with fish retina. Having embarked on this particular path, encountering John Dowling was of course inevitable. Intrigued by retinal fractionation studies underway in John's lab in 1981, I arranged to spend a six-month sabbatical in Cambridge where I planned to capitalize on the photoreceptor fractions they were throwing away. Those fractions did not work out as planned, but the stimulating interactions with John and the people in his lab permanently altered my perspective. Before, my interest had been narrowly focused on the photoreceptor cytoskeleton and its upstream regulation (a sort of "fish retina as white rat" prejudice). After my stay in John's lab, I was much more interested in the biology of the retina itself. For this celebratory occasion I will review here some of our efforts to understand how teleost retinomotor movements are regulated by light and circadian signals.

Intracellular regulation of photoreceptor retinomotor movements: the role of cyclic AMP

Our first efforts sought to identify intracellular signal pathways affecting retinomotor movements. Since both light and circadian signals trigger retinomotor movements, we surmised that their intracellular signaling pathways were likely to converge somewhere upstream of the cytoskeletal machinery responsible for movement. Since cyclic AMP (cAMP) was known to affect cell motility in several cell types, and since retinal cyclic nucleotide levels were known to be altered by light (see Lolley, 1980), we immediately examined the roles of cyclic nucleotides. Using intraocular injections and cultured retinas we showed that treatments that elevate intracellular cAMP (but not cGMP) produced retinomotor positions characteristic of darkness (night) in teleost rods, cones and RPE cells (Burnside et al., 1982; Burnside and Basinger, 1983; Burnside and Ackland, 1984).

Similar effects were obtained using isolated RPE cells, permeabilized cones, and isolated fragments (inner/outer segments) of rods and cones (RIS–ROS and CIS–COS), suggesting that increasing cytoplasmic cAMP levels had a local and direct effect in each cell type (Gilson et al., 1986; Burnside et al., 1993; Liepe and Burnside, 1993a; Garcia and Burnside, 1994).

These findings, along with many other reports in the literature, suggested that elevated cAMP levels in the dark (at night) might be a general feature of cyclic diurnal and circadian signaling in vertebrate photoreceptors. Direct measurements have shown that whole retinal cAMP levels are higher in the dark than in the light in many species (Burnside et al., 1982; Iuvone, 1986; Cohen and Blazynski, 1990), but total cAMP levels include contributions from all retinal neurons. Studies of light and circadian control of retinal melatonin release more specifically argue that photoreceptor cAMP levels are elevated in vertebrate photoreceptors in darkness (night) (cf. Cahill and Besharse, 1991, 1995). Cyclic AMP regulates melatonin synthesis by influencing the activity of the rate-limiting enzyme in melatonin production, arylalkylamine *N*-acetyltransferase. In the vertebrate retina this enzyme is localized in photoreceptors. Since retinal melatonin release is elevated at night in both cyclic light and constant dark conditions, higher dark (night) levels of cAMP are implicated (Iuvone and Besharse, 1986; Cahill and Besharse, 1991, 1995; Hasegawa and Cahill, 1998). Photoreceptor cAMP levels rise in the dark due to the activity of Ca^{++}-calmodulin-dependent adenylate cyclase (Willardson et al., 1996). Since cAMP levels are elevated in the dark (night) in both cyclic light (LD) and constant darkness (DD), and since cAMP induces dark-adaptive retinomotor positions in photoreceptors, we suggested that retinomotor movements are coupled to the diurnal and circadian cycle by cAMP.

Since inhibitors of cAMP-dependent protein kinase (PKA) block dark-adaptive retinomotor movements in both cone and rod isolated inner/outer segment preparations (CIS–COS and RIS–ROS) (Liepe and Burnside, 1993a; Rey and Burnside, 1999), it seems likely that cAMP mobilizes the photoreceptor cytoskeleton by protein phosphorylation. The observation that cAMP can trigger

elongation in detergent-permeabilized models of cones in situ, further suggests that critical targets of PKA are detergent-insoluble, and thus associated with the cytoskeleton itself (see Burnside, 1988). The cone protein targets of these regulatory mechanisms are not yet known.

Pharmacological studies of RIS–ROS motility (Liepe and Burnside, 1993a) suggested that phosphorylation of mediator proteins by PKA is enhanced in darkness, and that dephosphorylation is required for light-induced RIS–ROS elongation. As pure preparations of rod inner/outer segments (RIS–ROS) can be more readily obtained than CIS–COS, we have used RIS–ROS to attempt to identify targets of cAMP-dependent phosphorylation (Pagh-Roehl and Burnside, 1995). Although pharmacological studies showed cAMP and cGMP to be similarly effective in promoting and maintaining dark-adaptive myoid movements in RIS–ROS (Liepe and Burnside, 1993a), cAMP and cGMP both appear to act through PKA in RIS–ROS homogenates (Pagh-Roehl et al., 1993). Both cAMP and cGMP stimulate phosphorylation of identical proteins; however cGMP-stimulated phosphorylation requires 1000-fold higher concentrations, and is inhibited by the PKA inhibitor PKI. Thus our results concur with previous reports that photoreceptors lack PKG (Hamm, 1990).

Using isolated retinas for in vivo phosphorylation experiments we identified two phosphoproteins, phosducin and PP33 (probably phosducin-like protein, see Thulin et al., 1999) as primary targets of PKA in RIS–ROS (Pagh-Roehl et al., 1993, 1995). Phosducin is a photoreceptor specific protein which binds the βγ subunits of transducin with high affinity, competitively excluding the binding of the α subunit and formation of the transduction competent heterotrimer (Lee et al., 1992). Phosducin is phosphorylated by PKA in the dark (Lee et al., 1990) and phosphorylated phosducin no longer blocks association of α and βγ transducin subunits (Gaudet et al., 1999). Phosducin is phosphorylated by Ca^{++} calmodulin kinase as well as by PKA in RIS–ROS homogenates, suggesting coordinated regulation of this protein by cAMP and calcium signaling pathways. In the light photoreceptor Ca^{++} and cAMP concentrations decrease and phosducin is dephosphorylated by phosphatases (Pagh-Roehl et al., 1995). Pharmacological manipulation of kinases and phosphatases has parallel effects on upon RIS–ROS elongation and on phosphorylation of PKA and P33, suggesting that there is a strong correlation between the dark-adapted retinomotor position and phosphorylation of these two rod proteins. This correlation may infer causality or it might simply reflect the fact that both are strongly regulated by PKA. We have no direct evidence that they are causally related. However, most of the phosducin in rods localizes to the inner segment (Thulin et al., 1999) where it may be expected to modulate adenylate cyclase and phopsholipasse C-β (see Yoshida et al., 1994).

Light-activation of RIS–ROS elongation in vitro requires relatively high light intensities (20% bleach) (Liepe and Burnside, 1993b). The photoreceptive mechanism responsible for this activation can accurately count quanta for light pulse durations up to at least 10 min, suggesting that the critical factor in light-activation of RIS–ROS elongation is quantum catch, rather than duration of the light stimulus. Photon counting can clearly take place within the rod outer and inner segment, in the absence of interneuronal signaling. Similar high intensity thresholds and photon counting mechanisms have been reported to mediate entrainment of the activity rhythm in hamsters (Nelson and Takahashi, 1991) and cone contraction in *Xenopus* (Besharse and Witkovsky, 1992). High intensity threshold and the ability to count quanta over long durations may be common denominators of photoreceptive functions that attune the organism to the daily light-dark cycle, rather than mediate vision.

Since inhibition of phosphatases blocks light activation of RIS–ROS elongation, it seems likely that protein dephosphorylation plays a critical role in regulating light-adaptive rod retinomotor movements. Pharmacological studies using selective kinase and phosphatase inhibitors suggest that multiple kinases and phosphatases participate in the pathway between light and RIS–ROS elongation (Pagh-Roehl et al., 1996). Three classes of inhibitors promoted elongation in the dark: PKA inhibitors, PKC inhibitors and one inhibitor, H85, which blocks neither of these types of kinases. These findings suggest that rod elongation is inhibited both by PKA and an unidentified kinase or kinases, possibly a diacylglycerol-independent form of PKC. The PKC inhibitor effect was not blocked by PMA, suggesting

a role for calcium-lipid-independent PKCs recently shown to be present in rod inner segments.

Extracellular regulation of photoreceptor retinomotor movements: roles for dopamine and adenosine

Observations from studies using intraocular injection in vivo, isolated retinas in culture, and isolated cone inner-outer segment fragments (CIS–COS) all point to a role for dopamine in regulating teleost cone retinomotor movements. Darkness or forskolin promoted cone myoid elongation, whereas light or dopamine promoted cone myoid contraction (Dearry and Burnside, 1988, 1989; Burnside et al., 1993; Hillman et al., 1995). Dark-induced CIS–COS elongation could also be inhibited by dopamine agonists and antagonists with a pharmacological profile most closely resembling that of the dopamine D4 receptor (Hillman et al., 1995). Rat photoreceptors have also been shown to possess D4-like receptors (Tran and Dickman, 1992). D4 receptors are members of the D2 family of receptors, which inhibit adenylate cyclase and thus reduce intracellular cAMP levels. Our finding that dopamine blocked forskolin-induced but not dibutyrl cAMP-induced cone elongation further suggests that dopamine is acting via inhibiting adenylate cyclase. Both light and dopamine reduce photoreceptor cAMP levels in retinas of several species (see Iuvone, 1986; Cohen and Blazinski, 1990; Cahill and Besharse, 1995; Hasegawa and Cahill, 1998).

The ability of light and dopamine to control retinomotor movements in isolated CIS–COS indicates that these agents can act directly on cones. In the teleost retina, the source of retinal dopamine is the interplexiform cell whose projections extend into the outer plexiform layer (see Wagner and Wulle, 1990; Wagner et al., 1992). If the D4 receptors regulating retinomotor movement are on the inner (and/or outer) segments as suggested by our CIS–COS results, released dopamine would have to diffuse over tens of microns to reach the inner segments in vivo. The very high affinity of the D4 receptors (Kds in the nM range) may facilitate this paracrine mode of signaling.

A role for dopamine in circadian regulation of cone retinomotor movement was suggested by studies employing intraocular injection of dopamine agonists and antagonists in animals maintained in constant darkness (DD) (McCormack and Burnside, 1992; Wagner et al., 1992). Cone myoid contraction was induced at midnight by intraocular injection of dopamine or D2 receptor agonists. The partially contracted cones of DD animals at subjective midday were induced to fully contract by intraocular injection of dopamine or D2 agonists, or to elongate by injection of the D2 antagonist sulpiride. Also the predawn cone contraction observed in DD animals in response to circadian signals was completely eliminated by intraocular injection of the D2 antagonist shortly before the expected time of light onset. These observations suggest that ciracadian regulation of cone myoid length is mediated by endogenous dopamine, acting via D2 family receptors. Similar effects were observed in another teleost, the blue acara (Kolbinger et al., 1990; Douglas et al., 1991). Dopamine is unlikely, however, to be the sole circadian regulator, since both light-induced and circadian cone movements persisted (at reduced amplitude) after lesion of interplexiform cells by 6-hydoxydopamine (Douglas et al., 1991; Wagner et al., 1992).

Interestingly, cones appear to be much more sensitive to dopamine than rods. Dopamine is much more effective than light at producing light-adaptive myoid contraction in CIS–COS (Dearry and Burnside, 1988; Burnside et al., 1993), whereas light is much more effective than dopamine in RIS–ROS (Liepe and Burnside, 1993b). Dopamine is much more effective at producing light-adaptive movement in CIS–COS than in RIS–ROS, suggesting that rods are relatively insensitive to dopamine. This insensitivity of rods to dopamine was also observed in the blue acara (Kolbinger et al., 1996), where regulation of rod movement by light and by circadian signals was unaffected by 6-hydroxydopamine lesion of dopaminergic interplexiform cells.

The relative effectiveness of dopamine and light in triggering CIS–COS contraction is consistent with spectral sensitivity studies of cone retinomotor movements in intact fish and frog retinas (see Besharse and Witkovsky, 1992; Wagner et al., 1992). These studies suggest that in vivo cone retinomotor movements are not triggered directly by light, but indirectly via a rod mediated pathway. In both fish and frog, the action spectrum for triggering light adaptive cone retinomotor movements most closely fits the absorption curve of the rod photopigment. Since light induction of teleost cone retinomotor movements can be blocked by dopamine D2 antagonists in vivo (see Dearry and Burnside, 1988; Wagner et al., 1992), it seems likely that rods affect teleost cone reitnomotor movements in vivo by stimulating the release of dopamine from interplexiform cells (see Wagner et al., 1992 for discussion).

Recent observations indicate that the neuromodulator adenosine can also influence cone retinomotor movements. In isolated CIS–COS, myoid elongation can be induced by activation of adenosine A2 receptors and inhibited by A2-receptor antagonists (Rey and Burnside, 1999). Since A2 receptors are positively coupled to adenylate cyclase, this finding corroborates previous results with agents that elevate cAMP. Since adenosine agonists trigger movement in isolated CIS–COS, it is clear that the receptors are present on cone inner and/or outer segments. Since cones elongate at subjective dusk in fish maintained in constant darkness, and since adenosine stimulates cone elongation, adenosine might function as an endogenous circadian signal for expected dark onset. Alternatively, adenosine effects on cone movements could be a local effect, reflecting photoreceptor metabolic activity. A dark-associated increase in the adenosine level in the subretinal space would be predicted from light/dark changes in photoreceptor Na^+/K^+-ATPase activity in the photoreceptor inner segments (Torre, 1982), since an adenosine transporter is present in photoreceptors (Ehinger and Perez, 1984). Thus adenosine is likely to be exported into the extracellular space along its concentration gradient in darkness. Thus the onset of darkness and the associated increase in Na^+,K^+-ATPase activity in the photoreceptor inner segments are likely to be accompanied by an increase in intracellular adenosine levels, and consequently, increased release of adenosine into the subretinal space. The binding of released adenosine to photoreceptor A2 receptors could then enhance dark adaptation of photoreceptors by stimulating adenylate cyclase, thereby reinforcing the dark signal.

Together our studies suggest that dopamine and adenosine have antagonistic effects on cone retinomotor movements: dopamine triggers light-adaptive whereas adenosine triggers dark-adaptive cone retinomotor responses. Although adenosine may also inhibit retinal dopamine release (Crosson et al., 1994), our CIS–COS results show that both adenosine and dopamine can directly influence light-dark intracellular signaling pathways by interacting with receptors residing on cone inner and/or outer segments. Of course these observations do not rule out the possibility that adenosine affects cone movement indirectly via effects on dopamine release in vivo.

Regulation of retinomotor movements in the RPE

Pigment granule aggregation and dispersion can be induced in isolated teleost RPE sheets and dissociated RPE cells (Dearry and Burnside, 1988, 1989; Garcia and Burnside, 1994). Regulation of RPE movement can thus be studied in vitro in the absence of influences from the retina or choroid. Light has no effect on pigment position in isolated RPE sheets or cells; however, pigment granule dispersion can be induced by dopamine or D2 family agonists, and aggregation can be induced by treatments which elevate cAMP, such as forskolin and cAMP analogs (Dearry and Burnside, 1988; Garcia and Burnside, 1994). In isolated RPE cells aggregated in cAMP, pigment dispersion can be induced by microinjection of the PKA inhibitors PKI or H-89, suggesting that continuous phosphorylation of PKA targets is required to maintain the aggregated state. Since aggregation can also be induced by the phosphatase inhibitor okadaic acid, these observations suggest that PKA and phosphatases are simultaneously active in RPE cells, and that their relative activities are altered by light and/or dark signals from the retina. In a survey of agents reported to elevate cAMP in RPE cells of other species, we found none that produced a significant effect on fish RPE pigment position; those tested were adenosine, ATP, prostaglandins E_1 and D_2, melatonin, iodomelatonin, histamine, or vasointestinal peptide (Garcia and Burnside, 1994).

Surprisingly, we found that underivatized cAMP was as effective as membrane permeant cAMP analogs at activating pigment granule aggregation in isolated RPE sheets in the presence of IBMX, (Garcia and Burnside, 1994). Washout of exogenous cAMP induced dispersion. Thus underivitized cAMP appears to either bind to surface receptors or enter the cells via organic ion transporters. Since ATP and adenosine were ineffective, it seemed unlikely that cAMP was acting on purinergic receptors. The organic ion transport inhibitors probenecid and sulfinpyrazone blocked cAMP- but not forskolin-induced pigment aggregation, suggesting that exogenous cAMP can actually enter the cells via these channels to activate pigment aggregation. These observations suggest that increased dark levels of cAMP in the subretinal space could trigger pigment granule aggregation in the RPE. Cyclic AMP efflux has been reported from many cell types, including pinealocytes (Nikaido and Takahashi, 1989), and has been shown to be related to intracellular cAMP accumulation (Barber and Butcher, 1983). Thus elevated levels of cAMP in photoreceptors in darkness might be expected to produce cAMP efflux into the subretinal space. If retinal photoreceptors produce diurnal or circadian cycles of cAMP efflux as previously reported for pinealocytes (Nikaido and Takahashi, 1989), then released cAMP could serve as a retina to RPE signal for darkness. Not only light but also dark signals may be transmitted from the retina to the RPE across the subretinal space via first messengers.

Dopamine and alpha adrenergic agonists can induce pigment dispersion (the light adaptive retinomotor movement) in isolated RPE of both sunfish (Dearry and Burnside, 1988) and bullfrog (Dearry et al., 1990). We were surprised to find that in fish RPE, dopamine triggers dispersion via D2-family receptors (and is opposed by forskolin), while in frog RPE, dopamine triggers dispersion via D1 receptors (and is mimicked by forskolin). These findings suggest that although the light-adaptive effect of dopamine has been conserved, different receptors and intracellular pathways have evolved in fish and amphibians to harness retinomotor movements to light-driven changes in dopamine release from the retina.

The action spectrum for light-adaptive melanin pigment dispersion in teleost RPE in vivo also matches the absorption spectrum for the visual pigment of rods (Ali and Crouzy, 1968), suggesting that RPE retinomotor movements, like those of cones, may also be regulated by a rod-mediated dopaminergic pathway. Furthermore, medium from light-cultured sunfish retinas induced pigment dispersion in isolated RPE sheets, and this effect was blocked by D2-family dopamine receptor antagonists, suggesting that light stimulates release of endogenous retinal dopamine which then promotes RPE pigment dispersion (Dearry and Burnside, 1989). Dopamine overflow is approximately 3 fold higher from light-cultured sunfish retinas than from dark-cultured retinas (Dearry and Burnside, 1989). These observations led us to hypothesize that dopamine could act as a retina to RPE signal for light onset. More recently, light-adaptive movements have been shown to recover in fish whose interplexiform cells have been lesioned by intraocular injections of 6-hydroxydopamine, thus eliminating the sole retinal source of dopamine (Douglas et al., 1992). Since intraocular injections of dopamine antagonists do block light-induced pigment migration in unlesioned retinas, dopamine appears to play a role in regulating these movements under normal conditions. However, some other mechanism can apparently take over in the chronic absence of dopamine in the lesioned retinas (Wagner et al., 1992). Clearly, dopamine is not the only mechanism by which the retina can communicate a light onset signal to the RPE. Perhaps cycles of cAMP release from the retina as described above could provide an alternative light–dark signal to the RPE in 6-hydroxydopamine-lesioned animals.

Conclusions

Our studies suggest that there is a complex interplay of signaling mechanisms responsible for controlling retinomotor movements in photoreceptors and RPE cells. In the teleost retina, dark-adaptive retinomotor positions are produced by elevating cAMP in rods, cones, and RPE cells. Thus elevated cAMP appears to be a fundamental darkness signal in all three cell types. The observation that cAMP-dependent protein kinase inhibitors block dark-adaptive movements in all three cell types suggests that the dark signal entails

phosphorylation of specific mediator proteins. Since different cytoskeletal mechanisms are activated in each cell type to effect the dark-adaptive retinomotor movements, it seems likely that critical protein targets of cAMP-dependent protein kinase are unique to each cell type. The specific protein mediators that regulate the cytoskeletal responses have not yet been identified.

Light is highly effective at triggering retinomotor movements in isolated RIS–ROS, while dopamine is much more effective than light itself at triggering the light-adaptive retinomotor movements of CIS–COS. These observations are consistent with spectral sensitivity reports suggesting that light-adaptive retinomotor movements in both cones and RPE are activated by a rod-triggered signaling pathway. The effectiveness of dopamine D2 antagonists in blocking light-induced movements in both cones and RPE in vivo further suggest that dopamine is an important extracellular messenger in this rod signaling pathway. Nonetheless, 6-hydroxydopamine lesion studies indicate that light-induced retinomotor movements can still occur (though at reduced amplitude) in the chronic absence of dopamine. Since D2 antagonists do block light-induced cone and RPE movements in acute experiments, it seems likely that some other cyclic signaling mechanism is upregulated to replace dopamine in chronically dopamine-depleted retinas.

Since adenosine can induce dark-adaptive movements in cones, and since underivatized cAMP can trigger dark-adaptive pigment aggregation in RPE cells, it seems likely that messengers signifying darkness are also released into the subretinal space. These messengers may act as primary signals for darkness, or they may serve to reinforce other signals and thus facilitate the maintenance of high intracellular cAMP levels throughout an extended period of darkness.

Only cones exhibit circadian changes in retinomotor position in constant darkness in sunfish. D2 antagonist studies suggest that dopamine participates in circadian regulation of these movements, but dopamine depletion experiments make it clear that other signals can suffice in the absence of dopamine. Perhaps the circadian oscillator can influence intracellular cAMP levels directly, or perhaps other signals, like adenosine, can signal alternating day–night cycles in the absence of dopamine. Further studies are required to fully understand these mechanisms.

484

Acknowledgments

This work has been supported by grants from the National Eye Institute (EY03575). The author wishes to thank Kerri Rollins for her assistance in the preparation of the manuscript.

Reference

Ali, M.A. (1975) Retinomotor responses. In: Ali, M.A. (Ed.), *Vision in Fishes*. Plenum Press, New York, pp. 313–355.

Ali, M.A. and Crouzy A.R. (1968) Action spectrum and quantal thresholds of retinomotor responses in the brook trout. *Salvelinus fontinalis* (Mitchill). *Z. Vergl. Physiol.*, 59: 86–89.

Arey, L.B. (1915) The occurrence and significance of photomechanical changes in the vertebrate retina—a historical survey. *J. comp. Neurol.*, 25: 535–554.

Arey, L.B. (1916) Movements in the visual cells and retinal pigment of the lower vertebrates. *J. Comp. Neurol.*, 26: 121–201.

Barber, R. and Butcher, R.W. (1983) The egress of cAMP from metazoan cells. *Adv. Cyclic Nuc. Res.*, 15: 119–138.

Besharse, J.C. and Witkovsky, P. (1992) Light-evoked contraction of red absorbing cones in the *Xenopus* retinal is maximally sensitive to green light. *Vis. Neurosci.*, 8: 243–249.

Burnside, B. (1988) Photoreceptor contraction and extension: calcium and cAMP regulation of microtubule- and actin-dependent changes in cell shape. In: Lasek, R.J. (Ed.), *Intrinsic Determinant of Neuronal Cell Form*. Alan R. Liss, Inc., New York, pp. 323–359.

Burnside, B. and Ackland, N. (1984) Effects of circadian rhythm and cAMP on retinomotor movements in the green sunfish. *Lepomis cyanellus. Invest. Ophthalmol. Vis. Sci.*, 25: 539–545.

Burnside, B. and Basinger, S. (1983) Retinomotor pigment migration in the teleost retinal pigment epithelium. II. Cyclic-3',5'-adenosine monophosphate induction of dark-adaptive movement in vitro. *Invest. Ophthalmol. and Vis. Sci.*, 24: 16–23.

Burnside, B., Evans, M., Fletcher, T. and Chader, G.J. (1982) Induction of Dark-Adaptive Retinomotor Movement (Cell Elongation) in Teleost Retinal Cones by Cyclic Adenosine 3',5'-Monophosphate. *J. Gen. Physiol.*, 79: 759–774.

Burnside, B. and Nagle, B. (1983) Retinomotor movements of photoreceptors and retinal pigment epithelium: mechanisms and regulation. In: Osborne, N. and Chader, G. (Eds.), *Progress in Retinal Research*, Vol. 2, Pergamon Press, Oxford, pp. 67–109.

Burnside, B., Wang, E., Pagh-Roehl, K. and Rey, H. (1993) Retinomotor movements in isolated teleost retinal cone inner-outer segments preparations (CIS–COS): effects of light, dark and dopamine. *Exp. Eye Res.*, 57: 709–722.

Cahill, G.M. and Besharse, J.C. (1991) Resetting the circadian clock in cultured *Xenopus* eyecups: regulation of retinal melatonin rhythms by light and D2 dopamine receptors. *J. Neurosci.*, 11: 2959–2971.

Cahill, G.M. and Besharse, J.C. (1995) Circadian rhythmicity in vertebrate retinas: regulation by a photoreceptor oscillator. *Prog. Retinal Eye Res.*, 14: 267–291.

Cohen, A.I. and Blazynski, C. (1990) Dopamine and its agonists reduce a light-sensitive pool of cyclic AMP in mouse photoreceptors. *Vis. Neurosci.*, 4: 43–52.

Crossen, C.E., Debenedetto, R. and Gidday, J.M. (1994) Functional evidence for retinal adenosine receptors. *J. Ocul. Pharmacol.*, 10: 499–507.

Dearry, A. and Burnside, B. (1988) Stimulation of distinct D2 dopaminergic and alpha2-adrenergic receptors induces light-adaptive pigment dispersion in teleost retinal pigment epithelium. *J. Neurochem.*, 51: 1516–1523.

Dearry, A. and Burnside, B. (1989) Light-induced dopamine release from teleost retinas acts as a light-adaptive signal to the retinal pigment epithelium. *J. Neurochem.*, 53: 870–878.

Dearry, A., Edelman, J.L., Miller, S. and Burnside, B. (1990) Dopamine induces light-adaptive retinomotor movements in bullfrog cones via D2 receptors and in retinal pigment epithelium via D1 receptors. *J. Neurochem.*, 54: 1367–1378.

Detwiler, S.R. (1943) *Vertebrate Photoreceptors*. Macmillan, New York, p. 184.

Douglas, R.H. (1982) The function of photomechanical movements in the retina of the rainbow trout *(Salmo gairdneri)*. *J. Exp. Biol.*, 96: 389–403.

Douglas, R.H., Wagner, H.J. and Zaunreiter, M. (1991) Dopamine is not required for light induced or endogenous photomechanical movements in teleost fish. *Invest. Ophthalmol. Vis. Sci.*, 32: 2903.

Douglas, R.H., Wagner H.-J., Zaunreiter, M., Behrens, U.D. and Djamgoz, M.B. (1992) The effect of dopamine depletion on light-evoked and circadian retinomotor movements in the teleost retina. *Vis. Neurosci.*, 9: 335–343.

Ehinger, B. and Perez, M.T.R. (1984) Autoradiography of nucleoside uptake into the retina. *Neurochem. Int.*, 6: 369–381.

García, D.M. and Burnside, B. (1994) Suppression of cAMP-induced pigment granule aggregation in RPE by organic anion transport inhibitors. *Invest. Ophthalmol. Vis. Sci.*, 35: 178–188.

Garten, S. (1907) Die veranderungen der Netzhaut durch Licht. Graefe-Saemisch handbuch der gesamten. *Augenheilkunde, Leipzig 2*, Chapter 12, 250–280.

Gaudet, R., Savage, J.R., McLaughlin, J.N., Willardson, B.M. and Sigler, P.B. (1999) A molecular mechanism for the phosphorylation-dependent regulation of heterotrimeric G proteins by posducin. *Mol. Cell*, 3: 649–660.

Gilson, C.A., Ackland, N. and Burnside, B. (1986) Regulation of reactivated elongation in lysed cell models of teleost retinal cones by cAMP and calcuim. *J. Cell Biol.*, 103: 1047–1059.

Hamm, H. (1990) Regulation by light of cyclic nucleotide-dependent protein kinases and their substrates in frog rod outer segments. *J. Gen. Phys.*, 95: 545–567.

Hasegawa, M. and Cahill, G. (1998) Cyclic AMP Resets the Circadian Clock in Cultured *Xenopus* Retinal Photoreceptor Layers. *J. Neurochem.*, 70: 1523–1531.

Hillman, D., Li, D. and Burnside, B. (1995) Evidence for D_4 receptor regulation of retinomotor movement in isolated teleost cone inner-outer segments. *J. Neurochem.*, 64: 1326–1335.

Iuvone, P.M. (1986) Evidence for a d2 dopamine receptor in frog retina that decreases cyclic AMP accumulation and serotonin N-acetyltransferase activity. *Life Sci.*, 38: 331–342.

Iuvone, P.M. and Besharse, J.C. (1986) Cyclic AMP stimulates serotonin N-acetyltransferase activity in *Xenopus* retina in vitro. *J. Neurochem.*, 46: 33–36.

Kolbinger, W., Kohler, K., Oetting, H. and Weiler, R. (1990) Endogenous dopamine and cyclic events in the fish retina. I. HPLC assay of total content, release, and metabolic turnover during different light/dark cycles. *Vis. Neurosci.*, 5: 595–602.

Kolbinger, W., Wagner, D. and Wagner, H.J. (1996) Control of rod retinomotor movements in teleost retinae: the role of dopamine in mediating light-dependent and circadian signals. *Cell Tissue Tes.*, 285: 445–451.

Lee, R.H., Brown, B.M. and Lolley, R.N. (1990) Protein kinase A phosphorylates retinal phosducin on serine 73 in situ. *J. Biol. Chem.*, 265: 15860–15866.

Lee, R.H., Ting, T.D., Lieberman, B.S., Tobias, D.E., Lolley, R.N. and Ho, Y.K. (1992) Regulation of retinal cGMP cascade by phosducin in bovine rod photoreceptor cells. Interaction of phosducin and transducin. *J. Biol. Chem.*, 267: 25104–25112.

Liepe, B.A. and Burnside, B. (1993a) Cyclic nucleotide regulation of teleost rod photoreceptor inner segment length. *J. Gen. Physiol.*, 102: 75–98.

Liepe, B.A. and Burnside, B. (1993b) Light-activation of teleost rod photoreceptor elongation. *Exp. Eye Res.*, 57: 117–126.

Lolley, R.N. (1980) Cyclic nucleotide metabolism in the vertebrate retina. In: Zadunaisky, J.A. and Davson, H. (Eds.), *Current Topics in Eye Research*, Academic Press, New York.

McCormack, C.A. and Burnside, B. (1992) A role for endogenous dopamine in circadian regulation of retinal cone movement. *Exp. Eye Res.*, 55: 511–520.

Mueller, H. (1856) Anatomisch—physiogische untersuchungen uber die retina bei nemschen und wirbelthieren. *Z. Wiss. Zool.*, 8: 1–122.

Nelson, D.E. and Takahashi, J.S. (1991) Comparison of visual sensitivity for suppression of pineal melatonin and circadian phase-shifting in the golden hamster. *Brain Res.*, 554: 72–277.

Nikaido, S.S. and Takahashi, J.S. (1989) Twenty-four hour oscillation of cAMP in chick pineal cells: role of cAMP in the acute and circadian regulation of melatonin production. *Neuron*, 3: 609–619.

Pagh-Roehl, K., Han, E. and Burnside, B. (1993) Identification of cyclic nucleotide- regulated phosphoproteins, including phosducin, in motile rod inner/outer segments of teleosts. *Exp. Eye Res.*, 57: 679–691.

Pagh-Roehl, K. and Burnside, B. (1995) Preparation of teleost rod inner and outer segments, In: Dentler, W.L. and Whitman, G.B. (Eds.), *Methods in Cell Biology: Cilia and Eukaryotic Flagella*. Academic Press, New York, pp. 83–92.

Pagh-Roehl, K., Lin, D., Su, L. and Burnside, B. (1995) Phosducin and P33 are in vivo targets of PKA and Type 1 of 2A Phosphatases, regulators of cell elongation in teleost rod outer segments. *J. Neurosci.*, 15: 6475–6488.

Pagh-Roehl, K., Lin, D. and Burnside, B. (1996) Stimulation of cell elongation in teleost rod photoreceptors by distinct protein kinase inhibitors. *J. Neurochem.*, 66: 2311–2319.

Parker, G.H. (1932) The movements of the retinal pigment. *Ergeb. Biol.*, 9: 239–292.

Rey, H. and Burnside, B. (1999) Adenosine stimulates cone photoreceptor myoid elongation via an adenosine A2-like receptor. *J. Neurochem.*, 72: 2345–2355.

Thulin, C.D, Howes, K., Driscoll, C.D., Savage, J.R., Rand, T.A., Baehr, B.M. and Willardson, B.M. (1999) The immunolocalization and divergent roles of phosducin and phosducin-like protein in the retina. *Mol. Vis.*, 5: 40.

Torre, V. (1982) The contribution of the electrogenic sodium-potassium pump to the electrical activity of toad rods. *J. Physiol. (Lond.)*, 333: 315–341.

Tran, V.T. and Dickman, M. (1992) Differential localization of dopamine D1 and D2 receptors in rat retina. *Invest. Ophthalmol. Vis. Sci.*, 33: 1620–1626.

Wagner, H.J. and Wulle, I. (1990) Dopaminergic interplexiform cells contact photoreceptor terminals in catfish retina. *Cell Tissue Res.*, 359–365.

Wagner, H.J., Kirsch, M. and Douglas, R.H. (1992) Light dependent and endogenous circadian control of adaptation in teleost retinae. In: Ali, M.A. (Ed.), *Rhythms in Fishes Plenum*. New York, pp. 255–291.

Walls, G.L. (1942) *The Vertebrate Eye*. Hafner, New York, p. 780

Welsh, J.H. and Osborne, C.M. (1937) Diurnal changes in the retina of the catfish. Ameiurus nebulosis. *J. comp. Neurol.*, 66: 349–359.

Willardson, B.M., Wilkins, J.F., Yoshida, T. and Bitensky, M.W. (1996) Regulation of phosducin phosphorylation in retinal rods by Ca2+/calmodulin-dependent adenylyl cyclase. *Proc. Natl. Acad. Sci. USA*, 93: 1475–1479.

Yoshida, T., Willardson, B.M., Wilkins, J.F., Jensen, G.J., Thornton, B.D. and Bitensky, M.W. (1994) The phosphorylation state of phosducin determines its ability to block transducin subunit interactions and inhibit transducin binding to activated rhodopsin. *J. Biol. Chem.*, 269: 24050–24057.

H. Kolb, H. Ripps and S. Wu (Eds.)
Progress in Brain Research, Vol. 131

CHAPTER 35

Circadian and efferent modulation of visual sensitivity

Robert Barlow*

Center for Vision Research, Department of Ophthalmology, Upstate Medical University, 750 Adams Street, Syracuse, NY 13210, USA

Introduction

Animals adapt their visual sensitivity by responding to changes in ambient lighting and, in many cases, anticipating them. Studies by John Dowling, his students and colleagues have contributed significantly toward understanding how light-dependent as well as endogenous circadian and efferent mechanisms modulate the sensitivity of the retina.

Cajal (1892) first identified efferent inputs to the vertebrate retina at the end of the last century. In 1966 Dowling and Cowan showed that the centrifugal fibers entering the bird retina terminate on cell bodies of the inner nuclear layer. Dowling and Ehinger (1975) then showed that a recently detected interretinal cell, the interplexiform cell, carries information from the inner to the outer plexiform layers of fish and primate. Zucker and Dowling (1987) later found that the centrifugal fibers entering the fish retina terminate on the interplexiform cells. With these studies John Dowling and his colleagues uncovered a curious property of the fish visual system: a centrifugal input from the brain terminates on a second centrifugal pathway in the retina. They further showed that the second centrifugal component, the interplexiform cell, contains dopamine, and that dopamine strongly modulates the circuitry of the

outer retina (Lasater and Dowling, 1985; Mangel and Dowling, 1985; Dowling, 1991). Centrifugal innervation and dopamine appear to be related in another teleost, the zebrafish where a dominant mutation in zebrafish, *night blindness b*, raises visual thresholds in prolonged darkness, disrupts the centrifugal innervation to the retina, and reduces the number of retinal dopaminergic interplexiform cells (Li and Dowling, 2000a). These studies from John's laboratory have uncovered intriguing properties of the brain's efferent input to the retina in some species, but how they influence visual sensitivity is not clear.

Recently John Dowling and his colleagues turned their attention towards the circadian modulation of visual function. Using a behavioral paradigm, Li and Dowling (1998) found that a circadian clock decreases the visual sensitivity of zebrafish rather than increases it as has been found in most other animals. They then showed that dopamine, which they had already coupled with the centrifugal input to the retina, appears to mediate the effect of the circadian clock on visual sensitivity of the fish retina (Li and Dowling, 2000b). In addition to pioneering studies on light-triggered mechanisms of retinal adaptation, John Dowling and colleagues have provided important insights about how circadian and efferent mechanisms may modulate visual sensitivity. Taken together, their studies underscore the variety of physiological processes that have evolved to modulate the function of the visual system.

* Tel.: 315-464-7770; Fax: 315-464-7712;
E-mail: barlowr@upstate.edu

In this chapter I review the range of circadian rhythms detected in various visual systems, focus on a few of them and consider the modulation of retinal sensitivity by efferent signals from the brain. As noted above much has been learned from research on fish, the primary animal model in John Dowling's laboratory. I will present the results of research carried out in my laboratory on two other animal models: an invertebrate, the horseshoe crab *Limulus polyphemus*, and a vertebrate, the Japanese quail *Coturnix coturnix japonica*. I will also mention briefly preliminary results from studies of *Xenopus laevis* and humans.

Circadian rhythms characterize most visual systems

Circadian oscillators are intimately related with the visual systems of most, if not all, animals. Entrained by visual inputs, the oscillators modulate the function of the visual system at the level of the retina and higher pathways. The range of properties that exhibit circadian changes is truly remarkable. Table 1 list those detected in vertebrates and Table 2 gives those found in the well-studied invertebrate, *Limulus* (review of other invertebrates: Barlow et al., 1989). They extend from changes in photoreceptors, the most distal cells in the visual system, to more proximal levels both in the retina and in higher visual centers. A number of species share circadian rhythms such as the daily the synthesis of rhodopsin (toad, fish and mouse) the shedding of rod disc membranes (frogs and rats), and cone disc membranes (chicks and squirrels). Interestingly in *Limulus*, a circadian oscillator controls the priming of the processes that shed rhodopsin-containing membrane (rhabdom) but not the shedding event itself. Important to this chapter is that the synthesis of two ubiquitous neuromodulators, dopamine and melatonin, undergo circadian rhythms in many vertebrate retinas. Most important is that the output of the visual system—behavior—undergoes circadian changes in *Limulus*, fish and mammals. How circadian changes at various levels of the visual system influence behavior is not known.

Where are the circadian oscillators that affect the visual system located? Those that modulate retinal function can be located either in the brain as in

Limulus (Barlow et al., 1977; Calman and Battelle, 1991) or in the retina itself as in quail (Underwood et al., 1988) and hamster (Tosini and Menaker, 1996). In *Xenopus* circadian oscillators are located in the photoreceptors themselves (Cahill and Besharse, 1993).

Circadian rhythms in the sensitivity of the *Limulus* lateral eye

A clear example of the circadian modulation of the visual system is the horseshoe crab, *Limulus*. At dusk a circadian oscillator in the brain transmits efferent optic-nerve activity to the lateral eyes influencing most every physiological and anatomical property of the retina (Table 2). The endogenous rhythms of the retina combine with mechanisms of light and dark adaptation to increase visual sensitivity by $\sim 10^6$ from day to night nearly compensating for the shift in the intensity of ambient illumination after sunset.

The centrally located clock increases visual sensitivity primarily by acting on the most distal cell of the visual system, the photoreceptor. Efferent optic nerve fibers from the circadian clock terminate on individual photoreceptor cells. At night efferent signals carried by the fibers change the "noise", gain and photon catch of single cells which in turn changes their intensity coding properties. At night a single photoreceptor cell recorded over a two-day period from an unanesthetized *Limulus* in darkness (Fig. 1, left) reveals an increase in its receptor potential evoked by a test flash ("signal") and a decrease in the rate of quantum bumps generated in the absence of light ("noise"). During the day, its "signal" declined and "noise" increased. These circadian changes in activity are transmitted to the second-order eccentric cell of an ommatidium. Their effects on retinal sensitivity can be studied by recording the output of a single optic nerve fiber (Fig. 1, right). First, the intensity–response function of the discharge of a single optic nerve fiber was measured with the ommatidium in its natural daytime state, i.e. adapted to a background intensity equal to that measured in the animal's underwater environment during the day (Log I = −2). The monotonically shaped intensity–response function (unfilled circles) encoded a range of ~ 4 log units of light intensity. Then the animal was

Table 1. Circadian rhythms in the vertebrate visual system

	Time	Animal
Anatomy		
Rod: disc shedding	day	rat (LaVail, 1976, Tierstein et al., 1980), *Xenopus*(Pierce and Besharse, 1986)
myoid contraction	night	fish (Levinson and Burnside, 1981)
Cone: disc shedding	night	squirrel (Young, 1967), chick (Young, 1978)
myoid contraction	day	fish (Levinson and Burnside, 1981), *Xenopus* (Pierce and Besharse, 1985)
synaptic ribbon increase	day	fish (Kohler et al., 1990), newt (Wulle et al., 1990)
RPE pigment migration	day	fish (Kohler et al., 1990), *Xenopus* (Pierce and Besharse, 1985)
Horizontal-cell spinule formation	day	fish (Weiler et al., 1988; Douglas and Wagner, 1983)
Corneal epithelium thickness increase	night	quail (Oishi and Matsumoto, 1985), human (Fujita, 1980)
Metabolism		
Rod opsin synthesis	day	toad and fish (Korenbrot and Fernald, 1989), mouse (vonSchantz et al., 1999)
Cone opsin synthesis	night	chick (Pierce et al., 1993; vonSchantz et al., 1999)
Retinal dopamine synthesis	day	rat (Wirz-Justice et al., 1984), fish (Wulle et al., 1990), quail (Manglapus et al., 1999)
Retinal melatonin synthesis	night	*Xenopus* (Cahill and Besharse, 1990), birds (Zawilska and Iuvone, 1992; Underwood et al., 1988; Thomas and Iuvone, 1991; Manglapus et al., 1999), hamster (Tosini and Menaker, 1996)
Retinal tryptophan hydroxylase synthesis	night	*Xenopus* (Green et al., 1995) and chicken (Chong et al., 1998)
Retinal tyrosine hydroxylase activity increase	day	fish (McCormack and Burnside, 1993)
Retinal serotonin NAT activity increase	night	chicken (Hamm and Menaker, 1980), *Xenopus* (Besharse and Iuvone, 1983)
Physiology		
Cone dominance of ERG b-wave	day	quail (Manglapus et al., 1998), pigeon (Barattini et al., 1981)
Rod dominance of cone H-cell response	night	fish (Mangel and Wang, 1996)
ERG b-wave increase	night	rabbit (Brandenburg et al., 1983; Manglapus et al., 1998)
	day	zebrafish (Li and Dowling, 1998), lizard (Fowlkes et al., 1984), *Xenopus* (Barlow et al., 2000)
Electro-oculogram increase	day	human (Anderson and Purple, 1980)
Lateral geniculate nucleus response increase	night	rat (Hanada and Kawamura, 1984)
Visually-evoked cortical potential increase	night	rabbit (Bobbert et al., 1978)
Intraocular pressure increase	night	human (Boyd and McLeod, 1964), rabbit (Katz et al., 1975)
Behavior		
Visual sensitivity increase	night	rat (Rosenwasser et al., 1979; Reme et al., 1991), goldfish (Bassi and Powers, 1987)
	day	zebrafish (Li and Dowling, 1998), human (Bassi and Powers, 1987; Barlow et al., 1997)

dark adapted during the day and the I-R function was remeasured. It acquired a nonmonotonic shape (dashed curve) revealing a second encoding mechanism (Kaplan and Barlow, 1975) that increased sensitivity by ~4 log units to the lower range of light intensities. Dark adapting the eye also caused spontaneous optic nerve spiking (~0.6 ips) in the dark (Log $I = -\infty$). The animal remained in darkness until the clock shifted the eye into its nighttime state and a third I-R function was measured (filled circles). Its monotonic shape "Night" function reveals a remarkable increase in gain (impulses/s/photon) at low light intensities and a decrease in spontaneous spiking activity in the dark (Barlow and Kaplan, 1993). The clock's circadian input combined with dark adaptation to shift the

490

Table 2. Circadian rhythms in the *Limulus* lateral eye

Retinal property	Day	Night	Reference
Efferent input	absent	present	Barlow et al., 1977; Barlow, 1983
Gain	low	high	Renninger et al., 1984; Barlow et al., 1987
Noise	high	low	Barlow et al., 1977; Kaplan and Barlow, 1980; Barlow et al., 1993
Quantum bumps	short	long	Kaplan et al., 1990
Frequency response	fast	slow	Batra and Barlow, 1990
Dark adaptation	fast	slow	Kass and Berent, 1988
Lateral inhibition	strong	weak	Renninger and Barlow, 1979; Ruta et al., 1999
Cell position	proximal	distal	Barlow and Chamberlain, 1980; Barlow et al., 1980
Pigment granules	clustered	dispersed	Barlow and Chamberlain, 1980
Aperture	constricted	dilated	Chamberlain and Barlow, 1977, 1987
Acceptance angle	6°	13°	Barlow et al., 1980
Photomechanical movements	trigger	prime	Chamberlain and Barlow, 1987
Photon catch	low	high	Barlow et al., 1980
Membrane shedding	trigger	prime	Chamberlain and Barlow, 1979, 1984
Arrestin mRNA level	high	low	Battelle et al., 2000
Intense light effects	protected	labile	Barlow et al., 1989
Visual sensitivity	low	high	Powers and Barlow, 1985; Herzog et al., 1996

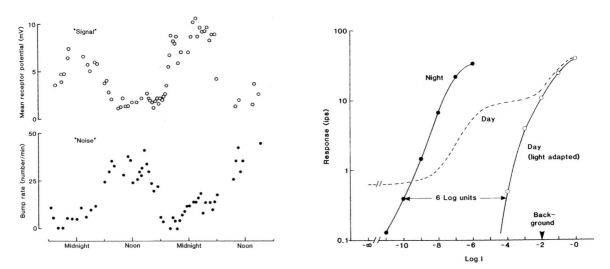

Fig. 1. *Left:* Circadian rhythms in response and noise recorded over a 2-day period from a single *Limulus* photoreceptor cell in situ. Open circles give the mean amplitudes of the receptor potential ("signal") in response to 6-s test flashes. Light intensity incident on the single ommatidium was 10^6 photons/s (400–700 nm). Filled circles give the rates of quantum bumps ("noise") generated spontaneously in darkness. (Barlow et al., 1987). *Right:* Intensity-response functions for a single optic nerve fiber of the *Limulus* lateral eye. The steady-state firing rate is plotted on a log scale on the ordinate as a function of log light intensity plotted on the abscissa. Steady-state rates are the average rates the last 7 s of 10 s flashes. Unfilled circles give light-adapted function (background intensity: LogI = −2), and dashed curve gives dark-adapted function measured during the day. Filled circles give function measured in darkness at night. Light intensity incident on the single ommatidium at Log I = 0 was 10^{12} photons/s (400–700 nm).

I-R function ~6 log units to the left: an approximate million-fold increase in retinal sensitivity.

Part of the nighttime increase in sensitivity results from a >10-fold increase in photon catch caused by a distal shift in the position of photoreceptor cells and dilation of the aperture that limits the light absorbed

by photoreceptors (Table 2). As indicated above part results from an increase in the gain of the photoreceptor response (membrane depolarization/photon; Barlow et al., 1987) which is influenced by a voltage-dependent conductance that repolarizes the photoreceptor membrane during light stimulation

(Pepose and Lisman, 1978). Reducing the efficacy of this membrane mechanism of light adaptation appears to be one way the clock increases photoreceptor gain at night (Barlow et al., 1987). The clock also increases gain by increasing the duration of quantum bumps, the elemental responses to single photons (Kaplan et al., 1990). The temporal change may result from decreased nighttime levels of arrestin, the molecule that deactivates activated rhodopsin (Battelle et al., 2000).

How does the clock reduce "dark noise" in Limulus photoreceptors? Dark noise, which limits visual sensitivity, is a ubiquitous property of both vertebrate and invertebrate photoreceptors. It has been attributed to thermal isomerizations of native rhodopsin (Barlow, 1988), but the Arrhenius energy we measure for dark noise ($\sim$27 kcal/mole; Barlow et al., 1993) is far less than that required for isomerization ($\sim$45 kcal/mole; Birge, 1990). An alternative explanation is that dark noise results from the thermal isomerization of an unstable form of rhodopsin, one in which the Schiff-base linkage is unprotonated. Theoretical studies indicate that deprotonation lowers the energy barrier for isomerization from $\sim$45 to 23 kcal/mole which is near the Arrhenius energies we measured (Barlow et al., 1993; Birge and Barlow, 1995). Indeed, mutations of rhodopsin that completely or partially deprotonate the Schiff base activate transduction mechanisms in darkness (for example: Sakmar et al., 1989; Robinson et al., 1992). We hypothesize that during the day not all of the large number of rhodopsin molecules ($\sim$10^9) within the photoreceptors of a *Limulus* ommatidium are protonated. A small population is unprotonated and can thermally isomerize to produce spontaneous quantum bumps that mimic photon absorption events. We further hypothesize that the circadian clock decreases pH in the vicinity of photoreceptors at night which in turn decreases the small population of unstable rhodopsin molecules and thus reduces dark noise (Barlow et al., 1993). Interestingly, a circadian clock decreases the pH of the fish retina at night that, in turn, may modulate synaptic transmission to suppress cone horizontal cell responses (Mangel, this volume).

The circadian clock's influence on retinal sensitivity can also be assessed by the day-night changes in signal-to-noise (S:N) properties of single photoreceptor cells. At night the S:N properties of the dark-adapted reticular cell recorded in Fig. 1 (left) increased approximately 50-fold. Remarkably signal increased and noise decreased at night. This is not unique to *Limulus*. Somatostatin has the same effect in the rabbit retina: it increases the signal and decreases the noise of ganglion cells (Zalutsky and Miller, 1990). Low concentrations of somatostatin (1 nM) increased the S:N characteristic about 6-fold. Higher concentrations (200 nM) completely suppressed spontaneous activity, yielding infinite sensitivity as measured by S:N properties. This is also the case for *Limulus* where the clock suppresses noise and increases signal in the early evening between 2100 h and 2400 h. Interestingly, this is the time of day when the animals search for mates.

Octopamine is the primary transmitter of the clock's actions on the retina (Battelle et al., 1982; Kass and Barlow, 1984). It acts via the second messenger cAMP to increase the gain and photon catch of photoreceptors but not to decrease their noise (Schneider et al., 1987). As noted above the nighttime decrease in noise appears to require a clock dependent reduction in retinal pH. Octopamine and protons may not be the only mediators of the clock's action. Experiments with retinal slices point to the existence of a third substance (Pelletier et al., 1984) that participates in a "push-pull" mechanism for controlling the circadian changes in retinal structure (Barlow et al., 1989). In this scheme the clock's release of octopamine "pushes" the structure of the retina to the nighttime state increasing photon catch and the acceptance angle (Table 2). The third substance, perhaps a circulating hormone, "pulls" retinal structure back to the daytime state after the cessation of efferent input at dawn. The push-pull actions appear coordinated and interdependent (Chamberlain and Barlow, 1987).

How do the circadian rhythms in retinal sensitivity effect Limulus behavior? The animals use vision to find mates (Barlow et al., 1982). Each spring they migrate to protected beaches from Maine to Mexico, pair off and build nests near the water's edge at high tide (Barlow et al., 1986). We studied their visual performance in the vicinity of underwater mate-like objects and found that they could see them about equally well day and night (Herzog et al., 1996). Their outstanding nighttime vision is consistent with our observation that the circadian increase in retinal sensitivity at night about compensates for the reduction in ambient lighting after sunset. The circadian changes in visual sensitivity serve an essential function: they enable animals to detect mates at night.

What is the neural code underlying mate detection in Limulus? Using neural mechanisms generally found in more complex retinas, the lateral eye converts the responses of photoreceptor cells into trains of optic nerve impulses and transmits them to the brain and to neighboring retinal receptors to mediate lateral inhibition. The entire ensemble of responses across the array of ~1,000 optic nerve fibers yields a "neural image" that encodes what the animal sees. We examined how the eye encodes natural scenes by using a cell-based model of the eye together with a shell-mounted camera (CrabCam; Passaglia et al., 1998). Computed ensembles of optic nerve activity ("neural images") reveal a robust encoding of moving mate-like objects during the day (Passaglia et al., 1997). At night the neural images are less clear. They are dominated by bursts of spikes apparently triggered by random photon events at the low nighttime light levels (Hitt et al., 2000). How does the brain decipher a reliable signal from such a noisy input? "Slow" synapses at the first synaptic level in the brain (lamina) integrate the optic nerve input with a time constant of ~400 ms. This lowpass temporal filtering suppresses the burstiness of the optic nerve input and enhances the coding of a mate-like object in the neural image but not to daytime levels. Additional lowpass spatial filtering appears necessary although laminar receptive fields have not been mapped with precision. In sum, circadian increases in the sensitivity of the lateral eye in combination with lowpass spatial and temporal filtering of its input to the brain explains in part how Limulus can see so well at night.

Circadian rhythms in retinal sensitivity of the Japanese quail

We extended our study of the circadian rhythms in *Limulus* to a vertebrate model, the Japanese quail, because its retina exhibits a circadian modulation of melatonin synthesis (Underwood et al., 1988, 1990) and receives an extensive efferent optic-nerve input from the brain (Uchiyama, 1989). Surprisingly, the

efferent and circadian systems in quail are not related as they are in *Limulus*. Rather than mediating circadian rhythms, the efferent optic-nerve input from the quail brain rapidly increases retinal sensitivity regardless of the time of day (Uchiyama and Barlow, 1994). The circadian oscillators that modulate retinal sensitivity in quail are located in the eyes themselves (Manglapus et al., 1998a). The suprachaismatic nucleus and pineal body also contain circadian oscillators. The circadian organization of quail is truly remarkable with four distinct circadian oscillators in the animal's head!

The influence of the ocular circadian oscillators on retinal function was investigated by recording the amplitude of the b-wave of the electroretinogram (ERG) when an animal is maintained in constant darkness (Manglapus et al., 1998a). Under these conditions the b-wave increases during the animal's subjective night and decreases during its subjective day. The latency to the peak of the b-wave decreases with as intensity increases, from ~80 ms to 40 ms, but does not change significantly from day to night. Reflecting postphotoreceptor activity, the corneal positive b-wave provides a convenient measure of retinal sensitivity (Dowling, 1960). The ERG a-wave reflects photoreceptor activity and was isolated by blocking the b-wave with APB producing the PIII component of the ERG. PIII also changes with time of day when an animal is kept in constant darkness. For unknown reasons the day–night changes are generally more robust over the first but not the second day. Entraining animals to a light–dark cycle shifted by 4 h from the solar cycle yielded an endogenous rhythm in the a- and b-waves that was shifted by 4 h. This and the ~24 h period of the endogenous rhythm of the ERG components are two hallmarks of a process controlled by a circadian oscillator.

The circadian rhythm of the ERG b-wave is associated with a shift in the spectral sensitivity of the retina (Fig. 2A). During the day, the sensitivity of the b-wave response is maximal in the range of 550 to 600 nm. At night the sensitivity increases about six fold and its maximum shifts to shorter wavelengths (~500 nm). Greater increases in sensitivity are detected at shorter wavelengths (<470 nm). The nighttime data are well fit with a nomogram for a rod photopigment ($\lambda_{max} = 506$ nm)

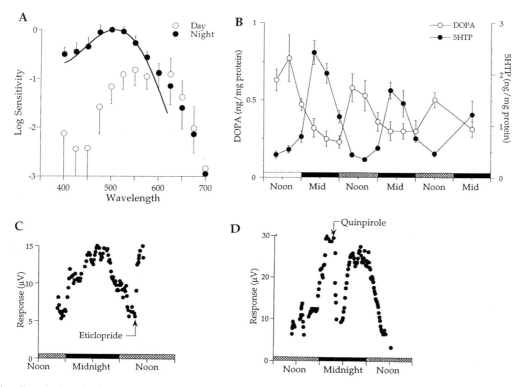

Fig. 2. Circadian rhythms in the Japanese quail retina. (**A**) Spectral sensitivity of the ERG b-wave is high at night (filled circles; $\lambda_{max} \sim 500$ nm) and low during the day (unfilled circles; $\lambda_{max} \sim 550-600$ nm). Circadian changes are maximal for short wavelength stimuli. Smooth curve is a monogram for a rod photopigment ($\lambda_{max} = 506$ nm) based on microspectrophotometric measurements. (Manglapus et al., 1998) (**B**) Retinal concentrations of DOPA (left y-axis) and 5-HTP (right y-axis) as a function of time. Measurements began every 4 h in cyclic lighting and continued into constant darkness. Noon is the middle of the subjective day, and midnight (Mid) is the middle of the subjective night. (**C**) Amplitude of the ERG b-wave in response to 470 nm flashes. Eticlopride, a dopamine D2 receptor antagonist, injected during the day (0935 h; arrow) rapidly increased the b-wave amplitude to nighttime levels. (**D**) Quinpirole, a dopamine D2 receptor agonist, injected at night (arrow; 2150 h) reduced the b-wave amplitude to low daytime levels. After midnight, the quinpirole effect subsided, and the b-wave amplitude returns to its high nighttime state (Manglapus et al., 1999).

derived from microspectrophotometric measurements. Thus rods dominate retinal sensitivity at night and cones dominate sensitivity during the day. This endogenous day–night change resembles the Purkinje shift of human vision but, unlike the Purkinje shift, it does not require a change in ambient light intensity. The spectral sensitivity of the isolated a-wave (PIII) does not change with time of day. It remains maximal at ~ 520 nm and may reflect multiple receptor mechanisms. The rhythmic changes in the a- and b-wave amplitudes have periods of ~ 24 h. They represent a circadian rhythm in the functional organization of the retina: a shift in rod–cone dominance.

In most studies of retinal circadian rhythms the action of clocks is to increase sensitivity at night. The

clock in the Japanese quail eye, however, acts to decrease sensitivity during the day. Li and Dowling (1998) reported a similar result in zebrafish. They found that that a circadian oscillator decreases the visual sensitivity of zebrafish during the day rather than increasing it at night.

Dopamine appears to be the neuromodulator of circadian rhythms in the quail retina (Manglapus et al., 1999). The activity of tyrosine hydroxlyase, the rate-limiting enzyme of dopamine synthesis, correlates with the circadian rhythm in retinal sensitivity (Fig. 2B). At night, dopamine levels are low, and the retina is rod dominated; during the day, dopamine levels are high and the retina is cone dominated. Blocking dopamine D2-like receptors during the day with eticlopride increases the sensitivity of the retina shifting it to the rod-dominated nighttime state (Fig. 2C). Activating dopamine D2-like receptors with quinpirole at night decreases the sensitivity (Fig. 2D) and shifts the retina to the cone-dominated daytime state. Haloperidol, a general blocker of both D1 and D2 receptors, mimics the effects of eticlopride by shifting the retina to the rod-dominated nighttime state. A selective antagonist for D1 dopamine receptors has no effect on retinal sensitivity or rod-cone dominance. Depleting retinal dopamine with 6-OHDA abolishes rhythms in sensitivity and yields a rod-dominated retina regardless of the time of day. Dopamine thus appears to mediate the circadian clock's action on the functional organization of the retina. Increased levels of dopamine during the day appear to block rod signals at the outer retina, allowing only cone signals to be transmitted to the inner retina.

Dopamine also mediates circadian rhythms in retinal physiology and morphology. Mangel reports in this book that dopamine mediates a circadian rhythm in the rod–cone dominance of fish cone horizontal cells via a subclass of D2 receptors termed D4 receptors. Applied at night, it produces cone-like responses typical of those observed during the day. Blocking D4 receptors during the day results in nighttime, rod-dominated responses (Mangel and Wang, 1996). The role of dopamine in the circadian rod-cone shift in fish retina strongly parallels it action in the quail retina. With regard to the circadian modulation of retinal structure, dopamine mediates circadian changes in horizontal spinule formation in fish (Wagner et al., 1992) and causes cone contraction and retinomotor movements in fish (Burnside, this book) and *Xenopus* (Pierce and Besharse, 1985). It is interesting to note that removing dopamine from the fish retina does not inhibit circadian retinomotor movements (Douglas et al., 1992).

Dopamine is a ubiquitous retinal neuromodulator. It not only mediates circadian rhythms in a wide range of species; it exerts both morphological and physiological adaptive effects in most (Dowling, 1991; Besharse and Iuvone, 1992; Witkovsky and Dearry, 1992). Often it appears to adapt retinas for daytime function, that is, serve as a light signal. For example, light releases dopamine in the retinas of *Xenopus* (Witkovsky et al., 1993) and rabbit (Bauer et al., 1980). It can induce light-adaptive cone contraction

via a D2 receptor mechanism in *Xenopus* (Pierce and Besharse, 1985) and fish (Burnside, this book) as well as decrease gap junctional coupling between horizontal cells in fish via a cAMP mechanism (Lasater and Dowling, 1985). It appears to uncouple amacrine cells via the same mechanism (Hampson et al., 1994). It modulates rod–cone coupling in *Xenopus*, enhancing cone signals and suppressing rod signals (Witkovsky et al., 1988), and does so via gap junctions (Krizaj and Witkovsky, 1993). It mimics the effects of light on rod–cone coupling in salamader (Yang and Wu, 1989). However, there is evidence that dopamine can increase sensitivity as if to adapt retinas for nighttime function. For example, in an elegant behavioral experiment Lin and Yazulla (1994) showed that dopamine increases brightness perception in fish. Li and Dowling (2000b) provide evidence that dopamine is required for maintaining light sensitivity in zebrafish and its depletion effects rod pathways in the inner retina. They found that abolishing dopaminergic cells with ocular injections of 6-OHDA blocks circadian rhythms and maintains the retina in its sensitive daytime state.

Regarding the site of action of dopamine, its receptors have been found in both the inner and outer plexiform layers of the retina (Kebabian and Calne, 1979). D1 receptors are located on horizontal cells and D2 receptors on both photoreceptors and amacrine cells (see Manglapus et al., 1999; Witkovsky and Dearry, 1992). The detection of D2 receptors in the outer retina is consistent with our observation in quail that dopamine acts at this level to modulate the transmission of rod signals to the inner retina.

Do the dopaminergic mechanisms described above function in the quail retina? We do not yet have an answer, but whatever mechanisms underlie the endogenous rod–cone shift in quail they must be (1) located in the outer plexiform layer because ON bipolar cells (b-waves) and not photoreceptors exhibit a rod–cone shift (Manglapus et al., 1998a); (2) triggered by cone responses because rod signals are not blocked below cone threshold (Manglapus et al., 1998a) and (3) mediated by dopamine via D2 receptors (Manglapus et al., 1999).

Does dopamine act alone in the quail retina? Interestingly, the circadian rhythm of dopamine synthesis is reciprocally related to that of melatonin in the quail retina (Fig. 2B). Also, the expression of mRNAs encoding two enzymes in the synthesis of melatonin, tryptophan hydroxylase and *N*-acetyltransferase, parallels the circadian rhythm in melatonin synthesis (Manglapus et al., 1998b); however, rhythmic changes in melatonin synthesis by itself does not modulate retinal sensitivity (Manglapus et al., 1998c). Melatonin levels have been linked with retinal function in darkness in at least two studies. In one, Pierce and Besharse (1985) found that melatonin mimics the effects of darkness on cone elongation in *Xenopus*. In the other, Mangel and Wang (1996) found that exogenous melatonin shifts cone horizontal cells to rod dominance in the fish retina in vivo. Inspired by these results, we tested the influence of melatonin on the quail retina following techniques used for dopamine. Although our studies are preliminary in nature, they have yet to show a direct effect of melatonin on either retinal sensitivity or rod-cone dominance (Manglapus et al., 1998a).

However, melatonin may have an indirect role in mediating circadian rhythms in the quail retina. Circadian rhythms in retinal melatonin have been found in a number of animals (see Table 1). Particularly interesting is melatonin's inhibition of dopamine release in rabbit, *Xenopus* and chicken retinas (Dubocovich, 1988; Boatright et al., 1994), and conversely dopamine's inhibition of melatonin release in both *Xenopus* and chicken (Cahill and Besharse, 1992; Zawilska, 1994). These two neuromodulators form a mutual inhibitory or "push-pull" biosynthetic mechanism in chick and *Xenopus*.

Our working hypothesis is that at night melatonin, under direct control of a retinal circadian clock, reduces dopamine levels and shifts the retina to rod dominance and increases its sensitivity. During the day, the clock-controlled melatonin levels decrease and dopamine levels increase to reduce the sensitivity of the retina and prepare it for visual processing during the day. In short, melatonin and dopamine interact at dawn and dusk to change the organization of the retina for optimal function day and night.

Circadian rhythm in the sensitivity of the *Xenopus* retina

Do the circadian rhythms in anatomy and metabolism of the *Xenopus* retina listed in Table 1 influence its sensitivity? To try to answer this question we recorded the ERG of an adult eye while the animal remained in darkness for several days. Although this approach was successful with *Limulus* and quail, it proved difficult with *Xenopus* because of the animal's poor tolerance to anesthesia. In most experiments the animal did not remain stable long to determine whether the ERG amplitude exhibited a circadian rhythm. In the few cases when it stabilized, the b-wave amplitude was lower at night than during the day. Although these results must be considered very preliminary, they suggest that a circadian oscillator either increases retinal sensitivity during the day or depresses it at night. *Limulus* is opposite: a circadian efferent input to the retina at night increases its sensitivity (Fig. 2). Also in quail, if our hypothesis is correct, a circadian increase in retinal melatonin at night inhibits dopamine release, shifting the retina to rod dominance and increasing its sensitivity. How circadian mechanisms may modulate the sensitivity of the *Xenopus* retina is not known, but its higher sensitivity during the day is reminiscent of what Li and Dowling (1998) reported in a behavioral study of the visual sensitivity of zebrafish. Thus circadian increases in sensitivity do not necessarily occur at night in all animals. In some, clocks may modulate visual sensitivity at the times of dawn or dusk when animals often search for prey.

Do circadian rhythms exist in human vision?

Electrophysiological studies have reported diurnal variations in the amplitude of the human ERG (Nozaki et al., 1983) and in its temporal response properties (Hankins et al., 1998). Psychophysical studies have found similar diurnal variations in human scotopic sensitivity (Bassi and Powers, 1986) and in chromatic sensitivity (Roenneberg et al., 1992). Interestingly, blood glucose levels influence human visual sensitivity (McFarland and Forbes, 1940; McFarland et al., 1945) and the hormonal control of glucose homeostasis changes with time of day (Agren et al., 1931; Aschoff, 1979a) with glucose utilization decreasing at night (Van Cauter et al., 1988). Are these daily changes in human vision and metabolism related?

In a preliminary psychophysical study we measured both contrast sensitivity and blood sugar levels of subjects over a period of several days (Barlow et al., 1993). Subjects were exposed to diurnal changes in environmental illumination, but their tested eye was patched at all times except when contrast thresholds were being measured at 2 h intervals using the Quest algorithm (Watson and Pelli, 1983). Subjects slept at night except when being tested. Under these conditions we found that contrast sensitivity decreases as much as four times at night, and the decreases were roughly correlated with decreases in blood glucose levels that naturally occur at night. Ingestion of fixed amount of glucose at night (Trutol) increased blood sugar levels (average increase: 74 ± 7 to 135 ± 14 mg/dl) and elevated contrast sensitivity to normal levels. To further test the influence of blood sugar level on visual sensitivity we reduced it artificially by injecting insulin during the day. Lowering blood glucose from normal levels to the range of 50–60 mg/dl reduced contrast sensitivity $\sim$10-fold. Levels below 50 mg/dl occasionally produced a transient visual scotoma lasting about 5 min and covering about $20°$ of the central visual field. The reason for this is not known.

The site of glucose action may be the retina. Ames and Gurian (1963) and later Winkler (1981) showed in mammal that glucose and oxygen are necessary for optimal retinal function: low glucose and/or oxygen decreases optic-nerve action potentials within minutes, and glucose perfusion and/or reoxygenation produce rapid and complete recovery. Also the sensitivity of cat eyes as assessed by the ERG b-wave increased when perfused with glucose (Macaluso et al., 1992) and when made hypoxic (Linsenmeier et al., 1983). The retina is not the only glucose dependent part of the visual system. We used functional magnetic resonance imaging (fMRI) to examine higher levels and in initial studies found that physiological changes in blood glucose levels changed the hemodynamic responses of the visual cortex (Barlow et al., 1997). fMRI also revealed significant time-of-day changes in cortical activity.

Effects of metabolism on vision date back to the early days of aviation when pilots flying at altitudes (>18,000 ft) reported darkened visual fields. Related research carried out during World War II showed that both hypoxia and hypoglycemia decreased visual sensitivity, as assessed by dark adaptation and that glucose ingestion could counter the effects of hypoxia on visual sensitivity and visa versa (McFarland and Forbes, 1940; McFarland et al., 1945). Our preliminary studies confirm this earlier work showing that glucose, a major energy source for CNS function, can modulate human contrast sensitivity. We hypothesize that the changes in sensitivity with time of day we detected result from daily changes in blood sugar level. Because our studies were not carried out under constant conditions, the daily changes in sensitivity cannot be considered as evidence for a circadian rhythm in visual sensitivity.

Efferent modulation of retinal sensitivity

Circadian oscillators, metabolism, and adaptation are not the only modulators of retinal sensitivity. As noted at the beginning many animals have evolved centrifugal pathways that can modulate retinal function via efferent signals transmitted either from the brain or from within the retina. Centrifugal pathways from the brain are known to exist in fish, birds and mammals (Uchiyama, 1989) and invertebrates (Barlow et al., 1989). Their functional organization can be classified as either "local" or "global". An example of "global" is the *Limulus* visual system in which a few efferent fibers enter the retina, branch profusely and influence the entire retina. An example of "local" is the retinotopic arrangement of the centrifugal input from the isthmo-optic nucleus (ION) in Japanese quail. It provides the circuitry for modulating the properties of specific regions of the quail retina.

We studied the influence of the centrifugal pathway in quail and found that it can increase the response of ganglion cells without changing the configuration of their receptive fields (Uchiyama and Barlow, 1994). Specifically, stimulating the ION with a brief train of 10 impulses (pulse duration: 100 μs; pulse frequency: 200 Hz) immediately preceding the onset of a 1 s drifting sine wave grating enhanced the response of a ganglion cell >60% (Fig. 3A–C). Both with and without ION input the response was maximal for sine-wave grating with spatial frequencies in the range of 1–2 cycles/deg

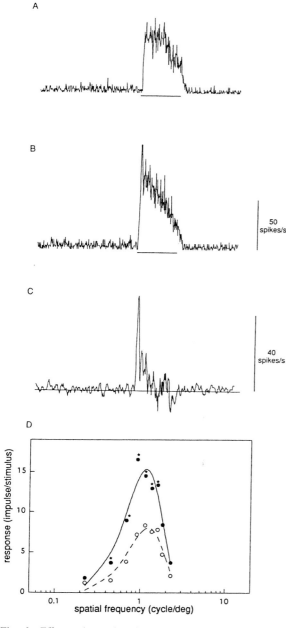

Fig. 3. Efferent input increases the response of a retinal ganglion cell in Japanese quail. (A–C): Histograms of spikes evoked by drifting gratings (horizontal bars) for 1 s without (A) and with (B) stimulation of the ION. The difference in the two histograms (A–B) is plotted in (C) after time averaging. 50 sweeps were averaged for this ON-OFF direction-selective cell. (D): Spatial frequency tuning curves of a retinal ganglion cell with (filled circles) and without (open circles) ION stimulation. Smooth curves were fitted using the DOG. Temporal frequency was maintained at 5 Hz for ON non-direction-selective cell.

(Fig. 3D). The data when normalized overlap indicating that the ION input increased response without changing the shape of the spatial frequency tuning curve. We conclude that efferent inputs from the midbrain can enhance retinal responses without affecting the center-surround organization of their receptive fields.

The feedback system in quail is retinotopically organized—retina to tectum to ION to retina—with about 10,000 centrifugal fibers projecting from the ION to the retina in a point-to-point manner. This "local" organization may enable single ION fibers to assist in shifting visual attention in space by changing ganglion cell responses in a specific region of the retina. Such a selective attention mechanism would be consistent with the known role of the optic tectum in orienting behavior (Uchiyama, 1989). It is also reminiscent of the "searchlight hypothesis" proposed for the cortical feedback to the lateral geniculate nucleus (Crick, 1984; Koch, 1987). Although centrifugal fibers innervate the mammalian retina, the most abundant efferent pathway is the cortical feedback to the LGN. Recent studies suggest that the cortical feedback to LGN cells may have a role in the generation of orientation tuning (Murphy et al., 1999), may increase their responses by disinhibition (Wörgötter et al., 1998), may enhance their contrast gain (Przybyszewski et al., 2000) and may operate via metabotropic receptors (McCormack and vonKrosigk, 1992). In sum, there is much more to learn about this massive and intriguing efferent pathway of the mammalian visual system (Crick and Koch, 1998).

The efferent input to the retina of teleost fish from the olfactory bulb terminates on other efferent neurons: the dopaminergic interplexiform cells (DA-IPCs; Zucker and Dowling, 1987). Having a mutual interest in efferent pathways, John Dowling and I attempted to do with the green sunfish retina what my laboratory had done earlier with the *Limulus* eye, namely drive efferent inputs by shocking the optic nerve trunk and monitoring their effect on retinal sensitivity. We used an isolated eyecup preparation but unfortunately could not maintain

Asterisks show responses under ION stimulation that are statistically higher ($p < 0.05$) than control responses (Uchiyama and Barlow, 1994).

its viability, as assessed by the ERG, and thus could not determine the effect of shocking. A more recent study by John and Lei Li revealed a possible role of centrifugal inputs in the regulation of visual sensitivity of zebrafish. They found that a dominant mutation, *night blindness b*, suppresses visual sensitivity, reduces the number of DA-IPCs, and disrupts both the centrifugal input to the retina and the circadian modulation of visual sensitivity, (Li and Dowling, 2000a). Taken together these effects suggest that the centrifugal input excites DA-IPCs which, in turn, raises dopamine levels enhancing the transmission of rod signals to the inner retina which then reduces visual threshold. Other than this possibility the function of the centrifugal input to the fish retina remains unknown.

Conclusions and future perspectives

The ultimate goal of neuroscience is to understand how the brain works. In his book, *The Retina: An Approachable Part of the Brain* (1987) John Dowling suggests that we can gain important information about brain function by analyzing a small piece of brain tissue, the retina. Our challenge then is to understand how the retina works, that is, how its circuitry produces a "neural image" of the visual world.

Analyzing a relatively simple retina may yield important insights about the function of more complex ones. Indeed that of the horseshoe crab, *Limulus*, has proven complex enough to be interesting, yet simple enough to be understood. Using a computational approach we unraveled its coding properties and determined the neural image it sends to the brain about visual stimuli that are behaviorally relevant, namely mates. We were surprised to discover that this retina is not so "simple" after all. A circadian clock increases its sensitivity at night enabling the animal to detect potential mates as well as it does during the day. We have not yet deciphered the eye's neural code for nighttime vision but have uncovered some of the remarkable cellular mechanisms that produce the highly sensitive nighttime state. This is an extremely sophisticated eye that modulates most every property of the retina, to gain sensitivity at night. The challenge is to understand how it efficiently encodes information about potential mates under the photon-limited conditions of the animal's marine habitat at night. The lesson learned as Keffer Hartline noted: "if it's simple, it's not an eye."

This brings us to the vertebrate eye, a far more complex organ than that of *Limulus*. With tens of millions of cells, numerous cell types, dendritic processes and synaptic contacts, the task of deciphering its neural code is indeed taunting. How to meet John's challenge? Is the vertebrate retina truly approachable? Developing a cell-based, realistic computational model as we did for *Limulus* appears unrealistic. A different computational approach is needed, one that by necessity models ensembles of neurons. The danger is that such modeling overlooks details in the neural circuitry and "the truth is in the details". As was the case for *Limulus* insights can come from understanding how the retina adapts or is modulated to function optimally under different conditions. Much has been learned from studies by John Dowling, his colleagues and others about the endogenous mechanisms that adapt the retina to function under various lighting regimes. Also we are gaining a better appreciation of the modulatory influences of efferent inputs and circadian oscillators. But we have yet to put all the pieces together.

Major challenges are to understand how circadian changes at various levels of the visual system influence visually guided behavior, how efferent signals from the brain are triggered, and how do they influence the signals the brain receives from the retina.

Doing so requires a multidisciplinary approach, one that combines the power of molecular biology with that of animal psychophysics as well as the tools of electrophysiology, neuroanatomy and computational neuroscience. Insight about the function of a normal visual system can often be gained by mutating the system and carefully investigating the resulting phenotype with a variety of techniques. Here again John Dowling has pointed the way by establishing an ambitious research program that uses the zebrafish to study the cellular basis of visual function with mutagenic techniques. It is an ideal model system as John and his colleagues have demonstrated. The research is tedious and laborious, but some of the contributions to this book underscore its benefits.

The numerous cellular mechanisms that adapt and modulate retinal function provide important clues about its function. They underscore the retina's critical role as the interface between the brain and the constantly changing visual world. Although we ultimately strive to learn how the brain in all its complexity works, understanding first how the retina in all of its altered states works may prove equally challenging.

Acknowledgments

Supported by grants from the National Eye Institute, National Institute of Mental Health, National Science Foundation and by Research to Prevent Blindness and the Lions of Central New York.

References

Agren, G., Wilander, O. and Jorpes, E. (1931) Cyclic changes in the glycogen content of the liver and muscles of rats and mice. Biochem. J., 25: 777–785.

Ames, A., III and Gurian, B.S. (1963) Effects of glucose and oxygen deprivation on function of isolated mammalian retina. J. Neurophysiol., 26: 617–634.

Anderson, M.L. and Purple, R.L. (1980) Circadian rhythms and variability of the clinical electro-oculogram. Invest. Ophthalmol. Vis. Sci., 19: 278–288.

Aschoff, J. (1979a) Circadian rhythms: general features and endocrinological aspects. In: Krieger, D.T. (Eds.), Endocrine Rhythms. Raven Press, New York, pp. 1–6.

Barattini, S., Battisti, B., Cervetto, L. and Marroni, P. (1981) Diurnal changes in the pigeon electroretinogram. Rev. Can. Biol., 40: 133–137.

Barlow, H.B. (1988) Thermal limit to seeing. Nature, 334: 296–297.

Barlow, R.B., Jr., Boudreau, E.A. and Pelli, D.G. (1993) Metabolic modulation of human visual sensitivity. Invest. Ophthalmol. Vis. Sci., 34(4): 785.

Barlow, R.B. and Kaplan, E. (1993) Intensity Coding and Circadian Rhythms in the Limulus Lateral Eye. In: Verrillo, R.T. (Eds.), Sensory Research: Multimodal Perspectives, L. Erlbaum Assoc., pp. 55–73.

Barlow, R.B., Birge, R.R., Kaplan, E. and Tallent, J.R. (1993) On the molecular origin of photoreceptor noise retinas. Nature, 366: 64–66.

Barlow, R.B., Boudreau, E.A., Moore, D.C., Huckins, S.C., Lindstrom, A.M. and Farell, B. (1997) Glucose and time of day modulate human contrast sensitivity and fMRI signals from visual cortex. Invest. Ophthalmol. Vis. Sci., 38: S735.

Barlow, R.B., Jr. (1983) Circadian rhythms in the Limulus visual system. J. Neurosci., 3: 856–870.

Barlow, R.B., Jr., Kaplan, E., Renninger, G.H. and Saito, T. (1987) Circadian rhythms in Limulus photoreceptors. I. Intracellular recordings. J. Gen. Physiol., 89: 353–378.

Barlow, R.B., Jr., Ireland, L.C. and Kass, L. (1982) Vision has a role in Limulus mating behavior. Nature, 296: 65–66.

Barlow, R.B., Jr., and Chamberlain, S.C. (1980) Light and circadian clock modulate structure and function in Limulus photoreceptors. In: Williams, T.P. and Baker, B.N. (Eds.), The Effects of Constant Light on Visual Processes. Plenum Press, NY, pp. 247–269.

Barlow, R.B., Jr., Powers, M.K., Howard, H. and Kass, L. (1986) Migration of Limulus for mating: Relation to lunar phase, tide height, and sunlight. Bio. Bull., 171: 310–329.

Barlow, R.B., Jr., Chamberlain, S.C. and Lehman, H.K. (1989) Circadian rhythms in invertebrate vision. In: Stavenga, D.C. and Hardie, R.C. (Eds.), Facets of Vision. Springer-Verlag, Berlin, pp. 257–280.

Barlow, R.B., Jr., Chamberlain, S.C. and Levinson, J.Z. (1980) The Limulus brain modulates the structure and function of the lateral eyes. Science, 210: 1037–1039.

Barlow, R.B., Jr., Bolanowski, S.J. and Brachman (1977) Efferent optic nerve fibers mediate circadian rhythms in the Limulus eye. Science, 197: 86–89.

Barlow, R.B., Parshley, M.R., Kelly, M.J. and Knox, B.E. (2000) Visual sensitivity of Xenopus. Invest. Ophthalmol. Vis. Sci., 41: S715.

Bassi, C.J. and Powers, M.K. (1986) Daily fluctuations in the detectability of dim lights by humans. Physiol. Behav., 38: 871–877.

Bassi, C.J. and Powers, M.K. (1987) Circadian rhythm in goldfish visual sensitivity Invest. Opthal. Vis. Sci., 28: 1811–1815.

Batra, R. and Barlow, R.B., Jr. (1990) Circadian rhythms in the temporal response of the Limulus lateral eye. J. Gen. Physiol., 95: 229–244.

Battelle, B.A., Williams, C.D., Schremser-Berlin, J.L. and Cacciatore, C. (2000) Regulation of arrestin mRNA levels in Limulus lateral eye: Separate and combined influences of circadian efferent input and light. Vis. Neurosci., 17: 217–227.

Battelle, B.A., Evans, J.A. and Chamberlain, S.C. (1982) Efferent fibers to Limulus eyes synthesize and release octopamine. Science, 216: 1250–1252.

Bauer, B., Ehinger, B. and Aberg, L. (1980) 3h-dopamine release from the rabbit retina. Albrecht von Graefee's Arch. Klin. Exp. Oph., 215: 71–78.

Besharse, J. and Iuvone, P.M. (1992) Is dopamine a light-adaptive or a dark-adaptive modulator in retina? Neurochem. Int., 20(2): 193–199.

Besharse, J. and Iuvone, P.M. (1983) Circadian clock in Xenopus eye controlling retinal serotonin N-acetyltransferase. Science, 305: 133–135.

Besharse, J. and Iuvone, P.M. (1983) Circadian clock in Xenopus eye controlling retinal serotonin N-acetyltransferase. Nature, 305: 133–135.

Birge, R.R. (1990) Nature of the primary photochemical events in rhodopsin and bacteriorhodopsin. Biochim. Biophys. Acta, 1016: 293–327

500

Birge, R.R. and Barlow, R.B. (1995) On the molecular origins of thermal noise in vertebrate and invertebrate photoreceptors. *Biophys. Chem.*, 55: 115–126.

Boatright, J., Rubim, N.M. and Iuvone, P.M. (1994) Regulation of endogenous dopamine release in amphibian retina by melatonin: the role of GABA. *Vis. Neurosci.*, 11: 1013–1018.

Bobbert, A.C., Krul, W.H. and Brandenburg, J. (1978) Photoperiodic programming of diurnal changes in rabbit visual eboked potentials. *Int. J. Chrono.*, 5: 307–325.

Boyd, T.A.S. and McLeold, L.E. (1964) Circadian rhythm of plasma corticoid levels, intraocular pressure and aqueous outflow facility in normal and glaucomatous eyes. *Ann. NY. Acad. Sci.*, 117: 567–613.

Brandenburg, J., Bobbert, A.C. and Eggelmeyer, E. (1983) Circadian changes in the response of the rabbit's retina to flashes. *Behav. Brain Res.*, 7: 113–123.

Cajal, S.R. (1892) La rétine des zertébrés. *La cellule*, 9: 119–257.

Cahill, G.M. and Besharse, J.C. (1993) Circadian clock functions localized in Xenopus retinal photoreceptors. *Neuron*, 10: 573–577.

Cahill, G.M. and Besharse, J.C. (1990) Circadian regulation of melatonin in the retina of *Xenopus laevis*: limitation by serotonin availability. *J. Neurochem.*, 54: 716–719.

Cahill, G.M. and Besharse, J.C. (1992) Light-sensitive melatonin synthesis by *Xenopus* photoreceptors after destruction of the inner retina. *Vis. Neurosci.*, 8: 487–490.

Calman, B.G. and Battelle, B.A. (1991) Central origin of the efferent neurons projecting to the eyes of *Limulus polyphemus. Vis. Neurosci.*, 6: 481–495.

Chamberlain, S.C. and Barlow, R.B., Jr. (1987) Controls of structural rhythms in the lateral eye of *Limulus*: Interactions of diurnal lighting and circadian efferent activity. *J. Neurosci.*, 7: 2135–2144.

Chamberlain, S.C. and Barlow, R.B., Jr. (1977) Morphological Correlates of Efferent Circadian Activity and Light Adaptation in the *Limulus* Lateral Eye. *Biol. Bull.*, 153: 418–419.

Chamberlain, S.C. and Barlow, R.B., Jr. (1979) Light and efferent activity control rhabdom turnover in *Limulus* photoreceptors. *Science*, 206: 361–363.

Chamberlain, S.C. and Barlow, R.B., Jr. (1984) Transient membrane shedding in *Limulus* photoreceptors: Control mechanisms under natural lighting. *J. Neurosci.*, 4: 2792–2810.

Chong, N.W., Cassone, V.M., Bernard, M., Klein, D.C. and Iuvone, P.M. (1998) Circadian expression of tryptophan hydroxylase mRNA in chicken retina. *Mol. Brain Res.*, 61: 243–250.

Crick, F. (1984) Function of the thalamic reticular complex: The searchlight hypothesis. *Proc. Natl. Acad. Sci. USA*, 81: 4586–4590.

Crick, F. and Koch, C. (1998) Constraints on cortical and thalamic projections: the no-strong-loops hypothesis. *Nature*, 391: 245–250.

Douglas, R., et al. (1992) The effect of dopamine depletion on light-evoked and circadian retinomotor movements in the teleost retina. *Vis. Neurosci.*, 9(3–4): 335–343.

Douglas, R.H. and Wagner, H.-J. (1983) Endogenous control of spinule formation in horizontal cells of the teleost retina. *Cell Tissue Res.*, 229: 443–449.

Dowling, J.E. (1960) The chemistry of visual adaptation in the rat. *Nature*, 188: 114–118.

Dowling, J.E. (1987) *The retina: an approachable part of the brain.* Harvard University Press, Cambridge, MA.

Dowling, J.E. (1991) Retinal neuromodulation: the role of dopamine. *Vis. Neurosci.*, 7: 87–97.

Dowling, J.E. and Cowan, W.M. (1966) An electron microscope study of normal and degenerating centrifugal fiber terminals in the pigeon retina. *Z. Zellforsch. Mikrosk. Anat.*, 71: 14–28.

Dowling, J.E. and Ehinger, B. (1975) Synaptic organization of thalmic-containing interplexiform cells of the goldfish Cebus monkey retinas. *Science*, 188: 270–273.

Dubocovich, M.L. (1988) Role of melatonin in retina. In: Osborne, N.N. and Chader, G.J. (Eds.), *Progress Retinal Research*, 8: 129–151.

Fowkles, D.H., Karwoski, C.J. and Proenza, L.M. (1984) Endogenous circadian rhythm in electroretinogram of free-moving lizards. *Invest. Ophthalmol. Vis. Sci.*, 25: 121–124.

Fujita, S. (1980) Diurnal variations in human corneal thickness. *Jpn. J. Ophthalmol.*, 24: 444–456.

Green, C., Cahill, G.M. and Besharse, J.C. (1995) Regulation of tryptophan hydroxylase expression by a retinal circadian oscillator in vitro. *Brain Res.*, 667: 283–290.

Hamm, H.E. and Menaker, M. (1980) Retinal rhythms in chicks—circadian variation in melatonin and serotonin N-acetyltransferase activity. *Proc. Natl. Acad. Sci.*, 77: 4998–5002.

Hampson, E.C., Weiler, R. and Vaney, D.I. (1994) pH-gated dopaminergic modulation of horizontal cell gap junctions in mammalian retina. *Proc. Roy. Soc. Lond. B Biol. Sci.*, 255: 67–72.

Hanada, Y. and Kawamura, H. (1984) Circadian rhythms in synaptic excitability of the dorsal lateral geniculate nucleus in the rat. *Int. J. Neurosci.*, 22: 253–261.

Hankins, M.W., Jones, R.J. and Ruddock, K.H. (1998) Diurnal variation in the b-wave implicit time of the human electroretinogram. *Vis. Neurosci.*, 15: 55–67.

Herzog, E.H., Powers, M.K. and Barlow, R.B. (1996) *Limulus* vision in the ocean day and night: effects of image size and contrast. *Vis. Neurosci.*, 13: 31–41.

Hitt, J.M., Ruta, V., Dodge, F.A. and Barlow, R.B. (2000) Explaining night vision in *Limulus. Invest. Ophthamol. Vis. Sci.*, 41: S28.

Kaplan, E. and Barlow, R.B. (1975) Properties of visual cells in the lateral eye of *Limulus in situ*. Extracellular recordings. *J. Gen. Physiol.*, 66: 303–326.

Kaplan, E. and Barlow, R.B., Jr. (1980) Circadian clock in *Limulus* brain increases response and decreases noise of retinal photoreceptors. *Nature*, 286: 393–395.

Kaplan, E., Barlow, R.B., Renninger, G. and Purpura, K. (1990) Circadian rhythms in *Limulus* photoreceptors. II. Quantum bumps. *J. Gen. Physiol.*, 96: 665–685.

Kass, L. and Barlow, R.B., Jr. (l984) Efferent neurotransmission of circadian rhythms in *Limulus* lateral eye. I. Octopamine-induced increases in retinal sensitivity *J. Neurosci.*, 4: 908–917.

Kass, L. and Berent, M. (1988) Circadian rhythms in adaptation to light of *Limulus* photoreception. *Comp. Biochem. Physiol.*, C91: 229–239.

Katz, R.S., Henkind, P. and Weitzman, E.D. (1975) the circadian rhythm of th einterocular pressure in the New Zealand white rabbit. *Inv. Oph.*, 14: 775–780.

Kebabian, J.W. and Calne, D.B. (1979) Multiple receptors for dopamine. *Nature*, 277: 493–498.

Koch, C. (1987) The action of the corticofugal pathway on sensory thalamic nuclei: A hypothesis. *Neuroscience*, 23: 399–406.

Kohler, K., Kolbinger, W., Kurz-Isler, G. and Weiler, R. (1990) Endogenous dopamine and cyclic events in the fish retina, II: Correlation of retinomotor movement, spinule formation, and connexon density of gap junctions with dopamine activity during light/dark cycles. *Vis. Neurosci.*, 5: 417–428.

Korenbrot, J.I. and Fernald, R.D. (1989) Circadian rhythm and light regulate opsin mRNA in rod photoreceptors. *Nature*, 337: 454–457.

Krizaj, D. and Witkovsky, P. (1993) Effects of submicromolar concentration of dopamine on photoreceptor to horizontal cell communication. *Brain Res.*, 627: 122–128.

Lasater, E.M. and Dowling, J.E. (1985) Dopamine decreases conductance of the electrical junctions between cultured retinal horizontal cells. *Proc. Natl. Acad. Sci.*, 82: 3025–3029.

LaVail, M.M. (1976) Rod Outer Segment Disc Shedding in the Rat Retina: Relationship to Cyclic Lighting. *Science*, 194: 1071–1073.

Levinson, G. and Burnside, B. (1981) Circadian rhythms in teleost retinomotor movements. *Invest. Ophthalmol. Vis. Sci.*, 20: 294–303.

Li, L. and Dowling, J.E. (1998) Zebrafish visual sensitivity is regulated by a circadian clock. *Vis. Neurosci.*, 15: 851–857.

Li, L. and Dowling, J.E. (2000a) Disruption of the olfactoretinal centrifugal pathway may relate to the visual system defect in *night blindness b* mutant zebrafish. *J. Neurosci.*, 20: 1883–1892.

Li, L. and Dowling, J.E. (2000b) Effects of dopamine depletion on visual sensitivity of zebrafish. *J. Neurosci.*, 20: 1893–1903.

Lin, Z.-S. and Yazulla, S. (1994) Depletion of retinal dopamine increases brightness perception in goldfish. *Vis. Neurosci.*, 11: 683–693.

Linsenmeier, R.A., Mines, A.H. and Steinberg, R.H. (1983) Effects of Hypoxia and Hypercapnia on the light peak and electroretinogram of the cat. *Invest. Opthalmol. Vis. Sci.*, 24: 37–46.

Macaluso, C., Onoe, S. and Niemeyer, G. (1992) Changes in glucose level affect rod function more han cone function in the isolated, perfused cat eye. *Invest. Opthalmol. Vis. Sci.*, 33: 2798–2807.

Mangel, S. and Wang, Y. (1996) Circadian clock regulates rod and cone input to fish retinal cone horizontal cells. *PNAS*, 93: 4655–4660.

Mangel, S. and Dowling, J.E. (1985) Responsiveness and receptive field size of carp horizontal cells are reduced by prolonged darkness and dopamine. *Science*, 229: 1107–1109.

Manglapus, M.K., Barlow, R.B and Pierce, M.E. (1998b) Daily Rhythms of mRNA Expression in the Japanese Quail Retina. *Invest. Ophthalmol. Vis. Sci.*, 39: S237.

Manglapus, M.K., Iuvone, P.M., Underwood, H., Pierce, M.E. and Barlow, R.B. (1999) Dopamine mediates a circadian rhythm in rod-cone dominance in the Japanese quail retina. *J. Neurosci.*, 19: 4132–4141.

Manglapus, M.K., Pierce, M.E. and Barlow, R.B. (1998c) Rhythmic Expression of Melatonin Does Not Influence Rod-Cone Dominance in the Quail Retina. *Soc. Neurosci. Abstrs.*, 24: 1872.

Manglapus, M.K., Uchiyama, H., Buelow, N. and Barlow, R.B. (1998a) Circadian rhythms of rod-cone dominance in the Japanese quail retina. *J. Neurosci.*, 18: 4775–4784.

McCormack, C. and Burnside B. (1993) Light and circadian modulation of teleost retinal tyrosine hydroxylase activity. *Invest. Ophthalmol. Vis. Sci.*, 34(5): 1853–1860.

McCormack, D.A. and vonKrosigk, M. (1992) Corticothalamic activation modulates thalamic firing through glutamate metabotropic receptors. *Proc. Natl. Acad. Sci. USA*, 89: 2774–2778.

McFarland, R.A. and Forbes, W.H. (1940) The effects of variations in the concentration of oxygen and of glucose on dark adaptation. *J Gen. Physiol.*, 24: 69.

McFarland, R.A., Halperin, M.H. and Niven, J.I. (1945) Visual thresholds as an index of the modification of the effects of anoxia by glucose. *Am. J. Physiol.*, 144: 378.

Murphy, P.C., Duckett, S.G. and Sillito, A.M. (1999) Feedback connections to the lateral geniculate nucleus and cortical response properties. *Science*, 286: 1552–1554.

Nozaki, S., Wakakurua, M. and Ishikawa, S. (1983) Circadian rhythm of human electroretinogram. *Jpn. J. Opthalmol.*, 27: 346–352.

Oishi, T. and Matsumoto, M. (1985) Circadian mitotic rhythm in the corneal epithelium of Japanese quail: Intraocular initiation of the rhythm. In: Hiroshige, T. and Honma, K. (Eds.), *Circadian Clocks and Zeitgebers*. Hokkaido University Press, pp. 45–54.

Passaglia, C.L., Dodge, F.A., Herzog, E.H., Jackson, S. and Barlow, R.B. (1997) Deciphering a neural code for vision. *Proc. Natl. Acad. Sci.*, 94: 12649–12654.

Passaglia, C.L., Dodge, F.A. and Barlow, R.B. (1998) A cell-based model of the *Limulus* lateral eye. *J. Neurophysiol.*, 80: 1800–1815.

Pelletier, J.L., Kass, L., Renninger, G.H. and Barlow, R.B., Jr. (1984) cAMP to Octopamine Partially Mimic a Circadian Clock's Effect on *Limulus* Photoreceptors. *Invest. Ophthamol. Vis. Sci.*, (Suppl. 25): 288.

Pepose, J.S. and Lisman, J.E. (1978) Voltage-sensitive potassium channels in *Limulus* ventral photoreceptors. *J. Gen. Physiol.*, 71: 101–120.

502

Pierce, M.E., Sheshberaadaran, H., Zhang, Z., Fox, L.E., Applebury, M.L. and Takahashi, J.S. (1993) Circadian regulation of iodopsin gene expression in embryonic photoreceptors in retinal cell culture. *Neuron*, 10: 1–20.

Pierce, M.E. and Besharse, J.C. (1985) Circadian regulation of retinomotor movements I. Interaction of melatonin and dopamine in the control of cone length. *J. Gen. Physiol.*, 86: 671–689.

Pierce, M.E. and Besharse, J.C. (1986) Melatonin and dopamine interactions in the regulation of rhythmic photoreceptor metabolism. In: O'Brien, P.J. and Klein, D.C. (Eds.), *Pineal and Retinal Relationships*. Academic Press, NY, pp. 219–237.

Powers, M.K. and Barlow, R.B., Jr. (1985) Behavioral correlates of circadian rhythms in *Limulus* visual system. *Biol. Bull.*, 169: 578–591.

Przybyszewski, A.W., Gaska, J.P., Foote, W. and Pollen, D.A. (2000) Striate cortex increases contrast gain of macaque LGN neurons. *Vis. Neurosci.*, 17: 485–494.

Reme, C.E., Wirz-Justice, A. and Terman, M. (1991) The visual input stage of the mammalian circadian pacemaking system: I. Is there a clock in the mammalian eye? *J. Biol. Rhythms*, 6: 5–29.

Renninger, G.H. and Barlow, R.B., Jr. (1979) Lateral Inhibition, Excitation, and the Circadian Rhythm of the *Limulus* Compound Eye. *Soc. Neurosci. Abstr.*, 5: 804.

Renninger, G.H., Kaplan, E. and Barlow, R.B., Jr. (1984) A Circadian Clock Increases the Gain of Photoreceptor Cells of the *Limulus* Lateral Eye. *Biol. Bull.*, 167: 532.

Robinson, P.R., Cohen, G.B., Zhukovsky, E.A. and Oprian, D.D. (1992) Constitutive activation of rhodopsin by mutation of LYS296. *Neuron*, 9: 719–725.

Roenneberg, T., Lotze, M. and vonSteinbüchel, N. (1992) Diurnal variation in human visual sensitivity dertemined by incremental thresholds. *Clin. Vis. Sci.*, 7: 83–91.

Rosenwasser, A.M., Raibert, M., Terman, J.S. and Terman, M. (1979) Circadian rhythm of luminance detectability in the rat. *Physiol. Behav.*, 23: 17–21.

Ruta, V.J., Dodge, F.A. and Barlow, R.B. (1999) Evaluation of circadian rhythms in the Limulus Eye. *Bio. Bull.*, 197: 233–234.

Sakmar, T.P., Franke, R.R. and Khorana, H.G. (1989) Glutamic acid-113 serves as the retinylidene Schiff base counterion in bovine rhodopsin. *Proc. Natl. Acad. Sci.*, 86: 8309–8313.

Schneider, M., Lehmen, H.K. and Barlow, R.B., Jr. (1987) Efferent Neurotransmitters Mediate Differential Effects in the *Limulus* Lateral Eye. *Invest. Ophthalmol. Vis. Sci.*, (Suppl. 28): 186.

Teirstein, P.S., Goldman, A.I. and O'Brien, P.J. (1980) Local and central regulation of ROS disc shedding. *Invest. Ophthalmol. Vis. Sci.*, 19: 1268–1273.

Thomas, K. and Iuvone, P.M. (1991) Circadian rhythm of tryptophan hydroxylase activity in chicken retina. *Cell. Mol. Neurobiol.*, 11(5): 511–527.

Tosini, G. and Menaker, M. (1996) Circadian rhythms in cultured mammalian retina. *Science*, 272: 419–421.

Uchiyama, H. (1989) Centrifugal pathways to the retina: Influence of the optic tectum. *Vis. Neurosci.*, 3: 183–206.

Uchiyama, H. and Barlow, R.B. (1994) Centrifugal inputs enhance responses of retinal ganglion cells in the Japanese quail without changing their spatial coding coding properties. *Vision Res.*, 34: 2189–2194.

Underwood, H., Siopes, T. and Barrett, R.K. (1988) Does a biological clock reside in the eye of quail? *J. Biol. Rhythms*, 3: 323–331.

Underwood, H., Barrett, R.K. and Siopes, T. (1990) Melatonin does not link the eyes to the rest of the circadian system in quail: A neural pathway is involved. *J. Biol. Rhythms*, 5: 349–361.

Van Cauter, E., Desir, D., Decoster, C., Fery, F. and Balasse, E.O. (1988) Nocturnal decrease in glucose tolerance during constant glucose infusion. *J. Clin. Endocrinol. Metab.*, 69: No. 3, 604–610.

VonSchantz, M., Lucas, R.J. and Foster, R.G. (1999) Circadian oscillation of photopigment transcript levels in the mouse retina. *Mol. Brain Res.*, 72: 108–114.

Wagner, H.-J., Behrens, U.D., Zaunreiter, M. and Douglas, R.H. (1992) The circadian component of spinule dynamics in teleost retinal horizontal cells is dependent on the dopaminergic system. *Vis. Neurosci.*, 9(3–4): 345–351.

Watson, A.B. and Pelli, D. (1983) A Bayesian adaptive psychometric method. *Percept. Psychophys.*, 33: 113–120.

Weiler, R., Kohler, K., Kirsch, M. and Wagner, H.-J. (1988) Glutamate and dopamine modulate synaptic plasticity in horizontal cell dendrites of fish retina. *Neurosci. Lett.*, 87: 205–209.

Winkler, B.S. (1981) Glycolytic and oxidative metabolism in relation to retinal function. *J. Gen. Physiol.*, 77: 667–692.

Wirz-Justice, A., DaPrada, M. and Reme, C. (1984) Circadian rhythm in rat retinal dopamine. *Neurosci. Lett.*, 45: 21–25.

Witkovsky, P., Stone, S. and Besharse, J.C. (1988) Dopamine modifies the balance of rod and cone inputs to horizontal cells of the *Xenopus* retina. *Brain Res.*, 449: 332–336.

Witkovsky, P. and Dearry, A. (1992) Functional roles of dopamine in the vertebrate retina. *Prog. Ret. Res.*, 11: 247–292.

Witkovsky, P., Nicholson, C., Rice, M., Bohmmaker, K. and Meller, E. (1993) Extracellular dopamine concentration in the retina of the clawed frog, *Xenopus laevis*. *Proc. Natl. Acad. Sci. USA*, 90: 5667–5671.

Wörgötter, F., Nelle, E., Li, B. and Funke, J. (1998) The influence of corticofugal feedback on the temporal structure of visual response of cat thalamic relay cells. *J. Physiol.*, 509: 797–815.

Wulle, I., Kirsch, M. and Wagner, H.-J. (1990) Cyclic changes in dopamine and DOPAC content, and tyrosine hydroxylase activity in the retina of a cichlid fish. *Brain Res.*, 515: 163–167.

Yang, X.-L. and Wu, S. (1989) Modulation of rod-cone coupling by light. *Science*, 224: 352–354.

Young, R.W. (1967) The renewal of photoreceptor cell outer segments. *J. Cell. Biol.*, 33: 61–72.

Young, R.W. (1978) The daily rhythm of shedding and degradation of rod and cone outer segment membranes in the chick retina. *Invest. Ophthalmol. Vis. Sci.*, 17: 105–116.

Zalutsky, R.A. and Miller, R.F. (1990) The physiology of somatostatin in the rabbit retina. *J. Neurosci.*, 10: 383–393.

Zawilska, J. (1994) The role of dopamine in the regulation of melatonin biosynthesis in vertebrate retina. *Acta Neurobiol. Exp.*, (Suppl. 54): 47–56.

Zawilska, J.B. and Iuvone, P.M. (1992) Melatonin synthesis in chicken retina: Effect of kainic acid-induced lesions on the diurnal rhythm D2 dopamine receptor-mediated regulation of serotonin *N*-acetyltransferase activity. *Neurosci. Lett.*, 135: 71–74.

Zucker, C.L. and Dowling, J.E. (1987) Centrifugal fibres synapses on dopamine interplexiform cells in the teleost retina. *Nature*, 300: 166–168.

H. Kolb, H. Ripps and S. Wu (Eds.)
Progress in Brain Research, Vol. 131

CHAPTER 36

Circadian clock regulation of neuronal light responses in the vertebrate retina

Stuart C. Mangel*

Department of Neurobiology, University of Alabama School of Medicine, CIRC 425, 1719 6th Avenue South, Birmingham, AL 35294, USA

Introduction

The retina is able to respond to visual images in starlight and in the midday sun, and at all times in between, during which changes in ambient illumination of approximately eight orders of magnitude can occur (Munz and MacFarland, 1977; Reme et al., 1991). In most vertebrate retinas, two types of photoreceptor cell, rods and cones, provide visual sensitivity throughout this range. Rods mediate vision in dim light, whereas cones operate in bright light and provide color vision and high visual acuity.

Since the pioneering work almost three decades ago that revealed the basic circuitry and light responses of neurons in the vertebrate retina (Dowling and Werblin, 1969; Werblin and Dowling, 1969; Kaneko, 1970), it has become apparent that the retina is a dynamic system in which the response properties of retinal neurons are influenced by a variety of adaptive mechanisms. These adaptive mechanisms enable the retina to respond to visual images both in starlight and in the midday sun. The plasticity of retinal light sensitivity derives from at least two kinds of adaptive mechanisms (Dowling and Ripps, 1970; Dowling, 1987). The first adaptive mechanism, photoreceptor adaptation, is determined by the relative degree of visual pigment bleaching or regeneration in photoreceptors (Dowling, 1963, 1987) and

by the regulatory role of Ca^{2+} in the phototransduction process (Lagnado and Baylor, 1992). The second adaptive mechanism, network or neural adaptation, is mediated by cellular and synaptic mechanisms of retinal networks or circuits (Dowling, 1987; Wu, 1991).

Research in John Dowling's laboratory has been focused for many years on understanding how light and dark adaptation alter the light responses of retinal neurons (Dowling, 1987, 1991). When I joined his lab as a postdoctoral fellow in 1981, much of the interest in network adaptation centered on the role of dopamine, a retinal neurotransmitter, in regulating adaptation in horizontal cells, a type of second order neuron in the retina that receives synaptic contacts from cone and/or rod photoreceptor cells. While in John's laboratory, I studied the effects of light and dark adaptation on fish horizontal cells, as well as the roles of glutamate and dopamine and their respective receptors in these adaptive phenomena (Ariel et al., 1984, 1986; Mangel and Dowling, 1985, 1987; Mangel et al., 1985, 1989).

As an independent investigator with my own laboratory at the University of Alabama at Birmingham, I have continued to study adaptive phenomena in the vertebrate retina. Although it has been clear for many years that neuronal light responses can be modulated by environmental factors (e.g. the level of ambient illumination), little was known until recently concerning how factors intrinsic

*E-mail: mangel@nrc.uab.edu

to the retina (e.g. a circadian oscillator or clock) modulate neuronal light responses. In the past few years, we have studied circadian clock regulation of the light responses of fish horizontal cells in my laboratory.

A circadian clock is a type of biological oscillator that has persistent rhythmicity with a period of approximately 24 h in the absence of external timing cues (e.g. constant darkness). In addition, a circadian clock can be entrained by cyclic environmental stimuli, such as light (Pittendrigh, 1981). It is now clear that vertebrate circadian oscillator systems are located in the retinas of amphibia (Besharse and Iuvone, 1983; Cahill and Besharse, 1993), mammals (Tosini and Menaker, 1996), and possibly birds (Underwood et al., 1990), in the pineal gland (Robertson and Takahashi, 1988), and in the suprachiasmatic nucleus (Welsh et al., 1995). In vertebrate retinas, a variety of cellular phenomena are regulated by a circadian clock, including melatonin production and release (Besharse and Iuvone, 1983; Tosini and Menaker, 1996), dopamine content and release (Wirz-Justice et al., 1984; Kolbinger et al., 1990), retinomotor movements (Burnside and Nagle, 1983), horizontal cell spinule formation (Wagner et al., 1992), opsin synthesis (Korenbrot and Fernald, 1989), gene transcription (Pierce et al., 1993; Green and Besharse, 1994), photoreceptor disk shedding (LaVail and Ward, 1978), and neuronal activity (Wang and Mangel, 1996). In addition, circadian and diurnal rhythms of visual sensitivity, as measured by psychophysical detectability and by the electroretinogram, have been found in many vertebrate species, including fish, rabbit and human (Brandenburg et al., 1983; Fowlkes et al., 1984; Terman and Terman, 1985; Bassi and Powers, 1986, 1987; Schaeffel et al., 1991; Li and Dowling, 1998; Manglapus et al., 1998).

The purpose of the present paper is to summarize recent work in my lab that has examined the effects of a circadian clock on the light responses of fish horizontal cells. I will show that a circadian clock regulates rod and cone input to fish cone horizontal cells, a type of horizontal cell in the goldfish retina that receives synaptic contact from cones, but not from rods. I will then show that the clock achieves its effects by raising dopamine levels in the day so that dopamine D2-like receptors are activated. Finally,

I will summarize other recent work in my lab which shows that a clock regulates the pH of the retina.

A circadian clock regulates the light responses of horizontal cells

A few years after I had set up my own laboratory at the University of Alabama at Birmingham, John asked me to join him at the Marine Biological Labs, Woods Hole, MA, to reinvestigate the role of dopamine in light and dark adaptation of fish horizontal cells. I was happy to do so, and we were joined by Reto Weiler and Bill Baldridge. We decided to begin by studying the effects of dark adaptation on horizontal cells. To our surprise we found that when the fish retina was strictly maintained in a dark-adapted state, the light responses of cone horizontal cells were dominated by rod input (Mangel et al., 1994).

When I returned to Birmingham, Yu Wang, a postdoctoral fellow in my lab, and I investigated this phenomenon further and discovered that the light responses of fish cone horizontal cells depend on the time of day. Specifically, we found that the light responses of goldfish retinal L-type cone horizontal cells exhibited a circadian rhythm when the fish were maintained in constant darkness (Fig. 1). During the subjective day, the responses were cone-mediated and similar to classic responses previously reported for these cells. In contrast, during the subjective night, the responses were rod-dominated. Compared to the day, the responses at night were slower, smaller in size, longer in duration, and response threshold was considerably lower (Wang and Mangel, 1996). Although the light responses of rod horizontal cells resembled those of cone horizontal cells at night with respect to threshold, waveform and kinetics, the responses of rod horizontal cells did not depend on the time of day (Wang and Mangel, 1996). Thus, although the clock regulates the light responses of cone horizontal cells, it may not affect rod horizontal cells.

The effects of the clock at night occurred in the presence of scotopic background illumination, but were not observed when the background illumination was in the photopic range. In fact, a dim light background in the scotopic range was continuously present for the cells shown in Fig. 1. In addition,

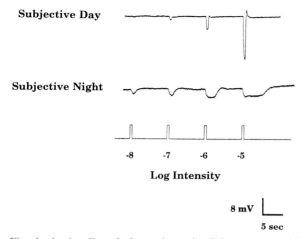

Subjective Day

Subjective Night

-8   -7   -6   -5

Log Intensity

8 mV

5 sec

Fig. 1. A circadian clock regulates the light responses of goldfish cone horizontal cells. Cone input to L-type cone horizontal cells predominates during the subjective day and rod input predominates during the subjective night. Compared to the day, the responses at night are slower, smaller in size, longer in duration, and response threshold is approximately a hundred times lower. Similar results were obtained from 43 other cells.

repeated flashes of a dim light in the scotopic to low mesopic range did not prevent the occurrence of the effects of the clock at night, nor did it produce light sensitization. In contrast, repetitive flashing of a light in the high mesopic to photopic range at night overrode the effects of the clock and produced light sensitization. That is, a rod-dominated response at night can be changed into a cone-dominated response by bright light stimulation (Wang and Mangel, 1996).

A circadian rhythm in cone input to cone horizontal cells is illustrated in Fig. 2a, which depicts average responses to a bright light stimulus ($-2 \log I_o$) as a function of time in the dark. Following constant darkness, average responses to a bright stimulus were greater during the subjective day (Zeitgeber time (ZT) 0–12, first and second cycles, where ZT 0 is dawn) than during the subjective night (ZT 12–24, first and second cycles). The presence of an endogenous circadian oscillator that regulates cone input to cone horizontal cells is also shown (Fig. 2b) in the

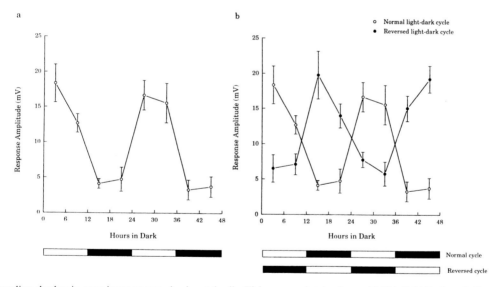

Fig. 2. Circadian rhythm in cone input to cone horizontal cells. Fish were maintained on a 12:12 h light/dark cycle for at least 14 days and then placed in the dark for 3–48 h. (a) Average responses to a bright stimulus ($-2 \log I_o$) as a function of time in the dark are greater during the subjective day than during the subjective night. (b) Following prior reversal of the light/dark cycle for at least 14 days, the circadian rhythm of responses to a bright stimulus ($-2 \log I_o$) was reversed. In parts a and b, the presence of a recording from a cone horizontal cell was confirmed following cell impalement by flashing a series of dim ($\leq -6 \log I_o$) lights. Following this, a single bright ($-2 \log I_o$) light was flashed. In parts a and b, data were averaged only from responses to this single bright light stimulus (one bright light stimulus/retina). In each case, a response to a single bright light stimulus ($-2 \log I_o$) was obtained at the circadian time indicated. Surgical isolation of the retina occurred approximately 2 h before this bright light response was recorded. The maximum, unattenuated intensity (I_o) of full field white light stimuli from a 100 W tungsten-halogen lamp was $1.0 \times 10^3 \ \mu W \ cm^{-2}$. Intensity values indicated in the text are relative to I_o. Each data point represents averages obtained from 6 to 21 cells (1 cell/retina). Reprinted with permission from *Proc. Natl. Acad. Sci. USA*.

508

reversal of the 24 h rhythm of cone horizontal cell light responses induced by prior reversal of the light–dark cycle. The ability to reverse a 24 h rhythm exhibited in constant darkness by prior reversal of the light–dark cycle not only demonstrates that the circadian clock can be entrained by light (Pittendrigh, 1981), but is also an essential manipulation to demonstrate circadian rhythmicity. This is because reversal of the rhythm by reversal of the light–dark cycle demonstrates that other diurnal environmental cues, such as diurnal changes in ambient temperature, are not responsible for the circadian rhythmicity. These results together thus demonstrate that a circadian clock regulates the responses of cone horizontal cells to bright light stimulation and indicate that cone input to cone horizontal cells is greatly reduced during the subjective night.

A circadian rhythm in rod and cone input to cone horizontal cells is shown in Fig. 3. Following one full cycle of constant darkness, average cone horizontal cell spectral sensitivity during the subjective night (ZT 15, second cycle) closely matched that of rod horizontal cells (and rods) for wavelengths ≤ 600 nm. In contrast, average cone horizontal cell spectral sensitivity during the subjective day (ZT 3, second cycle) was similar to that of red (625 nm) cones (Harosi and MacNichol, 1974), as was the spectral sensitivity of light-sensitized cone horizontal cells during the subjective night (data not shown). Interestingly, the greater relative spectral sensitivity of cone horizontal cells in the far red region of the spectrum during the subjective night, compared to rod horizontal cells, may indicate that cone horizontal cells still receive some input from red (625 nm) cones at night. The relative spectral sensitivity of rod horizontal cells closely resembled that of goldfish rods (cf. Schwanzara, 1967).

These findings indicate that a circadian clock regulates the light responses of goldfish cone horizontal cells. During the day, L-type cone horizontal cell light responses are driven primarily by red (625 nm) cones, but during the night, cone horizontal cell light responses are driven primarily by rods and light responsiveness to bright lights is greatly reduced. Because of the action of the circadian clock, cone input to cone horizontal cells predominates during the day and rod input predominates during the night. Therefore, under starlight conditions, rod input

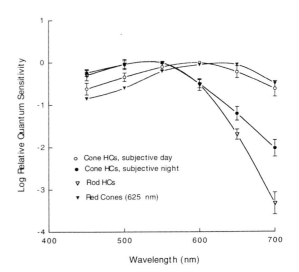

Fig. 3. Spectral sensitivity measurements demonstrate a circadian rhythm of rod and cone input to cone horizontal cells (HCs). Following one full cycle of constant darkness, average L-type cone horizontal cell spectral sensitivity during the subjective night (Zeitgeber (ZT) 15, where ZT 0 corresponds to dawn; second cycle) closely matched that of rod horizontal cells (and rods) for wavelengths ≤ 600 nm. In contrast, average L-type cone horizontal cell spectral sensitivity during the subjective day (ZT 3, second cycle) was similar to that of red (625 nm) cones. The relative spectral sensitivity of rod horizontal cells closely resembled that of goldfish rods. Each data point represents averages obtained from 6 to 12 cells (1 cell/retina). Reprinted with permission from *Proc. Natl. Acad. Sci. USA.*

to fish cone horizontal cells will predominate and cone input will be significantly reduced, but present.

The regulation of rod and cone input to fish cone horizontal cells may be a primary function of the retinal circadian clock. The data suggest that dark-adapted, cone-connected bipolar and ganglion cell surrounds in the fish will be rod-dominated at night due to action of the circadian clock, because horizontal cells contribute to bipolar and ganglion cell surrounds in the fish (Naka and Nye, 1971; Toyoda and Tonosaki, 1978). If a circadian clock in other vertebrates, such as mammals, also regulates rod and cone input to cone-connected horizontal cells, then one would expect dark-adapted ganglion cell surrounds at night to be rod-dominated in these species as well, since horizontal cells contribute to ganglion cell surrounds in mammals (Mangel, 1991). Interestingly, recent observations of cat ganglion cells indicate that dark-adapted surrounds are rod-dominated (Guenther and Zrenner, 1993). In fact, electroretinogram studies in the intact quail have also indicated that a clock regulates rod and cone pathways (Manglapus et al., 1998). Such a circadian clock-induced functional reorganization of neuronal receptive fields may underlie the circadian rhythm in visual sensitivity that has been seen in many vertebrates, including humans (Fowlkes et al., 1984; Bassi and Powers, 1986, 1987; Reme et al., 1991), especially if there is circadian clock control of bipolar and ganglion cell centers as well.

In summary, a circadian clock regulates the light responses of goldfish cone horizontal cells. Because of the action of the clock, cone input to cone horizontal cells predominates in the day and rod input predominates in the night. Circadian clock regulation of rod and cone pathways should enhance visual sensitivity at dusk and visual acuity at dawn, as well as enhance contrast sensitivity at night. The adaptational state of the retina is therefore not simply a reflection of environmental cues, such as the onset of day or night, or the level of ambient illumination, but is also regulated by a circadian clock.

The clock utilizes dopamine to regulate rod and cone inputs to cone horizontal cells

In addition to receiving synaptic input from cones, cone horizontal cells in the fish also receive synaptic contact from a dopaminergic neuron, the interplexiform cell (Dowling and Ehinger, 1978; Yazulla and Zucker, 1988). Because (1) retinal dopamine levels in a number of species, including fish, are higher in the day, than in the night (Wirz-Justice et al., 1984; Kolbinger et al., 1990); and (2) dopamine modulates rod and cone input to horizontal cells (Witkovsky et al., 1988), Yu Wang and I investigated whether the clock regulates rod and cone input to fish cone horizontal cells through dopamine pathways.

Superfusion of dopamine (1–5000 nM) during the subjective night increased cone input and eliminated rod input to the cells (Fig. 4a), a state typically observed during the subjective day. In contrast, dopamine application during the subjective day had no effect (1–10 nM) or increased (100–5000 nM) responses slightly (Fig. 4b). Destruction of dopaminergic cells following 6-hydroxydopamine (6-OHDA)

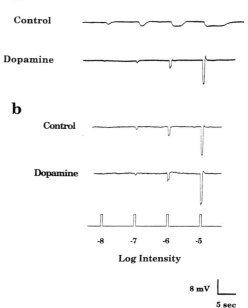

Fig. 4. Exogenous dopamine application increases cone input and decreases rod input to goldfish retinal L-type cone horizontal cells. (a) Superfusion of dopamine (100 nM) during the subjective night increased cone input and eliminated rod input to the cells, so that light responses closely resembled those typically observed during the day. (b) Superfusion of dopamine (100 nM) during the subjective day produced a slight increase in the size of the light responses. Similar results were obtained from 9 (a) and 8 (b) cells. Subjective day data in this figure were obtained under conditions of constant darkness during the second cycle at ZT3. Subjective night data were obtained at ZT15.

pretreatment increased rod input and decreased cone input during the subjective day and had no effect during the subjective night. Prior injection of saline as a control had no effect on the light responses of horizontal cells in the day or night (data not shown). These results strongly suggest that the clock increases endogenous dopamine levels in the day, compared to the night.

Extensive studies in my lab have also characterized the type of dopamine receptor and second messenger pathway activated by the clock (Mangel and Wang, 1996). As summarized in Fig. 5, the increased level of endogenous dopamine during the day activates D2-like, and not D1-like, receptors. For example,

DAY:

Clock → ↑ DA → ↑ D2 Receptor → ↓ cAMP → ↓ PKA → ↓ Rod-Cone → Cone Input
                Activation   Gap Junctional Predominates
                                                         Conductivity

NIGHT:

Clock → ↓ DA → ↓ D2 Receptor → ↑ cAMP → ↑ PKA → ↑ Rod-Cone → Rod Input
                Activation   Gap Junctional Predominates
                                                         Conductivity

Fig. 5. Proposed circadian clock pathway in the fish retina. The clock raises dopamine (DA) levels in the day so that D2-like receptors on photoreceptor cells are activated. This in turn lowers intracellular cAMP levels and protein kinase A (PKA) activation in photoreceptors, decreasing the conductance between rod–cone gap junctions so that cone input dominates cone horizontal cells. At night, rod input dominates cone horizontal cells, because the clock has lowered dopamine levels below the threshold of activation of the D2-like receptors. As a result, intracellular cAMP levels and PKA activation in photoreceptors increase, raising the conductance between rod–cone gap junctions. See the text for details.

application of quinpirole, a D2-like receptor agonist, during the subjective night increased cone input and eliminated rod input to the cells, an effect similar to that of dopamine. In contrast, application of spiperone, a general D2-like receptor antagonist, during the subjective day reduced cone input and introduced rod input. SCH23390, a D1 antagonist, had no effect during the subjective day. Application of spiperone alone or in conjunction with SCH23390 during the subjective night had no effect on the light responses, indicating that the level of endogenous dopamine at night was below the threshold of dopamine receptor activation.

Dose-response data for dopamine in the day and night obtained in my lab (Mangel and Wang, 1996) further suggest that dopamine has little or no effect on the amplitude of light responses during the day, because endogenous dopamine is already bound to its receptors. In contrast, at night the level of endogenous dopamine is below the threshold of dopamine receptor activation, as indicated by the lack of effect of the D2-like antagonist, spiperone, at night. Specifically, the dose-response data suggest that the circadian-induced dopamine concentration in the outer retina is approximately 20 nM during the day and less than 0.5 nM during the night. In addition, the fact that exogenous dopamine at very low concentrations (1–5 nM) can affect horizontal cells at night, but not in the day, strongly suggests that the

results cannot be explained by a hyperactive dopamine transporter at night.

The decreased activation of D2-like receptors during the night, which increases the level of cAMP and the activation of protein kinase A, enhances rod input and decreases cone input to cone horizontal cells (Mangel and Wang, 1996). For example, experiments in my lab have shown that application of forskolin, an activator of adenylate cyclase, during the subjective day reduced cone input and introduced rod input to cone horizontal cells. In contrast, application of Rp-CAMPS, an inhibitor of cAMP-dependent protein kinase, during the subjective night, or octanol, an alcohol that uncouples gap junctions, increased cone input and decreased rod input.

These findings thus suggest that dopamine acts as a circadian clock signal for the day by increasing cone input and decreasing rod input to fish cone horizontal cells. During the day, an increased level of dopamine activates D2-like receptors, but during the night, dopamine levels are too low to activate the receptors. Activation of D2-like receptors during the day decreases rod input and increases cone input to cone horizontal cells via decreases in intracellular cyclic AMP and protein kinase A activation (see Fig. 5). Moreover, it is likely that the D2-like receptors that are involved with this circadian phenomenon are located on photoreceptor cells, because D2-like receptors are found on photoreceptors, and not on horizontal cells (Dearry and Burnside, 1986; Harsanyi and Mangel, 1992; Cohen et al., 1992; Rashid et al., 1993; Yazulla and Lin, 1995; Wang et al., 1997). Moreover, the effects of exogenous dopamine and quinpirole persist following destruction of dopaminergic cells with 6-OHDA (Mangel and Wang, 1996). The clock thus regulates rod and cone input to cone horizontal cells by activating postsynaptic D2-like receptors on photoreceptor cells and not by activating D2 autoreceptors on dopaminergic cells (Harsanyi and Mangel, 1992; Rashid et al., 1993; Yazulla and Lin, 1995; Wang et al., 1997). It has also been reported that circadian clock regulation of the amplitude of the electroretinogram in the quail retina is mediated by activation of D2 receptors (Manglapus et al., 1999).

The release of dopamine depends on distinct circadian and light adaptive processes. The circadian clock, which is likely intrinsic to the retina itself (Besharse and Iuvone, 1983; Underwood et al., 1990; Cahill and Besharse, 1993; Tosini and Menaker, 1996), modulates the dopamine concentration in the fish outer retina from less than 0.5 nM during the night to approximately 20 nM in the day, as noted above. Flickering and sustained light stimuli in the photopic range may then further increase dopamine concentration during the day to the high nanomolar/low micromolar level (Kirsch and Wagner, 1989; Harsanyi and Mangel, 1992; Witkovsky et al., 1993; Harsanyi et al., 1996; Weiler et al., 1997). It is at this higher dopamine level (high nanomolar/low micromolar) that D1 receptors are activated. In the vertebrate retina (Harsanyi and Mangel, 1992; Wang and Mangel, 2001), as in other intact neural tissue (Kebabian and Calne 1979; Civelli et al., 1993; Missale et al., 1998), D1 receptors are two to three orders of magnitude less sensitive to dopamine than D2 receptors.

The effects of dopamine that are reported here were observed in retinas kept in constant darkness, that is, no light stimuli were flashed before horizontal cell impalement. It has recently been reported that dark-adapted retinas possess a high degree of sensitivity to light stimuli in the low photopic range and brighter (Morgan and Boelen, 1996; Wang and Mangel, 1996). In fact, we have found that a single flash of light at night brighter than -4.5 log I_o

(i.e. low photopic range) can significantly increase fish cone horizontal cell response size, as well as eliminate rod input to the cells.

Earlier studies (Mangel and Dowling, 1985, 1987; Yang et al., 1988), which had reported that dopamine release was higher in the dark than in the light, were performed before it was known that dark-adapted retinas were highly sensitive to stimuli in the photopic range or that the actions and release of dopamine are dependent on the time of day. It thus seems likely that the discrepancy between these earlier findings and those reported here may be due to the fact that the retinas in the earlier studies were light-sensitized, because occasional flashes of light in the photopic range were used to facilitate cell impalement. Thus, the apparent discrepancy between the present work and these earlier studies may be explained by differences in the level of adaptation.

A complete description of the processes that result from the actions of dopamine and lead to the modulation of rod and cone input to cone horizontal cells is not yet available. When dopamine levels are low at night, it is unclear how rod input reaches cone horizontal cells or how the efficacy of cone input to the cells decreases. However, the following scenario can account for our findings in part (Fig. 5). Because (1) goldfish cone horizontal cells receive synaptic contact from cones and not from rods (Stell, 1967); and (2) rod–cone gap junctions are present in numerous vertebrates (Raviola and Gilula, 1973), including fish (Witkovsky et al., 1974), it is possible that dopamine mediates circadian clock regulation of rod and cone input to cone horizontal cells by modulating rod–cone coupling. Specifically, the clock increases dopamine levels during the day so that D2-like receptors on photoreceptor cells are activated. This in turn decreases rod–cone coupling via decreases in cyclic AMP and protein kinase A activation. Thus, it is possible that rod input reaches cone horizontal cells at night because of a circadian clock-induced decrease in dopamine concentration that increases the conductivity of rod–cone gap junctions. The finding that octanol, an alcohol that uncouples gap junctions, acts like dopamine (Mangel and Wang, 1996) supports this suggestion. In addition, the finding that octanol increases cone input to cone horizontal cells, in addition to decreasing rod input, supports the previous suggestion (Mangel et al., 1994) that cone-mediated signals are shunted at cone pedicles at night when rod–cone coupling is high, because rods outnumber cones in the goldfish retina by an average of about 12 fold (Stell and Harosi, 1976). It should be noted that there is precedence to suggest that cAMP increases the coupling between rods and cones at night. Although the gap junctions between retinal horizontal cells are uncoupled by cAMP (Lasater, 1987; DeVries and Schwartz, 1989), gap junctional coupling is enhanced by cAMP in liver, heart and other systems (Dermietzel and Spray, 1993), presumably due to differences in connexin type in horizontal cells, compared to liver and heart.

It is important to note that circadian and light-adaptive phenomena are different and may utilize different mechanisms. Although it has been reported that light adaptation during the day increases the conductivity of rod–cone gap junctions (Yang and Wu, 1989) through activation of dopamine D2-like receptors (Krizaj et al., 1998), it is possible that the clock, in contrast to light stimulation, increases the conductivity of rod–cone gap junctions at night. In fact, as shown in Fig. 1 of Wang and Mangel (1996) and elsewhere (Witkovsky et al., 1988; Yang and Wu, 1989), bright light stimulation of dark-adapted, but not light-adapted, retinas produces rod-mediated responses in horizontal cells during the day. In contrast, the clock produces rod-mediated responses in fish horizontal cells to dim, but not to bright, light at night. It is thus likely that the underlying dopamine-mediated circadian and light-evoked processes are different. In fact, the effects of exogenous dopamine application in the fish retina clearly depend on both the state of adaptation and the time of day. That is, dopamine reduces cone input to fish cone horizontal cells when applied to light-adapted retinas in the day (Mangel and Dowling, 1985, 1987; Harsanyi and Mangel, 1992; Wang et al., 1997), but as shown here (Fig. 4), dopamine increases cone input to cone horizontal cells when applied to dark-adapted retinas at night, and has little or no effect, when applied to dark-adapted retinas in the day. These differences suggest that the effects of dopamine on cone horizontal cells are modulated by some other factor(s) and that day and night retinas are profoundly different neural tissues.

A second, but not necessarily mutually-exclusive explanation for the day–night actions of dopamine must first hypothesize that rods make direct synaptic contacts onto cone horizontal cells in the goldfish retina that have yet to be observed. According to this view, a circadian-induced increase in dopamine levels during the day would somehow suppress rod to cone horizontal cell transmission (Akopian and Witkovsky, 1996) and augment cone to cone horizontal cell transmission. However, the means by which D2 receptor activation would augment a cone pathway while simultaneously suppressing a rod pathway is presently not clear.

Light-sensitization of fish cone horizontal cell light responses (Fig. 1 in Wang and Mangel, 1996) and the effects of dopamine on cone horizontal cell light responses (Fig. 4 here) can occur during the night about 10 times faster than retinomotor movements (Burnside and Nagle, 1983) or horizontal cell spinule formation (Douglas and Wagner, 1983). Thus, dopamine-mediated transmission from cones to cone horizontal cells can occur even when cones are elongated and horizontal cell spinules are relatively sparse. This suggests that retinomotor movements and horizontal cell spinule formation and dissolution do not themselves underlie the circadian clock effects of dopamine on transmission from rods and cones to cone horizontal cells.

Our findings demonstrate at the single cell level that a circadian clock utilizes dopamine to modulate neuronal activity and connections in the vertebrate retina. It is possible that similar circadian effects occur in other regions of the central nervous system, such as the basal ganglia, limbic system, and suprachiasmatic nucleus (Viswanathan et al., 1994; Missale et al., 1998), where dopamine functions as a transmitter. Disruptions in circadian clock pathways and in the circadian regulation of dopamine action may contribute in part to diurnal aspects of Parkinson's disease, schizophrenia, and seasonal affective disorder.

A circadian clock regulates extracellular pH in the fish retina

Although it is generally accepted that the acid-base ratio of tissue, as represented by the pH, is strictly regulated to maintain normal function, recent studies in the nervous system have shown that neuronal activity can result in significant shifts in pH (Chesler and Kaila, 1992). Because many retinal phenomena, including neuronal activity (Wang and Mangel, 1996), are regulated by a circadian clock, Andrey Dmitriev, a postdoctoral fellow in my lab, and I investigated whether a circadian clock regulates the pH of the retina. We measured the pH_o of the goldfish retina in the subjective day and night, using H^+-selective microelectrodes (Dmitriev and Mangel, 2000). The electrodes were placed in the Ringer above the retina and moved toward the tissue in 100 μm steps. A clear pH gradient was always recorded in the solution above the retina (Fig. 6a). The pH always reached a minimum value when the electrode reached the retina.

Retinal pH_o was lower than Ringer pH (7.60) in both the subjective day and night, but lowest during the subjective night. During the subjective day, the average difference between the retinal pH_o and the Ringer pH was 0.21 ± 0.01 (SEM) ($n = 34$), whereas during the subjective night the average difference between the retinal pH_o and the Ringer pH was 0.31 ± 0.01 ($n = 34$; $p < 0.01$). This day (7.39)/night (7.29) pH difference indicates that the retina produces more acid at night than in the day, that is, the mass metabolic activity of the retina is higher during the night.

The difference between retinal pH_o and Ringer pH exhibited a circadian rhythm for more than two full circadian cycles (Fig. 6b). The difference between retinal pH_o and Ringer pH was greater during the subjective night (ZT15 and 21), than during the subjective day (ZT3 and 9). In addition, the day–night difference between retinal pH_o and Ringer pH could be entrained by altering the previous light–dark cycle. The data shown (Fig. 6b) were obtained from animals maintained for two weeks in a visual environment phase-advanced by 6 h.

The circadian rhythm in retinal pH_o was independent of the Ringer pH. When Ringer pH was 7.60 (Fig. 6), the pH gradient at night was 36% greater than the pH gradient during the day, and when Ringer pH was set at 7.30 by increasing the proportion of CO_2 in the O_2/CO_2 gas mixture, the pH gradient at night was 36% greater than the pH gradient during the day.

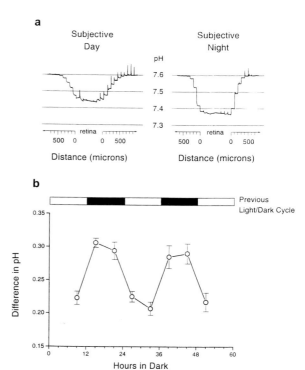

Fig. 6. (a) A circadian clock regulates the extracellular pH of the fish retina. Extracellular pH (pH_o) as a function of distance (μm) from a superfused goldfish retina in the subjective day and night. pH-sensitive microelectrodes were advanced through the Ringer to the retina, then through the retina, and finally withdrawn. Retinal pH_o was always lower than Ringer pH and the difference between retinal and Ringer pH was larger in the subjective night, than in the subjective day. The electrodes were moved in 100 μm steps every 30 s. Fast "spikes" on the records are movement artifacts. (b) The average difference between retinal and Ringer pH exhibits a circadian rhythm. Before the fish were maintained in constant darkness, they were entrained to a 12 h light/12 h dark cycle for at least 14 days. The light/dark cycle is indicated at the top of the figure. Retinae were prepared in either the subjective day or night. The time of subjective day or night indicated corresponds to the time that pH measurements were made. Each data point represents mean value ± SEM for 7–12 measurements. Modified from Dmitriev and Mangel (2000).

The magnitude of the circadian-induced change in retinal pH_o is large enough to influence synaptic transmission between retinal neurons. A decrease in Ringer pH from 7.6 to 7.4, which will reduce retinal pH_o by approximately 0.1 pH units, reduces the size of cone horizontal cell light responses by about 50% (Fig. 4 of Harsanyi and Mangel, 1993; Dmitriev and Mangel, 2000).

Although light stimulation modulates retinal pH_o, as mentioned previously, circadian-induced changes in retinal pH_o are several times greater than light-induced changes. The amplitude of the light-induced pH changes in the isolated goldfish retina was dependent on retinal depth and was largest in the most distal portion of the retina, namely, the subretinal space, the extracellular space surrounding the photoreceptors. However, in no case did light stimulation increase retinal pH_o by more than 0.02 pH units. These results thus indicate that circadian clock regulation of the metabolic activity of the retina, as represented by retinal pH_o, is several times greater than light–dark-induced changes.

The findings indicate that a circadian clock regulates the pH of the fish retina so that retinal pH_o is lower in the night, compared to the day. The clock-induced shift in pH is several times greater than light-induced pH changes and large enough to influence synaptic transmission between cones and cone horizontal cells, the first synapse of the retina. These results are the first demonstration that pH_o in the central nervous system can be modulated by a circadian clock, an endogenous neural process.

The finding that the clock decreases retinal pH_o at night suggests that the clock increases the production of acid in the retina at night in a sustained manner over the course of many hours. Such a sustained increase in acid production at night is most likely due to an increase in energetic metabolism at night and in fact, an increase in lactic acid at night has been demonstrated recently (Dmitriev et al., 1999). Moreover, a sustained increase in acid production requires an intracellular source, suggesting that there is one or more type of neuron in the retina that produces more acid at night. A change in acid-base transport, for example, can probably not account for a sustained decrease in pH_o, because such a change would result in substantial depletion of intracellular acid, leading to neuronal dysfunction. In contrast, light-evoked changes in pH_o, which are smaller in size and more transient, and often of mixed polarity (Oakley and Wen, 1989; Borgula et al., 1989; Yamamoto et al., 1992; Dmitriev and Mangel, 2000), might be due to changes in acid-base transport or carbonic anhydrase activity.

Although the clock-induced decrease in retinal pH at night likely reflects a clock-induced increase in retinal metabolic activity (Dmitriev et al., 1999), the processes whereby the clock affects pH and metabolic activity are not known. The decrease in pH and the increase in metabolic activity at night may be due to clock-induced ionic conductance changes and/or to clock-induced changes in acid-base transport that result from the action of neurotransmitters such as melatonin (Cassone et al., 1988; Cosci et al., 1997) and dopamine (Shulman and Fox, 1996). Alternatively, the clock may be directly increasing the activity of specific enzymes in retinal metabolic pathways at night.

A circadian clock-induced increase in the concentration of protons during the night may serve as a clock signal for the night. Recent work has shown that a circadian clock regulates the light responses of goldfish cone horizontal cells (see above; Wang and Mangel, 1996). Due to the action of the clock, the responses are cone-mediated during the day and rod-mediated, slower, and smaller in size during the night. A decrease in Ringer pH from 7.6 to 7.4, which reduces retinal pH_o by approximately 0.1 pH units, an amount comparable to the extent of circadian regulation, reduces the size of fish cone horizontal cell light responses by about 50% (Dmitriev and Mangel, 2000; Harsanyi and Mangel, 1993). A decrease in retinal pH_o may reduce cone horizontal cell light responses by decreasing transmitter release from cones (Barnes et al., 1993). Thus, the clock-induced decrease in retinal pH_o during the night may contribute to the suppression of cone horizontal cell light responses observed during the night. Circadian clock regulation of the pH and metabolic activity of the retina may therefore modulate synaptic transmission in the retina. The clock-induced decrease in retinal pH_o during the night may also increase rod photoreceptor sensitivity by stabilizing rhodopsin (Barlow et al., 1993). Studies which have used 2-deoxyglucose to measure metabolic activity have indicated that a circadian clock also regulates metabolic activity in the suprachiasmatic nucleus (Schwartz and Gainer, 1977). Thus, it is possible that circadian clock regulation of pH and metabolic activity is a general property of neural circadian clock tissue.

In summary, a circadian clock regulates the extracellular pH of the fish retina so that the pH is lower at night than in the day. The clock-induced shift in pH is several times greater than light-induced pH changes and large enough to influence synaptic transmission between retinal neurons. Thus, an intrinsic oscillator in neural tissue may modulate metabolic activity and pH as part of normal daily function.

Conclusions and future perspectives

Retinal neurons are affected by an endogenous circadian clock, as well as by light. Our experiments on fish cone horizontal cells indicate that a circadian clock increases the extent of rod pathways at night and increases the extent of cone pathways during the day. The clock uses specific diffusible factors, such as dopamine and protons, to regulate rod and cone pathways. The clock activates specific dopamine D2-like receptors during the day by increasing endogenous dopamine levels. Activation of D2-like receptors increases cone pathway function via a decrease in intracellular cAMP in photoreceptor cells. The clock also increases the metabolic activity of the retina at night, as revealed by a decrease in retinal pH and an increase in lactic acid at night. The decrease in pH at night may then decrease synaptic transmission from cones to cone horizontal cells.

Circadian clock regulation of rod and cone pathways should enhance visual sensitivity at dusk and visual acuity at dawn. In addition, rod access to cone pathways at night might enhance contrast sensitivity at night. The adaptational state of the retina therefore is not simply a reflection of environmental cues, such as the onset of day or night or the magnitude of ambient illumination, but is also regulated by an endogenous circadian clock. Future studies, which examine clock effects on other retinal neurons, such as ganglion cells, or clock effects on visual sensitivity (e.g. Li and Dowling, 1998), should be able to elucidate more completely how the circadian clock in the retina affects retinal function.

Because neurons in the retina and in other brain regions share common cellular and molecular mechanisms, our research can provide insights not only into how the retina functions, but also into how other neurons function and adapt. In addition, because disruption of circadian clock processes and light–dark-adaptive mechanisms may mediate photoreceptor cell degeneration, our research will likely increase understanding of retinal disease states, as well as of normal retinal function.

Acknowledgments

Supported in part by grants to S.C.M. from the National Institutes of Health (EY05102), the National Science Foundation (IBN-9819981), and the Plum Foundation, and by a National Eye Institute CORE Grant (P30 EY03039) to the University of Alabama at Birmingham.

References

Akopian, A. and Witkovsky, P. (1996) D2 dopamine receptor-mediated inhibition of a hyperpolarization-activated current in rod photoreceptors. J. Neurophysiol., 76: 1828–1835.

Ariel, M., Lasater, E.M., Mangel, S.C. and Dowling (1984) On the sensitivity of H1 horizontal cells of the carp retina to glutamate, aspartate and their agonists. Brain Res., 295: 179–183.

Ariel, M., Mangel, S.C. and Dowling, J.E. (1986) N-methyl-D-aspartate acts as an antagonist of the photoreceptor transmitter in the carp retina. Brain Res., 372: 143–148.

Barlow, R.B., Birge, R.R., Kaplan, E. and Tallent, J.R. (1993) On the molecular origin of photoreceptor noise. Nature, 366: 64–66.

Barnes, S., Merchant, V. and Mahmud, F. (1993) Modulation of transmission gain by protons at the photoreceptor output synapse. Proc. Natl. Acad. Sci. USA, 90: 10081–10085.

Bassi, C.J. and Powers, M.K. (1986) Daily fluctuations in the detectability of dim lights by humans. Physiol. Behav., 38: 871–877.

Bassi, C.J. and Powers, M.K. (1987) Circadian rhythm in goldfish visual sensitivity. Invest Ophthalmol. Vis. Sci., 28: 1811–1815.

Besharse, J.C. and Iuvone, P.M. (1983) Circadian clock in Xenopus eye controlling retinal serotonin N-acetyltransferase. Nature, 305: 133–135.

Borgula, G.A., Karwoski, C.J. and Steinberg, R.H. (1989) Light-evoked changes in extracellular pH in frog retina. Vision Res., 29: 1069–1077.

Brandenburg, J., Bobbert, A.C. and Eggelmeijer, F. (1983) Circadian changes in the response of the rabbit's retina to flashes. Behav. Brain Res., 7: 113–123.

Burnside, B. and Nagle, B. (1983) Retinomotor movements of photoreceptors and retinal pigment epithelium: mechanisms and regulation. Prog. Retinal Res., 2: 67–109.

516

Cahill, G.M. and Besharse, J.C. (1993) Circadian clock functions localized in *Xenopus* retinal photoreceptors. *Neuron*, 10: 573–577.

Cassone, V.M., Roberts, M.H. and Moore, R.Y. (1988) Effects of melatonin on 2-deoxy-14C-glucose uptake within rat suprachiasmatic nucleus. *Am. J. Physiol.*, 255: R332–R337.

Chesler, M. and Kaila, K. (1992) Modulation of pH by neuronal activity. *Trends Neurosci.*, 15: 396–402.

Civelli, O., Bunzow, J.R. and Grandy, D.K. (1993) Molecular diversity of the dopamine receptors. *Ann. Rev. Pharmacol. Toxicol.*, 32: 281–307.

Cohen, A.I., Todd, R.D., Harmon, S. and O'malley, K.L. (1992) Photoreceptors of mouse retinas possess D4 receptors coupled to adenylate cyclase. *Proc. Natl. Acad. Sci. USA*, 89: 12093–12097.

Cosci, B., Longoni, B. and Marchiafava, P.L. (1997) Melatonin induces membrane conductance changes in isolated retinal rod receptor cells. *Life Sci.*, 60: 1885–1889.

Dearry, A. and Burnside, B. (1986) Dopaminergic regulation of cone retinomotor movement in isolated teleost retinas. I. Induction of cone contraction is mediated by D2 receptors. *J. Neurochem.*, 46: 1006–1031.

Dermietzel, R. and Spray, D.C. (1993) Gap junctions in the brain: where, what type, how many and why? *Trends Neurosci.*, 16: 186–192.

De Vries, S.H. and Schwartz, E.A. (1989) Modulation of an electrical synapse between solitary pairs of catfish horizontal cells by dopamine and second messengers. *J. Physiol.*, 414: 351–375.

Dmitriev, A.V. and Mangel, S.C. (2000) A circadian clock regulates the pH of the fish retina. *J. Physiol.*, 522: 77–82.

Dmitriev, A.V., Nagy, T.R. and Mangel, S.C. (1999) A circadian clock regulates the metabolic activity of the fish retina. *Invest. Ophthalmol. Vis. Sci.*, (Suppl. 40): S611.

Douglas, R.H., Wagner, H.-J. (1983) Endogenous control of spinule formation in horizontal cells of the teleost retina. *Cell Tissue Res.*, 229: 443–449.

Dowling, J.E. (1963) Neural and photochemical mechanisms of visual adaptation in the rat. *J. Gen. Physiol.*, 46: 459–474.

Dowling, J.E. (1987) *The Retina: an Approachable Part of the Brain*. Harvard University Press, Cambridge, MA.

Dowling, J.E. (1991) Retinal neuromodulation: the role of dopamine. *Vis. Neurosci.*, 7: 87–97.

Dowling, J.E. and Ehinger, B. (1978) The interplexiform cell system. I. Synapses of the dopaminergic neurons of the goldfish retina. *Proc. R. Soc. Lond. B*, 201: 7–26.

Dowling, J.E. and Ripps, H. (1970) Visual adaptation in the retina of the skate. *J. Gen. Physiol.*, 56: 491–520.

Dowling, J.E. and Werblin, F.S. (1969) Organization of retina of the mudpuppy, Necturus maculosus. I. Synaptic structure. *J. Neurophysiol.*, 32: 315–338.

Fowlkes, D.H., Karowski, C.J. and Proenza, L.M. (1984) Endogenous circadian rhythm in electroretinogram of free-moving lizards. *Invest. Ophthalmol. Vis. Sci.*, 25: 229–232.

Green, C.B. and Besharse, J.C. (1994) Tryptophan hydroxylase expression is regulated by a circadian clock in *Xenopus laevis* retina. *J. Neurochem.*, 62: 2420–2428.

Guenther, E. and Zrenner, E. (1993) The spectral sensitivity of dark- and light-adapted cat retinal ganglion cells. *J. Neurosci.*, 13: 1543–1550.

Harosi, F.I. and Macnichol, E.F. (1974) Visual pigments of goldfish cones. *J. Gen. Physiol.*, 63: 279–304.

Harsanyi, K. and Mangel, S.C. (1992) Activation of dopamine D2 receptors increases the electrical coupling between fish horizontal cells by inhibiting dopamine release. *Proc. Natl. Acad. Sci. USA*, 89: 9220–9224.

Harsanyi, K. and Mangel, S.C. (1993) Modulation of cone to horizontal cell transmission by calcium and pH in the fish retina. *Vis. Neurosci.*, 10: 81–91.

Harsanyi, K., Wang, Y. and Mangel, S.C. (1996) Activation of NMDA receptors produces dopamine-mediated changes in fish retinal horizontal cell light responses. *J. Neurophysiol.*, 75: 629–639.

Kaneko, A. (1970) Physiological and morphological identification of horizontal, bipolar and amacrine cells in goldfish retina. *J. Physiol. (Lond.)*, 207: 623–633.

Kebabian, J.W. and Calne, D.B. (1979) Multiple receptors for dopamine. *Nature*, 277: 93–96.

Kirsch, M. and Wagner, H.-J. (1989) Release pattern of endogenous dopamine in teleost retinae during light adaptation and pharmacological stimulation. *Vision Res.* 29: 147–154.

Kolbinger, W., Kohler, K., Oetting, H. and Weiler, R. (1990) Endogenous dopamine and cyclic events in the fish retina, 1: HPLC assay of total content, release, and metabolic turnover during different light/dark cycles. *Vis. Neurosci.*, 5: 143–149.

Korenbrot, J.I. and Fernald, R.D. (1989) Circadian rhythm and light regulate opsin mRNA in rod photoreceptors. *Nature*, 337, 454–457.

Krizaj, D., Gabriel, R., Owen, W.G. and Witkovsky, P. (1998) Dopamine D2 receptor-mediated modulation of rod–cone coupling in the Xenopus retina. *J. Comp. Neurol.*, 398: 529–538.

Lagnado, L. and Baylor, D. (1992) Signal flow in visual transduction. *Neuron*, 8: 995–1002.

Lasater, E.M. (1987) Retinal horizontal cell gap junctional conductance is modulated by dopamine through a cyclic AMP-dependent protein kinase. *Proc. Natl. Acad. Sci. USA*, 84: 7319–7323.

Lavail, M.M. and Ward, P.A. (1978) Studies on the hormonal control of circadian outer segment disc shedding in the rat retina. *Invest. Ophthalmol.*, 17: 1189–1193.

Li, L. and Dowling, J.E. (1998) Zebrafish visual sensitivity is regulated by a circadian clock. *Vis. Neurosci.*, 15: 851–857.

Mangel, S.C. (1991) Analysis of the horizontal cell contribution to the receptive field surround of ganglion cells in the rabbit retina. *J. Physiol.*, 442, 211–234.

Mangel, S.C. (1999) Activation of adenosine A2a receptors mediates circadian clock regulation of rod and cone input to fish cone horizontal cells. *Invest. Ophthalmol. Vis. Sci.*, (Suppl. 40): S386.

Mangel, S.C., Ariel, M. and Dowling, J.E. (1985) Effects of acidic amino acid antagonists upon the spectral responses of carp horizontal cells: circuitry of the outer retina. *J. Neurosci.*, 5: 2839–2850.

Mangel, S.C., Ariel, M. and Dowling, J.E. (1989) D-aspartate potentiates the effects of both L-aspartate and L-glutamate on horizontal cells in the carp retina. *Neuroscience*, 32: 19–26.

Mangel, S.C., Baldridge, W.H., Weiler, R. and Dowling, J.E. (1994) Threshold and chromatic sensitivity changes in fish cone horizontal cells following prolonged darkness. *Brain Res.*, 659: 55–61.

Mangel, S.C. and Dowling, J.E. (1985) Responsiveness and receptive field size of carp horizontal cells are reduced by prolonged darkness and dopamine. *Science*, 229: 1107–1109.

Mangel, S.C. and Dowling, J.E. (1987) The interplexiform-horizontal cell system of the fish retina: effects of dopamine, light stimulation and time in the dark. *Proc. Roy. Soc. Lond. B*, 231: 91–121.

Mangel, S.C. and Wang, Y. (1996) Circadian clock regulation of rod and cone pathways in the vertebrate retina. *Invest. Ophthalmol. Vis. Sci.*, Suppl. 37: S17.

Manglapus, M.K., Uchiyama, H., Buelow, N.F. and Barlow, R.B. (1998) Circadian rhythms of rod–cone dominance in the Japanese quail retina. *J. Neurosci.*, 18, 4775–4784.

Manglapus, M.K., Iuvone, P.M., Underwood, H., Pierce, M.E. and Barlow, R.B. (1999) Dopamine mediates circadian rhythms of rod–cone dominance in the Japanese quail retina. *J. Neurosci.*, 19: 4132–4141.

Missale, C., Nash, S.R., Robinson, S.W., Jaber, M. and Caron, M.G. (1998) Dopamine receptors: From structure to function. *Physiol. Rev.*, 78: 189–225.

Morgan, I.G. and Boelen, M.K. (1996) A retinal dark-light switch: a review of the evidence. *Vis. Neurosci.*, 13: 399–409.

Munz, F.W. and Macfarland, W.N. (1977) Evolutionary adaptations of fishes to the photic environment. In: Crescitelli, F. (Ed.), *Handbook of Sensory Physiology. The Visual System in Vertebrates*. Springer-Verlag, Berlin, pp. 193–274.

Naka, K.-I. and Nye, P.W. (1971) Role of horizontal cells in organization of the catfish retina receptive field. *J. Neurophysiol.*, 34: 785–801.

Oakley, B. and Wen, R. (1989) Extracellular pH in the isolated retina of the toad in darkness and during illumination. *J. Physiol.*, 419: 353–378.

Pierce, M.E., Sheshberadaran, H., Zhang, Z., Fox, L.E., Applebury, M.L. and Takahashi, J.S. (1993) Circadian regulation of iodopsin gene expression in embryonic photoreceptors in retinal cell culture. *Neuron*, 10: 579–584.

Pittendrigh, C.S. (1981) Circadian systems: General Perspective. In: Aschoff J. (Ed.), *Handbook of Behavioral Neurobiology*, Biological Rhythms, Vol. 4, Plenum, New York, pp. 57–80.

Rashid, K. Baldridge, W.H. and Ball, A.K. (1993) Evidence for D2 receptor regulation of dopamine release in the goldfish retina. *J. Neurochem.*, 61: 2025–2033.

Raviola, E. and Gilula, N.B. (1973) Gap junctions between photoreceptor cells in the vertebtate retina. *Proc. Natl. Acad. Sci. USA*, 70: 1667–1681.

Reme, C., Wirz-Justice, A., Terman, M. (1991) The visual input stage of the mammalian circadian pacemaking system: I. Is there a clock in the mammalian eye? *J. Biol. Rhythms*, 6: 5–29.

Robertson, L.M. and Takahashi, J.S. (1988) Circadian clock in cell culture: II. In vitro photic entrainment of melatonin oscillation from dissociated chick pineal cells. *J. Neurosci.*, 8: 22–30.

Schaeffel, F., Rohrer, B., Lemmer, T. and Zrenner, E. (1991) Diurnal control of rod function in the chicken. *Vis. Neurosci.*, 6: 641–653.

Schwanzara, S.A. (1967) The visual pigments of fresh water fishes. *Vision Res.*, 7: 121–148.

Schwartz, W. and Gainer, J.H. (1977) Suprachiasmatic nucleus: use of 14C-labeled deoxyglucose uptake as a functional marker. *Science*, 197: 1089–1091.

Shulman, L.M. and Fox, D.A. (1996) Dopamine inhibits mammalian photoreceptor Na^+, K^+-ATPase activity via a selective effect on the alpha 3 isozyme. *Proc. Natl. Acad. Sci. USA*, 93: 8034–8039.

Stell, W.K. (1967) The structure and relationship of horizontal cells and photoreceptor-bipolar synaptic complexes in goldfish retina. *Am. J. Anat.*, 121: 401–424.

Stell, W.K. and Harosi, F.I. (1976) Cone structure and visual pigment content in the retina of the goldfish. *Vision Res.*, 16: 647–657.

Terman, M. and Terman, J. (1985) A circadian pacemaker for visual sensitivity? *Ann. N.Y. Acad. Sci.*, 453: 147–161.

Tornqvist, K., Yang, X.-L. and Dowling, J.E. (1988) Modulation of cone horizontal cell activity in the teleost fish retina, III: Effects of prolonged darkness and dopamine on electrical coupling between horizontal cells. *J. Neurosci.*, 8: 2279–2288.

Tosini, G. and Menaker, M. (1996) Circadian rhythms in cultured mammalian retina. *Science*, 272: 419–421.

Toyoda, J.-I. and Tonosaki, K. (1978) Effect of polarisation of horizontal cells on the on-centre bipolar cell of carp retina. *Nature*, 276: 399–400.

Underwood, H., Barrett, R.K. and Siopes, T. (1990) The quail's eye: A biological clock. *J. Biol. Rhythms*, 5: 257–265.

Viswanathan, N., Weaver, D.R., Reppert, S.M. and Davis, F.C. (1994) Entrainment of the fetal circadian pacemaker by prenatal injections of the dopamine agonist SKF38393. *J. Neurosci.*, 14: 5393–5398.

Wagner, H.-J., Behrens, U.D., Zaunreiter, M. and Douglas, R.H. (1992) The circadian component of spinule dynamics in teleost retinal horizontal cells is dependent on the dopaminergic system. *Vis. Neurosci.*, 9: 345–351.

Wang, Y. and Mangel, S.C. (1996) A circadian clock regulates rod and cone input to fish retinal cone horizontal cells. *Proc. Natl. Acad. Sci. USA*, 93: 4655–4660.

Wang, Y., Harsanyi, K. and Mangel, S.C. (1997) Endogenous activation of dopamine D2 receptors regulates dopamine release in the fish retina. *J. Neurophysiol.*, 78: 439–449.

Weiler, R., Baldridge, W.H., Mangel, S.C. and Dowling, J.E. (1997) Modulation of endogenous dopamine release in the fish retina by light and prolonged darkness. *Vis. Neurosci.*, 14: 351–356.

518

Welsh, D.K., Logothetis, D.E., Meister, M. and Reppert, S.M. (1995) Individual neurons dissociated from rat suprachaismatic nucleus express independently phased firing rhythms. *Neuron*, 14: 697–706.

Werblin, F.S. and Dowling, J.E. (1969) Organization of the retina of the mudpuppy, Necturus maculosis. II. *J. Neurophysiol.*, 32: 339–355.

Wirz-Justice, A., Da Prada, M. and Reme, C.E. (1984) Circadian rhythm in rat retinal dopamine. *Neurosci. Lett.*, 45: 21–25.

Witkovsky, P., Shakib, M. and Ripps, H. (1974) Interreceptoral junctions in the teleost retina. *Invest. Opthalmol.*, 13(12): 996–1009.

Witkovsky, P., Nicholson, C., Rice, M.E., Bohmaker, K. and Meller, E. (1993) Extracellular dopamine concentration in the retina of the clawed frog, *Xenopus laevis*. *Proc. Natl. Acad. Sci. USA*, 90: 5667–5671.

Witkovsky, P., Stone, S. and Besharse, J.C. (1988) Dopamine modifies the balance of rod and cone inputs to horizontal cells of the *Xenopus* retina. *Brain Res.*, 449: 332–336.

Wu, S.M. (1991) Signal transmission and adaptation-induced modulation of photoreceptor synapses in the retina. *Prog. Ret. Res.*, 10: 27–44.

Yamamoto, F., Borgula, G.A. and Steinberg, R.H. (1992) Effects of light and darkness on pH outside rod photoreceptors in the cat retina. *Exp. Eye Res.*, 54: 685–697.

Yang, X.-L., Tornqvist, K. and Dowling, J.E. (1988) Modulation of cone horizontal cell activity in the teleost fish retina, II: Role of interplexiform cells and dopamine in regulating light responsiveness. *J. Neurosci.*, 8: 2269–2278.

Yang, X.-L. and Wu, S.M. (1989) Modulation of rod-cone coupling by light. *Science*, 244: 352–354

Yazulla, S. and Lin, Z.-S. (1995) Differential effects of dopamine depletion on the distribution of 3H-SCH23390 and 3H-spiperone binding sites in the goldfish retina. *Vision Res.*, 35: 2509–2514.

Yazulla, S. and Zucker, C.L. (1988) Synaptic organization of dopaminergic interplexiform cells in the goldfish retina. *Vis. Neurosci.*, 1: 13–29.

H. Kolb, H. Ripps and S. Wu (Eds.)
Progress in Brain Research, Vol. 131
© 2001 Elsevier Science B.V. All rights reserved

CHAPTER 37

Spinules and nematosomes in retinal horizontal cells: a "thorny" issue

Joaquín De Juan* and Magdalena García

Departamento de Biotecnología, Facultad de Ciencias, Universidad de Alicante, Apdo. Correos 99, Alicante 03080, Spain

Introduction

A striking feature in teleost retinas, is the presence of protrusions, called spinules, on horizontal cell lateral elements that contact cone pedicles. Spinules are dynamic structures, which form during light adaptation and disappear during dark adaptation. Although the role of spinules is still unclear, the combination of intracellular recording and quantitative ultrastructural analysis has suggested that they may be involved in some way in feedback transmission from cone horizontal cells (HCs) to cone pedicles. In addition to spinules, teleost external HCs exhibit cytoplasmic inclusions named nematosomes. These structures decrease in size as the number of spinules increases, suggesting an inverse relationship between them. The function of nematosomes also remains unknown. The aims of this chapter are to summarize our present understanding of the structure and plasticity of spinules and nematosomes in HCs of teleost retinas and to see if we can come to any conclusions as to their roles in information processing in these retinas. Important aspects of these studies were initiated when the first author spent one year in John Dowlings laboratory at Harvard University.

Spinules in retinal horizontal cells: concept and morpho-functional characteristics

In teleosts, the synaptic connections between photoreceptors and cone horizontal cells (HCs) undergo a morphological re-arrangement, depending on the state of ambient illumination and experimental conditions (Fig. 1). During light adaptation (Fig. 1, Protocol II), the lateral elements of HCs extend finger-like spinules (Wagner, 1980) into the central cavity of the cone pedicle (Fig. 2A): these spinules disappear during dark adaptation (Fig. 1, Protocol VII; Fig. 2B). Spinules are typically 0.5 μm in length and 0.1 μm in width, and are characterized by electron-dense triangular and periodic densities, which line the tips beneath the membrane and serves as a marker for them. The densities show a positive ethanolic phosphotungstic acid (EPTA) reaction, suggesting their possible synaptic nature (Wagner, 1980). Unlike HCs dendrites at either position around synaptic ribbons, the E-face intramembraneous particles are not noticably specialised at spinules. The spinule cytosol is typically clear without vesicles and organelles. The extracellular space has no intracleft matrix (Fig. 2C).

The spinules are dynamic structures, which form during light adaptation, and disappear almost completely during dark adaptation (Raynauld et al., 1979; Wagner, 1980; Weiler and Wagner, 1984; Djamgoz et al., 1985b, 1988; Downing and Djamgoz, 1989; Kirsch et al., 1990; De Juan et al., 1991, 1996;

---
* Corresponding author: Joaquín De Juan, Tel.: 96-590-3848; Fax: 96-590-3965; E-mail: jdj@ua.es

520

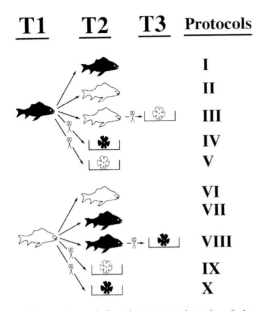

T1 T2 T3 Protocols

I
II
III
IV
V

VI
VII
VIII
IX
X

Fig. 1. Protocols used for ultrastructural study of the fish retinas. Left side represents the initial state of illumination: dark (black fish) or light (white fish) adaptation for long-time (T1 > 2 h). Protocols I and VI represents the "in vivo" maintenance of the fish in constant dark or light adaptation respectively. The only change between T1 and T2 are the experimental manipulations (i.e. dopamine intraocular injection). Protocols II and VII are the normal change to light or dark adaptation respectively. In protocols IV, V, IX, and X the eyes were removed (scissors) and theirs eyecups superfused in light- (white retina) or dark- (black retina) conditions for 60 min (T2). In protocols III and VIII, after a long-time of dark or light adaptation (T1), the animals were light (white fish) and dark (black fish) adapted for a short time (T2 = 10 min respectively), with the eyes then being removed (scissors) and their eyecups superfused in dark (black retina) or light (white retina) conditions for 60 min (T3).

De Juan and García, 1998; García and De Juan, 1999). In several species (Wagner, 1980; Wagner and Douglas, 1983), the time course of formation or disappearance is between 45 to 60 min. Following full light adaptation, the formation of spinules means an increase of about 25% of contact area between the HCs dendrites and the cone plasmalemma (Wagner, 1990). In addition, during light and dark adaptation spinules undergo some morphological changes. Light adapted spinules have a slender shape, whereas dark adapted ones are rounder. Spherical spinules contain the same kind of triangular membrane thickenings observed in slender ones (Wagner, 1980).

The number of spinules per pedicle in light adapted retinas is greater in some teleosts than in others. In *Micropterus salmoides* (De Juan et al., 1996; De Juan and García, 1998; García and De Juan, 1999) and *Roccus americana* (De Juan and Dowling, 1987; De Juan et al., 1991), the number of spinules per pedicle profile is double that in *Carassius auratus, Tinca tinca* and *Cyprinus carpio* (Wagner and Douglas, 1983). In dark adapted retinas, this number is close to zero in *Micropterus salmoides* (De Juan et al., 1996; De Juan and García, 1998; García and De Juan, 1999) and *Roccus Americana* (De Juan and Dowling, 1987; De Juan et al., 1991), whereas in other teleosts this number ranges from one to two spinules per pedicle (Wagner, 1980). Histological sectioning methods cannot account for these numerical differences, since the use of tangential or transversal section gives the same spinule number (Wagner, 1980). We determine spinule frequency as spinule/pedicle (De Juan et al., 1996; De Juan and García, 1998; García and De Juan, 1999), other authors habitually use the ratio spinules/synaptic ribbon (S/R). In our opinion, the use of the S/R ratio has disadvantages, because the number of synaptic ribbons is variable, depending on ambient illumination and the species of fish. For instance, in *Sparus auratus*, the number of synaptic ribbons is unaffected by light conditions, whereas in *Dicentrarchus labrax*, synaptic ribbons show a striking decrease to about 50% after 1 h of dark adaptation (García et al., 1998a). In the example of *Rocus americana*, the number of synaptic ribbon per pedicle shows a decrease to about 25% after 2 h of dark adaptation, but in *Micropterus salmoides*, there is no difference in ribbon number between light and dark adapted retinas for 2 h at a time. However, in both species, the number of synaptic ribbons exhibits a striking decrease to about 50% at midnight (García et al., 1998b).

When serial-sections have been used in the reconstruction of cone pedicles, the number of spinules per HC's dendrite is about 29 (Wagner and Speck, 1983). It has been observed that older fish generally have more spinules than younger ones (Douglas and Wagner, 1983). In general, we deduced from several data sets that predator fishes have more intense cone retinomotor movements (RMM) and number of spinules than non-predator fishes. When fish are reared for 1 year in white or monochromatic

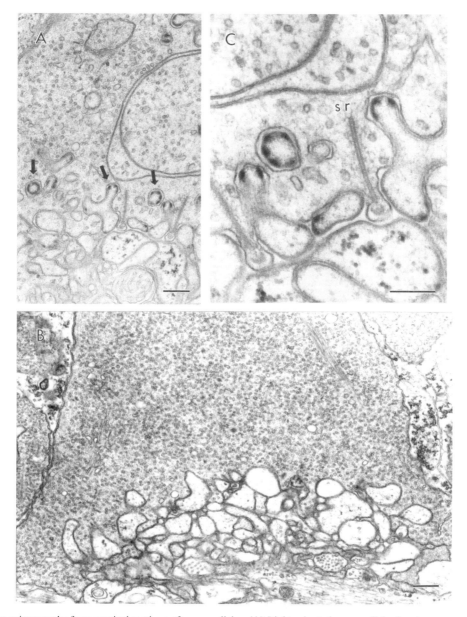

Fig. 2. Electron micrographs from vertical sections of cone pedicles. (A) Light adapted cone pedicle showing many spinules (arrows). (B) Dark adapted cone pedicle without spinules. (C) Magnification of electron micrograph A showing spinules around the synaptic ribbon (sr). Note the electron densities beneath the membrane and the spinule cytosol without vesicles and organelles. Bar: 0.5 μm.

"red", "green", or "blue" light, the S/R ratio in light adapted retinas falls with decreasing wavelength in all cone types. In addition, there are more incompletely formed spinules in the blue light group (Kröger and Wagner, 1996).

The combination of intracellular recording and quantitative ultrastructural analysis has suggested that spinules may be the sites of feedback transmission from cone horizontal cells (HCs) to pedicles of cones (Raynauld et al., 1979; Wagner, 1980; Weiler and Wagner, 1984; Djamgoz et al., 1985a, 1985b, 1988; Downing and Djamgoz, 1989; Kirsch et al., 1990). The primary neural control for the photoreceptor synapses is the negative feedback synapse between HCs and cone photoreceptors. Light hyperpolarizes the HCs and their response feeds back to cones through the sign-inverting synapse, resulting in a depolarizing response in the cones (Wu, 1992). In darkness, HCs are despolarized by the continuous flow of photoreceptor neurotransmitter glutamate. GABA released by HCs in darkness opens Cl-channels in cones and hyperpolarizes them tonically in darkness. In the presence of light stimuli, HCs are hyperpolarized, and the GABA release is suppressed. Thus, both HCs spinules and HCs feedback are suppressed in the dark and activated by light adaptation (Wu, 1991).

In this sense, when spinules are absent from the retina, color opponent responses in HCs and ganglion cells, believed to depend on HCs-cone feedback, are also suppressed. There is a correlation between chromaticity HC responses and spinule numbers (Raynauld et al., 1979; Weiler and Wagner, 1984; Djamgoz et al., 1988, 1989; Kirsch et al., 1990) however it has been difficult to prove a role in the processing that leads directly to color vision. HCs spinules are not required for wavelength discrimination (Yazulla et al., 1996). HCs spinules are not needed for the transmission of photopic (red cone) luminosity signals through the ON pathway of the retina. Thus, although HCs spinule formation is correlated with light adaptation in fish retinas its function in luminosity coding is still undetermined (Yazulla et al., 1996). Another possible role is in dealing with optical blur to enhance signal edges or contours, or compute contrast in the image (Balboa and Grzywacz, 2000). Spinules have in general been considered as sites of dual function, pre- and post-synaptic, between cone pedicles and HCs (Downing and Djamgoz, 1989). However the significance of these structures is still uncertain.

Spinules and nematosomes

Cytoplasmic inclusions resembling nucleoli, and termed nucleolus-like bodies or nematosomes (Hindelang-Gertner et al., 1974), were originally described a century ago in ganglionic nerve cells. Since then, these structures have been found in different areas of the central (Le Beux, 1972; Katoth and Shimizu, 1982) and peripheral (Grillo, 1970)

nervous system. They are particularly numerous in the hypothalamus and circumventricular organs (Santolaya, 1973; Anzil et al., 1973; Hindelang-Gertner et al., 1974; Katoth and Shimizu, 1982; Fechner, 1986), but were not described in the retina until 1987 when they were seen in HCs of *Roccus americana* (De Juan and Dowling, 1987) (Fig. 3). Since then, we have observed them in external HCs from several teleosts, including *Dicentrarchus labrax*, *Sparus aurata Linnaeus* and *Micropterus salmoides*.

Nematosomes are composed of granular and filamentous electron-dense material within a more electron lucent matrix. They are generally located near mitochondria or the cell membrane (Fig. 4). The nematosomes have no limiting membrane, and appear more often spherical or ovoid than polygonal or elongated. As in other locations, nematosomes appear as a thread-like structure. In thin cross-sections, nematosomes present their fibers arranged in parallel fashion and the fibers are united by spicules that project perpendicularly to the fiber edge (Fig. 3 and 4).

In HCs from long-term dark adapted retinas, nematosomes are significantly larger and more numerous than in long-term light adapted ones (Fig. 5a). We suggested that the electron-dense material lining the spinules resembles the material observed in the nematosomes. We suggested inverse relationship (Fig. 5b) between the incidence of electron-dense material in spinules and the size and number of nematosomes (De Juan et al., 1991, 1996; De Juan and García, 1998). Although this inverse correlation does not prove that the spinules' electron-dense material belongs to the nematosomes, we have ultrastructural evidence suggesting a connection between them. In effect, as shown in Fig. 3, it is possible to observe nematosomel material "travelling" through the dendrites of HCs near cone pedicles. On occasions, we also observe nematosomes near the curved and thick plasmalemma. Moreover, we have observed plasmalemmal infolding of HCs with electron-dense material that resembles immature spinules (Fig. 6).

Although nematosomes were first described a century ago, their functions are still unclear. Grillo (1970) speculated that nematosomes may be an intermediary in the transfer of nuclear-derived material to synapses. Presumably, this material plays a role in the

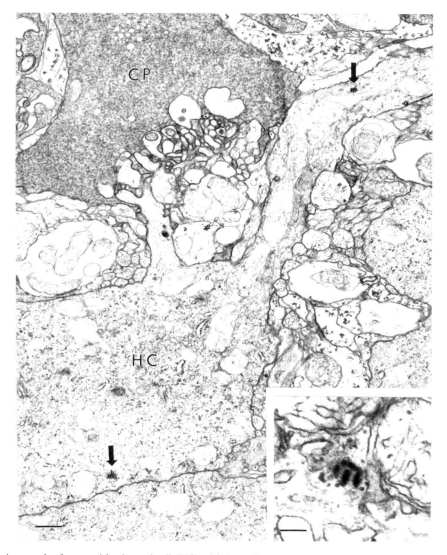

Fig. 3. Electron micrograph of external horizontal cell (HC) with 2 small nematosomes (arrows). A nematosome is also seen in the dendrite of horizontal cell near the cone pedicle (CP). *Inset*: higher magnification of a small nematosome to show the spicules between the fibers. Bar: 1 μm (0.1 μm).

intercellular adhesion or in the control of synaptic transmission by providing receptors, enzymes, or other substances essential for synaptic function. Several authors (Grillo, 1970; Santolaya, 1973; Hindelang-Gertner et al., 1974; Katoth and Shimizu, 1982) have found evidence for RNA in these nucleolus-like bodies and have suggested that they could synthesise proteinaceous substances. Halkka and Halkka (1975), studying chromosomes of the oocytes of the dragonfly, have suggested that

nematosomes are storage structures for long-lived informational RNA. These nematosomes are later found adjacent to the mitochondria and undergo transformations that are synchronized with changes in oocyte activity. Ockleford et al. (1987) also proposed that nematosomes could be related to the neuronal cytoskeleton and play a role in the maintenance of the shape of the axons and synaptic terminals. These hypotheses are consistent with data reported by Hámori and Lakos (1980) who, after

524

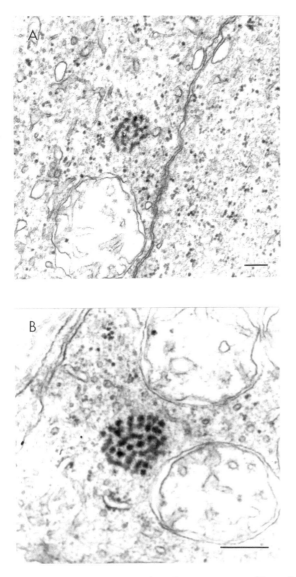

Fig. 4. Electron micrographs of nematosomes. Note the granular and filamentous electron dense material within the more electron lucent matrix. Observe the fibers united by spicules that run perpendicular to the fiber edge. (A) Nematosome located near mitochondria and the cell membrane. (B) Nematosome located near mitochondria. Bar: 0.3 μm.

transecting Purkinje cell axons in adult rats, found a regular presence of nematosomes in the synaptic terminals of the hypertrophied branches.

Recently, a close relationship has been established between the nematosomes and the neural protein HAP1, which interacts with huntington protein of

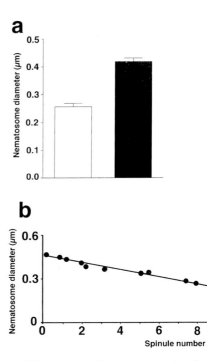

Fig. 5. (a) Histogram showing changes in size of nematosomes in the horizontal cells after long-term light (open bar) and dark (black bar) adaptation of the retinas (Mean ± S.E.M.). (b) Regression analysis of the mean values of spinule number and nematosome size from short-term light or dark adapted retinas.

Huntington's disease (Li et al., 1998). These authors propose that HAP1 isoforms are involved in the formation of HAP1-immunoreactive nematosomes in the neuronal cytoplasm. Furthermore, nematosomes have been linked to a 165 kDa protein expressed in the visual system during the critical period of development (Kind et al., 1997).

Finally, there are data that show a close relationship between nematosomes, aromatases, and estrogens (Leranth et al., 1985; Leranth et al., 1991). In estrogen-treated African green monkeys (*Cercopithecus aethiops*), a large number of nematosomes are found in neurons with progesterone receptors and glutamic acid decarboxylase (GAD). These neurons are located in the arcuate and ventromedial hypothalamic nuclei (Leranth et al., 1991). This association between nematosomes and neurons which are sensitive to estrogen is interesting, because in teleosts retinas (see below), centrifugal fibers that originate from ganglion cells adjacent to the olfactory bulb (Zucker and Dowling, 1987) make conventional synapses on interplexiform

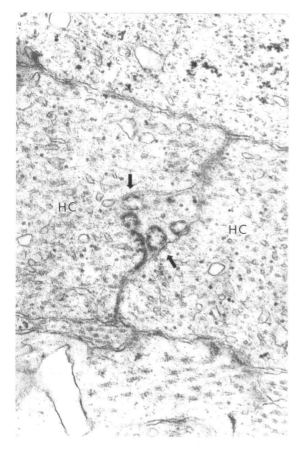

Fig. 6. Electron micrograph of two external horizontal cells (HC) showing plasmalemmal enfolding with electron dense material resembling immature spinules (arrows).

dopaminergic cells (DA-IPC) and contain gonado-tropin hormone-releasing hormone (GnRH)-like. In this way, we know today that estrogens also have a very important function on the CNS of vertebrates (Callard et al., 1995).

If spinules represent a type of synapse as proposed by Wagner (1980), then electron-dense material could relate to synaptic transmission or synaptic attachment. The increase in size and number of nemato-somes in dark adapted retinas suggests that this material becomes condensed in nematosomes during dark adaptation, and is dispersed and migrates towards the spinule tips during light adaptation. Our findings are reminiscent of the increase in the number of nucleolus-like bodies found by Fechner (1986) in the pinealocytes of short-day animals as compared with long-day ones.

Mechanisms underlying the formation and disruption of spinules

The molecular motors in spinule formation and dissolution

Little is known about the mechanisms underlying the formation and dissolution of HC's spinules. From a theoretical point of view, three basic mechanisms can be considered in spinule formation and dissolution: (1) an active cone pedicle traction and repulsion of spinules; (2) a protrusion and retraction of spinules into the cone; and (3) a combination of the two. Studies of morphological changes in spines on pyramidal cells of the cortex look at cytoskeleton proteins such as actin and tubulin, as well as associated proteins. Many authors (Crick, 1982; Fifková and Delay, 1982; Fischer et al., 1998; van Rossum and Hanisch, 1999; Halpain, 2000) have described contractile proteins associated with each spine, suggestive of a role in changing the spine's shape during neural activity. Thus, in the formation and dissolution of HCs' spinules, cytoskeletal elements such as the actin and microtubules are probably also involved (Ter-Margarian and Djamgoz, 1992; Schmitz and Köhler, 1993; Weiler and Janssen-Bienhold, 1993; De Juan and García, 1998).

Regarding actin's presence in spinules, published data are controversial. Whereas some authors have reported actin in spinules (Weiler and Janssen-Bienhold, 1993), others could not detect it either in pedicles or in the spinules themselves, but have detected it in the HCs' dendrites (Schmitz and Kohler, 1993). Several experiments have shown a significant reduction in the number of spinules in pedicles after application of Cytochalasin B (Ter-Margarian and Djamgoz, 1992; Weiler and Janssen-Bienhold, 1993) or Cytochalasin D (Ter-Margarian and Djamgoz, 1992; Schmitz and Kohler, 1993; De Juan and García, 1998) (Fig. 7, 8 and 9) probably because of the inhibition of actin polymerization (Casella et al., 1981). In these experiments, other actin-dependent retinal functions can also be affected, such as cone contraction (Burnside and Nagle, 1983), rod elongation (O'Connor and Burnside, 1982), and the dispersion of pigment granules of the retinal pigment epithelium (Burnside et al., 1982). Hence, Cytochalasin B or D transforms the retina into the

526

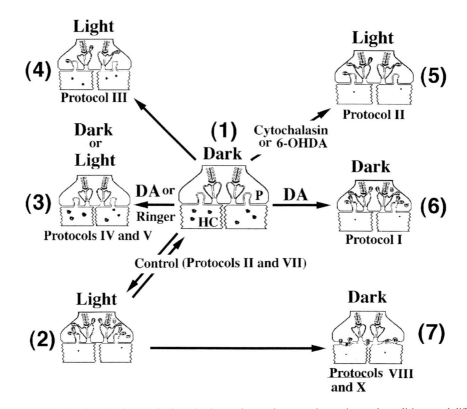

Fig. 7. Experimental models showing the changes in the spinule number under several experimental conditions and different protocols (see Fig. 1) applied. (1) The drawing represents the junction zone between pedicle (P) and horizontal cell (HC) in a normal dark-adapted retina. In the P spinules are absent and HC show several large nematosomes. (2) Normal light-adapted retina with numerous spinules. Relationships between (1) and (2) and vice versa (double arrows) represent the normal cycle of light and dark adaptation and correspond to Protocols II and VII in Fig. 1. (3) In this model the isolation of the retina in the dark impairs spinule formation at light and at dark with DA addition (see Protocols IV and V in Fig. 1). (4) As in the previous model, one observes the need for optic nerve integrity for spinule formation. However, the spinule number is proportional to the time that the retina is in the living animal. (5) Treatment with Cytochalasin or 6-OHDA causes significant reduction in spinule formation "in vivo". (6) Intraocular injection of DA at dark induces normal spinule formation. Compare with Model 3 where the retina has been isolated. (7) Optic nerve integrity is also needed for dissolution when fish change from light adaptation to dark adaptation.

equivalent of a partially dark adapted retina. However, spinule densities were seen after Cytochalasin D-treatment although the protrusion of processes was inhibited. This suggests that the formation of spinules consists of two components: the formation of membrane densities and the protrusion of processes, which may be separately controlled (Schmitz and Kohler, 1993).

Intraocular injection of colchicine produces a marked inhibition of spinule formation during light adaptation (Schmitz and Kohler, 1993). Tubulin can be detected in the OPL in rat, mouse and fish retinas by anti-tubulin immunoreactivity

(Woodford and Blanks, 1989; Schmitz and Kohler, 1993). However, alpha- and beta-tubulin antibodies label neither the photoreceptor terminals nor the distal end of HC dendrites that invaginate into cone pedicles. This disruption could lead to insufficient transport of material into the dendritic terminals, thereby preventing spinule formation. Furthermore, the distributions of tubulin label suggests that mechanism of dendritic transport may differ in the proximal and distal portions of the dendrites. In distal dendrites the transport may be independent of microtubules (Schmitz and Kohler, 1993).

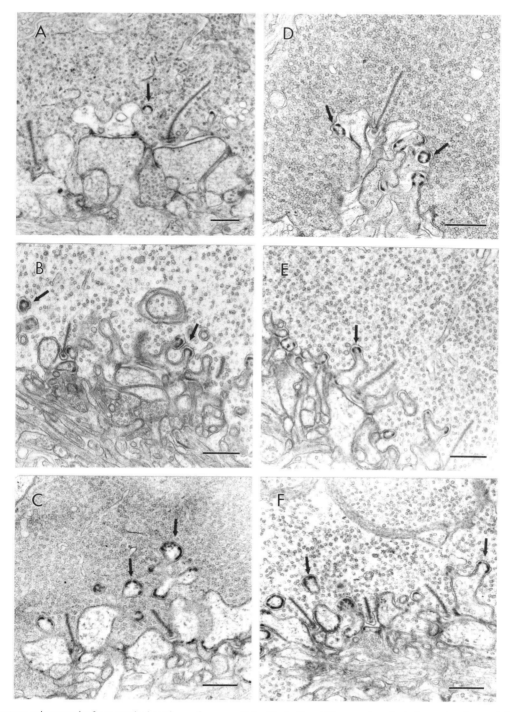

Fig. 8. Electron micrographs from vertical sections of cone pedicles illustrating differences in spinule formation (arrows) depending of experimental conditions. (A) Light-adapted retinas from Cytochalasin-treated eyes have reduced numbers of spinules. (B) Dark-adapted dopamine-treated retinas show some spinules. (C) 6-OHDA-treated light-adapted. (D) Dark-adapted retina studied according to protocol X. The spinules do not disappear but are not invaginated into the cone pedicle. (E) Contralateral DA-untreated dark-adapted retina. (F) The contralateral 6-OHDA-untreated retina appears similar to the 6-OHDA-treated retina. Bar: 0.5 μm.

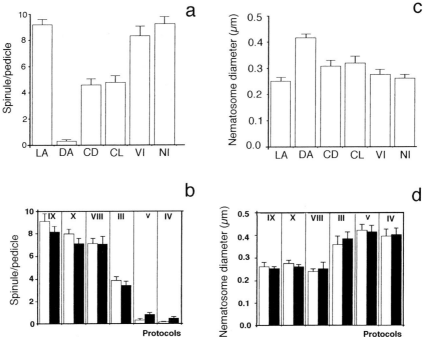

Fig. 9. (a) Histogram showing the effects of intraocular injection of cytochalasin D in one eye (CD) and vehicle in the contralateral eye (CL), compared with vehicle-injected (VI) eyes and non-injected (NI) fellow eyes in control animals. All are compared with control light-adapted (LA) or dark-adapted (DA) eyes. Cytochalasin D injection reduced the number of spinules per pedicle both in the injected eye (CD) and the contralateral (CL) one. This number reached values intermediate between light-adapted (LA) and dark-adapted (DA) retinas for 1 h. (From De Juan and García, 1998). (b) Histograms show the changes in the number of spinules per pedicle. The roman numeral atop each pair of bins indicate the protocols employed (see Fig. 1 and 7). Dopamine superfusion (black bars) does not modify the number of spinules in comparison to the controls (open bars) (From De Juan et al., 1996). (c) Cytoclasin D increased the nematosome size in both the cytochalasin-injected eye (CD) and the contralateral (CL) vehicle-injected eye. This size was between those obtained in light-adapted (LA) and dark-adapted (DA) retinas. The results of vehicle-injected eyes (VI) and non-injected (NI) fellow eyes in control animals were similar to those in light-adapted eyes (LA) (From De Juan and García, 1998). (d) Histograms show the sizes of nematosomes under the protocols the same as in (b) (From De Juan et al., 1996).

The retraction of spinules is neither affected by colchicine nor by Cytochalasin B or D. Therefore, the mechanism for retraction does not seem to require a functional network of actin and may be driven by passive forces such as cell turgor (Schmitz and Kohler, 1993).

Neuractive substances involved in spinule formation and dissolution

(A) Glutamate induces spinule dissolution during dark adaptation

For more than a decade, there are data that link glutamate to spinule degradation during dark adaptation (Weiler et al., 1988). Several experiments have shown that spinule dissolution is determined by a massive entrance of Ca^{2+} into HCs. It is unlikely that voltage-gated calcium channels are involved in the spinule retraction though, because the presence of cobalt does not impair their dissolution (Weiler et al., 1996). The Ca^{2+} entrance is triggered by glutamate action over AMPA-receptors and the subsequent activation of calmodulin and Ca/Calmoduline dependent Proteinkinase II (CaMkII). When retinas are kept under continuous illumination, the dissolution of spinules can be triggered by actions of glutamate analogues on AMPA/kainate receptors. Activation of AMPA and kainate receptors, but not NMDA receptors, increase intracellular Ca^{2+} in the presence of agonists (Okada et al., 1999) and trigger the spinules retraction. However, some experiments have shown that kainate-preferring receptors contribute little or nothing to the observed intracellular increase of Ca^{2+} (Weiler et al., 1995; Okada et al., 1999).

(B) Dopamine as co-regulator of spinule formation

We now address the literature's controversy on dopamine's role in spinule formation (Wagner and Djamgoz, 1993, 1994; Weiler, 1994; Baldridge and Ball, 1994; De Juan et al., 1996). It has been reported that spinule formation in light adaptation is mimicked by exogenously applied DA (Weiler et al., 1988; Köhler and Weiler, 1990), and partially inhibited in retinas lesioned with 6-hydroxydopamine (6-OHDA) (Köhler and Weiler, 1990; De Juan et al., 1990; Kirsch et al., 1991; Wagner et al., 1992), and inhibited by dopamine D1 antagonists (Kirsch et al., 1991). These data suggest that DA released by DA-IPCs in teleost fish induces light-dependent spinule formation (Weiler et al., 1988; Köhler and Weiler, 1990; Kirsch et al., 1991; Wagner et al., 1992). However, there are several results in conflict with this hypothesis. Neither in the isolated retina nor in vivo is DA a very potent signal for the induction of spinule formation. The number of spinules induced by light is two to five times higher than the number induced by DA (Weiler, 1994). Furthermore, DA depletion or dopaminergic antagonists do not prevent spinule formation during light adaptation although spinules do not persist in the light adapted retina in the presence of DA antagonists (Weiler et al., 1988; Köhler and Weiler, 1990).

Behavior of spinule formation is different in isolated dark adapted retinas superfused with DA than in retinas from dark adapted fishes whose eyes were injected with DA. Sixty min of DA superfusion in the dark does not produce spinules in an isolated eyecup and its nematosomes are as large as in the normal dark adapted condition (Fig. 1, Protocol IV; Figs. 7 and 9) (De Juan et al., 1996). By contrast, intraocular injection of DA in dark adapted fish produces an increase in the density of spinules and a reduction in the nematosome's diameters (Fig. 1, Protocol 1; Figs. 7 and 8B) (De Juan et al., 1990) as in

normal light adaptation. This suggests an essential role for DA in the induction of spinules. However, in agreement with results reported earlier, depletion of retinal DA with intraocular injections of 6-OHDA produces only a partial (albeit significant) reduction (Figs. 7 and 8C) in spinule formation (Köhler and Weiler, 1990; De Juan et al., 1990; Kirsch et al., 1991; Wagner et al., 1992; Yazulla and Studholme, 1995; Yazulla et al., 1996). In support, DA injected into an eye previously depleted of dopaminergic cells could not form spinules (Köhler and Weiler, 1990). Hence, these data suggest that DA is not the only signal for the appearance of spinules in the light (Köhler and Weiler, 1990; De Juan et al., 1990, 1996; Kirsch et al., 1991; Yazulla and Studholme, 1995). It appears, that DA is needed far more for the persistence of spinules than as a signal for the induction of spinules (Weiler, 1994).

(C) Second messengers and spinule formation:

The signals and intracellular cascades underlying spinule formation and dissolution are still only partially understood. There is special interest in the involvement of second messengers that link superficial receptors with intracellular proteins involved in spinule formation and dissolution, such as cyclic adenosine monophosphate (cAMP), protein kinase C (PKC) and Ca^{2+}/calmodulin-dependent protein kinase II (CaMkII).

Several studies have analyzed the possible influence of cAMP on spinule formation. However, the results obtained are contradictory and the discrepancies may be attributed to differences in experimental design (Behrens et al., 1992). In some experiments, the increase of intracellular cAMP mediated by DA through D1 receptors in isolated dark-adapted retinas produces an increase in the number of spinules (Behrens et al., 1992; Wagner and Djamgoz, 1993). By contrast, in other similar experiments using isolated retinas, increases in the concentration of cAMP or the injection of dibutyryl-cAMP does no result in spinule formation (Köhler and Weiler, 1990). These data seriously question the involvement of this second messenger in spinule formation (Köhler and Weiler, 1990; Weiler, 1994).

PKC has not been localized by immunocytochemical methods to HCs of teleost retinas (Kato et al., 1990). However, its activation using esters of phorbol promotes the formation of new spinules in dark-adapted animals. This activation also induces spinule formation in a retina depleted of DA-IPCs, thus excluding the possibility that PKC activation causes the release of DA. On the other hand, synaptically isolated HCs form spinules vigorously upon activation of PKC, and exhibit strong binding of phorbol esters, supporting a localization of PKC activity in these neurons (Weiler et al., 1991).

In spinule retraction during dark adaptation, the activation of CaMkII is an important step. As Weiler et al. (1995) demonstrated, spinule retraction is prevented in vivo by injection of calmidazolium (an inhibitor of calmodulin) into the eyeball. The same happens by injection of KN-62, an CaMkII inhibitor. These also show that lowering the external calcium concentration prevents dark- and AMPA-induced retraction of spinules in an eyecup preparation. The phosphorylation patterns of phosphoproteins derived from purified horizontal cells are affected by inhibitors of camodulin and CaMkII respectively. Some of the affected phosphoproteins appear to be cytoskeleton-associated proteins, including GAP-43.

(D) Nitric oxide (NO) triggers spinule formation

The possible involvement of nitric oxide (NO) gas in light adaptive morphological changes in the outer retina of a cyprinid fish has been studied by Greenstreet and Djamgoz (1994). Isolated retina were treated in the dark by either of two NO-donor compounds (S-nitroso-n-acetylpenicillamine and sodium nitroprusside) and then studied by light and electron microscopy. Application of NO induced contraction of cone photoreceptor myoids and formation of horizontal cell spinules. Accordingly, the cone index and the S/R ratio showed 15–20% and 49–95% changes, respectively, compared with controls. These data are consistent with the involvement of NO in the light adaptation process in the outer retina of teleost fish. However, the inhibitor of endogenous NO synthesis L-nitroarginine (0.1 mM) had not influence on the formation or retraction of spinules (Pottek et al., 1997).

(E) The argued effect of Ethambutol in spinule formation

For Köhler et al. (1995), a high dose of Ethambutol (10 mM) reduced the number of spinules by 30% in previously light adapted retinas. When Ethambutol was applied in the dark with subsequent light adaptation, the result was an intense reduction of light-induced spinule formation. The inhibition of spinule formation was dose dependent. Low doses (0.1 mM) of Ethambutol caused 40% inhibition and high doses (10 mM) caused 70% inhibition. Besides affecting spinules, Ethambutol occasionally induced a degeneration of cone pedicles and altered synaptic connections between horizontal cells and cones in a dose-related fashion. This indicated that Ethambutol can influence the color-coding process already at the level of the cone-horizontal cell synapse (Köhler et al., 1995).

For other authors (Wietsma et al., 1995), the effects of Ethambutol was not as dramatic. It changed only transiently the receptive field size and spectral sensitivity of horizontal cells. The spectral characteristics of horizontal cells did not change in long-term Ethambutol-treated goldfish. Spinule formation on HC dendrites remained unaffected by Ethambutol. These authors concluded that Ethambutol did not induce functional dark adaptation of horizontal cells and that the Ethambutol-induced red-green color vision deficiency does not originate in the HC layers.

(F) Retinoic acid induced formation of spinules

Intraocular injection of retinoic acid in dark-adapted carps produces the formation of numerous spinules at the dendrites of HCs, as in light adapted retinas. By contrast, the addition of citral, a competitive inhibitor of the dehydrogenase responsible for the production of retinoic acid in vivo, impairs spinule formation during light adaptation. When HCs are recorded intracellularly in preparations superfused with retinoic acid, the HC's spatial properties are those of light adapted retinas. Therefore, retinoic acid acts as a light signaling modulator. Its activity appears not to be at the transcriptional level because its action was not blocked by actinomysin (Weiler et al., 1998).

Central control in formation/disruption of spinules

It has been reported that dopamine (DA) influences spinule formation (Kirsch et al., 1988; Weiler et al., 1988; Djamgoz et al., 1989; Köhler and Weiler, 1990). In teleost fish, DA is released by the DA-IPCs (Ehinger et al., 1969; Dowling and Ehinger, 1978; Dowling, 1986, 1987, 1989, 1991; Umino and Dowling, 1991), which provide an intraretinal centrifugal pathway from the inner to the outer plexiform layer, where these cells make abundant synapses on cone-related HCs. The DA-IPCs receive all their input in the inner plexiform layer from amacrine cells and centrifugal fibers (Dowling and Ehinger, 1975; Zucker and Dowling, 1987). In this way, the Central Nervous System (CNS) may act directly upon the retinal modulation of the HCs' in response to changes in the light environment (Stell et al., 1984, 1987; Walker and Stell, 1986; Umino and Dowling, 1991). The idea of a central control of spinule formation and retraction is supported by five lines of evidence:

Spinule outgrowth needs light adaptation and optic nerve integrity

By means of an ultrastructural and morphometric study, we showed that spinule formation and dissolution, and changes in nematosomes size were impaired in isolated eyecups, during light adaptation (Fig. 1, Protocol V; Figs. 7 and 9). Moreover, for an isolated retina, DA did not produce any effects over spinule formation (Fig. 1, Protocols IV and V; Figs. 7 and 9). Consequently, optic nerve integrity was necessary for spinule formation and disruption (De Juan et al., 1996). This suggested a central influence, probably through centrifugal fibres, on spinule formation. However, cone contraction was absolutely independent of central influence as in other species (Dearry and Barlow, 1987). A related aspect of optic nerve integrity on the physiology of HC, is that optic nerve crush influences the density of gap junctions between HCs (Kurz-Isler et al., 1992).

It was reported that spinule formation and cone contraction are independent processes that can be triggered by only a brief (1–2 min) exposure to light (Wagner and Douglas, 1983; Weiler and Wagner, 1984; Dearry and Burnside, 1986). In a series of experiments, we analyzed the influence of a short light exposure (10 min) on spinule formation. In these experiments, long-term dark-adapted fishes (> 2 h) were exposed to light for 10 min before eyecup isolation (Fig. 1, Protocol III; Fig. 9). In this case, the number of spinules did not reach the values of light adapted retinas, rising to only 30% of these values. This suggests that, although spinule formation has an endogenous control (Douglas and Wagner, 1983) and can be started by only a brief exposure to light, optic nerve integrity is necessary for total spinule formation. However, cones contracted as expected.

Spinule retraction needs dark adaptation and optic nerve integrity

Similarly, the dissolution of spinules needs optic nerve integrity. In long-term light adapted retinas, which were isolated and dark adapted for 1 h (Fig. 1, Protocol X; Figs. 7–9), spinules did not decrease, but spinules did not invaginate into cone pedicles (Fig. 8D). In other experiments, long-term light adapted fish (> 2 h) were exposed to dark for 10 min before eyecup isolation and then dark adapted for 60 min (Fig. 1, Protocol VIII; Figs. 7 and 9). In this case, spinules did not disappear as in dark adapted retinas and numbers remained close to those in light adapted retinas. In this case, the spinules did not invaginate into the cone pedicles either.

Centrifugal fibers project into the retina and release neuropeptides onto DA-IPC

In a number of non-mammalian species, DA release seems to be influenced by centrifugal fibers projecting to the retina (Ramón y Cajal, 1892; Stell et al., 1987; Réperant et al., 1989). In teleost retinas, this efferent pathway originates in ganglion cells adjacent to the olfactory bulb (Zucker and Dowling, 1987). In this respect, an interesting observation concerns the mutant *noseless* (*nos*) zebrafish (*nos*/+) which has visual defects due to altered olfactory inputs perhaps through DA-IPCs (Li and Dowling, 1998). This group of olfactory neurons and their axons is known as the *nervus terminalis* (Stell et al., 1984; Stell et al., 1987). In the retina, the centrifugal fibers have been observed by electron microscopy (Zucker and Dowling, 1987), and make conventional synapses on DA-IPC, and contain FMRFamide-like and gonadotropin hormone-releasing hormone (GnRH)-like and peptides (Münz et al., 1982; Stell et al., 1984). DA-IPCs in turn make synapses onto HCs.

The neuropeptide GnRH, closely mimicks the effects of DA on HCs indicating that GnRH acts by stimulating the release of DA from DA-IPC. In contrast, FMRF-amide-like peptides suppress the effects of GnRH on horizontal cells (Stell et al., 1984; Umino and Dowling, 1991). There are experiments that suggest a role for the centrifugal fibers in spinule formation. In effect, it has been reported that GnRH induces light adaptive spinule formation in dark adapted retinas (Behrens et al., 1993), and we have observed (see above) that formation and dissolution of spinules need the integrity of the optic nerve, and consequently the efferent fibers (De Juan et al., 1996).

Spinule formation is subject to a circadian rhythm

Spinule formation and dissolution shows a circadian rhythm. This is at least partially endogenously controlled because the rythmical changes continue in total darkness (Douglas and Wagner, 1983; Wagner et al., 1992). However, complete spinule formation requires some exogenous light stimulation because the dark rhythm exhibits reduced spinule density compared with a normal light/dark cycle (Douglas and Wagner, 1982; Wagner et al., 1992). Moreover, when a fish is exposed to continuous light, the spinules do not show an endogenous circadian rhythm. Spinules gradually decreased until reaching an intermediate level after 30 h.

Consensual response in the spinule formation

Finally, we have reported a direct interocular effect on spinule formation. Thus, intraocular injections of Cytochalasine D in *Micropterus salmoides* (De Juan and García, 1998), 6-OHDA, and DA in *Roccus americana* (unpublished data) produced parallel changes on spinule number and nematosome sizes in both injected and contralateral eyes. Intraocular injection of cytochalasin D into the right eye of

dark-adapted fish produces a 55% reduction in the number of spinules when the fish is adapted to light for one hour (Fig. 1, Protocol II; Figs. 7, 8A and 9a). The contralateral untreated eye (vehicle-injected eye) shows also a surprising reduction in spinule density of similar magnitude as in the treated eye (cytochalasin-injected eye). Nematosomes in both eyes are significantly increased in size in comparison to control retinas adapted to the light (Figs. 7 and 9b). In contrast, Cytochalasin D prevents the normal contraction of cones in the right eye during light, while the contralateral eye has cones that contract normally.

In a similar way, the monocular intravitreal injection of DA into the right eye of dark adapted fish causes a significant increase in the density of spinules (Figs. 7 and 8B) not only in the injected eye, (Fig. 1, Protocol I) but also in the contralateral untreated eye (vehicle-injected eye) (Fig. 8E). However, nematosomes in the dopamine-injected eyes adapted to darkness show a reduction in size, which becomes closer to the size in light-adapted eyes. The size of the nematosome in the contralateral untreated eye remains close to that in dark adaptation.

In eyes previously treated with 6-OHDA, we observed a significant reduction of the spinules' density when the eyes were light adapted (Fig. 1, Protocol II; Figs. 7 and 8C). This spinule reduction was also observed in the contralateral, untreated retina (Figs. 7 and 8F). However, 6-OHDA did not produce changes in nematosome size during light adaptation, since nematosome size was similar in control and 6-OHDA-injected light adapted retina.

In addition to a consensual response in spinule formation, the influence of one eye on the contralateral eye has been shown in other physiological aspects of the retina. Owusu-Yaw et al. (1992) have reported that the removal of one eye, a monocular optic nerve crush, and lesions of the optic tectum and *nervus terminalis* induce rod-precursor proliferation in ipsi and contralateral eyes of goldfish. Similarly, Negishi et al. (1991) have shown that unilateral intravitreal injection of 6-OHDA or tunicamycin produces a slow increase of rod precursor proliferation in both retinas. Similarly, a variety of consensual retinal effects have been described in humans. In particular, changes in retinal sensitivity during light adaptation. (Denny et al., 1991; Auerbach et al., 1992).

These interocular effects may be essential for matching the inputs from both eyes to higher visual centers so that the eyes could function cooperatively (Schütte, 1995). We propose a similar explanation for the consensual response in spinule formation. Finally, our data must serve as a cautionary reminder that for many experimental manipulations of the eye, the fellow eye cannot serve as a control.

To explain this interocular phenomenon, we can consider three possibilities (De Juan and García, 1998): first, there is a direct interaction between both eyes mediated by the centrifugal fibers. Second, we cannot rule out the possibility that intraocular injection of drugs may cause the release of a diffusible, blood-borne factor, which acts on spinule formation and dissolution. In a similar way, a humoral mechanism for explaining a contralateral effect in RMM has been suggested (Ali, 1975). This factor when released into the circulatory system can perhaps produce the same effects in the untreated retina as in the treated. For instance, the factor could activate higher visual pathways which project through centrifugal fibers to the contralateral retina (Negishi et al., 1991). Third, the possibility exists that drugs injected intraocularly may be transported by the blood and cause, in a humoral way, the same effects on spinule formation in the contralateral retina as in the treated. Although we cannot completely rule out this explanation, our data suggest that it is unlikely. In effect, the injection of Cytochalasin D into the right eye prevents the normal contraction of the cones during light adaptation. However, in the left untreated eye, the cones contract normally like in retinas from control light-adapted fish (De Juan and García, 1998). Furthermore, the injection of DA in the dark into an eye induces the normal contraction of the cones as in light adaptation. In contrast, in the contralateral, untreated eye, the cones elongated normally, as in retinas from control dark-adapted fish. Contralateral effects of 6-OHDA intraocular injections, are not attributable to the 6-OHDA transported by the blood to the untreated eye. In effect, while the treated eye shows a loss of TOH-IR, the contralateral untreated eye is not directly affected by the drug as evidenced by the presence of TOH-IR in this eye.

The possibility remains that the threshold concentration for the effect of drugs on cone contraction is higher than for the effect on spinule formation. We do not believe that this is likely. This is because the drug concentration in the blood stream is diluted to a level below that of the least effective concentration, since the volume of blood in fish is about 0.03 ml/g (Randall, 1970). Hence, drugs would be diluted to a concentration 300 times lower.

Conclusion and future perspectives

The spinules of HCs appeared probably 300 millions years ago in teleost fish. They were observed for the first time by Stell in 1966 in *Carassius auratus*. In 1980, Wagner presented the first complete description of these curious processes. In the last twenty years, about a hundred of papers have described several aspects of the structure and function of spinules, yet their role is still uncertain. We can summarize the state of our knowledge of spinules in the following ways:

(1) Spinules and nematosomes of HCs are retinal structures exclusive to teleost fish. In our opinion, these structures represent the over-expression of a more general process normally not detectable in other cells. The functions of the spinules are still not well known today.

(2) The feedback transmission from cone HCs to pedicles of cones through sign-inverting synapses does not need the integrity of optic nerve fibers and works in isolated retinas. However, the formation and dissolution of spinules need a central control through centrifugal fibers, probably by means of GnRH and and FMRF-amide peptide. There is no formation and dissolution of HC spinules in isolated retinas.

(3) Dopamine release from DA-IPCs is probably stimulated by GnRH and contributes to spinule formation. However, DA is not the only factor responsible for triggering spinule formation.

(4) We have observed that the more predatorial a fish is and the less clear its underwater environment, the more cone RMM, spinules in light adaptation, and large nematosomes in dark adaptation occur.

(5) HCs spinules are required neither for wavelength discrimination nor for the transmission of photopic-luminosity signals through the

534

ON pathway of the retina. Spinules could help the retina to deal with noise without missing relevant clues from the visual world, most prominently, occlusion boundaries between objects.

(6) Finally, we think that the spinule's electron-dense material originates in nematosomes, which represent a ribonucleoprotein storage needed for the modulation of spinule synapses.

Concerning nematosomes, our starting point is the thought that they represent morphological expressions of storage of ribonucleoproteins related to the spinule densities. As has been argued by Steward (1995), an important aspect of neuronal function involves the delivery of mRNAs to subcellular domains. The specialized region of cytoplasm that lies beneath the postsynaptic membrane is one such subcellular domain. In this way, neurons may sort mRNA into different subcellular domains using the same mechanisms that are employed during embryonic differentiation to establish polarity. In the case of neurons, it is clear that some of the dendritically localized mRNAs encode proteins that are important for synaptic junction and that they play a role in intercellular signalling cascades and synaptic plasticity.

Acknowledgments

We wish to thank Dr. Norberto M. Grzywacz for improving the English. This research was supported by DGICYT PB-96–0414 to JDJ.

References

Ali, M.A. (1975) Retinomotor responses. In: Ali, M.A. (Ed.), "Vision in Fishes". Plenum, New York, pp. 313–355.

Anzil, A.P., Herrlinger, H. and Blinzinger, K. (1973) Nucleolus-like in neuronal perikarya and processes: phase and electron microscope observations on the hypothalamus of the mouse. Z. Zellforsch, 146: 329–337.

Auerbach, E., Dörrenhaus, A. and Cavonius, C.R. (1992) Changes in sensitivity of the dark-adapted eye during concurrent light adaptation of the other eye. Vis. Neurosci., 8: 359–363.

Balboa, R.M. and Grzywacz, N.M. (2000) The role of early retinal lateral inhibition: More than maximizing luminance information. Vis. Neurosci., 17: 77–89.

Baldridge, W.H. and Ball, A.K. (1994) Spinules: a case for retinal synaptic plasticity. TINS, 17: 6–7.

Behrens, U.D., Wagner, H.J. and Kirsch, M. (1992) cAMP-mediated second messenger mechanisms are involved in spinule formation in teleost cone horizontal cells. Neurosci. Lett., 147: 93–96.

Behrens, U.D. Douglas, R.H. and Wagner, H.J. (1993) Gonadotropin-releasing hormone, a neuropeptide of efferent projections to the teleost retina induces light-adaptive spinule formation on horizontal cell dendrites in dark-adapted preparations kept in vitro. Neurosci. Lett., 164: 59–62.

Burnside, B., Adler, R.A. and O'Connor, P. (1982) Pigment migration in the teleost retinal pigment epithelium: I. Roles for actin and microtubules in pigment granule transport and cone movement. Invest. Ophtalmol. Vis. Sci., 24: 1–15.

Burnside, B. and Nagle, B. (1983) Retinomotor movements of photoreceptors and retinal pigment epithelium: mechanisms and regulation. In: Osborn N. and Chader G. (Eds.), "Progress in Retinal Research", Vol. 2, Pergamon, Oxford, pp. 67–109.

Callard, G.V., Kruger, A. and Betka, M. (1995) The goldfish as a model for studying neuroestrogen synthesis, localization, and action in the brain and visual system. Environ. Health Perspect., 103(7): 51–57.

Casella, J.F., Flanagan, M.D. and Lin, S. (1981) Cytochalasin-D inhibits actin polymerization and induces depolymerization of actin filaments formed during platelet cell shape change. Nature, 293: 302–305.

Crick, R. (1982) Do dendritic spines twitch? TINS, 5: 44–46.

De Juan, J. and Dowling, J.E. (1987) Structural Changes in photoreceptor terminals and horizontal cells in the White perch following prolonged dark adaptation. Invest. Ophthalmol. Vis. Sci., (Suppl.) 28(3): 238.

De Juan, J., Iñiguez, C. and Dowling, J.E. (1990) Influence of dopamine on spinules, synaptic ribbons and nematosomes in white perch retina. Invest. Ophthalmol. Vis. Sci., (Suppl. 31): 333.

De Juan, J., Iñiguez. and Dowling, J.E. (1991) Nematosomes in external horizontal cells of white perch (Roccus americana) retina: changes during dark and light adaptation. Brain Res., 546: 176–180.

De Juan, J., García, M. and Cuenca, N. (1996) Formation and dissolution of spinules and changes in nematosome size require optic nerve integrity in black bass (Micropterus salmoides) retina. Brain Res., 707: 213–220.

De Juan, J. and García, M. (1998) Interocular effect of actin depolymerization on spinule formation in teleost retina. Brain Res., 792: 173–177.

Dearry, A. and Burnside, B. (1986) Dopaminergic regulation of cone retinomotor movement in isolated teleost retinas. I. Induction of cone contraction is mediated by D2 receptors. J. Neurochem., 46: 1006–1021.

Dearry, A. and Barlow, R.B. (1987) Circadian rhythms in the green sunfish retina. J. Gen. Physiol., 89: 745–770.

Denny N., Frumkes, T.E., Barris, M.C. and Eysteinsson, T. (1991) Tonic interocular supression and bionocular summation in human vision. J. Physiol., 437: 449–460.

Djamgoz, M.B.A., Downing, J.E.G. and Wagner, H.J. (1985a) The cellular origin of an unusual type of S-potential: an intracellular horseradish peroxidase study in a cyprinid retina. *J. Neurocytol.*, 14: 469–486.

Djamgoz, M.B.A., Downing, J.E.G., Prince, D.J. and Wagner, H.J. (1985b) Physiological and ultrastructural evidence for light-dependent plasticity of cone photoreceptor horizontal cell feed-back interactions in the isolated retinas of cyprinid fish. *J Physiol.*, 362: 20.

Djamgoz, M.B.A., Downing, J.E.G., Kirsch, M., Prince, D.J. and Wagner, H.J. (1988) Plasticity of cone horizontal cell function in cyprinid fish retina: effects of background illumination of moderate intensity. *J. Neurocytol.*, 17: 701–710.

Djamgoz, M.B.A., Kirsch, M. and Wagner, H.J. (1989) Haloperidol suppresses light-induced spinule formation and biphasic responses of horizontal cells in fish (roach) retina. *Neurosci. Lett.*, 107: 200–204.

Douglas, R.H. and Wagner, H.J. (1982) Endogenous patterns of photomechanical movements in teleosts: their relation to activity rhythms. *Cell Tissue Res.*, 226: 133–144.

Douglas, R.H. and Wagner, H.J. (1983) Endogenous control of spinule formation in horizontal cells of the teleost retina. *Cell Tissue Res.*, 229: 443–449.

Dowling, J.E. and Ehinger, B. (1975) Synaptic organization of the amine-containing interplexiform cells of the goldfish and Cebus monkey retinas. *Science*, 188: 270–273.

Dowling, J.E. and Ehinger, B. (1978) The interplexiform cell system. I. Synapses of the dopaminergic neurons of the goldfish retina. *Proc. Roy. Soc. Lond.*, 201: 7–26.

Dowling, J.E. (1986) Dopamine: a retinal modulator? *TINS*, 9: 236–240.

Dowling, J.E. (1987) In xxx *The retina. An approachable part of the brain.* Harvard University Press, Cambridge, M.A., pp. 48.

Dowling, J.E. (1989) Neuromodulation in the retina: the role of dopamine. *Sem. Neurosci.*, 1: 35–43.

Dowling, J.E (1991) Retinal neuromodulation: the role of dopamine. *Vis. Neurosci.*, 7: 87–97.

Downing, J.E.G. and Djamgoz, M.B.A. (1989) Quantitative analysis of cone photoreceptor-horizontal cell connectivity patterns in the retina of a cyprinid fish: electron microscopy of functionally identified and HRP-labelled horizontal cells. *J. Comp. Neurol.*, 289: 537–553.

Ehinger, B., Falck, B. and Laties, A.M. (1969) Adrenergic neurons in teleost retina. *Z. Zellforsch. Mikrosk. Anat.*, 97: 285–297.

Fechner, F. (1986) Nucleolus-like bodies in the pineal gland of the Djungarian hamster (*Phodopus sungorus*). *Cell Tissue Res.*, 243: 441–443.

Fifková, I. and Delay, R.J. (1982) Cytoplasmic-actin in neuronal processes as a possible mediator of synaptic plasticity. *J. Cell Biol.*, 95: 345–350.

Fischer, M., Kaech, S., Knutti, D. and Matus, A. (1998) Rapid actin-based plasticity in dendritic spines. *Neuron*, 20: 847–854.

García, M., Guardiola, J.V. and De Juan, J. (1998a) Plasticity of synaptic ribbon and synaptic vesicle densityafter short-term dark-adaptation. *Ophthal. Res.*, 30(S1): 16.

García, M., Guardiola, J.V. and De Juan J. (1998b) Plasticity of synaptic ribbon and synaptic vesicle density in photoreceptor terminals of two teleost species. *Invest. Opthalmol. Vis. Sci.*, (Suppl.) 39(4): S1058.

García, M. and De Juan, J. (1999) Fine structure of the retina of black bass, *Micropterus salmoides*, (Centrarchidae, teleostei). *Histol. Histopathol.*, 14(1999): 1053–1065.

Greenstreet, E.H. and Djamgoz, M.B.A. (1994) Nitric oxide induces light-adaptive morphological changes in retinal neurones. *Neuroreport*, 6(1): 109–112.

Grillo, M.A. (1970) Cytoplasmic inclusions resembling nucleoli in sympathetic neurons of adults rats. *J. Cell Biol.*, 45: 100–117.

Halkka, L. and Halkka, O. (1975) Accumulation of gene products in the oocytes of the dragonfly Crodulia aenea L. I. The nematosomes. *J. Cell Sci.*, 19, 103–115.

Halpain, S. (2000) Actin and the agile spine: how and why do dendritic spines dance? *TINS*, 23(4): 141–146.

Hámory, J. and Lakos, I. (1980) Ultrastructural alterations in the initial segments and in the recurrent collateral terminals of Purkinje cells following axotomy. *Cell Tissue Res.*, 212: 415–427.

Hindelang-Gertner, C., Stoeckel, M.E., Porte, A., Dellman, H.D. and Madarász, B. (1974). *Cell Tissue Res.*, 155: 211–219.

Kato, S., Ishita, S., Mawatari, K., Matsukawa, T. and Negishi, K. (1990) Dopamine release via protein kinase C activation in the fish retina. *J. Neurochem.*, 54: 2082–2090.

Katoth, Y. and Shimizu, N. (1982) The light and electron microscopic localization of intracytoplasmic nucleolus-like bodies in the mouse brain stained by Holmes' silver method. *Arch. Histol. Jap.*, 45: 325–333.

Kind, P.C., Kelly, G.M., Fryer, H.J.L., Blakemore, C. and Hockfieldf, S. (1997) Phospholipase C-beta 1 is present in the botryosome, an intermediate compartment-like organelle, and is regulated by visual experience in cat visual cortex. *J. Neurosci.*, 17(4): 1471–1480.

Kirsch, M., Wagner, H.J. and Djamgoz, M.B.A. (1988) Dopamine and plasticity of horizontal cell function in teleost retina: regulation of a spectral mechanism through D1-receptors. *Brain Res.*, 31: 401–412.

Kirsch, M., Djamgoz, M.B.A. and Wagner, H.J. (1990) Correlation of spinule dynamics and plasticity of the horizontal cell spectral response in cyprinid fish retina: quantitative analysis. *Cell Tissue Res.*, 260: 123–130.

Kirsch, M., Wagner, H.J. and Djamgoz, M.B.A. (1991) Dopamine and plasticity of horizontal cell function in the teleost retina: regulation of a spectral mechanism through D1-receptors. *Vision Res.*, 31: 401–412.

Köhler, K. and Weiler, R. (1990) Dopaminergic modulation of transient neurite outgrowth from horizontal cells of the fish retina is not mediated by cAMP. *Eur. J. Neurosci.*, 2: 788–794.

536

Köhler, K., Zrenner, E. and Weiler, R. (1995) Ethambutol alters spinule-type synaptic connections and induces morphologic alterations in the cone pedicles of the fish retina. *Invest.Ophthalmol. Vis. Sci.*, 36(6): 1046–1055.

Kröger, R.H.H. and Wagner, H.J. (1996) Horizontal cell spinule dynamics in fish are affected by rearing in monochromatic light. *Vision Res.*, 36(24): 3879–3890.

Kurz-Isler, G., Voigt, T. and Wolburg, H. (1992) Modulation of connexon densities in gap junctions of horizontal cell perikarya and axon terminals in fish retina: effects of light/dark cycles, interruption of the optic nerve and application of dopamine. *Cell Tissue Res.*, 268: 267–275.

Le Beux, Y.N. (1972) An ultrastructural study of a cytoplasmic filamentous body, termed nematosome, in the neurons of the rat and cat substantia nigra. *Z. Zellforsch.*, 133: 289–325.

Leranth, C., Sakamoto, H., MacLusky, N.J., Shanabrough, M. and Naftolin, F. (1985) Estrogen responsive cells in the arcuate nucleus of the rat contain glutamic acid decarboxylase (GAD): an electron microscopic immunocytochemical study. *Brain Res.*, 331(2): 376–381.

Leranth, C., Shanabrough, M. and Naftolin, F. (1991) Estrogen induces ultrastructural changes in progesterone receptor-containing GABA neurons of the primate hypothalamus. *Neuroendocrinol.*, 54(6): 571–579.

Li, L. and Dowling, J.E. (1998) Olfactory inputs are required for normal visual funciton in zebrafish. *Invest. Ophthalmol. Vis. Sci.*, (Suppl.) 39(4): S433.

Li, S.H., Gutekunst, C.A., Hersch, S.M. and Li, X.J. (1998) Association of HAP1 Isoforms with a Unique Cytoplasmic structure. *J. Neurochem.*, 71: 2178–2185.

Münz, H., Class, B., Stumpf, W.E. and Jennes, L. (1982) Centrifugal innervation of the retina by luteinizing hormone releasing hormone (LHRH-immunoreactive telencephalic neurons in teleostean fishes). *Cell Tissue Res.*, 222: 313–323.

Negishi, K., Stell, W.K., Teranishi, T., Karkhanis, A., Owusu-Yaw, V. and Takasaki, Y. (1991) Induction of proliferating cell nuclear antigen (PCNA)-immunoreactive cells in goldfish retina following intravitreal injection with 6-hydroxydopamine. *Cell. Mol, Neurobiol.*, 11: 639–659.

Ockleford, C.D., Nevard, C.H.F., Indans, I. and Jones, C.J.P. (1987) Structure and function of the nematosome, *J. Cell Sci.*, 87:27–44.

O'Connor, P.M. and Burnside, B. (1982) Elevation of cyclic AMP activates an actin-dependent contraction in teleost retinal rods. *J. Cell. Biol.*, 95: 445–452.

Okada, T., Schultz, K., Geurtz, W., Hatt, H. and Weiler, R. (1999) AMPA-preferring receptors with high Ca2+ permeability mediate dendritic plasticity of retinal horizontal cells. *Eur. J. Neurosci.*, 11(3): 1085–1095.

Owusu-Yaw, V., Kyle, A.L. and Stell, W.K. (1992) Effects of lesions of the optic nerve, optic tectum and nervus terminalis on rod precursor proliferation in the goldfish retina. *Brain Res.*, 576: 220–230.

Pottek, M., Schultz, K. and Weiler, R. (1997) Effects of nitric oxide on the horizontal cell network and dopamine release in the carp retina. *Vision Res.*, 37(9): 1091–1102.

Ramón y Cajal, S. (1892) La rétine des vertebrés. *La Cellule*, 9: 119–257.

Randall, D.J. (1970) The circulatory system. In: Hoar, W.S. and Randall, D.J. (Eds.), *Fish Physiology*. Academic Press, London, pp. 133–172.

Raynauld, J.P., Laviolette, J.R. and Wagner, H.J. (1979) Goldfish retina: a correlate between cone activity and morphology of the horizontal cell in cone pedicles. *Science*, 204: 1436–1438.

Repérant, J., Miceli, D., Vesselkin, N.P. and Molotchnikoff, S. (1989) The centrifugal visual system of vertebrates: a centuries-old search reviewed. *Int. Rev. Cytol.*, 118: 115–171.

Santolaya, R.C. (1973) Nucleolus-like bodies in the neuronal cytoplasm of the mouse arcuate nucleus. *Z. Zellforsch.*, 146: 318–328.

Schmitz, Y. and Köhler, K. (1993) Spinule formation in the fish retina: is there an involvement of actin and tubulin? An electromicroscopic immunogold study. *J. Neurocytol.*, 22: 205–214.

Schütte, M. (1995) Centrifugal innervation of the rat retina. *Vis. Neurosci.*, 12: 1083–1092.

Stell, W.K., Walker, S.E., Chohan, K.S. and Ball, A.K. (1984) The goldfish nervus terminalis: a luteinizing hormone-releasing hormone and molluscan cardioexcitatory peptide immunoreactive olfactoretinal pathway. *Proc. Natl. Acad. Sci. USA*, 81: 940–944.

Stell, W.K., Walker, S.E. and Ball, A.K. (1987) Functional-anatomical studies in the terminal nerve projection to the retina of bony fishes. *Ann. NY. Acad. Sci.*, 519: 80–96.

Steward, O. (1995) Targeting of mRNAs to subsynaptic microdomains in dendrites. *Curr. Opin. Neurobiol.*, 5: 55–61.

Ter-Margarian, A. and Djamgoz, M.B.A. (1992) Cytochalasin inhibits light-dependent synaptic plasticity of horizontal cells in teleost retina. *Neurosci. Lett.*, 147: 131–135.

Umino, O. and Dowling, J.E. (1991) Dopamine release from interplexiform cells in the retina: effects of GnRH, FMRFamide, bicuculline and enkephalin on horizontal cell activity. *J. Neurosci.*, 11: 3034–3046.

Van Rossum, D. and Hanisch, U.K. (1999) Cytoskeletal dynamics in dendritic spines: direct modulation by glutamate receptors? *TINS*, 22(7): 290–295.

Wagner, H.J. (1980) Light-dependent plasticity of the morphology of horizontal cell terminals in cone pedicles of fish retinas. *J. Neurocytol.*, 9: 573–590.

Wagner, H.J. and Speck, P.T. (1983) Ein mikrocomputergestütztes System zur graphischen Rekonstruktion von Serienschnitten. *Verh. Anat. Ges. Fena.*, 77: 187–188.

Wagner, H.J. and Douglas, R.H. (1983) Morphologic changes in teleost primary and secondary retinal cells folowing brief exposure to light. *Invest. Ophthalmol. Vis. Sci.*, 24: 24–29.

Wagner, H.J. (1990) Retinal structure of fishes. In: Ron. H. Douglas and Mustafa B.A. Djamgoz (Eds.), *The visual system of fish*, Chapman and Hall, pp. 109–157.

Wagner, H.J., Behrens, U.D., Zaunreiter, M. and Douglas, R.H. (1992) The circadian component of spinule dynamics in teleost retinal horizontal cells is dependent on the dopaminergic system. *Vis. Neurosci.*, 9: 345–351.

Wagner, H.J. and Djamgoz, M.B.A. (1993) Spinules: a case for retinal synaptic plasticity. *TINS*, 16: 201–206.

Wagner, H.J. and Djamgoz, M.B.A. (1994) Spinules: a case for retinal synaptic plasticity. *TINS*, 17: 7–8.

Walker, S. and Stell, W.K. (1986) Gonadotropin-releasing hormone (GnRH), molluscan cardioexcitatory peptide (FMRF)amide), enkephalin and related neruopeptides affect goldfish retinal ganglion cell activity. *Brain Res.*, 384: 262–273.

Weiler, R. and Wagner, H.J. (1984) Light-dependent change of cone horizontal cell interactions in carp retina. *Brain Res.*, 298: 1–9.

Weiler, R., Köhler, K., Kirsch, M., and Wagner, H.J. (1988) Glutamate and dopamine modulate synaptic plasticity in horizontal cell dendrites of fish retina. *Neurosci. Lett.*, 87: 205–209.

Weiler, R., Köhler, K. and Janssen-Bienhold, U. (1991) Protein kinase C mediates transient spinule-type neurite outgrowth in the retina during light adaptation. *Proc. Natl. Acad. Sci. USA*, 88: 3603–3607.

Weiler, R. and Janssen-Bienhold, U. (1993) Spinule-type neurite outgrowth from horizontal cells during light adaptation in the carp retina: an actin-dependent process. *J. Neurocytol.*, 22: 129–139.

Weiler, R. (1994) Spinules: a case for retinal synaptic plasticity. *TINS*, 17(1): 6.

Weiler, R., Schultz, K. and Janssen-Bienhold, U. (1995) Dendrites during dark adaptation involves the activation of Ca-2+/Calmodulin-dependent Protein Kinase II. *Eur. J. Neurosci.*, 7(9): 1914–1919.

Weiler, R., Schultz, K. and Janssen-Bienhold, U. (1996) Ca-2+-dependency of spinule plasticity at dendrites of retinal horizontal cells and its possible implication for the functional role of spinules. *Vision Res.*, 36(24): 3891–3900.

Weiler, R., Schultz, K., Pottek, M., Tieding, S. and Janssen-Bienhold, U. (1998) Retinoic acid has light-adaptive effects on horizontal cells in the retina. *Proc. Natl. Acad. Sci. USA*, 95(12): 7139–7144.

Wietsma, J.J., Kamermans, M. and Spekreijse, H. (1995) Horizontal cells function normally in ethambutol-treated goldfish. *Vision Res.*, 35(12): 1667–1674.

Woodford, B.J. and Blanks, J.C. (1989) Localization of actin and tubulin in developing and adult mammalian photoreceptors. *Cell Tissue Res.*, 256: 495–505.

Wu, S.M. (1991) Input-Output relations of the feedback synapse between horizontal cells and cones in the tiger salamander retina. *J. Neurophysiol.*, 65: 1197–1206.

Wu, S.M. (1992) Feedback connections and operation of the outer plexiform layer of the retina. *Curr. Opin. Neurobiol.*, 2: 462–468.

Yazulla, S. and Studholme, K.M. (1995) Volume transmission of dopamine may modulate light-adaptive plasticity of horizontal cell dendrites in the recovery phase following dopamine depletion in goldfish retina. *Vis. Neurosci.*, 12: 827–836.

Yazulla, S. and Lin, Z.S. and Studholme, K.M. (1996) Dopaminergic control of light-adaptive synaptic plasticity and role in goldfish visual behavior. *Vision Res.*, 36: 4045–4057.

Zucker, C.L. and Dowling, J.E. (1987) Centrifugal fibres synapse on dopaminergic interplexiform cells in the teleost retina. *Nature*, 300: 166–168.

SECTION VI

Retinal development and genetics

H. Kolb, H. Ripps and S. Wu (Eds.)
Progress in Brain Research, Vol. 131

CHAPTER 38

Understanding retinal cell fate determination through genetic manipulations

James M. Fadool*

Department of Biological Science and Program in Neuroscience, Florida State University, 235 Biomedical Research Facility, Tallahassee, FL 32306-4340, USA

The histology, physiology and biochemistry of the retina are strikingly conserved among most classes of vertebrate (Grun, 1982; Dowling, 1987). Not surprising, therefore, were the observations that development of the retina also proceed in very similar manners. The eye develops from no less than three distinct embryological tissues, neuroectoderm, skin ectoderm, and head mesenchyme of neural crest cell origin, through highly coordinated, inductive interactions. Today, the molecular basis of the inductive interactions is being elucidated through the cloning and analysis of genes based upon the gene expression patterns and the analysis of mutations affecting development. This chapter will provide an introduction to the molecular embryology regulating the development of the vertebrate neural retina with particular emphasis on current genetic strategies using the zebrafish as a model organism.

Early embryonic development

The development of the neural retina originates during the early stages of neurulation (Coulombre, 1965; Jean et al., 1998). Following specification of the eye field, bilateral protrusions within the forebrain mark the initiation of morphogenesis of the optic vesicles. The optic vesicles continue to extend towards the surface ectoderm inducing the formation of the lens placodes (Fig. 1). Through reciprocal interactions, the distal region of optic vesicle invaginates, and the lateral portions constrict forming the bilayered optic cup that remains attached to the forebrain via the optic stalk. The neural retina and the retinal pigment epithelium (RPE) differentiate from the inner and outer layers of the optic cup respectively. The margins of the optic cup differentiate into the ciliary apparatus and posterior iris. The stalk, initially functions as a pathway for ganglion cell axon outgrowth, and later provides the progenitors for glia of the optic nerve.

Experimental embryology has demonstrated a great deal of plasticity in the developmental potential of the regions of the optic cup (Detwiler and Van Dyke, 1953, 1954; Coulombre, 1965; Guillemot and Cepko, 1992; Pittack et al., 1997; Hyer et al., 1998; Nguyen and Arnheiter, 2000). Differentiation of the neural retina and RPE from the optic vesicle requires contact with the head ectoderm and neural crest-derived mesenchyme respectively. Following the removal of the overlying skin ectoderm, the distal region of the optic cup differentiates into pigmented epithelium. Likewise, if the optic vesicle is removed from the embryo and adjacent ectoderm or surrounded with head mesenchyme, a pigmented epithelium forms. Later in development, loss of signaling from the lens results in abnormal development of the neural retina. The genetic disorder resulting in the loss of eyes in the blind cavefish has been attributed

* Tel.: 850-644-3550; Fax: 850-644-0989;
E-mail: jfadool@bio.fsu.edu

542

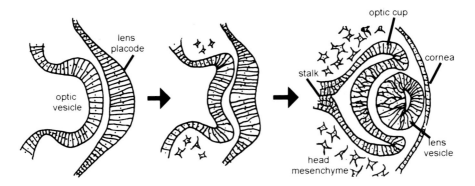

Fig. 1. Diagram of the steps in the development of the optic cup. **A.** Induction of the lens placode by the optic vesicle. **B.** Reciprocal interactions leading to invagination of the optic cup and lens vesicle. **C.** The neural epithelium of the optic cup develops into the neural retina, retinal pigmented epithelium, ciliary apparatus and glial cells of the optic nerve.

to defective signaling between the lens and the retina (Yamamoto et al., 2000). The deficit can be rescued by grafting head ectoderm from wild type into blind cavefish embryos.

The RPE also retains some degree of plasticity to differentiate as neural retina. In amphibians, grafting the otic vesicle or the nasal placode behind the eye can induce a secondary neural retina from the pigmented epithelium and the RPE can transdifferentiate into a neural retina following ablation of the neural retina (Detwiler and Van Dyke, 1953, 1954; Coulombre, 1965). Thus, the induction and maintenance of the neural versus pigmented epithelial cell fate arises from local cellular interactions. However, when most of the early embryological manipulations were conducted little was known about the molecules involved in these events and the molecular tools were not yet available.

Recent experiments indicate that fibroblast growth factors are important to the induction of neural retina from the neuroepithelium (Guillemot and Cepko, 1992; Hyer et al., 1998). Both FGF1 and FGF2 are expressed in the skin ectoderm and their receptors are expressed in the developing optic vesicle. FGF8 is temporally expressed in the distal part of the optic vesicle at the time of contact with the skin ectoderm (Vogel-Hopker et al., 2000). Experimentally, FGF can replace the neural retinal-inducing signal although the rescue of morphogenesis is incomplete (Pittack et al., 1997; Hyer et al., 1998; Nguyen and Arnheiter, 2000). In the chick embryo, following removal of the skin ectoderm, normal differentiation of the neural retina can be maintained by transplantation of FGF secreting cells or infection

of the surrounding tissue with an FGF retrovirus vector. In vitro, application of FGF neutralizing antibodies blocks differentiation of the neural retina demonstrating that FGFs are indeed necessary for induction to occur.

The exposure of RPE to FGFs in vitro or ectopic application of FGFs in vivo results in transdifferentiation into neural retina. Both the nasal placode and optic vesicle are potent sources of FGFs explaining the induction of neural tissue from the RPE (Detwiler and Van Dyke, 1953, 1954; Coulombre, 1965). The mode of action of FGFs in partitioning the optic primordia into RPE and neural retina is thought to be through the down regulation of expression of the transcription factor *Mitf* in the distal optic vesicle, while *Mitf* expression is maintained in the RPE and head mesenchyme (Nguyen and Arnheiter, 2000). Mutations of *Mitf* (mouse microphthalmia, *Mi*) results in poorly developed eyes stemming from alterations in the RPE (Graw, 1996). It has also been proposed that signaling by BMP7 or related members of the transforming growth factor beta family antagonize endogenous FGFs, inhibits neural induction and permits differentiation as RPE. It would be interesting to examine if the competence of some tissues to form ectopic retina and lens structures following misexpression of *Rx-Six* gene family members or *Pax-6* is somehow biased to regions of the neural tube exposed to an endogenous source of those growth factors (Oliver and Gruss, 1997; Jean et al., 1998).

The most proximal parts of the optic vesicle give rise to the optic stalk, an embryological structure with a fate clearly different than that of the neural retina and RPE. Expression of the paired-domain transcription factor *Pax-2* is thought to be an important step in the positioning of the optic stalk and optic nerve relative to the neural retina and RPE (Macdonald et al., 1995; Masai et al., 2000). Mutation of *Pax-2* in mouse, zebrafish (*Noi*) and humans results in expansion of the neural retina and RPE into the optic stalk leading to colobomas. Experimentally, the over expression of *Pax-2* in zebrafish embryos leads to an expansion of ventral midline structures and a decrease in the size of the retina. *Pax-2* expression is regulated in part by ventral midline signaling with one of the key regulators being *sonic hedgehog* (*shh*). *Shh* is a potent signaling molecule for pattern formation in numerous systems including the neural tube and limb bud. Mice or zebrafish homozygous for the null mutation in *shh* and zebrafish homozygous for either the *cyclops*, *squint* or *one eyed pinhead* mutations, which disrupt signaling in the ventral midline, display a dramatic reduction of *Pax-2* gene product (Masai et al., 2000). Over expression of *shh* in zebrafish embryos results in an expansion of the expression domain of *Pax-2* into the optic cup at the expense of expression of *Pax-6* (Macdonald et al., 1995; Masai et al., 2000). Thus, in vertebrate embryogenesis, mid-line signaling acts to position the expression domain of *Pax-2* such that *Pax-2* and *Pax-6* partition the optic vesicle into proximal (optic stalk) and distal (retinal) structures.

Retinal progenitor cells

Following the induction of a neural fate, the cells of the inner layer of the optic cup, called neuroblasts, continue to divide forming a multilayered neuro-epithelium that differentiates into all retinal cells. During the process of neurogenesis, several hurdles must be overcome, namely, the genesis of the appropriate ratio of cells, migration of cells to the appropriate laminar position within the epithelium and establishment of the synaptic connections with neighboring cells. Most current models suggest that at the first stage in the process, local extracellular signals act upon the cells to either direct or inhibit a particular cell fate. Simultaneously, intrinsic properties of the progenitor cells change with the effect

that, over developmental time, the potential of the neuroblasts become restricted to fewer cell fates (Belliveau and Cepko, 1999; Cepko, 1999; Adler, 2000; Belliveau et al., 2000; Perron and Harris, 2000).

Titiated-thymidine incorporation has demonstrated a relationship between the timing of terminal mitosis (birth date) and cell fate (Sidman, 1961; Kahn, 1974; Carter-Dawson and LaVail, 1979; Stiemke and Hollyfield, 1995). In all species examined, the initial post-mitotic cells differentiate as ganglion cells. Other early cell types include horizontal cells, cones, and amacrine cells, while rods, Muller glia and bipolar cells are born last. As in other regions of the brain, retrovirus vectors, lineage-tracking dyes and embryo chimeras have conclusively demonstrated that retinal cells are generated by a lineage-independent mechanism (Price et al., 1987; Turner and Cepko, 1987; Holt et al., 1988; Wetts et al., 1989; Turner et al., 1990). Retinal progenitors can generate combinations of neurons, photoreceptor cells and Muller glia. Even very late in development, individual progenitors maintain the potential to give rise to clones of as few as two cells containing neurons and glia. These data argue against a stem cell population for each cell type, but suggest that environmental signals act upon progenitors cells to direct cell fate. The knowledge that the seven major classes are generated in sequential pattern, enables the search for molecular regulators of neurogenesis.

Lateral inhibition through the Notch-Delta pathway may play a general role in the production of neuronal diversity by timing the differentiation of neuroblast. In the retina, expression of the *Notch* and the ligands encoded by the *Delta* and *Jagged* gene families are spatially and temporally related, with overlapping domains first in the central retina and as neurogenesis continues becoming restricted to the retinal margins (Perron et al., 1998; see Perron and Harris, 2000). Transfection of an activated Notch receptor into retinoblasts inhibit their normal differentiation into mature neurons. Conversely, over-expression of a dominant negative form of Delta pushes cells into a differentiated state. The Notch signaling pathway has been implicated as a factor in ganglion cell differentiation (Austin et al., 1995). Diminishing Notch expression in chick retinoblast early in cell fate determination leads to an increase in the number of differentiating ganglion cells.

Conversely, activation of Notch signaling decreases the number of ganglion cells. It is likely, however, that Notch signaling is involved in the generation of all retinal neurons not just ganglion cells. The release from the Notch-signaling early in development should yield ganglion cells or amacrine cells while release from inhibition at later stages of development should generate bipolar cells or rods.

One exception to this pattern may be in the generation of radial glia. Endogenous Notch protein continues to be expressed in radial glial fibers of the central nervous system including radial glia of the developing forebrain and Muller glia of the retina (Furukawa et al., 2000; Giano et al., 2000). The role of Notch signaling in promoting radial glia identity was examined by over expression of constitutively active Notch in the embryonic forebrain and retina using retrovirus vectors (Bao and Cepko, 1997; Furukawa et al., 2000; Giano et al., 2000). In these studies, virus-infected cells had a morphology and gene expression profile consistent with radial glial phenotypes. Expression of *Hes1*, a basic helix-loop-helix transcription factor and a down-stream effector of Notch signaling, produces similar results. Surprisingly, Muller glia are one of the last cell types born in the retina and differentiation requires cell-to-cell interactions with neurons (Linser and Moscona, 1979) while radial glia of the forebrain are one of the first cell types present. Thus, in addition to inhibiting neuronal differentiation, Notch signaling appears to promote a radial glial phenotype (also see section below).

Regulators of neurogenesis

The specific cellular and environmental factors (intrinsic versus extrinsic factors) that influence cell fate continue to be the subject of intense investigation. In vitro analysis has been one method for examining the action of putative ligands in cell fate determination (Watanabe and Raff, 1990, 1992; Altshuler and Cepko, 1992). Under various culture conditions, specific ligands have been attributed with the differentiation of specific cell types. Laminin and FGFs have ben found to promote the differentiation of ganglion cells (Guillemot and Cepko, 1992). FGF-2, taurine and retinoic acid appear to influence rod

cell differentiation while thyroid hormone may induce a cone fate (Altshuler et al., 1993; Kelley et al., 1994; Kelley et al., 1995; Levine et al., 2000b). It has also been considered that in the absence of environmental signals, the cells will adopt a default pathway (Adler, 2000).

Just as some environmental signals may induce neuroblasts to adopt a specific cell fate, progenitor cells or newly post-mitotic cells may be inhibited from adopting a particular cell fate. Several lines of evidence indicate a feed back mechanism by which differentiated neurons produce a signal to inhibit neighboring cells from expressing a similar fate. It would follow that removal or dilution of the feed back signals would result in overproduction of the class of cell producing that signal. Waid and McLoon (1998) demonstrated that in coculture experiments, ganglion cells from older retina secrete factors that cause progenitors in younger population to produce other cell types. Feedback inhibition was also proposed for the regulating amacrine cell number (Belliveau and Cepko, 1999). In the amphibian, which maintains a modest capacity to regenerate the neural retina, the experimental ablation of tyrosine-hydroxylase containing amacrine cells with the neurotoxin 6-hydroxydopamine (Reh and Tulley, 1986), leads to a higher density of new tyrosine hydroxylase containing cells at the retinal margin. Thus, there exists a balance between instructive and inhibitory signals to collectively direct neuronal diversity in the retina.

Intrinsic differences

The response of progenitors to intercellular signals changes during the course of development (Watanabe and Raff, 1990, 1992). Coculture of cells from pre- and post-natal rat retinas demonstrates that cells in S-phase at the time of culture continue to differentiate on a built in time course (Belliveau et al., 2000). A fifty-fold excess of post-natal versus embryonic cells does not alter the timetable of differentiation of the embryonic cells into rods, a post-natal phenotype. Similarly, a fifty-fold excess of embryonic cells to post-natal cells does not alter post-natal cell differentiation as rods. Although, fewer cells differentiated as rods and the number of bipolar cells increases.

However, there is no production of embryonic cell types such as cones. The true test of restriction in cell fate is through transplantation experiments of progenitors between embryos of different stages. This has not been closely examined in the retina, however in ferret embryos, age specific bias of progenitors has been documented in the cortex (Desai and McConnell, 2000). Thus the restriction of the potential of progenitor cells may be a common factor in neurogenesis in the central nervous system.

The population of progenitor cells may not be homogenous but composed of cells intrinsically biased in their ability to generate cells types. In a statistical analysis of the published data, Williams and Goldowitz (1992) demonstrate that progenitor cells are biased in their ability to generate cell types. Taking advantage of the ability to consistently identify blastomeres in Xenopus embryos, a lineage dependent mechanism in the formation of dopamine and neuropeptide-Y amacrine cell subtypes has been identified (Moody et al., 2000).

Recent experiments demonstrate that transcription factors of several families regulate various aspects of cell fate determination in the retina (Graw, 1996; Jean et al., 1998; Cepko, 1999; Ohnuma et al., 1999; Furukawa et al., 2000, 1997; Perron and Harris, 2000). For example, *Brn3b* and *atonal*-related gene have been implicated in ganglion cell differentiation (Erkman et al., 1996; Masai et al., 2000). Expression of *Hes1* and *Hes5* promote Muller glia differentiation, while *neuroD* promotes amacrine and rod cell production at the expense of Muller glia and bipolar cells (Cepko, 1999; Furukawa et al., 2000; Hojo et al., 2000; Perron and Harris, 2000). Similarly, factors with roles in patterning of the optic tissue have additional roles in the differentiation of specific cell types at later stages of retinal development (Graw, 1996; Jean et al., 1998; Mathers and Jamrich, 2000).

Another area that has recently come under investigation is the role of cell cycle withdrawal in cell differentiation. Two cyclin-dependent kinase inhibitors, p27Kip1\\p27/Xip1 and p57kip2 have been implicated in neuronal differentiation (Ohnuma et al., 1999; Dyer and Cepko, 2000; Levine et al., 2000a). The expression of both proteins is upregulated in retinal progenitors coincident with exit from the cell cycle and the onset of differentiation. Overexpression leads to cell cycle withdrawal and

loss-of-function is associated with continued cellular proliferation. During neurogenesis in the retina, expression of the two proteins differs. Expression of p27Kip1 is coincident with the onset of differentiation of most retinal cell types but is maintained only in Muller glia (Levine et al., 2000a) and in Xenopus, appears to act in concert to promote the determination of the Muller cell phenotype (Ohnuma et al., 1999). Expression of p57Kip2, however, was upregulated in a subpopulation of progenitors during early stages of neurogenesis and was maintained in a subpopulation of amacrine cells (Dyer and Cepko, 2000). It was concluded that the late expression has a direct albeit unknown role in the development or maintenance of these two cell types. Thus intrinsic differences include the mechanisms that regulate cell cycle withdrawal of progenitors. But the question of how the expression of cyclin-dependent kinase inhibitors or other regulators of cell cycle progression dovetails with environmental factors and expression of transcription factors, remains to be answered.

The zebrafish as a genetic and cellular model

The zebrafish (*Danio rerio*) fulfills the criterion as a suitable model for study of many aspects of vertebrate development (Nuesslein-Volhard, 1994). The zebrafish is a fresh water teleost, that is easily reared in the laboratory. A breeding pair of fish can produce > 100 fertilized eggs per mating. Fertilization is external, and the egg and embryo are transparent facilitating visual observation. Development is rapid: the larvae hatch in 3 days post fertilization (dpf), and the fish reach sexual maturity in several months. The zebrafish embryo provides access to developing systems unparalleled by avian and mammalian models.

The zebrafish is proving an attractive vertebrate model for genetic analysis of eye development. The expression of transcription factors, eye and lens morphogenesis and retinal histogenesis exhibit a great deal of consistency with other vertebrates (Pueschel et al., 1992; Schmitt and Dowling, 1994, 1996, 1999; Hu and Easter, 1999). Cellular differentiation is first identifiable at 36 hpf (hour postfertilization), with the histogenesis of ganglion cells in the ventronasal aspect of the eye. Differentiation progresses in a wave-like fashion across the nasal retina into the dorsal then temporal retina. By 48 hpf, lamination has spread across most of the retina and most major classes of cells can be identified by morphological or cytochemical criterion by 72–96 hpf (Fig. 2) (Larison and Bremiller, 1990; Raymond et al., 1995; Schmitt and Dowling, 1996).

The first experiments conducted on zebrafish in John Dowling's laboratory were aimed at identifying molecules that altered patterning of the optic primordial. Experiments by Hyatt et al. (1992) demonstrated that retinoic acid (RA) treatment of embryos had clear and reproducible effects upon eye development. In zebrafish, treatment of the early embryo with RA results in duplication of the ventral retina or expansion of the ventral region of the optic primordia (Hyatt et al., 1992). Conversely, decreasing the endogenous pool of RA, through inhibition of the retinal dehydrogenase with citral, results in loss of the ventral aspect of the eye (Marsh-Armstrong et al., 1994; Hyatt et al., 1996b). An effect of RA upon the developing eye should not have been too surprising since experiments conducted in the 1930s through the 1960s conclusively demonstrated characteristic pattern of ocular defects in the offspring of female rats deprived of vitamin A (reviewed in Hyatt and Dowling, 1997). However, the phenomenon of duplication of the ventral retina could not have been predicted. These and other examples of the role of RA in patterning the retinal tissue are discussed in greater detail by Drager et al. (this volume).

At later stages of embryogenesis (48 hpf), treatment with RA or citral, has specific but opposite effects upon the maturation of rods and cones (Hyatt et al., 1996a). Embryos treated with increasing concentrations of RA demonstrate an expansion of the rhodopsin positive cells in all regions of the retina compared to untreated-controls. Labeling of mitotic cells with BrdU demonstrates that the effects of RA are on a post mitotic population. Conversely, treatment with citral, decreases the distribution and intensity of staining with rod specific markers. Surprisingly, these changes in rod development are paralleled by the opposite effect upon cones. RA treatment leads to decrease staining for the cone opsins and fewer profiles of cones in histological sections. These data suggest that the RA signaling pathway is involved in the differentiation and maturation of both rod and cone photoreceptor cells within the developing zebrafish retina, similar to in vitro and in vivo data in rodents (Kelley et al., 1994, 1995; Levine et al., 2000b).

Mutations affecting eye development

Much of our knowledge of genes important to development has come from the analysis of spontaneous or induced mutations. One common approach for identifying genes involved in vertebrate development is based upon homology screens for genes previously identified in invertebrate model organisms such as *Drosophila* or *Caenorhabditis elegans*. Many vertebrate genes exhibit structural and functional similarities to *Drosophila* genes required for neuronal determination, differentiation and function (Graw, 1996; Salzberg and Bellen, 1996; Oliver and Gruss, 1997; Jean et al., 1998). The wave-like progression of neurogenesis in the zebrafish retina (Schmitt and Dowling, 1996; Hu and Easter, 1999; Marcus et al., 1999) is reminiscent of the progression of the morphogenetic furrow in the *Drosophila* ommatidium. In *Drosophila*, secretion of hedgehog from mature ommatidial neurons initiates neurogenesis through induction of the bHLH transcription factor *atonal* in immature neurons. Recently, a wave of *shh* expression has also been demonstrated in the patterning of the zebrafish retina (Neumann and Nuesslein-Volhard, 2000) and the initiation of neurogenesis follows expression of the atonal family member, *ath5* (Masai et al., 2000), suggesting an even greater degree of evolutionary conservation during visual system development than anticipated.

Classical (forward) genetic screens are considered unbiased methods for uncovering gene functions, since no prior assumptions about the nature of the gene product are unnecessary. Genetic screens of *Drosophila* have uncovered many mutations affecting the structure, function and development of the compound eye. However, the systematic screen for genes involved in vertebrate eye development had been limited (reviewed in Graw, 1996). Genetic analysis of existing mouse populations have identified numerous mutations and loci affecting eye development (Williams et al., 1998; Munroe et al., 2000), however until recently, the expense and logistics

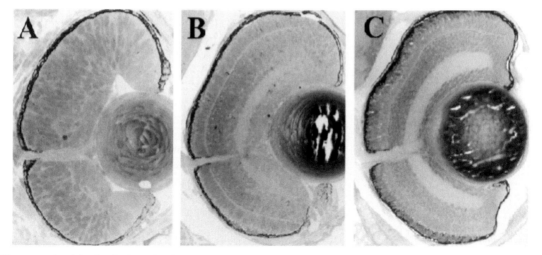

Fig. 2. Neurogenesis of the developing zebrafish retina. **A.** 40 hpf, differentiation of ganglion cells in the inner retina and formation of the optic nerve is evident. **B.** 52 hpf, differentiation of cellular layers of the inner and outer retina and two synaptic layers is evident. **C.** 120 hpf, morphological differentiation of photoreceptor cell outer segments is pronounced with large rod segments present in the ventral retina and teiring of cone photoreceptors in the central retina prominently displayed.

of a large-scale screen was deemed impractical (Hawes et al., 1999).

Two groups have developed the methods for efficient and large-scale chemical mutagenesis of zebrafish for the express purpose of identifying loci essential to embryological development (Driever et al., 1996; Haffter et al., 1996). Both screens use the alkylating agent *N*-ethyl-*N*-nitrosourea (ENU) to induce point mutations in the zebrafish spermatagonia. Numerous mutations affecting the retina, retinal tectal projections and vision have been isolated. Malicki et al. (1996), identified 49 mutations at 38 loci that affected the development of the retina: mutations affecting retinal lamination, specification of the eye anlagen, loss of photoreceptors, reduced eye size, retinal degeneration, eye pigmentation and the ventral retina. Analysis of retinal-tectal projection using fluorescent tracers DiO and DiI has identified 114 mutations in 35 genes (Baier et al., 1996; Karlstrom et al., 1996; Trowe et al., 1996). Subsequent behavioral analysis of the 400 loci identified as essential to zebrafish embryogenesis revealed 25, that when mutated result in visual impairment (Neuhauss et al., 1999). The existing mutations continue to serve as a resource to test new hypotheses or uncover loci essential to newly defined processes.

The effectiveness of the ENU mutagenesis has also enabled the success of several smaller scale highly focused screens to uncover genes affecting specific organ systems including the visual system. In Dr. John Dowling's laboratory, these techniques, in conjunction with behavioral and morphological screens, have been used to identify dominant and recessive mutations affecting visual function and retinal development (Brockerhoff et al., 1995, 1997; Fadool et al., 1997; Li and Dowling, 1997; Link et al., 2000; see accompanying chapters).

The mutagenesis can be outlined as follows (Fig. 3). Male zebrafish, exposed to the potent mutagen ENU, are out-crossed to wild-type females to produce an F1-generation. Each F1 fish represents the mutagenized haploid genome of a single sperm. Individual F1 fish are either out-crossed or pairs are crossed to each other producing an F2 family. Pairs of F2 siblings are inbred, and recessive mutations are uncovered in the F3 generation. At 24 h intervals, the third generation larvae are viewed under a stereomicroscope and scored for developmental abnormalities. Morphological defects in the lens, retina pigmented epithelium, eye size and shape, and forebrain are reserved.

In the morphological screen, non-specific retinal degenerations constitute the largest group of

548

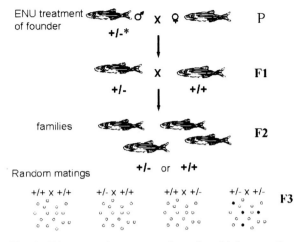

ENU treatment of founder +/-* ♂ X ♀ P

+/- X +/+ F1

families F2

+/- or +/+

Random matings

+/+ X +/+   +/- X +/+   +/+ X +/-   +/- X +/-   F3

Fig. 3. Diagrammatic representation of a third generation screen of chemically mutagenized zebrafish. Spermatogonial cells of male zebrafish of the parental generation (P) are mutated by exposure to ethyl-nitrosyl urea. Fish are mated to wild-type female fish. Each fish of the resulting F1 generation represent the mutagenized genome of a single sperm. F1 fish are mated to produce an F2 family half of which are heterozygous for any loci present in the mutagenized sperm. Mutations are uncovered in the F3 progeny from approximately one quarter of the sibling matings of the F2 families.

mutations affecting eye development (Fadool et al., 1997). These are characterized by a small eye phenotype appearing between 1.5 and 3 dpf. Histological analysis reveals prominent cell death across the entire retina. Nuclei have condensed chromatin, with no vacuolization or swelling of the cytoplasm or organelles, typical of apoptotic cell death. In most mutants, RPE hyperplasia is observed. A number of the retinal degenerations is associated with moderate brain degeneration though not all areas of the CNS are affected. These data suggest an effect upon neurotrophic factors necessary for neuron survival, their receptors and/or transduction cascades.

Other mutations result in the degeneration of specific cells in the neural retina. Mutations that affect the ganglion cell layer, inner nuclear layer, photoreceptor cell layer and proliferative zone have been identified. The ganglion cell mutant has been studied in greatest detail (Fig. 4). In the wild-type retina, the ganglion cells begin to differentiate between 34 and 36 hpf (Schmitt and Dowling, 1996; Hu and Easter, 1999). By 60 hpf, the ganglion cell layer is approximately 3–4 nuclei in thickness and the other layers of the retina have differentiated. In the mutant animals, called *archie*, the ganglion cell layer is greatly reduced with zero or one layer of nuclei and a very thin optic nerve observed 120 hpf. Surprisingly, the lamination of the retina and differentiation of other cell types appear relatively normal. Histological and cytochemical analyses at earlier time points, reveal many apoptotic cells in the ganglion cell layer and the presumptive inner nuclear layer, and delayed development of the other retinal cell types. However, those ganglion cells that do survive make the appropriate retinal-tectal projects as visualized with DiI and DiO. Eventually, the ganglion cells that do form inhibit neighboring cells from adopting a similar fate, and specification of other cell types continues. These data suggest that the *archie* gene product functions during differentiation but not specification of ganglion cells. However, it is unclear whether it affects all types of ganglion cells or results in the loss of specific subclasses of ganglion cells.

The *archie* phenotype most closely resembles the targeted disruption of the murine gene *Brn-3b*, a member of the POU-domain family of transcription factors (Erkman et al., 1996). *Brn-3b* is associated with differentiation of ganglion cells of the retina. The knock-out mouse lacks two-thirds of its ganglion cells but other retinal layers are intact. This is consistent with a role in ganglion cell maturation but not specification. The *archie* phenotype also resembles the *lakritz* mutant identified by behavioral screening of the mutant loci identified in the Tubigen morphological screen (Neuhauss et al., 1999). However, differences are observed. In the *archie* phenotype, the surviving ganglion cells do make the appropriate retinal-tectal projection which is not observed in *lakritz*. Secondly, *archie* demonstrates greater plieotropy, affecting the skeleton and gill arches. Complementation studies need to be preformed between these lines as well as others with similar phenotypes to determine if multiple loci are involved in ganglion cell survival as preliminary comparisons suggest. With improved mapping techniques, finer resolution of the genetic map, and assignment of cloned genes to genetic loci, an increasing number of previously identified mutations will be cloned by positional or candidate gene approach.

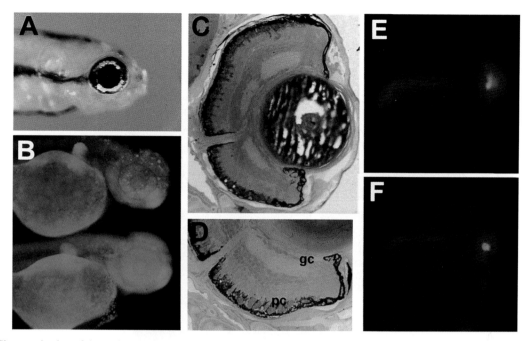

Fig. 4. Characterization of the *archie* mutant phenotype. **A.** Lateral view of archie larva characterized by a slightly reduced eye size and enlarged pupil. **B.** Live embryo staining for apoptotic cells using acridine orange labeling and viewed with an FITC filter set in archie (upper) and wild-type (lower) sibling embryos at 36 hpf. Note the numerous fluorescent profiles in the retina and optic tectum of the mutant embryo. **C.** Transverse section of a 120 hpf archie eye. Relatively normal lamination of the retina and tiering of the photoreceptor cells in the central retina are present. Note the incomplete formation of the inner plexiform layer. **D.** A higher magnification image demonstrates a single layer of cells in the ganglion cell layer compared to 3–4 cells observed in wild-type (see Fig. 2). **E** and **F.** Retinotectal projections in wild type (**E**) and archie mutant larvae (**F**) visualized with DiO. Dio was injected into the eye and projections to the contralateral eye were labeled in both mutant and wild-type larvae although there was a considerable decrease in labeling intensity in mutant larvae.

Molecular markers of differentiation

The process of neurogenesis and cellular differentiation can be defined by the timely expression of specific cellular markers either by in situ hybridization or immunocytochemistry. To generate cell specific markers for the zebrafish retina, a series of monoclonal antibodies was generated in collaboration with Dr. Paul J. Linser, of the University of Florida. The hybridoma supernatants were screened by Western blot analysis and immunohistochemical labeling of retina. From the initial fusion, 36 clones were identified that label cells of the retina. The labeling specificity can be subdivided into: (a) 18 photoreceptor cell specific with possibly 10 of those recognizing opsins; (b) 5 Muller cell and glia-specific; (c) two plexiform specific; and (d) 3 label the RPE and blood vessels of the brain. Individual clones that label amacrine cells of the inner nuclear layer, cytoskeletal elements of some neurons, and mitochondria have also been identified. Labeling by the 1D1 Mab, which recognizes an epitope on rhodopsin, may provide a useful marker for differentiation of rods (Fig. 5).

Gene expression can also be studied in transient and stable transgenic lines of zebrafish. First demonstrated over a decade ago, the production of transgenic zebrafish was hindered by several technical difficulties. However, many recent advances in the technologies for the generation of transgenic fish have overcome many of the obstacles (reviewed in Lin, 2000). The use of retrovirus vectors results in a dramatic increase in the number of germline integrations and is the basis for an insertional mutagenesis screen (Becker et al., 1998; Amsterdam et al., 1999). The recent use of cell specific promoters and green

550

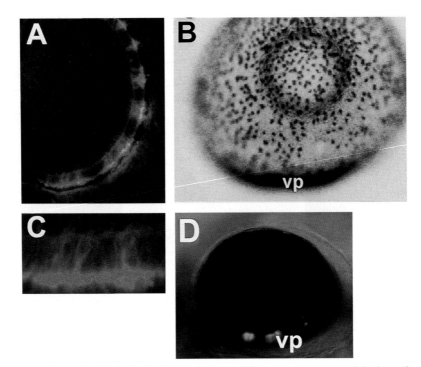

Fig. 5. Rhodopsin expression in the larval zebrafish retina. **A**, **B** and **C**. Rhodopsin immunoreactivity in sections (**A** and **B**) and whole mount (**C**) larval zebrafish eyes localized with the 1D1 monoclonal antibody. Dense labeling of the outer nuclear layer cells within the ventral patch (vp) and scattered across the retina is consistent with rhodopsin gene expression. At a higher magnification, labeling of the plasma membrane and outer segment material of immature photoreceptor cells. **D.** Green fluorescent protein expression in live zebrafish embryos under the control of the *Xenopus* rhodopsin promoter. Labeling of the ventral patch (vp) was consistent with 1D1 immunoreactivity at 3 dpf. Later examination revealed a pattern similar to endogenous rhodopsin expression (not shown) indicating the specificity of the *Xenopus* rhodopsin promoter.

fluorescent protein as a reporter gene, has overcome many of the original pitfalls associated with loss of reporter gene expression following germ line transmission of the transgene (Amsterdam et al., 1995; Higashijima et al., 1997; Long et al., 1997; Lin, 2000). We have recently generated transgenic zebrafish with retina-specific expression of GFP using the Xenopus opsin promoter (Knox et al., 1998). This promoter drives expression in a spatial and temporal pattern consistent with opsin expression (Fig. 5D). The generation of transgenic lines of zebrafish with cell specific expression of GFP opens many new avenues of investigation. As GFP expression can be observed in living embryos, highly focused genetic screens to identify mutations altering the expected pattern of gene expression are now possible. Cell specific promoters can be used to drive the expression or misexpression of dominant negative forms of signaling molecules, or transcription factors to investigate their roles in normal development. And the recent development of transposon technologies for the generation of transgenic zebrafish (Fadool et al., 1998; Raz et al., 1998), increase the feasibility of alternative genetic screens, such as gene traps and enhancer-traps, to identify genes involved in retinal development and function. With the advent of genomic resources, the zebrafish is filling the need as a model organism for the study of vertebrate development.

Conclusions and future perspectives

The integration of genetics, cellular methods and experimental embryology has furthered our understanding of the mechanisms underlying development of the vertebrate retina. Taken as a whole, the literature demonstrates that cell fate in the neural retina is regulated by inductive interactions as well as intrinsic properties of the progenitor cells. Recent evidence also demonstrates the progenitor cell populations to be heterogeneous and implicate specific molecular factors in the bias of progenitors towards specific cellular phenotypes. However, few studies have attempted to elucidate the mechanisms regulating differentiation of the many subtypes of neurons in the retina, and fewer have attempted to understand the mechanisms that guide the formation of functional circuits. Whether the observed heterogeneity in progenitor cells represents the first stage towards development of subclasses of neurons is unclear. What is certain, is that our understanding of the underlying mechanisms can only benefit by the current trend towards integrating genetic methods with more detailed physiological analysis of retinal function.

Acknowledgments

The data described in this work was initiated in the laboratory of John E. Dowling and is currently supported by grant EY13020 to JMF.

References

Adler, R. (2000) A model of retinal cell differentiation in the chick embryo. *Prog. Retin. Eye Res.*, 19: 529–557.

Altshuler, D. and Cepko, C. (1992) A temporally regulated, diffusible activity is required for rod photoreceptor development in vitro. *Development*, 114: 947–957.

Altshuler, D., Lo-Turco, J.J., Rush, J. and Cepko, C. (1993) Taurine promotes the differentiation of a vertebrate retinal cell type in vitro. *Development*, 119: 1317–1328.

Amsterdam, A., Burgess, S., Golling, G., Chen, W., Sun, Z., Townsend, K., Farrington, S., Haldi, M. and Hopkins, N. (1999) Large-scale insertional mutagenesis screen in zebrafish. *Genes Dev.*, 13: 2713–2724.

Amsterdam, A., Lin, S. and Hopkins, N. (1995) The *Aequorea victoria* green fluorescent protein can be used as a reporter in live zebrafish embryos. *Dev. Biol.*, 171: 123–129.

Austin, C.P., Feldman, D.E., Ida, J.A. and Cepko, C.L. (1995) Vertebrate retinal ganglion cells are selected from competent progenitors by the action of Notch. *Development*, 121: 3637–3650.

Baier, H., Klostermann, S., Trowe, T., Karlstrom, R.O., Nusslein-Volhard, C. and Bonhoeffer, F. (1996) Genetic dissection of the retinotectal projection. *Development*, 123: 415–425.

Bao, Z.Z. and Cepko, C.L. (1997) The expression and function of Notch pathway genes in the developing rat eye. *J. Neurosci.*, 17: 1425–1434.

Becker, T.S., Burgess, S.M., Amsterdam, A.H., Allende, M.L. and Hopkins, N. (1998) Not really finished is crucial for development of the zebrafish outer retina and encodes a transcription factor highly homologous to human Nuclear Respiratory Factor-1 and avian Initiation Binding Repressor. *Development*, 125: 4369–4378.

Belliveau, M.J. and Cepko, C.L. (1999) Extrinsic and intrinsic factors control the genesis of amacrine and cone cells in the rat retina. *Development*, 126: 555–566.

Belliveau, M.J., Young, T.L. and Cepko, C.L. (2000) Late retinal progenitor cells show intrinsic limitations in the production of cell types and the kinetics of opsin synthesis. *J. Neurosci.*, 20: 2247–2254.

Brockerhoff, S.E., Hurley, J.B., Janssen-Bienhold, U., Neuhauss, S.C.F., Driever, W. and Dowling, J.E. (1995) A behavioral screen for isolating zebrafish mutants with visual system defects. *Proc. Natl. Acad. Sci. USA*, 92: 10545–10549.

Brockerhoff, S.E., Hurley, J.B., Niemi, G.A. and Dowling, J.E. (1997) A new form of inherited red-blindness identified in zebrafish. *J. Neurosci.*, 17: 4236–4242.

Carter-Dawson, L.D. and LaVail, M.M. (1979) Rods and cones in the mouse retina: autoradiographic analysis of cell generation using tritiated thymidine. *J. Comp. Neurol.*, 188: 263–272.

Cepko, C.L. (1999) The roles of intrinsic and extrinsic cues and bHLH genes in the determination of retinal cell fates. *Curr. Opin. Neurobiol.*, 9(1): 37–46.

Coulombre, A.J. (1965) The Eye. In: DeHaan, R.L. and Urspring, H. (Eds.), *Organogenesis*. Holt, Rinehart and Winston, New York, pp. 219–251.

Desai, A.R. and McConnell, S.K. (2000) Progressive restriction in fate potential by neural progenitors during cerebral cortical development. *Development*, 127: 2863–2872.

Detwiler, S.R. and Van Dyke, R.H. (1953) The induction of neural retina from the pigment epithelial layer of the eye. *J. Exp. Zool.*, 122: 367–383.

Detwiler, S.R. and Van Dyke, R.H. (1954) Further experimental observations on retinal inductions. *J. Exp. Zool.*, 126: 135–156.

Dowling, J.E. (1987) The retina, an approachable part of the brain. Belknap, Harvard University Press, Cambridge, MA.

Driever, W., Solnica-Krezel, L., Schier, A.F., Neuhauss, S.C., Malicki, J., Stemple, D.L., Stainier, D.Y., Zwartkruis, F., Abdelilah, S., Rangini, Z., Belak, J. and Boggs, C. (1996) A genetic screen for mutations affecting embryogenesis in zebrafish. *Development*, 123: 37–46.

Dyer, M.A. and Cepko, C.L. (2000) p57(Kip2) regulates progenitor cell proliferation and amacrine interneuron development in the mouse retina. *Development*, 127: 3593–3605.

Erkman, L., McEvilly, R.J., Luo, L., Ryan, A.K., Hooshmand, F., O'Connell, S.M., Keithley, E.M., Rapaport, D.H., Ryan, A.F. and Rosenfeld, M.G. (1996) Role of the

552

transcription factors Brn3.1 and Brn3.2 in auditory and visual system development. *Nature*, 381: 603–606.

Fadool, J.M., Brockerhoff, S.E., Hyatt, G.A. and Dowling, J.E. (1997) Mutations affecting eye morphology in the developing zebrafish (Danio rerio). *Dev. Genet.*, 20(3): 288–295.

Fadool, J.M., Hartl, D.L. and Dowling, J.E. (1998) Transposition of the mariner element from Drosophila mauritiana in zebrafish. *Proc. Natl. Acad. Sci. USA*, 95: 5182–5186.

Furukawa, T., Morrow, E.M. and Cepko, C.L. (1997) Crx, a novel otx, like homeobox gene, shows photoreceptor, specific expression and regulates photoreceptor differentiation. *Cell*, 91: 531–541.

Furukawa, T., Mukherjee, S., Bao, Z.Z., Morrow, E.M. and Cepko, C.L. (2000) rax, Hes1, and notch1 promote the formation of Muller glia by postnatal retinal progenitor cells. *Neuron*, 26: 383–394.

Gaiano, N., Nye, J.S. and Fishell, G. (2000) Radial glial identity is promoted by Notch1 signaling in the murine forebrain. *Neuron*, 26: 395–404.

Graw, J. (1996) Genetic aspects of embryonic eye development in vertebrates. *Develop. Genet.*, 18: 181–197.

Grun, G. (1982) The development of the vertebrate retina: a comparative study. *Adv. Anat. Embry. Cell Biol.*, 78: 1–83.

Guillemot, F. and Cepko, C.L. (1992) Retinal fate and ganglion cell differentiation are potentiated by acidic FGF in an in vitro assay of early retinal development. *Development*, 114: 743–754.

Haffter, P., Granato, M., Brand, M., Mullins, M.C., Hammerschmidt, M., Kane, D.A., Odenthal, J., van Eeden, F.J., Jiang, Y.J., Heisenberg, C.P., Kelsh, R.N., Furutani, Seiki M., Vogelsang, E., Beuchle, D., Schach, U., Fabian, C. and Nusslein-Volhard, C. (1996) The identification of genes with unique and essential functions in the development of the zebrafish, Danio rerio. *Development*, 123: 1–36.

Hawes, N.L., Smith, R.S., Chang, B., Davisson, M., Heckenlively, J.R. and John, S.W. (1999) Mouse fundus photography and angiography: a catalogue of normal and mutant phenotypes. *Mol. Vis.*, 5: 22.

Higashijima, S., Okamoto, H., Ueno, N., Hotta, Y. and Eguchi, G. (1997) High-frequency generation of transgenic zebrafish which reliably express GFP in whole muscles or the whole body by using promoters of zebrafish origin. *Dev. Biol.*, 192: 289–299.

Hojo, M., Ohtsuka, T., Hashimoto, N., Gradwohl, G., Guillemot, F. and Kageyama, R. (2000) Glial cell fate specification modulated by the bHLH gene Hes5 in mouse retina. *Development*, 127: 2515–2522.

Holt, C.E., Bertsch, T.W., Ellis, H.M. and Harris, W.A. (1988) Cellular determination in the Xenopus retina is independent of lineage and birth date. *Neuron*, 1: 15–26.

Hu, M. and Easter, S.S. (1999) Retinal neurogenesis: the formation of the initial central patch of postmitotic cells. *Dev. Biol.*, 207: 309–321.

Hyatt, G.A. and Dowling, J.E. (1997) Retinoic acid: A key molecule for eye and photoreceptor development. *Invest. Ophthal. Vis. Neurosci.*, 38: 1471–1475.

Hyatt, G.A., Schmitt, E.A., Fadool, J.M. and Dowling, J.E. (1996a) Retinoic acid alters photoreceptor development in vivo. *Proc. Natl. Acad. Sci. USA*, 93: 13298–13303.

Hyatt, G.A., Schmitt, E.A., Marsh-Armstrong, N. and Dowling, J.E. (1992) Retinoic acid induces duplication of the zebrafish retina. *Proc. Natl. Acad. Sci. USA*, 89: 8293–8297.

Hyatt, G.A., Schmitt, E.A., Marsh-Armstrong, N., McCaffery, P., Drager, U.C. and Dowling, J.E. (1996b) Retinoic acid establishes ventral retinal characteristics. *Development*, 122: 195–204.

Hyer, J., Mima, T. and Mikawa, T. (1998) FGF1 patterns the optic vesicle by directing the placement of the neural retina domain. *Development*, 125(5): 869–877.

Jean, D., Ewan, K. and Gruss, P. (1998) Molecular regulators involved in vertebrate eye development. *Mech. Dev.*, 76(1–2): 3–18.

Kahn, A.J. (1974) An autoradiographic analysis of the time of appearance of neurons in the developing chick neural retina. *Dev. Biol.*, 38: 30–40.

Karlstrom, R.O., Trowe, T., Klostermann, S., Baier, H., Brand, M., Crawford, A.D., Grunewald, B., Haffter, P., Hoffmann, H., Meyer, S.U., Muller, B.K., Richter, S., van Eeden, F.J., Nusslein-Volhard, C. and Bonhoeffer, F. (1996) Zebrafish mutations affecting retinotectal axon pathfinding. *Development*, 123: 427–438.

Kelley, M.W., Turner, J.K. and Reh, T.A. (1994) Retinoic acid promotes differentiation of photoreceptors in vitro. *Development*, 120: 2091–2102.

Kelley, M.W., Turner, J.K. and Reh, T.A. (1995) Ligands of steroid/thyroid receptors induce cone photoreceptors in vertebrate retina. *Development*, 121: 3777–3785.

Knox, B.E., Schlueter, C., Sanger, B.M., Green, C.B. and Besharse, J.C. (1998) Transgene expression in Xenopus rods. *FEBS Lett.*, 423: 117–121.

Larison, K.D. and Bremiller, R. (1990) Early onset of phenotype and cell patterning in the embryonic zebrafish retina. *Development*, 109: 567–576.

Levine, E.M., Close, J., Fero, M., Ostrovsky, A. and Reh, T.A. (2000a) p27 (Kipl) regulates cell cycle withdrawal of late multipotent progenitor cells in the mammalian retina. *Dev. Bio.*, 219(2): 299–314.

Levine, E.M., Fuhrmann, S. and Reh, T.A. (2000b) Soluble factors and the development of rod photoreceptors. *Cell Mol. Life Sci.*, 57(2): 224–234.

Li, L. and Dowling, J.E. (1997) A dominant form of inherited retinal degeneration caused by a non-photoreceptor cell-specific mutation. *Proc. Natl. Acad. Sci. USA*, 94: 11645–11650.

Lin, S. (2000) Transgenic zebrafish. *Methods Mol. Biol.*, 136: 375–383.

Link, B.A., Fadool, J.M., Malicki, J. and Dowling, J.E. (2000) The zebrafish young mutation acts non-cell-autonomously to uncouple differentiation from specification for all retinal cells. *Development*, 127: 2177–2188.

Linser, P.J. and Moscona, A.A. (1979) Induction of glutamine synthetase in the embryonic neural retina: localization in

Muller fibers and dependence on cell interactions. *Proc. Natl. Acad. Sci. USA*, 76: 6476–6480.

Long, Q., Meng, A., Wang, H., Jessen, J.R., Farrell, M.J. and Lin, S. (1997) GATA-1 expression pattern can be recapitulated in living transgenic zebrafish using GFP reporter gene. *Development*, 124: 4105–4111.

Macdonald, R., Barth, K.A., Xu, Q., Holder, N., Mikkola, I. and Wilson, S.W. (1995) Midline signalling is required for Pax gene regulation and patterning of the eyes. *Development*, 121: 3267–3278.

Malicki, J., Neuhauss, S.C., Schier, A.F., Solnica-Krezel, L., Stemple, D.L., Stainier, D.Y., Abdelilah, S., Zwartkruis, F., Rangini, Z. and Driever, W. (1996) Mutations affecting development of the zebrafish retina. *Development*, 123: 263–273.

Marcus, R.C., Delaney, C.L. and Easter, S.S., Jr. (1999) Neurogenesis in the visual system of embryonic and adult zebrafish (Daniorerio). *Vis. Neurosci.*, 16: 417–424.

Marsh-Armstrong, N., McCaffery, P., Gilbert, W., Dowling, J.E. and Drager, U.C. (1994) Retinoic acid is necessary for development of the ventral retina in zebrafish. *Proc. Natl. Acad. Sci. USA*, 91: 7286–7290.

Masai, I., Stemple, D.L., Okamoto, H. and Wilson, S.W. (2000) Midline signals regulate retinal neurogenesis in zebrafish. *Neuron*, 27: 251–263.

Mathers, P.H. and Jamrich, M. (2000) Regulation of eye formation by *Rx* and *pax6* homeobox genes. *Cell. Mol. Life Sci.*, 57: 186–194.

Moody, S.A., Chow, I. and Huang, S. (2000) Intrinsic bias and lineage restriction in the phenotype determination of dopamine and neuropeptide Y amacrine cells. *J. Neurosci.*, 20(9): 3244–3253.

Munroe, R.J., Bergstrom, R.A., Zheng, Q.Y., Libby, B., Smith, R., John, S.W., Schimenti, K.J., Browning, V.L. and Schimenti, J.C. (2000) Mouse mutants from chemically mutagenized embryonic stem cells. *Nat. Genet.*, 24: 318–321.

Neuhauss, S.C., Biehlmaier, O., Seeliger, M.W., Das, T., Kohler, K., Harris, W.A. and Baier, H. (1999) Genetic disorders of vision revealed by a behavioral screen of 400 essential loci in zebrafish. *J. Neurosci.*, 19: 8603–8615.

Neumann, C.J. and Nuesslein-Volhard, C. (2000) Patterning of the zebrafish retina by a wave of sonic hedgehog activity. *Science*, 289: 2137–2139.

Nguyen, M. and Arnheiter, H. (2000) Signaling and transcriptional regulation in early mammalian eye development: a link between FGF and MITF. *Development*, 127(16): 3581–3591.

Nuesslein-Volhard, C. (1994) Of flies and fishes. *Science*, 266: 572–574.

Ohnuma, S., Philpott, A., Wang, K., Holt, C.E. and Harris, W.A. (1999) p27Xic1, a Cdk inhibitor, promotes the determination of glial cells in Xenopus retina. *Cell*, 99: 499–510.

Oliver, G. and Gruss, P. (1997) Current views on eye development. *Trends Neurosci.*, 20(9): 415–421.

Perron, M. and Harris, W.A. (2000) Determination of vertebrate retinal progenitor cell fate by the Notch pathway and basic helix-loop-helix transcription factors. *Cell Mol. Life Sci.*, 57(2): 215–223.

Perron, M., Kanekar, S., Vetter, M.L. and Harris, W.A. (1998) The genetic sequence of retinal development in the ciliary margin of the Xenopus eye. *Dev. Biol.*, 199(2): 185–200.

Pittack, C., Grunwald, G.B. and Reh, T.A. (1997) Fibroblast growth factors are necessary for neural retina but not pigmented epithelium differentiation in chick embryos. *Development*, 124: 805–816.

Price, J., Turner, D. and Cepko, C. (1987) Lineage analysis in the vertebrate nervous system by retrovirus-mediated gene transfer. *Proc. Natl. Acad. Sci. USA*, 84: 156–160.

Pueschel, A.W., Gruss, P. and Westerfield, M. (1992) Sequence and expression pattern of pax-6 are highly conserved between zebrafish and mice. *Development*, 114: 643–651.

Raymond, P.A., Barthel, L.K. and Curran, G.A. (1995) Developmental patterning of rod and cone photoreceptors in embryonic zebrafish. *J. Comp. Neurol.*, 359: 537–550.

Raz, E., van Luenen, H.G., Schaerringer, B., Plasterk, R.H.A. and Driever, W. (1998) Transposition of the nematode Caenorhabditis elegans Tc3 element in the zebrafish Danio rerio. *Curr. Biol.*, 8: 82–88.

Reh, T.A. and Tulley, T. (1986) Regulation of tyrosine hydroxylase-containing amacrine cell number in larval frog retina. *Develop. Biol.*, 114: 463–469.

Salzberg, A. and Bellen, H.J. (1996) Invertebrate and vertebrate neurogenesis: Variations on the same theme. *Develop. Gen.*, 18: 1–10.

Schmitt, E.A. and Dowling, J.E. (1994) Early eye morphogenesis in the zebrafish, Brachydanio rerio. *J. Comp. Neurol.*, 344: 532 542.

Schmitt, E.A. and Dowling, J.E. (1996) Comparison of topographical patterns of ganglion and photoreceptor cell differentiation in the retina of the zebrafish, Danio rerio. *J. Comp. Neurol.*, 371: 222–234.

Schmitt, E.A. and Dowling, J.E. (1999) Early retinal development in the zebrafish, Danio rerio: light and electron microscopic analyses. *J. Comp. Neurol.*, 404: 515–536.

Sidman, R.L. (1961) Histogenesis of the mouse retina studied with tritiated thymadine. In: *The Structure of the Eye*. Academic Press, New York, pp. 487–506.

Stiemke, M.M. and Hollyfield, J.G. (1995) Cell birthdays in *Xenopus laevis* retina. *Differentiation*, 58: 189–193.

Trowe, T., Klostermann, S., Baier, H., Granato, M., Crawford, A.D., Grunewald, B., Hoffmann, H., Karlstrom, R.O., Meyer, S.U., Muller, B., Richter, S., Nusslein-Volhard, C. and Bonhoeffer, F. (1996) Mutations disrupting the ordering and topographic mapping of axons in the retinotectal projection of the zebrafish, Danio rerio. *Development*, 123: 439–450.

Turner, D.L. and Cepko, C.L. (1987) A common progenitor for neurons and glia persists in rat retina late in development. *Nature*, 328: 131–136.

Turner, D.L., Snyder, E.Y. and Cepko, C.L. (1990) Lineage-independent determination of cell type in the embryonic mouse retina. *Neuron*, 4: 833–845.

Vogel-Hopker, A., Momose, T., Rohrer, H., Yasuda, K., Ishihara, L. and Rapaport, D.H. (2000) Multiple functions of fibroblast growth factor-8 (FGF-8) in chick eye development. *Mech. Develop.*, 94: 25–36.

554

Waid, D.K. and McLoon, S.C. (1998) Ganglion cells influence the fate of dividing retinal cells in culture. *Development*, 125(6): 1059–1066.

Watanabe, T. and Raff, M.C. (1990) Rod photoreceptor development in vitro: intrinsic properties of proliferating neuroepithelial cells change as development proceeds in the rat retina. *Neuron*, 2: 461–467.

Watanabe, T. and Raff, M.C. (1992) Diffusable rod-promoting signals in the developing rat retina. *Development*, 114: 899–906.

Wetts, R., Serbedzija, G.N. and Fraser, S.E. (1989) Cell lineage analysis reveals multipotent precursors in the ciliary margin of the frog retina. *Develop. Biol.*, 136: 254–263.

Williams, R.W. and Goldowitz, D. (1992) Lineage versus environment in embryonic retina: a revisionist perspective. *Trends Neurosci.*, 15(10): 368–373.

Williams, R.W., Strom, R.C. and Goldowitz, D. (1998) Natural variation in neuron number in mice is linked to a major quantitative trait locus on Chr 11. *J. Neurosci.*, 18(1): 138–146.

Yamamoto, Y. and Jeffery, W.R. (2000) Central role for the lens in cave fish eye degeneration. *Science*, 289: 631–633.

Young, R.W. (1985) Cell proliferation during postnatal development of the mouse. *Dev. Brain Res.*, 21: 229–239.

H. Kolb, H. Ripps and S. Wu (Eds.)
Progress in Brain Research, Vol. 131

CHAPTER 39

Genetic and epigenetic analysis of visual system functions of zebrafish

Lei Li*

Department of Physiology, University of Kentucky College of Medicine, 800 Rose Street, Lexington, KY 40536, USA

Introduction

In early 1996, after finishing my Ph.D. work, I joined the Dowling laboratory at Harvard as a postdoctoral fellow. Taking advantage of my previous training in mutational screening of locomotory deficit mutants in *C. elegans*, John and I decided to initiate a search for dominant visual system mutations in zebrafish. We hoped that zebrafish mutations such as those causing slow retinal degeneration would provide a tool for genetic studies of human retinal diseases, i.e. retinitis pigmentosa. At that time, the optokinetic response test was used in the Dowling lab to evaluate visual responses of larval zebrafish, yet methods used for measuring quantitatively the visual sensitivity of adult zebrafish were lacking. The first task I embarked upon was to develop an assay that would be robust enough to distinguish visual system mutants from their normal siblings in adult zebrafish. John spent hours with me explaining the basics of vertebrate visual function and encouraging me to try various types of test to get the best screening conditions. After spending three months in our zebrafish facility dark room observing fish behavior, I developed a behavioral assay, based on the visually mediated escape response of

the fish to a threatening object, that permits a quantitative analysis of visual sensitivity of adult zebrafish (Li and Dowling, 1997).

As John predicted, this behavioral assay is exceptionally useful. The first set of experiments I performed using this assay is to measure the course of dark adaptation of adult zebrafish. When I compared data that were obtained from experiments conducted between early morning and late afternoon hours, I found that thresholds of both the cone and rod systems were significantly higher in early morning than in late afternoon. I showed the data to John, and he suggested repeating the threshold measurement every 2–3 h in a 24-h period. From there, John introduced me to circadian biology. It turned out that the threshold difference between early morning and late afternoon is controlled by an endogenous circadian clock (Li and Dowling, 1998).

In the past four years, using this assay we have measured in zebrafish both cone and rod sensitivity, the time course of cone and rod dark adaptation, and the effects of circadian clock and dopamine depletion on behavioral visual function. We have also screened the F1 generation of mutagenized zebrafish for visual system mutations (Li and Dowling, 1997, 1998, 2000a, 2000b). I review here the usefulness of zebrafish as a model for genetic and epigenetic studies of vertebrate visual system functions.

---

* Tel.: 859-323-4757; Fax: 859-323-1070;
E-mail: leili@pop.uky.edu

Zebrafish as a genetic model for vertebrate vision research

Dominant retinal degenerations have been described in many vertebrates including man. In humans, for example, approximately 40% of retinitis pigmentosa (RP) cases are dominantly inherited (Bunker et al., 1984). We know most about dominant RP where mutations have been found in photoreceptor cell-specific genes such as the rhodopsin or peripherin genes (Dryja et al., 1990, 1991; Kemp et al., 1994; Stone, 1998). However, it is estimated that only about half of the dominant RP cases can be accounted for by the mutations so far discovered (Berson, 1993). Thus, our understanding of the genetic mechanisms of dominant RP is still only in its infancy.

To gain a better understanding of dominant RP, mutational approaches using other organisms have attempted to identify genes that are involved in RP-like dominant retinal degenerations. A number of fly mutations, such as *rdgB* and *rdgC*, have been isolated and characterized. These mutations have proven to be exceptionally useful for molecular genetic studies of dominant retinal degeneration (Harris and Stark, 1977; Steele and O'Tousa, 1990). However, vertebrate models that are suitable for mutational screening of retinal degeneration genes have been lacking. The *rd* mouse and Irish setter dog that has rod–cone dysplasia have been used for molecular and cellular studies of vertebrate retinal degeneration (Olsson et al., 1992; Roof et al., 1994; Farber, 1995). However, these animals are not suited for genetic screening because of their large space requirement and long generation time.

Zebrafish (*Danio rerio*) have recently become a mainstream genetic model for vertebrate vision research (Brockerhoff et al., 1995; Malicki et al., 1996; Li and Dowling, 1997). Zebrafish are small tropical fresh-water fish that have been inbred in many laboratories (Streisinger et al., 1981; Nusslein-Volhard, 1994; Westerfield, 1995; Kimmel et al., 1995). Zebrafish are highly visual animals, exhibiting behavioral responses to visual stimuli as early as 3 days of age (Brockerhoff et al., 1995; Easter and Nicola, 1996). They are tetrachromatic, possessing ultraviolet-, red-, green-, and blue-sensitive cones, as well as abundant rods (Branchek and Bremiller, 1984; Robinson et al., 1993; Raymond et al., 1995;

Schmitt and Dowling, 1996, 1999; Vihtelic et al., 1999). Recently, mutations that affect zebrafish retinal development and function have been identified (Brockerhoff et al., 1995; Baier et al., 1996; Malicki et al., 1996; Li and Dowling, 1997, 2000a; Neuhauss et al., 1999). For example, by examining the size and the shape of developing retinas, Malicki et al. (1996) identified 49 mutations that affect zebrafish retinal development. These include mutations that affect retinal neuronal differentiation, proliferation, patterning, or degeneration. Among those mutations, 7 are photoreceptor cell-specific. By tracing fluorescent labeled retinal ganglion cell axons, Baier et al. (1996) uncovered 114 mutations that affect zebrafish retinotectal pathfinding. Most of these mutations cause defects in retinal ganglion cell pathfinding from eye to tectum or fiber sorting in the optic tract (Karlstrom et al., 1996; Trowe et al., 1996). Using a behavioral assay based on optokinetic response, Brockerhoff et al. (1995, 1997) has identified zebrafish mutants that show normal eye or retinal morphology but are blind. Among them are one that is completely blind, and one that is red-light blind.

Zebrafish mutations have proven to be very useful in our understanding of the genetic mechanisms of vertebrate retinal development and function. However, the use of zebrafish recessive mutations to study age-related retinal disease in adult animals is limited. One of the drawbacks in the screening of recessive mutations is the relatively long generation time of zebrafish. For example, it takes approximately 8–10 months to generate F3 generation from mutagenized founders (Mullins et al., 1994; Solnica-Krezel et al., 1994). Furthermore, virtually all of the currently available zebrafish recessive mutants demonstrate defects other than the retinal defects, and they tend to develop abnormally and die between 5 and 8 days of age (Brockerhoff et al., 1995; Karlstrom et al., 1996; Malicki et al., 1996; Trowe et al., 1996). Thus, it has not been generally possible to study age-related eye diseases in adult zebrafish.

Behavioral analysis of visual sensitivity of adult zebrafish

The behavioral assay, based on the visually mediated escape response, permits a rapid screening of non-lethal dominant visual system mutations in adult zebrafish (Li and Dowling, 1997). It works as follows. Normally, zebrafish swim slowly in circles when confined to a circular container. However, when challenged by a threatening object, i.e. a black segment rotating outside the container, the fish display a robust escape response: as soon as the black segment comes into view, the fish immediately turn and rapidly swim away (Fig. 1). Usually, a judgement of whether the fish is seeing the black segment can be made in less than 5 s.

We have analyzed the escape response of zebrafish to the black segment somewhat quantitatively. In two one-minute trials in which the drum rotates first clockwise and then counterclockwise, the fish encounter the black segment about 50 times. The fish typically display robust escape responses to the approach of the black segment on 40–45 occasions. By varying the light intensity that illuminates the black segment, we are able to evaluate the threshold light that is needed for the fish to see the black segment. Following bright light adaptation, for example, we measure at different times during dark

adaptation the threshold light intensities required to evoke escape responses when the fish is challenged by the black segment. This provides data with regard the absolute sensitivity levels of the both cone and rod systems, as well as the time course of dark adaptation (Li and Dowling, 1997; see also Dowling, 1987).

Zebrafish cone and rod sensitivities are influenced by a circadian clock

We evaluated zebrafish visual sensitivity behaviorally as a function of time of the day. Under a normal light/dark (14/10 h) cycle, visual thresholds of rod and cone systems are 2.2 and 1.4 log units lower, respectively, in late afternoon hours than in early morning hours. Over a 24-h period, zebrafish are most sensitive to light prior to light off (subjective dusk) and least sensitive prior to light on (subjective dawn). This rhythm of visual sensitivity persists in constant lighting conditions and can be phase shifted by a light pause (Fig. 2).

The circadian rhythm of visual sensitivity persists for 6–7 days in constant dark and 1–2 days in constant light. Thereafter, visual thresholds at all

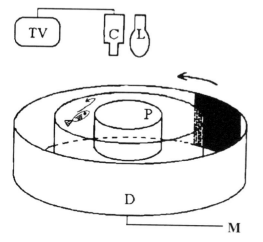

Fig. 1. Apparatus used for behavioral analysis of visual sensitivity of adult zebrafish. The apparatus consists of an immobilized circular container, surrounded by a rotating drum (D) covered with white paper. A black segment is marked on the paper that serves as a threatening object. A post (P) is placed in the center of the container to prevent the fish from swimming directly from one side of the container to the other. The drum is illuminated from above with a light source (L) and turned at 10 rpm by a motor (M). The fish is viewed by a television (TV) monitor attached to an infrared video camera (C) (Permitted by *Proc. Natl. Acad. Sci. USA*).

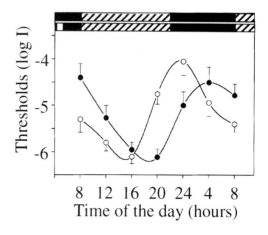

Fig. 2. Circadian rhythm of behavioral visual sensitivity during a 24-h period in constant darkness in control (filled circles) and phase shifted animals (open circles). In controls, thresholds are higher in early morning (subjective 4 a.m.) and lower in late afternoon (subjective 6 p.m.). In the experimental group, following a light pause at 4 a.m, the rhythm of sensitivity advances by 4 h. As a consequence, thresholds are higher at subjective midnight and lower at subjective 2 p.m. (Permitted by *Vis. Neurosci.*).

times converge at a level similar to thresholds measured in late afternoon hours in controls. These latter data suggest that the circadian clock functions to decrease the visual sensitivity. This rhythm of visual sensitivity is also observed in electroretinographic (ERG) recordings in animals kept in constant darkness. However, the threshold difference between early morning and late afternoon is only about 1.2 log unit as measured by the ERG. These data suggest that there is some circadian regulation of visual sensitivity downstream from the site of generation of the ERG, i.e. in the inner retina (Li and Dowling, 1998).

Isolation of visual system mutations in zebrafish

Using our behavioral assay, we have so far screened approximately 1,000 F1 generation fish mutagenized with N-ethyl-N-nitrosourea (ENU). For mutant screening, the rotating black segment is illuminated with light approximately 1.0 log unit above the absolute visual sensitivity level of the wild-type fish. At this intensity of illumination, the fish that demonstrate escape responses to the black segment are considered normal. On the other hand, individuals that fail the escape response test are isolated as night blind. So far we have isolated seven dominant mutants that failed the escape response test. All these mutations have been rescreened and outcrossed with wild-type zebrafish. Two of these mutants, *night blindness a* (*nba*) and *night blindness b* (*nbb*), have been further characterized (Table 1).

The nba *mutation*

The heterozygous *nba* (*nba*$^{+/-}$) mutants show normal behavioral visual sensitivity levels during the first 2–3 months of age, but thereafter, they become night blind. By 4 months, the visual threshold of *nba*$^{+/-}$ mutants is about 1.5 log units above the threshold level of control animals. The loss of *nba*$^{+/-}$ visual sensitivity is progressive with age. Between 5.5 and 9.5 months of age, for example, the average threshold of *nba*$^{+/-}$ mutants rises by 0.7 log units to reach levels about 2.5 log units above the absolute threshold level of wild-type zebrafish. The loss of visual sensitivity of *nba*$^{+/-}$ fish is also evident in ERG recordings, indicating that the defect caused by the *nba*$^{+/-}$ mutation is in the outer retina (Fig. 3).

Histological examination showed that *nba*$^{+/-}$ mutants undergo late onset photoreceptor cell degeneration involving initially the rods but eventually the

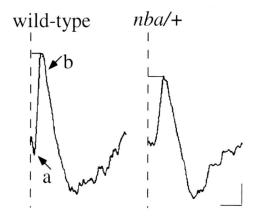

Fig. 3. Full-field ERGs recorded from 13-month-old wild-type (left) and *nba*$^{+/-}$ (right) fish in responding to a medium level white flash. The fish were dark-adapted approximately one hour prior to recordings. a, a-wave; b, b-wave. Note the reduction of b-wave amplitude and the increase of b-wave implicit time in the mutant. The vertical dashed lines indicate the onset of the 10 ms light stimuli, and the horizontal lines indicated the implicit times of the b-waves. Calibration bars (right lower) signify 200 ms horizontally and 50 μV vertically (Permitted by *Proc. Natl. Acad. Sci. USA*).

Table 1. Night blind mutants isolated from mutagenized zebrafish

Mutation	Heterozygotes		Homozygotes	
	Photoreceptors	INL neurons	CNS	Lethality
nba	Degenerate	Degenerate	Degenerate	Yes
nbb	Normal	Degenerate	Degenerate	Yes

Both *nba* and *nbb* mutations were isolated from a F1 generation of ENU treated zebrafish. Both mutants have been outcrossed with wild-type fish for at least four times. INL, inner nuclear layer; CNS, central nervous system.

cones as well. The photoreceptor degeneration of $nba^{+/-}$ mutants, however, is not uniform over the retina but tends to be patchy. Cones generally are preserved better than rods, but areas of cone degeneration are also observed (Fig. 4). Degeneration of inner retinal neurons is occasionally observed in $nba^{+/-}$ mutants. As a consequence, the thickness of $nba^{+/-}$ retina is somewhat reduced as compared to controls (Li and Dowling, 1997).

Whereas heterozygous *nba* mutants are viable to adulthood and show age-related retinal degeneration, homozygous *nba* ($nba^{-/-}$) fish display early onset neural degeneration throughout the brain which is obvious by 2 days post-fertilization (dpf). By 3 dpf, the $nba^{-/-}$ retinas as well as the central nervous system (CNS) are virtually destroyed. Abnormalities are also observed in other organs of developing $nba^{-/-}$ embryos, including the heart (Fig. 4). By 5 dpf, all homozygous *nba* fish die. These data suggest that the *nba* mutation is not in a photoreceptor cell-specific gene, but may represent a new form of inherited retinal degeneration (Li and Dowling, 1997).

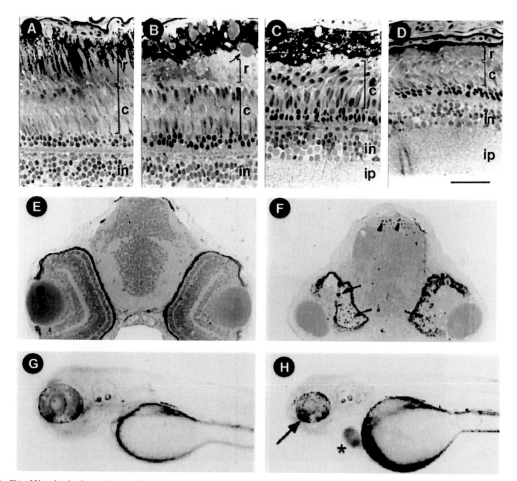

Fig. 4. (A–D): Histological sections of 13-month-old wild-type (A) and *nba* fish (B–D) retinas. Panels B–D show central retinal sections from a single $nba^{+/-}$ retina. Note the variability of cone (c) and rod (r) degeneration in $nba^{+/-}$ fish (stained by methylene blue). in, inner nuclear layer; ip, inner plexiform layer. (E–F): Histological sections that cross the CNS and retinas of 3-day-old wild-type (E) and homozygous *nba* (F) fish. Note the apoptotic cells in the $nba^{-/-}$ CNS and retinas (stained by methylene blue). (G–H): Photographs of 2.5-day-old wild-type (G) and *nba* (H) embryos. Note the small eye (arrow) and blood cells that have pooled in the heart (asterisk) in $nba^{-/-}$ mutant. Calibration bar: A, 100 μm; B–D, 80; E and F, 100 μm; G and H, 250 μm (Permitted by *Proc. Natl. Acad. Sci. USA*).

The nbb *mutation*

The *nbb* mutation presents another type of dominant retinal degeneration. As adults, $nbb^{+/-}$ mutants show abnormal visual threshold fluctuations when measured following prolonged dark adaptation. After 2 h of dark adaptation, for example, visual thresholds of $nbb^{+/-}$ mutants fluctuate by up to 3–4 log units, unlike control animals in which visual thresholds are maintained at a constant level. Light sensitizes $nbb^{+/-}$ animals; thus, early dark adaptation of $nbb^{+/-}$ fish is virtually normal. Using phototopically-matched red and green illumination, we demonstrated that in $nbb^{+/-}$ mutants the rod system function is absent behaviorally. This suggests the *nbb* mutation selectively blocks the rod-signal pathway (Li and Dowling, 2000a).

We further evaluated the visual defect of $nbb^{+/-}$ fish using electrophysiological methods. ERGs recorded from $nbb^{+/-}$ mutants are normal in terms of waveform and a- and b-wave light thresholds. This suggests that the outer retina of $nbb^{+/-}$ mutants is functional and reasonably normal. However, the light thresholds required to elicit ganglion cell discharges in $nbb^{+/-}$ fish are raised as compared to those of controls, suggesting that the defect of $nbb^{+/-}$ mutants is in the inner retina. Using histological and immunocytochemical methods, we found that in $nbb^{+/-}$ mutants the olfactory centrifugal projection to the retina is disrupted and reduced (Fig. 5) and

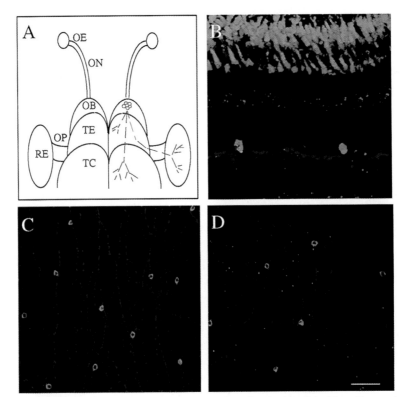

Fig. 5. (A) Schematic drawing of olfactoretinal centrifugal input to the retina in zebrafish. The olfactoretinal centrifugal pathway originates from the terminalis neurons (TNs, red circles) that are located in the olfactory bulb. OE, olfactory epithelium; ON, olfactory nerve; OB, olfactory bulb; OP, optic nerve; RE, retina; TE, telencephalon; TC, tectum. (B) A double-labeled retinal section showing the centrifugal fibers (red) and DA-IPCs (green, arrows). Centrifugal fibers and DA-IPCs are identified using antibodies against FMRFamide and tyrosine hydroxylase, respectively. (C–D) Confocal images taken from nasal/ventral regions of double-labeled wild-type (C) and $nbb^{+/-}$ (D) retinas. Centrifugal fibers are shown in red and DA-IPCs are shown in green. Note the disruption and reduction of centrifugal fibers and the reduction of DA-IPCs in the $nbb^{+/-}$ retina. Calibration bar: B, 100 μm; C and D, 30 μm (Permitted by *J. Neurosci.*).

Table 2. The number of centrifugal fiber varicosity (per mm^2) and DA-IPC (per retina) in wild-type and mutant retinas

	Varicosity	DA-IPC
Wild-type	3,086 ± 457	1,116 ± 40
nbb$^{+/-}$	1,471 ± 485	885 ± 67

Data were obtained from 11.5 months old whole-mount double-labeled retinas (with antibodies against FMRFamide and tyrosine hydroxylase).

the number of the retinal dopaminergic interplexiform cells (DA-IPCs) is decreased (Table 2).

To test the hypothesis that olfactoretinal centrifugal input to the retina is required for visual system function, we measured visual sensitivity of zebrafish in which the olfactoretinal centrifugal pathway is lesioned. In animals in which the olfactory epithelium was ablated, the behavioral visual thresholds are normal in the first 20 min of dark adaptation. However, threshold fluctuations are observed when animals are kept in prolonged darkness, mimicking the visual defects observed in nbb$^{+/-}$ mutants (Li and Dowling, 2000a). These data suggest that the defect of nbb is not retinal-specific but may be in the olfactory system as well.

Dopamine depletion blocks selectively the rod pathway

One of the conclusions drawn from the nbb mutation is that dopamine is required for rod signal transmission (Li and Dowling, 2000a). To test this hypothesis, we measured visual sensitivity of zebrafish in which the DA-IPCs were depleted by intraocular injections of 6-hydroxydopamine (6-OHDA). During the first 6–8 min of dark adaptation following bright light adaptation, visual thresholds of DA-IPC-depleted animals are similar to those of control animals. Thereafter, visual thresholds are elevated such that by 14–18 min of dark adaptation, thresholds of DA-IPC-depleted animals are 2–3 log units above levels of control animals. The loss of behavioral visual sensitivity of DA-IPC-depleted animals is likely due to a rod system dysfunction: using phototopically matched color lights the Purkinje shift normally observed in controls is not evident in the 6-OHDA treated animals (Li and Dowling, 2000b; Fig. 6).

In DA-IPC depleted animals, the ERGs are normal in terms of light sensitivity and waveform,

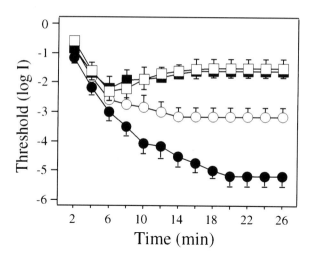

Fig. 6. Dark adaptation curves of control (circles) and DA-IPC-depleted (squares) animals using red (625 nm, open symbols) and green (500 nm, filled symbols) illumination. Note that no red–green threshold differences are observed in 6-OHDA-treated fish at 6 and 20 min of dark adaptation, unlike controls in which the thresholds determined by red light are 0.3 and 2.0 log units higher than thresholds determined by green light when measured at these two time points (Permitted by *J. Neurosci.*).

but the light threshold for eliciting a ganglion cell discharge is raised by 1.8 log units as compared to controls. This suggests that the defect caused by dopamine depletion is in the inner retina. Partial rescue of the behavioral visual sensitivity loss in DA-IPC-depleted animals occurred when dopamine or a long-acting dopamine agonist, ADTN, is intraocularly injected (Fig. 7).

Conclusions and future perspectives

Zebrafish have proven to be an excellent model for genetic and epigenetic studies of vertebrate vision. Our research has been focusing on the behavioral, physiological, and genetic studies of zebrafish visual system function and disease. Using a behavioral assay based on the visually mediated escape responses, we have evaluated visual sensitivity of both the cone and rod systems, the effect of circadian clock, dopamine, and olfactoretinal centrifugal input in the regulation of zebrafish visual sensitivity. In a search of F1 generation of mutagenized zebrafish, we have identified seven dominant mutations that cause slow retinal degeneration, such as nba and nbb.

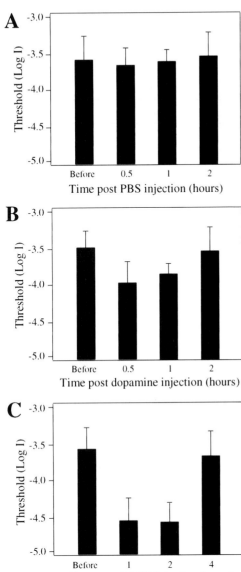

Fig. 7. Behaviorally measured visual thresholds of DA-IPC depleted animals before and after intraocular injections of PBS (A), dopamine (B), and a dopamine receptor agonist, ADTN (C). (A) As a control, zebrafish are sham-injected with PBS. (B) Dopamine injected at a concentration of 200 μM. Note the threshold decreases at 30 min and 1 h post dopamine injection. At 2 h post-injection, the thresholds of DA-IPC-depleted animals return to levels similar to those measured prior to dopamine injections. (C) ADTN injected at a concentration of 10 μM. At 1 and 2 h post-injection, visual thresholds of DA-IPC-depleted animals are significantly decreased. The effect of ADTN on behavioral visual sensitivity is insignificant at 4 h post-injection (Permitted by *J. Neurosci.*).

At the present time, the genetic mechanism and cell specificity of *nba* and *nbb* genes are unknown. In heterozygotes, both *nba* and *nbb* are viable to adulthood and show only retinal defects. However, when bred to homozygosity, they cause entire CNS degeneration and embryonic lethality. These data suggest that neither *nba* nor *nbb* are retinal specific genes, instead, they are expressed beyond the eye.

In the years to come, we will extend our studies to isolate and characterize dominant mutations, gene alleles, and extragenic suppressors that affect zebrafish visual system development and function. In doing so, we hope to gain a better understanding of the genetic basis of vertebrate dominant retinal degeneration, and hopefully, to provide tools for human RP research.

References

Baier, H., Klostermann, S., Trowe, T., Karlstrom, R.O., Nusslein-Volhard, C. and Bonhoeffer, F. (1996) Genetic dissection of the retinotectal projection. *Development*, 123: 415–425.

Berson, E.L. (1993) Retinitis Pigmentosa. *Invest. Ophthalmol. Vis. Sci.*, 34: 1659–1676.

Branchek, T. and Bremiller, R. (1984) The development of photoreceptors in the zebrafish, *Branchydanio rerio*. I. Structure. *J. Comp. Neurol.*, 224: 107–115.

Brockerhoff, S.E., Hurley, J.B., Janssen-Bienhold, U., Neuhauss, S.C.F., Driever, W. and Dowling J.E. (1995) A behavioral screen for isolating zebrafish mutants with visual system defects. *Proc. Natl. Acad. Sci. USA*, 92: 10545–10549.

Brockerhoff, S.E., Hurley, J.B., Niemi, G.A. and Dowling, J.E. (1997) A new form of inherited red-blindness identified in zebrafish. *J. Neurosci.*, 17: 4236–4242.

Bunker, C.H., Berson, E.L., Bromley, W.C., Hayes, R.P. and Roderick, T.H. (1984) Prevalence of retinitis pigmentosa in Maine. *Am. J. Ophthalmol.*, 97: 357–365.

Dowling, J.E. (1987) *The retina: An approachable part of the brain*. Harvard University Press. Cambridge, MA.

Dryja, T.P., McGee, T.L., Reichel, E., Hahn, L.B., Cowley, G.S., Yandell, D.W., Sandberg, M.A. and Berson, E.L. (1990) A point mutation of the rhodopsin gene in one form of retinitis pigmentosa. *Nature*, 343: 364–399.

Dryja, T.P., Hahn, L.B., Cowley, G.S., McGee, T.L. and Berson, E.L. (1991) Mutation spectrum of the rhodopsin gene among patients with autosomal dominant retinitis pigmentosa. *Proc. Natl. Acad. Sci. USA*, 88: 9370–9374.

Easter, S.S. and Nicola, G.N. (1996) The development of vision in the zebrafish, *Danio rerio*. *Dev. Biol.*, 180: 646–663.

Farber, D.B. (1995) From mice to men: The cyclic GMP phosphodiesterase gene in vision and disease. *Invest. Ophthalmol. Vis. Sci.*, 36: 263–275.

Harris, W.A. and Stark, W.L. (1977) Hereditary retinal degeneration in Drosophila melanogaster. A mutant defect associated with phototransduction process. *J. Gen. Physiol.*, 69: 261–291.

Karlstrom, R.O., Trowe, T., Klostermann, S., Baier, H., Brand, M., Crawford, A.D., Grunewald, B., Haffter, P., Hoffmann, H., Meyer, S.U., Muller, B.K., Richter, D., Van Eeden, F.J.M., Nusslein-Volhard, C. and Bonhoeffer, F. (1996) Zebrafish mutations affecting retinotectal axon pathfinding. *Development*, 123: 427–438.

Kemp, C.M., Jacobson, S.G., Cideciyan, A.V., Kimura, A.E., Sheffield, V.C. and Stone, E.M. (1994) RDS gene mutations causing retinitis pigmentosa or macular degeneration lead to the same abnormality in photoreceptor function. *Invest. Ophthalmol. Vis. Sci.*, 35: 3154–3162.

Kimmel, C.B., Ballard, W.W., Kimmerl, S.R., Ullmann, B. and Schilling, T.F. (1995) Stages of embryonic development of the zebrafish. *Dev. Dyn.*, 203: 253–310.

Li, L. and Dowling, J.E. (1997) A dominant form of inherited retinal degeneration caused by a non-photoreceptor cell-specific mutation. *Proc. Natl. Acad. Sci. USA*, 94: 11645–11650.

Li, L. and Dowling, J.E. (1998) Zebrafish visual sensitivity is regulated by a circadian clock. *Vis. Neurosci.*, 15: 851–857.

Li, L. and Dowling, J.E. (2000a) Disruption of the olfactoretinal centrifugal pathway may relate to the visual system defect in *night blindness b* mutant zebrafish. *J. Neurosci.*, 20: 1883–1892.

Li, L. and Dowling, J.E. (2000b) Effects of dopamine depletion on visual sensitivity of zebrafish. *J. Neurosci.*, 20: 1893–1903.

Malicki, J., Neuhauss, S.C.F., Schier, A.F., Solnica-Krezel, L., Stemple, D.L., Stainier, D.Y.R., Abdelilah, S., Zwartkruis, F., Rangini, Z. and Driever, W. (1996) Mutations affecting development of the zebrafish retina. *Development*, 123: 263–273.

Mullins, M.C., Hammerschmidt, A., Haffter, P. and Nusslein-Volhard, C. (1994) Large-scale mutagenesis in the zebrafish: in search of genes controlling development in a vertebrate. *Curr. Biol.*, 4: 189–202.

Nusslein-Volhard, C. (1994) Of flies and fishes. *Science*, 266: 572–574.

Neuhauss, S.C.F., Biehlmaier, O., Seeliger, M.W., Das, T., Kohler, K., Harris, W.A. and Baier, H. (1999) Genetic disorders of vision revealed by a behavioral screen of 400 essential loci in zebrafish. *J. Neurosci.*, 19: 8603–8615.

Olsson, J.E., Gordon, J.W., Pawlyk, B.S., Roof, D., Hayes, A., Molday, R.S., Mukai, S., Cowley, G.S., Berson, E.L. and Dryja, T.P. (1992) Transgenic mice with a rhodopsin mutation (Pro23His): A mouse model of autosomal dominant retinitis pigmentosa. *Neuron*, 9: 815–830.

Raymond, P.A., Barthel, L.K. and Curran, G.A. (1995) Developmental patterning of rod and cone photoreceptors in embryonic zebrafish. *J. Comp. Neurol.*, 359: 537–550.

Roof, D.J., Adamian, M. and Hayes, A. (1994) Rhodopsin accumulation at abnormal sites in retinas of mice with a human P23H rhodopsin transgene. *Invest. Ophthalmol. Vis. Sci.*, 35: 4049–4062.

Robinson, J., Schmitt, E.A., Harosi, F.I., Reece, R.J. and Dowling, J.E. (1993) Zebrafish ultraviolet visual pigment: Absorption spectrum, sequence and localization. *Proc. Natl. Acad. Sci. USA*, 90: 6009–6012.

Schmitt, E.A. and Dowling, J.E. (1996) Comparison of topographical patterns of ganglion and photoreceptor cell differentiation in the retina of the zebrafish. *J. Comp. Neurol.*, 371: 222–234.

Schmitt, E.A. and Dowling, J.E. (1999) Early retinal development in the zebrafish, Danio rerio: Light and electron microscopic analyses. *J. Comp. Neurol.*, 404: 515–536.

Solnica-Krezel, L., Schier, A.F. and Driever, W. (1994) Efficient recovery of ENU-induced mutations from the zebrafish germline. *Genetics*, 136: 1401–1420.

Steele, F. and O'Tousa, J.E. (1990) Rhodopsin activation causes retinal degeneration in Drosophila *rdgC* mutant. *Neuron*, 4: 883–890.

Stone, E.M. (1998) Expanding the repertoire of RP genes. *Nat. Genet.*, 19: 311–313.

Streisinger, G., Walker, C., Dower, N., Knauber, D. and Singer, F. (1981) Production of clones of homozygous diploid zebra fish (Brachydanio rerio). *Nature*, 291: 293–296.

Trowe, T., Klostermann, S., Baier, H., Granato, M., Crawford, A.D., Grunewald, B., Hoffmann, H., Karlstrom, R.O., Meyer, S.U., Muller, B., Richter, S., Nusslein-Volhard, C. and Bonhoeffer, F. (1996) Mutations disrupting the ordering and topographic mapping of axons in the retinotectal projection of the zebrafish, *Danio rerio. Development*, 123: 439–450.

Vihtelic, T.S., Doro, C.J. and Hyde, D.R. (1999) Cloning and characterization of six zebrafish photoreceptor opsin cDNAs and immunolocolization of their corresponding proteins. *Vis. Neurosci.*, 16: 571–585.

Westerfield, M. (1995) The zebrafish book: A guide for the laboratory use of zebrafish (*Danio rerio*). University of Oregon Press, Eugene, OR.

H. Kolb, H. Ripps and S. Wu (Eds.)
Progress in Brain Research, Vol. 131

CHAPTER 40

Genetic analysis of initial and ongoing retinogenesis in the zebrafish: comparing the central neuroepithelium and marginal zone

Brian A. Link* and Tristan Darland

Department of Molecular and Cellular Biology, Harvard University, 16 Divinity Avenue, Cambridge, MA 02135, USA

Overview

The vertebrate eye develops from highly coordinated inductive and migratory events involving cells derived from multiple embryonic origins. The retina forms from the inner most layer of the optic cup and is thus derived from diencephalic neuroectoderm. Just as highly coordinated inductive and migratory events establish the various components of the eye, similar regulatory events are involved in establishing the various cell types and the multi-layered organization of the retina. Following differentiation of the nascent retina in several vertebrates, the eye continues to grow throughout the life of the animal. Ongoing differentiation has been long established for amphibians and fish (Hollyfield, 1968; Johns, 1977; Wetts and Fraser, 1988) and more recently this phenomenon has been described for avians (Fischer and Reh, 2000). New retinal cells are added at the distal-most edge of the retina from a specialized area termed the marginal zone. In this paper we summarize the salient features of initial or central retinal differentiation, as well as ongoing or marginal zone differentiation. Particular attention is paid to one model organism—*Danio rerio*, the zebrafish. We then present genetic data from zebrafish that

lends insight into both central and marginal zone differentiation and the interactions between the two processes. We conclude by outlining questions that remain to be addressed for retinal development and highlight the experimental utility of model organisms that display robust proliferative marginal zones.

Central retinal differentiation

Central retinal differentiation is the culmination of a series of cellular events common to the development of other regions in the central nervous system: proliferation, cell cycle withdrawal, specification, migration and differentiation. At the earliest stages of retinal development, all of the neuroepithelial cells that line the optic cup are proliferative. These multipotent progenitor cells give rise to all cell types found within the retina. The elongated progenitor cells span the width of the neuroepithelium. The nuclear position of each cell correlates to the stage of the mitotic cycle. Neuroepithelial cells undergo cellular division at the apical boarder, near the retinal pigmented epithelium. DNA synthesis occurs more basally, towards the vitreal surface. Because the neuroepithelial cells of the optic cup divide asynchronously, the structure appears psuedostratified. In zebrafish, the first cells to permanently withdraw from the cell cycle do so around 28 h post fertilization (hpf)

---

* Corresponding author: Brian A. Link, Tel.: 617-495-2599; Fax: 617-496-3321; E-mail: Blink@fas.harvard.edu

within the nasal region of the ventral retina (Hu and Easter, 1999; Schmitt and Dowling, 1999). Similar to other vertebrates, ganglion cells are the first cell-type born in zebrafish. Cell cycle withdrawal of ganglion cells advances laterally from this initiation site—often referred to as the ventral patch—sweeping nasally towards the dorsal retina before returning to the ventral retina through the temporal sector. Within a vertical column of cells, inner nuclear types are the next to stop dividing, followed by photoreceptors in the outer nuclear layer. Therefore, viewing the processes of terminal mitosis within the central retina as a whole, three fan-like waves initiate terminal mitosis in an inside-to-outside gradient (Hu and Easter, 1999).

Cellular specification, the commitment of a progenitor cell to differentiate as one particular cell type, can occur just prior to cell cycle withdrawal or after the terminal mitosis during migration. Cell type specification within the retina is not fully understood, but current ideas have recently been reviewed (Cepko et al., 1996; Harris, 1997). In brief, data from multiple labs support a model where both intrinsic and extrinsic factors contribute to restrictions in a progenitors repertoire of possible cell fates, until finally, it is restricted to differentiate as one cell type. During specification of the central retina, there is a phylogenetically conserved birth-order of cell types. Subtle differences among species do exist, but ganglion cells are invariably the first cell-type born and rod photoreceptor, bipolar and Müller glial cells are among the last. These temporal biases suggest that either specification cues and/or the progenitor cells' competence to respond to such signals, change throughout development.

While the mode of retinoblast migration remains relatively uncharacterized, it is clear that the path is radial away from the apical ventricular zone. In this way, columns of clonally related cells are formed. Unlike other regions of the central nervous system, such as the cerebral cortex and cerebellum where neuroblasts migrate along radially spanning glial cells, there are no obvious guidance cells for retinoblasts (Hatten, 1999). The mode of retinal precursor cell migration has been proposed to occur by one of two different methods. In the first method, following final mitosis, precursor cells re-establish apical and basal processes and the nucleus translocates to the appropriate laminar position. In the second proposed method, the rounded retinal precursor cells migrate through extracellular matrix until reaching the proper layer. Assessment of retinal precursor migration in birds by in vivo cell-labeling and histological inspection suggests that both migratory modes are employed during central retinal differentiation (Snow and Robson, 1995). Perhaps a better understanding of retinal precursor cell migration can give insights into the cellular interactions that contribute to cell-type specification. The zebrafish may serve as an excellent model to study these cell movements owing to rapid development and embryonic transparency allowing access for time-lapse analysis.

Once a retinal precursor cell has finished migration, it begins (or perhaps continues) the process of cellular differentiation. Defined in the broadest terms, differentiation is the execution of genetic pathways that lead to the structural and biochemical specializations which enable a particular cell type to perform it's unique functions. Retinal cell differentiation, as with other cell types, has been defined largely by marker expression, morphological criteria, and for neurons, electrophysiological properties. While the mechanisms that regulate retinal cell differentiation remain incompletely uncharacterized, it is clear that intrinsic genetic programs as well as cell–cell and cell–matrix interactions together determine the differentiation state of retinal cells.

The marginal zone: stem cells and ongoing retinal differentiation

One of the many reasons that fish, and for that matter amphibians, are popular experimental model systems in vision research is because their retinas contains self-renewing populations of neuronal stem cells. In this respect, the fish retina joins a growing list of areas in the adult vertebrate central nervous system (CNS) with stem cell populations (Brock et al., 1998). Understanding the dynamics and regulation of such stem cells has obvious clinical relevance for the treatment of neural injury and degenerative disorders. Zebrafish have proven especially amenable for studying neuronal development because of the relative ease of stock maintenance, accessibility of the embryo, and the potential for genetic analysis.

Zebrafish grow as much as 100 fold in length and 1,000,000 fold in volume during their lifetime. Such prolonged and extensive growth throughout life requires continual expansion and modification of the visual field. Labeling mitotically active cells using tritiated-thymidine demonstrated that the growth of the eye and expansion of the visual field in the adult goldfish is accomplished by cell addition to the retina (Fernald, 1990). Cell addition occurs at the peripheral edge of the retina, a region referred to as the marginal zone. Other studies have demonstrated that in addition to the marginal zone, neuronal progenitor cells are sparsely scattered throughout the outer and inner nuclear layers of the fish retina and are induced to rapidly proliferate in response to injury (Raymond and Hitchcock, 1997). These cells which include the rod progenitors are in large measure responsible for the regenerative capacity of the fish retina. Retinal regeneration, though an extremely interesting topic of research, is beyond the scope of this chapter.

Recently, studies in zebrafish using 5′-bromo-2′-deoxyuridine (BrdU) to label mitotically active cells have demonstrated that the marginal zone actively produces neurons throughout embryogenesis and adulthood (Hu and Easter, 1999; Marcus et al., 1999). At 24 hpf, all cells of the retina are labeled, indicating that the entire neuroepithelium is actively dividing (see Figs. 2G and 3G). By 48 hpf, proliferating cells are restricted to the outer nuclear layer and the peripheral retina. Proliferating cells are considerably reduced in number by 72 hpf as nearly all DNA synthesis has ceased in the outer nuclear layer. Only cells in the marginal zone and a few progenitors in the inner nuclear layer incorporate BrdU at this time point (see Figs. 2H and 3H).

How neurogenesis is maintained in the marginal zone after it stops in the central retina is unknown. Furthermore, it is not certain whether development of cells originating in the marginal zone proceeds along a distinct pathway or recapitulates the process that occurs earlier in the central retina. Efforts to understand how marginal zone cells develop have involved examination of expression patterns for neurogenic, proneural and transcription factor genes.

Marker gene expression in the marginal zone

The advantage of using the marginal zone as a model of neurogenesis is that cells are arranged spatially in a manner reflecting their stage of development. Thus, a cross-section of the eye is in effect a time-lapse picture of how retinal cells develop and differentiate, with the youngest cells positioned most peripherally. Recently, an important study in *Xenopus* used the marginal zone to examine the timing of proneural and neurogenic gene expression with respect to proliferation during retinal development (Perron et al., 1998). Genes expressed in more peripheral regions compared to those expressed more centrally, were hypothesized to function earlier in the course of progenitor cell differentiation. Results from these studies defined regions in the marginal zone with distinct yet overlapping patterns of gene expression. For example, Pax6, a paired-type homeodomain protein critical for eye development for all species examined, showed an expression pattern which began in the most peripheral region of the marginal zone (Hitchcock et al., 1996). The expression domain of neurogenic genes such as the *deltas*, which are required for proliferating neuroepithelium, began in a region more central than *pax6*. Likewise, proneural gene expression, required for proliferating neuroblasts, began in a region more central than *delta*. In addition, subsets of these markers are expressed by fully differentiated neurons in specific cell layers of the mature retina. The conclusion reached by the investigators was that in retinal development, genes such as *pax6*, the neurogenic and proneural genes act sequentially in hierarchical pathways. Underlying these experiments is the assumption that development in the marginal zone reflects that occurring earlier in the central retina.

Comparison of initial central and marginal zone gene expression

An exhaustive study similar to that described above has not yet been performed on the marginal zone of the zebrafish. However, information gleaned from the literature and from our own experiments indicate that homologs for most of the genes described in the *Xenopus* study are also expressed in the marginal zone of the zebrafish. Furthermore, expression patterns for some of these genes reflect an expression hierarchy maintained in both the early central retina and later in the marginal zone. One example is the paired-type homeodomain genes *vsx-1* and *vsx-2* characterized in the goldfish and zebrafish (Passini et al., 1997). *Vsx-2* is expressed in proliferating cells of the early retina and later within the marginal zone. *Vsx-1*, on the other hand is expressed by cells as they exit the cell cycle, with message being detected early in the central retina after *vsx-2* is turned off. Later, *vsx-1* is found in a region just outside the marginal zone where newly post-mitotic cells are beginning to differentiate. Interestingly, the expression of both genes is retained in fully differentiated bipolar cells. The maintained expression in specific cell types appears to be a common theme among early expressed retinal genes. For example, *six3* and *rx* genes are expressed throughout the proliferating neuroepithelium and then later restricted to specific cell types including amacrine and photoreceptors cells, respectively (Oliver et al., 1995; Mathers et al., 1997). Despite dynamic and often complex expression patterns for genes expressed in the initial central retina, similarities can be found in the marginal zone which suggests a common pathway of development for the two cell populations.

In our experiments we have investigated a number of previously identified genes that are expressed during initial differentiation in the central retina. Similar to the studies cited above, we find that expression patterns of each is reiterated in specific regions of the marginal zone. For example, *pax6.1* shows expression throughout the retinal neuroepithelium at 24 hpf during proliferative expansion of the retinoblast pool. By 48 hpf, expression has been refined to those cells in the prospective inner two nuclear layers of the retina (Fig. 1A). Eventually, *pax6* expressing cells are found only in the inner portion of the inner nuclear layer and in the ganglion cell layer where amacrine and ganglion cells reside (Fig. 1B; Hitchcock et al., 1996). Within the marginal zone, expression is maintained in proliferating progenitor cells, similar to the central neuroepithelium at earlier times.

The gene *delta D*, which encodes a ligand that stimulates Notch receptor activity, is also expressed in neuroepithelial cells during initial central differentiation. Within the retina, Notch activity is thought to negatively regulate the competence of retinal precursor cells for responding to specification signals (Lewis, 1998; Rapaport and Dorsky, 1998). In support of this function, *delta D* is expressed in only a subset of cells at 48 hpf, presumably those yet to be specified to a particular cell type (Fig. 1C). At later times, following specification and differentiation in the central retina, a zone of *delta D*-positive cells can be seen in the marginal zone. Interestingly, the region of *delta D* expressing cells does not encompass the distal-most marginal zone cells, perhaps distinguishing those being primed for cellular specification from those simply undergoing stem-cell renewal.

Islet proteins, LIM-type homeodomain transcription factors, are first expressed within the zebrafish retina in post-mitotic ganglion, bipolar and horizontal cells (Fig. 1E; Korzh et al., 1993). Islet expression is maintained into adulthood. At the marginal zone of juvenile zebrafish (15 dpf), elongated cells are void of Islet-immunoreactivity, but similar to initial central differentiation, expression is found just as ganglion, bipolar and horizontal cells become post-mitotic and migrate into the appropriate lamina (Fig. 1F).

These expression patterns serve as three examples of genes that define distinct stages in initial, central retina development that are mirrored in the ongoing development of the marginal zone. The majority of markers investigated in species with continuous retinal development share similarities in central versus marginal zone expression. However, the bulk of markers that have been investigated during marginal zone development are transcription factors and members of the Notch-Delta family. Other types of regulatory factors such as soluble secreted factors, their receptors, and extra cellular matrix components, have not been assessed. In addition, marker analyses tend to ignore quantitative aspects of expression, and perhaps critical and distinct levels of regulator factors differ between central and marginal zone development.

While the similarities are most often noted, there are some obvious differences between initial and ongoing retinal development. Chief among these differences is that initial central differentiation begins from a group of approximately equivalent cells—although subtle inequalities between retinal

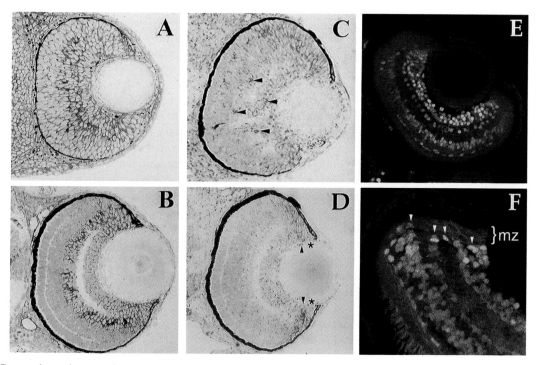

Fig. 1. Gene and protein expression patterns during retinal development. In situ hybridization for *pax6* mRNA at 2 dpf (**A**) and 4 dpf (**B**). *delta D* mRNA at 2 dpf (**C**). Note the strongly *delta-D* positive cells scattered throughout the central retina (arrowheads, C). *delta D* mRNA at 4 dpf (**D**) Note the strong band of *delta-D* positve cells (arrowheads D) in the proximal marginal zone, while those in the distal tip of the marginal zone are negative (asterisks D). Islet-immunoreactivity at 2 dpf (**E**) and within the marginal zone of 15 dpf juvenile fish (**F**). Note those cells recently incorporated into their lamina are strongly immunoreactive for Islet (arrowheads F). For in situ hybridizations, mRNA stains purple and the sections were counter-stained with methylene blue. For immunostaining, Islet is green-yellow and the sections were counterstained red with the nuclear dye propidium iodide. Green found in the photoreceptor outersegments is due to auto-flourescence. mz, marginal zone.

neuroepithelial cells likely exist (Jasoni and Reh, 1996; Jensen and Raff, 1997; Cepko, 1999). The situation is quite different for marginal zone progenitors where an established template of well differentiated cell types exist in close proximity. The differences in the local environments between central and marginal zone retinoblasts may impact the way in which these cells differentiate. One other difference worth noting is the timing of cell differentiation. Initial central development occurs in three pulsetile bursts (Hu and Easter, 1999). It is unclear whether cell cycle withdrawal in the marginal zone is regulated in a similar fashion. Clearly, progenitors are maintained in a proliferative state for much greater lengths of time as compared to the neuroepithelial cells of the optic cup and the overall process occurs more slowly. In order to further probe and compare the mechanisms of initial central and marginal zone

retinal development, we have employed forward genetics in zebrafish.

Forward genetics to investigate central and marginal zone retinal development

For a number of years, the Dowling lab has conducted an ongoing screen in zebrafish for mutations that affect visual development and function (Brockerhoff et al., 1995; Fadool et al., 1997). As part of this screen, we have isolated recessive mutations that affect initial differentiation of the central retina, and therefore disrupt retinal lamination, as well as mutations that perturb ongoing peripheral development and thus distort the marginal zone. Recessive mutations have been identified based on morphological and histological examination.

Mutagenesis was preformed using established protocols: a founding population of male fish (F_0-generation) were treated with the point-mutagen ENU and through successive incrossing, recessive mutations were revealed in F_3-generation embryos (Solinca-Krezel et al., 1994).

This forward genetic approach is advantageous for several reasons in defining critical components of either initial central retinal or marginal zone development. A prime advantage to forward genetics is the unbiased selection of genes with essential functions in the processes under investigation. In theory, a forward genetic approach will identify essential genes—regardless of preconceived ideas and models—in all relevant gene families including transcriptional regulators, competence factors, soluble secreted factors and their receptors, signal transduction molecules, as well as extracellular matrix components. Another advantage to this approach is that the genetic alterations are heritable, facilitating mosaic analyses to define cell–cell and cell–environment interactions. Heritable genetic alterations also enable epistasis experiments to define genetic signaling pathways. Zebrafish are a choice model organism in which to conduct our screen owing to rapid central retinal development and an easily identifiable and robust marginal zone. In addition, the high genetic conservation and structural homology within the eyes of vertebrates makes these studies germain to human development and pathogeneis.

Mutations that affect initial, central retinal development

Young

Zebrafish with the *young* (*yng*) mutation are defective in retinal differentiation (Link et al., 2000). Neuroepithelial cells appear normal, although those of the central retina remain proliferative for a greater period of time than those in wild type embryos. However, the pattern of cell cycle withdrawal is similar to wild types (Fig. 2A and C). Post-mitotic retinal progenitors can become specified to each of the cell classes normally found in the retina. These cells, though, irrespective of type, do not express markers for a fully differentiated state nor undergo morphological specializations (Fig. 2D). This lack of differentiation prevents the retina from gaining its characteristic laminations (Fig. 2B). BrdU studies demonstrate the marginal zone remains proliferative and the cells of this region appear morphologically normal (Link et al., 2000). This observation suggests that a differentiated central retina is not required in order to maintain the marginal zone. Similar to the central retina, marginal zone precursor cells are unable to fully differentiate. This result suggests that the *yng* gene product is likely required for retinal differentiation in both regions. An alternative interpretation is that a fully differentiated central retina is necessary to direct the differentiation of marginal zone precursor cells. Identification of the gene affected by the *yng* mutation and assessment of the distribution of the protein will distinguish between these two possibilities.

Bewildered

The *bewildered* (*bwd*) mutation, similar to *yng*, prevents retinal lamination. At the optic cup stage, the *bwd* retina appears morphologically normal. Later, from approximately 56 hpf and beyond, the eye is clearly smaller than wild types. Differences are first noted in retinal histology when neuroepithelial cells begin to exit the cell cycle in normal embryos. At this time within the mutant retina, an increase in pyknotic cells is observed (Fig. 2A and E). By 4 dpf, cell death is very obvious (Fig. 2F). The cells that remain appear elongated and neuroepithelial. BrdU-incorporation studies demonstrate two points. One is that proliferation is normal at early stages of development, and the decreased eye size is likely due to increased cell death. Second, nearly all of the surviving cells remain BrdU-positive. Cumulatively, these observations suggest that the *bwd* mutation causes the retina to maintain a neuroepithelial state. Perhaps the dying cells are newly post-mitotic and defective in the differentiation process. With this arrest in retinal development, a defined marginal zone is never formed. It will be interesting to test whether the *bwd* gene product is necessary for cell cycle withdrawal of neuroepithelial cells or whether it is essential for the specification, differentiation, and/or survival of post-mitotic retinal cells.

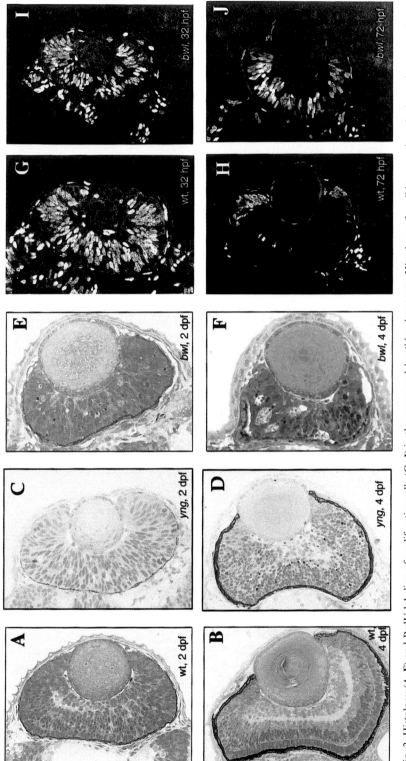

Fig. 2. Histology (A–F) and BrdU labeling of proliferative cells (G–J) in the *young* and *bewildered* mutants. Histology of a wild type embryo is shown for comparison at 2 days (A) and 4 days (B). Histology for the *young* (C, D) and *bewildered* (E, F) mutants at 2 and 4 days, respectively. Immunolabeling for BrdU in wild type and *bewildered* embryos was performed at 32 hpf after a 1 h pulse (G) and at 72 hpf after a 12 h pulse (H). Note that morphology and proliferation of cells in the central retina at the earlier time points is essentially normal. Later, the central retina maintains neuroepithelial characteristics and exhibits increased cell death. The marginal zone in these mutants appears relatively normal.

Mutations that affect the marginal zone

Round eye

Given the evidence from marker expression studies suggesting that neurogenesis in the marginal zone is a recapitulation of events in the central retina, it was surprising that mutations affecting zebrafish eye morphology were discovered that specifically disrupted development in the periphery (Fadool et al., 1997). One of these mutations, *round eye (rde)*, is shown at 32 and 96 hpf in Fig. 3C and D respectively. During the earliest stages, the retina develops normally with respect to gross morphology of the neuroepithelium (Fig. 3D). Also, BrdU labeling indicates that the central region of *rde* retina proliferates normally (data not shown). At early stages, less than 3 dpf, *rde* mutants can be identified only by a very subtle difference in the size of the eye. The difference in eye size is more apparent by 72 hpf and histological examination reveals the appearance of pyknotic cells adjacent to the marginal zone (Fadool et al., 1997). The central retina displays normal lamination and all cell types appear to be present. By 96 hpf the mutant eye is more spherical in shape and much smaller in total size than wild types. Upon histological inspection, the *rde* marginal zone is clearly reduced in size; however, the central retina still displays normal lamination (Fig. 3D). Labeling studies with BrdU indicate that there are proliferating cells in the marginal zone at 96 hpf, although the number of labeled cells is considerably less than in wild type (data not shown). Since the initial characterization of *rde*, other similar mutations have been discovered.

Marginal zone deficient

Marginal zone deficient (mzd) is another example of a mutation that affects peripheral retinal development, but does not inhibit initial central differentiation. Similar to *rde*, retinal development appears normal in *mzd* mutants up to 32 hpf, although the eyes are noticeably smaller than those of *rde* mutants (Fig. 3E). BrdU labeling at this time shows that most cells of central retina of *mzd* are proliferating normally (Fig. 3I). By 72 h, again as seen in *rde*, cell death becomes apparent near the marginal zone, particularly in the ganglion cell layer (data not shown). Otherwise, the central retina appears normal. At 96 h, the marginal zone is obviously smaller than in wild type as determined by histology (Fig. 3F) and BrdU labeling (Fig. 3J). By this time some defects in the central retina can be detected as well, particularly in the outer nuclear layer, which displays some delamination. This defect in the photoreceptor layer is reflected too by the increase in BrdU-labeled cells in the central retina. These cells are presumably rod progenitors that may be attempting to repair the damage.

Despite the effect in the outer nuclear layer, the outstanding characteristic of the *mzd* mutation is the reduced development in the peripheral retina. As is the case for *rde*, there are proliferating cells in the marginal zone at 96 hpf. Evidently, the peripheral stem cells themselves are not affected by the mutation. The narrowing of the proliferating zone, as well as the prevalence of cell death at the marginal zone border, suggests that *rde* and *mzd* mutations affect a later stage of development. Interestingly, these mutations do not affect the same process during development of the central retina. The existence of these mutations suggests that some aspects in the development of cells from the marginal zone are distinct from those of the central retina.

What do the mutants tell us?

In the *yng* and *bwd* mutations, the proliferating neuroepithelium of the optic cup appears normal. However, with either mutation, the optic cup neuroepithelium is defective in differentiation. This failure to fully develop eventually results in extensive cell death by 96 h (data not shown). Interestingly, in *yng* and *bwd* the marginal zone appears morphologically normal. Because the health of the eye is compromised at later time points it is difficult to test whether cells arising from the marginal zone in these mutants develop properly. Analysis of the *yng* and *bwd* mutations, therefore, does not provide definitive evidence for differences in the development of the central and peripheral retina. Analysis of these mutants, however, does suggest that a differentiated

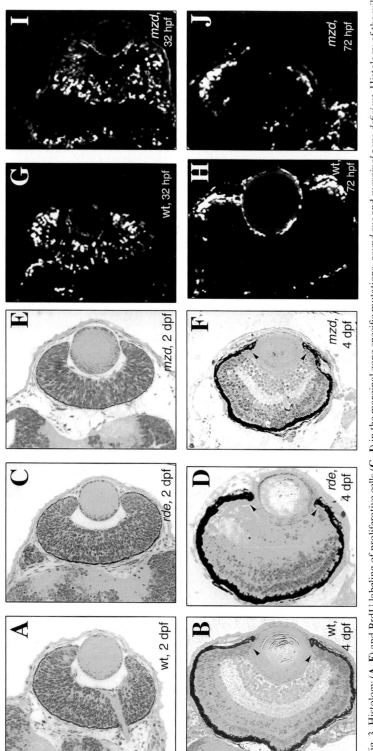

Fig. 3. Histology (**A–F**) and BrdU labeling of proliferative cells (**G–J**) in the marginal zone specific mutations, *round eye* and *marginal zone deficient*. Histology of the wild type at 2 days (**A**) and 4 days (**B**) is compared to that of *round eye* (**C**, **D**) and *marginal zone deficient* in the wild type and *marginal zone deficient* embryos was performed after a 1 h pulse at 32 h (**G** and **I** respectively) and a 24 h pulse at 72 h (**H** and **J** respectively). Note the normal morphology and lamination of cells in the central retina, but the reduced size and number of proliferating cells in the marginal cells.

central retina is not required for maintenance of the marginal zone.

The marginal zone mutations strongly suggest that there are differences in the regulatory pathways governing initial development of the retina and the processes operating later in the periphery. Both *rde* and *mzd* mutants have proliferative cells in the marginal zone as late as 96 h. The defects therefore do not appear to affect the status of the peripheral-most cells, which presumably include the neural stem cells. Instead, cell death at the border of the marginal zone and the initial central retina indicates that the two mutations are involved at some later stage of development. The zone of BrdU-labeled cells appears narrower in both mutations. These mutations may therefore affect the transition of proliferative neuroepthilial cells to post-mitotic retinal precursors. Alternatively, these mutations may affect the pathway of neural specification and the increased cell death adjacent to the proliferating marginal zone cells is due to apoptosis of abnormal cells. In support of this, preliminary data suggests that some neurogenic markers, specifically *delta B* and *delta D*, are not expressed in the *rde* marginal zone. It is unclear, however, if the absence of *delta* expression is the primary defect caused by the mutation, or a secondary effect created by the death of cells that help maintain the marginal zone. In any event, it is clear that the defects in *rde* and *mzd*, do not affect the central retina. The specificity of these mutations suggests that there are some fundamental differences between initial development of the central retina and ongoing development in the marginal zone.

Multidisciplinary approaches to study retinal development

While past studies and the experiments described above have given insights into much of the fundamentals of developmental retinal biology, much is yet to be discovered. In particular, our understanding of specific cellular behaviors and the underlying molecular mechanisms that facilitate key processes such as cell cycle withdrawal, cell-type specification, migration, differentiation, and the maintenance of stem cells and progenitors remains limited. In order to better understand the relationships between these key processes, and how the cells and molecules which mediate them interact, we and others are now using multidisciplinary strategies in our research. Zebrafish retinal development is particularly well suited for cellular and molecular dissection. Differentiation initiates in a predictable and well characterized region (a site termed the nasoventral patch), proceeds rapidly in a organized fashion (the fan-like wave), and is marked by robust ongoing differentiation where stem cell biology can be studied (the marginal zone). In addition, the zebrafish is a powerful experimental system in which mutational analyses and gene or protein expression studies can be combined. Further sophistication in experimental approach is possible through over-expression of specific molecules by transient or transgenic methods (Meng et al., 1999). The demonstration of RNA interference in zebrafish (by anti-sense or double-stranded approaches) now provides a tool for targeted gene knockdown studies (Barabino et al., 1997; Li et al., 2000). Lastly, embryonic accessibility and established cell transplantation methods are useful to test for critical cell or tissue interactions (Malicki, 1999). For these reasons, we are enthusiastic about using zebrafish to study retinal development.

Extending the comparison to gain further insight into central and marginal zone development

The gene expression patterns and mutations that have been discussed provide insights into initial development in the central retina as well as ongoing retinogenesis within the marginal zone. To date, several observations in initial development of the central retina have not been investigated in marginal zone differentiation. For example, are the specific cellular behaviors that occur in initial central development occurring during marginal zone differentiation? Are the three consecutive waves of cell cycle withdrawal described by Hu and Easter (1999) happening within the periphery? Evidence has been provided in support of a conserved birth-order within the adult marginal zone that is similar to that during initial differentiation (Marcus et al., 1999). Another question that remains to be fully answered is whether the cell types are generated in equal proportions during central and marginal zone development. Potentially, terminal mitosis occurs as rhythmic pulses within the marginal zone and this ensures the generation of correct cell type proportions as the retina grows. In such a model, the rate of growth would be proportional to the frequency of consecutive bursts of terminal mitoses, where each round of bursts results in a set of appropriately specified cells. Regardless, the mechanisms and significance of the central terminal differentiation waves have yet to be realized. Interestingly, a genetic approach to study the morphogenic furrow, an analogous wave of differentiation in *Drosophila* eye development, has proven to be a rich source for discovery of key factors in retinal development in both invertebrates and vertebrates (Heberlein and Moses, 1995).

Regionally patterned gene expression found during central retinal development is another observation worth testing in the marginal zone. Several genes are expressed within the undifferentiated neuroepithelium in either a dorsal-ventral pattern or in a nasal-temporal way, presumably encoding axial identity (Hyatt et al., 1996; Yuasa et al., 1996; Schulte et al., 1999). Are "ventral" genes expressed in the undifferentiated neuroepithelium restricted to the ventral portion of the marginal zone? One exciting insight into this question of whether the marginal zone is regionally patterned comes from work in *Xenopus*. Investigating the disproportional growth of the ventral retina during metamorphosis, Marsh-Armstrong and colleagues have recently shown that an enzyme which inactivates thyroid hormone, known to be responsible for the ventral cellular proliferation, is limited to the dorsal retina (Marsh-Armstrong et al., 1999).

How regional patterns are established is unknown, but differences may depend on an undifferentiated retinal cell's surrounding tissues. Differences in the surrounding environment between undifferentiated, central neuroepithelial cells and those in the marginal zone could impact their development. Possible influential tissues include the lens, periocular mesenchyme, the optic stalk, the retinal pigmented epithelium, and the neural retina itself. Indeed, in zebrafish the retinal pigmented epithelium has been demonstrated to be a source of Hedgehogs, potent secreted signaling molecules, that are produced in a wave that closely precedes that of initial retinal

differentiation. Through a combination of genetics and gene knockdown experiments, Stenkamp et al. (2000) have shown that Hedgehogs are important for photoreceptor differentiation. It will be interesting to see if and where hedgehog signaling components are expressed in the marginal zone and the associated retinal pigmented epithelium. Finally, the retina itself may underlie differences in central and marginal zone differentiation. Several examples for the influence of differentiated retinal cells directing the fate of yet unspecified cells have been described. Such interactions have been studied in the context of feed-back inhibition for ganglion and amacrine cell fates (Waid and McLoon, 1998; Belliveau and Cepko, 1999). As the retinal cell composition changes during initial central differentiation, so too does the signaling microenvironment. Are the same temporal changes in signals preserved in spatial microenvironments within the marginal zone? The eventual identification of the genes responsible for central retinal and marginal zone mutations will aid in addressing these and related questions of initial and ongoing retinal development.

Conclusions and future prospects

The traditional view of neurobiology has held that, with some exceptions, the proliferative capacity of the adult vertebrate nervous system is extremely limited. The constant turnover of the olfactory epithelium in most vertebrates is perhaps the most widely cited exception. More recently, experiments have shown that the vertebrate forebrain has populations of self-renewing stem cells that can be induced to differentiate in a manner reflecting the environment in which they are placed (Luskin, 1998). It is now becoming clear that similar stem cell populations exist throughout the mammalian central nervous system. Most relevant to retinal biology is the identification of stem cells that reside within the mammalian pigmented epithelium of the ciliary margin (Ahmad et al., 2000; Tropepe et al., 2000). This population of cells can differentiate into multiple retinal cell types under experimental conditions. These findings argue that the cells in the mammalian ciliary margin represent an evolutionary counterpart to those in the marginal zone of aquatic vertebrates

(Tropepe et al., 2000). However, the mammalian ciliary stem cells do not possess regenerative capacity under normal conditions. The eye of the zebrafish has considerable regenerative capability, with stem cells concentrated in the marginal zone. The robust nature of this regenerative ability as well as the convenience of maintaining zebrafish colonies make this animal an ideal organism for studying the dynamics of neuronal stem cell behavior. More importantly, the genetic analyses possible with zebrafish allows the identification of genes that regulate and maintain these stem cells. An understanding of the genetic basis of retinal differentiation in experimental organisms, particularly with regard to the similarities and differences between initial and ongoing development, may enable strategies for clinical intervention in human retinal disease.

Acknowledgments

We are indebted to the guidance, encouragement, and support of our mentor, John Dowling. All of the work presented here was accomplished during post-doctoral fellowships in the Dowling laboratory. We gratefully acknowledge all of the members of the Dowling lab for helpful suggestions and excellent comradery. Special thanks go to Pam Kainz for critically reading working drafts. Finally, we acknowledge those whose work we have built on and collaborators for generously providing tools (Catherine Haddon in Julian Lewis' Laboratory, *delta* genes; James M. Fadool, who originally identified the *young* and *round eye* mutations while a post-doc in the Dowling Lab).

References

Ahmad, I., Tang, L. and Pham, H. (2000) Identification of neural progenitors in the adult mammalian eye. *Biochem. Biophys. Res. Commun.*, 270: 517–521.

Barabino, S.M.L., Spada, F., Cotelli, F. and Boncinelli, E. (1997) Inactivation of the zebrafish homologue of *Chx10* by anitsense oligonucleotides causes eye malformations similar to the ocular retardation phenotype. *Mech. Dev.*, 63: 133–143.

Belliveau, M.J. and Cepko, C.L. (1999) Extrinsic and intrinsic factors control the genesis of amacrine and cone cells in the rat retina. *Development*, 126: 555–566.

Brock, S.C., Bonsall, J. and Luskin, M.B. (1998) The neural progenitor cells of the forebrain subventricular zone: intrinsic properties in vitro and following transplantation. *Methods*, 16: 268–281.

Brockerhoff, S.E., Hurley, J.B., Janssen-Bienhold, U., Neuhauss, S.C.F., Driever, W. and Dowling, J.E. (1995) A behavioral screen for isolating zebrafish mutants with visual system defects. *Proc. Natl. Acad. Sci. USA*, 92: 10545–10549.

Cepko, C.L. (1999) The roles of intrinsic and extrinsic cues and bHLH genes in the determination of retinal cell fates. *Curr. Opin. Neurobiol.*, 9: 37–46.

Cepko, C.L., Austin, C.P., Yang, X., Alexiades, M. and Ezzeddine, D. (1996) Cell fate determination in the vertebrate retina. *Proc. Natl. Acad. Sci. USA*, 93: 589–595.

Fadool, J.M., Brockerhoff, S.E., Hyatt, G.A. and Dowling, J.E. (1997) Mutations affecting eye morphology in the developing zebrafish. *Developmental Genetics*, 20: 1–8.

Fernald, R.D. (1990) Teleost vision: seeing while growing. *J. Exp. Zool.*, (Suppl. 5): 167–180.

Fischer, A.J. and Reh, T.A. (2000) Identification of a proliferating marginal zone of retinal progenitors in postnatal chickens. *Dev. Biol.*, 220: 197–210.

Harris, W.A. (1997) Cellular diversification in the certebrate retina. *Curr. Opin. Genet. Dev.*, 7: 651–658.

Hatten, M.E. (1999) Central nervous system neuronal migration. *Ann. Rev. Neurosci.*, 22: 511–539.

Heberlein, U. and Moses, K. (1995) Mechanisms of *Drosophila* retinal morphogenesis: the virtues of being progressive. *Cell*, 81: 987–990.

Hitchcock, P.F., Macdonald, R.E., VenDeRyt, J.T. and Wilson, S.W. (1996) Antibodies against Pax6 immunostain amacrine and ganglion cells and neuronal progenitors, but not rod precursors, in the normal and regenerating retina of the goldfish. *Neurobiology*, 29: 399–413.

Hollyfield, J.G. (1968) Differential addition of cells to the retina in *Rana pipiens* tadpoles. *Dev. Biol.*, 18: 163–179.

Hu, M. and Easter, S.S. (1999) Retinal neurogenesis: the formation of the intial central patch of postmitotic cells. *Dev. Biol.*, 207: 309–321.

Hyatt, G.A., Schmitt, E.A., Fadool, J.M. and Dowling, J.E. (1996) Retinoic acid alters photorector development in vivo. *Proc. Natl. Acad. Sci. USA*, 93: 13298–13303.

Jasoni, C.L. and Reh, T.A. (1996) Temporal and spatial pattern of MASH-1 expression in the developing rat retina demonstrates progenitor cell heterogeneity. *J. Comp. Neurol.*, 369: 319–327.

Jensen, A.M. and Raff, M.C. (1997) Continuous observation of multipotential retinal progenitors cells in clonal density culture. *Dev. Biol.*, 188: 267–279.

Johns, P.R. (1977) Growth of the adult goldfish eye:III. Source of new retinal cells. *J. Comp. Neurol.*, 176: 343–358.

Korzh, V., Edlund, T. and Thor, S. (1993) Zebrafish primary neurons initiate expression of the LIM homeodomain protein Isl-1 at the end of gastrulation. *Development*, 118: 417–425.

Lewis, J. (1998) Notch signalling and the control of cell fate choices in vertebrates. *Cell Dev. Biol.*, 9: 583–589.

Li, Y.-X., Farrell, M.J., Ruiping, L., Mohanty, N. and Kirby, M.L. (2000) Double-stranded RNA injection produces null phenotypes in zebrafish. *Dev. Biol.*, 217: 394–405.

Link, B.A., Fadool, J.M., Malicki, J. and Dowling, J.E. (2000) The zebrafish *young* mutation acts non-cell-autonomously to uncouple differentiation from specification for all retinal cells. *Development*, 127: 2177–2188.

Luskin, M.B. (1998) Neuroblasts of the postnatal mammalian forebrain: their phenotype and fate. *J. Neurobiol.*, 36: 221–233.

Malicki, J. (1999) The zebrafish: biology. In: Detrich, H.W. Westerfield, M. and Zon, L.I. (Eds.), *Methods in Cell Biology*, Vol. 59, Academic Press, pp. 273–295.

Marcus, R.C., Delaney, C.L. and Easter, S.S., Jr. (1999) Neurogenesis in the visual system of embryonic and adult zebrafish (*Danio rerio*). *Vis. Neurosci.*, 16: 417–424.

Marsh-Armstrong, N., Huang, H., Remo, B.F., Liu, T.T. and Brown, D.D. (1999) Asymmetric growth and development of the Xenopus laevis retina during metamorphosis is controlled by type III deiodinase. *Neuron*, 24: 871–878.

Mathers, P.H., Grinberg, A., Mahon, K.A. and Jamrich, M. (1997) The *rx* homeobox gene is essential for vertebrate eye development. *Nature*, 387: 603–607.

Meng, A., Jessen, J.R. and Lin, S. (1999) The zebrafish: genetics and genomics. In: Detrich, H.W. Westerfield, M. and Zon, L.I. (Eds.), *Methods in Cell Biology*, Vol. 60, Academic Press, pp. 133–147.

Oliver, G., Mailhos, A., Wehr, R., Copeland, N.G., Jenkins, N.A. and Gruss, P. (1995) *Six3*, a murine homologue of the *sine oculis* gene, demarcates the most anterior border of the developing neural plate and is expressed during eye development. *Development*, 121: 4045–4055.

Passini, M.A., Levine, E.M., Canger, A.K., Raymond, P.A. and Schechter, N. (1997) *Vsx-1* and *vsx-2*: differential expression of two *paired*-like homeobox genes during zebrafish and goldfish retinogenesis. *J. Comp. Neurol.*, 388: 495–505.

Perron, M., Kanekar, S., Vetter, M.L. and Harris, W.A. (1998) The genetic sequence of retinal development in the ciliary margin of the *Xenopus* eye. *Dev. Biol.*, 199: 185–200.

Rapaport, D.H. and Dorsky, R.I. (1998) Inductive competence, its significance in retinal cell fate determination and a role for Delta-Notch signaling. *Semin. Cell Dev. Biol.*, 9: 241–247.

Raymond, P.A. and Hitchcock, P.F. (1997) Retinal regeneration: common principles but a diversity of mechanisms. *Adv. Neurol.*, 72: 171–184.

Schmitt, E.A. and Dowling, J.E. (1999) Early retinal development in the zebrafish, *Danio rerio*: light and electron microscopic analyses. *J. Comp. Neurol.*, 404: 515–536.

Schulte, D., Furukawa, T., Peters, M.A., Kozak, C.A. and Cepko, C.L. (1999) Misexpression of the Emx-related homeobox genes cVax adn mVax2 ventralizes the retina and perturbs the retinotectal map. *Neuron*, 24: 541–553.

Snow, R.L. and Robson, J.A. (1995) Migration and differentiation of neurons in the retina and optic tectum of the chick. *Exp. Neurol.*, 134: 13–24.

Solnica-Kretzel, L., Schier, A.F. and Driever, W. (1994) Efficient recovery of ENU-induced mutations from the zebrafish germline. *Genetics*, 136: 1401–1420.

Stenkamp, D.L., Frey, R.A., Prabhudesai, S.N. and Raymond, P.A. (2000) Function for *hedgehog* genes in zebrafish retinal development. *Dev. Biol.*, 220: 238–252.

Tropepe, V., Coles, B.L.K., Chiasson, B.J., Horsford, D.J., Elia, A.J., Mcinnes, R.R. and van der Kooy, D. (2000) Retinal stem cells in the adult mammalian eye. *Science*, 287: 2032–2036.

Waid, D.K. and McLoon, S.C. (1998) Ganglion cells influence the fate of dividing retinal cells in culture. *Development*, 125: 1059–1066.

Wetts, R. and Fraser, S.E. (1988) Multipotent precursors can give rise to all major cell types of the frog retina. *Science*, 239: 1142–1145.

Yuasa, J., Hirano, S., Yamagata, M. and Noda, M. (1996) Visual projection map specified by topographic expression of transcription factors in the retina. *Nature*, 382: 632–635.

H. Kolb, H. Ripps and S. Wu (Eds.)
Progress in Brain Research, Vol. 131
© 2001 Elsevier Science B.V. All rights reserved

CHAPTER 41

Retinoic acid synthesis and breakdown in the developing mouse retina

Ursula C. Dräger*, Huanchen Li, Elisabeth Wagner and Peter McCaffery

*Developmental Neuroscience, Eunice Kennedy Shriver Center, Waltham, MA 02452, USA
and Department of Psychiatry, Harvard Medical School, Boston, MA 02115, USA*

Functions of retinoids

Vitamin A (= retinol) is necessary for function and survival of adult vertebrates, and it is even more critical for embryonic development. Eye development is most sensitive to vitamin A deficiency. When a pregnant animal is partially deprived of vitamin A, the offspring may appear more-or-less normal, but its eyes are too small or missing (Hale, 1937). More severe vitamin A deficiency affects many organs in the developing embryo, including the heart and brain. Practically all vitamin A actions are mediated by two metabolites (Dowling and Wald, 1960): retinaldehyde forms the light-sensitive chromophore bound to opsin, and retinoic acid (RA) regulates gene transcription. Whereas the visual function of retinoids is evolutionarily ancient—it is present in all animal classes—the transcriptional role is much more recent: it is fully evolved only in vertebrates (Laudet, 1997). RA acts by binding to nuclear receptors which are members of a large family that includes, among many others, the steroid and thyroid hormone receptors (Mangelsdorf et al., 1995). The RA receptors fall into two classes, RAR and RXR, and each class comprises three different forms (α, β, γ). They function either as homodimers or as heterodimers (Mangelsdorf and Evans, 1995). Since the RXR class forms, in addition, obligatory heterodimers with several other nuclear receptors, including those for thyroid hormone, vitamin D and prostaglandin, the multitude of possible combinatorial constellations of the RA receptors is staggering.

The expression of well over 300 proteins, found in every organ of the body, can be regulated by RA (Gudas et al., 1994; Quadro et al., 1999; McCaffery and Dräger, 2000). This includes a majority of growth factors and receptors, transcription factors and enzymes, and a long list of ion-channel, structural and extracellular matrix proteins. In fact, the expression of a large portion of the factors involved in neuronal growth, migration and differentiation has been shown to be influenced by RA. Although the large diversity of RA-regulated proteins appears bewildering, there is some order in RA actions, which renders them often physiologically predictable. RA effects generally follow similar themes, and RA tends to function as a higher-order switch for the control of complex cellular programs. In many cases, RA terminates cell proliferation and activates differentiation programs. Early in embryogenesis, RA can induce a precursor region to advance developmentally towards its destined fate, and it can impart vectorial information onto an organ anlage, such as the antero-posterior axis onto the limb bud (Tickle et al., 1982) and the dorso-ventral axis on the eye anlage (Hyatt et al., 1996).

*Corresponding author: Ursula C. Dräger, Developmental Neuroscience, E. Kennedy Shriver Center, Waltham, MA 02452, USA; Tel.: 781-642-0174; Fax: 781-894-9968; E-mail: UDrager@shriver.org

Identification of retinaldehyde dehydrogenases in the embryonic mouse

We became interested in the RA field by accident and through a backwards approach. In a search for the mechanisms that create axial asymmetry in the embryonic retina, we identified the aldehyde dehydrogenase AHD2 in the dorsal part of the embryonic retina (McCaffery et al., 1991). AHD2 was previously studied as an adult liver enzyme, and it was the only identified enzyme that was implicated in RA synthesis (Lee et al., 1991). All excitement in the retinoid field had focused on the RA receptors and the retinoid binding proteins, and very little detail was known about RA synthesis. Metabolic studies that require large amounts of tissue were usually done on crude extracts from adult organs, which contain a mixture of enzymes (Napoli, 1990). It was known that the last step in RA synthesis, the irreversible oxidation of retinaldehyde to RA, can be catalyzed by aldehyde dehydrogenases as well as by aldehyde oxidases. Apart from AHD2, it was not known what other members of the large enzyme families act on retinoids, and nothing was known about RA synthesis in the embryo.

We developed novel techniques for the detection of RA-synthesizing enzymes, which make it possible to analyze minute amounts of tissue dissected from early embryos (McCaffery et al., 1992). These are zymographic techniques, based on the analysis of isoelectric focusing gels for enzyme function with RA-reporter cells (Wagner et al., 1992; McCaffery and Dräger, 1997). By zymography on the early embryonic eye, we found that practically all RA synthesis is mediated by aldehyde dehydrogenases (rather than oxidases) (McCaffery et al., 1993). Comparisons of RA synthesis in dorsal and ventral retina halves confirmed a high rate in dorsal retina, but showed even higher synthesis ventrally (McCaffery et al., 1992). The zymographic analysis revealed a new retinaldehyde dehydrogenase (RALDH) activity in the ventral retina, which was provisionally named V1 (McCaffery et al., 1992); the cloned enzyme has now been renamed RALDH3 (Li et al., 2000). With the same zymographic technique we found another retinaldehyde dehydrogenase, named first V2 and then RALDH2, when we cloned it (McCaffery et al., 1992; McCaffery et al., 1993; Zhao et al., 1996).

These three retinaldehyde dehydrogenases are the only RA-generating enzymes detectable in the very early mouse embryo, and they account for much of the RA synthesis later on. Because their names vary (Greenfield and Pietruszko, 1977; Lee et al., 1991; McCaffery et al., 1992; McCaffery et al., 1993; Zhao et al., 1993; Hsu et al., 1994; Labrecque et al., 1995; Wang et al., 1996; Zhao et al., 1996; Ang and Duester, 1997; Petersen and Lindahl, 1997; Yoshida et al., 1998), the following table defines the nomenclature used here:

Name used here	Characteristic expression site	Other names
RALDH1	dorsal retina	AHD2, E1, ALDH1
RALDH2	embryonic trunk	V2, ALDH11
RALDH3	ventral retina	V1, ALDH6

RALDH2

The RALDH2 enzyme is the first enzyme expressed in the embryo. In the mouse it becomes detectable at embryonic day 7.5 (E7.5) (Dräger and McCaffery, 1995; Zhao et al., 1996; Niederreiter et al., 1997). It appears first in the midportion of the embryo in the mesoderm surrounding Hensen's node, and high enzyme expression persists in the trunk region throughout development. In the eye anlage, RALDH2 is expressed transiently only for a few hours during the first part of E8 (Wagner et al., 2000). Its expression is restricted to the ventral rim of the eyefield, as is visible in the left embryo of Fig. 1, which is viewed from its ventral side. Later during E8, and early on E9, all RALDH2 mRNA disappears from the head (Fig. 1, right). A few days later, however, RALDH2 reappears here. In the eye, it is expressed in the surrounding tissue, but not the neural retina; its main localization in the brain is in the meninges (Yamamoto et al., 1996; Niederreiter et al., 1997).

RALDH3

The second RA-generating enzyme expressed in the embryo is the V1 activity. We cloned it from

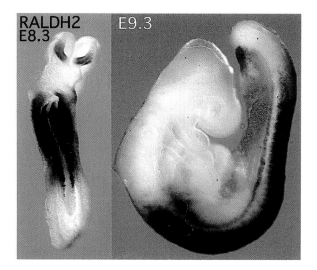

Fig. 1. In situ hybridizations for RALDH2 mRNA on two young mouse embryos, shown at same scale. The younger one, about at embryonic day 8.3 (~E8.3), is viewed from its ventral side, and the older one, at ~E9.3, from laterally. Note the transient strong labeling at the ventral edge of the forebrain plate, which is the ventral rim of the optic recess.

the mouse embryo, by using its restricted and differential expression patterns as a screening tool (Li et al., 2000). Its sequence shows it to be a mouse homologue to ALDH6, an enzyme cloned from adult human salivary gland (Hsu et al., 1994). Recently ALDH6 was found to act as a retinaldehyde dehydrogenase (Yoshida et al., 1998). For this reason, we call the mouse enzyme RALDH3. Its expression in the developing eye region is illustrated in Fig. 2, which shows closely timed whole mount preparations treated by in situ hybridizations for RALDH3 mRNA. RALDH3 expression begins in the eye region slightly before E8.5, about a third of a day after RALDH2. It appears first in the surface epithelium covering the eye field and surrounding face. Over the following three days, the shape of the surface labeling changes very rapidly in patterns that indicate beginning morphogenetic events of the ectoderm. In the earlier ages shown in Fig. 2, the formations of the lens and the olfactory organ from ectodermal placodes are marked by RALDH3. After E11, the beginning eye lid system with the naso-lacrimal groove is delineated by a rectangular-shaped, oblique RALDH3 pattern. In the optic vesicle, RALDH3 expression is restricted to the

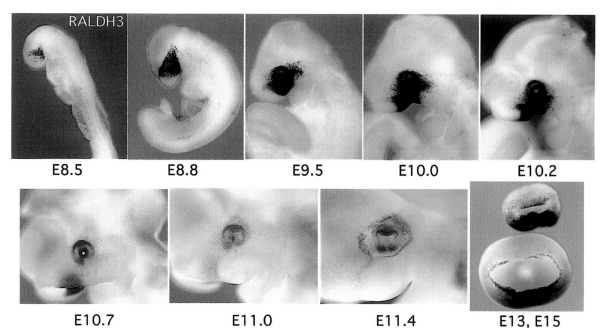

Fig. 2. In situ hybridizations for RALDH3 mRNA on a series of mouse embryos, heads and isolated retina cups, all shown at same scale. In the retinas, up is dorsal and down ventral.

dorsal retinal pigment epithelium and the ventral neural retina. In addition to the developing eye and olfactory organ, RALDH3 is transiently expressed at high levels in the lateral division of the ganglionic eminence (McCaffery and Dräger, 1994; Li et al., 2000). The ganglionic eminence is a transient embryonic structure in the ventral telencephalon, a large germinal mass which gives rise to the corpus striatum and to GABAergic interneurons throughout the cerebral cortex (Anderson et al., 1997; Tamamaki et al., 1997; Tan et al., 1998). This telencephalic RALDH3 site represents a major source of RA for the early embryonic forebrain.

CYP26

The third enzyme that modulates RA levels in the retina (McCaffery et al., 1999) is CYP26, a member of the cytochrome P450-linked oxidase family (Roberts et al., 1992). CYP26 has been identified in screens for factors whose expression is upregulated by RA, and it has been shown to degrade RA through oxidation (White et al., 1996; Fujii et al., 1997; Ray et al., 1997). During the first part of E8 in the mouse, all CYP26 expression in the head is limited to neural crest cells that migrate from segmental subdivisions of the rhombencephalon into the face (Fig. 3, left). Activity of CYP26 in these cells will create locally very low RA levels, which are likely to be required for the normal formation of neural-crest derived structures. This is indicated by the known teratogenic effects of RA on the neural crest: exposure of very early embryos to high levels of exogenous RA results

in neural-crest linked malformations such as cleft palate (Shenefelt, 1972; Lammer et al., 1985). When the eye begins to form, CYP26 appears first in the dorsal pole of the optic vesicle, as shown here for ~E8.6 (Fig. 3). Its expression at this location intensifies, and, when the neural retina forms, it shifts ventrally to form a horizontal stripe that runs across the retina above the optic disc (Fig. 3, right).

RALDH1

The last retinoid metabolizing enzyme that is activated in the eye region is the RA-synthesizing RALDH1 (McCaffery et al., 1991; McCaffery et al., 1999). It appears first in the dorsal pole of the eye vesicle in a location that overlaps partially with the RA-degrading CYP26, but a few hours later (Fig. 4, left). This order of succession can be interpreted to indicate that CYP26 creates the local conditions for activation of RALDH1. Such an interpretation is consistent with teratogenic actions of RA on early eye formation in zebrafish: exposure to an excess of RA prevents expression of the dorsal-retina enzyme zRALDH1 (Hyatt et al., 1996). Whereas CYP26 expression shifts downwards over the following days, RALDH1 expression persists in the dorsal retina (Fig. 4, right). In the embryonic retina, very high RALDH1 levels mark the dorsal third. Postnatally and throughout adult life, RALDH1 continues to be expressed in the same retinal region but at lower levels than in the embryo. By contrast, both CYP26 and RALDH3 disappear postnatally from the retina (McCaffery et al., 1993; McCaffery et al., 1999).

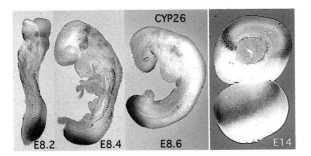

Fig. 3. In situ hybridizations for CYP26 mRNA on three mouse embryos during E8 and of isolated E14 retina cups, shown from front and back.

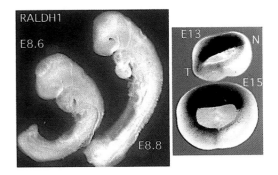

Fig. 4. In situ hybridizations for RALDH1 mRNA on two mouse embryos during E8, and of isolated E13 and E15 retina cups. T, temporal retina; N, nasal.

In addition to the strong expression in dorsal retina, the isolated retina cups reveal a more subtle feature of RALDH1 (Fig. 4, right): it extends along the temporal margin of the retina all the way ventrally to the remnant of the optic fissure (Wagner et al., 2000). In the retina of the later embryo, the three retinoid-metabolizing enzymes are segregated into three non-overlapping territories: RALDH1 in the dorsal third, CYP26 in a horizontal border and RALDH3 in the ventral two-thirds. Thus the only location where two enzymes overlap is the peripheral temporo-ventral retina, containing both RALDH3 and RALDH1. This retinal region also stands out functionally: it contains two separate but overlapping population of retinal ganglion cells, one giving rise to crossed and the other to uncrossed retinofugal projections (Dräger and Olsen, 1980).

RA reporter mouse

The arrangement of three retinoid-metabolizing enzymes creates three RA concentration zones along the dorso-ventral retina axis: high RA zones in dorsal and ventral retina separated by a horizontal RA-poor stripe (McCaffery et al., 1999). These RA differences are directly visible in retinas of a RA reporter mouse strain, which is transgenic for β-galactosidase expression activated by a sensitive RA response element (Rossant et al., 1991). Local expression of β-galactosidase in this mouse requires two conditions: (1) the cells have to be RA-responsive, i.e. they have to express RA receptors; and (2) the cells have to be exposed to endogenously synthesized RA. The RA reporter retina in Fig. 5A shows the RA concentration zones along the dorso-ventral axis; in

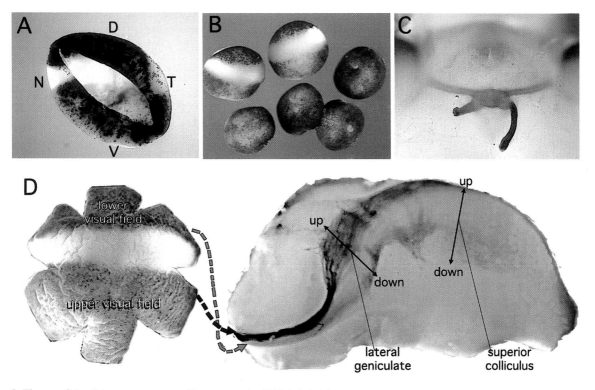

Fig. 5. Tissues of the RA reporter mouse (Rossant et al., 1991) labeled for β-galactosidase. **A.** Isolated retina cup from postnatal day 10. **B.** Retinas from E18 embryos. The two retinas with stripes are normal controls. The solidly labeled retinas are from embryos whose mother was injected intraperitoneally with RA. **C.** Optic chiasm of an E14 embryo viewed from below. The optic nerves (down in the figure) are torn off from the eyes, and the optic tracts (up) curve around the hypothalamus towards the diencephalic targets. Note that the optic tracts appear as two parallel bundles. **D.** Schematic composite of RA reporter tissues to illustrate how the visual field projects onto the di- and mesencephalon. The dorsal and ventral visual fields are traced out from the retina whole mount to the chiasm area in a brain whole mount, from which the telencephalon has been dissected away.

addition, even the narrow temporal RALDH1 expression is visible as a blue border at the temporal ciliary edge (Wagner et al., 2000). Retina cells within the white horizontal stripe have the potential to respond to RA, or they can rapidly gain it: when a pregnant mouse is injected with an excess of RA, the capacity of CYP26 in the embryonic retinas becomes transiently overloaded, and the white stripe fills in rapidly (see the solidly labeled retinas in Fig. 5B). Soon after the excess RA is eliminated, the stripe reappears (not shown).

High levels of β-galactosidase are transported anterogradely along the optic axons in the RA reporter mouse (Wagner et al., 2000). Because the retina is exceptionally rich in retinaldehyde dehydrogenases and RA, and levels in the brain are overall low, the heavily labeled optic axons stand out on the pale surface of the brain. This is visible in Fig. 5C for the optic chiasm. When the optic axons have passed through the chiasm to form the optic tract, the projections from dorsal and ventral retina sort into separate bundles. The gap between the bundles is due to unlabeled optic axons projecting from the horizontal stripe. Over the primary optic targets in the di- and mesencephalon, including the lateral geniculate nucleus and the superior colliculus, the two bundles spread out to match the retinotopic maps in these regions (Fig. 5D) (Wagner et al., 2000). Like in Xenopus (Holt and Harris, 1983), the dorsal and ventral retinofugal projections in mice are clearly separated in the di- and mesencephalon from the earliest stage of axon ingrowth.

In adult mice, the eyes are positioned partly laterally and partly on top of the head, which allows them to view a large portion of their surroundings simultaneously (Dräger and Olsen, 1980). The midline of the visual field extends from in front of the head to above beyond the zenith. This geometry results in retinal coordinates that appear backwards tilted. However, when the retinal projections in the RA reporter mouse are compared with electrophysiologically determined visual maps, it becomes evident that the embryonic RA compartments match precisely the conditions of the visual world (Fig. 5D): the ventral retina, marked originally by RALDH3, sees the upper visual field towards the sky, the dorsal RALDH1-labeled retina sees the ground, and the CYP26 stripe runs parallel to the optic projection of the horizon (Wagner et al., 2000). An experimental benefit of the RA reporter labeling is that it propagates an image of the dorso-ventral axis formation from the eye anlage stage all the way to the adult retina. The match between the reporter labeling and the functional visual coordinates indicates that the orientation of the retina axes in the early embryo predicts the functional conditions of the visual system in the adult.

Possible developmental roles of RALDHs in development of the retina and its central projections

The subdivision of the developing retina into dorsal and ventral retinaldehyde-dehydrogenase compartments separated by a horizontal border is probably conserved throughout vertebrates (McCaffery et al., 1999). Most surprisingly, even the eye disc of the insect embryo is subdivided into a geometrically similar pattern, although this is not formed by retinoid metabolizing enzymes (Brodsky and Steller, 1996). In Drosophila, no RA receptors have yet been found, but both vertebrates and invertebrates use the potential RA precursor retinaldehyde as visual chromophore bound to opsin. Because in the vertebrate visual cycle bleached free retinaldehyde is released from opsin, the primary role of retinaldehyde dehydrogenases was probably a protection from an excess of free retinaldehyde in bright light. The by-product RA may then have taken control over more ancient molecular mechanisms in eye formation. The reason why RA became integrated in the process of dorso-ventral eye formation, might be related to dorso-ventral differences in retinaldehyde forms used as visual chromophore in some insects (Seki et al., 1989) and some vertebrates (Reuter et al., 1971). Because the division of the developing retina into compartments is highly conserved, such a geometric arrangement must provide optimal conditions for the expression of spatial patterning mechanisms. These include morphogenetic gradients of cell-surface factors for the guidance of retinal axons to their targets (Sperry, 1963; Drescher, 1997).

The retina is unique in its high concentration of RA and its intricate patterns of RA-metabolizing enzymes. No similar or complementary conditions exist in the primary optic targets. Rather, the optic axons grow into brain regions that contain no (or very little) detectable endogenous RA-synthesizing enzymes. The early optic tectum contains, however, populations of cells that are sensitive to RA (Wagner et al., 2000). The high expression of retinaldehyde dehydrogenases in the developing retina provides a potential mechanism through which the eye can influence the optic targets in the brain. Retinaldehyde dehydrogenases expressed in neurons are transported anterogradely within axons; this includes the optic axons (McCaffery et al., 1992; McCaffery and Dräger, 1994; Berggren et al., 1999). In the nigro-striatal projection, where a subpopulation of the dopaminergic cells in the substantia nigra are rich in RALDH1, practically all measurable RA production takes place in the synaptic terminal region in the striatum. RA produced by the retinaldehyde dehydrogenases in retinal growth cones and axons is likely to act on RA-responsive cells along the optic pathway. Such a mechanism could account, for instance, for the known trophic effects of the retinal innervation on optic targets.

Conclusions and future prospects

The eyes, like the cerebral hemispheres, develop as part of the forebrain in the early embryo. Many of the patterning molecules involved in the morphogenesis of the eyes are also expressed in the brain, consistent with the eyes being integral components of the rostral central nervous system. A major distinguishing feature is the transcriptional activator RA: whereas the eyes are unusually rich in RA, overall brain levels are rather low. In the emerging eye anlage, three RA-synthesizing enzymes and one RA-degrading oxidase are expressed in tight and dynamically regulated patterns. Retina cells that express retinaldehyde dehydrogenases are also highly responsive to RA. By contrast, in the brain the cellular sites of RA synthesis and RA response tend to be spatially separated. Although the teratogenic effects of vitamin-A deficiency or excess show that formation of the brain depends on RA, most of its tissues are completely devoid of RA-synthesizing enzymes. In addition to low RA levels distributed uniformly by the circulation, RA for the embryonic brain is supplied by three local sources of very high retinaldehyde dehydrogenase expression: the ganglionic eminence, the meninges and the optic axons. Because RA is a small acidic lipid, it can diffuse for some distance through solid tissue or across fluid-filled spaces. Its range of action is bound to be considerably farther than diffusible protein morphogens, a feature that makes RA a patterning tool for longer dimensions. RA concentration gradients through the early neural tube, set up by diffusion, are likely of significance for neurogenesis. A major topic that needs to be addressed is how the RA effects are integrated into other morphogenetic events, i.e. what factors activate expression of retinaldehyde dehydrogenases, and whose expression in turn is regulated by RA.

Acknowledgments

The work described in this review was supported by N.I.H. grants EY01938, HD05515 and HD01179. We thank J. Rossant and N. Rosenthal for the RA reporter mice, M. Petkovich for the CYP26 probe, and D. Smith for technical assistance.

References

Anderson, S.A., Eisenstat, D.D., Shi, L. and Rubenstein, J.L. (1997) Interneuron migration from basal forebrain to neocortex: dependence on Dlx genes. *Science*, 278: 474–476.

Ang, H.L. and Duester, G. (1997) Initiation of retinoid signaling in primitive streak mouse embryos: spatiotemporal expression patterns of receptors and metabolic enzymes for ligand synthesis. *Dev. Dyn.*, 208: 536–543.

Berggren, K., McCaffery, P., Dräger, U.C. and Forehand, C.J. (1999) Differential distribution of retinoic acid synthesis in the chicken embryo as determined by immunolocalization of the retinoic acid synthetic enzyme RALDH-2. *Dev. Biol.*, 210: 288–304.

Brodsky, M.H. and Steller, H. (1996) Positional information along the dorsal-ventral axis of the *Drosophila* eye: graded expression of the *four-jointed* gene. *Dev. Biol.*, 173: 428–446.

Dowling, J.E. and Wald, G. (1960) The biological function of vitamin A acid. *Proc. Natl. Acad. Sci. USA*, 46: 587–608.

Dräger, U.C. and McCaffery, P. (1995) Retinoic-acid synthesis in the developing spinal cord. *Adv. Exp. Med. Biol.*, 372: 185–192.

Dräger, U.C. and Olsen, J.F. (1980) Origins of crossed and uncrossed retinal projections in pigmented and albino mice. *J. Comp. Neurol.*, 191: 383–412.

586

Drescher, U. (1997) The Eph family in the patterning of neural development. *Curr. Biol.*, 7: 799–807.

Fujii, H., Sato, T., Kaneko, S., Gotoh, O., Fujii-Kuriyama, Y., Osawa, K., Kato, S. and Hamada, H. (1997) Metabolic inactivation of retinoic acid by a novel P450 differentially expressed in developing mouse embryo. *EMBO J.*, 16: 4163–4173.

Greenfield, N.J. and Pietruszko, R. (1977) Two aldehyde dehydrogenases from human liver. *Biochim. Biophys. Acta*, 483: 35–45.

Gudas, L.J., Sporn, M.B. and Roberts, A.B. (1994) Cellular biology and biochemistry of the retinoids. In: Sporn, M.B., Roberts, A.B. and Goodman, D.S. (Eds.), *The Retinoids: Biology, Chemistry, and Medicine*. Raven Press, New York.

Hale, F. (1937) The relation of maternal vitamin A deficiency to microphthalmia in pigs. *Texas State J. Med.*, 33: 228–232.

Holt, C. and Harris, W.A. (1983) Order in the initial retinotectal map in Xenopus: a new technique for labelling growing nerve fibers. *Nature*, 301: 150–152.

Hsu, L.C., Chang, W.-C., Hiraoka, L. and Hsien, C.-L. (1994) Molecular cloning, genomic organization, and chromosomal localization of an additional human aldehyde dehydrogenase gene, ALDH6. *Genomics*, 24: 333–341.

Hyatt, G., Schmitt, E.A., Marsh-Armstrong, N., McCaffery, P., Dräger, U.C. and Dowling, J.E. (1996) Retinoic acid establishes ventral retinal characteristics. *Development*, 122: 195–204.

Labrecque, J., Dumas, F., Lacroix, A. and Bhat, P.V. (1995) A novel isoenzyme of aldehyde dehydrogenase specifically involved in the biosynthesis of 9-*cis* and all-*trans* retinoic acid. *Biochem. J.*, 305: 681–684.

Lammer, E.J., Chen, D.T., Hoar, R.M., Agnish, N.D., Benke, P.J., Braun, J.T., Curry, C.J., Fernhoff, P.M., Grix, A.W., Lott, I.T., Richard, J.M. and Sun, S.C. (1985) Retinoic acid embryopathy. *N. Engl. J. Med.*, 313: 837–841.

Laudet, V. (1997) Evolution of the nuclear receptor super-family: early diversification from an ancestral orphan receptor. *J. Mol. Endocrinol.*, 19: 207–226.

Lee, M.-O., Manthey, C.L. and Sladek, N.E. (1991) Identification of mouse liver aldehyde dehydrogenases that catalyze the oxidation of retinaldehyde to retinoic acid. *Biochem. Pharmacol.*, 42: 1279–1285.

Li, H., Wagner, E., McCaffery, P., Smith, D., Andreadis, A. and Dräger, U.C. (2000) A retinoic acid synthesizing enzyme in ventral retina and telencephalon of the embryonic mouse. *Mech. Dev.*, 95: 283–289.

Mangelsdorf, D.J. and Evans, R.M. (1995) The RXR hetero-dimers and orphan receptors. *Cell*, 83: 841–850.

Mangelsdorf, D.J., Thummel, C., Beato, M., Umesono, K., Blumberg, B., Kastner, P., Mark, M., Chambon, P. and Evans, R.M. (1995) The nuclear receptor superfamily: the second decade. *Cell*, 83: 835–839.

McCaffery, M. and Dräger, U.C. (1997) A sensitive bioassay for enzymes that synthesize retinoic acid. *Brain Res. Protocols*, 1: 232–236.

McCaffery, P. and Dräger, U.C. (1994) High levels of a retinoic-acid generating dehydrogenase in the meso-telence-phalic dopamine system. *Proc. Natl. Acad. Sci. USA*, 91: 7772–7776.

McCaffery, P. and Dräger, U.C. (2000) Regulation of retinoic acid signaling in the embryonic nervous system: a master differentiation factor. *Cytokine Growth Factor Rev.*, 11: 233–249.

McCaffery, P., Lee, M.-O., Wagner, M. A., Sladek, N. E. and Dräger, U.C. (1992) Asymmetrical retinoic acid synthesis in the dorso-ventral axis of the retina. *Development*, 115: 371–382.

McCaffery, P., Posch, K.C., Napoli, J.L., Gudas, L. and Dräger, U.C. (1993) Changing patterns of the retinoic acid system in the developing retina. *Dev. Biol.*, 158: 390–399.

McCaffery, P., Tempst, P., Lara, G. and Dräger, U.C. (1991) Aldehyde dehydrogenase is a positional marker in the retina. *Development*, 112: 693–702.

McCaffery, P., Wagner, E., O'Neil, J., Petkovich, M. and Dräger, U.C. (1999) Dorsal and ventral retinal territories defined by retinoic acid synthesis, break-down and nuclear receptor expression. *Mech. Dev.*, 82: 119–130. Corrections 85: 203–214.

Napoli, J.L. (1990) In vitro synthesis of retinoic acid from retinol and β-carotene. In: Packer, L. (Ed.), *Methods in Enzymology*, pp. 470–482.

Niederreither, K., McCaffery, P., Dräger, U.C., Chambon, P. and Dollé, P. (1997) Restricted expression and retinoic acid-induced downregulation of the retinaldehyde dehydrogenase type 2 (RALDH-2) gene during mouse development. *Mech. Dev.*, 62: 67–78.

Petersen, D. and Lindahl, R. (1997) Aldehyde dehydrogenases. In: Guingerich, F.P. (Ed.), *Comprehensive Toxicology: Biotransformations*, Elsevier Science, Oxford.

Quadro, L., Blaner, W.S., Salchow, D.J., Vogel, S., Piantedosi, R., Gouras, P., Freeman, S., Cosma, M.P., Colantuoni, V. and Gottesman, M.E. (1999) Impaired retinal function and vitamin A availability in mice lacking retinol-binding protein. *EMBO J.*, 18: 4633–4644.

Ray, W.J., Bain, G., Yao, M. and Gottlieb, D.I. (1997) CYP26, a novel mammalian cytochrome P450, is induced by retinoic acid and defines a new family. *J. Biol. Chem.*, 272: 18702–18708.

Reuter, T.E., White, R.H. and Wald, G. (1971) Rhodopsin and porphyropsin fields in the adult bullfrog retina. *J. Gen. Physiol.*, 58: 351–371.

Roberts, E.S., Vaz, A.D.N. and Coon, M.J. (1992) Role of isozymes of rabbit microsomal cytochrome P-450 in the metabolism of retinoic acid, retinol and retinal. *Mol. Pharmacol.*, 41: 427–433.

Rossant, J., Zirngibl, R., Cado, D., Shago, M. and Giguère, V. (1991) Expression of a retinoic acid response element-hsplacZ transgene defines specific domains of transcriptional activity during mouse embryogenesis. *Genes Dev.*, 5: 1333–1344.

Seki, T., Fujishita, S. and Obana, S. (1989) Composition and distribution of retinal and 3-hydroxyretinal in the compound eye of the dragonfly. *Exp. Biol.*, 48: 65–75.

Shenefelt, R.E. (1972) Morphogenesis of malformations in hamsters caused by retinoic acid. *Teratology*, 5: 403–418.

Sperry, R.W. (1963) Chemoaffinity in the orderly growth of nerve fiber patterns and connections. *Proc. Natl. Acad. Sci. USA*, 50: 703–710.

Tamamaki, N., Fujimori, K.E. and Takauji, R. (1997) Origin and route of tangentially migrating neurons in the developing neocortical intermediate zone. *J. Neurosci.*, 17: 8313–8323.

Tan, S.S., Kalloniatis, M., Sturm, K., Tam, P.P., Reese, B.E. and Faulkner-Jones, B. (1998) Separate progenitors for radial and tangential cell dispersion during development of the cerebral neocortex. *Neuron*, 21: 295–304.

Tickle, C., Alberts, B., Wolpert, L. and Lee, J. (1982) Local application of retinoic acid to the limb bud mimics the action of the polarizing region. *Nature*, 296: 564–566.

Wagner, E., McCaffery, P. and Dräger, U.C. (2000) Retinoic acid in the formation of the dorso-ventral retina and its central projections. *Dev. Biol.*, 222: 460–470.

Wagner, M., Han, B. and Jessell, T.M. (1992) Regional differences in retinoid release from embryonic neural tissue detected by an in vitro reporter assay. *Development*, 116: 55–66.

Wang, X., Penzes, P. and Napoli, J.L. (1996) Cloning of a cDNA encoding an aldehyde dehydrogenase and its expression in Escherichia coli. Recognition of retinal as substrate. *J. Biol. Chem.*, 271: 16288–16293.

White, J.A., Guo, Y.D., Baetz, K., Beckett-Jones, B., Bonasoro, J., Hsu, K. E., Dilworth, F.J., Jones, G. and Petkovich, M. (1996) Identification of the retinoic acid-inducible all-trans-retinoic acid 4-hydroxylase. *J. Biol. Chem.*, 271: 29922–29927.

Yamamoto, M., McCaffery, P. and Dräger, U.C. (1996) Influence of the choroid plexus on cerebellar development: analysis of retinoic acid synthesis. *Dev. Brain Res.*, 93: 182–190.

Yoshida, A., Rzhetsky, A., Hsu, L.C. and Chang, C. (1998) Human aldehyde dehydrogenase gene family. *Eur. J. Biochem.*, 251: 549–557.

Zhao, D., McCaffery, P., Ivins, K.J., Neve, R.L., Hogan, P., Chin, W.W. and Dräger, U.C. (1996) Molecular identification of a major retinoic-acid synthesizing enzyme: a retinaldehyde-specific dehydrogenase. *Eur. J. Biochem.*, 240: 15–22.

Zhao, D., McCaffery, P., Neve, R.L., Hogan, P., Chin, W.W. and Dräger, U.C. (1993) Molecular cloning of a major retinoic-acid synthetic enzyme: a retinaldehyde-specific dehydrogenase. *Soc. Neurosci. Abstr.*, 19: 218.

H. Kolb, H. Ripps and S. Wu (Eds.)
Progress in Brain Research, Vol. 131
© 2001 Elsevier Science B.V. All rights reserved

CHAPTER 42

Postnatal development of the rat retina and some of its neurotransmitter systems in vitro

Kjell Johansson and Berndt Ehinger*

The Wallenberg Retina Center, Department of Ophthalmology, Lund University Hospital, SE-221 85 Lund, Sweden

Introduction

Most living tissues are constantly remodeled, and it appears likely that this is not a random event but that it is strictly monitored and governed by different signal systems. Several types of control systems (including conventional neurotransmitters and hormones) are possible and needed for this, and several are governed at least in part by a variety of microenvironmental factors, including retinoic acid, basic fibroblast growth factor, ciliary neurotrophic factor and taurine (see e.g. Reichenbach and Robinson, 1995; Hyatt and Dowling, 1997; Ezzeddine et al., 1997). John Dowling has participated in many pioneering studies on such factors, on retinal microcircuits and on retinal neurotransmitters (Dowling, 1996, 1999), and his influence can be seen in any modern textbook (e.g. Rodieck, 1998). However, it has also long been felt that there must be different short-range circuits acting at the cell-to-cell level. Less is known about them, but the rod and cone photoreceptors in the retina form a system that is a good example. In many tapetoretinal diseases, the error has been located to the rods. Nevertheless, cones also succumb when the rods disappear, and it is apparent that the rods have some trophic influence that is required for the proper maintenance of cones. The nature of this system is not known. Different kinds of process guidance systems have also been extensively studied, and the knowledge evolving on netrin and ephrin systems can be used as examples (Tessier-Lavigne and Goodman, 1996; Frisén et al., 1998, 1999).

Signal systems at the cell-to-cell level are often best studied in vitro, where the tissue can be directly observed and readily influenced by exposure to appropriate concentrations of different substances. However, only recently have techniques become available for maintaining mammalian retinas in good condition in vitro. Both tissue explants and slice cultures have been described in which neurons express several immunohistochemically detectable neurotransmitters (Sparrow et al., 1990; Feigenspan et al., 1993a; Gähwiler et al., 1997; recent review: Seigel, 1999). Mouse photoreceptor cells have been shown to express transduction enzymes also in long-term cultures (weeks; Caffé et al., 1993; Söderpalm et al., 1994). Much of the long-term work has been done on mouse retina. Noting the usefulness of an explant for studying the influence of substances on the development of the retina, we have extended the technique to fetal rat retina and examined the structure of the developing explants as well as certain aspects of its function. We here review our work on establishing a procedure for maintaining rat newborn rat retinas in culture for up to three weeks and the first results with it. Again, we find ourselves in a field, development, where John Dowling's work has had considerable impact.

---

* Corresponding author: Berndt Ehinger, Tel.: +46 46 17 16 90; Fax: +46 46 211 50 74; E-mail: Berndt.Ehinger@oft.lu.se

590

The design of the experiments summarized here and the animal care were according the ARVO convention for ophthalmologic animal experimentation and approved by the Swedish Government Committee for Animal Experimentation Ethics. The work is being or will be published in more detail elsewhere (e.g. Johansson et al., 2000a,b).

A fetal rat retina culture system

Retinas were obtained from PVG rats (which are pigmented) and cultured with a technique modified after Stoppini and colleagues (1991). Freshly enucleated eyes PVG rats were immersed in cold CO_2-independent medium (Gibco, Paisley, UK) while trimming away external muscle and connective tissue. Immediately before further dissection, they were incubated for 17–18 min at 37°C in CO_2-independent medium supplemented with proteinase K, 0.5 mg/ml (Sigma, St Louis, MO). The treatment made it possible to dissect off the retina with its pigment epithelium attached. The proteinase K incubation time is critical and has to be adjusted to fit the tissue handling of the person doing the dissection. The tissue was gently explanted onto Millicell®-PCF 3.0 μm inserts with the vitreal side up, and the inserts were placed in tissue culture plates (Fig. 1A and B). It is critically important that the handling is gentle.

The retina explants were maintained in Dulbecco's modified Eagle's medium (DMEM; Sigma) supplemented with 10% fetal calf serum at 37°C with 99%

humidity and 5% CO_2 L-glutamine, penicillin and streptomycin were added to the medium. The specimens were cultured for up to 3 weeks, changing the medium every second day.

Results and discussion

Overall morphology of cultured rat retina explants

Cryostat sections of the tissues were examined with routine immunohistochemical methods as described elsewhere (Johansson et al., 2000a,b). Double-labeled sections were examined with a Bio-Rad MRC1024 confocal imaging system. Standard procedures were used for electron microscopy on tissue specimens fixed in glutaraldehyde and osmium tetroxide. The recoverin antiserum was a kind gift from Dr. A.M. Dizhoor of Kresge Eye Institute in Detroit, Mich.

The nuclear and plexiform layers of the inner retina were found to develop best in culture when the retinal pigment epithelium faced the culture membrane. The tissue then and survived for at least 3 weeks with only minor deviations from litter-matched retinas. Rosette formation was not prominent and did not appear to affect the organization of the inner retina (Fig. 2), even though the photoreceptor layer at times was somewhat uneven. Retinal blood vessels did not develop.

At the electron microscopic level, several of the characteristics present in the plexiform layers of P21

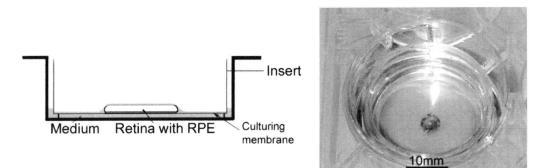

Fig. 1A and B. Schematic illustration and photograph of the retina culture system. The retina with its pigment epithelium attached is carefully placed on the filter membrane of a 30 mm Millicell®-PCF 3.0 μm insert in a culturing well. The pigment epithelium faces the filter, and the retina is only partially immersed in the culture medium, which covers the tissue by capillary action. The system is kept at 37°C in an incubator with 99% humidity and 5% CO_2.

retina were also observed after 3 weeks in vitro. Numerous terminals with dense-cored vesicles and/or small clear vesicles were observed throughout the entire inner plexiform layer. Some of the terminals established conventional synapses and, to a lesser extent, ribbon synapses typical for bipolar cells (Fig. 3A). In photoreceptor terminals, ribbon synapses appeared in the normal triad arrangement (Fig. 3B). Synaptophysin, a marker protein for synapses, was abundantly present in both plexiform layers (Johansson et al., 2000b), possibly even overexpressed.

Already from plain morphology, it thus appears that explants from newborn rat retinas can be maintained in culture for up to 3 weeks. At the time of explantation, the tissue is undifferentiated, but it can develop and become well differentiated with the expected layering, when compared with litter-matched normal retinas of the same age.

However, some morphological deviations are also evident already by routine microscopy. The photoreceptor outer segments and ganglion cells do not develop well. Developing inner retinal neurons, including ganglion cells are readily stained with antibodies directed against the Hu family of RNA-binding proteins in immature neurons (Barami et al., 1995), and the latter are clearly reduced in number (Fig. 4A and B). When explanted, ganglion cells become axotomized and in our culture they are deprived of their target and its trophic influences, which likely explains why they do not develop well (Germer et al., 1997). The lack of ganglion cells in vitro is thus not of the type seen in adults after axotomy, but rather a failure to develop normal contacts which leads to apoptotic removal of them. Naturally occurring cell death among postnatal

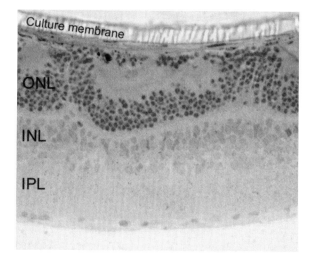

Fig. 2. Light micrograph of a PVG rat retina explanted on its third postnatal day (P3) and kept in culture for 18 days, resulting in a 21 postnatal days (P21) retina. Note the good layering of the retina even though the photoreceptor layer is slightly irregular, the underdeveloped photoreceptor outer segments and the paucity of large neurons in the ganglion cell layer. The culture membrane usually bends slightly in the histotechnical processing, like in this image. ONL, outer nuclear layer; INL, inner nuclear layer; IPL, inner plexiform layer. Toluidine blue, ×310.

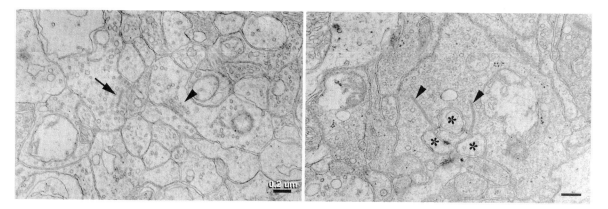

Fig. 3A and B. Electron micrographs showing synaptic structures in the plexiform layers of retina cultured to P21. A. Both conventional and ribbon synapses (arrowhead and arrow, respectively) with associated clear vesicles were identified in the inner plexiform layer. B. A photoreceptor terminal invagination in the outer plexiform layer with synaptic ribbons (arrowhead) contacting post-synaptic structures (asterisks). Scale bars: 0.2 μm.

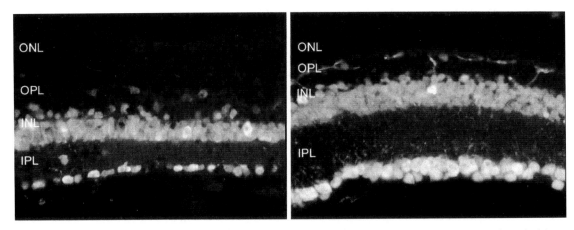

Fig. 4A and B. Cultured and normal P21 PVG rat retinas showing the distribution of Hu-positive somata in the retinal layers. Left, retina cultured from P3 to P21; right, litter-matched control. The number of Hu-positive somata in the ganglion cell layer of cultured retinas was strongly reduced (A) compared to the litter-matched normal retina (B). ONL, outer nuclear layer; INL, inner nuclear layer; IPL, inner plexiform layer. Adapted from Johansson et al., 2000b. Fluorescence micrographs, ×290.

ganglion cells peaks at around P3 and may continue at a lower rate for 1 week (Dreher et al., 1983; Maslim et al., 1986, 1995).

The middle layers of the retina (including the outer nuclear layer, the outer plexiform layer, the inner nuclear layer and the inner plexiform layer) regularly appeared to have a regular overall organization in our explants, despite at times a modest rosette formation in the photoreceptor layer and always an extensive loss of ganglion cells. The latter is a likely cause for the irregularities in the neuron contacts in the inner plexiform layer, which are further described below.

Cone and rod bipolar cells and AII amacrine cells

Rod bipolar cells synapse on AII amacrine cells which in turn contact ganglion cells via the ON- and OFF-cone pathway (review: Vaney, 1997). Protein kinase C (PKC) and parvalbumin immunoreactivity was seen in rod bipolar and AII amacrine cells, respectively, in retinas cultured to P14 or P21 (Fig. 5A; Johansson et al., 2000b). The number of PKC and parvalbumin somata, their position and arborization patterns were similar in cultured and litter-matched retinas. Terminals of AII amacrine cells in cultured retinas extended into the inner plexiform layer but were less developed in the cultured retinas than in normal tissue of the same

age. Confocal microscopy showed that their terminals came close to the rod bipolar cell terminals (Fig. 5B).

Recoverin immunoreactivity is a marker for two types of cone bipolar cells with terminals in two sublayers of the inner plexiform layer of the normal retina (Fig. 6B; Chun et al., 1999a). As expected, strong immunoreactivity appeared in the photoreceptor layer of both normal and cultured retinas, as well as in cone bipolar cells ending in the outermost part of the inner plexiform layer (type 2) and in its innermost part (type 8). In cultured retinas (Fig. 6A), there was a strong reduction in terminals in the innermost part of the inner nuclear layer (type 8). They extensively contact GABA amacrine cells as both pre- and postsynaptic elements. Like the NOS immunoreactive neurons (Johansson et al., 2000b), their processes in the innermost part of the inner plexiform layer are thus sensitive to the conditions prevailing in cultured retinas, of which the most apparent is the lack of ganglion cells.

Nitrergic neurons

Neuronal NOS immunolabeling was observed in retinas cultured up to P21 (Johansson et al., 2000b). Like in normal retina, their perikarya appeared in amacrine cells and displaced amacrine cells, respectively. There were two types of NOS immunoreactive amacrine cells with slightly different labeling and

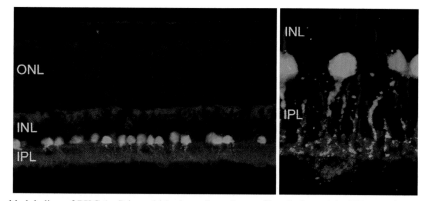

Fig. 5A and B. Double labeling of PKC (red) in rod bipolar cells and parvalbumin (green) in AII amacrine cells in a PVG rat retina explanted at P3 and kept in culture until P21. Note the relatively normal appearance of the processes from both rod bipolar cells and the AII amacrine cells. The high power confocal microscope image (B) has been enhanced to show how the processes of the two cell types regularly appear in close proximity to each other. When the green parvalbumin terminals are superimposed on the red rod bipolar cell terminals, the net result is a yellow spot. ONL, outer nuclear layer; INL, inner nuclear layer; IPL, inner plexiform layer. Adapted from Johansson et al., 2000b. Left, ×250, Right ×890.

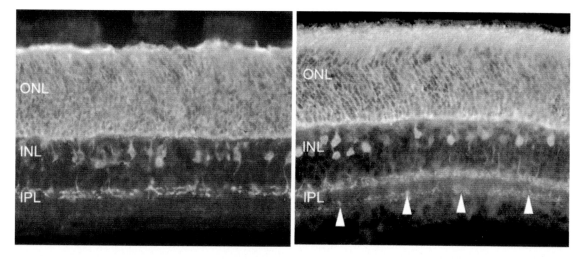

Fig. 6A and B. Recoverin immunoreactivity in PVG rat retina cultured from P3 to P14 (A) and a P14 littermate (B). Recoverin is abundantly present in photoreceptors and in cone bipolar cells in the inner nuclear layer. Note that the type 8 cone bipolar cell terminals, forming the inner sublamina in the control retina (B, arrowheads) are absent in the cultured retina (A). ONL, outer nuclear layer; INL, inner nuclear layer; IPL, inner plexiform layer. Fluorescence micrographs, ×290.

morphological characteristics were distinguishable, as seen also in normal retinas (Perez et al., 1995; Chun et al., 1999b). The processes of both types ramified in the outer sublaminas of the inner plexiform layer, and the innermost parts of this layer were almost devoid of NOS immunoreactive fibers. When compared with litter-matched P14 and P21 retinas, the NOS labeling appeared similar but not identical. Both the intensity and distribution of NOS labeling within the inner plexiform layer of normal retinas appeared to be more pronounced (Johansson et al., 2000b).

For studying NO-receptive neurons, exogenous NO was added directly in the culture wells with the following protocol. The retinas were first incubated with medium containing 1 mM isobutyl methylxantine (IBMX) and 0.1 mM zaprinast for 30 min in a

594

CO$_2$ incubator at 37°C, and NO stimulation was then achieved by adding 1 mM sodium nitroprusside to the medium for 10 min with the phosphodiesterase inhibitors still present (Johansson and Ehinger, 1999; Johansson et al., 2000b). In order to be able to make appropriate comparisons, tissues from age- and litter-matched rats of the same strain were like cultured retinas mounted on a Millicell® insert and concomitantly and identically stimulated with NO.

When the retina is challenged by NO generated from sodium nitroprusside, cGMP immunohistochemistry will reveal bipolar cells as well as amacrine cells and some ganglion cells (Gotzes et al., 1998; Johansson et al., 2000c). In retina cultured to P14 and P21 and stimulated with sodium nitroprusside, we found numerous cGMP immunolabeled cell somata that were distributed throughout the inner nuclear layer. Both amacrine cells and bipolar cells were observed and several of them developed distinct processes that terminated within the inner plexiform layer (Fig. 7A and B). The inner plexiform layer appeared well developed and two sublaminas of cGMP labeling were discernible. The outermost sublamina appeared close to the inner nuclear layer and may correspond to sublamina 1, and the other lamina was observed in close proximity to the ganglion cell layer and may correspond to sublamina 4 or 5.

Comparisons with NO stimulated litter-matched P14 and P21 retinas revealed large similarities

in staining properties of cell bodies and their distribution patterns. However, there were also some remarkable differences, most conspicuously a reduction in the number of cGMP immunoreactive sublaminas in the inner plexiform layer. Two sublaminas were easily observed in the ON and OFF-region of the cultured retina whereas four sublaminas were present within the inner plexiform layer of the litter-matched P14 retina (Fig. 7B). The innermost sublamina in the ON-region was well developed in cultured retinas and displayed heavy cGMP labeling characteristics, especially in comparison with normal P14 retinas. As the retina matured, the cGMP labeling in outermost sublamina was strongly reduced in the normal retina, but less so in culture (Johansson et al., 2000b). As will be further discussed, we assume that this relative upregulation of NO receptors is due to a loss of NO-releasing terminals.

Cholinergic neurons

ChAT and VAChT immunolabeling was examined in retinas cultured to P14 and P21. Both were colocalized in subsets of amacrine cells located in the inner nuclear layer and displaced amacrine cells distributed in the ganglion cell layer, which is the distribution seen in normal retinas (Johansson et al., 2000b). This distribution pattern was similar to that observed in

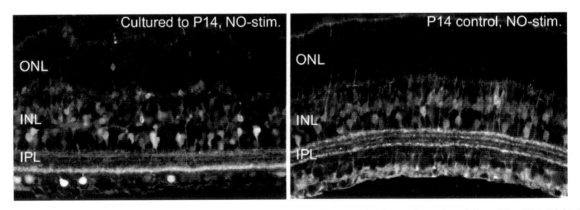

Fig. 7A and B. cGMP immunoreactivity in PVG rat retinas stimulated with NO. Left (A), a retina cultured from P3 to P14. Right (B), the corresponding littermate. Note that there are four sublayers in the inner plexiform layer in the normal P14 retina, but only two in the cultured, in which also the innermost is much stronger than the other. Adapted from Johansson et al., 2000b. ONL, outer nuclear layer; INL, inner nuclear layer; IPL, inner plexiform layer. Fluorescence micrographs, ×290.

litter-matched P14 and P21 retina, except that the number of ChAT immunolabeled amacrine cells in some of the cultured specimens appeared to be higher (Johansson et al., 2000b). ChAT and VACht also colocalized in two distinct sublaminas within the inner plexiform layer, as is typical of cholinergic amacrine cell processes in the inner plexiform layer (Koulen, 1997; Wassélius et al., 1998), but there was in retinas cultured to P14 also an additional third layer of ChAT immunoreactive processes in the middle of the inner plexiform layer. There thus appears to be an upregulation of the number of cholinergic neurons at about P14 in cultured retinas.

The distribution of cholinergic receptors of the mAChR2 type was also examined in retinas cultured to P14 and P21 (Johansson et al., 2000b). They appeared predominantly at and in the inner plexiform layer, but with marked differences from the in vivo situation. The general mAChR2 pattern at P14 and P21 is characterized by sub-populations of distinctly labeled amacrine cell somata located in the inner nuclear layer and a centrally located lamina within the inner plexiform layer that is surrounded by diffuse labeling (Fig. 8B). Contrasting, the inner plexiform layer of cultured retinas displayed intense mAChR2 immunolabeling in both the ON- and OFF-laminas, particularly in retina cultured to P21 (Fig. 8A).

In all developing retinas examined, the outer plexiform layer also displayed distinct mAChR2 labeled processes derived from cell somata located close to this layer (Fig. 8A). A thin process extended from some of somata and terminated in the inner plexiform layer, giving these cells morphological characteristics similar to a bipolar cell (see Euler and Wässle, 1995).

The increased mAChR2 labeling was most striking, both in the number of cell somata and in the intensity and distribution of the immunoreactivity in the inner plexiform layer. The presynaptic cholinergic marker, ChAT, also showed extra cholinergic processes in the inner parts of the retina. The mAChR2 labeling was most obviously increased in the outer and inner thirds of the inner plexiform layer, whereas the labeling in the middle of the layer appeared normal and as previously described (Wassélius et al., 1998; Johansson and Ehinger, 1999). Complex interactions between muscarinic receptors and growth factors in development and plasticity have previously been noted, but they are not well understood (Hohmann and Berger-Sweeney, 1998). Further, the expression of muscarinic receptors, particularly mAChR2, appears to be increased by developmentally regulated factors which have only partially been identified (McKinnon et al., 1998; Nadler et al., 1999). We assume that the upregulation of mAChR2 in rat retina explants has a corresponding background. The details remain to be worked out.

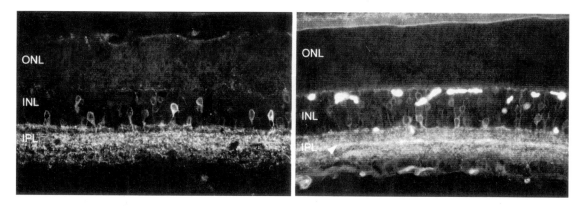

Fig. 8A and B. Muscarinic acetylcholine receptor (mAChR2) in a PVG rat retina cultured from P3 to P21 (A) with a corresponding littermate control (B). Note the increased density of the cholinergic receptor subunit in particularly the cultured retina. The arrowhead in the right panel points to the central sublamina, which is normally seen in adult retina. There is strong non-specific staining of the capillaries in the right hand panel (B). The cultured retina (A) does not contain any capillaries. Adapted from Johansson et al., 2000b. ONL, outer nuclear layer; INL, inner nuclear layer; IPL, inner plexiform layer. Fluorescence micrographs, ×290.

Development of the innermost retinal layers in vitro

True ganglion cells are axotomized in explanted retinas, and we expected major ganglion cell degeneration after 2–3 weeks in culture. This could be suspected already from simple stainings, and the lack of Hu immunoreactive cells in cultured retinas shows that there is indeed a lack of ganglion cells. It is usually assumed that amacrine cells do not die after axotomy in adult animals (see Huxlin and Bennett, 1995), but we nevertheless found some morphological differences in the inner plexiform layer of cultured retina that directly or indirectly seem to relate to the large ganglion cell death.

It is apparent that most of the changes noted in this study affects the inner half of the retina, and most notably the innermost layer (sublamina b, or the ON lamina) of the inner plexiform layer. As will be discussed, we suspect the lack of ganglion cells partly causes the deviations.

NOS positive amacrine cell processes distribute in both the ON and OFF-regions in the inner plexiform layer (Perez et al., 1995; Kim et al., 1999; Chun et al., 1999b). In cultured fetal rat retina, there was a significant reduction of such processes, predominantly in the ON-region but also in the OFF-region. Nitrergic amacrine cells located in the inner nuclear layer either are unaffected (Huxlin and Bennett, 1995) or increase in number and labeling intensity following axotomy (Klöcker et al., 1999), and NOS neurons in fetal developing tissue thus respond differently. The lack of ganglion cells in cultured retinas is a possible reason for the down-regulation of NOS-positive fibers, and our results suggest that it is particularly the NOS-positive terminals in the ON-region, which are dependent on the presence of ganglion cell dendrites during development. It remains to be established whether the NOS amacrine cells are dependent on direct cell–cell contacts with ganglion cell dendrites, or if the ganglion cells release a factor that promote amacrine cell survival (see Waid and McLoon, 1998; Belliveau and Cepko, 1999).

Nitric oxide (NO) is known to affect a number of different kinds of neurons in the retina, including certain amacrine and bipolar cells, and this can be visualized as a change in their cGMP content (Gotzes et al., 1998; Johansson et al., 2000c). If NOS labeled terminals in the inner plexiform layer disappear, one might expect changes of soluble guanylate cyclase and perhaps also cGMP. An up-regulation of cGMP labeling was indeed observed, and the effect was most predominant in sublamina 4. By inhibiting the production of NO with L-arginine analogs, small increases in cGMP immunolabeling have been noted, which was explained as an increased sensitivity to soluble guanylate cyclase activity (Prickaerts et al., 1998). It is possible that the decreased NOS innervation in the ON-lamina in cultured fetal rat retina results in such increased sensitivity of soluble guanylate cyclase, which would lead to increased cGMP levels following NO stimulation.

It is remarkable how several neuron systems of the inner plexiform layer are upregulated in cultured fetal retinas, most notably the nitrergic and cholinergic ones. The detailed reasons for this may vary with the circumstances, but the connexion with development seems clear enough. It may be noted that neurotransmitters like GABA, NO and acetylcholine have been suspected to be developmental regulators (e.g. Redburn and Rowe-Rendleman, 1996; Fletcher and Kalloniatis, 1997). There is a similar and remarkable upregulation of the GluR2 receptor during the normal development of the rat retina (Johansson et al., 2000a).

Conclusions

With the procedure described, it is possible to maintain developing rat retinas in culture for up to 3 weeks with only minor morphological deviations. We have demonstrated the appearance of several neuronal classes, using different neurotransmitters and other markers in the cultured retinas (synaptophysin, recoverin, PKC, parvalbumin, ChAT, VAChT, mAChR2, NOS and Hu). Except for ganglion cells and photoreceptor outer segments, the overall morphology of all neurons was like in the normal retina. Specific neural populations in retinas cultured for 2 or 3 weeks thus exhibit immunoreactivities to various components of the cholinergic, glutamatergic and nitrergic signaling pathways. With certain exceptions, the individual labeling pattern in each of these pathways developed in a manner that is comparable with that observed in litter-matched P14 and P21 retinas. Thus, each of these pathways seems to have the same temporal expression pattern as in vivo, and neural interactions should be possible between the major cell populations in our cultured retinas. From the present and previous immunohistochemical work in rats and other species (Feigenspan et al., 1993b; Rowe Rendleman et al., 1996), we conclude that several sub-populations of amacrine, bipolar and horizontal cells develop in vitro, and display the same phenotypic morphology and biochemistry as in vivo.

There is a lack of ganglion cells in the cultured retinas, and this seems to affect the distribution of both amacrine and bipolar cell processes as well as the expression of receptors and other cell markers in the inner plexiform layer. On the basis of available in vitro data we propose that ganglion cell survival is a prerequisite for the development of neurons associated with particularly the ON part of the inner plexiform layer. Ganglion cell loss during culture appear to induce conditions that alter the physiological environment for neuronal populations that develop and differentiate later than ganglion cells. The mechanisms behind this feature are currently unknown.

Acknowledgments

The work summarized here was supported by the Swedish Medical Research Council (13012-01A and 14X-2321), the Foundation Fighting Blindness, BioMed, Crown Princess Margaret's Committee for the Blind, the Knut and Alice Wallenberg, the Crafoord, the Clas Groschinsky and the Vårdal Foundations. We acknowledge Drs. J. deVente and A.M. Dizhoor for the generous gift of the cGMP and recoverin antibodies, respectively.

References

Barami, K., Iversen, K., Furneaux, H. and Goldman, S.A. (1995) Hu protein as an early marker of neuronal phenotypic differentiation by subependymal zone cells of the adult songbird forebrain. *J. Neurobiol.*, 28: 82–101.

Belliveau, M.J. and Cepko, C.L. (1999) Extrinsic and intrinsic factors control the genesis of amacrine and cone cells in the rat retina. *Development*, 126: 555–566.

Caffé, A.R., Szél, A., Juliusson, B., Hawkins, R. and van Veen, T. (1993) Hyperplastic neuroretinopathy and disorder of

pigment epithelial cells precede accelerated retinal degeneration in the SJL/N mouse. *Cell Tissue Res.*, 271: 297–307.

Chun, M.H., Kim, I.B., Oh, S.J. and Chung, J.W. (1999a) Synaptic connectivity of two types of recoverin-labeled cone bipolar cells and glutamic acid decarboxylase immunoreactive amacrine cells in the inner plexiform layer of the rat retina. *Vis. Neurosci.*, 16: 791–800.

Chun, M.H., Oh, S.J., Kim, I.B. and Kim, K.Y. (1999b) Light and electron microscopical analysis of nitric oxide synthase-like immunoreactive neurons in the rat retina. *Vis. Neurosci.*, 16: 379–389.

Dowling, J.E. (1996) Retinal processing of vision. In: Greger, R. and Windhorst, U. (Eds.), *Comprehensive Human Physiology*, Vol. 1. Springer-Verlag, Berlin Heidelberg, pp. 773–788.

Dowling, J.E. (1999) Retinal processing of visual information. *Brain Res. Bull.*, 50: 317.

Dreher, B., Potts, R.A. and Bennett, M.R. (1983) Evidence that the early postnatal reduction in the number of rat retinal ganglion cells is due to a wave of ganglion cell death. *Neurosci. Lett.*, 36: 255–260.

Euler, T. and Wässle, H. (1995) Immunocytochemical identification of cone bipolar cells in the rat retina. *J. Comp. Neurol.*, 361: 461–478.

Ezzeddine, Z.D., Yang, X., Dechiara, T., Yancopoulos, G. and Cepko, C.L. (1997) Postmitotic cells fated to become rod photoreceptors can be respecified by CNTF treatment of the retina. *Development*, 124: 1055–1067.

Feigenspan, A., Bormann, J. and Wässle, H. (1993b) Organotypic slice culture of the mammalian retina. *Vis. Neurosci.*, 10: 203–217.

Feigenspan, A., Wässle, H. and Bormann, J. (1993a) Pharmacology of GABA receptor Cl-channels in rat retinal bipolar cells. *Nature*, 361: 159–162.

Fletcher, E.L. and Kalloniatis, M. (1997) Localisation of amino acid neurotransmitters during postnatal development of the rat retina. *J. Comp. Neurol.*, 380: 449–471.

Frisén, J., Holmberg, J. and Barbacid, M. (1999) Ephrins and their Eph receptors: multitalented directors of embryonic development. *EMBO J.*, 18: 5159–5165.

Frisén, J., Yates, P.A., McLaughlin, T., Friedman, G.C., O'Leary, D.D. and Barbacid, M. (1998) Ephrin-A5 (AL-1/RAGS) is essential for proper retinal axon guidance and topographic mapping in the mammalian visual system. *Neuron*, 20: 235–243.

Gähwiler, B.H., Capogna, M., Debanne, D., McKinney, R.A. and Thompson, S.M. (1997) Organotypic slice cultures: a technique has come of age. *Trends Neurosci.*, 20: 471–477.

Germer, A., Kuhnel, K., Grosche, J., Friedrich, A., Wolburg, H., Price, J., Reichenbach, A. and Mack, A.F. (1997) Development of the neonatal rabbit retina in organ culture. 1. Comparison with histogenesis in vivo, and the effect of a gliotoxin (alpha-aminoadipic acid). *Anat. Embryol. (Berlin)*, 196: 67–79.

Gotzes, S., De Vente, J. and Muller, F. (1998) Nitric oxide modulates cGMP levels in neurons of the inner and outer retina in opposite ways. *Vis. Neurosci.*, 15: 945–955.

598

Hohmann, C.F. and Berger-Sweeney, J. (1998) Cholinergic regulation of cortical development and plasticity. New twists to an old story. *Perspect. Dev. Neurobiol.*, 5: 401–425.

Huxlin, K.R. and Bennett, M.R. (1995) NADPH diaphorase expression in the rat retina after axotomy—a supportive role for nitric oxide. *Eur. J. Neurosci.*, 7: 2226–2239.

Hyatt, G.A. and Dowling, J.E. (1997) Retinoic acid. A key molecule for eye and photoreceptor development. *Invest. Ophthalmol. Vis. Sci.*, 38: 1471–1475.

Johansson, K., Bruun, A., deVente, J. and Ehinger, B. (2000c) Immunohistochemical analysis of the developing inner plexiform layer in postnatal rat retina. *Invest. Ophthalmol. Vis. Sci.*, 41: 305–313.

Johansson, K., Bruun, A., Grasbon, T. and Ehinger, B. (2000b) Growth of postnatal rat retina *in vitro*. Development of neurotransmitter systems. *J. Chem. Neuroanat.*, 19: 117–128.

Johansson, K., Bruun, A., Törngren, M. and Ehinger, B. (2000a) Development of glutamate receptor subunit 2 immunoreactivity in postnatal rat retina. *Vis. Neurosci.*, 17: 737–742.

Johansson, K. and Ehinger, B. (1999) Nitric oxide/cyclic GMP and the development of neural circuits in the postnatal rat retina. FASEB Summer Research Conference, 1999.

Kim, I.B., Lee, E.J., Kim, K.Y., Ju, W.K., Oh, S.J., Joo, C.K. and Chun, M.H. (1999) Immunocytochemical localization of nitric oxide synthase in the mammalian retina. *Neurosci. Lett.*, 267: 193–196.

Klöcker, N., Kermer, P., Gleichmann, M., Weller, M. and Bahr, M. (1999) Both the neuronal and inducible isoforms contribute to upregulation of retinal nitric oxide synthase activity by brain-derived neurotrophic factor. *J. Neurosci.*, 19: 8517–8527.

Koulen, P. (1997) Vesicular acetylcholine transporter (VAChT): a cellular marker in rat retinal development. *NeuroReport*, 8: 2845–2848.

Maslim, J., Webster, M. and Stone, J. (1986) Stages in the structural differentiation of retinal ganglion cells. *J. Comp. Neurol.*, 254: 382–402.

Maslim, J., Egensperger, R., Holländer, H., Humphrey, M. and Stone, J. (1995) Receptor degeneration is a normal part of retinal development. In: Anderson, R.E., LaVail, M.M. and Hollyfield, J.G. (Eds.), *Degenerative Diseases of the Retina*. Plenum Press, New York, pp. 187–193.

McKinnon, L.A., Gunther, E.C. and Nathanson, N.M. (1998) Developmental regulation of the cm2 muscarinic acetylcholine receptor gene: selective induction by a secreted factor produced by embryonic chick retinal cells. *J. Neurosci.*, 18: 59–69.

Nadler, L.S., Rosoff, M.L., Hamilton, S.E., Kalaydjian, A.E., McKinnon, L.A. and Nathanson, N.M. (1999) Molecular analysis of the regulation of muscarinic receptor expression and function. *Life Sci.*, 64: 375–379.

Perez, M.T., Larsson, B., Alm, P., Andersson, K.E. and Ehinger, B. (1995) Localisation of neuronal nitric oxide synthase-immunoreactivity in rat and rabbit retinas. *Exp. Brain Res.*, 104: 207–217.

Prickaerts, J., De Vente, J., Markerink-van Ittersum, M. and Steinbusch, H.W. (1998) Behavioural, neurochemical and neuroanatomical effects of chronic postnatal N-nitro-L-arginine methyl ester treatment in neonatal and adult rats. *Neuroscience*, 87: 181–195.

Redburn, D.A. and Rowe-Rendleman, C. (1996) Developmental neurotransmitters; signals for shaping neuronal circuitry. *Invest. Ophthalmol. Vis. Sci.*, 37: 1479–1482.

Reichenbach, A. and Robinson, S.R. (1995) Phylogenetic constrains on retinal organisation and development. *Prog. Retin. Eye Res.*, 15: 139–171.

Rodieck, R.W. (1998) *The First Steps in Seeing*. Sinauer Associates, Inc., Sunderland, Massachussetts.

Rowe Rendleman, C., Mitchell, C.K., Habrecht, M. and Redburn, D.A. (1996) Expression and downregulation of the GABAergic phenotype in explants of cultured rabbit retina. *Invest. Ophthalmol. Vis. Sci.*, 37: 1074–1083.

Seigel, G.M. (1999) The golden age of retinal cell culture. *Mol. Vis.*, 5(4): electronic citation. http://www.molvis.org/molvis/v5/p4

Sparrow, J.R., Hicks, D. and Barnstable, C.J. (1990) Cell commitment and differentiation in explants of embryonic rat neural retina. Comparison with the developmental potential of dissociated retina. *Brain Res. Dev. Brain Res.*, 51: 69–84.

Stoppini, L., Buchs, P.A. and Muller, D. (1991) A simple method for organotypic cultures of nervous tissue. *J. Neurosci. Methods*, 37: 173–182.

Söderpalm, A., Szél, À., Caffé, A.R. and van Veen, T. (1994) Selective development of one cone photoreceptor type in retinal organ culture. *Invest. Ophthalmol. Vis. Sci.*, 35: 3910–3921.

Tessier-Lavigne, M. and Goodman, C.S. (1996) The molecular biology of axon guidance. *Science*, 274: 1123–1133.

Vaney, D.I. (1997) Neuronal coupling in rod-signal pathways of the retina. *Invest. Ophthalmol. Vis. Sci.*, 38: 267–273.

Waid, D.K. and McLoon, S.C. (1998) Ganglion cells influence the fate of dividing retinal cells in culture. *Development*, 125: 1059–1066.

Wassélius, J., Johansson, K., Bruun, A., Zucker, C. and Ehinger, B. (1998) Correlations between cholinergic neurons and muscarinic m2 receptors in the rat retina [published erratum appears in *NeuroReport* 1998 Jul 13; 9(10): 2436]. *NeuroReport*, 9: 1799–1802.

H. Kolb, H. Ripps and S. Wu (Eds.)
Progress in Brain Research, Vol. 131
© 2001 Elsevier Science B.V. All rights reserved

CHAPTER 43

The function of the cholinergic system in the developing mammalian retina

Z. Jimmy Zhou*

Departments of Physiology and Biophysics and Ophthalmology, University of Arkansas for Medical Sciences, Little Rock, AR 72205, USA

Introduction

Acetylcholine is a classic neurotransmitter present in all vertebrate retinas studied to date (Brecha, 1983). In the adult mammalian retina, cholinergic neurons represent a unique class of amacrine cells synonymously known as the "starburst" (Famiglietti, 1983), which exist at both sides of the inner plexiform layer (IPL) as two mirror-symmetric populations (Hayden et al., 1980; Vaney et al., 1981; Famiglietti, 1983, 1985). Starburst cells are perhaps the best characterized of all amacrine cells. They have a number of distinctive characteristics (for review, Masland and Tauchi, 1986; Vaney, 1990; Wassle and Boycott, 1991), which are consistent across species, suggesting a highly conserved role of the cholinergic system in the retina.

The development of cholinergic neurons in the retina has also been studied in a rich variety of vertebrate species. Cholinergic markers, including choline acetyltransferase (ChAT), acetylcholinesterase (AChE) and cholinergic receptors, appear at the earliest stages of retinal development when precursors of cholinergic amacrine cells begin to differentiate in the neuroblastic layer of the developing retina (Sugiyama et al., 1977; Spira et al., 1987; Hamassaki-Britto et al., 1994; Matter et al., 1995;

Prada et al., 1999). It has been proposed that ACh is released as a developmental cue by the cholinergic neuroblasts as they migrate through the ventricular zone to the IPL (Redburn and Rowe-Rendleman, 1996). After entering the IPL, as shown in the chick retina (Prada et al., 1999), the differentiating cholinergic amacrine cells initially exist as a single population of ACh- and GABA-containing cells but then polarize and separate into two mirror-symmetric populations in their final destinations in the amacrine and ganglion cell layers.

Although the developmental role of the cholinergic system in the retina is still poorly understood, studies in many vertebrate species at various developmental stages have implicated ACh as a critical neurotransmitter for retinal development (Ramoa et al., 1987; Lipton et al., 1988; Lipton and Kater, 1989; Lauder, 1993; Sernagor and Grzywacz, 1996; Feller et al., 1996; Zhou, 1998; Penn et al., 1998; Zhou and Zhao, 2000). It is thought that at least two broad and separate cholinergic mechanisms are involved in retinal development: one is in the early phases of neuronal genesis and cell migration, whereas the other occurs during neuronal growth and synaptogenesis (Redburn and Rowe-Rendleman, 1996); however, the exact nature of cholinergic actions in either of these mechanisms is still unclear.

Recently, there has been a swell of interest in the functional role of the cholinergic system in the developing visual system. In the mammalian retina,

*Tel.: 501-686-8128; Fax: 501-686-8167;
E-mail: zhoujimmy@uams.edu

many recent studies have focused on the physiology of the developing cholinergic system, especially in relation to rhythmic spontaneous retinal waves and activity-dependent visual system development. These studies have provided important information about anatomical and physiological properties of cholinergic neurons in the developing retina, as well as new insights into the role of the cholinergic system in visual development. This chapter reviews some of these recent findings with an emphasis on functional properties of the cholinergic system around the time of synaptogenesis in the IPL. Although many of the findings in this research area were first reported in several different species, illustrations given in this chapter are adapted exclusively from results obtained from the rabbit retina, in which the cholinergic system has been best described both during development and in adulthood.

Properties of the cholinergic system in the developing mammalian retina

Anatomical characteristics of cholinergic retinal neurons during development

In the mammalian retina, immunohistochemistry with antiserum against ChAT or vesicular acteycholine transporter (VAChT) has identified cholinergic retinal neurons in early postnatal rat (Mitrofanis and Stone, 1988; Koulen, 1997), cat (Dann, 1989), ferret (Feller et al., 1996), tree shrew (Sandmann et al., 1997), rabbit (unpublished observation by S.J. Bakewell and Z.J. Zhou) and opossum (Camargo De Moura Campos and Hokoc, 1999). In general, the distribution pattern of cholinergic neurons in the inner mammalian retina remains consistent across species. By the age when conventional synapses in the IPL just begin to form (about 45–65% of the caecal period[1]), two bands of narrowly stratifying cholinergic plexuses are already present in the developing IPL, and two populations of immunoreactive

cholinergic cell bodies are found adjacent to the IPL in the amacrine and ganglion cell layers, respectively. These putative cholinergic amacrine cells attain their adult-like branching pattern early in development. In rabbit, the characteristic "starburst" morphology (Fig. 1) is seen with Lucifer-yellow-staining at least as early as embryonic day E29 (unpublished observation by Z.J. Zhou). The presence of the narrowly stratifying, radially symmetric pattern of starburst dendrites at this early age is remarkable, especially given that the IPL is still poorly developed and that ribbon synapses from bipolar cells have not begun to form (McArdle et al., 1977). It remains an intriguing question as to what instructs the formation of this highly restricted dendritic stratification pattern during early development.

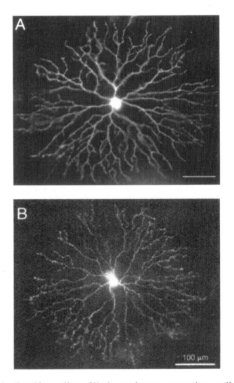

Fig. 1. Lucifer-yellow-filled starburst amacrine cells. (**A**) Displaced starburst cell in the inferior mid-periphery of a flat mount newborn rabbit retina photographed immediately after whole-cell patch-clamp recordings (figure adapted from Zhou, 1998). Notice the numerous dendritic spines and the lack of varicosities in distal dendrites. Scale bars: 50 μm. (**B**) Starburst amacrine cell from an adult rabbit retina showing varicosities in distal dendrites and a lack of dendritic spines (adapted from Tauchi and Masland, 1984). Scale bar: 100 μm.

---

[1]The caecal period is defined as the time between conception and eye opening. Many of the developmental events involved in the establishment of the visual pathways occur at about the same stage of the caecal period in all mammalian retinas (Dreher and Robinson, 1988).

Despite their similar dendritic branching patterns and mirror-symmetric distribution across the IPL, early developing (Fig. 1A) and adult (Fig. 1B) starburst cells differ at least in two important morphological aspects (Wong and Collin, 1989; Sandmann et al., 1997; Zhou, 1998). First, there are numerous dendritic spines in the developing but not the adult starburst cell, indicating a high degree of modification and plasticity of the starburst dendritic structure during development. Second, unlike the mature starburst cell whose output synapses are confined to the varicose zone in the distal dendritic field (Famiglietti, 1992), the early developing starburst cell lacks concentrated varicosities in distal dendrites (Fig. 1), suggesting major differences in synaptic organization between the developing and the mature cholinergic system. These anatomical differences are consistent with the belief that the role of the cholinergic system changes during retinal development (Zhou and Fain, 1996; Zhou and Zhao, 2000).

In addition to the strong immunostaining of cholinergic amacrine cells in the inner retina, weak ChAT- and VAChT-like immunoreactivities have also been found in putative horizontal cells of the rat retina during a transient developmental period between postnatal days P4 and P10 (Kim et al., 1998). The nature of these ChAT- and VAChT-like immunoreactivities in the developing outer retina is unclear, but they seem consistent with the presence of immunoreactivity to muscarinic antibodies in the outer plexiform layer of the developing mammalian retina (Hutchins, 1994). Thus, the cholinergic system may play a role in the development of the outer retina as well (Redburn and Rowe-Rendleman, 1996).

Voltage-gated currents and membrane excitability of starburst amacrine cells

With the development of mammalian retinal slice and wholemount preparations, it has recently become possible to investigate cellular physiological properties of morphologically identified cholinergic amacrine cells, especially the displaced population, in the developing rabbit retina with patch-clamp and calcium imaging techniques (Zhou and Fain, 1995, 1996; Zhou, 1998; Butts et al., 1999). In the adult rabbit retina, displaced starburst cells can be selectively labeled with the fluorescent dye DAPI (Masland et al., 1984). This method also works quite well in P18 and older postnatal rabbits (Fig. 3) (Zhou and Fain, 1995), but it is not reliable in rabbits younger than two weeks old. Definitive identification of starburst cells during physiological recordings was made morphologically, for example, by including Lucifer yellow (0.1–1%) in the whole-cell pipette solution to label the dendrites (Zhou and Fain, 1996; Zhou, 1998).

When recorded under whole-cell voltage clamp in a wholemount preparation superfused with Ames medium (Ames and Nesbett, 1981) at 37°C, displaced starburst cells in the newborn rabbit retina displayed a number of voltage-gated currents with a characteristic profile (Fig. 2A). Inward, TTX-sensitive Na^+ currents were found in most of the displaced starburst cells tested between the age of E29 (two days before birth) and P11 (time of eye opening). However, the peak Na^+ current amplitude was typically much smaller (by at least two-fold) than that of outward K^+ currents. This current profile was in contrast to that of ganglion cells, whose peak Na^+ current amplitude was usually equivalent to or larger than that of outward K^+ currents (Fig. 2C). Similarly, voltage responses of starburst cells under current-clamp were also characteristically different from those of ganglion cells (Fig. 2B,D). Starburst cells usually generated a single spike in response to a prolonged current pulse. The threshold for somatic action potentials in the starburst cell was above -35 mV (Fig. 1B), as opposed to about -45 mV in the ganglion cell (Fig. 2D). Action potentials elicited in ganglion cells were also considerably larger and narrower than those elicited in starburst cells (Fig. 2B,D) and often consisted of multiple spikes during prolonged depolarizing current injections. On the other hand, the resting membrane potential of displaced starburst cells was typically below -70 mV, about 20 mV more hyperpolarized than that of ganglion cells. This combination of low resting membrane potential and high action potential threshold suggests that it would be difficult to elicit somatic action potentials from the developing starburst cell under physiological conditions. Indeed, spontaneous generation of somatic action potentials has never been observed from neonatal starburst cells even during rhythmic spontaneous excitation

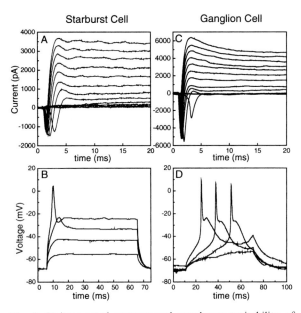

Fig. 2. Voltage-gated currents and membrane excitability of displaced starburst (A, B; from a P0 rabbit retina) and ganglion cell (C, D; from a P3 rabbit retina). Currents shown here have been corrected for membrane leakage. (A) Whole-cell currents elicited by depolarizing voltage steps (13 steps in 10 mV increments) under voltage clamp from a holding potential of −70 mV. (B) Voltage responses from the same starburst cell to depolarizing current pulses of 200-pA increments under current clamp. (C) Whole-cell currents from a ganglion cell voltage-clamped at −70 mV in response to the same voltage protocol as in A. (D) Voltage responses of the same ganglion cell to depolarizing current pulses of 80, 100, 140 and 160 pA. Recordings were made in Ames medium at 37°C with a pipette solution containing (in mM): 110 KCl, 5 NaOH, 0.5 $CaCl_2$, 2 $MgCl_2$, 5 EGTA, 10 HEPES, 2ATP, 0.5 GTP and 2 ascorbic acid. (Adapted from Zhou, 1998.)

(see section below) (Zhou, 1998). Furthermore, spontaneous retinal waves in the early postnatal ferret, which are believed to be driven mainly by ACh, persisted in the presence of TTX (Stellwagen et al., 1999). Similar results were also obtained in embryonic day E26 rabbit retina, although TTX blocked Ca^{2+} waves in E30 and older rabbits (unpublished observation by Z.J. Zhou).

As retinal development proceeded, action potential generation in starburst cells became even more difficult because the Na^+ current amplitude quickly diminished to an undetectable level shortly after eye opening (Zhou and Fain, 1995). The functional role of Na^+ currents in starburst cells is presently unclear. In the mature rabbit retina, there have been conflicting results and interpretations as to whether starburst cells are capable of firing action potentials (Bloomfield, 1992; Jensen, 1995; Taylor and Wassle, 1995; Peters and Masland, 1996; Zhou and Fain, 1996; Cohen, 1999). In the early postnatal rabbit retina, there is no doubt that starburst cells can be driven to spike by extrinsic depolarizing currents (Zhou and Fain, 1996), but, as mentioned above, somatic action potentials have never been observed during spontaneous, rhythmic excitation (Zhou, 1998).

Neurotransmitter receptors of the developing starburst cell

Physiological and pharmacological properties of amino acid receptors on displaced starburst cells have been characterized in rabbits from the early age of synaptogenesis (E29) (Paul and Zhou, 2000) to P28 (Zhou and Fain, 1995), an age when retinal structure and ganglion cell light responses appeared adult-like (Masland, 1977; McArdle et al., 1977). Starting from the earliest age tested (E31), pressure injection of glutamate and its analogs elicited robust responses from displaced starburst cells under patch clamp in the wholemount retina in saline containing 1 mM Cd^{2+} (Zhou, 2001a), suggesting that functional glutamate receptors were present on these cells long before the onset of bipolar cell synaptogenesis in the IPL. The glutamate-evoked response in newborn starburst cells was mediated mainly by nonNMDA receptors, but a small NMDA receptor-mediated component could not be ruled out. Neonatal starburst cells also responded to GABA and glycine with pharmacological characteristics consistent with the presence of $GABA_A$ and glycine receptors. Similar experiments also identified NMDA and nonNMDA receptors, as well as $GABA_A$ and glycine receptors on ganglion cells in the newborn rabbit retina (Paul and Zhou, 2000).

The presence of excitatory and inhibitory amino acid receptors on displaced starburst cells persisted throughout the postnatal development of the rabbit retina. Figure 3 shows voltage-clamp records from DAPI-labeled displaced starburst cells in a slice preparation of P14–28 rabbit (Zhou and Fain, 1995). In the presence of 1 mM Cd^{2+}, every starburst cell tested had robust responses to GABA.

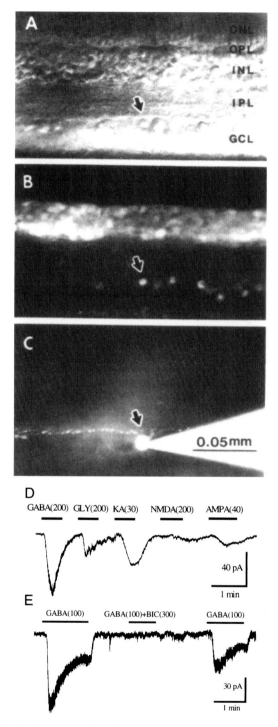

D

GABA(200) GLY(200) KA(30) NMDA(200) AMPA(40)

40 pA

1 min

E

GABA(100) GABA(100)+BIC(300) GABA(100)

30 pA

1 min

Fig. 3. Responses of starburst amacrine cells to amino acid agonists and antagonists. (A) A 150 μm thick slice from a 3-week-old rabbit retina photographed with Hoffman modulation contrast optics. (B) Epifluorescence image of the same slice

The responses could be completely blocked by high concentrations (100–300 μM) of bicuculline, suggesting the presence of $GABA_A$ but not $GABA_C$ receptors. Strychnine-sensitive glycine receptors, and CNQX-sensitive nonNMDA receptors were also found in nearly every starburst cell recorded. NMDA responses were recorded from many starburst cells, but they were generally small and somewhat variable in amplitude from cell to cell (Zhou and Fain, 1995).

In the adult rabbit retina, there is some anatomical evidence that cholinergic amacrine cells make synapses onto each other (Brandon, 1987; Millar and Morgan, 1987; Famiglietti, 1991). However, it has remained unclear whether starburst cells directly communicate among themselves physiologically and, if they do, whether ACh and/or GABA is used at the synapses between starburst cells. This question becomes particularly important during development because of the possibility that a lateral network of recurrent cholinergic connections may play an important role in the formation of spontaneous retinal waves (Feller et al., 1997; Zhou, 1998).

Patch-clamp experiments have recently indicated that displaced starburst cells in the newborn rabbit retinal wholemount responded to exogenously applied ACh and its nicotinic analog DMPP with inward, desensitizing currents (Zhou, 2001a). These currents persisted in the presence of 1 mM Cd^{2+} to block Ca^{2+}-dependent release of endogenous neurotransmitters. The current–voltage curve showed strong inward rectification, typical of neuronal nicotinic receptors. These results suggest that the developing starburst cells communicate with each other using nicotinic receptors, although it is also possible that nicotinic receptors are used as auto receptors.

as in A, showing the selective staining of displaced starburst cells in the GCL one day after an intravitreal injection of DAPI. (C) Fluorescence micrograph of the dendritic morphology of a displaced starburst cell after whole-cell patch clamp with a Lucifer-yellow-filled pipette. Arrows in A–C indicate same starburst cell. (D) Whole-cell current responses of a starburst cell to batch-applied GABA, glycine, kainate, NMDA (coapplied with 1 μM glycine), and AMPA. (E) Bicuculline (BIC) completely abolished GABA-evoked responses in starburst cells. Recordings were made in the presence of 1 mM Cd^{2+} at a holding potential of −70 mV. Numbers in parentheses indicate the concentration of drugs in μM. (Adapted from Zhou and Fain, 1995.)

The function of the cholinergic system during retinal development

The development of precise neuronal circuits in the visual system often requires electric activity (Kalil, 1990; Constantine-Paton et al., 1990; Cook, 1991; Goodman and Shatz, 1993; Katz and Shatz, 1996). Depending on the stage of development, such neuronal activity may be either spontaneously generated within the developing network or driven by visual input. In the vertebrate retina, correlated bursts of electric activity occur spontaneously during certain developmental periods prior to eye opening, and they are believed to play an important role in the refinement of specific neuronal connectivity in both the central visual pathway (Cline, 1991; Goodman and Shatz, 1993; Shatz, 1996) and the retina itself (Sernagor and Grzywacz, 1996). Although the exact cellular mechanism responsible for the generation of spontaneous retinal activity is still not known, it has become increasingly clear that rhythmic spontaneous activities are a general phenomenon in the developing nervous system and occur in more than just one developmental period. At different stages of visual development, spontaneous retinal activities are believed to play different functional roles, and the cellular mechanism for the generation of such activities may be different as well.

In the developing mammalian retina, bursts of spontaneous excitation have been found in ganglion (Masland, 1977; Maffei and Galli-Resta, 1990; Meister et al., 1991) and amacrine cells (Wong et al., 1993; Zhou, 1998) from the age immediately before synaptogenesis in the IPL (60–70% caecal period) to shortly before eye opening (93–98% caecal period). These bursts occur in local retinal domains at a frequency of 0.2–2/min and propagate tangentially in the form of waves at a speed of one to several hundred microns per second (Feller et al., 1996; Zhou and Zhao, 2000; Bansal et al., 2000; Zhou, 2001b). The developmental course of the wave can be divided into at least two broad stages. During the early stage (60–80% caecal period), the wave is believed to provide important developmental cues for the segregation of eye-specific layers in the LGN (Shatz and Stryker, 1988; Penn et al., 1998). It has been proposed that the late wave, which occurs during 80–95% of caecal period, may be important for the segregation of ON and OFF layers in the LGN (Wong and Oakley, 1996). In addition to a role in the development of the retinogeniculate pathway, the spontaneous retinal activity may be also important for neuronal development in other areas of the visual system, particularly the retina itself (Bodnarenko and Chalupa, 1993; Sernagor and Grzywacz, 1996).

Cholinergic neurotransmission is required for spontaneous retinal waves

Recent studies from the mammalian retina suggest that spontaneous retinal waves between the ages of 60% and 98% caecal period rely critically on neurotransmitter-mediated interactions (for review, Feller, 1999; Wong, 1999). Feller and colleagues (1996) provided the first evidence that the generation of the early spontaneous retinal wave in the mammalian retina requires nicotinic cholinergic neurotransmission because antagonists to nicotinic receptors completely blocked the wave. Similar results have also been reported in rabbits during a specific period between E26 and P2 (Zhou and Zhao, 2000), and in the developing mouse retina (Bansal et al., 2000).

In the mammalian species so far studied, spontaneous retinal waves share a basic spatiotemporal pattern, even though detailed differences in wave property do exist among different species. Figure 4 shows spontaneous bursting activities in the ganglion cell layer of a P0 rabbit retina measured with Ca^{2+} imaging. These activities were highly rhythmic, occurring at a frequency of 0.2–2/min and propagating at a speed of 100–300 µm/s. During each passing of a wave, ganglion cells fired a burst of action potentials in response to a burst of synaptic input. The rhythmic input to ganglion cells could be completely blocked by curare (Fig. 5A), indicating that the synaptic input depended critically on nicotinic interactions. Detailed analysis of the current–voltage relation suggested that a major part of the input to ganglion cells during the wave was mediated by nicotinic receptors, but glycinergic input also played an essential role in the rabbit retina (Paul and Zhou, 2000). These results are consistent with the finding (Paul and Zhou, 2000) that neonatal

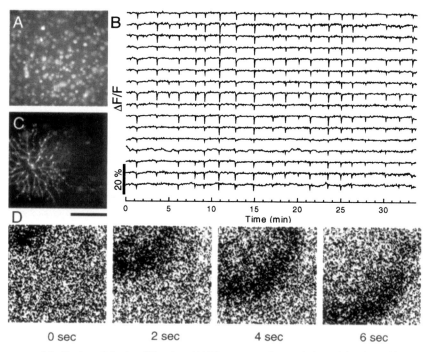

0 sec   2 sec   4 sec   6 sec

Fig. 4. Spontaneous waves of rhythmic activity in a P0 retina. (A) Fluorescence image (taken with a 40× objective lens) of Fura-2-AM-loaded cells in the ganglion cell layer of a neonatal rabbit retina (excitation wavelength: 380 nm; long-pass emission filter: 500 nm). (B) Relative (%) changes in fluorescence intensity from 16 cells randomly selected from the field of view shown in A. Each downward deflection in the traces indicates a transient increase in intracellular free Ca^{2+} concentration associated with the passing of a spontaneous wave. (C) Lucifer-yellow-filled displaced starburst amacrine cell from another retina photographed at the same magnification as in A. The cell body, which was pulled way after patch clamp, is not shown here. (D) Sequential difference images (ΔF) of a spontaneous wave recorded with a 10× objective lens. The dark region indicates the wavefront where Ca^{2+} concentration is elevated. Scale bar: 100 μm in A and C; 400 μm in D. (Adapted from Zhou and Zhao, 2000.)

rabbit ganglion cells express nicotinic receptors and respond to puffs of cholinergic agonists in the presence of Cd^{2+} (Fig. 5).

Direct participation of starburst cells in spontaneous retinal waves

In order to understand how the cholinergic system contributes to the generation and propagation of spontaneous retinal waves, patch-clamp recordings were made from morphologically identified displaced starburst cells in the wholemount retina of perinatal rabbits (Zhou, 1998). When current-clamped at their resting membrane potential, displaced starburst cells displayed spontaneous, rhythmic bursts of sub-threshold depolarization. The frequency of these bursts was similar to that of spontaneous waves, indicating that cholinergic amacrine cells directly

participated in retinal waves (Fig. 6). These results also suggest that ACh is released in rhythmic bursts.

The finding that starburst cells directly participate in the spontaneous rhythmic excitation also provides the first convincing evidence that retinal interneurons play an integral role in the generation and propagation of retinal waves. Moreover, it has been suggested that the spontaneous excitation may be generated first among developing interneurons in the inner retina and then "read out" by ganglion cells (Feller et al., 1997). A recent report that spontaneous bursts of excitation persisted even after ganglion cells have undergone apoptosis following axotomy (Stellwagen et al., 2000) seems to support this hypothesis. Regardless whether this hypothesis will prove to be true, an important question is how ganglion cells interact with retinal interneurons to produce propagating bursts of spikes.

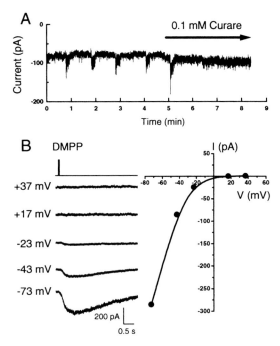

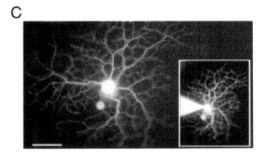

A
0.1 mM Curare

B
DMPP

+37 mV

+17 mV

-23 mV

-43 mV

-73 mV

200 pA
0.5 s

I (pA)

V (mV)

C

Fig. 5. (A) Rhythmic bursts of synaptic input recorded from a ganglion cell under voltage-clamp in a P0 rabbit retinal wholemount preparation. The bursts occurred at a frequency of ~1/min, similar to that of spontaneous waves, and could be completely blocked by curare. (B) Responses of a ganglion cell to puffs of the nicotinic agonist DMPP (1 mM) in physiological saline supplemented with 1 mM Cd^{2+}. (C) An example of a ganglion cell responding to DMPP. The dendritic morphology suggests a putative ON-OFF direction selective ganglion cell in the neonatal rabbit retina. Inset in D shows the same cell before the removal of the patch pipette. Scale bar: 50 μm.

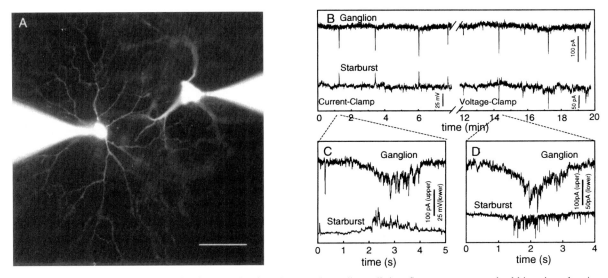

Fig. 6. Simultaneous patch-clamp recording from a pair of starburst and ganglion cells in a flat-mount neonatal rabbit retina, showing close correlation between spontaneous activities in the two cells. (A) Example of a pair of neighboring starburst and ganglion cells recorded simultaneously with pipettes filled with Lucifer yellow. Scale bar: 50 μm. (B) A 20-min-long segment of dual recording from a ganglion cell under voltage-clamp at −70 mV (upper trace) and a nearby displaced starburst cell under currant- (lower left trace) and voltage-clamp (V_h = −70 mV, lower right trace). Spontaneous bursts of excitation in the ganglion cell are shown as brief inward synaptic currents (downward deflections), and those from the starburst cell are shown as bursts of either membrane depolarization (upward deflections under current-clamp, lower left) or inward synaptic currents (downward deflections under voltage-clamp, lower right). (C) and (D) Expanded views of two pairs of bursts. (Adapted from Zhou, 1998.)

In an attempt to understand how ganglion cells interact with cholinergic amacrine cells during retinal waves, dual patch-clamp recordings were performed successfully from pairs of displaced starburst and neighboring ganglion cells in the wholemount newborn rabbit retina (Zhou, 1998). These recordings showed that the rhythmic excitation in these two cell types was highly correlated (Fig. 6), suggesting that starburst and ganglion cells participated in same retinal waves. Similar results were also obtained by measuring changes in intracellular Ca^{2+} in morphologically identified displaced starburst amacrine cells and their neighboring ganglion cells in the newborn rabbit retina (unpublished observation by Z.J. Zhou). Thus, it appears that the "read out" of the bursting cholinergic activity by ganglion cells is quite direct, as opposed to being heavily filtered (Feller et al., 1997).

Transition from a nicotinic to a muscarinic role in spontaneous retinal waves

Because spontaneous retinal waves exist over an extended developmental period during which the retinal circuitry itself is changing dramatically, it is expected that the cellular mechanism underlying the wave may also change significantly as new circuits and synapses are recruited into the network. As discussed earlier, the nicotinic system provides a major fast excitatory drive for the early (< 80% caecal period) spontaneous wave in the mammalian retina. At this developing stage, the glutamatergic system contributes little to the wave, consistent with the fact that bipolar cells differentiate and form synapses in the IPL much later than do ganglion and amacrine cells (McArdle et al., 1977; Greiner and Weidman, 1982; Stone et al., 1985). However, as the bipolar cell input to the IPL develops, the balance of excitatory inputs to amacrine and ganglion cells is expected to shift from the cholinergic to the glutamatergic system. Indeed, in ferrets older than P15 (Wong et al., 2000) and rabbits older than P1 (Zhou and Zhao, 2000) spontaneous retinal waves became increasingly insensitive to nicotinic antagonists. Instead, the waves were completely blocked by glutamate receptor antagonists CNQX and AP7 (Fig. 7). Thus the major excitatory drive for the wave

underwent a dramatic transition from the cholinergic to the glutamatergic system at ~75–80% caecal period in mammals.

More interestingly, it was also found that the transition between the cholinergic and glutamatergic systems was closely correlated with a second, rather surprising transition within the cholinergic system itself, namely, a transition from a nicotinic to a muscarinic drive for the wave (Zhou and Zhao, 2000). Before the transition, retinal waves were blocked by nicotinic but not muscarinic antagonists. After the transition, however, the waves were completely blocked by antagonists to M1 or M3 type muscarinic receptors, but not by nicotinic antagonists. Figure 7C summarizes developmental changes in the effects of nicotinic, muscarinic and glutamatergic antagonists on the spontaneous wave in rabbits between E26 and P6. The emergence of muscarinic and glutamatergic inputs occurred during a similar developmental period (P1–3), with the glutamatergic drive appearing first at ~P1, followed by a muscarinic drive starting at ~P2. The decline of the nicotinic drive also began at ~P2 but had a slightly slower time course, so that the complete withdraw of the nicotinic drive occurred at ~P4–P5, after the muscarinic and glutamatergic inputs were securely established. Thus, the transitions in the cholinergic and glutamatergic systems were highly coordinated, reflecting a profound and interrelated change in the role of these neurotransmitter systems in spontaneous retinal waves.

Possible functional role of the nicotinic, muscarinic and glutamatergic systems in the initiation and propagation of spontaneous retinal waves

Given the drastic transitions in the excitatory drives for spontaneous retinal waves, one might expect that the spateotemporal dynamics of the wave would also be fundamentally different after the transitions. Surprisingly, a comparison between the wave frequency, speed and size obtained from rabbits before and after the transitions did not show drastic differences in basic characteristics of the wave (Zhao et al., 1999). Similar results have also been found in the developing ferret retina (Feller, 1999),

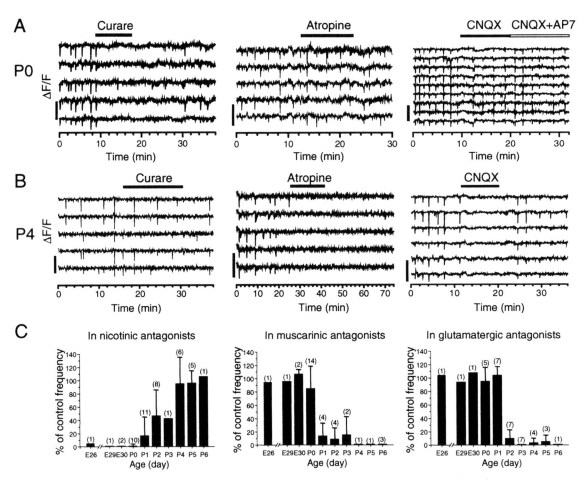

Fig. 7. Transitions in neurotransmitter systems underlying the spontaneous retinal wave in rabbits. (A) Early spontaneous waves in P0 retinas were reversibly blocked by d-tubocurare (curare, 25 μM), but not by atropine (2 μM), CNQX (4 μM), or CNQX (4 μM)+D-AP7 (200 μM). (B) The late spontaneous activity in P4 retinas was no longer sensitive to curare (100 μM). Instead, it could be blocked by atropine (0.5 μM) and CNQX (4 μM). Scale bar: 20%. (C) Summary of the inhibitory effect (expressed in % of control wave frequency) of nicotinic, muscarinic and glutamatergic receptor antagonists between E26 and P6. Error bars indicate S.E. Numbers in parentheses indicate the total number of experiments pooled at each age. (Adapted from Zhou and Zhao, 2000.)

although more detailed properties (e.g. burst frequency in ON and OFF ganglion cells, see Wong and Oakley, 1996) were altered considerably after the transitions. Consistent patterns of spontaneous activity have also been found following transitions between completely different neurotransmitter systems in other regions of the developing nervous system, including the hippocampus and spinal cord (for review, Feller, 1999). These observations have led to the hypothesis (for review, O'Donovan et al., 1998; Feller, 1999) that spontaneous, rhythmic activities in these developing regions may be dictated mainly by homeostatic

mechanisms. According to this theory, the threshold and the refractoriness of the spontaneous excitation are determined by the overall excitatory input from a number of mutually compensating transmitter systems and the efficacy of each system, but not by the detailed identity or circuitry of the excitatory drive. Thus, one may speculate that the transition from the fast cholinergic to the fast glutamatergic drive in spontaneous retinal waves may not drastically change the overall excitability of the network, so that the threshold and the refractory process of the spontaneous excitation remain quite similar.

On the other hand, it is well known that the cholinergic and glutamatergic circuits in the vertebrate retina differ completely (Dowling, 1987). In particular, the glutamatergic system is believed to mediate information flow mainly in the vertical direction from the outer to the inner retina (Wassle and Boycott, 1991) whereas the cholinergic system is formed by starburst amacrine cells, whose processes extend laterally and widely in the IPL (Masland and Tauchi, 1986; Vaney, 1990). Thus, in the above homeostatic model, it seems difficult to imagine that the glutamatergic system can completely replace the cholinergic system without causing drastic changes at least in the propagation pattern of the wave. It remains an intriguing puzzle as to what enables the glutamatergic system to replace the cholinergic system as the primary fast excitatory drive without fundamentally changing the macroscopic properties of the wave, particularly the characteristics of wave propagation.

One possible clue to this puzzle may be provided by the above finding that the transition between the fast cholinergic and fast glutamatergic drives was correlated with the transition between a nicotinic and a muscarinic role of the cholinergic system in the wave (Zhou and Zhao, 2000). Because the late retinal wave is critically dependent on muscarinic transmission, it is almost certain that the starburst network remains essential for the late spontaneous wave. Thus, even after the glutamatergic input replaces the nicotinic system as the major fast excitatory drive for the wave, the cholinergic system, through the activation of muscarinic receptors, continues to play a critical role in wave propagation, perhaps by providing a similar lateral cholinergic network to mediate the propagation of local glutamatergic excitation.

An indirect support for the above notion comes from the finding that partial blockade of muscarinic receptors led to smaller and slower waves whereas a partial block of AMPA/KA receptors reduced the wave frequency and amplitude, but not the size or the speed of the wave (Fig. 8) (Zhou and Zhao, 2000). Thus, glutamate released from bipolar cells might be more suited for strong but more localized excitation in ganglion and amacrine cells, whereas the cholinergic system might be particularly important for lateral propagation of this excitation. Recent

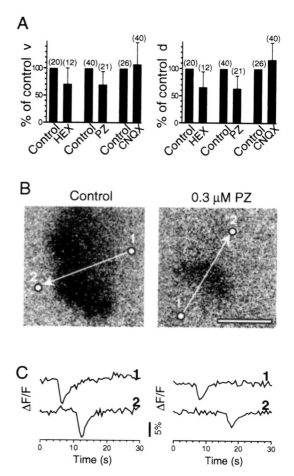

Fig. 8. Effects of nicotinic, muscarinic and glutamatergic antagonists on the speed (v) and the radial dimension (d) of the wavefront. (A) Relative (percent of control) v and d under partial blockade by sub-saturating concentrations of hexamethoniusm (HEX , 0.1–2 μM, or 1–3 μM in 100 μM picrotoxin), pirenzepine (PZ, 0.1–0.3 μM, or 1–2 μM in 100 μM picrotoxin) and CNQX (0.2 μM, or 2 μM in 100 μM picrotoxin). In some of the experiments, picrotoxin was included in both control and test solutions to enhance the wave so that partial blockade of the wave by HEX, PZ and CNQX was more attainable. Numbers in parentheses indicate the number of waves included in the analysis. Error bars indicate S.E. (B) Representative waves recorded from a P3 retina in control and the presence of 0.3 μM PZ, respectively. Arrows indicate the direction of wave propagation. Scale bar: 500 μm. (C) Relative changes in the fluorescence intensity from the circles in B marked with "1" and "2", respectively. The distance between each pair of circles is 932 μm. The speed v, calculated from the time delay between the two peaks in traces 1 and 2, is 167 μm/s in control and 93 μm/s in PZ. The radial dimension d, calculated from the product of v and the mean half-amplitude width of the peaks, is 474 μm in control and 233 μm in PZ. (Adapted from Zhou and Zhao, 2000.)

results from the developing turtle and chick retina also showed that partial nicotinic blockade led to spatial shrinkage of waves, whereas partial blockade of glutamatergic input reduced the overall excitability but not the spatial extent of the wave (Sernagor and Grzywacz, 1999; Sernagor et al., 2000).

Thus, in the early developing mammalian retina, the cholinergic system, through the activation of nicotinic receptors, seems to provide the primary excitatory drive for both the initiation and propagation of spontaneous waves (the wave is also mediated by additional transmitter systems, see below). However, after the emergence of the glutamatergic drive, the cholinergic network for the wave switches to a muscarinic receptor-mediated system, which probably takes over the role of the early nicotinic system in mediating wave propagation. Because the muscarinic system also uses the starburst network, this could provide an efficient mechanism for preserving the basic pattern of wave propagation.

Another possible explanation for the above puzzle is that the propagation of the wave may be mediated not so much by synaptic interactions but rather by diffusion of excitable substances, such as neurotransmitters. This idea is similar to the K^+ diffusion model (Burgi and Grzywacz, 1994), although there has been little evidence for K^+ itself being the diffusing agent important for wave propagation. Furthermore, there is evidence in the rabbit (unpublished results by Z.J. Zhou) and chick (Wong et al., 1998) retina that gap junction blockers inhibit the wave. Possible contributions of neurotransmitter diffusion and electric synapses to the wave pattern remain to be investigated.

Contribution of other neurotransmitter systems to spontaneous retinal waves

While the cholinergic system plays an essential role in early spontaneous waves in the mammalian retina, it should be pointed out that other transmitters, such as glycine (Zhou, 2001b), GABA (Fischer et al., 1998), and adenosine (Stellwagen et al., 1999), also contribute to wave generation and propagation. In the rabbit retina, glycine provided an essential excitatory drive for early retinal waves, because the glycine receptor antagonist strychnine completely blocked

the early wave (Zhou, 2001b). As development proceeded, the glycinergic contribution changed from excitation to inhibition, presumably as a result of a reduction in intracellular Cl^- concentration caused by an increased expression of K-Cl cotransporters. This transition occurred at P0–1 in the rabbit and was concomitant with the appearance of the glutamatergic drive for the wave, the transition from an excitatory to an inhibitory glycinergic contribution also occurred at ~P0–1 in rabbit (unpublished observation by Z.J. Zhou), demonstrating yet another correlated transition among neurotransmitter systems for the wave (Zhou, 2001b).

In the early (<P10) developing ferret retina, GABA is thought to be excitatory as well (Fischer et al., 1998). However, it remains controversial whether GABA exerts a significant influence on early spontaneous waves (Fischer et al., 1998; Stellwagen et al., 1999). In the rabbit retina, GABA significantly reduced the frequency and the speed of the late (>P0) wave (Zhou and Zhao, 2000) but had little effect on the early spontaneous wave (unpublished observation by Z.J. Zhou). It remains to be seen how the cholinergic system interacts with glycinergic, GABAergic, adenosinergic and other transmitter systems in mediating the spontaneous wave at various stages of development.

Conclusions and future prospects

As a classic excitatory neurotransmitter used by an extraordinarily well-conserved and well-organized cell class in the retina, ACh undoubtedly plays a vital role in retinal function. In the adult mammalian retina, ACh is thought to be important for maintaining adequate light response sensitivity of ganglion cells, especially those involved in detecting object motion and motion direction, although a specific role of cholinergic interactions in retinal processing is still poorly understood. In the developing retina, it has become increasingly clear that ACh is a transmitter critical for many aspects of neuronal development. Recent studies have shed important light on basic cellular physiology of cholinergic amacrine cells during development. We now know that the nicotinic system provides an essential excitatory drive for early retinal waves, and that the cholinergic function during development is extremely dynamic, involving transitions both within the cholinergic system and between different neurotransmitter systems. These dynamic interactions and transitions help to shape the characteristic features of the spontaneous retinal excitation at different stages of visual development.

Like in the adult retina, detailed and specific physiological functions of the cholinergic system in the developing retina remain to be revealed. Future research should determine the functional role and the cellular mechanism of the cholinergic system in the formation of spontaneous retinal waves, as well as in other aspects of retinal development. It will be important to understand the function of both nicotinic and muscarinic systems and their interactions with various neurotransmitter systems in the context of synaptogenesis and circuit formation in the developing retina.

After decades of studies of the cholinergic amacrine cell using immunochemical, anatomical, pharmacological, electrophysiological, optical, computational and molecular genetic methods, the future prospect is truly excellent that the starburst network may be used as a useful model system for understanding mechanisms of synaptogenesis, synaptic function and modification, as well as dendritic structure-function relationship and network processing.

Acknowledgments

Part of this work is supported by grants from NIH (EY10894) and Research to Prevent Blindness, Inc. The author would like to thank Gordon L. Fain, Dichen Zhao, Sunil S. Paul and Suzanne J. Bakewell for past research collaboration and Kris Morgan for assistance with the manuscript.

References

Ames, A.D. and Nesbett, F.B. (1981) In vitro retina as an experimental model of the central nervous system. J. Neurochem., 37: 867–877.

Bansal, A., Singer, J.H., Hwang, B.J., Xu, W., Beaudet, A. and Feller, M.B. (2000) Mice lacking specific nicotinic acetylcholine receptor subunits exhibit dramatically altered spontaneous activity patterns and reveal a limited role for retinal waves in forming ON and OFF circuits in the inner retina. J. Neurosci., 20: 7672–7681.

Bloomfield, S.A. (1992) Relationship between receptive and dendritic field size of amacrine cells in the rabbit retina. J. Neurophysiol., 68: 711–725.

Bodnarenko, S.R. and Chalupa, L.M. (1993) Stratification of ON and OFF ganglion cell dendrites depends on glutamate-mediated afferent activity in the developing retina. Nature, 364: 144–146.

Brandon, C. (1987) Cholinergic neurons in the rabbit retina: dendritic branching and ultrastructural connectivity. Brain Res., 426: 119–130.

Brecha, N. (1983) A review of retinal neurotransmitters: histochemical and biochemical studies. In: Emson, P.C. (Ed.), Chemical Neuroanatomy. Raven Press, New York, pp. 85–129.

Burgi, P.Y. and Grzywacz, N.M. (1994) Model for the pharmacological basis of spontaneous synchronous activity in developing retinas. J. Neurosci., 14: 7426–7439.

Butts, D.A., Feller, M.B., Shatz, C.J. and Rokhsar, D.S. (1999) Retinal waves are governed by collective network properties. J. Neurosci., 19: 3580–3593.

Camargo De Moura Campos, L. and Hokoc, J.N. (1999) Ontogeny of cholinergic amacrine cells in the oppossum (Didelphis aurita) retina. Int. J. Dev. Neurosci., 17: 795–804.

Cline, H.T. (1991) Activity-dependent plasticity in the visual systems of frogs and fish. Trends Neurosci., 14: 104–111.

Cohen, E.D. (1999) Calcium currents in starburst amacrine cells of the rabbit retina. Society for Neuroscience Abstracts, 25: 1041.

Constantine-Paton, M., Cline, H.T. and Debski, E. (1990) Patterned activity, synaptic convergence, and the NMDA receptor in developing visual pathways. Annu. Rev. Neurosci., 13: 129–154.

Cook, J.E. (1991) Correlated activity in the CNS: a role on every timescale? Trends Neurosci., 14: 397–401.

Dann, J.F. (1989) Cholinergic amacrine cells in the developing cat retina. J. Comp. Neurol., 289: 143–155.

Dowling, J.E. (1987) The retina. The Belknap Press, Cambridge.

Dreher, B. and Robinson, S.R. (1988) Development of the retinofugal pathways in birds and mammals: Evidence for a common 'time-table'. Brain Behav. Evol., 31: 369–390.

Famiglietti, E.V. (1985) Starburst amacrine cells: morphological constancy and systematic variation in the anisotropic field of rabbit retinal neurons. J. Neurosci., 5: 562–577.

Famiglietti, E.V. (1991) Synaptic organization of starburst amacrine cells in rabbit retina: analysis of serial thin sections by electron microscopy and graphic reconstruction. J. Comp. Neurol., 309: 40–70.

Famiglietti, E.V. (1992) Dendritic co-stratification of ON and ON-OFF directionally selective ganglion cells with starburst amacrine cells in rabbit retina. J. Comp. Neurol., 324: 322–335.

Famiglietti, E.V., Jr. (1983) 'Starburst' amacrine cells and cholinergic neurons: mirror-symmetric on and off amacrine cells of rabbit retina. Brain Res., 261: 138–144.

612

Feller, M.B. (1999) Spontaneous correlated activity in developing neural circuits. *Neuron*, 22: 653–656.

Feller, M.B., Wellis, D.P., Stellwagen, D., Werblin, F.S. and Shatz, C.J. (1996) Requirement for cholinergic synaptic transmission in the propagation of spontaneous retinal waves. *Science*, 272: 1182–1187.

Feller, M.B., Butts, D.A., Aaron, H.L., Rokhsar, D.S. and Shatz, C.J. (1997) Dynamic processes shape spatiotemporal properties of retinal waves. *Neuron*, 19: 293–306.

Fischer, K.F., Lukasiewicz, P.D. and Wong, R.O. (1998) Age-dependent and cell class-specific modulation of retinal ganglion cell bursting activity by GABA. *J. Neurosci.*, 18: 3767–3778.

Goodman, C.S. and Shatz, C.J. (1993) Developmental mechanisms that generate precise patterns of neuronal connectivity. *Cell*, (Suppl. 72): 77–98.

Greiner, J.V. and Weidman, T.A. (1982) Embryogenesis of the rabbit retina. *Exp. Eye Res.*, 34: 749–765.

Hamassaki-Britto, D.E., Gardino, P.F., Hokoc, J.N., Keyser, K.T., Karten, H.J., Lindstrom, J.M. and Britto, L.R. (1994) Differential development of alpha-bungarotoxin-sensitive and alpha- bungarotoxin-insensitive nicotinic acetylcholine receptors in the chick retina. *J. Comp. Neurol.*, 347: 161–170.

Hayden, S.A., Mills, J.W. and Masland, R.M. (1980) Acetylcholine synthesis by displaced amacrine cells. *Science*, 210: 435–437.

Hutchins, J.B. (1994) Development of muscarinic acetylcholine receptors in the ferret retina. *Brain Res. Dev. Brain Res.*, 82: 45–61.

Jensen, R.J. (1995) Receptive-field properties of displaced starburst amacrine cells change following axotomy-induced degeneration of ganglion cells. *Vis. Neurosci.*, 12: 177–184.

Kalil, R.E. (1990) The influence of action potentials on the development of the central visual pathway in mammals. *J. Exp. Biol.*, 153: 261–276.

Katz, L.C. and Shatz, C.J. (1996) Synaptic activity and the construction of cortical circuits. *Science*, 274: 1133–1138.

Kim, I.B., Park, D.K., Oh, S.J. and Chun, M.H. (1998) Horizontal cells of the rat retina show choline acetyltransferase- and vesicular acetylcholine transporter-like immunoreactivities during early postnatal developmental stages. *Neurosci. Lett.*, 253: 83–86.

Koulen, P. (1997) Vesicular acetylcholine transporter (VAChT): a cellular marker in rat retinal development. *Neuroreport*, 8: 2845–2848.

Lauder, J.M. (1993) Neurotransmitters as growth regulatory signals: role of receptors and second messengers. *Trends Neurosci.*, 16: 233–240.

Lipton, S.A. and Kater, S.B. (1989) Neurotransmitter regulation of neuronal outgrowth, plasticity and survival. *Trends Neurosci.*, 12: 265–270.

Lipton, S.A., Frosch, M.P., Phillips, M.D., Tauck, D.L. and Aizenman, E. (1988) Nicotinic antagonists enhance process outgrowth by rat retinal ganglion cells in culture. *Science*, 239: 1293–1296.

Maffei, L. and Galli-Resta, L. (1990) Correlation in the discharges of neighboring rat retinal ganglion cells during prenatal life. *Proc. Natl. Acad. Sci. USA*, 87: 2861–2864.

Masland, R. and Tauchi, M. (1986) The cholinergic amacrine cells. *Trends Neurosci.*, 9: 218–223.

Masland, R.H. (1977) Maturation of function in the developing rabbit retina. *J. Comp. Neurol.*, 175: 275–286.

Masland, R.H., Mills, J.W. and Hayden, S.A. (1984) Acetylcholine-synthesizing amacrine cells: identification and selective staining by using radioautography and fluorescent markers. *Proc. R. Soc. Lond. B Biol. Sci.*, 223: 79–100.

Matter, J.M., Matter-Sadzinski, L. and Ballivet, M. (1995) Activity of the beta 3 nicotinic receptor promoter is a marker of neuron fate determination during retina development. *J. Neurosci.*, 15: 5919–5928.

McArdle, C.B., Dowling, J.E. and Masland, R.H. (1977) Development of outer segments and synapses in the rabbit retina. *J. Comp. Neurol.*, 175: 253–274.

Meister, M., Wong, R.O., Baylor, D.A. and Shatz, C.J. (1991) Synchronous bursts of action potentials in ganglion cells of the developing mammalian retina. *Science*, 252: 939–943.

Millar, T.J. and Morgan, I.G. (1987) Cholinergic amacrine cells in the rabbit retina synapse onto other cholinergic amacrine cells. *Neurosci. Lett.*, 74: 281–285.

Mitrofanis, J. and Stone, J. (1988) Distribution of cholinergic amacrine cells in the retinas of normally pigmented and hypopigmented strains of rat and cat. *Vis. Neurosci.*, 1: 367–376.

O'Donovan, M.J., Chub, N. and Wenner, P. (1998) Mechanisms of spontaneous activity in developing spinal networks. *J. Neurobiol.*, 37: 131–145.

Paul, S.S. and Zhou, Z.J. (2000) The essential role of cholinergic and glycinergic inputs in spontaneous waves in the early developing rabbit retina. *Society for Neuroscience Abstracts*, 26: 1078.

Penn, A.A., Riquelme, P.A., Feller, M.B. and Shatz, C.J. (1998) Competition in retinogeniculate patterning driven by spontaneous activity. *Science*, 279: 2108–2112.

Peters, B.N. and Masland, R.H. (1996) Responses to light of starburst amacrine cells. *J. Neurophysiol.*, 75: 469–480.

Prada, F., Medina, J.I., Lopez-Gallardo, M., Lopez, R., Quesada, A., Spira, A. and Prada, C. (1999) Spatiotemporal gradients of differentiation of chick retina types I and II cholinergic cells: identification of a common post-mitotic cell population. *J. Comp. Neurol.*, 410: 457–466.

Ramoa, A.S., Campbell, G. and Shatz, C.J. (1987) Transient morphological features of identified ganglion cells in living fetal and neonatal retina. *Science*, 237: 522–525.

Redburn, D.A. and Rowe-Rendleman, C. (1996) Developmental neurotransmitters. Signals for shaping neuronal circuitry. *Invest. Ophthalmol. Vis. Sci.*, 37: 1479–1482.

Sandmann, D., Engelmann, R. and Peichl, L. (1997) Starburst cholinergic amacrine cells in the tree shrew retina. *J. Comp. Neurol.*, 389: 161–176.

Sernagor, E. and Grzywacz, N.M. (1996) Influence of spontaneous activity and visual experience on developing retinal receptive fields. *Curr. Biol.*, 6: 1503–1508.

Sernagor, E. and Grzywacz, N.M. (1999) Spontaneous activity in developing turtle retinal ganglion cells: pharmacological studies. *J. Neurosci.*, 19: 3874–3887.

Sernagor, E., Eglen, S.J. and O'Donovan, M.J. (2000) Differential effects of acetylcholine and glutamate blockade on the spatiotemporal dynamics of retinal waves. *J. Neurosci. (Online)*, 20: RC56.

Shatz, C.J. (1996) Emergence of order in visual system development. *J. Physiol. Paris*, 90: 141–150.

Shatz, C.J. and Stryker, M.P. (1988) Prenatal tetrodotoxin infusion blocks segregation of retinogeniculate afferents. *Science*, 242: 87–89.

Spira, A.W., Millar, T.J., Ishimoto, I., Epstein, M.L., Johnson, C.D., Dahl, J.L. and Morgan, I.G. (1987) Localization of choline acetyltransferase-like immunoreactivity in the embryonic chick retina. *J. Comp. Neurol.*, 260: 526–538.

Stellwagen, D., Shatz, C.J. and Feller, M.B. (1999) Dynamics of retinal waves are controlled by cyclic AMP [see comments]. *Neuron*, 24: 673–685.

Stellwagen, D., Goldberg, J.L., Shatz, C.J. and Barres, B.A. (2000) Activity changes in axotomized rat retinal ganglion cells before programmed cell death. *Society for Neuroscience Abstracts*, 26: 330.

Stone, J., Egan, M. and Rapaport, D.H. (1985) The site of commencement of retinal maturation in the rabbit. *Vision Res.*, 25: 309–317.

Sugiyama, H., Daniels, M.P. and Nirenberg, M. (1977) Muscarinic acetylcholine receptors of the developing retina. *Proc. Natl. Acad. Sci. USA*, 74: 5524–5528.

Tauchi, M. and Masland, R.H. (1984) The shape and arrangement of the cholinergic neurons in the rabbit retina. *Proc. R. Soc. Lond. B*, 233: 101–119.

Taylor W.R. and Wassle, H. (1995) Receptive field properties of starburst cholinergic amacrine cells in the rabbit retina. *Eur. J. Neurosci.*, 7: 2308–2321.

Vaney, D.I. (1990) The mosaic of amacrine cells in the mammalian retina. *Prog. Ret. Res.*, 9: 49–100.

Vaney, D.I., Peichi, L. and Boycott, B.B. (1981) Matching populations of amacrine cells in the inner nuclear and ganglion cell layers of the rabbit retina. *J. Comp. Neurol.*, 199: 373–391.

Wassle, H. and Boycott, B.B. (1991) Functional architecture of the mammalian retina. *Physiol. Rev.*, 71: 447–480.

Wong, R.O. (1999) Retinal waves and visual system development. *Annu. Rev. Neurosci.*, 22: 29–47.

Wong, R.O. and Collin, S.P. (1989) Dendritic maturation of displaced putative cholinergic amacrine cells in the rabbit retina. *J. Comp. Neurol.*, 287: 164–178.

Wong, R.O. and Oakley, D.M. (1996) Changing patterns of spontaneous bursting activity of on and off retinal ganglion cells during development. *Neuron*, 16: 1087–1095.

Wong, R.O., Meister, M. and Shatz, C.J. (1993) Transient period of correlated bursting activity during development of the mammalian retina. *Neuron*, 11: 923–938.

Wong, W.T., Sanes, J.R. and Wong, R.O. (1998) Developmentally regulated spontaneous activity in the embryonic chick retina. *J. Neurosci.*, 18: 8839–8853.

Wong, W.T., Myhr, K.L., Miller, E.D. and Wong, R.O. (2000) Developmental changes in the neurotransmitter regulation of correlated spontaneous retinal activity. *J. Neurosci.*, 20: 351–360.

Zhao, D., Cornett, L. and Zhou, Z.J. (1999) Consistency and modulation of spontaneous waves of excitation in the developing rabbit retina. *Society for Neuroscience Abstracts*, 25: 1806.

Zhou, Z.J. (1998) Direct participation of starburst amacrine cells in spontaneous rhythmic activities in the developing mammalian retina. *J. Neurosci.*, 18: 4155–4165.

Zhou, Z.J. (2001a) Cholinergic responses from starburst amacrine cells of the developing rabbit retina. *Invest. Ophthalmol. Vis. Sci.* (Suppl.), in press.

Zhou, Z.J. (2001b) A critical role of the glycinergic system in spontaneous retinal waves of the developing rabbit. *J. Neurosci.*, in press.

Zhou, Z.J. and Fain, G.L. (1995) Neurotransmitter receptors of starburst amacrine cells in rabbit retinal slices. *J. Neurosci.*, 15: 5334–5345.

Zhou, Z.J. and Fain, G.L. (1996) Starburst amacrine cells change from spiking to nonspiking neurons during retinal development. *Proc. Natl. Acad. Sci. USA*, 93: 8057–8062.

Zhou, Z.J. and Zhao, D. (2000) Coordinated transitions in neurotransmitter systems for the initiation and propagation of spontaneous retinal waves. *J. Neurosci.*, 20: 6570–6577.

Retinal degenerations

H. Kolb, H. Ripps and S. Wu (Eds.)
Progress in Brain Research, Vol. 131

CHAPTER 44

Legacy of the RCS rat: impact of a seminal study on retinal cell biology and retinal degenerative diseases

Matthew M. LaVail*

Beckman Vision Center, University of California San Francisco, San Francisco, CA 94143-0730, USA

Introduction

In the field of retinal degenerations, we now take for granted that much information is known about many different aspects of the diseases known collectively as retinitis pigmentosa (RP) and age-related macular degeneration (AMD), and numerous variants of these blinding disorders. This includes areas such as definition of the phenotypes and molecular characterization of the genotypes, as well as a number of potential therapeutic approaches for these heretofore untreatable diseases. We recognize that much of this new information has been made possible by the availability of numerous animal models of the diseases which are found in many species, most widely studied in the mouse, rat, dog and cat. Moreover, many basic principals of retinal cell biology have also come from studies of these animal models.

The ready availability of many animal models obviously did not always exist. In the early 1920s, Keeler discovered the first mutant model, the "rod-less" mouse (Keeler, 1924), which was much later shown to be the same as the widely distributed retinal degeneration mutation (*rd*) in mice (Pittler et al., 1993). Bourne et al. (1938a,b) discovered a second

model, an inherited retinal degeneration in rats that appeared to resemble human RP. This degeneration in the rat received relatively little attention (Lucas et al., 1955) during the next 20 years. Then, in 1962, a paper appeared by Dowling and Sidman that characterized the disease in this rat model as an inherited retinal dystrophy using a multidisciplinary approach with state of the art tools of the time: electron microscopy, rhodopsin biochemistry and electroretinograpy (ERG). In this case, John Dowling, who as a young scientist working with Professor George Wald at Harvard University in the late 1950s had defined the relationship between vitamin A deficiency and night blindness (Dowling and Wald, 1958) and explored a number of features of visual adaptation in the rat (Dowling, 1960), began collaborating with a young physician scientist, Richard Sidman, at nearby Harvard Medical School. Sidman, who had first clearly identified the interphotoreceptor matrix histochemically (Sidman and Wislocki, 1954), defined the histogenetic pattern of retinal cell genesis autoradiographically (Sidman, 1961a) and had carried out tissue culture analyses of degenerating retinas (Sidman, 1961b), had obtained some of the originally described dystrophic rats. He was in the process of inbreeding them and later named the inbred strain "RCS" in recognition of the original source of the rats, the Royal College of Surgeons (Sidman and Pearlstein, 1965).

*Tel.: 415-476-4233; Fax: 415-476-0709;
E-mail: mmlv@itsa.ucsf.edu

618

The collaboration between Dowling and Sidman was highly successful because both of these young scientists had a passion for the retina, were interested in the causes of retinal degenerations, were highly skilled and experienced in their respective areas and were extremely creative individuals. Without question, their paper in 1962 is a classic in the field of retinal degeneration. It could be argued, as I shall do here, that the work either directly or indirectly led to many of the basic cell biological principals dealing with photoreceptors and the retinal pigment epithelium (RPE) that we know today, and that it and the retinal dystrophic rat stimulated the development of many key tenants that are known and experimental therapeutic approaches that are currently being studied in the field of retinal degeneration. Their study in 1962 stimulated hundreds of cytopathologic, electrophysiologic, biochemical, genetic, nutritional and behavioral studies on the retinal dystrophic rats (LaVail, 1979, 1981a). In addition to the many positive aspects of this study, the paper illustrates how a scholarly work can stimulate new questions and directions of research even if some of the interpretations

later prove to be incorrect. Following brief descriptions of the phenotype and genotype, the areas of and reasons for the impact of the paper by Dowling and Sidman, and of the RCS rat, itself, will be given.

Definition of the phenotype

Superficial similarities between the rat disease and RP in man were pointed out in the initial description of the rats in 1938 (Bourne et al., 1938a). Dowling and Sidman (1962) clarified many aspects of the phenotype. This included the overproduction of rhodopsin (up to twice normal values), which was associated with abundant, abnormal lamellar membranes located between the developing rod outer segments and the RPE. The photoreceptors achieved virtually adult form and ERG function before degenerating, which began about 3 weeks of age (Fig. 1A), leading to the loss of ERG sensitivity and selective depression of the a-wave at high luminances. At later stages, as photoreceptors disappeared (Fig. 1B and C) and rhodopsin was lost, RPE cells were said

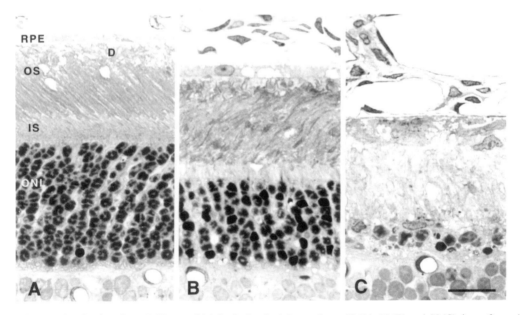

Fig. 1. Light micrographs of retinas from RCS rats with inherited retinal dystrophy at 20 (**A**), 32 (**B**) and 55 (**C**) days of age. At day 20, outer segment debris membranes (**D**) have accumulated at the surface of the retinal pigment epithelium (RPE). At day 32, the outer segment zone has become a disorganized debris zone, and many photoreceptor nuclei are degenerating. By day 55, most of the photoreceptor nuclei have disappeared, but the debris zone remains. *IS*, inner segments; *OS*, outer segments. (Bar = 15 μm). (From LaVail, M.M. and Battelle, B.A.: *Exp. Eye Res.* 21:167, 1975. Reprinted with permission; © Academic Press Inc., London, Ltd.)

to de-differentiate, detach and migrate through the outer segment-debris zone. Eventually, the b-wave of the ERG entirely disappeared by 2–3 months of age. Remarkably, long after most photoreceptors degenerated, at 8–12 months of age, the dystrophic rats could still respond to visually guided stimuli, presumably through the very few surviving photoreceptor cells that were still connected synaptically to inner retinal neurons (LaVail et al., 1974). As discussed below, the most remarkable phenotypic characteristic of the dystrophic rat is the failure of its RPE cells to phagocytize shed rod outer segment membranes (Herron et al., 1969; Bok and Hall 1971; LaVail et al., 1972), which results in the accumulation of outer segment debris membranes (Herron et al., 1969; Bok and Hall, 1971; LaVail and Battelle, 1975). Significantly, when the dystrophic rats were reared in the darkness the rate of degeneration was slowed, as measured by anatomical, biochemical and ERG parameters (Dowling and Sidman, 1962).

Definition of the genotype

In early mammalian genetic studies, the retinal dystrophy in the rat was shown to be inherited as an autosomal recessive disorder (Bourne and Grüneberg, 1939). Several strains and stocks of rats with inherited retinal dystrophy descended from the original animals (LaVail, 1981a), but the most widely studied and most genetically well-defined line was the inbred RCS strain developed by Sidman (Sidman and Pearlstein, 1965), as noted above. Congenic (genetically similar) strains of RCS rats were later developed with different pigmentation types (LaVail, et al., 1975) that gave different rates and hemispheric distributions of degeneration (LaVail and Battelle, 1975), and congenic control rats (+/+ at the retinal dystrophy locus) were also produced (LaVail, 1981c). Through conventional mammalian linkage testing, the mutant gene was localized to linkage group IV in the rat and formally given the gene symbol "rdy" for retinal dystrophy (LaVail, 1981b). As discussed below, the mutant gene was found to be expressed in the RPE cell. Most recently, through a positional cloning approach the rdy gene mutation has been demonstrated to be a deletion in the receptor tyrosine kinase gene Mertk (D'Cruz et al., 2000).

Validity of retinal degeneration research

One of the less tangible but very important features of the Dowling and Sidman study in 1962 was that it not only was of excellent technical quality and a scholarly work, but that it was published in the most prestigious general cell biological journal of the time. Most studies on retinal degenerations had previously been published only in specialty journals, and the Dowling and Sidman work took direct aim at the legitimacy of pathological processes for general cell biological audiences by stating in their introduction, "Cell biology has many facets, including the study of cell reactions in disease." They further pointed out to the more general audience that "more information is available on function, chemistry and structure of photoreceptors than of most cell types." The study was highly visible in the *Journal of Cell Biology*, and as such, it stimulated considerable interest in the field of retinal degeneration research. Moreover, it demonstrated that studies on retinal degenerations carried out with state of the art methods and concepts could have acceptance in the most significant journals of the day.

Light deprivation and role of environmental light in retinal degenerations

One of the most remarkable findings of Dowling and Sidman (1962) was that photoreceptor degeneration is slowed considerably when the pink-eyed dystrophic rats are reared in the dark. This environmental modification of the genetic disorder led, in part, to the experimental therapeutic measure of light deprivation for patients with early stages of retinitis pigmentosa (Berson, 1971, 1980) and emphasized the possible role of environmental light in retinal degenerations. Dark-rearing has not been successful in slowing photoreceptor degeneration in many other animal models, except in those cases where genetic mutations result in defects in rhodopsin shut off, such as arrestin knockouts (Chen et al., 1999) or in some rhodopsin mutations (Naash et al., 1996). The concept of light deprivation slowing degenerations gave emphasis to the corollary that excessive light might accelerate the degenerations, and many ophthalmologists have recommended dense sunglasses for their patients. Excessive light has also been implicated in the etiology of age-related macular degeneration (Young, 1988). In experimental animals with inherited retinal degenerations, six different models have a greater susceptibility to light damage than that seen in normal control animals (LaVail et al., 1999), including the RCS rat (Noell, 1965). Increased susceptibility to light damage in a relatively wide range of different mutations and, presumably, cytopathologic processes, suggests that photoreceptors undergoing hereditary degenerations may be at greater risk than normal photoreceptors to the damaging effects of a second insult such as excessive environmental light (LaVail et al., 1999).

Role of the RPE in rod outer segment renewal

In the late 1950s and early 1960s, the source of rod outer segment membranes was conjectured to be from the infolding of outer segment membranes, based on static electron micrographs. In the RCS rat, the source of the rhodopsin-containing extracellular lamellae was unclear to Dowling and Sidman (1962), who thought that one source might even be the RPE. This provocative idea, and the overall question of the source of the extra membranes, stimulated thought on the subject of outer segment and rhodopsin biosynthesis. The question of outer segment synthesis was answered by Richard Young's autoradiographic demonstration in 1967 that outer segment discs were continually renewed at the base of the outer segment (Young, 1967). Soon thereafter it was discovered by Young and Bok (1969) that the retinal pigment epithelium (RPE) in normal animals phagocytizes and degrades outer segment membranes that are shed each day. With this information in hand, several groups immediately turned to the RCS rat where it was found that the RPE of the dystrophic rat fails to phagocytize outer segment membranes, resulting in an accumulation of these membranes at the surface of the RPE (Bok and Hall, 1969, 1971; Herron et al., 1969; LaVail et al., 1972). This defect has led to the widespread use of the mutant rats as a tool to explore photoreceptor–RPE cell interactions and mechanisms of phagocytosis in both normal and diseased retinas (Burnside, 1976; Mullen and LaVail, 1976; Edwards and Szamier, 1977;

Essner, et al., 1978; Goldman and O'Brien, 1978; Chaitin and Hall, 1983a,b; Seyfried-Williams and McLaughlin, 1983; Seyfried-Williams et al., 1984; Tarnowski and McLaughlin, 1987; Tarnowski et al., 1988; Heth and Schmidt, 1992; McLaren, et al., 1993; Heth et al., 1995).

The RCS rat emphasized the need for a balance between synthesis and disposal of outer segment membranes in order to maintain a normal adult rod outer segment length. Ripps (1982) and others have pointed out that the basis for some forms of retinal degeneration may be an imbalance in the disk synthesis and shedding rates, resulting in a progressive shortening that is seen in some forms of RP. This has led several laboratories to develop methods such as fundus reflectometry to measure rhodopsin content and kinetics in very small regions of the retina and thereby correlate the visual fields with the status of visual pigments in the retina. Thus, the example of abnormal disk turnover of the RCS rat stimulated questions about the general role of outer segment renewal and turnover in retinal degenerations.

RPE as the cellular site of mutant gene expression in retinal degenerations

By the use of experimental chimeras, Mullen and LaVail (1976) found that the primary site of mutant gene expression in the RCS rat is the RPE cell rather than the photoreceptor cell. In the chimeric retinas, the mutant RPE cells virtually always appeared adjacent to degenerating photoreceptors, and surviving photoreceptors were always found adjacent to normal RPE cells. This was the first case in which the primary cellular site of mutant gene expression could be identified in any inherited or degenerative disorder of the central nervous system in mammals, and it heightened the awareness of the vision research community to the possibility that RPE defects may be involved more generally than previously suspected in photoreceptor degenerations.

For a number of years following the advent of molecular genetics, numerous genes that caused retinal degenerations were discovered and many were cloned. These represented mutations in genes that coded for many different molecules that were either photoreceptor-specific structural proteins or were involved in the visual transduction (Dryja and Li, 1995; Molday, 1998). It appeared that perhaps the RCS rat was an anomaly, that RPE gene defects would not play a significant role in retinal degenerations. Then, several key studies demonstrated that mutations in molecules found in the RPE can, indeed, lead to retinal degenerations. Defects in RPE65 result in early onset severe retinal dystrophy/Leber's congenital amaurosis (Gu et al., 1997; Marlhens et al., 1997), and defects in cellular retinaldehyde-binding protein leads to an autosomal recessive form of RP (Maw et al., 1997). The discovery of an RPE mutation in *Mertk* in the RCS rat (D'Cruz et al., 2000) heralds the increase in the number of RPE-specific gene defects and, therefore, the likelihood that more retinal degenerations will be found that are due to mutated genes expressed in RPE cells.

Circadian rhythmicity in rod outer segment disk shedding

Since the discovery that rod outer segment disc shedding is under circadian control in the rat retina (LaVail, 1976), numerous metabolic processes in photoreceptors and the RPE have been found to occur rhythmically, either under diurnal or circadian control (Besharse, 1982). The question that stimulated the initial study that started this field was generated while analyzing the RCS rat, or at least experimental chimeras with a mixture of RCS embryos. This is detailed elsewhere (LaVail, 1981a), but briefly, the fact that some phagosomes containing shed rod outer segment discs were seen in RPE cells from RCS rats in the chimeras suggested a possible "curing" of the phagocytosis defect by neighboring wild-type cells. This raised the question of how many phagosomes are normally seen in wild-type retinas? In other words, what was the baseline with which to compare the potentially "cured" RCS RPE cells in the chimeras? An assessment of the published works of many investigators revealed far fewer phagosomes than should have been seen, given the number of discs degraded each day. This led to the possibility that most investigators were not looking at the correct time of day to see the majority of phagosomes, which ultimately was found to be 0.5–2 h after the onset of light in the morning

(LaVail, 1976). This is an example of how the analysis of mutants almost inevitably raises questions about the wild-type.

Role of the interphotoreceptor matrix in normal and degenerating retinas

Through the use of histochemical methods, it was discovered that in RCS rats a defect exists in the interphotoreceptor matrix (IPM) as early as a week before the onset of photoreceptor cell loss which may, in part, explain the reason for photoreceptor cell death (LaVail et al., 1981). Until this time, relatively little attention had been paid to the IPM. This observation in RCS rats, along with the discovery of interphotoreceptor retinoid binding protein by four laboratories in the same year, helped focus the attention of vision scientists on the importance of the IPM (Bridges and Adler, 1985), in general, and stimulated studies on the role of the IPM in hereditary retinal degenerations (Gonzalez-Fernandez et al., 1984, 1985; Eisenfeld et al., 1985; LaVail et al., 1985a,b, 1993; Schmidt et al., 1988; van Veen et al., 1988; Johnson et al., 1989; Tawara and Hollyfield, 1990; Uehara et al., 1991; Lazarus et al., 1993; Mieziewska et al., 1993a,b).

RPE transplantation and photoreceptor/retinal transplantation

The successful transplantation of normal, wild-type RPE cells into the subretinal space of RCS rats resulted in the remarkable rescue of photoreceptor cells adjacent to and nearby the transplanted RPE cells (Li and Turner, 1988; Gouras et al., 1989; Lopez et al., 1989). By every metabolic parameter tested, the rescued photoreceptors were identical to normal, wild-type photoreceptors (LaVail et al., 1992). The initial transplantation studies with RCS rats opened an important new research area with significant therapeutic ramifications, particularly in the area of AMD, where the RPE is often atrophied, or following surgery for choroidal neovascularization in AMD where the RPE is inadvertently removed. Indeed, based on reviews (Milam, 1993; Litchfield et al., 1997) and literature searches, there have been more than 75 published studies of RPE cell transplantation in the past 10 years that have involved the RCS rat or been stimulated by studies on this animal model. Moreover, the success of RPE transplantation stimulated the field of photoreceptor or retinal transplantation which has had more limited success, given the more complex tissue and cellular interactions than with RPE transplantation (Milam, 1993; Litchfield et al., 1997). Nevertheless, the field offers a potential therapeutic approach for sight restoration that is independent of gene mutation or degeneration etiology.

Pharmacological therapy for retinal degenerations

In 1990, it was found that photoreceptor degeneration in RCS rats can be delayed significantly with the intraocular injection of the peptide, basic fibroblast growth factor (bFGF) (Faktorovich et al., 1990). This finding has led to the new field of study of survival factor rescue (Steinberg, 1994) and provided hope that a pharmacological therapeutic approach may be successful for some forms of retinal degenerative diseases. It now appears that some survival factors, such as ciliary neurotrophic factor, can successfully slow photoreceptor degeneration in a number of different types of genetic disorders (LaVail et al., 1998), so the rescue effect may be on the apoptotic cell death process, itself, and the protection may be mutation-independent. Here, as in the area of RPE and photoreceptor transplantation, studies first carried out successfully on the RCS rat have opened a potential new field of therapy for blinding diseases.

Ubiquity of the RCS rat in retinal cell biological and degeneration research

The importance of the RCS rat in vision research can also be demonstrated in another way. In 1995 and 1999, computer searches using Medline for studies were carried out on inherited retinal degenerations in laboratory animals. The searches revealed that the number of papers dealing with the RCS rat almost outnumbered the combined total of papers on all mouse, dog and cat forms of retinal degeneration mutants. This comparison does not diminish the importance of the mouse, dog and cat models, since

each has some advantages that the others do not have, but the results clearly document the substantial current interest in the RCS rat as a laboratory animal.

Perhaps the most significant way to illustrate the importance of the RCS rat in retinal degeneration research is to consider it's role in the ultimate goal in this research field, the elucidation of means to delay, halt or prevent photoreceptor degenerations. Quite simply, 8–10 years ago there were no obvious, realistic ways to achieve this goal. Now there are three that offer promise—gene therapy, transplantation and growth factors—although the feasibility of each requires substantially more research effort. As noted above, the RCS rat is responsible for and continues to play a major role in the latter two of these three areas of research.

It should also be noted that the RCS rat has and continues to serve as an experimental model for several other important areas of visual science, either independently or in conjunction with inherited retinal degenerations. These include: (1) phagocytic mechanisms of RPE cells (Burnside, 1976; Hall, 1978; Essner et al., 1978; Seyfried-Williams and McLaughlin, 1983; Chaitin and Hall, 1983b; Seyfried-Williams et al., 1984; Hall and Abrams, 1987; Tarnowski and McLaughlin, 1987; Tarnowski et al., 1988; Heth and Schmidt, 1992; McLaren et al., 1993; Heth et al., 1995); (2) degradative processes and lysosomal enzymes in the RPE (El-Hifnawi et al., 1994; El-Hifnawi, 1995); (3) barrier functions of the RPE and their disruption (Caldwell et al., 1982, 1984; Caldwell and McLaughlin, 1983; Organisciak and Winkler, 1994; Wroblewski et al., 1994); (4) cellular and molecular properties of the RPE (Gregory et al., 1992; Strauss and Wienrich, 1993; Malecaze et al., 1993) and photoreceptors (Boesze-Battaglia et al., 1994; Mirshahi et al., 1994); (5) growth factor and receptor expression and localization in the retina (Connolly et al., 1991; Malecaze et al., 1993; Rakoczy et al., 1993); (6) properties of the electroretinogram (Sandberg et al., 1988; Hawlina et al., 1992; Deshpande et al., 1992); (7) neovascularization and proliferative vitreoretinopathy (El-Hifnawi, 1987; Caldwell, 1989; Caldwell et al., 1989; Weber et al., 1989; Roque and Caldwell, 1990, 1991; Seaton and Turner, 1992; Seaton et al., 1994); (8) cataracts in retinal degenerations

(Hess et al., 1982, 1985, 1991; Zigler and Hess, 1985; Dovrat et al., 1993); (9) ciliary body anomalies in retinal degenerations (Yamaguchi et al., 1991); (10) corneal abnormalities in retinal degenerations (Yamaguchi et al., 1990); (11) rescue mechanisms in retinal degeneration (Humphrey et al., 1993; Nir et al., 1999; Akimoto et al., 1999; Lawrence et al., 2000); (12) the role of microglia in retinal degenerations (Thanos, 1992; Thanos and Richter, 1993); (13) changes in the inner retina following photoreceptor cell loss (Villegas-Pérez et al., 1998); (14) immunological properties of the RPE (Zhang and Bok, 1998); (15) regulatory mechanisms of light damage (Organisciak et al., 1999); (16) metabolism of the retina and RPE in retinal degeneration, including the role of such molecules as glutathione peroxidase (Akeo et al., 1999), oxygen (Valter et al., 1998) and caspase-like proteases (Katai et al., 1999) and (17) function of bipolar cells and other inner retinal neurons in retinal degenerations (Bush et al., 1995; Hanitzsch et al., 1998). Thus, the RCS rat continues to be one of the most important tools in vision science.

Conclusions and future perspective

Recent positional cloning of the *rdy* gene in the RCS rat (D'Cruz et al., 2000), and the even more recent finding of human retinal degeneration patients with mutations in the same gene (Gal et al., 2000), will almost certainly make the RCS rat an even more important model for the study of retinal cell biology, retinal degenerative disease processes and therapeutic applications for blinding diseases. The advances that have been made and continue to come from the study of the RCS rat are a fitting tribute to John Dowling and his colleague, Richard Sidman. Without their seminal experiments in 1962, it is problematic whether our knowledge would have advanced nearly so far in many areas of retinal cell biology and in causative and therapeutic aspects of retinal degenerative diseases.

Acknowledgments

Supported by NIH Research Grants EY01919 and EY06842, Core Grant EY02162 and funds from the Foundation Fighting Blindness, Research to Prevent Blindness, Macula Vision Research Foundation and That Man May See, Inc. MML is an RPB Senior Scientist Investigator.

References

Akeo, K., Tsukamoto, H., Okisaka, S., Hiramitsu, T. and Watanabe, K. (1999) The localization of glutathione peroxidase in the photoreceptor cells and the retinal pigment epithelial cells of Wistar and Royal College of Surgeons dystrophic rats. *Pigment Cell Res.*, 12: 107–117.

Akimoto, M., Miyatake, S., Kogishi, J., Hangai, M., Okazaki, K., Takahashi, J.C., Saiki, M., Iwaki, M. and Honda, Y. (1999) Adenovirally expressed basic fibroblast growth factor rescue photoreceptor cells in RCS rats. *Invest. Ophthalmol. Vis. Sci.*, 40: 273–279.

Berson, E.L. (1971) Light deprivation for early retinitis pigmentosa. A hypothesis. *Arch. Ophthalmol.*, 85: 521–529.

Berson, E.L. (1980) Light deprivation and retinitis pigmentosa. *Vision Res.*, 20: 1179–1184.

Besharse, J.C. (1982) The daily light-dark cycle and rhythmic metabolism in the photoreceptor-pigment epithelial complex. In: Osborne, N. and Chader, G. (Eds.), *Progress in Retinal Research*. Pergamon Press, Oxford, pp. 81–124.

Boesze-Battaglia, K., Organisciak, D.T. and Albert, A.D. (1994) RCS rat retinal rod outer segment membranes exhibit different cholesterol distributions than those of normal rats. *Exp. Eye Res.*, 58: 293–300.

Bok, D. and Hall, M.O. (1969) The etiology of retinal dystrophy in RCS rats. *Invest. Ophthalmol.*, 6: 649–650.

Bok, D. and Hall, M.O. (1971) The role of the pigment epithelium in the etiology of inherited retinal dystrophy in the rat. *J. Cell Biol.*, 49: 664–682.

Bourne, M.C., Campbell, D.A. and Tansley, K. (1938a) Heriditary degeneration of the rat retina. *Brit. J. Ophthalmol.*, 22: 613–623.

Bourne, M.C., Campbell, D.A. and Tansley, K. (1938b) Retinitis pigmentosa in rats. *Trans. Ophthalmol. Soc. UK*, 58: 234–245.

Bourne, M.C. and Grüneberg, H. (1939) Degeneration of the retina and cataract, a new recessive gene in the rat. *J. Hered.*, 30: 130–136.

Bridges, C.D. and Adler, A.J. (1985) *The Interphotoreceptor Matrix in Health and Disease*. Alan R. Liss Inc., New York.

Burnside, M.B. (1976) Possible roles of microtubules and actin filaments in retinal pigmented epithelium. *Exp. Eye Res.*, 23: 257–275.

Bush, R.A., Hawks, K.W. and Sieving, P.A. (1995) Preservation of inner retinal responses in the aged Royal College of Surgeons rat. *Invest. Ophthalmol. Vis. Sci.*, 36: 2054–2062.

Caldwell, R.B. (1989) Extracellular matrix alterations precede vascularization of the retinal pigment epithelium in dystrophic rats. *Curr. Eye Res.*, 8: 907–921.

624

Caldwell, R.B. and McLaughlin, B.J. (1983) Permeability of retinal pigment epithelial cell junctions in the dystrophic rat retina. *Exp. Eye Res.*, 36: 415–427.

Caldwell, R.B., McLaughlin, B.J. and Boykins, L.G. (1982) Intramembrane changes in retinal pigment epithelial cell junctions of the dystrophic rat retina. *Invest. Ophthalmol. Vis. Sci.*, 23: 305–318.

Caldwell, R.B., Roque, R.S. and Solomon, S.W. (1989) Increased vascular density and vitreo-retinal membranes accompany vascularization of the pigment epithelium in the dystrophic rat retina. *Curr. Eye Res.*, 8: 923–937.

Caldwell, R.B., Wade, L.A. and McLaughlin, B.J. (1984) A quantitative study of intramembrane changes during cell junctional breakdown in the dystrophic rat retinal pigment epithelium. *Exp. Eye Res.*, 150: 104–117.

Chaitin, M.H. and Hall, M.O. (1983a) Defective ingestion of rod outer segments by cultured dystrophic rat pigment epithelial cells. *Invest. Ophthalmol. Vis. Sci.*, 24: 812–820.

Chaitin, M.H. and Hall, M.O. (1983b) The distribution of actin in cultured normal and dystrophic rat pigment epithelial cells during the phagocytosis of rod outer segments. *Invest. Ophthalmol. Vis. Sci.*, 24: 821–831.

Chen, J., Simon, M.I., Matthes, M.T., Yasumura, D. and LaVail, M.M. (1999) Increased susceptibility to light damage in an arrestin knockout mouse model of Oguchi disease (stationary night blindness). *Invest. Ophthalmol. Vis. Sci.*, 40: 2978–2982.

Connolly, S.E., Hjelmeland, L.M. and LaVail, M.M. (1991) Localization of bFGF in developing retinas of normal and RCS rats. *Invest. Ophthalmol. Vis. Sci.*, (Suppl. 32): 754.

D'Cruz, P.M., Yasumura, D., Weir, J., Matthes, M., Abderrahim, H., LaVail, M.M. and Vollrath, D. (2000) Mutation of the receptor tyrosine kinase gene *Mertk* in the retinal dystrophic RCS rat. *Hum. Mol. Genet.*, 9: 645–651.

Deshpande, S., Thompson, M., Parker, J.A. and Abrahamson, E.W. (1992) Study of retinal dystrophy in RCS rats: a comparison of Mg-ATP dependent light scattering activity and ERG b-wave. *Vision Res.*, 32: 425–432.

Dovrat, A., Ding, L.L. and Horwitz, J. (1993) Enzyme activities and crystallin profiles of clear and cataractous lenses of the RCS rat. *Exp. Eye Res.*, 57: 217–224.

Dowling, J.E. (1960) The chemistry of visual adaptation in the rat. *Nature*, 188: 114–118.

Dowling, J.E. and Sidman, R.L. (1962) Inherited retinal dystrophy in the rat. *J. Cell Biol.*, 14: 73–109.

Dowling, J.E. and Wald, G. (1958) Vitamin A deficiency and night blindness. *Proc. Natl. Acad. Sci. USA*, 44: 648–661.

Dryja, T.P. and Li, T. (1995) Molecular genetics of retinitis pigmentosa. *Hum. Mol. Genet.*, 4: 1739–1743.

Edwards, R.B. and Szamier, R.B. (1977) Defective phagocytosis of isolated rod outer segments by RCS rat retinal pigment epithelium in culture. *Science*, 197: 1001–1003.

Eisenfeld, A.J., Bunt-Milam, A.H. and Saari, J.C. (1985) Immunocytochemical localization of interphotoreceptor retinol-binding protein in developing normal and RCS rat retinas. *Invest. Ophthalmol. Vis. Sci.*, 26: 775–778.

El-Hifnawi, E. (1995) Localization of cathepsin D in rat ocular tissues. An immunohistochemical study. *Anat. Anzeig.*, 177: 11–17.

El-Hifnawi, E., Kuhnel, W., El-Hifnawi, A. and Laqua, H. (1994) Localization of lysosomal enzymes in the retina and retinal pigment epithelium of RCS rats. *Anat. Anzeig.*, 176: 505–513.

El-Hifnawi, E.S. (1987) Pathomorphology of the retina and its vasculature in hereditary retinal dystrophy in RCS rats. In: Zrenner, E., Krastel, H. and Goebel, H.H. (Eds.), *Research in Retinitis Pigmentosa*. Pergamon Journals Ltd., London, pp. 417–434.

Essner, E., Roszka, J.R. and Schreiber, J.H. (1978) Phagocytosis and surface morphology in cultured retinal pigment epithelial cells. *Invest. Ophthalmol. Vis. Sci.*, 17: 1040–1048.

Faktorovich, E.G., Steinberg, R.H., Yasumura, D., Matthes, M.T. and LaVail, M.M. (1990) Photoreceptor degeneration in inherited retinal dystrophy delayed by basic fibroblast growth factor. *Nature*, 347: 83–86.

Gal, A., Li, Y., Thompson, D.A., Weir, J., Orth, U., Jacobson, S.G., Apfelstedt-Sylla, E. and Vollrath, D. (2000) Mutations in *MERTK*, the human orthologue of the RCS rat retinal dystrophy gene, cause retinitis pigmentosa. *Nat. Genet.* 26: 270–271.

Goldman, A.I. and O'Brien, P.J. (1978) Phagocytosis in the retinal pigment epithelium of the RCS rat. *Science*, 201: 1023–1025.

Gonzalez-Fernandez, F., Fong, S.-L., Liou, G.I. and Bridges, C.D.B. (1985) Interstitial retinol-binding protein (IRBP) in the RCS rat: effect of dark-rearing. *Invest. Ophthalmol. Vis. Sci.*, 26: 1381–1385.

Gonzalez-Fernandez, F., Landers, R.A., Glazebrook, P.A., Fong, S.-L., Liou, G.I., Lam, D.M.K. and Bridges, C.D.B. (1984) An extracellular retinol-binding glycoprotein in the eyes of mutant rats with retinal dystrophy: development, localization and biosynthesis. *J. Cell Biol.*, 99: 2092–2098.

Gouras, P., Lopez, R., Kjeldbye, H., Sullivan, B. and Brittis, M. (1989) Transplantation of retinal epithelium prevents photoreceptor degeneration in the RCS rat. *Prog. Clin. Biol. Res.*, 314: 659–671.

Gregory, C.Y., Abrams, T.A. and Hall, M.O. (1992) cAMP production via the adenylyl cyclase pathway is reduced in RCS rat RPE. *Invest. Ophthalmol. Vis. Sci.*, 1992: 3121–3124.

Gu, S., Thompson, D.A., Srikumari, C.R.S., Lorenz, B., Finckh, U., Nicoletti, A., Murthy, K.R., Rathmann, M., Kumaramanickavel, G., Denton, M.J. and Gal, A. (1997) Mutations in RPE65 cause autosomal recessive childhood-onset severe retinal dystrophy. *Nature Genet.*, 17: 194–197.

Hall, M.O. (1978) Phagocytosis of light- and dark-adapted rod outer segments by cultured pigment epithelium. *Science*, 202: 526–528.

Hall, M.O. and Abrams, T. (1987) Kinetic studies of rod outer segment binding and ingestion by cultured rat RPE cells. *Exp. Eye Res.*, 45: 907–922.

Hanitzsch, R., Aeumer, C., Lichtenberger, T. and Wurziger, K. (1998) Impaired function of bipolar cells in the Royal College of Surgeons rat. *Acta Anat. (Basel)*, 162: 119–126.

Hawlina, M., Jenkins, H.G. and Ikeda, H. (1992) Diurnal variations in the electroretinographic c-wave and retinal melatonin content in rats with inherited retinal dystrophy. *Doc. Ophthalmol.*, 79: 141–150.

Herron, W.L., Riegel, B.W., Myers, O.E. and Rubin, M.L. (1969) Retinal dystrophy in the rat-a pigment epithelial disease. *Invest. Ophthalmol.*, 8: 595–604.

Hess, H.H., Knapka, J.J., Newsome, D.A., Westney, I.V. and Wartofsky, L. (1985) Dietary prevention of cataracts in the pink-eyed RCS rat. *Lab. Anim. Sci.*, 35: 47–53.

Hess, H.H., Newsome, D.A., Knapka, J.J. and Westney, G.E. (1982) Slitlamp assessment of age of onset and incidence of cataracts in pink-eyed, tan-hooded retinal dystrophic rats. *Curr. Eye Res.*, 2: 265–269.

Hess, H.H., O'Keefe, T.L., Kuwabara, T. and Westney, I.V. (1991) Numbers of cortical vitreous cells and onset of cataracts in Royal College of Surgeons Rats. *Invest. Ophthalmol. Vis. Sci.*, 32: 200–207.

Heth, C.A., Marescalchi, P.A. and Ye, L. (1995) IP3 generation increases rod outer segment phagocytosis by cultured Royal College of Surgeons retinal pigment epithelium. *Invest. Ophthalmol. Vis. Sci.*, 36: 984–989.

Heth, C.A. and Schmidt, S.Y. (1992) Protein phosphorylation in retinal pigment epithelium of Long-Evans and Royal College of Surgeons rats. *Invest. Ophthalmol. Vis. Sci.*, 33: 2839–2847.

Humphrey, M.F., Parker, C., Chu, Y. and Constable, I.J. (1993) Transient preservation of photoreceptors on the flanks of argon laser lesions in the RCS rat. *Curr. Eye Res.*, 12: 367–372.

Johnson, L.V., Blanks, J.C. and Hageman, G.S. (1989) Effects of retinal degenerations on the cone matrix sheath. In: LaVail, M.M., Hollyfield, J.G. and Anderson, R.E. (Eds.), *Inherited and Environmentally Induced Retinal Degenerations*. Alan R. Liss Inc., New York, pp. 217–232.

Katai, N., Kikuchi, T., Shibuki, H., Kuroiwa, S., Arai, J., Kurokawa, T. and Yoshimura, N. (1999) Caspaselike proteases activated in apoptotic photoreceptors of Royal College of Surgeons rats. *Invest. Ophthalmol. Vis. Sci.*, 40: 1802–1807.

Keeler, C.E. (1924) The inheritance of a retinal abnormality in white mice. *Proc. Natl. Acad. Sci.*, 10: 329–333.

LaVail, M.M. (1976) Rod outer segment disc shedding in rat retina: relationship to cyclic lighting. *Science*, 194: 1071–1074.

LaVail, M.M. (1979) The retinal pigment epithelium in mice and rats with inherited retinal degeneration. In: Zinn, K.M. and Marmor, M.F. (Eds.), *The Retinal Pigment Epithelium*. Harvard University Press, Cambridge, pp. 357–380.

LaVail, M.M. (1981a) Analysis of neurological mutants with inherited retinal degeneration. *Invest. Ophthalmol. Vis. Res.*, 21: 638–657.

LaVail, M.M. (1981b) Assignment of retinal dystrophy (rdy) to linkage group IV of the rat. *J. Hered.*, 72: 294–296.

LaVail, M.M. (1981c) Photoreceptor characteristics in congenic strains of RCS rats. *Invest. Ophthalmol. Vis. Sci.*, 20: 671–675.

LaVail, M.M. and Battelle, B.A. (1975) Influence of eye pigmentation and light deprivation on inherited retinal dystrophy in the rat. *Exp. Eye Res.*, 21: 167–192.

LaVail, M.M., Gorrin, G.M., Yasumura, D. and Matthes, M.T. (1999) Increased susceptibility to constant light in *nr* and *pcd* mice with inherited retinal degenerations. *Invest. Ophthalmol. Vis. Sci.*, 40: 1020–1024.

LaVail, M.M., Li, L., Turner, J.E. and Yasumura, D. (1992) Retinal pigment epithelial cell transplantation in RCS rats: normal metabolism in rescued photoreceptors. *Exp. Eye Res.*, 55: 555–562.

LaVail, M.M., Pinto, L.H. and Yasumura, D. (1981) The interphotoreceptor matrix in rats with inherited retinal dystrophy. *Invest. Ophthalmol. Vis. Sci.*, 21: 658–668.

LaVail, M.M., Sidman, M., Rauzin, R. and Sidman, R.L. (1974) Discrimination of light intensity by rats with inherited retinal degeneration: a behavioral and cytological study. *Vision Res.*, 14: 693–702.

LaVail, M.M., Sidman, R.L. and Gerhardt, C.O. (1975) Congenic strains of RCS rats with inherited retinal dystrophy. *J. Hered.*, 242–244.

LaVail, M.M., Sidman, R.L. and O'Neil, D.A. (1972) Photoreceptor-pigment epithelial cell relationships in rats with inherited retinal degeneration. Radioautographic and electron microscope evidence for a dual source of extra lamellar material. *J. Cell Biol.*, 53: 185–209.

LaVail, M.M., White, M.P., Gorrin, G.M., Porrello, K.V. and Mullen, R.J. (1993) Retinal degeneration in the nervous mutant mouse. I. Light microscopic cytopathology and changes in the interphotoreceptor matrix. *J. Comp. Neur.*, 333: 168–181.

LaVail, M.M., Yasumura, D. and Hollyfield, J. (1985a) The interphotoreceptor matrix in retinitis pigmentosa: preliminary observations from a family with an autosomal dominant form of disease. In: LaVail, M.M., Hollyfield, J.G. and Anderson, R.E. (Eds.), *Retinal Degeneration: Experimental and Clinical Studies*. Alan R. Liss Inc., New York, pp. 51–62.

LaVail, M.M., Yasumura, D., Matthes, M.T., Lau-Villacorta, C., Unoki, K., Sung, C.-H. and Steinberg, R.H. (1998) Protection of mouse photoreceptors by survival factors in retinal degenerations. *Invest. Ophthalmol. Vis. Sci.*, 39: 592–602.

LaVail, M.M., Yasumura, D. and Porrello, K. (1985b) Histochemical analysis of the interphotoreceptor matrix in hereditary retinal degenerations. In: Bridges, C.D. and Adler, A.J. (Eds.), *The Interphotoreceptor Matrix in Health and Disease*. Alan R. Liss Inc., New York, pp. 179–193.

Lawrence, J.M., Sauve, Y., Keegan, D.J., Coffey, P.J., Hetherington, L., Girman, S., Whiteley, S.J., Kwan, A.S., Pheby, T. and Lund, R.D. (2000) Schwann cell grafting into the retina of the dystrophic RCS rat limits functional deterioration. *Invest. Ophthalmol. Vis. Sci.*, 41: 518–528.

Lazarus, H.S., Sly, W.S., Kyle, J.W. and Hageman, G.S. (1993) Photoreceptor degeneration and altered distribution of interphotoreceptor matrix proteoglycans in the mucopolysaccharidosis VII mouse. *Exp. Eye Res.*, 56: 531–541.

Li, L. and Turner, J.E. (1988) Inherited retinal dystrophy in the RCS rat: prevention of photoreceptor degeneration by pigment epithelial cell transplantation. *Exp. Eye Res.*, 47: 911–917.

Litchfield, T., Whiteley, S. and Lund, R. (1997) Transplantation of retinal pigment epithelial, photoreceptor and other cells as treatment for retinal degeneration. *Exp. Eye Res.*, 64: 655–666.

Lopez, R., Gouras, P., Kjeldbye, H., Sullivan, B., Reppucci, V., Britis, M., Wapner, F. and Goluboff, E. (1989) Transplanted retinal pigment epithelium modifies the retinal degeneration in the RCS rat. *Invest. Ophthalmol. Vis. Sci.*, 30: 586–588.

Lucas, D.R., Attfield, M. and Davey, J.B. (1955) Retinal dystrophy in the rat. *J. Path. Bact.*, 70: 469–474.

Malecaze, F., Mascarelli, F., Bugra, K., Fuhrmann, G., Courtois, Y. and Hicks, D. (1993) Fibroblast growth factor receptor deficiency in dystrophic retinal pigmented epithelium. *J. Cell Physiol.*, 154: 631–642.

Marlhens, F., Bareil, C., Griffoin, J.-M., Zrenner, E., Amalric, P., Eliaou, C., Liu, S.-Y., Harris, E., Redmond, T.M., Arnaud, B., Claustres, M. and Hamel, C.P. (1997) Mutations in RPE65 cause Leber's congenital amaurosis. *Nature Genet.*, 17: 194–197.

Maw, M.A., Kennedy, B., Knight, A., Bridges, R., Roth, K.E., Mani, E.J., Mukkadan, J.K., Nancarrow, D., Crabb, J.W. and Denton, M.J. (1997) Mutation of the gene encoding cellular retinaldehyde-binding protein in autosomal recessive retinitis pigmentosa. *Nature Genet.*, 17: 198–200.

McLaren, M.J., Inana, G. and Li, C.Y. (1993) Double fluorescent vital assay of phagocytosis by cultured retinal pigment epithelial cells. *Invest. Ophthalmol. Vis. Sci.*, 34: 317–326.

Mieziewska, K., van Veen, T. and Aguirre, G.D. (1993a) Development and fate of interphotoreceptor matrix components during dysplastic photoreceptor differentiation: a lectin cytochemical study of rod-cone dysplasia 1. *Exp. Eye Res.*, 56: 429–441.

Mieziewska, K., van Veen, T. and Aguirre, G.D. (1993b) Structural changes of the interphotoreceptor matrix in an inherited retinal degeneration: a lectin cytochemical study of progressive rod-cone degeneration. *Invest. Ophthalmol. Vis. Sci.*, 34: 3056–3067.

Milam, A.H. (1993) Strategies for rescue of retinal photoreceptor cells. *Curr. Opin. Neurobiol.*, 3: 797–804.

Mirshahi, M., Thillaye, B., Tarraf, M., de Kozak, Y. and Faure, J.P. (1994) Light-induced changes in S-antigen (arrestin) localization in retinal photoreceptors: differences between rods and cones and defective process in RCS rat retinal dystrophy. *Europ. J. Cell Biol.*, 63: 61–67.

Molday, R.S. (1998) Photoreceptor membrane proteins, phototransduction, and retinal degenerative diseases. *Invest. Ophthalmol. Vis. Sci.*, 39: 2491–2513.

Mullen, R.J. and LaVail, M.M. (1976) Inherited retinal dystrophy: primary defect in pigment epithelium determined with experimental rat chimeras. *Science*, 192: 799–801.

Naash, M.I., Peachey, N.S., Li, Z.Y., Gryczan, C.C., Goto, Y., Blanks, J., Milam, A.H. and Ripps, H. (1996) Light-induced acceleration of photoreceptor degeneration in transgenic mice expressing mutant opsin. *Invest. Ophthalmol. Vis. Sci.*, 37: 775–782.

Nir, I., Liu, C. and Wen, R. (1999) Light treatment enhances photoreceptor survival in dystrophic retinas of Royal College of Surgeons rats. *Invest. Ophthalmol. Vis. Sci.*, 40: 2383–2390.

Noell, W.K. (1965) Aspects of experimental and hereditary retinal degeneration. In: Graymore, C.N. (Ed.), *Biochemistry of the Retina*. Academic Press, London, pp. 51–72.

Organisciak, D.T., Li, M., Darrow, R.M. and Farber, D.B. (1999) Photoreceptor cell damage by light in young Royal College of Surgeons rats. *Curr. Eye Res.*, 19: 188–196.

Organisciak, D.T. and Winkler, B.S. (1994) Retinal light damage: practical and theoretical considerations. In: Osborne, N. and Chader, G. (Eds.), *Prog. Retin. Eye. Res.*, Pergamon Press, Oxford, pp. 1–29.

Pittler, S.J., Keeler, C.E., Sidman, R.L. and Baehr, W. (1993) PCR analysis of DNA from 70-year-old sections of rodless retina demonstrates identity with the mouse *rd* defect. *Proc. Natl. Acad. Sci. USA*, 90: 9616–9619.

Rakoczy, P.E., Humphrey, M.F., Cavaney, D.M., Chu, Y. and Constable, I.J. (1993) Expression of basic fibroblast growth factor and its receptor in the retina of Royal College of Surgeons rats. A comparative study. *Invest. Ophthalmol. Vis. Sci.*, 34: 1845–1852.

Ripps, H. (1982) Night blindness revisited: from man to molecules. Proctor Lecture. *Invest. Ophthalmol. Vis. Sci.*, 23: 588–609.

Roque, R.S. and Caldwell, R.B. (1990) Muller cell changes precede vascularization of the pigment epithelium in the dystrophic rat retina. *Glia*, 3: 464–475.

Roque, R.S. and Caldwell, R.B. (1991) Pigment epithelial cell changes precede vascular transformations in the dystrophic rat retina. *Exp. Eye Res.*, 53: 787–798.

Sandberg, M.A., Pawlyk, B.S., Crane, W.G. and Berson, E.L. (1988) Diurnal rhythm in the electroretinogram of the Royal College of Surgeons (RCS) pigmented rat. *Exp. Eye Res.*, 46: 929–936.

Schmidt, S.Y., Heth, C.A., Edwards, R.B., Brandt, J.T., Adler, A.J., Spiegel, A., Shichi, H. and Berson, E.L. (1988) Identification of proteins in retinas and IPM from eyes with retinitis pigmentosa. *Invest. Ophthalmol. Vis. Sci.*, 29: 1585–1593.

Seaton, A.D., Sheedlo, H.J. and Turner, J.E. (1994) A primary role for RPE transplants in the inhibition and regression of neovascularization in the RCS rat. *Invest. Ophthalmol. Vis. Sci.*, 35: 162–169.

Seaton, A.D. and Turner, J.E. (1992) RPE transplants stabilize retinal vasculature and prevent neovascularization in the RCS rat. *Invest. Ophthalmol. Vis. Sci.*, 33: 83–91.

Seyfried-Williams, R. and McLaughlin, B.J. (1983) The use of sugar-coated beads to study phagocytosis in normal and dystrophic retina. *Vision Res.*, 23: 485–494.

Seyfried-Williams, R., McLaughlin, B.J. and Cooper, N.G.F. (1984) Phagocytosis of lectin-coated beads by dystrophic and normal retinal pigment epithelium. *Exp. Cell Res.*, 154: 500–509.

Sidman, R.L. (1961a) (Ed.) Histogenesis of mouse retina studied with thymidine-^{3}H. In: *The Structure of the Eye*, Academic Press, pp. 487–506.

Sidman, R.L. (1961b) Tissue culture studies of inherited retinal dystrophy. *Dis. Nerv. Sys.*, 22: 14–20.

Sidman, R.L. and Pearlstein, R. (1965) Pink-eyed dilution (*p*) gene in rodents: increased pigmentation in tissue culture. *Dev. Biol.*, 12: 93–116.

Sidman, R.L. and Wislocki, G.B. (1954) Histochemical observations on rods and cones in retinas of vertebrates. *J. Histochem. Cytochem.*, 2: 413–433.

Steinberg, R.H. (1994) Survival factors in retinal degenerations. *Curr. Opin. Neurobiol.*, 4: 515–524.

Strauss, O. and Wienrich, M. (1993) Cultured retinal pigment epithelial cells from RCS rats express an increased calcium conductance compared with cells from non-dystrophic rats. *Pflug. Archiv. Europ. Physiol.*, 425: 68–76.

Tarnowski, B.I. and McLaughlin, B.J. (1987) Phagocytic interactions of sialated glycoprotein, sugar, and lectin coated beads with rat retinal pigment epithelium. *Curr. Eye Res.*, 6: 1079–1089.

Tarnowski, B.I., Shepherd, V.L. and McLaughlin, B.J. (1988) Expression of mannose receptors for pinocytosis and phagocytosis on rat retinal pigment epithelium. *Invest. Ophthalmol. Vis. Sci.*, 29: 742–748.

Tawara, A. and Hollyfield, J.G. (1990) Proteoglycans in the mouse interphotoreceptor matrix. III. Changes during development and degeneration in the *rds* mutant. *Exp. Eye Res.*, 51: 301–315.

Thanos, S. (1992) Sick photoreceptors attract activated microglia from the ganglion cell layer: a model to study the inflammatory cascades in rats with inherited retinal dystrophy. *Brain Res.*, 588: 21–28.

Thanos, S. and Richter, W. (1993) The migratory potential of vitally labelled microglial cells within the retina of rats with hereditary photoreceptor dystrophy. *Int. J. Dev. Neurosci.*, 11: 671–680.

Uehara, F., Yasumura, D. and LaVail, M.M. (1991) Development of light-evoked changes of the interphotoreceptor matrix in normal and RCS rats with inherited retinal dystrophy. *Exp. Eye Res.*, 53: 55–60.

Valter, K., Maslim, J., Bowers, F. and Stone, J. (1998) Photoreceptor dystrophy in the RCS rat: roles of oxygen, debris and bFGF. *Invest. Ophthalmol. Vis. Sci.*, 39: 2427–2442.

van Veen, T., Ekstron, P., Wiggert, B., Lee, L., Hirose, Y., Sanyal, S. and Chader, G.J. (1988) A developmental study of interphotoreceptor retinoid-binding protein (IRBP) in single and double homozygous *rd* and *rds* mutant mouse retinae. *Exp. Eye Res.*, 47: 291–305.

Villegas-Pérez, M.P., Lawrence, J.M., Vidal-Sanz, M., LaVail, M.M. and Lund, R.D. (1998) Ganglion cell loss in RCS rat retina: a result of compression of axons by contracting intraretinal vessels linked to the pigment epithelium. *J. Comp. Neur.*, 392: 58–77.

Weber, M.L., Mancini, M.A. and Frank, R.N. (1989) Retinovitreal neovascularization in the Royal College of Surgeons rat. *Curr. Eye Res.*, 8: 61–74.

Wroblewski, J.J., Wells III, J.A., Eckstein, A., Fitzke, F., Jubb, C., Keen, T.J., Inglehearn, C., Bhattacharya, S., Arden, G.B., Jay, M. and Bird, A.C. (1994) Macular dystrophy associated with mutations at codon 172 in the human retinal degeneration slow gene. *Ophthalmology*, 101: 12–22.

Yamaguchi, K., Yamaguchi, K., Sheedlo, H.J. and Turner, J.E. (1991) Ciliary body degeneration in the Royal College of Surgeons rat. *Exp. Eye Res.*, 52: 539–548.

Yamaguchi, K., Yamaguchi, K. and Turner, J.E. (1990) Corneal endothelial abnormalities in the Royal College of Surgeons rat. *Cornea*, 9: 217–222.

Young, R.W. (1967) The renewal of photoreceptor cell outer segments. *J. Cell Biol.*, 33: 61–72.

Young, R.W. (1988) Solar radiation and age-related macular degeneration. *Surv. Ophthalmol.*, 32: 252–269.

Young, R.W. and Bok, D. (1969) Participation of the retinal pigment epithelium in the rod outer segment renewal process. *J. Cell Biol.*, 42: 392–403.

Zhang, X. and Bok, D. (1998) Transplantation of retinal pigment epithelial cells and immune response in the subretinal space. *Invest. Ophthalmol. Vis. Sci.*, 39: 1021–1027.

Zigler, J.J. and Hess, H.H. (1985) Cataracts in the Royal College of Surgeons rat: evidence for initiation by lipid peroxidation products. *Exp. Eye Res.*, 41: 67–76.

H. Kolb, H. Ripps and S. Wu (Eds.)
Progress in Brain Research, Vol. 131
© 2001 Elsevier Science B.V. All rights reserved

CHAPTER 45

Retinal disease in vertebrates

Susan E. Brockerhoff *

Department of Biochemistry, Box 357350, University of Washington, Seattle, WA 98195, USA

Introduction

The identification of heritable mutations affecting visual behavior is a powerful way to discover genes involved in the function of the retina. Three vertebrate organisms that play an important role in identifying disease genes affecting retinal function are humans, mice and zebrafish. This article summarizes some of the information learned from characterizing mutations affecting the outer retina in humans, mice and zebrafish. This article also compares the advantages/disadvantages of these three systems. The information provided here is not a complete review of all the information obtained from genetic studies using these systems, but rather select information is provided so that comparisons between the systems can be made.

Model organisms with heritable retinal disorders have played an important role in Dr. Dowling's research since early in his career (Dowling and Sidman, 1962). In recent years the Dowling laboratory has exploited zebrafish genetics to identify mutant fish with defects in both retinal function and development. As a postdoctoral fellow with Dr. Dowling, I participated in the genetic screen for visual mutations in zebrafish. The aspect of the zebrafish project that I participated in is summarized in the final section of this chapter.

Overview of retinal anatomy

The overall structure of the retina in mice, humans and zebrafish is similar. In all three organisms the retina

* Tel.: 206-616-9464; Fax: 206-685-2320;
E-mail: sbrocker@u.washington.edu

contains three nuclear layers and two synaptic layers. The outer most retinal layer contains the photoreceptors, rods and cones. Rods are responsible for vision in dim (scotopic) light whereas cones are responsible for color vision and vision in bright (photopic) light. Photoreceptors are highly specialized cells containing a large extension (the outer segment) on the apical side and an uncommon type of synapse, called a ribbon synapse, on the basal side. It is within the outer segment that the molecules involved in phototransduction reside. The middle (inner) nuclear layer contains bipolar cells, which transmit information vertically through the retina, and this layer also contains two cell types that transmit information laterally, horizontal cells and amacrine cells. The horizontal cells reside in the outer part of the inner nuclear layer (near the photoreceptors) whereas the amacrine cells reside in the inner part of this layer. Finally, the third cellular layer contains primarily ganglion cells, the output neuron of the retina, and some amacrine cells, referred to as displaced amacrine cells. The axons of ganglion cells make up the optic nerve. The optic nerve exits the eye and forms a cable connecting the eye with the brain (for review see, Dowling, 1987).

Organization of the human retina

There are some striking differences in the organization of the photoreceptor layer in mice, humans and zebrafish. This may also be true for other cellular layers within the retina, however, differences in the inner nuclear cell layer and the ganglion cell layer are not as well documented as the observed differences in the organization of photoreceptor cells. In the human retina, the highest concentration of cones is found in the macula. The center of the macula, called the fovea, contains exclusively cones and no rods. The distribution of rods is the reciprocal of cones; the rod concentration is highest in the periphery and decreases in density up to the macula. In total, the rods outnumber cones by 20 to 1. There are three types of cones, a blue wavelength sensitive ($\sim$420 nm), wavelength sensitive cone, a green ($\sim$530 nm) wavelength sensitive cone and a red ($\sim$560 nm) wavelength sensitive cone (Merbs and Nathans, 1992).

Organization of the mouse retina

Cone photoreceptors in mice display a dorsal-ventral asymmetry in topography. Mice contain two types of cone photoreceptors, often referred to as short wavelength and mid wavelength receptors. The ventral half of the retina contains only the short wavelength cone whereas the dorsal retina contains both the short wave and the mid wave cones (Sz'el et al., 1992, 1996). The short wave cones absorb light maximally at 355 nm (Lyubarsky et al., 1999) whereas the mid wave cones absorb maximally at 508 nm (Sun et al., 1997). Rods are distributed throughout the mouse retina and outnumber cones by more than 30–1 (Carter-Dawson and LaVail, 1979).

Organization of the zebrafish retina

In contrast to mice and humans, zebrafish contain five visual pigments (1 rod and 4 cone). The cone pigments are referred to as UV-sensitive, blue-sensitive, green-sensitive and red-sensitive, absorbing maximally at 362, 415, 480 and 560 nm respectively (Robinson et al., 1993). In zebrafish, cone photoreceptors are arranged in a row mosaic that remains largely constant across the entire retina. In the row, the UV-sensitive cone is always adjacent to a green cone, the blue-sensitive cone is always adjacent to a red cone, and the red and green cones are always next to each other. Alternate rows are reversed in sequence leading to red alternating with green and blue alternating with UV between rows (Robinson et al., 1993). The exact number of rods verses cones

has not been determined although histological analyses suggest that in the adult fish rods outnumber cones. However, during early development the rods mature more slowly than cones; prior to approximately 12 days postfertilization (dpf), dark adaptation does not significantly increase the sensitivity of visual responses (Clark, 1981; Branchek, 1984). By screening young larval zebrafish for defective visual responses, this property of photoreceptor maturation can be exploited to identify mutations affecting cone viability (Brockerhoff et al., 1997, 1998).

Phototransduction

Despite differences in photoreceptor organization, the proteins involved in photoreceptor responses to light are highly conserved among different vertebrates. In mice, humans and zebrafish, light photoactivates the visual pigment inducing a conformational change that leads to the activation of the G-protein transducin. The alpha subunit of transducin, with GTP bound, removes the inhibitory subunit from phosphodiesterase (PDE) resulting in its activation and the hydrolysis of cGMP. A cation channel in the outer segment, gated by cGMP, closes when cGMP is hydrolyzed, leading to a decrease in sodium and calcium influx and subsequent membrane hyperpolarization. This hyperpolarization of the cell membrane leads to a graded reduction in neurotransmitter release at the terminal. Lower intracellular calcium stimulates a negative feedback loop that restores the cell to its preactivated state (Palczewski and Saari, 1997).

We recently demonstrated that by modifying the biochemical assays designed for analyzing phototransduction in mouse retinas, we were able to biochemically analyze, in zebrafish larvae, the activity of the molecules involved in both phototransduction and the visual cycle (Taylor et al., 2000). One interesting finding from this study was that in contrast to the widely held notion that fresh water fish contain the A2 retinal chromophore (Dowling, 1987), the predominant chromophore in zebrafish is an A1 type. These biochemical assays are useful tools for studying zebrafish mutants with defects in phototransduction or visual pigment regeneration.

Retinal disease in humans

Human retinal diseases are categorized based on a number of criteria, such as fundus appearance, behavioral responses to visual stimuli (psychophysics) and electroretinographic responses. These methods are noninvasive, relatively precise, and enable ophthalmologists to classify diseases altering retinal morphology and function. Some of the major classifications that are not systemic (i.e. affect only the retina) are retinitis pigmentosa (RP), Leber's congenital amaurosis, cone dystrophy, cone-rod dystrophy, congenital stationary night blindness (CSNB) and macular degeneration. These diseases specifically affect photoreceptor cells and contain approximately half of all genes causing retinal disease identified to date.

A great on-line resource that summarizes current data regarding human genes that cause retinal disease is http://www.sph.uth.tmc.edu/Retnet/home.htm. Also, there are several recent reviews on human retinal diseases (Farber and Danciger, 1997; Gregory-Evans and Bhattacharya, 1998; Rattner et al., 1999; Phelan and Bok, 2000;). The description presented here is intended only to highlight some of the interesting patterns that have emerged from identifying human disease genes. The mechanisms by which the molecules listed here cause retinal disease is not yet clear, although mechanisms are starting to emerge for some (for review see, Rattner et al., 1999).

Approximately half of the currently identified genes associated with causing retinal disease have been cloned. Most cloned disease genes were first identified using molecular and biochemical methods and then were analyzed as potential candidates for human retinal disease either based on linkage or through random screening of families with a variety of different retinal disorders (Dryja, 1997). One of the most successful examples of this approach has been with genes involved in rod and cone phototransduction. Phototransduction components represent the largest single class of genes implicated in retinal diseases. The obvious reason for this success has been the major effort of researchers to identify the genes responsible for the photoresponse in humans. The effort devoted to understanding phototransduction, particularly in rods, has led to the isolation of the major components of this cascade and the subsequent identification of mutations within these genes that cause photoreceptor diseases.

Another interesting finding observed from analyzing the summary of cloned and mapped genes is that different mutations in a single gene can cause different diseases. For example, although the majority of mutations in rhodopsin lead to dominant RP (Rattner et al., 1999 and references therein), mutations in this gene also cause both dominant CSNB (Dryja et al., 1993) and recessive RP (rRP) (Rosenfeld et al., 1992). In another example, mutations in ABCR, a photoreceptor specific member of the ATP-binding family of transporters, cause several types of macular degeneration (Rozet et al., 1999b), cone–rod dystrophy combined with RP (Cremers et al., 1998), and rRP (Rozet et al., 1999a).

Perhaps an even more striking observation is that mutations in apparently very different genes can cause the same disease. Recessive RP has been associated with mutations in over a dozen different genes. The diversity of different genes causing this disease is evident from the following description of genes identified as containing mutations in patients with rRP. Five genes causing rRP are involved in phototransduction. These are rhodopsin, arrestin, the alpha and beta subunits of rod cGMP PDE, and the alpha-subunit of cGMP gated channels in rods (see, http://www.sph.uth.tmc.edu/Retnet/home.htm).

The second most abundant class of proteins responsible for rRP is involved in chromophore regeneration and transport. RPE65, an abundant membrane associated protein that is specifically expressed in the retinal pigmented epithelium, causes several forms of retinal dystrophy including rRP (Marlhens et al., 1997, 1998; Morimura et al., 1998). RPE65 has been implicated in retinoid isomerization within the RPE, but its exact role in this process is unknown (Redmond et al., 1998). The second gene, ABCR, encodes a photoreceptor specific member of the ATP-binding family of transporters (Martinez-Mir et al., 1998; Rozet et al., 1999a). ABCR is localized on the rim of the discs in outer segments and originally was thought to reside solely in rods (Sun and Nathans, 1997). It has recently been identified in cone photoreceptors as well (Molday et al., 2000). ABCR appears to be involved in transporting *all-trans* retinal from the inner side to the outer side of the disc membrane (Weng et al., 1999). A third member of this class is cellular retinaldehyde binding protein (CRALBP) (Maw et al., 1997). CRALBP is one of several retinoid binding proteins involved in the visual cycle. In vitro, CRALBP binds preferentially to 11-*cis* retinol and promotes its oxidation to 11-*cis* retinal (Saari et al., 1994). CRALBP is also required for efficient iso-mero-hydrolase activity (Winston and Rando, 1998). Finally, a fourth member of this class is the opsin-like molecule RGR (Morimura et al., 1999). Upon exposure to light, RGR converts all-*trans* retinal to the 11-*cis* isomer (Hao and Fong, 1999).

Five additional genes linked to rRP are each in a separate category: (1) Tulp1, is a member of a family of evolutionarily conserved proteins of unknown function (Banerjee et al., 1998; Gu et al., 1998; Hagstrom et al., 1998); (2) CRB1, is a homologue to the *Drosophila* crumbs protein. This protein may play a role in cell–cell interactions and the maintenance of cell polarity (den Hollander et al., 1999); (3) Mutations in alpha-tocopherol (Vitamin E) carrier protein also cause rRP (Yokota et al., 1996). Since vitamin E is an important antioxidant in photo-receptor outer segments, its poor absorption likely leads to increased photooxidative damage; (4 and 5) RP2 and 3 are both X-linked and were both positionally cloned. The function of both of these genes is unclear (Meindl et al., 1996; Schwahn et al., 1998).

Summary of human advantages and disadvantages

The previous paragraphs briefly describe genes identified as causing rRP in humans. The description of the information known about these genes is incomplete and rRP is only one disease of many that disrupt photoreceptor viability and function. However, what is hopefully evident from this limited description of human diseases is that human genetics has played a critical role in understanding the function of known as well as unknown retinal genes. The disadvantages with humans as a genetic system are that rare mutations are less likely to be discovered, small pedigrees often make mapping mutations difficult, and the inability to rescue mutations can make gene identification difficult

particularly if the mutation identified is conservative. Also, the study of the biology of human retinal disease is limited to noninvasive techniques.

Retinal disease in mice

The mouse has served as an important model for identifying and understanding genes essential for normal retinal morphology for quite some time (Keeler, 1966; van Nie et al., 1978; Sanyal et al., 1980). Two mouse mutants that have played a major role in the photoreceptor field are rd and rds, since in these mutants the photoreceptor cells degenerate. The analysis and subsequent identification of the genes altered in these mutants was the source of extensive studies for decades. Some important original studies on the rd mouse implicated cGMP levels as playing a critical role in cell death (Lolley et al., 1977, Lolley, 1994). The identification of peripherin as mutated in the rds mouse emphasized the critical role of outer segment disc morphology in photoreceptor cell viability (Travis et al., 1989; Connell et al., 1991). Furthermore, even though the genes defective in the rd and in the rds mouse have been known for several years, these mutants conti-nue to play an important role in research aimed at understanding photoreceptor cell death and at rescu-ing degenerating photoreceptors (for one example, see Nir et al., 2000).

Additional mice with retinal degeneration, rd3, rd6 and rd7, have been described (Chang et al., 1993; Akhmedov et al., 2000; Hawes et al., 2000). The genes altered in the rd3 and rd6 mice have not been determined. The rd7 gene has recently been identi-fied as a photoreceptor-specific nuclear receptor (Akhmedov et al., 2000). Future studies analyzing the function of this gene will be of great interest. Other mouse mutations that have retinal degenera-tion have also been described but these have additional defects such as Purkinje cell degeneration and motor neuron degeneration (Hawes et al., 1999). Finally, there is a spontaneous mutant, nob, that is an important model for CSNB (Candille et al., 1999). Unlike the rd mutants, the photoreceptors in nob do not degenerate. From electroretinogram (ERG) analysis, the primary defect appears to be in trans-mission to neurons downstream of photoreceptors;

the ERG waveform has a large a-wave and no b-wave. The phenotype of nob resembles CSNB1 in humans and the nob gene maps to a region of the X chromosome that is homologous to the human X chromosome where CSNB1 is located (Candille et al., 1999).

Although the retinal mutations in mice have been important for studying photoreceptor function, few genetic screens to identify novel retinal mutations have been conducted. The major contribution that mice have made in recent years is through analysis of gene knockouts. However, this topic will not be addressed in this article. In one unbiased screen intended to uncover important genes in the visual system, visually evoked eye movements were analyzed from a subset of the preexisting mouse mutations (Balkema et al., 1984). The reflexive optokinetic eye movements that are elicited by observing rotating stripes were examined in many hypopigmented mice and in mice with neuromuscular defects. To analyze eye movements, restrained mice were placed in an optokinetic drum that had alternating light/dark vertical stripes and smooth pursuit and saccade eye movements were analyzed in response to the stripe rotation.

The Balkema screen led to the identification of 23 different mutants with abnormal optokinetic responses and it highlighted the usefulness of screening existing stock centers. Thirteen of the 23 were hypopigmentation mutants and ten had neuromuscular defects. None of the mutants identified in this screen had retinal degeneration. Furthermore the ERG was recorded from five hypopigmentation mutants (albino, beige, maroon, pale ears and pearl) and all five had normal ERG waveforms at dim and bright light levels. Mutants with outer retinal defects were not identified in this screen.

Summary of mouse advantages and disadvantages

The availability of the human genome sequence is stimulating genetic approaches to identifying gene function. Genetic screens in mice using strategies such as gene trapping and chemical mutagenesis will identify a collection of genes important in many biological processes (Justice et al., 1999). A primary disadvantage of mice for identifying novel retinal

genes is that the retina is rod dominated at all stages of development so genes affecting the less well characterized cone system will not be identified easily.

Studying the retina in zebrafish

Zebrafish as a model genetically tractable organism is being actively developed because of the obvious utility of studying vertebrate biology using a genetic approach. With zebrafish it is possible for small labs to conduct genetic screens aimed at identifying novel molecules or regulatory pathways in biological cascades. Furthermore, genomic resources necessary to identify mutated genes are widely available and are improving rapidly. Although not quite as sophisticated as the transgenesis techniques in mice, the creation of transgenic zebrafish is an area of active research.

Our specific goal in using zebrafish to study the visual system is to identify important molecules involved in photoreceptor (particularly cone) structure and function. Components identified by such an approach will complement biochemical and physiological approaches to studying the visual system. Novel molecules will be candidates for photoreceptor disease causing genes in humans. Some of the particular questions that we are studying are: (1) what are the molecular explanations for the differences between rod and cone physiology; (2) what regulates photoreceptor synaptic function and formation; and (3) what molecules are unique between the different cone sub-types?

An effective way to identify zebrafish mutants with photoreceptor defects is to measure the visual behavior of mutagenized fish. The behavioral assay that I optimized for measuring visual function, while a postdoctoral fellow with Dr. Dowling, is the optokinetic response, which measures eye movements in response to rotating stripes (Brockerhoff et al., 1995, 1997, 1998). In this assay, zebrafish larvae are placed in a 16 mm petri dish containing methylcellulose. The methylcellulose partially immobilizes the larvae. The petri dish containing larvae is then placed in the center of a drum that has alternating black and white stripes. In response to the stripe rotation, normal larvae will move their eyes in the direction of rotation. Initially the eyes slowly follow the stripes and when the stripes leave the field of view, the fish's eyes quickly return to their original position. This assay is very reliable and since the width of the stripes can be altered, has been used to measure the development of visual acuity in zebrafish (Clark, 1981). Mutant larvae show an abnormal response such as no response under any conditions (Allwardt, 1999), no response only at a specific wavelength (Brockerhoff et al., 1997) or a reversed response (Rick et al., 2000).

We have measured visual behavior as a primary screen to examine larvae between 5 and 6 dpf for recessive defects in the visual system. Our secondary screen is to measure the ERG of mutants with defective visual behavioral responses to identify fish with defects in the outer retina. We screen mutagenized larvae that appear otherwise completely normal since our assumption is that many visual mutants will likely not have morphological abnormalities. One other study using a similar approach has been reported, however, the mutants isolated in this screen were first identified as abnormal by criteria other than visual behavior (Neuhauss et al., 1999). These behavioral screens have identified a small collection of mutations affecting different layers of the retina (Brockerhoff et al., 1998; Neuhauss et al., 1999). From the histological analysis and ERG studies it has been possible to partially categorize the different mutations.

The ERG methodology has taken some time to perfect since the eye of a larval zebrafish is approximately 300 μm in diameter and zebrafish larvae are generally rather fragile. There are several tricky factors for obtaining reliable ERG recordings. It is important to position a larva on its side without significant manipulations. If the larvae are poked repeatedly to adjust their position, they usually die within a few minutes. We found that placing larvae onto a moistened piece of a bird feather usually results in their lying on their sides facing the light source. Also, it is important to make the electrode opening as wide as possible (typically 10–30 μm) and also to make sure that it is polished so that the surface is smooth. The electrode is then gently placed on the center of the cornea. It is not necessary to push the electrode into the eye with much force and in fact doing this will lead to premature death of the specimen. Figure 1 shows a zebrafish larva positioned for recording ERGs.

We have recently started adding 2-amino-4-phosphonobutyric acid (APB) to zebrafish to uncover the a-wave of the ERG response. We have found that bathing larvae in 1 mM APB for 1 min uncovers the a-wave but does not affect the overall health or swimming behavior of the larvae. APB is an agonist of metabotropic glutamate receptors of ON-bipolar cells (Shiells et al., 1981; Slaughter and Miller, 1981, 1985).

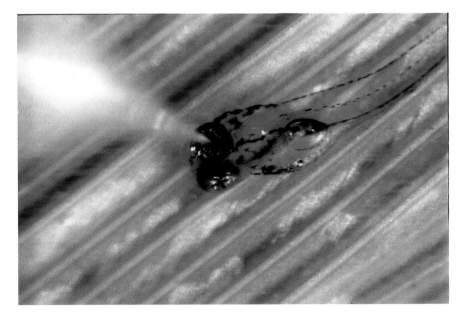

Fig. 1. Picture of a 5 dpf larval zebrafish lying on its side on a wet feather with a glass electrode sitting on the center of the cornea.

The initial slope of the a-wave has been attributed to photoreceptors (Lamb and Pugh, 1992). Figure 2 shows the ERG of a wild-type larva in the presence and absence of APB. Although APB may also affect other pathways such as On transmission from cones to horizontal (Nawy et al., 1989) it has no known effects on the early kinetics of the photoreceptor derived a-wave. We are using APB to characterize photoreceptor adaptation in zebrafish visual mutants.

To date five genes have been cloned in zebrafish based on position (Brownlie et al., 1998; Zhang et al., 1998; Donovan et al., 2000; Kupperman et al., 2000; Zhong et al., 2000). All of these reports were within the last two years and three were from the first half of this year suggesting that the identification of mutant genes through positional cloning is likely to increase exponentially during the next few years. Recent reviews summarize the different approaches that have been used to develop a high resolution genetic map, the genetic "tricks" available in zebrafish that aid in positional cloning, and the molecular

resources available for mapping and positional cloning (Beier, 1998; Talbot and Schier, 1999; Amemiya et al., 1999).

In addition to studies identifying and characterizing mutant zebrafish, several studies have been reported that characterize the development, morphology and physiology of the zebrafish retina (Robinson et al., 1993, 1995; Schmitt and Dowling, 1994, 1999; Raymond et al., 1995; Connaughton and Maguire, 1998; Schmitt et al., 1999; Connaughton and Nelson, 2000). The Dowling laboratory has also played a major role in these studies particularly in characterizing the anatomy of zebrafish retina during development. Furthermore, several papers characterizing the ERG response of larvae have been published (Branchek, 1984; Hughes et al., 1998; Saszik and Bilotta, 1999a, 1999b; Saszik et al., 1999). These studies provide information about the spectral sensitivity and color opponency of fish vision and also information about development of the scotopic and phototopic visual pathways. These studies are critical as a framework on which to analyze retinal mutants.

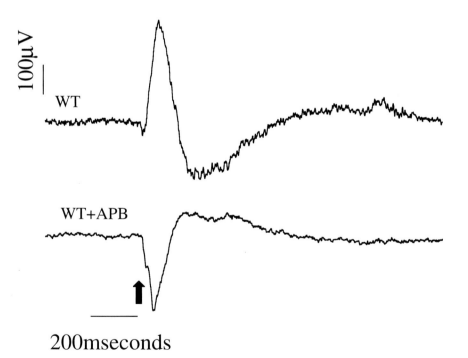

Fig. 2. Wild-type 5 dpf larval zebrafish ERG is the presence and absence of APB. The a-wave is uncovered by the application of 1 mM APB. The arrow indicates light onset. The flash stimulus was less than 1 ms in duration and was produced by a Canon 540EZ Speedlite flash set at 1/16 power. This figure is modified from Van Epps et al. (2001).

636

Conclusion and future perspectives for zebrafish

In zebrafish, genetic screens are done easily at low cost. This enables individual labs to conduct small-scale creative screens for specific types of mutations. Several such screens have been conducted in the Dowling laboratory (Li and Dowling, 1997; Brockerhof et al., 1997; Fadool et al., 1997; Link et al., 2000). I am now conducting similar screens at the University of Washington. For the studies I focus on, the abundance of cones in zebrafish makes it possible to identify mutations that specifically affect cone photoreceptors. These properties, combined with a rapidly improving genetic map, make zebrafish a very attractive model for identifying mutations disrupting cone photoreceptor structure and function. The use of zebrafish will complement genetic studies in mice and humans.

Acknowledgments

The author's research is supported in part by NIH grant EY12373.

References

Akhmedov, N.B., Piriev, N.I., Chang, B., Rapoport, A.L., Hawes, N.L., Nishina, P.M., Nusinowitz, S., Heckenlively, J.R., Roderick, T.H., Kozak, C.A., Danciger, M., Davisson, M.T. and Farber, D.B. (2000) A deletion in a photoreceptor-specific nuclear receptor mRNA causes retinal degeneration in the rd7 mouse. *Proc. Natl. Acad. Sci. USA*, 97: 5551–5556.

Allwardt, B.A. (1999) Ultrastructural analysis of photoreceptors in wildtype and mutant zebrafish larvae. In: *Neurobiology*, Harvard, Cambridge, Massachusetts, p. 211.

Amemiya, C.T., Zhong, T.P., Silverman, G.A., Fishman, M.C. and Zon, L.I. (1999) Zebrafish YAC, BAC, and PAC genomic libraries. *Methods Cell Biol.*, 60: 235–258.

Balkema, G.W., Mangini, N.J., Pinto, L.H. and Vanable, J.W., Jr. (1984) Visually evoked eye movements in mouse mutants and inbred strains. A screening report. *Invest. Ophthalmol. Vis. Sci.*, 25: pp. 795–800.

Banerjee, P., Kleyn, P.W., Knowles, J.A., Lewis, C.A., Ross, B.M., Parano, E., Kovats, S.G., Lee, J.J., Penchaszadeh, G.K., Ott, J., Jacobson, S.G. and Gilliam, T.C. (1998) TULP1 mutation in two extended Dominican kindreds with autosomal recessive retinitis pigmentosa. *Nat. Genet.*, 18: 177–179.

Beier, D.R. (1998) Zebrafish: genomics on the fast track. *Genome Res.*, 8: 9–17.

Branchek, T. (1984) The development of photoreceptors in the zebrafish, *brachydanio rerio*. II. Function. *J. Comp. Neurol.*, 224: 116–122.

Brockerhoff, S.E., Dowling, J.E. and Hurley, J.B. (1998) Zebrafish Retinal Mutants. *Vision Res.*, 38: 1335–1339.

Brockerhoff, S.E., Hurley, J.B., Janssen-Bienhold, U., Neuhauss, C.F., Driever, W. and Dowling, J.E. (1995) A behavioral screen for isolating zebrafish mutants with visual system defects. *Proc. Natl. Acad. Sci. USA*, 92: 10545–10549.

Brockerhoff, S.E., Hurley, J.B., Niemi, G.A. and Dowling, J.E. (1997) A new form of inherited red-blindness identified in zebrafish. *J. Neurosci.*, 20: 1–8.

Brownlie, A., Donovan, A., Pratt, S.J., Paw, B.H., Oates, A.C., Brugnara, C., Witkowska, H.E., Sassa, S. and Zon, L.I. (1998) Positional cloning of the zebrafish sauternes gene: a model for congenital sideroblastic anaemia [see comments]. *Nat. Genet.*, 20: 244–250.

Candille, S.I., Pardue, M.T., McCall, M.A., Peachey, N.S. and Gregg, R.G. (1999) Localization of the mouse nob (no b-wave) gene to the centromeric region of the X chromosome. *Invest. Ophthalmol. Vis. Sci.*, 40: 2748–2751.

Carter-Dawson, L.D. and LaVail, M.M. (1979) Rods and cones in the mouse retina. I. Structural analysis using light and electron microscopy. *J. Comp. Neurol.*, 188: 245–262.

Chang, B., Heckenlively, J.R., Hawes, N.L. and Roderick, T.H. (1993) New mouse primary retinal degeneration (rd-3). *Genomics*, 16: 45–49.

Clark, D.T. (1981) Visual responses in the developing zebrafish (*Brachydanio rerio*). In: *Biology*, University of Oregon, Eugene.

Connaughton, V.P. and Maguire, G. (1998) Differential expression of voltage-gated K+ and Ca2+ currents in bipolar cells in the zebrafish retinal slice. *Eur. J. Neurosci.*, 10: 1350–1362.

Connaughton, V.P. and Nelson, R. (2000) Axonal stratification patterns and glutamate-gated conductance mechanisms in zebrafish retinal bipolar cells [see comments]. *J. Physiol. (Lond.)*, 524(Pt 1): 135–146.

Connell, G., Bascom, R., Molday, L., Reid, D., McInnes, R.R. and Molday, R.S. (1991) Photoreceptor peripherin is the normal product of the gene responsible for retinal degeneration in the rds mouse. *Proc. Natl. Acad. Sci. USA*, 88: 723–726.

Cremers, F.P., van de Pol, D.J., van Driel, M., den Hollander, A.I., van Haren, F.J., Knoers, N.V., Tijmes, N., Bergen, A.A., Rohrschneider, K., Blankenagel, A., Pinckers, A.J., Deutman, A.F. and Hoyng, C.B. (1998) Autosomal recessive retinitis pigmentosa and cone-rod dystrophy caused by splice site mutations in the Stargardt's disease gene ABCR. *Hum. Mol. Genet.*, 7: 355–362.

den Hollander, A.I., ten Brink, J.B., de Kok, Y.J., van Soest, S., van den Born, L.I., van Driel, M.A., van de Pol, D.J., Payne, A.M., Bhattacharya, S.S., Kellner, U., Hoyng, C.B., Westerveld, A., Brunner, H.G., Bleeker-Wagemakers, E.M., Deutman, A.F., Heckenlively, J.R., Cremers, F.P. and Bergen, A.A. (1999) Mutations in a human homologue of Drosophila crumbs cause retinitis pigmentosa (RP12). *Nat. Genet.*, 23: 217–221.

Donovan, A., Brownlie, A., Zhou, Y., Shepard, J., Pratt, S.J., Moynihan, J., Paw, B.H., Drejer, A., Barut, B., Zapata, A., Law, T.C., Brugnara, C., Lux, S.E., Pinkus, G.S., Pinkus, J.L., Kingsley, P.D., Palis, J., Fleming, M.D., Andrews, N.C. and Zon, L.I. (2000) Positional cloning of zebrafish ferroportin1 identifies a conserved vertebrate iron exporter [see comments]. *Nature*, 403: 776–781.

Dowling, J.E. (1987) *The Retina: An Approachable Part of the Brain*. Belknap Press of Harvard University Press, Cambridge.

Dowling, J.E. and Sidman, R.L. (1962) Inherited Retinal Dystrophy in the Rat. *J. Cell Biol.*, 14: 73–109.

Dryja, T.P. (1997) Gene-based approach to human gene-phenotype correlations. *Proc. Natl. Acad. Sci., USA*, 94: 12117–12121.

Dryja, T.P., Berson, E.L., Rao, V.R. and Oprian, D.D. (1993) Heterozygous missense mutation in the rhodopsin gene as a cause of congenital stationary night blindness. *Nat. Genet.*, 4: 280–283.

Fadool, J.M., Brockerhoff, S.E., Hyatt G.A. and Dowing J.E. (1997) Mutation affecting eye morphology in the developing zebrafish *(Danio rerio)*. *Dev. Genet.*, 20: 1–8

Farber, D.B. and Danciger, M. (1997) Identification of genes causing photoreceptor degenerations leading to blindness. *Curr. Opin. Neurobiol.*, 7: 666–673.

Gregory-Evans, K. and Bhattacharya, S.S. (1998) Genetic blindness: current concepts in the pathogenesis of human outer retinal dystrophies. *Trends Genet.* 14: 103–108.

Gu, S., Lennon, A., Li, Y., Lorenz, B., Fossarello, M., North, M., Gal, A. and Wright, A. (1998) Tubby-like protein-1 mutations in autosomal recessive retinitis pigmentosa [letter]. *Lancet*, 351: 1103–1104.

Hagstrom, S.A., North, M.A., Nishina, P.L., Berson, E.L. and Dryja, T.P. (1998) Recessive mutations in the gene encoding the tubby-like protein TULP1 in patients with retinitis pigmentosa. *Nat. Genet.*, 18: 174–176.

Hao, W. and Fong, H.K. (1999) The endogenous chromophore of retinal G protein-coupled receptor opsin from the pigment epithelium. *J. Biol. Chem.*, 274: 6085–6090.

Hawes, N.L., Chang, B., Hageman, G.S., Nusinowitz, S., Nishina, P.M., Schneider, B.S., Smith, R.S., Roderick, T.H., Davisson, M.T. and Heckenlively, J.R. (2000) Retinal degeneration 6 (rd6): A new mouse model for human retinitis punctata albescens. *Invest. Opthalmol. Vis. Sci.*, 41: 3149–3157.

Hawes, N.L., Smith, R.S., Chang, B., Davisson, M., Heckenlively, J.R. and John, S.W. (1999) Mouse fundus photography and angiography: a catalogue of normal and mutant phenotypes. *Mol. Vis.*, 5: 22.

Hughes, A., Saszik, S., Bilotta, J., Demarco, P.J., Jr. and Patterson, W.F., 2nd (1998) Cone contributions to the photopic spectral sensitivity of the zebrafish ERG. *Vis. Neurosci.*, 15: 1029–1037.

Justice, M.J., Noveroske, J.K., Weber, J.S., Zheng, B. and Bradley, A. (1999) Mouse ENU mutagenesis. *Hum. Mol. Genet.*, 8: 1955–1963.

Keeler, C. (1966) Retinal degeneration in the mouse is rodless retina. *J. Hered.*, 57: 47–50.

Kupperman, E., An, S., Osborne, N., Waldron, S. and Stainier, D.Y. (2000) A sphingosine-1-phosphate receptor regulates cell migration during vertebrate heart development. *Nature*, 406: 192–195.

Lamb, T.D. and Pugh, E.N., Jr. (1992) A quantitative account of the activation steps involved in phototransduction in amphibian photoreceptors. *J. Physiol. (Lond.)*, 449: 719–758.

Li L. and Dowling, J.E. (1997) A dominant form of inherited retinal degeneration caused by a non-photoreceptor cell-specific mutation. *Proc. Natl. Acad. Sci. USA*, 94: 11645–11650.

Link, B.A., Fadool, J.M., Malicki, J., and Dowling, J.E. (2000). The Zebrafish young mutation acts non-cell-autonomously to uncouple differentiation from specification for all retinal cells. *Development* 127, 2177–88.

Lolley, R.N. (1994) The rd gene defect triggers programmed rod cell death. The Proctor Lecture [published erratum appears in *Invest. Ophthalmol.* 1995 Mar; 36(3): 520]. *Invest. Ophthalmol. Vis. Sci.*, 35: 4182–4191.

Lolley, R.N., Farber, D.B., Rayborn, M.E. and Hollyfield, J.G. (1977) Cyclic GMP accumulation causes degeneration of photoreceptor cells: simulation of an inherited disease. *Science*, 196: 664–666.

Lyubarsky, A.L., Falsini, B., Pennesi, M.E., Valentini, P. and Pugh, E.N., Jr. (1999) UV- and midwave-sensitive cone-driven retinal responses of the mouse: a possible phenotype for coexpression of cone photopigments. *J. Neurosci.*, 19: 442–455.

Marlhens, F., Bareil, C., Griffoin, J.M., Zrenner, E., Amalric, P., Eliaou, C., Liu, S.Y., Harris, E., Redmond, T.M., Arnaud, B., Claustres, M. and Hamel, C.P. (1997) Mutations in RPE65 cause Leber's congenital amaurosis [letter]. *Nat. Genet.*, 17: 139–141.

Marlhens, F., Griffoin, J.M., Bareil, C., Arnaud, B., Claustres, M. and Hamel, C.P. (1998) Autosomal recessive retinal dystrophy associated with two novel mutations in the RPE65 gene. *Eur. J. Hum. Genet.*, 6: 527–531.

Martinez-Mir, A., Paloma, E., Allikmets, R., Ayuso, C., del Rio, T., Dean, M., Vilageliu, L., Gonzalez-Duarte, R. and Balcells, S. (1998) Retinitis pigmentosa caused by a homozygous mutation in the Stargardt disease gene ABCR [letter; comment]. *Nat. Genet.*, 18: 11–12.

Maw, M.A., Kennedy, B., Knight, A., Bridges, R., Roth, K.E., Mani, E.J., Mukkadan, J.K., Nancarrow, D., Crabb, J.W. and Denton, M.J. (1997) Mutation of the gene encoding cellular retinaldehyde-binding protein in autosomal recessive retinitis pigmentosa. *Nat. Genet.*, 17: 198–200.

Meindl, A., Dry, K., Herrmann, K., Manson, F., Ciccodicola, A., Edgar, A., Carvalho, M.R., Achatz, H., Hellebrand, H., Lennon, A., Migliaccio, C., Porter, K., Zrenner, E., Bird, A., Jay, M., Lorenz, B., Wittwer, B., D'Urso, M., Meitinger, T. and Wright, A. (1996) A gene (RPGR) with homology to the RCC1 guanine nucleotide exchange factor is mutated in X-linked retinitis pigmentosa (RP3). *Nat. Genet.*, 13: 35–42.

Merbs, S.L. and Nathans, J. (1992) Absorption spectra of human cone pigments [see comments]. *Nature*, 356: 433–435.

Molday, L.L., Rabin, A.R. and Molday, R.S. (2000) ABCR, The ABC transporter implicated in Stargardt disease, is expressed in both rod and cone photoreceptor cells. *Nat. Genet.*, 25: 257–258.

Morimura, H., Fishman, G.A., Grover, S.A., Fulton, A.B., Berson, E.L. and Dryja, T.P. (1998) Mutations in the RPE65 gene in patients with autosomal recessive retinitis pigmentosa or leber congenital amaurosis. *Proc. Natl. Acad. Sci. USA*, 95: 3088–3093.

Morimura, H., Saindelle-Ribeaudeau, F., Berson, E.L. and Dryja, T.P. (1999) Mutations in RGR, encoding a light-sensitive opsin homologue, in patients with retinitis pigmentosa [letter]. *Nat. Genet.*, 23: 393–394.

Nawy, S., Sie, A. and Copenhagen, D.R. (1989) The glutamate analog 2-amino-4-phosphonobutyrate antagonizes synaptic transmission from cones to horizontal cells in the goldfish retina. *Proc. Natl. Acad. Sci. USA*, 86: 1726–1730.

Neuhauss, S.C., Biehlmaier, O., Seeliger, M.W., Das, T., Kohler, K., Harris, W.A. and Baier, H. (1999) Genetic disorders of vision revealed by a behavioral screen of 400 essential loci in zebrafish. *J. Neurosci.*, 19: 8603–8615.

Nir, I., Kedzierski, W., Chen, J. and Travis, G.H. (2000) Expression of Bcl-2 protects against photoreceptor degeneration in retinal degeneration slow (rds) mice. *J. Neurosci.*, 20: 2150–2154.

Palczewski, K. and Saari, J.C. (1997) Activation and inactivation steps in the visual transduction pathway. *Curr. Opin. Neurobiol.*, 7: 500–504.

Phelan, J.K. and Bok, D. (2000) A brief review of retinitis pigmentosa and the identified retinitis pigmentosa genes. *Mol. Vis.*, 6: 116–124.

Rattner, A., Sun, H. and Nathans, J. (1999) Molecular genetics of human retinal disease. *Annu. Rev. Genet.*, 33: 89–131.

Raymond, P.A., Barthel, L.K. and Curran, G.A. (1995) Developmental patterning of rod and cone photoreceptors in embryonic zebrafish. *J. Comp. Neurol.*, 359: 537–550.

Redmond, T.M., Yu, S., Lee, E., Bok, D., Hamasaki, D., Chen, N., Goletz, P., Ma, J.X., Crouch, R.K. and Pfeifer, K. (1998) Rpe65 is necessary for production of 11-*cis*-vitamin A in the retinal visual cycle. *Nat. Genet.*, 20: 344–351.

Rick, J.M., Horschke, I. and Neuhauss, S.C. (2000) Optokinetic behavior is reversed in achiasmatic mutant zebrafish larvae. *Curr. Biol.*, 10: 595–598.

Robinson, J., Schmitt, E.A. and Dowling, J.E. (1995) Temporal and spatial patterns of opsin gene expression in zebrafish *(danio rerio)*. *Vis. Neurosci.*, 12: 895–906.

Robinson, J., Schmitt, E.A., Harosi, F.I., Reece, R.J. and Dowling, J.E. (1993) Zebrafish ultraviolet visual pigment: absorption spectrum, sequence, and localization. *Proc. Natl. Acad. Sci., USA*, 90: 6009–6012.

Rosenfeld, P.J., Cowley, G.S., McGee, T.L., Sandberg, M.A., Berson, E.L. and Dryja, T.P. (1992) A null mutation in the rhodopsin gene causes rod photoreceptor dysfunction and

autosomal recessive retinitis pigmentosa. *Nat. Genet.*, 1: 209–213.

Rozet, J.M., Gerber, S., Ghazi, I., Perrault, I., Ducroq, D., Souied, E., Cabot, A., Dufier, J.L., Munnich, A. and Kaplan, J. (1999a) Mutations of the retinal specific ATP binding transporter gene (ABCR) in a single family segregating both autosomal recessive retinitis pigmentosa RP19 and Stargardt disease: evidence of clinical heterogeneity at this locus. *J. Med. Genet.*, 36: 447–451.

Rozet, J.M., Gerber, S., Souied, E., Ducroq, D., Perrault, I., Ghazi, I., Soubrane, G., Coscas, G., Dufier, J.L., Munnich, A. and Kaplan, J. (1999b) The ABCR gene: a major disease gene in macular and peripheral retinal degenerations with onset from early childhood to the elderly. *Mol. Genet. Metab.*, 68: 310–315.

Saari, J.C., Bredberg, D.L. and Noy, N. (1994) Control of substrate flow at a branch in the visual cycle. *Biochemistry*, 33: 3106–3112.

Sanyal, S., De Ruiter, A. and Hawkins, R.K. (1980) Development and degeneration of retina in rds mutant mice: light microscopy. *J. Comp. Neurol.*, 194: 193–207.

Saszik, S. and Bilotta, J. (1999a) Effects of abnormal light-rearing conditions on retinal physiology in larvae zebrafish. *Invest. Ophthalmol. Vis. Sci.*, 40: 3026–3031.

Saszik, S. and Bilotta, J. (1999b) The effects of temperature on the dark-adapted spectral sensitivity function of the adult zebrafish. *Vision Res.*, 39: 1051–1058.

Saszik, S., Bilotta, J. and Givin, C.M. (1999) ERG assessment of zebrafish retinal development. *Vis. Neurosci.*, 16: 881–888.

Schmitt, E.A. and Dowling, J.E. (1994) Early eye morphogenesis in the zebrafish, *Brachydanio rerio*. *J. Comp. Neurol.*, 344: 532–542.

Schmitt, E.A. and Dowling, J.E. (1999) Early retinal development in the zebrafish, *Danio rerio*: light and electron microscopic analyses. *J. Comp. Neurol.*, 404: 515–536.

Schmitt, E.A., Hyatt, G.A. and Dowling, J.E. (1999) Erratum: Temporal and spatial patterns of opsin gene expression in the zebrafish (*Danio rerio*): corrections with additions. *Vis. Neurosci.*, 16: 601–605.

Schwahn, U., Lenzner, S., Dong, J., Feil, S., Hinzmann, B., van Duijnhoven, G., Kirschner, R., Hemberger, M., Bergen, A.A., Rosenberg, T., Pinckers, A.J., Fundele, R., Rosenthal, A., Cremers, F.P., Ropers, H.H. and Berger, W. (1998) Positional cloning of the gene for X-linked retinitis pigmentosa 2 [see comments]. *Nat. Genet.*, 19: 327–332.

Shiells, R.A., Falk, G. and Naghshineh, S. (1981) Action of glutamate and aspartate analogues on rod horizontal and bipolar cells. *Nature*, 294: 592–594.

Slaughter, M.M. and Miller, R.F. (1981) 2-amino-4-phosphonobutyric acid: a new pharmacological tool for retina research. *Science*, 211: 182–185.

Slaughter, M.M. and Miller, R.F. (1985) Characterization of an extended glutamate receptor of the on bipolar neuron in the vertebrate retina. *J. Neurosci.*, 5: 224–233.

Sun, H., Macke, J.P. and Nathans, J. (1997) Mechanisms of spectral tuning in the mouse green cone pigment. *Proc. Natl. Acad. Sci. USA*, 94: 8860–8865.

Sun, H. and Nathans, J. (1997) Stargardt's ABCR is localized to the disc membrane of retinal rod outer segments [letter]. *Nat. Genet.*, 17: 15–16.

Sz'el, A., Rohlich, P., Caffe, A.R., Juliusson, B., Aguirre, G. and Van-Veen, T. (1992) Unique topographic separation of two spectral classes of cones in the mouse retina. *J. Comp. Neurol.*, 325: 327–342.

Sz'el, A., Rohlich, P., Caffe, A.R. and van, V.T. (1996) Distribution of cone photoreceptors in the mammalian retina. *Microsc. Res. Tech.*, 35: 445–462.

Talbot, W.S. and Schier, A.F. (1999) Positional cloning of mutated zebrafish genes. *Methods Cell Biol.*, 60: 259–286.

Taylor, M.R., van Epps, H.A., Kennedy, M.J., Saari, J.C., Hurley, J.B. and Brockerhoff, S.E. (2000) Biochemical analysis of phototransduction and visual cycle in zebrafish larvae. *Methods Enzymol.*, 316: 536–557.

Travis, G.H., Brennan, M.B., Danielson, P.E., Kozak, C.A. and Sutcliffe, J.G. (1989) Identification of a photoreceptor-specific mRNA encoded by the gene responsible for retinal degeneration slow (rds). *Nature*, 338: 70–73.

Van Epps, H. A., Yim, C. M., Hurley, J. B. and Brockerhoff, S.E. (2001). Investigations of photoreceptor synaptic transmission and light adapttion in the zebrafish visual mutant *nrc*. *Invest. Ophthalmol. Vis. Sci.*, 42: in press.

van Nie, R., Ivanyi, D. and Demant, P. (1978) A new H-2-linked mutation, rds, causing retinal degeneration in the mouse. *Tissue Antigens*, 12: 106–108.

Weng, J., Mata, N.L., Azarian, S.M., Tzekov, R.T., Birch, D.G. and Travis, G.H. (1999) Insights into the function of Rim protein in photoreceptors and etiology of Stargardt's disease from the phenotype in abcr knockout mice. *Cell*, 98: 13–23.

Winston, A. and Rando, R.R. (1998) Regulation of isomer-ohydrolase activity in the visual cycle. *Biochemistry*, 37: 2044–2050.

Yokota, T., Shiojiri, T., Gotoda, T. and Arai, H. (1996) Retinitis pigmentosa and ataxia caused by a mutation in the gene for the alpha-tocopherol-transfer protein [letter]. *N. Engl. J. Med.*, 335: 1770–1771.

Zhang, J., Talbot, W.S. and Schier, A.F. (1998) Positional cloning identifies zebrafish one-eyed pinhead as a permissive EGF-related ligand required during gastrulation. *Cell*, 92: 241–251.

Zhong, T.P., Rosenberg, M., Mohideen, M.A., Weinstein, B. and Fishman, M.C. (2000) gridlock, an HLH gene required for assembly of the aorta in zebrafish. *Science*, 287: 1820–1824.

H. Kolb, H. Ripps and S. Wu (Eds.)
Progress in Brain Research, Vol. 131
© 2001 Elsevier Science B.V. All rights reserved

CHAPTER 46

Photoreceptor rescue in an organotypic model of retinal degeneration

Judith Mosinger Ogilvie*

*Fay and Carl Simons Center for Biology of Hearing and Deafness, Central Institute for the Deaf,
4560 Clayton Avenue, and Department of Ophthalmology and Visual Sciences,
Washington University School of Medicine, St. Louis, MO 63110, USA*

Introduction

Retinitis pigmentosa (RP) is a genetically heterogeneous family of degenerative diseases in the retina. It is the leading cause of inherited blindness affecting 100,000 people worldwide. In 1958, results on dietary night blindness led Dowling and Wald (1958) to speculate, "that some forms of hereditary night blindness may possibly involve the failure to synthesize the specific protein of the rods—rod opsin." This observation foreshadowed recent discoveries of mutations in opsin and related genes. The progressive loss of RP was considered unstoppable. However, an explosion of research in this area has led to several possible treatments currently under investigation including transplantation, gene therapy, and trophic factor therapy. Studies using trophic factors may help us to understand the complex signaling pathways involved in the development and death of retinal neurons.

Many excellent genetic models of RP have been developed in the mouse retina, including the well characterized retinal dystrophy (*rd*) mouse (Farber et al., 1994). Rod photoreceptors in the *rd* mouse retina undergo a rapid degeneration within the first 3 weeks postnatal due to a mutation in the

* Tel.: 314-977-0280; Fax: 314-977-0030;
E-mail: jmo@cid.wustl.edu

β-subunit of the cyclic-GMP phosphodiesterase gene (Bowes et al., 1990; Pittler and Baehr, 1991). Cones degenerate more slowly during the lifetime of the animal. However, mouse models of RP present several difficulties for trophic factor studies. The small size of the mouse eye—especially in the young animal—can make intravitreal injections unreliable. Furthermore, metabolic turnover of the vitreous makes it difficult to maintain a known dosage of a drug for an extended time. Alternatively, isolated photoreceptor cell cultures have been used to investigate cell development and degeneration. However, they lack cell–cell interactions that may play an important role in cell survival. We have developed a long-term retinal organ culture model that presents several advantages for investigations of retinal degeneration, providing a controlled environment while maintaining cell–cell interactions (Ogilvie et al., 1999). In this model, postnatal day 2 eyes are enucleated, the retina is isolated from the eyecup and placed photoreceptor side down on a Millicell insert. Organ cultures are maintained in Dulbecco's modified Eagle's medium (DMEM), 10% fetal calf serum, and 1.25 µg/ml fungizone for 27 days in vitro (DIV) at 37°C, 5% CO_2 with feeding every 2–3 days. Overall, the retinal cultures appear healthy and maintain normal and reproducible retinal architecture with clearly distinguished inner and outer nuclear and plexiform layers. During 4 weeks in organ culture, the *rd* mouse retina undergoes photoreceptor degeneration comparable to that seen in vivo with only a monolayer of cell remaining in the outer nuclear layer. Organ cultures do differ from in vivo retinas in several aspects: ganglion cells are lost due to axotomy at the time of culture, outer segment development is incomplete, and the retinas appear thinner than in vivo due to spreading in the dish. Nevertheless, the reproducibility of this retinal organ culture model allows for quantitative analysis of photoreceptor survival in the outer nuclear layer as detailed elsewhere (Ogilvie et al., 1999). The *rd* mouse retinal organ culture has produced a number of interesting findings on inherited retinal degeneration as described below.

Caspase inhibitors diminish *rd* photoreceptor degeneration

Photoreceptor degeneration in the *rd* mouse bears the characteristic hallmarks of programmed cell death, including chromatin condensation and DNA laddering (Chang et al., 1993; Lolley, 1994; Portera-Cailliau et al., 1994). Programmed cell death resulting in apoptosis is characterized by a cascade of molecular events culminating in the activation of specific cysteine proteases known as caspases. Since caspase activation immediately precedes cell death in many models of neuronal degeneration, caspase inhibition could possibly prevent various forms of retinal dystrophy triggered by different genetic defects. *rd* mouse retinas were cultured in the presence of the general caspase inhibitor, boc-aspartyl(Ome)-fluoromethyl ketone (BAF). Fifty μM BAF significantly increased photoreceptor survival in *rd* organ cultures with approximately 50% of the photoreceptors remaining after 4 weeks compared to wild type control retinas (Fig. 1). Few pyknotic nuclei were seen in the BAF treated organ cultures, however many cells in the outer nuclear layer had lost the dense chromatin pattern that is characteristic of healthy, active photoreceptors. Since the initial insult to the photoreceptor cells (i.e. the *rd* mutation) remains unchanged, and since caspases act late in the process of programmed cell death, these results suggest that BAF may block the caspase-induced cell death and thereby delay, but not block, the

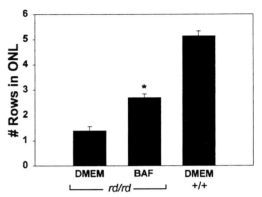

Fig. 1. Thickness of the outer nuclear layer in retinal organ cultures of *rd* and wild type (+/+) retinas treated with control media (DMEM) or with the caspase inhibitor, 50 μM BAF. BAF provided partial protection of *rd* photoreceptors, but showed significant loss compared to wild type controls. *$p<0.001$ vs. *rd* control and +/+ control. Standard error is indicated by bars.

degenerative process. Alternative caspase-independent mechanisms of cell death may be induced by the conditions of the mutant gene, in which case the increased photoreceptor cell survival seen at 27 DIV could disappear within another week. This is consistent with findings which indicate that caspase inhibitors may have therapeutic value where programmed cell death is a response to an acute insult, but are unlikely to be able to maintain the health of the cell in the presence of most chronic defects or injuries (Miller et al., 1997; Werth et al., 2000).

Trophic factor induced rescue of *rd* photoreceptors

Trophic factors are proteins that promote survival of specific cell populations during development and maintain the health of mature cells. They may act upstream in the programmed cell death molecular cascade to prevent or delay cell death. We have investigated the ability of 6 different growth factors individually and in combination to promote the survival of *rd* photoreceptors in retinal organ culture. Brain-derived neurotrophic factor (BDNF), ciliary neurotrophic factor (CNTF), fibroblast growth factor-2 (FGF2), glial cell line-derived neurotrophic factor (GDNF), neurturin, or persephon were added to the media of *rd* retinal organ cultures at a dose of 50 ng/ml each. As previously reported, none of the factors when used alone promoted photoreceptor

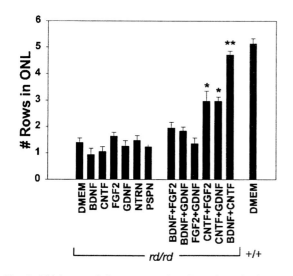

Fig. 2. Thickness of the outer nuclear layer in retinal organ cultures of *rd* and wild type (+/+) retinas treated with control media (DMEM) or with trophic factors for 27 DIV. Individual trophic factors and some combinations showed little effect on photoreceptor survival. CNTF added in combination with BDNF shows in extensive photoreceptor survival, comparable to that seen in wild type retinas. Significant survival was also seen with CNTF+FGF2 or CNTF+GDNF. BDNF, brain-derived neurotrophic factor; CNTF, ciliary neurotrophic factor; FGF2, fibroblast growth factor-2; GDNF, glial derived growth factor; NTRN, neurturin; PSPN, persephon. $*p < 0.001$ vs. *rd* control and +/+ control. $**p < 0.001$ vs. *rd* control but no significant difference from +/+ control. Standard error is indicated by bars.

survival (Ogilvie et al., 2000; Fig. 2). The combination of BDNF and CNTF, however, resulted in extensive photoreceptor survival, comparable to that seen in wild type retinal organ cultures after 27 DIV. CNTF combined with either FGF2 or GDNF produced partial rescue of the photoreceptors; other combinations had no significant effect. The trophic factors that interact to increase photoreceptor survival in the *rd* organ culture model also increase photoreceptor survival in other photoreceptor degeneration models, in many cases acting alone (Faktorovich et al., 1990; Faktorovich et al., 1992; LaVail et al., 1992; Caffé et al., 1993; Jing et al., 1996; Lambiase and Aloe, 1996; Cayouette and Gravel, 1997; Cayouette et al., 1998; Fontaine et al., 1998; LaVail et al., 1998). The synergistic action required in *rd* retinal organ cultures may reflect variation among species, different genetic or environmental models of light damage, and/or differences due to the organ

culture environment. Furthermore, most other models show a partial rescue of photoreceptors with trophic factor application over a period of 2 weeks or less. If the remaining photoreceptors degenerate after another 1–2 weeks, they would not be detected in the organ culture model at the end of the 4-week survival time.

Indirect actions of trophic factors.

The observation that CNTF and BDNF can promote photoreceptor survival is paradoxical in light of current evidence suggesting that the receptors for CNTF and BDNF (CNTFRα and trkB, respectively) are limited to the inner retina and are not expressed in photoreceptors (Perez and Caminos, 1995; Rickman and Brecha, 1995; Koide et al., 1995; Ugolini et al., 1995; Kirsch et al., 1997; Llamosas et al., 1997). This apparent inconsistency may be resolved by trophic factor activation of other retinal cells, which in turn may act indirectly on the photoreceptors (Harada et al., 2000; Ogilvie et al., 2000). For example, CNTF and BDNF may act on Müller cells and/or on retinal pigment epithelium since they interact directly with photoreceptors. Receptors for both trophic factors have also been identified on these cell types. In order to determine whether the trophic factors have an effect on Müller cells in organ culture, we cultured wild type and *rd* retinas with or without CNTF and BDNF for 27 DIV, fixed the tissue, and prepared 10 μm frozen sections for immunohistochemistry. Sections were treated with glial fibrillary acidic protein (GFAP) antiserum (1:1000), followed by incubation in goat-anti-rabbit serum conjugated to Cy3 (1:400). All organ cultures showed intense label of Müller cell processes in the inner retina due to gliosis resulting from the degeneration of ganglion cells following axotomy at the time of culturing (Fig. 3). The vertical Müller cell processes that span the retina were moderately labeled in wild type retinas. Extensive gliosis and intense GFAP immunoreactivity was evident throughout the untreated *rd* retinal culture, comparable to that seen in vivo (Bignami and Dahl, 1979). In contrast, both the wild type and *rd* retinal cultures treated with CNTF and BDNF showed intense labeling of Müller cells, but little or

644

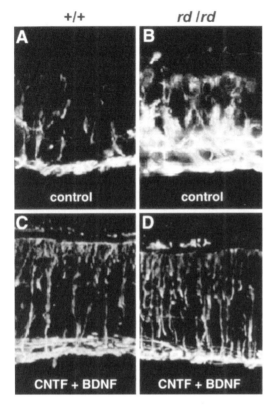

+/+   rd /rd

A   B
control   control

C   D
CNTF + BDNF   CNTF + BDNF

Fig. 3. Retinal organ cultures treated with control media (A, B) or with CNTF and BDNF (C, D) and stained with glial fibrillary acidic protein. All organ cultures show gliosis at the inner margin where ganglion cells have degenerated in vitro. (A) Control wild type organ cultures show moderate staining of Müller cells. (B) Control rd organ cultures show intense Müller cell labeling and extensive gliosis. Both wild type (C) and rd (D) organ cultures treated with growth factors show intense staining of Müller cells, but little gliosis.

no gliosis other than the innermost margin. These results are consistent with findings that CNTF induces GFAP activity in Müller cells and activates the STAT signaling cascade in vivo and in vitro (Peterson et al., 2000; Dudley et al., 2000). Other findings indicate neurotrophin receptor expression on Müller cells is modulated by photoreceptor injury and that subsequent glial-neuronal cell interactions may affect photoreceptor survival (Harada et al., 2000).

Role of dopamine on photoreceptor survival

In addition to Müller cells, CNTF and BDNF receptors have been identified on cells in the amacrine

cell layer. TrkB receptors in particular have been localized on dopaminergic cells (Cellerino and Kohler, 1997). Dopamine is a neuromodulator affecting most, if not all, cell types in the vertebrate retina. Dopamine acts directly on photoreceptor cells in a paracrine fashion through the D_4 receptor (D_2 family) on the inner segments (Cohen et al., 1992; Nguyen-Legros et al., 1999), although its function is still not well understood. We considered the possibility that the protective effects of BDNF and CNTF on photoreceptors in the rd organ culture could be produced by indirect action through a dopaminergic input. This hypothesis would predict that the addition of dopamine antagonists would block the protective effect of CNTF and BDNF on photoreceptors. For control experiments, rd retinal organ cultures were fed daily with media containing either a D_1 or a D_2 family dopamine antagonist (2 μM SCH-23390 or 0.1 μM sulpiride, respectively) for 27 DIV. Surprisingly, either antagonist induced complete survival of rd photoreceptors, despite the absence of the trophic factors (Ogilvie and Speck, 2000; Fig. 4). Since D_1 receptors are not known to be present on photoreceptors, the increased survival resulting from the D_1 antagonist may indicate an indirect pathway. In order to determine whether this result was due to a nonspecific pharmacological effect of the drugs, rd retinal cultures were treated with 100 μM 6-hydroxydopamine (6OHDA), a specific dopaminergic toxin, during the first 2 days in vitro and again with 50 μM 6OHDA on days 7–8. Photoreceptor survival was comparable to wild type controls (Fig. 4A, C). Furthermore, the addition of the dopamine agonist, 2-amino-6,7-dihydroxy-1,2,3,4-tetrahydronaphthalene (ADTN, 20 μM) to 6OHDA-treated cultures induced photoreceptor degeneration comparable to untreated rd organ cultures. These findings demonstrate that the endogenous neuromodulator dopamine is necessary for photoreceptor degeneration and that dopamine inhibition blocks photoreceptor degeneration in the rd organ culture model.

Photoreceptor development and survival

The rd mutation results in a rapid retinal degeneration that begins during the first postnatal week,

A

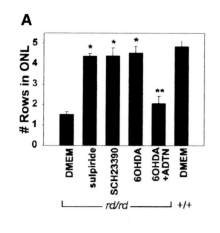

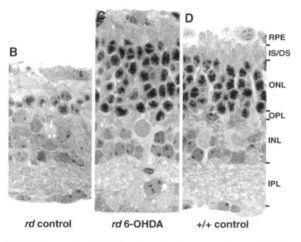

rd control   **rd 6-OHDA**   **+/+ control**

Fig. 4. Dopamine inhibition in retinal organ cultures. (A) The thickness of the outer nuclear layer in retinal organ cultures of *rd* retinas treated with the dopamine antagonists, sulpiride or SCH-23390, or the dopamine toxin, 6OHDA, show complete survival of photoreceptors, with no significant difference compared to wild type (+/+) controls. The addition of the dopamine agonist, ADTN, to 6OHDA treated retinas results in photoreceptor degeneration comparable to untreated *rd* organ cultures. (B–D) Photomicrographs of *rd* (B, C) or wild type (D) organ cultures. (B) The outer nuclear layer is reduced to a monolayer of photoreceptors in the untreated *rd* organ culture. (C) *rd* cultures treated with 6OHDA maintain photoreceptors with a robust appearance, morphologically indistinguishable from untreated wild type retinal cultures (D). RPE, retinal pigment epithelium; IS/OS, inner and outer segments; ONL, outer nuclear layer; OPL, outer plexiform layer; INL, inner nuclear layer; IPL, inner plexiform layer. $*p < 0.001$ vs. *rd* control but no significant difference from +/+ control. $**p < 0.001$ vs. wild type control but no significant difference from *rd* control. Standard error is indicated by bars.

with nearly complete loss of rod photoreceptors by maturity. Photoreceptors never develop normal outer segments in the *rd* mouse. This rapid degeneration provides a practical model for screening possible therapeutic agents. However many factors associated with neuronal survival also play significant roles in neuronal development or vice-versa. Dopamine decreases growth cone motility and neurite extension in retinal cells (Lankford et al., 1987; Lankford et al., 1988; dos Santos Rodrigues and Dowling, 1990). BDNF is necessary for normal development of retinal dopaminergic neurons (Cellerino et al., 1998). Exogenous CNTF has significant species-dependent effects on photoreceptor development and differentiation, although endogenous CNTF is quite low during this period. For example, embryonic chick retina responds to CNTF with a threefold increase in opsin-expressing cells (Fuhrmann et al., 1995), while neonatal rat retinas lose almost 90% of their opsin-expressing cells. Ezzeddine et al. (1997) have proposed that CNTF induces isolated rat rod precursors to transdifferentiate into bipolar cells as determined by immunolabeling of opsin and bipolar cell markers. In the *rd* organ culture treated with CNTF alone, photoreceptors clearly develop, differentiate, and degenerate just as seen in vivo. The addition of CNTF combined with other factors results in the development of an outer nuclear layer containing cells with morphological characteristics of photoreceptors. Thus, CNTF is unlikely to cause rod precursors to transdifferentiate in this system. However, recent evidence suggests that overexpression of the CNTF family member leukemia inhibitory factor during development of the mouse eye results in the inhibition or delay of photoreceptor terminal differentiation as indicated by outer segment assembly and opsin expression (Ash et al., 1997).

To further investigate a developmental role, *rd* retinas were grown in organ culture with or without the addition of CNTF and BDNF, or with dopamine antagonists, or 6OHDA as described above. After 27 DIV, the tissue was fixed and frozen sections were prepared for immunohistochemistry. The sections were incubated with Rho4D2 antibody to opsin (1:1000; kindly provided by Dr. David Hicks), washed, and stained with goat

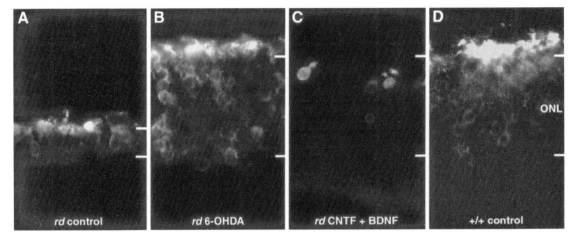

Fig. 5. Photomicrographs of organ cultures labeled with opsin after 27 DIV. (A) Opsin-like immunoreactivity was seen in the diminished outer nuclear layer of the control *rd* organ culture with a few residual inner segments. (B) Opsin-like immunoreactivity was seen throughout the outer nuclear layer with intense staining of inner/outer segment material in *rd* organ cultures treated with the dopamine toxin, 6OHDA. (C) Opsin-like immunoreactivity was limited to a few scattered cells in the outer nuclear layer of *rd* organ cultures treated with CNTF and BDNF. (D) Opsin-like immunoreactivity was seen throughout the outer nuclear layer of the control wild type organ cultures with intense staining of inner/outer segment material.

antiserum conjugated to mouse Cy3 (1:500). Untreated *rd* and wild type organ cultures showed intense labeling of remaining inner and outer segments as well as cells throughout the outer nuclear layer (Fig. 5A, D). The same labeling pattern was observed in cultures treated with 6OHDA (Fig. 5B) or dopamine antagonists (Ogilvie and Speck, 2000). Only a few intensely labeled cells were scattered through the outer nuclear layer in cultures treated with CNTF and BDNF suggesting that this combination of trophic factors decreases opsin expression in photoreceptors (Fig. 5C). These results indicate that CNTF and BDNF do not rescue rod photoreceptors from degeneration induced by the mutant cGMP-PDE gene, nor do they induce rod precursors to transdifferentiate into bipolar cells. Instead, they suppress or delay the expression of opsin and most likely other genes in the phototransduction pathway. If the mutant cGMP-PDE is not expressed in rod photoreceptors, it cannot cause cell death. A failure to express opsin, however, leads to the degeneration of photoreceptors over several months (Lem et al., 1999), as compared to several weeks in the *rd* retina. We predict that a similar fate would occur in immature photoreceptors treated with these trophic factors, if the opsin expression remains suppressed.

Conclusions and future perspectives

The *rd* retinal organ culture is a useful model to investigate the effects of exogenous and endogenous agents on photoreceptor development and degeneration. With this model we have found that caspase inhibitors can delay, but not block photoreceptor degeneration. CNTF and BDNF, and other trophic factor combinations, delay differentiation, which in turn, delays degeneration. Although this result does not support a therapeutic role for trophic factors, it presents new questions concerning the role of these factors in terminal differentiation of photoreceptors. If the neurotrophic factors act indirectly on photoreceptors, what other cell types are involved? What is the molecular mechanism underlying the suppression of opsin expression? How does this differ from the mature retina? What roles do endogenous CNTF and BDNF play in photoreceptor development?

Significantly, organ culture results suggest that dopamine inhibition does not delay terminal differentiation as indicated by opsin expression, but does block photoreceptor degeneration. The mechanism underlying photoreceptor survival induced by dopamine antagonists or dopamine depletion is currently under investigation.

More than 4 decades ago, Dowling and Wald made significant discoveries about dietary photoreceptor degeneration, which in turn led to important observations concerning hereditary photoreceptor degeneration. Later, as work in his lab shifted toward retinal circuitry, John Dowling and his colleagues identified the dopaminergic interplexiform cell, which initiated 25 years of investigation into the role of dopamine in the vertebrate retina. These two areas of investigation, which appeared to be independent, are now linked by the finding that dopamine plays a role in photoreceptor cell degeneration. Our ultimate understanding of the complex interactions within the retina will owe much to John's broad efforts to untangle retinal organization, function, and structure, and to his mentoring of generations of scientists working in this field.

Acknowledgments

I thank David Hicks for supplying the Rho4D2 antibody; Judith D. Speck, Jaclynn M. Lett, Albert Vinson, Jr., Alisen B. Huske for technical assistance. This work was supported in part by NIH grant NS01756 and the Foundation Fighting Blindness.

References

Ash, J.D., Rapp, L.M. and Overbeek, P.A. (1997) Photoreceptor development is blocked by the lens-specific expression of leukemia inhibitory factor (LIF). *Invest. Ophthalmol. Vis. Sci.*, 38: S226.

Bignami, A. and Dahl, D. (1979) The radial glia of Muller in the rat retina and their response to injury. An immunofluorescence study with antibodies to the glial fibrillary acidic (GFA) protein. *Exp. Eye Res.*, 28: 63–69.

Bowes, C., Li, T., Dancinger, M., Baxter, L.C., Applebury, M.L. and Farber, D.B. (1990) Retinal degeneration in the *rd* mouse is caused by a defect in the β subunit of rod cGMP-phosphodiesterase. *Nature*, 347: 677–680.

Caffé, A.R., Söderpalm, A. and van Veen, T. (1993) Photoreceptor-specific protein expression of mouse retina in organ culture and retardation of *rd* degeneration *in vitro* by a combination of basic fibroblast and nerve growth factors. *Curr. Eye Res.*, 12: 719–726.

Cayouette, M., Behn, D., Sendtner, M., Lachapelle, P. and Gravel, C. (1998) Intraocular gene transfer of ciliary neurotrophic factor prevents death and increases responsiveness of rod photoreceptors in the *retinal degeneration slow* mouse. *J. Neurosci.*, 18: 9282–9293.

Cayouette, M. and Gravel, C. (1997) Adenovirus-mediated gene transfer of ciliary neurotrophic factor can prevent photoreceptor degeneration in the retinal degeneration (*rd*) mouse. *Hum. Gene Ther.*, 8: 423–430.

Cellerino, A. and Kohler, K. (1997) Brain-derived neurotrophic factor/neurotrophin-4 receptor TrkB is localized on ganglion cells and dopaminergic amacrine cells in the vertebrate retina. *J. Comp. Neurol.*, 386: 149–160.

Cellerino, A., Pinzón-Duarte, G., Carroll, P. and Kohler, K. (1998) Brain-derived neurotrophic factor modulates the development of the dopaminergic network in the rodent retina. *J. Neurosci.*, 18: 3351–3362.

Chang, G.-Q., Hao, Y. and Wong, F. (1993) Apoptosis: final common pathway of photoreceptor death in *rd*, *rds*, and rhodopsin mutant mice. *Neuron*, 11: 595–605.

Cohen, A.I., Todd, R.D., Harmon, S. and O'Malley, K.L. (1992) Photoreceptors of mouse retinas possess D4 receptors coupled to adenylate cyclase. *Proc. Natl. Acad. Sci USA*, 89: 12093–12097.

dos Santos Rodrigues, P. and Dowling, J.E. (1990) Dopamine induces neurite retraction in retinal horizontal cells via diacylglycerol and protein kinase C. *Proc. Natl. Acad. Sci. USA*, 87: 9693–9697.

Dowling, J.E. and Wald, G. (1958) Vitamin A deficiency and night blindness. *Proc. Natl. Acad. Sci. USA*, 44: 648–661.

Dudley, V.J., Wang, Y., Li, C., Kuzmanovic, M., Smith, S., Ogilvie, J. and Sarthy, V. (2001) Jak-Stat-mediated regulation of GFAP expression in Müller cells. *Invest. Ophthalmol. Vis. Sci.*, Suppl. 42: in press.

Ezzeddine, Z.D., Yang, X., DeChiara, T., Yancopoulos, G. and Cepko, C.L. (1997) Postmitotic cells fated to become rod photoreceptors can be respecified by CNTF treatment of the retina. *Development*, 124: 1055–1067.

Faktorovich, E.G., Steinberg, R.H., Yasumura, D., Matthes, M.T. and LaVail, M.M. (1990) Photoreceptor degeneration in inherited retinal dystrophy delayed by basic fibroblast growth factor. *Nature*, 347: 83–86.

Faktorovich, E.G., Steinberg, R.H., Yasumura, D., Matthes, M.T. and LaVail, M.M. (1992) Basic fibroblast growth factor and local injury protect photoreceptors from light damage in the rat. *J. Neurosci.*, 12: 3554–3567.

Farber, D.B., Flannery, J.G. and Bowes-Rickman, C. (1994) The *rd* mouse story: seventy years of research on an animal model of inherited retinal degeneration. *Prog. Ret. Eye Res.*, 13: 31–64.

Fontaine, V., Kinkl, N., Sahel, J., Dreyfus, H. and Hicks, D. (1998) Survival of purified rat photoreceptors *in vitro* is stimulated directly by fibroblast growth factor-2. *J. Neurosci.*, 18: 9662–9672.

Fuhrmann, S., Kirsch, M. and Hofmann, H.-D. (1995) Ciliary neurotrophic factor promotes chick photoreceptor development in vitro. *Development*, 121: 2695–2706.

Harada, T., Harada, C., Nakayama, N., Okuyama, S., Yoshida, K., Kohsaka, S., Matsuda, H. and Wada, K. (2000) Modification of glial–neuronal cell interactions prevents photoreceptor apoptosis during light-induced retinal degeneration. *Neuron*, 26: 533–541.

Jing, S., Wen, D., Yu, Y., Holst, P.L., Luo, Y., Fang, M., Tamir, R., Antonio, L., Hu, Z., Cupples, R., Louis, J.-C., Hu, S., Altrock, B.W. and Fox, G.M. (1996) GDNF-induced activation of the ret protein tyrosine kinase is mediated by GDNFR-alpha, a novel receptor for GDNF. *Cell*, 85: 1113–1124.

Kirsch, M., Lee, M.-Y., Meyer, V., Wiese, A. and Hofmann, H.-D. (1997) Evidence for multiple, local functions of ciliary neurotrophic factor (CNTF) in retinal development: expression of CNTF and its receptors and in vitro effects on target cells. *J. Neurochem.*, 68: 979–990.

Koide, T., Takahashi, J.B., Hoshimaru, M., Kojima, M., Otsuka, T., Asahi, M. and Kikuchi, H. (1995) Localization of trkB and low-affinity nerve growth factor receptor mRNA in the developing rat retina. *Neurosci. Lett.*, 185: 183–186.

Lambiase, A. and Aloe, L. (1996) Nerve growth factor delays retinal degeneration in C3H mice. *Graefe's Arch. Clin. Exp. Ophthalmol.*, 234: S96–S100.

Lankford, K., De Mello, F.G. and Klein, W.L. (1987) A transient embryonic dopamine receptor inhibits growth cone motility and neurite outgrowth in a subset of avian retina neurons. *Neurosci. Lett.*, 75: 169–174.

Lankford, K.L., DeMello, F.G. and Klein, W.L. (1988) D1-type dopamine receptors inhibit growth cone motility in cultured retina neurons: evidence that neurotransmitters act as morphogenic growth regulators in the developing central nervous system. *Proc. Natl. Acad. Sci. USA*, 85: 4567–4571.

LaVail, M.M., Unok, K., Yasumura, D., Matthes, M.T., Yancopoulos, G.D. and Steinberg, R.H. (1992) Multiple growth factors, cytokines, and neurotrophins rescue photoreceptors from the damaging effects of constant light. *Proc. Natl. Acad. Sci. USA*, 89: 11249–11253.

LaVail, M.M., Yasumura, D., Matthes, M.T., Lau-Villacorta, C., Unoki, K., Sung, C.-H. and Steinberg, R.H. (1998) Protection of mouse photoreceptors by survival factors in retinal degenerations. *Invest. Ophthalmol. Vis. Sci.*, 39: 592–602.

Lem, J., Krasnoperova, N., Calvert, P., Kosaras, B., Cameron, D., Nicolo, M., Makino, C. and Sidman, R. (1999) Morphological, physiological, and biochemical changes in rhodopsin knockout mice. *Proc. Natl. Acad. Sci. USA*, 96: 736–741.

Llamosas, M., Cernuda-Cernuda, R., Huerta, J., Vega, J. and García-Fernández, J. (1997) Neurotrophin receptors expression in the developing mouse retina: an immunohistochemical study. *Anat. Embryol.*, 195: 337–344.

Lolley, R.N. (1994) The *rd* gene defect triggers programmed rod cell death. *Invest. Ophthalmol. Vis. Sci.*, 35: 4182–4191.

Miller, T.M., Moulder, K.L., Knudson, C.M., Creedon, D.J., Deshmukh, M., Korsmeyer, S.J. and Johnson, E.M., Jr. (1997) BAX deletion further orders the cell death pathway in cerebellar granule cells and suggests a caspase-independent pathway to cell death. *J. Cell Biol.*, 139: 205–217.

Nguyen-Legros, J., Versaux-Botteri, C. and Vernier, P. (1999) Dopamine receptor localization in the mammalian retina. *Mol. Neurobiol.*, 19: 181–204.

Ogilvie, J.M. and Speck, J.D. (2000) Dopamine inhibition increases photoreceptor survival in *rd* mouse retinal organ cultures. *Invest. Ophthalmol. Vis. Sci.*, Suppl. 41: S332.

Ogilvie, J.M., Speck, J.D. and Lett, J.M. (2000) Growth factors in combination, but not individually, rescue *rd* mouse photoreceptors in organ culture. *Exp. Neurol.*, 161: 676–685.

Ogilvie, J.M., Speck, J.D., Lett, J.M. and Fleming, T.T. (1999) A reliable method for organ culture of neonatal mouse retina with long-term survival. *J. Neurosci. Meth.*, 87: 57–65.

Perez, M.-T.R. and Caminos, E. (1995) Expression of brain-derived neurotrophic factor and of its functional receptor in neonatal and adult rat retina. *Neurosci. Lett.*, 183: 96–99.

Peterson, W., Wang, Q., Tzekova, R. and Wiegand, S. (2000) Ciliary neurotrophic factor and stress stimuli activate the Jak-STAT pathway in retinal neurons and glia. *J. Neurosci.*, 20: 4081–4090.

Pittler, S.J. and Baehr, W. (1991) Identification of a nonsense mutation in the rod photoreceptor cGMP phosphodiesterase β-subunit gene of the *rd* mouse. *Proc. Natl. Acad. Sci. USA*, 88: 8322–8326.

Portera-Cailliau, C., Sung, C.-H., Nathans, J. and Adler, R. (1994) Apoptotic photoreceptor cell death in mouse models of retinitis pigmentosa. *Proc. Natl. Acad. Sci. USA*, 91: 974–978.

Rickman, D.W. and Brecha, N.C. (1995) Expression of the proto-oncogene, trk, receptors in the developing rat retina. *Vis. Neurosci.*, 12: 215–222.

Ugolini, G., Cremisi, F. and Maffei, L. (1995) TrkA, TrkB, and p75 mRNA expression is developmentally regulated in the rat retina. *Brain Res.*, 704: 121–124.

Werth, J., Deshmukh, M., Cocabo, J., Johnson Jr., E. and Rothman, S. (2000) Reversible physiological alterations in sympathetic neurons deprived of NGF but protected from apoptosis by caspase inhibition or Bax deletion. *Exp. Neurol.*, 161: 203–211.

H. Kolb, H. Ripps and S. Wu (Eds.)
Progress in Brain Research, Vol. 131
© 2001 Elsevier Science B.V. All rights reserved

CHAPTER 47

Rod–cone interdependence: implications for therapy of photoreceptor cell diseases

José Alain Sahel*, Saddek Mohand-Said, Thierry Léveillard, David Hicks,
Serge Picaud and Henri Dreyfus

*Laboratoire de Physiopathologie Cellulaire et Moléculaire de la Rétine, EMI 9918 INSERM,
Université Louis Pasteur and Clinique Médicale A, Hôpitaux Universitaires de Strasbourg,
1 Place de l'Hôpital, 67091 Strasbourg Cedex, France*

Introduction

The retina, as an "approachable part of the brain", provides a unique site to explore the mechanisms of cell death and rescue in neuronal degeneration. Moreover, the number of currently untreatable blinding retinal conditions such as hereditary retinal degenerations has stimulated important research initiatives during the past decade. As a key researcher in the field John Dowling has described many relevant animal models and unravelled several mechanisms underlying retinal phototransduction and circuitry. These contributions are today crucial in understanding the pathogenesis of retinal diseases and designing pharmacological approaches to therapy. I remember proposing more than 10 years ago to John a hypothesis linking photoreceptor cell death in the *rd* mouse to the elevation of cGMP. His positive appreciation and further support at difficult periods have certainly been of utmost importance to the development, in line with these early discussions, of the research presented here.

Accumulating evidence from both molecular biology and physiological studies indicate that, in retinitis pigmentosa (RP), also termed rod–cone dystrophy,

not only are most mutations expressed exclusively in rods but also secondary degeneration of genetically normal cones occurs almost invariably after rod depletion. Loss of cone-mediated light adapted vision is actually the key event leading to blindness in these patients. For instance, patients affected with congenital stationary night blindness can still live a normal life in our modern artificially lit environment (Wright, 1997). Prevention of cone cell death and by inference retention of cone function might represent a very promising therapeutic approach for humans affected with this currently untreatable group of diseases. Among several putative mechanisms, the loss of trophic support occurring as a consequence of rod degeneration is now supported by experimental evidence. We describe herein alongside our studies, current knowledge and concepts on trophic rod–cone interactions during development and disease and their clinical significance.

Sequential degeneration of rods and cones in animal and human conditions

Photoreceptor cell interactions during development

Cell–cell interactions operate during cell specification, patterning and differentiation of the retina in both invertebrates and vertebrates. The role of cell–cell

* Corresponding author: José Alain Sahel, Tel.: + 333 88 11 61 37;
Fax: + 333 88 11 63 41; E-mail:sahel@neurochem.u-strasbg.fr

interactions and the signalling pathways involved in photoreceptor patterning have been most extensively studied in *Drosophila*, in which the analytical power of genetics coupled with the crystalline arrangement of the 750 ommatidia within the compound eye have been driving forces. A full treatment of the subject is beyond the scope of the present article (reviewed in Freeman, 1997) and we will only mention the major breakthroughs that have contributed to our current knowledge of photoreceptor development and differentiation.

Given the importance of *hh* in *Drosophila* eye development it was only natural that its role should be investigated in vertebrates. Jensen and Wallace (1997) showed that sonic hedgehog *Shh* was mitogenic for retinal precursors in reaggregate but not monolayer mouse embryonic retinal cultures, leading to increased numbers of many cell types. Corresponding temporal and spatial expression of *ptc* was also observed, and their results hence suggest a role for this pathway in regulating retinal cell numbers. Somewhat different results were obtained by Levine et al. (1997) using a mixed monolayer rat retinal culture system, in which selective stimulation of rod photoreceptor differentiation was observed. Furthermore this latter study demonstrated the presence of *Ihh* in the adjoining RPE, suggesting this may function in signalling between the RPE and photoreceptors. There are many further examples of the role of cell–cell interactions in determining cell fate within the retina. The epidermal growth factor receptor (EGFR) signalling pathway has been shown to be very important in retinal development both in invertebrates and vertebrates. Once again most detailed genetic analyses have been possible in *Drosophila*, where the crucial role of EGFR in retinal cell type determination and differentiation has been intensively investigated (Baker and Rubin, 1989; Freeman, 1996; Kumar et al., 1998). Within the rat retina, EGF can switch cell fates away from rods and towards Müller glia (Lillien, 1995). It has also been shown that EGF can delay rod differentiation through stimulating activation of a transcription factor, Mash-1 (Ahmad et al., 1998), and that EGF actually induces rod cell death at later developmental stages (Fontaine et al., 1998).

Considering in a stricter sense those interactions, which may occur between cones and rods, substantial

data are also available. In most species cone cells are among the first retinal cell types to leave the cell cycle, whereas rods are generally among the last to do so (Cepko et al., 1996). The concept that cones may constitute a default photoreceptor phenotype came from studies by Adler and Hatlee (1989), in which examination of monodispersed cultures established from early embryonic chick retinas revealed high numbers of cones, whereas this proportion decreased as a function of increasing embryonic age of the donor. Such data suggested that the cone phenotype would form in the absence of environmental cues, constituting a default pathway. Somewhat similar conclusions were reached by Harris and Messersmith (1992), using cultures of embryonic *Xenopus* retina in which two successive inductions were necessary to specify rod fate. However, evidence for a rather different scheme of events is also emerging, that rod differentiation is a necessary prerequisite for cone differentiation. In *Drosophila*, it has recently been shown that specification of opsin expression in R7 may occur autonomously, whereas this partner is responsible for the decision of R8 (the founder photoreceptor of the ommatidial unit and considered analogous to cones) to express either induced or default cell fates (Chou et al., 1999). Evidence from Stenkamp et al. (1996) and Raymond et al. (1995) suggests highly ordered inductive interactions occur between cones and rods to organise the differentiating photoreceptor mosaic in the goldfish retina. They showed that the first photoreceptors to differentiate are in fact a precocious population of rods, present in a small ventronasally located patch. Additional rods were recruited in proximity to this region, extending gradually across the retina. Cone opsin mRNA expression commenced after that of rod opsin, and followed a predictable order of spectral cell types: red followed by green followed by blue followed by ultraviolet (Raymond et al., 1995; Stenkamp et al., 1996). So despite the fact that cones leave the cell cycle earlier than rods in fish as in many other species (Raymond and Fernald, 1981), it appears to be the latter that trigger and coordinate photoreceptor differentiation. The authors additionally suggested that the precocious rod population may be distinct from rods generated later (Stenkamp et al., 1996). Similar conclusions for two distinct rod photoreceptor populations were drawn for differentiating rat retina (Morrow et al., 1998). The sequence of cone differentiation is thought to be due to either lateral cell–cell interactions or liberation of diffusible molecules. An analogous but controversial situation exists in mammals, since conflicting data in primate retinas have indicated the initial expression of either red-green cone (Wikler and Rakic, 1991) or rod and blue cone opsin (Bumsted et al., 1997). Additional data in bovine retina also indicates rods may trigger the onset of cone functionality. Although cones exit the cell cycle early in development of the bovine retina, the transcriptional levels of two cone-specific messenger RNAs (red cone opsin, blue cone γ sub-unit of cGMP phosphodiesterase) remain uniformly low for many weeks. It is not until rod photoreceptor precursors stop dividing much later in embryogenesis and commence their own differentiation (increased transcription of rod opsin, rod β sub-unit of cGMP phosphodiesterase mRNAs) that cones follow suit as though having waited for some inductive or permissive signal (DesJardin et al., 1993; van Ginkel and Hauswirth, 1994; van Ginkel et al., 1995). Finally, unidentified diffusible polypeptides secreted by quail embryonic neural retinal cultures specifically stimulate differentiation of the cone homologue within pineal glands (Araki 1997). It should be mentioned that recent data indicate that interactions might also exist in the opposite direction, and that in mice cones might be important for rod development. This stems from the observation that age-related rod degeneration was observed in coneless transgenic mice (Ying et al., 2000).

In summary to this section, one could speculate that crosstalk between rods and cones seems to be common place and occurs throughout the different steps of development, differentiation and maintenance.

Cone degeneration in retinitis pigmentosa

Mutations in virtually every identified protein of photoreceptor outer segments (OS) have been found associated with RP phenotypes. These include mutations in the visual pigment rhodopsin (Berson et al., 1991, Rosenfeld et al., 1992, Li et al., 1994), enzymes of the phototransduction cascade [transducin (Dryja et al., 1996), guanylate cyclase (Perrault et al., 1996), cGMP-dependent phosphodiesterase (McLaughlin et al., 1993)] and structural or trafficking proteins [peripherin/rds, ROM-1 (Kajiwara et al., 1994, Dryja et al., 1997), ABCR-RIM (Allikmets et al., 1997)]. Yet clues to understanding and eventually counteracting the events leading to photoreceptor cell death are still awaited. Most mutations selectively affect rods. These cells, which are responsible for peripheral and scotopic vision, die for unknown reasons by apoptosis (Chang et al., 1993), a mechanism of programmed cell death often related to growth factor deprivation and/or disorganization of the cell cycle. Cones, which are involved in color, photopic and high contrast vision, are rarely directly affected by the identified mutations, and yet in many cases these cells degenerate secondarily to rods, accounting for loss of central vision and blindness. Cideciyan et al. (1998) found that cone degeneration was observable in patients harbouring rhodopsin mutations once rod outer segment degeneration (as determined by physiological criteria) exceeded 75%. In this study, examination of rod and cone dysfunction in 18 different human rhodopsin mutations demonstrated that cone loss was spatially and temporally correlated to that of rods. The same sequence has been described in many animal models with spontaneous or targeted mutations leading to rod dysfunction and death. Animal models of inherited retinal degeneration show very similar aetiologies: the retinal degeneration (*rd*) mouse is a naturally occurring mutant strain exhibiting mutations in the gene coding for the β sub-unit of rod cGMP phosphosphodiesterase (Farber, 1995), as seen in some forms of human RP (McLaughlin et al., 1993). In this animal, rod degeneration is rapid and practically complete within one month of postnatal age, and is followed by more gradual progressive cone disappearance death (Carter-Dawson et al., 1978, Farber, 1995). Many transgenic strains have been prepared in which abnormal rhodopsin genes have been inserted, resembling the different forms of human RP. These include mice (Kedzierski et al., 1997), rats (Liu et al., 1999) and pigs (Petters et al., 1997), and invariably rod cells degenerate and die as a result of the mutation. In all these above examples for which data is available, subsequent to the initial phase of rod cell loss there is a second wave of cone cell loss. Transgenic mice in which rod photoreceptors are ablated with toxic transgenes also show secondary cone defects (McCall et al., 1996).

Ageing of the photoreceptor mosaic

The repercussion upon cones of pathogenic mechanisms initially affecting rods is not restricted to rod–cone dystrophies. Although the pathogenic events might be different in RP and macular degenerations, the importance of rod survival and function for RPE and cone physiology and survival is receiving increasing attention. This may even be relevant in the progression of age-related macular degeneration (ARMD), the leading cause of blindness after 50 years of age, affecting more than 8 million people in countries where epidemiological data are available. In a minority of patients with neovascular complications, ablative treatments (laser, photodynamic therapy, surgery or radiation therapy) can postpone the loss of central vision for an average interval of 18 months. No treatment is available for the more frequent atrophic form. Although most histopathologic and clinical studies incriminate RPE cells as the primary site of lesions in ARMD, some data point toward initial photoreceptor damage at the level of a dense rim of rods surrounding the fovea (5°). These include: (1) evidence by Curcio et al. (1993, 1996), from several carefully performed quantitative post-mortem studies, showing early rod cell death in ageing and ARMD; (2) the predictive value of scotopic functional testing in early ARMD (Sunness et al., 1989) and most recently by Owsley et al. (2000) finding regional differences in the retinal dark-adapted sensitivity loss of ARMD patients, incriminating rod vulnerability; (3) identification within retinal dystrophies displaying RPE alterations (pattern dystrophies, Stargardt's disease) of mutations in photoreceptors suggesting the primary defect does not occur at the level of the RPE (Bird et al., 1995; Allikmets et al., 1997). The sequence of events encountered in RP (i.e. cones die after rods) might therefore also be relevant to ARMD.

Putative mechanisms linking rod and cone cell death

In both ARMD and RP, prevention of cone cell death represents a very worthy and promising approach. Irrespective of the mutation the final common pathway of rod degeneration is apoptosis;

the mechanism underlying cone death remains unknown.

It is easy to imagine one of several non-mutually exclusive scenarios to account for this delayed cone loss (reviewed in Milam et al., 1998; Petters et al., 1997).

(a) In the first, rod breakdown would adversely affect neighbouring cones through non-specific environmental influences. The progressive disintegration of the surrounding far more numerous rods might leave the cone outer segments more vulnerable to toxic insults. Rods die by apoptosis, which normally avoids release of potentially toxic cellular metabolites, hence preventing extension of cellular breakdown to surrounding regions of tissues. It seems nevertheless possible that degeneration of the abundant rods (about twenty fold more numerous than cones in many mammalian species including man) could exert adverse effects upon the adjacent cones. Certainly, if rods were releasing general toxic by-products one would expect other nearby cell types, such as the immediately post-synaptic partners of photoreceptors, the bipolar cells, to die as well. Although there are some modifications of inner retinal neurones following photoreceptor loss they do not undergo widespread death. Preliminary data clearly indicate that excitotoxic mechanisms are present at early stages of the degenerative process in the *rd* mouse and that they account partially for inner retinal cell death loss and unexpectedly photoreceptor cell death (Meyer et al., submitted). Still, this mechanism of cone cell death should not persist once all rods have disappeared. Furthermore, each cone is individually surrounded by an insoluble glycocalyx that forms a privileged structural microdomain linking each cone to an RPE cell. Death by toxicity may therefore occur as an early limited event.

(b) Changes in the structural and biochemical microenvironment might also induce cone cell degeneration e.g. loss of structural support by neighbouring rods, alterations of the interphotoreceptor matrix, which contains factors promoting cone survival (Hewitt et al., 1990).

(c) Recent electrophysiological analyses of transgenic pigs containing mutant rhodopsin genes indicate failure of cone circuitry maturation, localised to hyperpolarizing cells post-synaptic to the middle wavelength-sensitive cones. These abnormalities occur prior to any alteration of cone photoreceptor physiology (Banin et al., 1999). These findings point towards a potential mechanism of cell–cell interaction that could be linked to the demonstration of intense neurite sprouting by rods, horizontal and bipolar cells in post-mortem retinas from patients with RP (Milam et al., 1998; Fariss et al., 2000). Failure to establish appropriate synaptic connections is a well known mechanism of neuronal degeneration (Oppenheim, 1991, Jacobson et al., 1997).

(d) Secondary changes at the level of the RPE and of glial cells including microglia (migration and proliferation) have been constantly described and could interfere with normal PR development, differentiation and survival.

Another explanation, which if true could have far-reaching implications, is that rods produce some kind of signal that is essential for maintaining cone viability, so that the disappearance of rods for whatever reason would deprive the cones of this signal and trigger their degeneration. We review here recent circumstantial evidence and experimental findings suggesting that not only do such rod–cone interactions exist but that moreover we can intervene to limit or prevent secondary cone death.

Lessons from retinal transplantation

During the last decade numerous animal studies concerning retinal transplantation have been published, and preliminary results led to human trials beginning in 1994. However many major questions remain unresolved and a lot of experimental work is required to conceive coherent strategies founded on scientific data in order to justify this new therapeutic approach and to validate it clinically. Within the retinal transplantation field, two different strategies can be distinguished, the first represented by RPE grafting which is proposed to exert beneficial effects upon the apposing photoreceptors, and the second by retinal neuronal transplantation hoping to directly replace defective tissue.

RPE transplantation

Publications concerning photoreceptor survival after RPE transplantation in animal models are numerous. Such surgery has already been performed in humans, although no objective functional or anatomical benefits have yet been reported. Some authors recommend this strategy as an adjuvant treatment in the surgery of neovascular membranes in complicated forms of the ARMD.

The first promising results were observed in the RCS rat, which carries a genetic disorder localised within the RPE manifested as phagocytic failure and rod degeneration (the mutation has recently been identified as a receptor tyrosine kinase, *Mertk* [D'Cruz et al., 2000]). Using this model of retinal degeneration Li and Turner (1988), Sheedlo et al. (1989) and Gouras and Lopez (1989) noted considerable delay in host retinal photoreceptor loss following transplantation of healthy RPE, and observed a correlation between the density of grafted cells and the number of surviving photoreceptors. Forty-eight hours after surgery phagosomal material was seen and normal metabolic parameters could be measured (LaVail et al., 1992; Sheedlo et al., 1989, 1991). Similar results were reported when human RPE was transplanted into the RCS retina. Some evidence of improvement in functional parameters was also recorded by the group of Coffey and Lund (Whiteley et al., 1996), and by Jiang et al. (1994). The effects provided by these transplantations in the RCS rat retina could possibly be due to release of trophic factors, since the extent of photoreceptor survival exceeded the borders of transplanted RPE. Some authors have reported defects in FGF receptor numbers in the RCS rat (Malecaze et al., 1993), and others have reported that FGF can stimulate OS phagocytosis (McLaren and Inana, 1997). It has been known for many years that protective effects are exerted by FGF-2 in the RCS rat (Faktorovich et al., 1990), and other neurotrophic factors such as CNTF, BDNF and interleukin-1β are also known to improve photoreceptor survival in animal models of phototoxicity and murine mutants (LaVail et al., 1992; 1998). The recent identification of the gene defect in RCS rats as the receptor tyrosine kinase *Mertk* lends further weight to the possibility that RPE exert trophic effects upon photoreceptors.

Nevertheless RPE transplantation presents some drawbacks, and application to human pathology should await progress in our understanding of the basic science prior to therapeutical use. If beneficial effects are mediated by trophic factors, such effects sometimes vary from one model to another. For example, FGF-2 promotes rat rod differentiation (Hicks and Courtois, 1992) and survival (Fontaine et al., 1998) in vitro, while it induces rod apoptosis in chicken photoreceptors (Yokoyama et al., 1997). Another important precaution in RPE transplantation is the need for permanent immunosupressive therapy to override rejection phenomena of these immune-competent cells and to permit graft survival.

Neuronal transplantation

Neuronal retinal transplantation has been geared essentially towards combating inherited retinal dystrophies such as RP, and transplantation of embryonic or adult retinal cells is used with integration and functional recovery as its main aim. Most experimental data have been provided by the laboratories of Del Cerro, Aramant and Gouras. They noted that injections of embryonic dissociated cells or embryonic retinal sheets into the subretinal space survived for long periods and exhibited a certain degree of differentiation (Del Cerro et al., 1985; Aramant et al., 1990; Gouras and Lopez, 1989). Recently Aramant recorded responses of the grafted tissue after light stimulation (Seiler et al., 1999), and the team of Lund reported graft integration with the host retina after injecting retinal cell suspensions from young donor mice into the sub-retinal space of aged *rd* mice (Kwan et al., 1999). They noted a new synaptic layer at the graft-host interface, containing substantial numbers of photoreceptor synapses that mediate a simple light-dark preference (Kwan et al., 1999). Unfortunately transplanted embryonic tissue develops many rosettes similar to those seen in retinoblastomas and retinal dysplasias. To avoid this, Ehinger's team used an approach consisting of implantation of entire retinas. In this case tissue organization was respected but connections with the host retina were prevented through the presence of all retinal layers (Ghosh et al., 1999). Most recently, this laboratory reported long term survival (10 months) of full-thickness embryonic transplants accompanied by the development of a normal laminated morphology in the host rabbit retina. In this recent study a few direct synaptic contacts between graft and host neuronal types were observed.

The majority of these studies were done using small animal models, essentially rats or mice. The inconvenience of these models is their small size, making surgery sometimes uncertain with frequent traumatic complications inducing great variability in the data. In addition ocular functional testing is complex and provides non-interpretable data. Fortunately other larger animal models are currently available, namely a strain of transgenic pig exhibiting dominant mutations of the rhodopsin gene (Petters et al., 1997). This animal not only carries a similar retinal disease to human RP sufferers, but its size allows comfortable, reproducible surgery and easy and reliable functional testing.

Paracrine effect of retinal neuronal transplantation

Although the concept of photoreceptor and/or RPE surgical replacement in retinal diseases is attractive, many functional aspects of the transplanted tissue and its integration into the complex visual chain have to be resolved before its routine applicability becomes feasible. An alternative scheme which does not require reconstruction of functional pathways is based on the hypothesis that transplanted rods act as reservoirs of trophic factors necessary for cone survival. The logical goal of such a precept is the purification and identification of such molecules, but in the short to mid-term it suggests that transplantation could be useful in limiting cone degeneration.

Using the *rd* mouse model we performed in vivo (transplantation) and in vitro (co-culture) studies. Our initial results indicated the existence of a link between secondary cone loss and lack of survival factor(s) provided by or requiring the presence of rods. Transplantation of rod-rich photoreceptor sheets, isolated by using the vibratome sectioning technique described by Silverman and Hughes (1989) (Fig. 1), into the subretinal space of 5 week old *rd* mice (an age when > 99% rods have disappeared) induced a significant increase in host cone survival

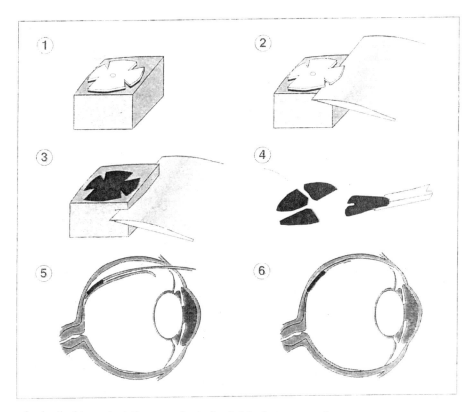

Fig. 1. Isolation and subretinal transplantation on a sheet of rod-rich photoreceptor layer.

2 weeks after surgery (Fig. 2) (Mohand Said et al., 1997). Compared to sham operated eyes, we observed increases of 30–40% in cone density within the central retina. In this study, pre-labeling of grafts in a subgroup of animals permitted verification of the reproducibility of the surgical technique, with correctly inserted grafts being identified in >90% of the cases. In addition, these studies excluded the possibility that increased cone numbers were due to an eventual colonization of the host retina by the few cones contained in the transplants. Comparison to sham operated controls ruled out the existence of non-specific effects related to release of trophic or inflammatory mediators induced by the surgical trauma itself.

The fact that the effect was recorded in the central part of the host retina, distant from the graft location, suggested a diffusible nature of the mediator(s) of the survival effect. We developed an organ co-culture model of whole retinas from 5 week old *rd* mice separated from test tissues by a semi-permeable

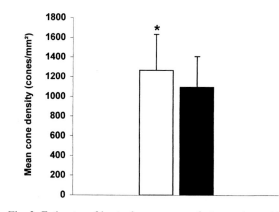

Fig. 2. Estimates of host *rd* mouse cone photoreceptors within the central field of paired transplanted and sham-operated animals after 2 weeks post-surgery. *, $p < 0.05$

membrane (Fig. 3). Since unequivocal demonstration of neuroprotective effects on cones by counting of thin sections was rendered very difficult by the extreme variability of cone cell distribution across the mouse retina (LaVail et al., 1997), we developed

656

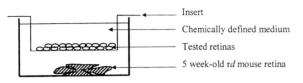

Fig. 3. Co-culture system: tested dissociated retinal cell, or retinal explants are cultured in the same medium than the 5 weeks rd mice retinal explants through an insert.

a more reliable stereological quantitative technique. Stereological counting is accepted as the most unbiased and reproducible method for enumerating neurones in the central nervous system (Gundersen et al., 1988; Coggeshall and Lekan, 1996), and its adaptation to the retina, based on a pseudo-random sampling of the total retinal surface (Fig. 4), allows an accurate and reproducible estimation of the total number of immunochemically identified cones. This method greatly reduced the large variation observed in other studies relying on the sampling of relatively few tissue sections (Farber, 1995; LaVail et al., 1997), and allows accurate estimations of cones and the detection of small changes in their numbers. Using this unbiased stereological approach, examination of organ cultured retinas after 1 week in vitro revealed significantly greater numbers of surviving cones, indicating prevention of around 50% expected cone loss if cultured in the presence of retinas containing rods (retinal cell cultures from young normal or rd mice, and retinal explants from adult normal mice) as compared to controls or co-cultures with rod-deprived retinas (retinal explants from aged rd mice) (Fig. 5) (Mohand Said et al., 1998). The fact that even non-functional rods improved the survival of cones (5 week rd retinas co-cultured with retinal cell cultures from 8 day rd mice) represents a result of capital importance, since it suggests approaches aimed at delaying secondary cone loss by maintaining alive non-functional rods might be advantageous. These approaches will be discussed below.

Recently we have extended our studies of transplantation effects on cone survival (Mohand Said et al., 2000). In order to see whether the survival of host cones is due specifically to rods or could be provided by other retinal cells, five groups of 5 weeks aged rd mice were used; non-operated controls, those grafted with pure sheets of rods isolated from young normal-sighted mice, those grafted with inner retinal cells from young normal donors, those receiving

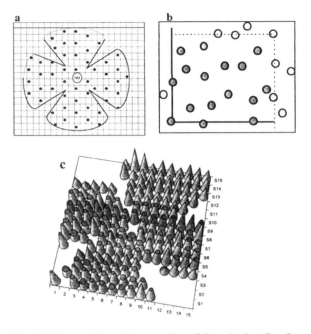

Fig. 4 (a) Systematic random sampling of the retinal surface for stereological counting. (b) Countings were performed using a stereological dissector (c) Example of a counted retina: distribution of the counted samples.

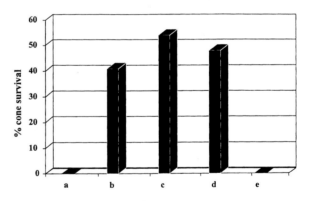

Fig. 5. Percentages of cone survival in rd retinas cultured alone (a) or co-culltured with dissociated retinal cell from 8 days rd mice (b), or from 8 days C57 mice (c), or with retinal explants from adult C57 mice (d), or adult rd mice (e) after one week.

transplants of entire retina from aged rd mice (rodless retina), and finally sham-operated controls receiving slabs of gelatin. Some methodological aspects of the procedures were improved, including the use of a calibrated trephine for transplant preparation and the development of a new subretinal injector based on mechanical, non-hydraulic pressure, which allows

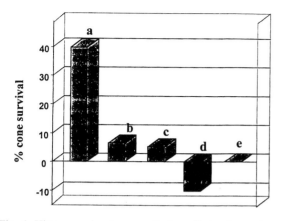

Fig. 6. Histogram showing quantitative effects of experimental treatments upon residual cone numbers in *rd* host retinas. Cone numbers are expressed as a percentage of the normal loss occuring during this period, relative to paired controls. Transplantation of rods preserves ~40% host cones destined to die. (**a**) C57 mouse photoreceptor grafted eyes, (**b**) C57 mouse inner retina grafted eyes, (**c**) *rd* mouse photoreceptor grafted eyes, (**d**) gelatin grafted eyes, (**e**) Paired non-operated eyes.

finer control of transplantation. Mice were allowed to survive 2 weeks post surgery, and the total cone numbers in their retinas were estimated by using the stereological method. Only mice receiving rod-rich transplants demonstrated statistically significant greater cone numbers, with rescue of 40% host cones normally destined to die during this period (Fig. 6). As in the initial study, pre-labeling of photoreceptor transplants with lipophilic fluorescent dyes confirmed the success (100%) of the surgical procedure. Photoreceptor grafts were of variable size and shape, routinely appearing as a sheet or scattered islands covering <10% of the total retinal surface, and were located in the mid- to far-periphery of the host retina. Label was always confined to the grafts, indicating that cells did not spread out to colonize host tissue (Fig. 7). The results of this study demonstrate that cone survival depends specifically on rods and showed that transplantation of normal rods allows histological neuroprotection against secondary cone death.

Indirect pharmacological neuroprotection of cones

The paracrine effect of rods on cone survival suggested that protecting rods may allow cone survival even if the rods are expressing the *rd* mutation. This hypothesis was supported by the observed cone neuroprotection in the organ co-culture model described above, suggesting that even rods carrying

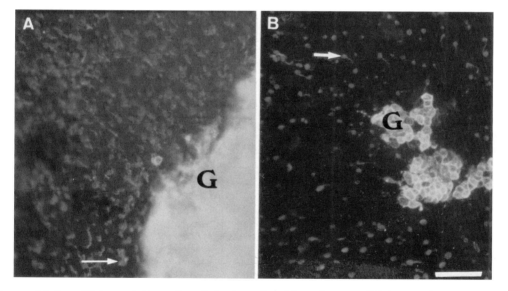

Fig. 7. Immunolabeling of flat-mounted transplanted *rd* retinas, viewed from above. (**A**) This large graft was pre-labeled with PKH26-GL fluorescing orange/red (G), clearly visible against the host retina in which green specks (arrow) are PNA-labeled cones. Scale bar = 20 μm.

658

mutations still stimulate increased cone survival. Such a mechanism may have occurred in previous reports describing rod photoreceptor rescue with trophic factors (LaVail et al., 1998). In our search for rod neuroprotective molecules, we showed that administration of GDNF can produce significant rod survival and delay the loss in cone function in the *rd* mouse (Fig. 8) (Frasson et al., 1999a). Another study from our group has established, in the same animal model, that a calcium-channel blocker can transiently rescue rod and cone photoreceptors with a preservation of cone function (Fig. 9) (Frasson et al., 1999b). Greater photoreceptor survival was also demonstrated by others (Liu et al., 1999) applying

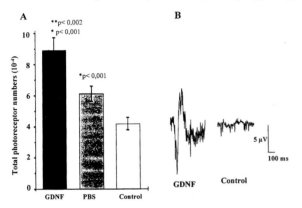

Fig. 8 (**A**) Rod numbers determined from transverse sections of GDNF, PBS, and non-injected *rd* retinas. * Comparison between non-injected retinas and GDNF or PBS treated retinas, ** comparison between GDNF and PBS treated retinas. (**B**) EGRs recorded from GDNF injected and (Control) non-injected eyes.

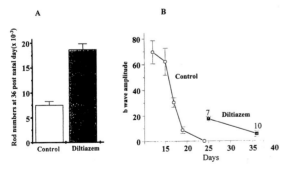

Fig. 9 (**A**) Quantification of diltiazem-induced rod cell rescue in flat mounted retinas of *rd* mice at post-natal day 36. (**B**) Diltiazem on the b-wave of ERG. In all control untreated *rd* mice, b-wave disappeared by post-natal day 24, whereas an ERG signal could still be mesured in all diltiazem treated *rd* mice on PND 24 and in some on PND 36.

an anti-capsase-3 inhibitor in transgenic rats with a rhodopsin mutation S334ter. These studies indicate that targeting common molecular events in rod degenerating pathways may provide pharmacological treatments applicable to different disease forms.

Perspectives and conclusions

Gene therapy, which theoretically represents the most logical and coherent approach to treating inherited retinal degenerations, will necessitate much time and effort to take its place among the panoply of therapeutic tools in medical practice. In the meantime, retinal transplantation could represent a rapidly accessible alternative. The demonstration by our studies of the paracrine effects of transplanted rods on host cones in the *rd* mouse, the lack of immune response to photoreceptors and the progress in retinal microsurgery (Kaplan et al., 1997) open the way to human clinical trials. Rescue of cones might not be affected by the type of mutation leading to rod cell death. In view of the number of mutations already described in RP this is no small advantage, since in most patients gene defects are not present in cones. Many issues, such as the long term survival of transplants, the duration of the effect and especially the functionality of surviving cones, remain currently unsolved. Larger animal models might provide decisive clues and will also offer the opportunity to extend these findings to different mutations and different species (e.g. rat, pig). The demonstration of the beneficial role of rods, even those themselves non-functional, in cone survival encourages strategies aimed at postponing or blocking rod cell death. Both trophic factors (LaVail et al., 1998; Frasson et al., 1999a) and pharmacological agents (Liu et al., 1999; Frasson et al., 1999b) have already been found to exert protective effects on rods. Cone survival could therefore also be obtained through such approaches, possibly using already existing drugs or via gene delivery of trophic factors.

References

Adler, R. and Hatlee, M. (1989) Plasticity and differentiation of embryonic retinal cells after terminal mitosis. *Science*, 243: 391–393.

Ahmad, I., Dooley, C. and Mand Afiat, S. (1998) Involvement of Mash-1 in EGF-mediated regulation of differentiation in the vertebrate retina. *Dev. Biol.*, 194: 86–98.

Allikmets, R., Shroyer, N.F., Singh, N., Seddon, J.M., Lewis, R.A., Berstein, P.S., Peiffer, A., Zabriskie, N.A., Li, Y., Hutchinson, A., Dean M., Lupski, R. and Leppert, M. (1997) Mutation of the Stargardt gene (ABCR) in age-related macular degeneration. *Science*, 277: 1805–1807.

Araki, M. (1997) Diffusible factors produced by cultured neural retinal cells enhance in vitro differentiation of pineal cone photoreceptors of developing quail retinas. *Dev. Brain Res.*, 104: 71–78.

Aramant, R., Seiler, M., Ehinger, B., Bergstrom, A., Gustavii, B., Brundin, P. and Adolph, A.R. (1990) Transplantation of human embryonic retina to adult rat retina. *Restorative Neurol Neurosci.*, 2: 9–22.

Baker, N.E. and Rubin, G.M. (1989) Effect on eye development of dominant mutations in Drosophila homologue of the EGF receptor. *Nature*, 340: 150–153.

Banin, E., Cideciyan, A.V., Aleman, T.S., Petters, R.M., Wong, F., Milam, A.H. and Jacobson, S.G. (1999) Retinal Rod Photoreceptor-Specific Gene Mutation Perturbs Cone Pathway Development *Neuron*, 223: 549–557.

Berson, E.L., Rosner, B., Sandberg, M.A. and Dryja, T.P. (1991) Ocular findings in patients with autosomal dominant retinitis pigmentosa and rhodopsin, proline-347-leucine. *Am. J. Ophthalmol.*, 111: 614–623.

Bird, A.C., Bressler, N.M., Bressler, S.B., Chisholm, I.H., Coscas, G., Davis, M.D., de Jong, P.T., Klaver, C.C., Klein, B.E., Klein, R. et al. (1995) An international classification and grading system for age-related maculopathy and age-related macular degeneration. The International ARM Epidemiolgial Study Group. *Surv. Ophthalmol.*, 39: 367–374.

Bumsted, K., Jasoni, C., Szel, A. and Hendrickson, A. (1997) Spatial and temporal expression of cone opsins during human retinal development. *J. Comp. Neurol.*, 378: 117–134. *Published erratum appears in J. Comp. Neurol.*, (1997) 380: 291.

Carter-Dawson, L.D., La Vail, M.M. and Sidman, R.L. (1978) Differential effect of the *rd* mutation on rods and cones in the mouse retina. *Invest. Ophthalmol. Vis. Sci.*, 17: 489–498.

Cepko, C.L., Austin, C.P., Yang, X., Alexiades, M. and Ezzedine, D. (1996) Cell fate determination in the vertebrate retina. *Proc. Natl. Acad. Sci. USA*, 93: 589–595.

Cideciyan, A.V., Hood, D.C., Huang, Y., Banin, E., Li, Z.Y., Stone, E.M., Milam, A.H. and Jacobson, S.G. (1998) Disease sequence from mutant rhodopsin allele to rod and cone photoreceptor degeneration in man. *Proc. Natl. Acad. Sci. USA*, 95: 7103–7108.

Chang, G.-Q., Hay, Y. and Wong, F. (1993) Apoptosis: Final common pathway of photoreceptor death in *rd*, *rds* and rhodopsin mutant mice. *Neuron*, 11: 595–605.

Cheng, T., Peachey, N.S., Li, S., Goto, Y., Cao, Y. and Naash, M.I. (1997) The effect of peripherin/*rds* haploinsufficiency on rod and cone photoreceptors. *J. Neurosci.*, 17: 8118–8128.

Chou, W.-H., Huber, A., Bentrop, J., Schulz, S., Schwab, K., Chadwell, L.V., Paulsen, R. and Britt, S.G. (1999) Patterning of the R7 and R8 photoreceptor cells of Drosophila: evidence for induced and default cell–fate specification. *Development*, 126: 607–616.

Coggeshall, R.E. and Lekan, H.E. (1996) Methods for determining numbers of cells and synapses: A case for more uniform standards of review. *J. Comp. Neurol.*, 364: 6–15.

Curcio, A., Millican, C.L., Allen, K.A. and Kalina, R.E. (1993) Ageing of the human photoreceptor mosaic: evidence for selective vulnerability of rods in central retina. *Invest. Ophthalmol. Vis. Sci.*, 34: 3278–3296.

Curcio, C.A., Medeiros, N.E. and Millican, C.J. (1996) Photoreceptor loss in Age-Related macular degeneration. *Invest. Ophthalmol. Vis. Sci.*, 37: 1236–1249.

D'Cruz, P.M., Yasumura, D., Weir, J., Matthes, M.T., Abderrahim, H., LaVail, M.M. and Vollrath, D. (2000) Mutation of the receptor tyrosine kinase gene Mertk in the retinal dystrophic RCS rat. *Hum. Mol. Genet.*, 9: 645–651.

Del Cerro, M., Gash, D.M., Rao, G.N., Notter, M.F., Wiegand, S.J. and Gupta, M. (1985) Intraocular retinal transplants. *Invest. Ophthalmol. Vis. Sci.*, 26: 1182–1185.

DesJardin, L.E., Timmers, A.M. and Hauswirth, W.W. (1993) Transcription of photoreceptor genes during foetal retinal development. Evidence for positive and negative regulation. *J. Biol. Chem.*, 268: 6953–6960.

Dryja, T.P., Hahn, L.B., Reboul, T. and Arnaud, B. (1996) Missense mutation in the gene encoding the alpha subunit of rod transducin in the Nougaret form of congenital stationary night blindness. *Nat. Genet.*, 13: 358–360.

Dryja, T.P., Hahn, L.B., Kajiwara, K. and Berson, E.L. (1997) Dominant and digenic mutations in the peripherin/*rds* and ROM1 genes in retinitis pigmentosa. *Invest. Ophthalmol. Vis. Sci.*, 38: 1972–1982.

Faktorovich, E.G., Steinberg, R.H., Yasumura, D., Matthes, M.T. and LaVail, M.M. (1990) Photoreceptor degeneration in inherited retinal distrophy delayed by fibroblast growth factor. *Nature*, 347: 83–86.

Farber, D.B. (1995) From mice to men: The cyclic GMP phosphodiesterase gene in vision and disease. *Invest. Ophthalmol. Vis. Sci.*, 36: 261–275.

Fariss, R.N., Zong-Yi, Li., Milam, A.H. (2000) Abnormalities in rod photoreceptors, amacrine cells, and horizontal cells in human retinas with retinitis pigmentosa. *Am. J. Ophthalmol.*, 129: 215–223.

Fontaine, V., Kinkl, N., Sahel, J., Dreyfus, H. and Hicks, D. (1998) Survival of purified rat photoreceptors in vitro is stimulated directly by Fibroblast Growth Factor-2. *J. Neurosci.*, 18: 9662–9672.

Frasson, M., Picaud, S., Léveillard, T., Mohand Said, S., Dreyfus, H., Hicks, D. and Sahel, J.A. (1999a) Glial cell line-derived neurotrophic factor promotes functional rescue of photoreceptors in a mouse model of inherited retinal degeneration. *Invest. Ophthalmol. Vis. Sci.*, 40: 2724–2734.

660

Frasson, M., Sahel, J.A., Fabre, M., Simonutti, M., Dreyfus, H. and Picaud, S. (1999b) Retinitis pigmentosa: rod Photoreceptor rescue by a calcium-channel blocker in the *rd* mouse. *Nat. Med.*, 10:1183–1187.

Freeman, M. (1996) Reiterative use of the EGF receptor triggers differentiation of all cell types in the *Drosophila* eye. *Cell*, 87: 651–660.

Freeman, M. (1997) Cell determination strategies in the Drosophila eye. *Development*, 124: 261–270.

Ghosh, F., Bruun, A. and Ehinger, B. (1999) Graft-Host connection in long-term full-thickness embryonic rabbit retinal transplant. *Invest. Ophthalmol. Vis. Sci.*, 40: 126–132.

Gouras, P. and Lopez, R. (1989) Transplantation of retinal epithelial cells. *Invest. Ophthalmol. Vis. Sci.*, 30: 1681–1683.

Gundersen, H.J.G., Bendtsen, T.F., Korbo, L., Marcussen, N., Moller, A., Nielsen, K., Nyengaard, J.R., Pakkenberg, B., Sorensen, F.B., Vesterby, A. and West, M.J. (1988) Some new simple and efficient stereological methods and their use in pathological research and diagnosis. *APMIS*, 96: 379–384.

Harris, W.A. and Messersmith, S.L. (1992) Two cellular inductions involved in photoreceptor determination in the Xenopus retina. *J. Neurosci.*, 9: 357–372.

Hewitt, A.T., Lindsey, J.D., Carbott, D. and Adler, R. (1990). Photoreceptor survival-promoting activity in interphotoreceptor matrix preparations: characterization and partial purification. *Exp. Eye Res.*, 50: 79–88.

Hicks, D. and Courtois, Y. (1992) Fibroblast growth factor stimulates photoreceptor differentiation in vitro. *J. Neurosci.*, 12: 2022–2033.

Jacobson, M.D., Weil, M. and Raff, M.C. (1997) Programmed cell death in animal development. *Cell*, 88: 347–354.

Jensen, A.M. and Wallace, V.A. (1997) Expression of sonic hedgehog and its putative role as a precursor cell mitogen in the developing mouse retina. *Development*, 124: 363–371.

Jiang, L.Q. and Hammasaki, D. (1994) Corneal electroretinographic function rescued by normal pigment epithelial grafts in retinal degenerative Royal College of Surgeons rats. *Invest. Ophthalmol. Vis. Sci.*, 35: 4300–4309.

Kajiwara, K., Berson, E.L. and Dryja, T.P. (1994) Digenic retinitis pigmentosa due to mutations at the unlinked peripherin/RD and ROM I loci. *Science*, 64: 1604–1608.

Kaplan, H.J., Tezel, T.H., Berger, A.S., Wolf, M.L. and Del Priore, L.V. (1997) Human photoreceptor transplantation in retinitis pigmentosa. A safety study. *Arch. Ophthalmol.*, 115: 1168–1172.

Kedzierski, W., Lloyd, M., Birch, D.G., Bok, D. and Travis, G.H. (1997) Generation and analysis of transgenic mice expressing P216L-substituted *rds*/peripherin in rod photoreceptors. *Invest. Ophthalmol. Vis. Sci.*, 38: 498–509.

Kumar, J.L., Tio, M., Hsiung, F., Akopyan, S., Gabay, L., Seger, R., Shilo, B.-Z. and Moses, K. (1998) Dissecting the roles of the Drosophila EGF receptor in eye development and MAP kinase activation. *Development*, 125: 3875–3885.

Kwan, A.S.L., Wang, S. and Lund, R.D. (1999) Photoreceptor layer reconstruction in a rodent model of retinal degeneration. *Exp. Neurol.*, 159: 21–33.

LaVail, M.M., Yasumura, D., Matthes, M.T., Lau-Villacorta, C., Unoki, K., Sung, C.H. and Steinberg, R.H. (1998) Protection of mouse photoreceptors by survival factors in retinal degenerations. *Invest. Ophthalmol. Vis. Sci.*, 39: 592–602.

LaVail, M.M., Matthes, M.T., Ysumura, D. and Steinberg, R.H. (1997) Variability in rate of cone degeneration in the retinal degeneration (*rd/rd*) mouse. *Exp. Eye Res.*, 65: 45–50.

LaVail, M.M., Unoki, K., Yasumura, D., Matthes, M.T., Yancopoulos, G.D. and Steinberg, R.H. (1992) Multiple growth factors, cytokines and neurotrophins rescue photoreceptors from the damaging effects of constant light. *Proc. Natl. Acad. Sci. USA*, 89: 11249–11253.

Levine, E.M., Roelink, H., Turner, J. and Reh, T.A. (1997) Sonic hedgehog promotes rod photoreceptor differentiation in mammalian retinal cells in vitro. *J. Neurosci.*, 17: 6277–6288.

Li, L. and Turner, J.E. (1988) Transplantation of retinal pigment epithelial cells to immature adult rat hosts: short- and long-term survival characteristics. *Exp. Eye Res.*, 47: 771–785.

Li, Z.Y., Jacobson, S.G. and Milam, A.H. (1994) Autosomal dominant retinitis pigmentosa caused by the threonine-17-methionine rhodopsin mutation: retinal histopathology and immunocytochemistry. *Exp. Eye Res.*, 58: 397–408.

Lillien, L. (1995) Changes in retinal cell fate induced by overexpression of EGF receptor. *Nature*, 377: 158–162.

Liu, C., Li, Y., Peng, M., Laties, A.M. and Wen, R. (1999) Activation of caspase-3 in the retina of transgenic rats with the rhodopsin mutation s334ter during photoreceptor degeneration. *J. Neurosci.*, 19: 4778–4785.

Malecaze, F., Mascarelli, F., Bugra, K., Fuhrmann, G., Courtois, Y. and Hicks, D. (1993) Fibroblast growth factor receptor deficiency in dystrophic retinal pigmented epithelium. *J. Cell Physiol.*, 154: 631–642.

McCall, M.A., Gregg, R.G., Merriman, K., Goto, Y., Peachey, N.S. and Stanford, L.R. (1996) Morphological and physiological consequences of the selective elimination of rod photoreceptors in transgenic mice. *Exp. Eye Res.*, 63: 35–50.

McLaren, M.J. and Inana, G. (1997) Inherited retinal degeneration: basic FGF induces phagocytic competence in cultured RPE cells from RCS rats. *FEBS Lett.*, 412: 21–29.

McLaughlin, M.E., Sandberg, M.A., Berson, E.L. and Dryja, T.P. (1993) Recessive mutations in the gene encoding the beta-subunit of rod phosphodiesterase in patients with retinitis pigmentosa. *Nat. Genet.*, 4: 130–134.

Milam, A.H., Li, Z.-H. and Fariss, R.N. (1998) Histopathology of the human retina in Retinitis Pigmentosa. *Prog. Retin. Eye Res.*, 17: 175–205.

Mohand Said, S., Hicks, D., Simonutti, M., Tran-Minh, D., Deudon-Combe, A., Dreyfus, H., Tenkova, T., Silverman, M., Mosinger, L., Ogilvie, J. and Sahel, J. (1997) Photoreceptor transplants increase host cone survival in the retinal degeneration (*rd*) mouse. *Ophthalmic Res.*, 29: 290–297.

Mohand Said, S., Deudon-Combe, A., Hicks, D., Fintz, A.C., Simonutti, M., Léveillard, T., Dreyfus, H. and Sahel, J.A. (1998) Normal rod photoreceptors increase cone survival in the retinal degeneration (*rd*) mouse. *Proc. Natl. Acad. Sci. USA*, 95: 8357–8362.

Mohand Said, S., Hicks, D., Léveillard, T., Dreyfus, H. and Sahel, J. (2000) Selective transplantation of rods delays cone loss in a retinitis pigmentosa model. *Arch. Ophthalmol.*, 118: 807–811.

Morrow, E.M., Belliveau, M.J. and Cepko, C.L. (1998) Two phases of rod photoreceptor differentiation during rat retinal development. *J. Neurosci.*, 18: 3738–3748.

Nir, I., Kedzierski, W., Chen, J. and Travis, G.H. (2000) Expression of Bcl-2 protects against photoreceptor degeneration in retinal degeneration slow (*rd*) mice. *J. Neurosci.*, 20: 2150–2154.

Oppenheim, R.W. (1991) Cell death during development of the nervous system. *Annu. Rev. Neurosci.*, 14: 453–501.

Owsley, C., Jackson, G.R., Cideciyan, A.V., Huang, Y., Fine, S.L., Ho, A.C., Maguire, M.G., Lolley, V. and Jacobson, S.G. (2000) Psychophysical evidence for rod vulnerability in age-related macular degeneration. *Invest. Ophthalmol. Vis. Sci.*, 41: 267–273.

Perrault, I., Rozet, J.M., Calvas, P., Gerber, S., Camuzat, A., Dollfus, H., Châtelin, S., Souied, E., Ghazi, I., Leowski, C., Bonnemaison, M., Le Paslier, D., Frézal, J., Dufier, J.L., Pittler, S., Munnich, A. and Kaplan, J. (1996) Retinal-specific guanylate cyclase gene mutations in Leber's congenital amaurosis. *Nat. Genet.*, 14: 461–464.

Petters, R.M., Alexander, C.A., Wells, K.D., Collins, B., Sommer, J.R., Blanton, M.R., Rojas, G., Hao, Y., Flowers, W.L., Banin, E., Cideciyan, A.V., Jacobson, S.G. and Wong, F. (1997) Genetically engineered large animal model for studying cone photoreceptor survival and degeneration in retinitis pigmentosa. *Nat. Biotech.*, 15: 965–970.

Raymond, P. and Fernald, R. (1981) Genesis of rods in teleost retina. *Nature*, 271: 360–362.

Raymond, P., Barthel, L.K. and Curran, G.A. (1995) Developmental patterning of rod and cone photoreceptors in embryonic zebrafish. *J. Comp. Neurol.*, 359: 537–550.

Rosenfeld, P.J., Cowley, G.S., McGee, T.L., Sandberg, M.A., Berson, E.L. and Dryja, T.P. (1992) A null mutation in the rhodopsin gene causes rod photoreceptor dysfunction and autosomal recessive retinitis pigmentosa. *Nat. Genet.*, 1: 209–213.

Seiler, M.J., Aramant, R.B. and Ball, S.L. (1999) Photoreceptor function of retinal transplants implicated by light-dark shift of S-antigen and rod transducin. *Vision Res.*, 39: 2589–2596.

Sheedlo, H.J., Li, L. and Turner, J.E. (1989) Functional and structural characteristics of photoreceptor cell rescued in RPE-cell grafted retinas of RCS dystrophic rats. *Exp. Eye Res.*, 47: 911–916.

Sheedlo, H.J., Gaur, V., Li, L., Seaton, A.D. and Turner, J.E. (1991) Transplantation to the disease and damaged retina. *Trends Neurosci.*, 14: 347–350.

Silverman, M.S. and Hughes, S.E. (1989) Transplantation of photoreceptors to light-damaged retina. *Invest. Ophthalmol. Vis. Sci.*, 30: 1684–1690.

Stenkamp, D.L., Hisatomi, O., Barthel, L.K., Tokunaga, F. and Raymond, P. (1996) Temporal expression of rod and cone opsins in embryonic goldfish retina predicts the spatial organization of the cone mosaic. *Invest. Ophthalmol. Vis. Sci.*, 37: 363–376.

Sunness, J.S., Massof, R.W., Johnson, M.A., Bressler, N.M., Bressler, S.B. and Fine, S.L. (1989) Diminished foveal sensitivity may predict the development of advanced age-related macular degeneration. *Ophthalmology*, 96: 375–381.

Van Ginkel, P.R. and Hauswirth, W.W. (1994) Parallel regulation of foetal gene expression in different photoreceptor cell types. *J. Biol. Chem.*, 269: 4986–4992.

Van Ginkel, P.R., Timmers, A.M., Szel, A. and Hauswirth, W.W. (1995) Topographical regulation of cone and rod opsin genes: parallel position dependent levels of transcription. *Dev. Brain Res.*, 89: 146–149.

Wikler, K.C. and Rakic, P. (1991) Relation f an array of early-differentiating cones to the photoreceptor mosaic in the primate retina. *Nature*, 351: 397–400.

Whiteley, S.J., Litchfield, T.M., Coffey, P.J. and Lund, R.D. (1996) Improvement of the pupillary light reflex of Royal College of Surgeons rats following RPE cell grafts. *Exp. Neurol.*, 140: 100–104.

Wright, A. (1997) A searchligth through the fog. *Nat. Genet.*, 17: 132–134.

Yokoyama, Y., Ozawa, S., Seyama, S., Namiki, H., Hayashi, Y., Kaji, K., Shirama, K., Shioda, M. and Kano, K. (1997) Enhancement of apoptosis in developing chick neural retina cells by basic fibroblast growth factor. *J. Neurochem.*, 68: 2212–2215.

Ying, S., Jansen, H., Lehman, M., Fong, S.-L. and Kao, W. (2000) Retinal degeneration in cone photorecptor cell–ablated transgenic mice. *Mol. Vis.*, 6: 101–108.

H. Kolb, H. Ripps and S. Wu (Eds.)
Progress in Brain Research, Vol. 131
© 2001 Elsevier Science B.V. All rights reserved

CHAPTER 48

Genes and diseases in man and models

Gustavo Aguirre*

James A. Baker Institute for Animal Health, College of Veterinary Medicine, Cornell University, Ithaca, NY 14853, USA

Introduction

In 1962 Dowling and Sidman carried out a now classical study on an inherited retinal dystrophy in the Royal College of Surgeons (RCS) rat (Dowling and Sidman, 1962). This study integrated with other work by Dowling and associates on the structure and function of retinal photoreceptors and pigment epithelium (RPE), and the effects of vitamin A deficiency on photoreceptor function and structure (Dowling and Wald, 1958; Dowling and Gibbons, 1962). Together, they showed the delicate balance that exists at the RPE-photoreceptor interface, and that any perturbation, whether inherited or experimentally induced, would result in the progressive structural and functional alterations that modify the beautifully organized photoreceptor cell, and ultimately result in visual cell degeneration and cell death. Blindness is the end-result of many of the diseases that affect the photoreceptor cells primarily, or secondarily as a result of RPE disease or dysfunction.

Since that time, the RCS rat, and a number of different animal models, including humans, have been used to study the cellular and molecular mechanisms of visual cell disease. These studies lead to a better understanding of how mutations in genes having a critical role in photoreceptor function, development, metabolism or viability result in visual cell dysfunction and degeneration. Some mutations in

photoreceptor specific genes were first identified and characterized in animals, e.g. the *rd* (PDE6B; Bowes et al., 1990; Pittler and Baehr, 1991) and *rds* (rds/peripherin; Travis et al., 1989) disorders in mice, before their recognition in human patients. Just recently a mutation in the *Mertk* gene, an RPE specific gene, has been found to be causally associated with the RCS retinal dystrophy (D'Cruz et al., 2000), thus bringing closure to the long search for the gene and mutation responsible for the disease in this animal model (see LaVail chapter "Legacy of the RCS Rat: Impact of a Seminal Study on Retinal Cell Biology and Retinal Degenerative Diseases" in this book for details on the history of the RCS rat in retinal research).

Using a combination of candidate gene, linkage and positional cloning approaches, great progress has been made in identifying human retinal disease genes or loci; to date (7/13/00), 123 retinal disease loci have been identified for which the gene and disease causing mutation has been identified in 57 (RetNet™ web page: http://www.sph.uth.tmc.edu/RetNet/). In regards to human retinal diseases, the animal models play critical roles. As illustrated with the *rd*, *rds* and more recently, RCS disorders, the models serve as an important gene discovery tool to identify novel retinal disease phenotypes and search for genes and mutations which can then be examined for causal association with disease in human patients. Additionally, since the animal models serve as homologues of human diseases, they serve to better characterize the molecular mechanisms of disease, and facilitate the development of experimental therapies useful in

---
*Tel.: 607-256-5620; Fax: 607-256-5689;
E-mail: gda1@cornell.edu

treatment strategies that will eventually be applicable to humans. Examples of some animal models that have been used in retinal disease research are presented in Table 1.

As a model for RP and allied retinal disorders, the dog is enjoying a renewed interest due to the variety of distinct retinal disease loci involved, the recent development of a framework genetic linkage map, and the resources to physically map and positionally clone the retinal diseases genes. In this chapter, I will review the retinal phenotypes of the different canine models, and discuss the evolving strategies that are used to find the genes and mutations responsible for these diseases.

Retinal disease phenotypes

There are a number of naturally occurring inherited diseases of dogs which primarily affect the photoreceptor cells and, to a lesser extent, the RPE. Most are progressive (see Aguirre et al., 1998a, for review),

Table 1. Selected examples of hereditary diseases of the RPE-photoreceptor complex in naturally occurring animal models

Disease name	Symbol	Human disease homologue	Gene mutation (locus*)	Reference**
Rat				
Retinal dystrophy	RCS		Mertk	D'Cruz et al., 2000
*Mice****				
retinal degeneration	*rd*	ARRP, CSNB	PDE6B	Bowes et al., 1990; Pittler and Baehr, 1991
retinal degeneration slow	*rds*	ADRP, Pattern Dystrophy, and Fundus Flavimaculatus	RDS/peripherin	Travis et al., 1989
retinal degeneration 7	*rd7*	Enhanced S-Cone syndrome	mPNR	Akhmedov et al., 2000
no observable b-wave	*nob*	X-linked CSNB1	(CSNB1)	Candille et al., 1999
Cat				
retinal dystrophy	*rdy*	ADRP	−	Barnett and Curtis, 1985
progressive rod–cone degeneration	*prcd*	ARRP	−	Narfström, 1983
Dog				
rod–cone dysplasia 1	*rcd1*	ARRP	PDE6B	Suber et al., 1993; Ray et al., 1994
rod–cone dysplasia 3	*rcd3*	ARRP	PDE6A	Petersen-Jones et al., 1999
early retinal degeneration	*erd*	Novel ARRP locus	(HSA 12p13q13)	Acland et al., 1999
congenital stationary nightblindness	*csnb*	CSNB, Lebers congenital amaurosis	RPE65	Aguirre et al., 1998b; Veske et al., 1999
progressive rod–cone degeneration	*prcd*	RP17	(HSA 17q23)	Acland et al., 1998
X-linked Progressive Retinal Atrophy	*XLPRA*	RP3	(HSA Xp21)	Zeiss et al., 2000
Achromatopsia	*cd*	Achromatopsia	(HSA 8q21–22)	Lowe et al., submitted
Chicken				
retinal degeneration	*rd*	Lebers congenital amaurosis	GC1	Semple-Rowland et al., 1998

* Comparative mapping of disease locus to human chromosome (HSA).
** Reference to most recent publications describing mutation and/or mapping of disease locus in animal model.
*** The Jackson Laboratory web page detailing the retinal degeneration mutants available: http://jaxmice.jax.org/jaxmicedb/html/model_130.shtml
ADRP: autosomal dominant retinitis pigmentosa; ARRP: autosomal recessive retinitis pigmentosa; CSNB: congenital stationary nightblindness; GC1: photoreceptor guanylate cyclase; PDE6A: cGMP phosphodiesterase alpha subunit; PDE6B: cGMP phosphodiesterase beta subunit; RPE65: retinal pigment epithelium 65 kDa protein.

although stationary disorders which selectively affect the function of rod and cone photoreceptors are recognized (Table 2). The progressive disorders, i.e. progressive retinal atrophy (PRA), represent a heterogeneous group of genetically different retinal diseases having similar phenotype. All show the same general ophthalmoscopic abnormalities, and visual deficits are characterized initially by rod dysfunction followed by loss of day vision; in the late stages of the disease the animals are blind, have end-stage retinal degenerative changes, and secondary cataracts. The clinical phenotype of PRA in dogs is similar to RP in man. Based on work in our laboratory, PRA is subdivided into developmental and degenerative diseases (Aguirre and Acland, 1988; Acland et al., 1989). The developmental class is characterized by dysplastic development of rod and/or cone photo-receptors, and represents a large aggregate of genetically distinct disorders which are expressed cytologically in the postnatal period, at the time that visual cells are beginning to differentiate. These include several gene loci among which are rod dysplasia (*rd*; Aguirre, 1978), rod–cone dysplasias 1–3 (*rcd1, rcd2, rcd3*; Ray et al., 1994; Wang et al., 1999b; Petersen-Jones et al., 1999), and early retinal degeneration (*erd*; Acland and Aguirre, 1987, and Acland et al., 1999). The salient functional (Fig. 1) and structural (Fig. 2) abnormalities for each of the disorders are quite specific, and have been used in assigning the gene locus designation (Fig. 3). In contrast, the degenerative class of diseases represent defects in photoreceptor maintenance, where the visual cells degenerate after having differentiated normally—this class includes mutations at the

Table 2. Inherited retinal and RPE disorders of dogs

Disease class and name	Gene or gene locus
Progressive Retinal Atrophy (PRA)	
Abnormal Development	
rod–cone dysplasia 1, 2 and 3	*rcd1, rcd2, rcd3*
rod dysplasia	*rd*
Early retinal degeneration	*erd*
Photoreceptor Degeneration	
progressive rod–cone degeneration	*prcd*
X-linked PRA 1 and 2	*XLPRA₁* and *XLPRA₂*
Non-progressive diseases	
cone degeneration	*cd*
congenital stationary nightblindness	*csnb*

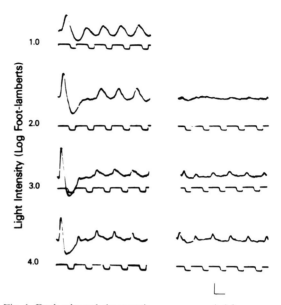

Fig. 1. Dark adapted electroretinograms recorded from normal (left) and *rd*-affected (right) dogs to 5 Hz flickering white light of variable intensity (1.0–4.0 log ft-L). No flicker responses are recorded from the *rd*-affected dog at intensities below 2 log ft-L. With the exception of the first response of a flicker series, which is a rod-dominated response, the affected dog follows the higher intensity flicker stimuli with responses similar in waveform, amplitude and peak latency to normal. Preservation of cones is also evident morphologically. Stimulus onset is the upward deflection of the baseline below each response series. Vertical calibration = 100 μV, horizontal calibration = 100 ms. (Figure adapted from Aguirre, 1978.)

progressive rod–cone degeneration (*prcd*; Aguirre and Acland, 1988; Acland et al., 1998) and XLPRA (Zeiss et al., 1999 and 2000) gene loci. Here, disease occurs more slowly, and is modified by temporal and topographic factors (Fig. 4). Different alleles have been identified at the *prcd* locus, and these segregate independently to regulate the rate, but not the phenotype, of photoreceptor degeneration (Acland and Aguirre, unpublished).

The gene locus designation noted above is used to identify those forms of PRA where extensive genetic, phenotypic and/or molecular studies have been carried out to identify the diseases as unique gene loci. In most cases, this conclusion has been based on classical genetic studies where intercrossing affected animals of different breeds establishes the non-allelic nature of the diseases (Acland et al., 1989). In addition, PRA is recognized as a clinically heritable disorder in another 70 or more breeds

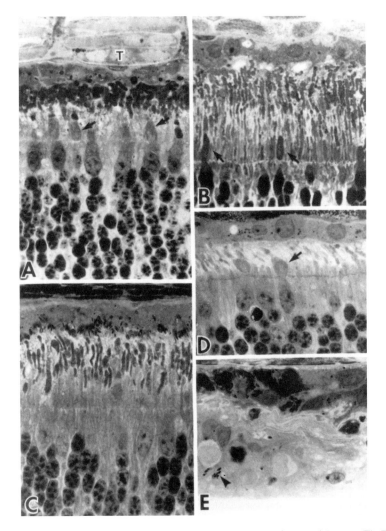

Fig. 2. Photoreceptor layer from *erd*-affected dogs at 30 (**A**), 54 (**B**), 98 (**C**), 140 (**D**) days, and 7 years (**E**). Early in development (**A**), cone photoreceptors (arrows) are prominent; by 54 days (**B**) the photoreceptor layer is wide and contains rod inner and outer segments of irregular lengths, but more normal cones (arrows). The lack of uniformity in rod inner and outer segment lengths is more clearly seen at 98 days (**C**), after loss of some photoreceptor cells. By 140 days (**D**) there is marked attenuation of the photoreceptor layer, and broad, prominent cones (arrows) are evident. End stage retinal atrophy and intraretinal pigment migration is present at 7 years (**E**) (arrowhead). T, tapetum lucidum. Original magnification, 1000×. (Reprinted from Acland and Aguirre, 1987.)

of dogs. Many of these breeds could have disease resulting from mutations of genes previously associated with inherited retinal disease in humans or other species, or, as well, resulting from mutations in novel genes. Thus molecular studies of this large group of breed-specific diseases is an important resource that may provide information on new genes or phenotypes that may be causally associated with photoreceptor disease.

The non-progressive disorders selectively affect the function of the rod or cone photoreceptors. They are considered "stationary" because the functional abnormality remains confined to one photoreceptor class, ophthalmoscopic evaluation shows a normal appearing retina throughout life, and morphologic examination confirms that the retina does not degenerate. Selective disease occurs in the cones of the cone degeneration mutant (*cd*; Gropp et al., 1996;

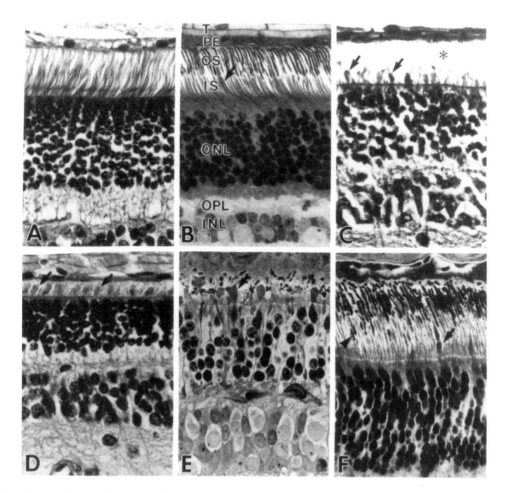

Fig. 3. Light micrographs of canine retina illustrating normal morphology (**A**, **B**), and the characteristic photoreceptor pathology found in different early-onset retinal diseases. The figure illustrates the optimal results obtained using paraffin (**A**, **C**, **D**) and plastic embedding (**B**, **E**, **F**) procedures. (**C**) *rcd2*-affected retina at 8 weeks of age shows extensive loss of photoreceptors which is more clearly visible because of artifactual separation (*) of RPE and retina. (**D**, **E**) *rcd1*-affected retinas at 6 and 8 weeks showing similar loss of rod photoreceptors, but better preservation of cones (arrows). (**F**) The *erd*-affected retina at 7.5 weeks of age shows more extensive development of rods and cones (arrows). However, there is loss of coordinate development between rods so that their inner and outer segments are distinct, but their proportions vary from cell to cell. T, tapetum lucidum; PE, pigment epithelium; OS, outer segment; IS, inner segment; ONL, outer nuclear layer; OPL, outer plexiform layer; INL, inner nuclear layer. Original magnification, 530×. (Reprinted from Acland et al., 1989.)

Lowe et al., submitted). Cone function is abnormal during retinal differentiation, and complete loss of cone mediated responses occurs within the first 2–3 months of life (Aguirre and Rubin, 1975). Cone disease and degeneration follows, but rod photoreceptors remain structurally (Fig. 5) and functionally normal (Aguirre and Rubin, 1974; Gropp et al., 1996). In contrast, congenital stationary nightblindness (*csnb*; Aguirre et al., 1998b) is named for the salient clinical visual deficit

exhibited by affected animals. This non-progressive disorder affects rod and, to a lesser extent cone function, although the site of the primary defect is in the RPE.

Once the phenotype and genetics were established for each of the diseases, we have used several approaches to identify the responsible gene and disease causing mutation. These have included candidate gene analysis and linkage/positional cloning; details are presented in the following sections.

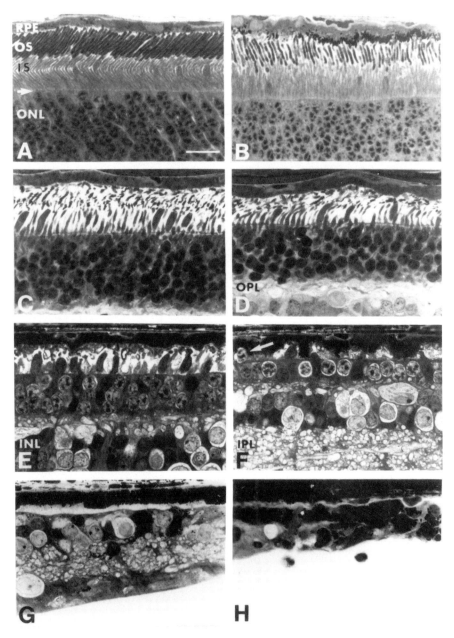

Fig. 4. Stages of retinal degeneration in males affected with X-linked progressive retinal atrophy (XLPRA). **A.** Normal retina; **B.** *Stage 1*: Outer segments have uneven borders and are faintly banded; **C.** *Stage 2*: Outer segments are fragmented and disorganized. Spaces between inner segments are due to photoreceptor loss, and cone inner segments are broader than normal. Apoptotic nuclei are present; **D.** *Stage 3*: Cone inner segments are broad, but cone outer segments are intact. Outer nuclear layer is reduced to 50% of its original width and the subretinal space is narrowed; **E.** *Stage 4*: Most outer segment material is absent. Remaining inner segments belong to cones. The outer nuclear layer is 2–3 nuclei thick with prominent pyknotic nuclei, and the outer plexiform layer is atrophic; **F.** *Stage 5*: Short stubs of inner segments are apposed to the RPE. The outer nuclear layer is reduced to a single layer of nuclei and is close to the inner nuclear layer due to atrophy of the outer plexiform layer. An extruded photoreceptor nucleus is present in the subretinal space (arrow); **G.** *Stage 6*: All inner and outer segment material is absent, and there is disorganization of retinal architecture; **H.** *Stage 7*: The neuroretina is reduced to a glial cord infiltrated with clusters of hypertrophic RPE cells. Anatomical regions of the retina are labeled as follows: RPE, Retinal pigment epithelium (note that the RPE is non-pigmented in tapetal regions in **A**, **C**, **D**, and pigmented in non-tapetal regions in **B**, **E**–**H**); OS, Outer segments; IS, Inner segments; Arrow (**A**) External limiting membrane; ONL, Outer nuclear layer; OPL, Outer plexiform layer; INL, Inner nuclear layer; IPL, Inner plexiform layer. Bar = 30 μm. (Reprinted from Zeiss et al., 1999.)

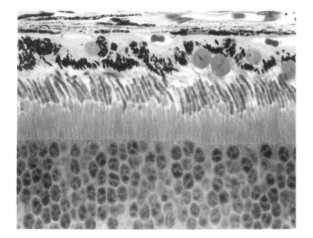

Fig. 5. Photomicrograph of the retina from an adult cone degeneration (*cd*)-affected dog. Cone disease results in degeneration and loss of cone photoreceptors. Two remaining cone nuclei have been extruded into the interphotoreceptor space, and now lie apposed to the RPE (right of center). The photoreceptor layer contains only rods which are structurally normal. Original magnification = 1450×.

Gene-based analysis

A gene-based approach to establish causal association between a gene mutation and an inherited retinal disease has been very successful in studies of RP and allied retinal diseases in man, particularly when only small pedigrees are available, or where a variety of simplex cases exist in the study population. Candidate genes are selected based on several considerations; e.g. genes which code for proteins that are involved in the phototransduction process, serve a critical structural role in the photoreceptor cell, are expressed exclusively or predominantly in the photoreceptor cells, are involved in biochemical pathways known to be abnormal in a hereditary retinal degeneration in any species, or are expressed abnormally in the photoreceptor cell. These are considered candidate genes for the diseases. Using such an approach, mutations in several genes, e.g. rhodopsin, RDS/peripherin, rom-1, α and β subunits of rod cyclic GMP-phosphodiesterase (PDE6A and PDE6B), the cyclic GMP-gated channel, guanylate cyclase, RPE65 and others have been shown to be causally associated with inherited retinal diseases (see Dryja, 1997, for review).

Molecular studies of inherited retinal diseases in dogs were initially limited to candidate gene analysis because of the lack of a canine genetic map, and the lack of comparative information between the canine, and the human and mouse maps. This prevented using the traditional positional cloning strategies which have been so successful in identifying retinal disease loci and genes in man. In addition, a gene based approach is the only one that can be used in dog breeds in which disease is ascertained in only a small number of animals, and informative pedigrees are not available for linkage analysis or genome scanning.

In order to carry out the candidate gene studies in dogs, however, it has been necessary to clone the canine specific genes and/or cDNAs, sequence the exons and scan for mutations in the coding region. In our lab, we have cloned several of the canine specific genes for many of the photoreceptor-specific or phototransduction proteins; some of these are RDS/peripherin (Ray et al., 1996a), transducin α1 (Ray et al., 1997), PDE6A (Wang et al., 1996a), PDE6G (Wang et al., 1996b), PDE6D (Wang et al., 1999a), phosducin (Zhang et al., 1998), the rod cyclic GMP-gated channel protein α subunit (Zhang et al., 1997), RPE65 (Aguirre et al., 1998b), RPGR (Zeiss et al., 2000). Other groups in the US, Germany, Finland and England have cloned most of the remaining canine-specific candidates for genes involved in the activation and de-activation phases of phototransduction or expressed in the photoreceptor cells (e.g. rom-1, rhodopsin, rod transducin-β and -γ, cone transducin-β and -γ, arrestin, PDE6B, rhodopsin kinase and recoverin), and these sequences have been deposited in GenBank. With this information, it is now possible to examine these candidate genes to determine if they are causally associated with any one of the forms of canine PRA.

The best example in the dog of using a candidate gene approach to identify a disease associated gene is rod-cone dysplasia1 (*rcd1*) in the Irish setter, a disease characterized by arrested differentiation of visual cells resulting from abnormal retinal cGMP metabolism (Aguirre, et al., 1978, 1982). Beginning at 10 days of age, deficient cyclic GMP-phosphodiesterase (cGMP-PDE) activity causes the retinal levels of cyclic GMP to rise sharply to concentrations up to 10-fold higher than normal;

these biochemical abnormalities are present before degenerative changes are observed in the photoreceptor cells. The morphologic and biochemical phenotype of the disease is similar to that present in the *rd* mouse (Farber and Lolley, 1974), and suggested that in the dog, like the mouse, the cGMP-phosphodiesterase subunits were reasonable candidate genes for analysis. The molecular identity between these two models of inherited retinal degeneration was subsequently confirmed by the identification of mutations in the beta subunit (PDE6B) of the cGMP-phosphodiesterase (Fig. 6) heterotrimeric complex (Bowes et al., 1990; Pittler and Baehr 1991; Suber et al., 1993; Ray et al., 1994). Mutations in this gene have also been found in human patients with autosomal recessive RP (McLaughlin et al., 1993).

Other successful candidate gene studies in dogs have resulted in identification of the PDE6A subunit gene (Petersen-Jones et al., 1999) as causally associated with early onset PRA, and a mutation in the RPE65 gene to result in *csnb* (Aguirre et al., 1998b; Veske et al., 1999). In neither case was there an a priori reason for selecting the candidate gene for

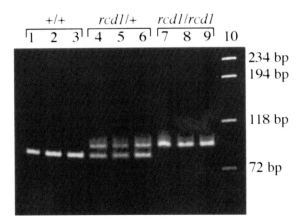

Fig. 6. Identification of the normal (+) and mutant (*rcd1*) alleles by allele-specific PCR (ASPCR) using allele-specific primers of different lengths. The sizes of the expected amplified product from the normal and mutant alleles are 81 and 90 bp, respectively. The product of ASPCR from normal (+/+; lanes 1, 2, and 3), *rcd1*-carrier (*rcd1*/+; lanes 4, 5, and 6), and *rcd1*-affected (*rcd1*/*rcd1*; lanes 7, 8, and 9) were analyzed by polyacrylamide gel electrophoresis. Lane 10 contains ϕx DNA digested with *Hae*III as a marker. Using this approach, it is possible to identify the specific codon 807 mutation in the PDE6B gene, and determine the genotype of dogs at the *rcd1* locus. (Figure adapted from Ray et al., 1996b.)

analysis, and it was part of a general screen for disease associated gene mutations. No mutations in the rhodopsin (Ray et al., 1999) or the rds/peripherin (Ray et al., 1996b) genes have been found in the multiple breeds of dogs with PRA that have been screened. This is surprising since mutations in these 2 genes account for a large proportion of the molecularly characterized forms of autosomal dominant RP (Dryja, 1997). A possible explanation for this difference is the selection pressure against disease phenotype that is used in breeding practices with dogs; this rapidly eliminates affected animals with dominant diseases while, at the same time, permitting those diseases caused by recessive gene defects to increase in frequency. To date, all autosomal retinal diseases in dogs that have been identified are recessively inherited.

A gene-based approach is not always successful in identifying the gene and disease causing mutation, even when there is very compelling biochemical or immunocytochemical evidence directing the candidate gene selection. For example, our laboratory has worked on another recessively inherited retinal degeneration found in collies, which has been termed rod–cone dysplasia 2 (*rcd2*) to differentiate it from the disease (*rcd1*) present in the Irish setter dogs (Woodford et al., 1982). Based on clinical, electrophysiological, morphological, and biochemical criteria, the two diseases are identical. In both, there is an equally rapid increase in retinal cGMP levels early in the postnatal period, and the magnitude of this elevation, as well as its time course, are very similar. In both *rcd1* and *rcd2* there is deficient cGMP-PDE activity. Using a combination of classical and molecular genetic analysis, we have conclusively excluded (Fig. 7) all the members of the cGMP-phosphodiesterase family (PDE6A, PDE6B, PDE6D, PDE6G) from association with the disease (Wang et al., 1999b). Similar compelling evidence for the involvement of the cone-specific transducin-β or -γ subunits has been found in the *cd* mutant retinas. In both cases, there is a dramatic decrease in expression of the gene product in the cone photoreceptors, and, that which is present, is no longer localized in the cone outer segments (Gropp et al., 1996; Akhmedov et al., 1997 and 1998). In both cases, however, involvement of these genes in the disease process has been convincingly ruled out. Details of the other

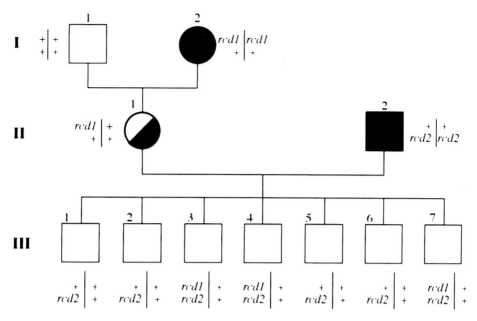

Fig. 7. Exclusion of PDE6B in rod–cone dysplasia 2 (*rcd2*) using a breeding strategy and molecular analysis that confirms nonallelism of *rcd1* (PDE6B nonsense mutation) and *rcd2*. Circles represent females, squares represent males, open symbols indicate normal phenotype, solid symbols indicate either *rcd1*-affected (I-2) or *rcd2*-affected (II-2) and half-filled symbol indicates *rcd1* heterozygous (II-1). The genotypes of the available animals are indicated next to each symbol (I and II), or underneath the symbols in generation III. Because of the mating pairs selected, all animals in generation III are heterozygous for *rcd2* (*rcd2/+*). Molecular analysis of all generation III dogs using the ASPCR method illustrated in Fig. 6 indicates that 3 animals (III-3, III-4, III-7) also are heterozygous for *rcd1*. Because of the normal phenotype status of all dogs in generation III, nonallelism of *rcd1* and *rcd2* is established. (Reprinted from Wang et al., 1999.)

candidate gene studies carried out in my laboratory are detailed in several additional publications (Ray et al., 1996a, 1997, 1999; Zhang et al., 1997, 1999)

Linkage/positional cloning

The candidate gene approach is ideally suited for mutation screening in different breeds of dogs where the number of affected animals is small, and informative pedigrees are not available for use in a genome wide screen and positional cloning. Where such pedigree resources are available, however, the gene based approach is of limited usefulness as each candidate excluded out of a potentially very large number does not result in moving closer to the identification of the disease causing gene; similarly, each new gene added to the list increases the effort needed to achieve success. Although the number of genes that cause retinal disease is finite, the upper limits of this number are difficult to define; presently

123 retinal disease loci have been identified for which the gene and disease causing mutation has been found in 57 (RetNet[TM] web page: http://www.sph.uth.tmc.edu/RetNet/). Based on the near linear rise in the number of new retinal disease loci and genes reported yearly since 1990, it is difficult to predict when the curve will level off to indicate that most of the genes involved in retinal disease phenotypes have been found.

In order to circumvent the limitations of working on a "genome-poor" species such a the dog, four years ago our laboratory undertook a collaborative effort with Elaine Ostrander's group at Fred Hutchinson Cancer Center to make a reference framework map of the dog using microsatellites generated in her lab (Ostrander et al., 1992; Francisco et al., 1996). For mapping, we used many 3 generation families which included 163 F_2 offspring from outcrossed and polymorphic individuals. The framework map generated has an average resolution of 13 cM, and covered greater than 60% of the genome (Mellersh et al., 1997).

Since then, the second and third generation maps have been completed, and a map resolution of 9.1 cM has been established with 341 markers which cover 2640 cM (Neff et al., 1999; Werner et al., 1999).

By itself, a microsatellite based linkage map of the dog is not sufficient to clone a disease gene. To circumvent this limitation, we assisted Ostrander's group to establish a panel of canine-rodent cell hybrids in which reference gene loci can be placed within the different linkage groups to help determine gene order and synteny between the human, mouse and dog maps for conserved regions of the genome. Initially, there were over 27 reference loci placed on this panel, at least 11 of which were photoreceptor genes (Langston et al., 1997). Since then a radiation hybrid (RH) map of the canine genome has been constructed (Priat et al., 1998), and, more recently, 2 canine BAC libraries have been made (Li et al., 1999). Lastly, the linkage and RH maps have been integrated with 724 unique markers (2/3 microsatellites, 1/3 genes) placed on 70 RH groups assigned to canine chromosomes or linkage groups; the unassigned RH groups cover less than1% of the genome (Mellersh et al., 2000). These resources, although modest in terms of the human genome project, will permit the mapping of disease genes or traits by cross-mapping from genome rich species such as man or mouse (Lyons et al., 1997).

In order to carry out a genome wide screen, it is essential that extensive 3 generation pedigrees be available for mapping. Because autosomal recessive diseases make the bulk of our disease pedigrees, informative pedigrees are created by breeding homozygous affected to non-affected heterozygous animals, and phenotype ascertainment is carried out after the age of risk for the disease using at least two independent criteria of which retinal histopathology of plastic embedded tissues is the most reliable. With such matings, all non-affected progeny are heterozygous, and all affected ones are homozygous for the disease; such phenotype/genotype correlation ascertains that all animals in the pedigree are informative for the mapping studies. With X-linked diseases, the strategy is similar, although the matings are usually between heterozygous females bred to either homozygous normal or hemizygous males.

Such pedigree and genetic resources have resulted in rapid progress in mapping several retinal disease loci. The first disease mapped was *prcd* (Fig. 8). Over 100 anchor loci and microsatellite based markers were used to map the disease to canine chromosome 9 (CFA9); identification of a linkage group flanking *prcd* ([TK1, GALK1, *prcd*]—[MYL4, C09.173, C09.2263]—RARA—C09.250—C09.474—NF1) localized *prcd* close to the centromeric end of the chromosome (Acland et al., 1998). Because of the conserved synteny of this region of CFA9 and distal human chromosome 17q, there is potential locus homology of *prcd* in the dog with RP17, a human retinitis pigmentosa locus for which no gene has yet been identified. Comparative genetic mapping of this region identified, as well, the homologous mouse chromosomal region (Werner et al., 1997). Since there are no mapped mouse retinal degeneration loci in the homologous region, the dog is, at present, the only model for this human retinal degenerative disorder. To identify the gene and mutation responsible for *prcd*, our studies are now directed at positionally cloning the gene by making an overlapping BAC contig over the minimal disease (zero recombination) interval, and testing positional candidates.

Similar rapid progress has been made with 3 other retinal disease loci, two autosomal and one X-linked. The autosomal disorder cone degeneration (*cd*) has been mapped to human chromosome (HSA) 8q21-22 (Lowe et al., submitted). This is the locus for a phenotypically similar disease in man (Pingelapese colorblindness; Winick et al., 1999) for which a mutation in the β-subunit of the cone cyclic nucleotide-gated cation channel gene has been recently identified (Sundin et al., 2000). Assuming that locus and genetic homology is established between the dog and human disorders, the dog will be the only model for this functionally devastating human retinal disorder. A second autosomal disorder, early retinal degeneration (*erd*), has been localized to canine radiation hybrid groups RH.34-a and RH.40-a. Multipoint analysis was used to place *erd* in the interval between two markers spanning a genetic distance of approximately 83 cM. Conserved synteny of this linkage group places *erd* in the chromosomal region homologous to HSA 12p13-q13, one for which there is no previously recognized human or animal retinal disease locus (Fig. 9, Acland et al., 1999). Further refinement of the disease locus, and positional cloning of the gene are

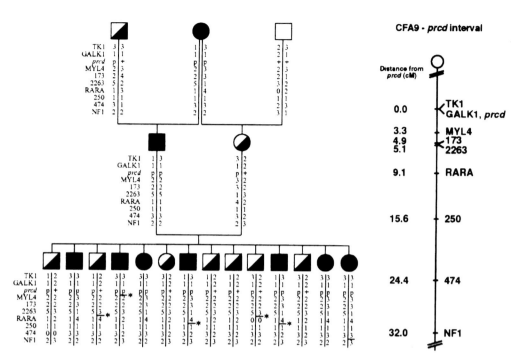

Fig. 8. *Left*: Pedigree informative for *prcd* with haplotype data. The order of loci is arranged according to results of 2 point linkage analyses. For the *prcd* locus, *p*, disease allele, +, wild-type allele. Loci 173, 2263, 474, and 250 represent microsatellite markers, and TK1, GALK1, MYL4, RARA and NF1 are genes located on CFA9. Haplotypes demonstrating recombination events are indicated (–*), although indicated position does not always correspond to the only possible site of the recombination. *Right*: Linkage map of the *prcd*-interval on canine chromosome 9 (CFA9). The location of *prcd* is shown relative to that of nine loci corresponding to type I and II markers. Loci listed on a single line indicate no recombinations observed between these markers. TK1 and GALK1/*prcd* are on separate lines but at a single location because, although no obligate recombinations were observed in this interval, indications of possible recombinations between TK1 and *prcd* were detected. Order and distances shown are based on 2-point linkage analyses of the data. (Reprinted with modification from Acland et al., 1998.)

now in progress. Thus *erd* represents a novel retinal disease locus, and, because of the very specific structural abnormalities expressed during the early differentiation of photoreceptors, identification of the gene responsible for the disease may yield new insights into the function of a new protein responsible for one critical aspect of photoreceptor development.

There is a lack of spontaneous animal models for X-linked retinal disease in general, and of X-linked retinitis pigmentosa (XLRP) in particular; currently, the Siberian husky dog is the only naturally occurring model of XLRP (Acland et al., 1994). This is a naturally occurring X-linked progressive retinal atrophy (XLPRA) closely resembling XLRP in humans. In affected males, initial degeneration of rods is followed by cone degeneration and complete retinal atrophy; carrier females have random patches of rod degeneration consistent with random X

chromosome inactivation. The disease was mapped by typing the XLPRA pedigree with 5 intragenic markers (DMD, RPGR, TIMP-1, Androgen Receptor, Factor IX) to establish a linkage map of the canine X chromosome, and confirms that the order of these 5 genes is identical to that on the human X. The disease in dogs was tightly linked to an intragenic polymorphism in the retinitis pigmentosa GTPase regulator (RPGR) gene (LOD 11.7, zero recombination), thus confirming locus homology with the RP3 form of XLRP in man (Fig. 10). To screen for disease causing mutations, we cloned the full-length canine RPGR cDNA and three additional splice variants, and quantitated the expression of each splice variant. No abnormalities were found by sequencing or expression (Zeiss et al., 2000). This finding is similar to what is found in approximately 80% of human XLRP patients whose disease maps to

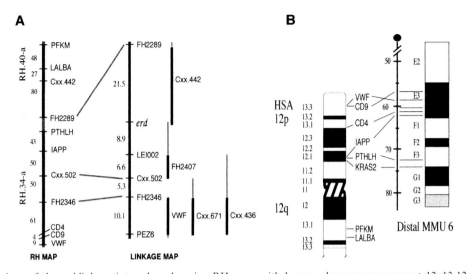

Fig. 9. Comparison of the *erd* linkage interval, and canine RH map, with human chromosome segment 12p13-12q13 (HSA12p), and distal mouse chromosome 6 (MMU6). Although the orientations of A and 3 are inverted relative to each other the order among corresponding loci is highly consistent. **A.** Comparison of the *erd* linkage interval with radiation hybrid (RH) mapping data (Priat et al., 1999) for the same region. The linkage map shows 6 loci (FH2289, *erd*, LEI002, Cxx.502, FH 2346 and PEZ6) in unique map positions, ordered with LOD ≥ 3.0. Additional markers Cxx.442, FH2407, Cxx.436, Cxx.671, and VWF, mapped to this interval but ordered with less precision, are displayed with range bars indicating their localization. Map distances are from MULTIMAP analysis of data in the present and additional studies (Mellersh et al., 1997; Neff et al., 1999). RH data confirms the ordering of the framework loci, and localizes the genes PFKM, LALBA, PTHLH, IAPP, CD4 and CD9 to the interval in addition to VWF, extending and confirming the conserved synteny of this linkage group with HSA12p13-12q13. **B.** Comparison of HSA12p (see Acland et al., 1999 for details) with distal MMU6 (data modified from *The Mouse Genome Informatics Web Site*, at The Jackson Laboratory, <http://www.informatics.jax.org>). The genes CD9, VWF, CD4, IAPP, PTHLH, and KRAS2 form a syntenic group that is conserved between these 2 species. This conserved syntenic group is clearly homologous to the *erd* linkage interval strongly suggesting that the human and murine homologs of the *erd* gene will be present on HSA12p and distal MMU 6, respectively. (Reprinted from Acland et al., 1999.)

the RP3 locus and no mutations in the RPGR gene have been detected (Meindl et al., 1996). More recently, a second XLPRA disorder (XLPRA$_2$) has been recognized in dogs (Aguirre et al., 2000). The disease also maps to the canine chromosomal region homologous to the RP3 interval. As with the disease in Siberian huskies, no disease causing mutations have been identified in the RPGR gene.

The studies in both the dog and human patients with X-linked retinal disease emphasize the importance for locus or genetic heterogeneity at the RP3 locus. On the one hand, it is possible that other retinal expressed genes which are located in the RP3 zero recombination interval are responsible for the disease. With the progress now being made in high throughput sequencing of this region of the X-chromosome in both species, it is likely that functionally relevant sequences will be identified which, when examined closely, will be found to

have gene mutations for some of the diseases that map to this interval. Alternatively, because of the complex splicing pattern of the RPGR gene, it is possible that yet to be characterized retinal-expressed transcripts exist, which when mutated cause photo-receptor degeneration. Comparative genomic studies between the human and dog for the RP3 and other regions will help identify the genes that are potentially involved in hereditary retinal diseases.

Conclusions and future perspectives

My work with the canine models was started in John Dowling's lab in the late 1960s, and was soon followed by the characterization of several diseases as distinct genetic disorders. Although superficially similar, each had very specific structural, functional and biochemical abnormalities. These differences

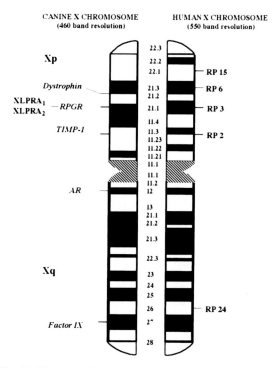

CANINE X CHROMOSOME
(460 band resolution)

HUMAN X CHROMOSOME
(550 band resolution)

Fig. 10. Ideogram of canine and human X chromosomes. The canine X chromosome, and locations of genes used to type the XLPRA pedigree are indicated on the left; the human X chromosome, and locations of the five X-linked RP loci are indicated on the right (adapted from RetNet http://www. sph.uth.tmc.edu/Retnet/). The physical locations of AR and Factor IX in the dog are known. There is no recombination between RPGR and XLPRA—as RPGR occupies a similar location on the canine X chromosome as on the human X chromosome, we can conclude that XLPRA is the locus homolog of RP3. Chromosome band patterns were adapted from published reports. (Reprinted from Zeiss et al., 2000.)

the molecular mechanisms of disease and developing therapeutic approaches for treatment of inherited retinal diseases. Both the human and its canine companion will benefit from the products of this research.

Acknowledgments

The studies described in this chapter represent the efforts of many individuals. In my laboratory, Drs. Greg Acland and Kunal Ray have played a pivotal role as have the many research associates, postdoctoral fellows, graduate students, research technicians and staff at the RDS facility. Other collaborators for different aspects of the research include Drs. Gene Anderson, Jerry Chader, Debora Farber, Paul O'Brien and Elaine Ostrander. I am most grateful to John Dowling for giving me the opportunity of working in his lab as a postdoctoral fellow, and for the high standards in research that he set for all who worked with him. These studies have been funded by NEI/NIH grants EY-01244, 06855, 13132, The Foundation Fighting Blindness, The Morris Animal Foundation/The Seeing Eye, and the AKC-Canine Health Foundation.

References

Acland, G.M. and Aguirre, G.D. (1987) Retinal degenerations in the dog: IV. Early retinal degeneration (erd) in Norwegian Elkhounds. *Exp. Eye Res.*, 44: 491.

Acland, G., Blanton, S.H., Hershfield, B. and Aguirre, G. (1994) XLPRA: A canine retinal degeneration inherited as an X-linked trait. *Am. J. Med. Gen.*, 52: 27–33.

Acland, G.M., Fletcher, R.T., Gentleman, S., Chader, G.J. and Aguirre, G.D. (1989) Non-allelism of three genes (rcd1, rcd2, erd) for early-onset hereditary retinal degeneration. *Exp. Eye Res.*, 49: 983–998.

Acland, G., Ray, K., Mellersh, C., Gu, W., Langston, A., Rine, J., Ostrander, E. and Aguirre, G. (1998) Linkage analysis and comparative mapping of canine progressive rod–cone degeneration (prcd) establishes potential locus homology with retinitis pigmentosa (RP17) in humans. *Proc. Natl. Acad. Sci. USA*, 95: 3048–3053.

Acland, G., Ray, K., Mellersh, C., Langston, A., Rine, J., Ostrander, E. and Aguirre, G. (1999) A novel retinal degeneration locus identified by linkage and comparative mapping of canine early retinal degeneration. *Genomics*, 59: 134–142.

were crucial in developing the concept of dividing retinal diseases into developmental and degenerative forms, and led to the genetic studies using intercross methods that identified allelism and non-allelism for diseases that had similar clinical phenotypes. Of the three diseases studied initially, *rd, prcd, cd*, the *rd* disorder no longer exists, but *cd* and *prcd* have now been mapped to canine chromosomal regions which indicate that they are homologous to human retinal diseases. The rapid progress that is now occurring in the field of canine genetics will expedite the identification of the genes underlying many of the inherited traits and diseases that make the dog a unique asset not only for gene discovery, but also for examining

Aguirre, G.D. (1978) Retinal degenerations in the dog. I. Rod dysplasia. *Exp. Eye Res.*, 26: 233.

Aguirre, G.D. and Acland, G.M. (1988) Variation in retinal degeneration phenotype inherited at the *prcd* Locus. *Exp. Eye Res.*, 46: 663–687.

Aguirre, G.D., Baldwin, B., Pearce-Kelling, S., Narfström, K., Ray, K. and Acland, G.M. (1998b) Congenital stationary night blindness in the dog: common mutation in the RPE65 gene indicates founder effect. *Mol. Vis.*, 4: 23–29.

Aguirre, G., Farber, D., Lolley, R., O'Brien, P., Alligood, J., Fletcher, R.T. and Chader, G. (1982) Retinal degenerations in the dog: III abnormal cyclic nucleotide metabolism in rod–cone dysplasia. *Exp. Eye Res.*, 35: 625–642.

Aguirre, G.D., Lolley, R., Farber, D., Fletcher, T. and Chader, G. (1978) Rod-cone dysplasia in Irish setter dogs: A defect in cyclic GMP metabolism in visual cells. *Science*, 201: 1133–1135.

Aguirre, G.D., Ray, J. and Stramm, L.E. (1998a) Diseases of the retinal pigment epithelium-photoreceptor complex in non-rodent animal models. In: Marmor, M.F. and Wolfensberger, T.J. (Eds.), *Retinal Pigment Epithelium-Current Aspects of Function and Disease*. Oxford University Press, New York, pp. 260–306.

Aguirre, G.D. and Rubin, L.F. (1974) Pathology of hemeralopia in the Alaskan Malamute dog. *Invest. Ophthalmol.*, 13: 231.

Aguirre, G.D. and Rubin, L.F. (1975) The electroretinogram in dogs with inherited cone degeneration. *Invest. Ophthalmol.*, 14: 840–847.

Aguirre, G.D., Zhang, Q., Zeiss, C.J. and Acland, G.M. (2000) Characterization of a second canine X-linked retinal degeneration (XLPRA2) which maps to the RP3 interval. *Invest. Ophthalmol. Vis. Sci.*, 41: S203.

Akhmedov, N.B., Piriev, N.I., Pearce-Kelling, S., Acland, G.M., Aguirre, G.D. and Farber, D.B. (1998) Evaluation of transducin γ-subunit as a candidate for inherited cone degeneration (*cd*) in the dog. *Invest. Ophthalmol. Vis. Sci.*, 39: 1775–1781.

Akhmedov, N.B., Piriev, N.I., Ray, K., Acland, G.M., Aguirre, G.D. and Farber, D.B. (1997) Structure and analysis of transducin β3-subunit, a candidate for inherited cone degeneration (*cd*) in the dog. *Gene*, 194: 47–56.

Akhmedov, N.B., Piriev, N.I., Rapoport, A.L., Hawes, N.L., Nishina, P.M., Nusinowitz, S., Heckenlively, J.R., Roderick, T.H., Kozak, C.A., Danciger, M., Davisson, M.T. and Farber, D.B. (2000) A deletion in a photoreceptor-specific nuclear receptor mRNA causes retinal degeneration in the *rd7* mouse. *Proc. Natl. Acad. Sci. USA*, 97: 551–555.

Barnett, K. and Curtis, R. (1985) Autosomal dominant progressive retinal atrophy in Abyssinian cats. *J. Hered.*, 76: 168–170.

Bowes, C., Li, T., Danciger, M., Baxter, L.C., Applebury, M.L. and Farber, D.B. (1990) Retinal degeneration in the rd mouse is caused by a defect in the β subunit of rod cGMP-phosphodiesterase. *Nature*, 347: 677–680.

Candille, S.I., Pardue, M.T., McCall, M.A., Peachey, N.S. and Gregg, R.G. (1999) Localization of the mouse nob (no b-wave) gene to the centromeric region of the X chromosome. *Invest. Ophthalmol. Vis. Sci.*, 40: 2748–2751.

D'Cruz, P.M., Yasumura, D., Weir, J., Matthes, M.T., Abderrahim, H., LaVail, M.M. and Vollrath, D. (2000) Mutation of the receptor tyrosine kinase gene *Mertk* in the retinal dystrophic RCS rat. *Hum. Mol. Genet.*, 9: 645–651.

Dowling, J. and Gibbons, I. (1962) The fine structure of the pigment epithelium in the albino rat. *J. Cell Biol.*, 14: 459–474.

Dowling, J.E. and Sidman, R.L. (1962) Inhereted retinal dystrophy in the rat. *J. Cell Biol.*, 14: 73–109.

Dowling, J.E. and Wald, G. (1958) Vitamin A deficiency and night blindness. *Proc. Natl. Acad. Sci. USA*, 46: 648–661.

Dryja, T.P. (1997) Gene-based approach to human gene-phenotype correlations. *Proc. Natl. Acad. Sci. USA*, 94: 12117–12121.

Farber, D.B. and Lolley, R.N. (1974) Cyclic guanosine monophosphate: Elevation in degenerating photoreceptor cells of the C3H mouse retina. *Science*, 186: 449–451.

Francisco, L.V., Langston, A.A., Mellersh, C.S., Neal, C.L. and Ostrander, E.A. (1996) A class of highly polymorphic tetranucleotide repeats for canine genetic mapping. *Mamm. Genome*, 7: 359–362.

Gropp, K.E., Szél, Á., Huang, J.C., Acland, G.M., Farber, D.B. and Aguirre, G.D. (1996) Selective absence of cone outer segment β3-transducin immunoreactivity in hereditary cone degeneration (*cd*). *Exp. Eye Res.*, 63: 285–296.

Langston, A.A., Mellersh, C.S., Neal, C.L., Ray, K., Acland, G.M., Gibbs, M., Aguirre, G.D., Fournier, R.E.K. and Ostrander, E.A. (1997) Construction of a panel of canine-rodent hybrid cell lines for use in partitioning of the canine genome. *Genomics*, 46: 317–325.

Li, R., Mignot, E., Faraco, J., Kadotani, H., Cantanese, J., Zhao, B., Lin, X., Hinton, L., Ostrander, E.A., Patterson, D.F. and de Jong, P.J. (1999) Construction and characterization of an eightfold redundant dog genomic bacterial artificial chromosome library. *Genomics*, 58: 9–17.

Lowe, J.K., Mellersh, C.S., Phippen, T., Aguirre, G.D., Ostrander, E.O. and Acland, G.M. Linkage and comparative mapping of canine cone degeneration: Locus homology to Pingelapese achromatopsia. (submitted, 7/00)

Lyons, L.A., Laughlin, T.F., Copeland, N.G., Jenkins, N.A., Womack, J.E. and O'Brien, S.J. (1997) Comparative anchor tagged sequences (CATS) for integrative mapping of mammalian genomes. *Nat. Genet.*, 15: 47–56.

McLaughlin, M.E., Sandberg, M.A., Berson, E.L. and Dryja, T.P. (1993) Recessive mutations in the gene encoding the β-subunit of rod phosphodiesterase in patients with retinitis pigmentosa. *Nat. Genet.*, 4: 130–134.

Meindl, A., Dry, K., Herrmann, K., Manson, F., Ciccodicola, A., Edgar, A., Carvalho, M.R., Achatz, H., Hellebrand, H., Lennon, A., Migliaccio, C., Porter, K., Zrenner, E., Bird, A., Jay, M., Lorenz, B., Wittwer, B., D'Urso, M., Meitinger, T. and Wright, A.A. (1996) A gene (RPGR) with homology to the RCC1 guanine nucleotide exchange factor is mutated in X-linked retinitis pigmentosa (RP3). *Nat. Genet.*, 13: 35–42.

Mellersh, C. S., Langston, A.A., Acland, G.M., Fleming, M.A., Ray, K., Weigand, N.A., Francisco, L.V., Gibbs, M., Aguirre, G.D. and Ostrander, E.A. (1997) A linkage map of the canine genome. *Genomics*, 46: 326–336.

Mellersh, C.S. Hitte, C., Richman, M., Vignaux, F., Priat, C., Jouquand, S., Werner, P., Andre, C., DeRose, S., Patterson, D.F., Ostrander, E.A. and Galibert, F. (2000) An integrated linkage-radiation hybrid map of the canine genome. *Mamm. Genome*, 11: 120–130.

Narfstrom, K. (1983) Hereditary progressive retinal atrophy in the Abyssinian cat. *J. Hered.*, 74: 273–276.

Neff, M.W., Broman, K.W., Mellersh, C.S., Ray, K., Acland, G.M., Aguirre, G.D., Ziegle, J.S., Ostrander, E.A. and Rine, J. (1999) A second-generation genetic linkage map of the domestic dog, *Canis familiaris*. *Genetics*, 151: 803–820.

Ostrander, E.A., Jong, P.M., Rine, J. and Duyk, G. (1992) Construction of small-insert genomic DNA libraries highly enriched for microsatellite repeat sequences. *Proc. Natl. Acad. Sci. USA*, 89: 3419–3423.

Petersen-Jones, S.M., Entz, D.D. and Sargan, D.R. (1999) cGMP phosphodiesterase-a mutation causes progressive retinal atrophy in the Cardigan Welsh Corgi dog. *Invest. Ophthalmol. Vis. Sci.*, 40: 1637–1644.

Pittler, S.J. and Baehr, W. (1991) Identification of a nonsense mutation in the rod photoreceptor cGMP phosphodiesterase β-subunit gene of the rd mouse. *Proc. Natl. Acad. Sci. USA*, 88: 8322–8326.

Priat, C., Hitte, C., Vignaux, F., Renier, C., Jiang, Z., Jouquand, S., Chéron, A., André, C. and Galibert, F. (1998) A whole-genome radiation hybrid map of the dog genome. *Genomics*, 54: 361–378.

Ray, K., Acland, G.M. and Aguirre, G.D. (1996a) Nonallelism of *erd* and *prcd* and exclusion of the canine RDS/peripherin gene as a candidate for both retinal degeneration loci. *Invest. Ophthalmol. Vis. Sci.*, 37: 783–795.

Ray, K., Lara Tejero, M.D., Baldwin, V.J. and Aguirre, G.D. (1996b) An improved diagnostic test for rod cone dysplasia 1 (*rcd1*) using allele-specific polymerase chain reaction. *Curr. Eye Res.*, 15: 583–587.

Ray, K., Baldwin, V.J., Acland, G.M., Blanton, S.H. and Aguirre, G.D. (1994) Cosegregation of codon 807 mutation of the canine rod cGMP phosphodiesterase β gene and *rcd1*. *Invest. Ophthalmol. Vis. Sci.*, 35: 4291–4299.

Ray, K., Baldwin, V.J., Zeiss, C.J., Acland, G.M. and Aguirre, G.D. (1997) Canine rod transducin α-1: Cloning of the cDNA and evaluation of the gene as a candidate for progressive retinal atrophy. *Curr. Eye Res.*, 16: 71–77.

Ray, K., Wang, W., Czarnecki, J., Acland, G. and Aguirre, G. (1999) Strategies for identification of mutations causing hereditary retinal diseases in dogs: evaluation of opsin as a candidate gene. *J. Hered.*, 90: 133–137.

Semple-Rowland, S.L., Lee, N.R., Van Hooser, J.P., Palczewski, K. and Baehr, W. (1998) A null mutation in the photoreceptor guanylate cyclase gene causes the retinal degeneration chicken phenotype. *Proc. Natl. Acad. Sci. USA*, 95: 1271–1276.

Suber, M.L., Pittler, S.J., Qin, N., Wright, G.C., Holcombe, V., Lee, R.H., Craft, C.M., Lolley, R.N., Baehr, W. and Hurwitz, R.L. (1993) Irish setter dogs affected with rod/cone dysplasia contain a nonsense mutation in the rod cGMP phosphodiesterase β subunit gene. *Proc. Natl. Acad. Sci. USA*, 90: 3968–3972.

Sundin, O.H., Yang, J.-M., Li, Y., Zhu, D., Hurd, J.N., Mitchell, T.N., Silva, E.D. and Maumenee, I.H. (2000) Genetic basis of total colourblindness among Pingelapese islanders. *Nat. Genet.*, 25: 289–293.

Travis, G.H., Brennan, M.B., Danielson, P.E., Kozak, C.A. and Sutcliffe, J.G. (1989) Identification of a photoreceptor-specific mRNA encoded by the gene responsible for retinal degeneration slow (*rds*). *Nature*, 338: 70–73.

Veske, A., Nilsson, S.E.G., Narfström, K. and Gal, A. (1999) Retinal dystrophy of Swedish Briard/Briard-Beagle dogs is due to a 4-bp deletion in RPE65. *Genomics*, 57: 57–61.

Wang, W., Acland, G., Ray, K. and Aguirre, G. (1999b) Evaluation of cGMP-phosphodiesterase (PDE) subunits for causal association with rod–cone dysplasia 2 (*rcd2*), a canine model of abnormal retinal cGMP metabolism. *Exp. Eye Res.*, 69: 445–453.

Wang, W., Zhang, Q., Acland, G., Mellersh, C., Ostrander, E., Ray, K. and Aguirre, G. (1999a) Molecular characterization and mapping of canine cGMP-phosphodiesterase delta subunit (*PDE6D*) Gene, 236: 325–332.

Wang, W., Acland, G.M., Aguirre, G.D. and Ray, K. (1996b) Cloning and characterization of the cDNA and gene encoding the γ-subunit of the cGMP-phosphodiesterase in canine retinal rod photoreceptor cells. *Gene*, 181: 1–5.

Wang, W., Acland, G.M., Aguirre, G.D. and Ray, K. (1996a) Cloning and characterization of the cDNA encoding the α-subunit of the cGMP-phosphodiesterase in canine retinal rod photoreceptor cells. *Mol. Vis.*, 2: 3–6.

Werner, P., Mellersh, C., Raducha, M., DeRose, S., Acland, G., Prociuk, U., Wiegand, N., Aguirre, G., Henthorn, P., Patterson, D. and Ostrander, E. (1999) Anchoring the canine linkage groups with chromosome-specific markers. *Mamm. Genome*, 10: 814–823.

Werner, P., Raducha, M.G., Prociuk, U., Henthorn, P.S. and Patterson, D.F. (1997) Physical and linkage mapping of human chromosome 17 loci to dog chromosomes 9 and 5. *Genomics*, 42: 74–82.

Winick, J.D., Blundell, M.L., Galke, B.L., Salam, A.A., Leal, S.M. and Karayiorgou, M. (1999) Homozygosity mapping of the achromatopsia locus in the Pingelapese. *Am. J. Hum. Genet.*, 64: 1679–1685.

Woodford, B.J., Liu, Y., Fletcher, R.T., Chader, G.J., Farber, D.B., Santos-Anderson, R. and Tso, M.O.M. (1982) Cyclic nucleotide metabolism in inherited retinopathy in collies: A biochemical and histochemical study. *Exp. Eye Res.*, 34: 703–714.

Zeiss, C.J., Acland, G.M. and Aguirre, G.D. (1999) Retinal pathology of canine X-linked progressive retinal atrophy, the locus homolog of RP3. *Invest. Ophthalmol. Vis. Sci.*, 40: 3292–3304.

Zeiss, C.J., Ray, K., Acland, G.M. and Aguirre, G.D. (2000) Mapping of X-linked progressive retinal atrophy (XLPRA), the canine homolog of retinitis pigmentosa 3 (RP3). *Hum. Mol. Genet.*, 9: 531–537.

Zhang, Q., Acland, G., Parshall, C.J., Haskell, J., Ray, K. and Aguirre, G. (1998) Characterization of canine photoreceptor phosducin cDNA and identification of a sequence variant in dogs with photoreceptor dysplasia. *Gene*, 215: 231–239.

Zhang, Q., Baldwin, V., Acland, G., Parshall, C.J., Haskell, J., Aguirre, G. and Ray, K. (1999) Photoreceptor dysplasia (*pd*) in miniature schnauzer dogs: evaluation of candidate genes by molecular genetic analysis. *J. Hered.*, 90: 57–61.

Zhang, Q., Pearce-Kelling, S., Acland, G.M., Aguirre, G.D. and Ray, K. (1997) Canine rod photoreceptor cGMP-gated channel protein α-subunit: studies on the expression of the gene and characterization of the cDNA. *Exp. Eye Res.*, 65: 301–309.

H. Kolb, H. Ripps and S. Wu (Eds.)
Progress in Brain Research, Vol. 131
© 2001 Elsevier Science B.V. All rights reserved

CHAPTER 49

Experimental retinal detachment: a paradigm for understanding the effects of induced photoreceptor degeneration

Steven K. Fisher[1,2,*], Jonathan Stone[3], Tonia S. Rex[2], Kenneth A. Linberg[1] and Geoffrey P. Lewis[1]

[1]*Neuroscience Research Institute, University of California, Santa Barbara, CA 93106, USA*
[2]*Molecular Cellular and Developmental Biology, University of California, Santa Barbara, CA 93106 USA*
[3]*NSW Retinal Dystrophy Research Center, Department of Anatomy and Histology, University of Sydney F13, NSW 2006, Australia*

Introduction

In 1961 Dowling and Gibbons reported that vitamin A deficiency caused rod outer segments to degenerate, and that restoring vitamin A to the diet would allow the outer segments to regenerate. This was a remarkable observation. It was the first real demonstration of vitamin A's ability to regulate the presence or absence of the outer segment, and showed unequivocally the cellular mechanism underlying blindness caused by vitamin A deficiency. It was also the first true experimental demonstration that photoreceptors, a sensory neuron, retain the ability to regenerate their outer segment in adult mammals. Interestingly, in a subsequent study they (Dowling and Gibbons, 1962) also reported the presence of lamellar inclusions in the RPE cells, paving the way to describing a mechanism for outer segment regeneration. As shown later by Young (1967) and others (Young and Bok, 1969), these bodies (phagosomes) are the end result of the disc shedding part of the renewal cycle for vertebrate photoreceptor outer segments (Fig. 1). Thus, these cells have evolved an elegant and highly efficient cellular machinery to assure the structural integrity of their outer segments throughout the lifetime of the animal, and one that allows for outer segment regeneration. New discs and plasma membrane are constantly produced at the base of the cell, and under normal conditions, these are assembled into an outer segment (Fig. 1; Steinberg et al., 1980; see http://insight.med.utah. edu/Webvision/). In 1968, Kroll and Machemer demonstrated that outer segments would also degenerate if the retina is detached from the retinal pigmented epithelium (RPE), and that the phagosomes disappear from the RPE in detached retina (Kroll and Machemer, 1968). Subsequently they also demonstrated that outer segments would regenerate when the retina was reattached, and the phagosomes would reappear, thus demonstrating that the renewal cycle was re-established (Kroll and Machemer, 1969). Retinal detachment is providing us with a method for studying the dynamics and mechanisms of induced outer segment degeneration and regeneration, as well as a model system for studying many other aspects of retinal degeneration. At the same time, it provides direct information on an important condition that causes significant visual impairment, and even loss of sight in humans.

* Corresponding author: Steven K. Fisher, Tel.: 805-893-3637; Fax: 805-893-2005; E-mail: fisher@lifesci.ucsb.edu

Photoreceptor Outer Segment Renewal Cycle

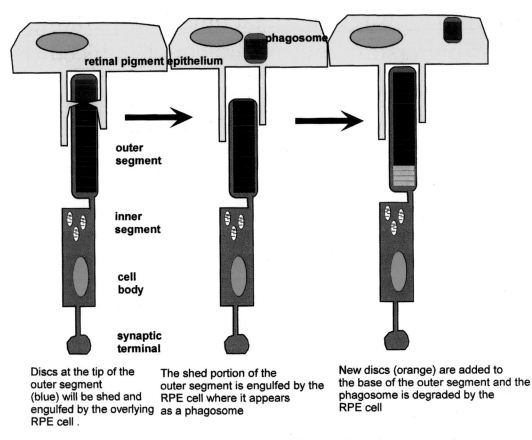

Fig. 1. A diagrammatic representation of the outer segment renewal cycle of vertebrate photoreceptor cells.

What is retinal detachment?

Under normal conditions the photoreceptor outer segments are in close apposition to the apical surface of the RPE (Fig. 2A). Indeed, this surface of the RPE extends long, and often quite elaborate processes that envelope the outer segments, often times reaching all the way to the inner segment (Steinberg and Wood, 1974; Steinberg et al., 1977; Anderson and Fisher, 1979; Fisher and Steinberg, 1982). It is these processes that participate actively in the phagocytosis of disc packets periodically shed from the outer segment. When this apposition is physically disrupted, and the sensory retina becomes separated from the apical surface, creating a new "subretinal"

space from the interphotoreceptor space, a retinal detachment occurs (Fig. 2B). This separation can occur due to various reasons (trauma and tearing of the retina, severe myopia, traction by foreign cells on the vitreal surface of the retina, etc.) but always results in the accumulation of fluid between the neural retina and RPE and a subsequent enlargement of the space between the two. Clinically there are different types of detachments (Hay and Landers, 1994), and these have different etiologies, different effects on vision and visual recovery, and are produced by different underlying mechanisms. In our studies we have modeled a rhegmatogenous detachment, or a condition in which there is a small hole across the retinal layers, therefore exposing the

Basic Cellular Responses to Retinal Detachment

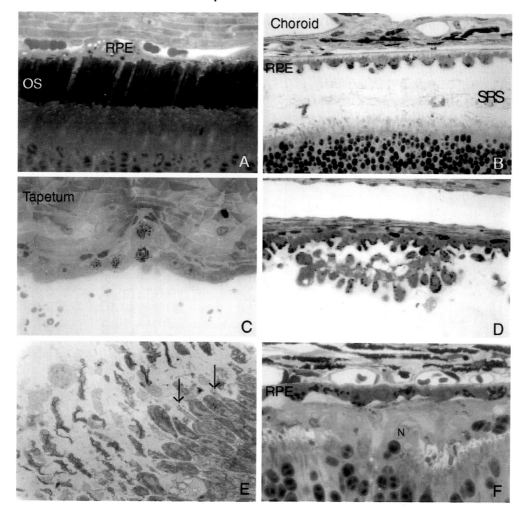

Fig. 2. Micrographs illustrating the basic cellular responses to retinal detachments: outer segment degeneration, RPE cell de-differentiation, proliferation, and gliosis. **A.** A light micrograph of the outer segment (OS)/RPE interface in normal cat retina. The "gaps" between the darkly stained rod outer segments mark the location of cone outer segments. The small, round inclusions in the RPE are phagosomes. A single phagosome appears just above the cone on the left. **B.** The interface shown in "A" after retinal detachment. There is now a subretinal space (SRS) measuring about 50 μm across, and this is filled with debris from degenerating outer segments. Note the scalloped appearance of the RPE and loss of apical processes. **C.** An autoradiogram showing tritiated-thymidine labeling of RPE cell nuclei 3 days after detachment. **D.** An assembly of RPE cells in the expanded subretinal space, a result of RPE proliferation. **E.** An electron micrograph of the interface shown in **B**, and showing that the debris in the space is composed of outer segment fragments. The 2 arrows mark photoreceptor cilia. Reprinted, with permission, from Lewis et al., 1999a. **F.** A light micrograph showing a large Müller cell scar in the subretinal space of a reattached cat retina. There is little outer segment regeneration on surviving photoreceptors beneath the scar. N, a Müller cell nucleus in the subretinal space.

subretinal space to components of vitreous and vice-versa. In some cases detachments occur when cells on the vitreal surface contract pulling the retina away from RPE, often times also leaving a tear across the retina. Such traction detachments often occur secondarily to successful surgical repair of a rhegmatogenous detachment, due to the proliferation of cells on the vitreal surface. In almost all cases this is a serious, nearly untreatable, ultimately blinding disease if the fovea is involved.

Why study retinal detachment?

Retinal detachment provides an experimental system in which to study many of the transformations that can occur between the biology of normal and abnormal retina. Our original intent was to use it as a method for studying the renewal cycle in cone outer segments. Understanding the capacity of cones for outer segment regeneration continues to be a significant problem. Young's original hypothesis of outer segment renewal excluded cones from the renewal cycle as described by rods and shown in Fig. 1, and postulated a different mechanism for them (Young, 1971). Rods were thought to construct new discs at the base of their outer segment. Cones were proposed to replace only "molecular components," of the outer segment and to not construct new discs nor dispose of packets of discs as phagosomes. This hypothesis was brought into question when Hogan et al. (1974) along with Anderson and Fisher (1975) demonstrated the presence of phagosomes in the human fovea and in species with cone-dominated retinas. Disc shedding from cones meant that they must also undergo disc morphogenesis in some form. The basic "mechanics" of these processes are now thought to be the same in rods and cones (Steinberg et al., 1980). Unlike the situation in rods, there was (and still is) no method available for quantifying the rate at which the cones renew their outer segment (Young, 1971; Anderson et al., 1978; Fisher et al., 1983). Thus, we reasoned, after failing to make cone-dominant species vitamin A deficient, that an animal model of retinal detachment and reattachment should provide the opportunity for measuring the rate at which cone outer segments re-grow, and thus, a measure of the rate at which these cells produce new membranes. In the course of the initial studies, it became obvious that the responses to retinal detachment are much more rich and interesting than we had anticipated. Indeed, the availability of antibody and molecular probes is now allowing us to continue identifying a host of cellular responses in addition to those initially identified in the early anatomic studies. These include: complex photoreceptor "deconstruction," proliferation of non-neuronal cells, changes in protein expression and amino acid profiles of most if not all retinal cell types, and plastic changes in second order neurons. Methods for altering these

responses may ultimately lead to ways of improving vision after reattachment surgery.

The retinopathy of detachment

Detachment initiates a "cascade" of events leading to numerous cellular changes that have recently been termed the "retinopathy of detachment" (Mervin et al., 1999), an apt term considering that every retinal layer is involved in the etiology of the response. Each cell-type studied so far has its own characteristic response signature.

RPE cell "de-differentiation"

The complex apical surface of the RPE cells assume a much "simpler" appearance as it loses the elaborate apical processes that ensheath the outer segments. These are replaced by a homogeneous fringe of microvilli-like processes (Fig. 2A). These cells also begin to proliferate, often forming mutiple layers adjacent to the original monolayer, or separate clusters or layers within the expanded subretinal space (Fig. 2C and D; Anderson et al., 1981, 1983). The presence of additional layers of RPE cells, especially when their apical surface does not face the photoreceptor layer, can result in areas in which photoreceptor outer segments do not regenerate even though the retina may be anatomically re-apposed (Anderson et al., 1986).

Photoreceptor cell deconstruction: the basic rod response

Photoreceptors ultimately respond to detachment in one of two ways: they die by apoptosis (Cook et al., 1995; Chang et al., 1996; Mervin et al., 1999) or they undergo a series of "deconstructive" changes (Fig. 3). These have been best characterized in rods and can be divided into several events involving different compartments of the cell.

Outer segment degeneration

Degeneration of the outer segment of the rods is the most dramatic and obviously rapid manifestation of

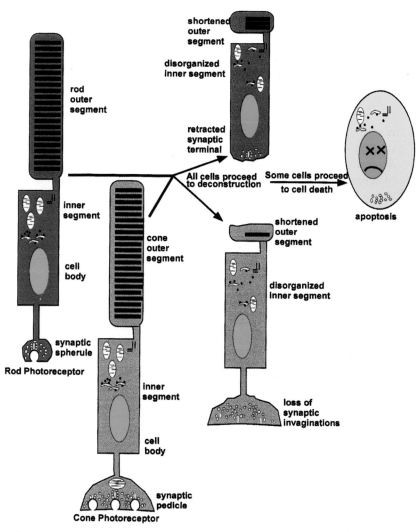

Fig. 3. A diagrammatic representation of the changes photoreceptor cells undergo after detachment. Almost immediately after separation from the RPE photoreceptors begin to undergo the process of "deconstruction." Some cells go on to survive in a highly modified state (cells in the middle) while other die by apoptosis. Cone outer segments appear to degenerate more quickly and completely than rods but their synaptic terminals do not retract.

detachment (Fig. 2B; Kroll and Machemer, 1968; Anderson et al., 1983). The outer segments of both rods and cones quickly shorten after detachment. In the cat retina, rod outer segments average 15–20 μm in length depending on retinal location, and within 7 days of detachment the average length will decrease to 4–5 μm (Lewis et al., 1999a). Even at 7 days, many photoreceptors will have no outer segment recognizable by light microscopy. In terms of outer segment regenerative capacity it is significant that the

connecting cilium never disappears from these cells (Fig. 2E). Autoradiographic studies show that newly synthesized proteins are still transported to the connecting cilium and surviving portion of the outer segment, which may consist of only a few disorganized discs (Lewis et al., 1991). Thus, the remaining discs do not appear to be remnants of the original outer segment, but are most likely new discs, representing an attempt by the rod to continue outer segment production. The rods may be able to add some new discs in the absence of RPE attachment, but they never construct a fully-formed outer segment. Why is this? Detached frog photoreceptors, which are probably more resistant to degeneration than their mammalian counterparts, in culture continue adding new discs in an apparently normal process and at a normal rate for several hours, but within 2 days, 75% of the cells are forming structurally abnormal discs at the outer segment base (Hale et al., 1991). Thus, the process of disc morphogenesis may eventually fail to produce normal discs in a photoreceptor detached from the RPE. There is a small but very specific aggregate of filamentous actin in the connecting cilium, in the region of disc morphogenesis (Vaughan and Fisher, 1987). The drug cytochalasin D disrupts this filamentous actin cytoskeleton, and treatment of photoreceptors with this drug produces abnormal discs (Williams and Fisher, 1987; Vaughan and Fisher, 1987). Hale et al (1996) showed that disrupting the filamentous actin cytoskeleton in the connecting cilium essentially stopped the cells from being able to construct new discs. Detachment also disrupts the f-actin cytoskeleton of the rod photoreceptor cell, and it may be this disruption that accounts for the inability of the cells to construct a normal outer segment (Lewis et al., 1995). In the presence of excess brain-derived neurotrophic factor (BDNF), the rods can construct surprisingly long and normal-appearing outer segments (Lewis et al., 1999a). It is possible that BDNF's action is to maintain the cytoskeleton of these cells, allowing normal outer segment formation to occur.

By what mechanism does the actual degeneration of the outer segment occur? Fragments of outer segments, and even individual discs can be recognized by TEM in the expanded subretinal space (Fig. 2E). Phagosomes are often observed within macrophages lying over the shortened outer segments (Anderson et al., 1983; Lewis et al., 1991), but are absent from the RPE. Although the dynamics of outer segment loss have not been studied, it seems unlikely that there is a simple "disintegration" of the outer segment, but rather a progressive shortening. Does the cell "release" packets of the outer segment in an organized/regulated manner such as occurs during the normal disc shedding cycle? The major evidence against this method of deconstruction is a lack of observed, regular packets of discs in the subretinal space, and the experimental evidence that normal rod disc shedding cannot occur in the absence of attachment to the RPE (Williams and Fisher, 1987). Does the outer segment degeneration proceed until the metabolic load on the cell is reduced to a level that compensates for the reduced availability of oxygen and other metabolites across the expanded subretinal space (see Linsenmeier and Padnick-Silver, 2000). When detached, does the rod cell actually regulate the number of new discs produced to match the availability of oxygen, or has the detachment simply disrupted the cytoskeleton (as discussed above), so that the cell can no longer form discs at its normal rate? These questions are yet to be answered experimentally. Experiments in which animals are kept in a hyperoxic (70% oxygen) environment however, do suggest a relationship between these events, i.e. the availability of oxygen may prevent the deconstruction of the cytoskeleton and thus allow outer segment formation (Mervin et al., 1999). On the other hand, the two may be independent of one another.

Inner segment de-compartmentalization

Inner segments are the home of an immense population of mitochondria as well as most of the machinery for protein synthesis and processing, with organelles being organized into compartments (the ellipsoid and myoid). Upon detachment this organization is disrupted, and the organelles intermingle (Erickson et al., 1983). Labeling with an antibody to the protein cytochrome oxidase confirms the ultrastructural observation that mitochondria are rapidly lost from these cells (Fig. 4D, E; Mervin et al., 1999). This is an important issue since these cells have a metabolic rate much higher than that of other neurons (Winkler, 1983). When animals are kept in an increased oxygen environment after detachment the mitochondria are preserved (Fig. 4D–F, J–L) suggesting that their loss is regulated by the lack of available oxygen from the choroidal circulation (Mervin et al., 1999). Disruption of the tubulin cytoskeleton, and its maintenance in hyperoxia is also easily observed in the inner segment and connecting cilium, although the tubulin cytoskeleton is actually lost throughout the rod cell (Fig. 4G–I).

Photoreceptor Deconstruction

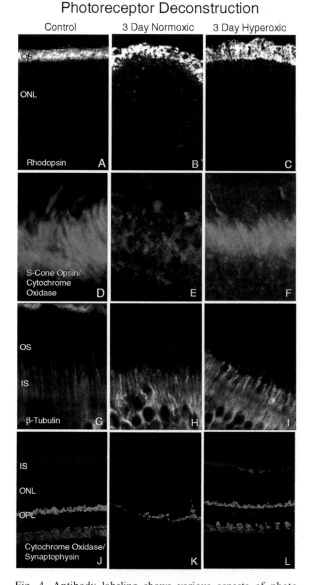

Fig. 4. Antibody labeling shows various aspects of photoreceptor deconstruction after detachment in normoxia (2 left columns) and their mitigation by oxygen therapy (right column). ONL, outer nuclear layer; OS, outer segment layer. **A,B,C.** Labeling with a rod-opsin antibody (kindly provided by Dr. R. Molday). In the control eyes (**A**) labeling is limited to the rod outer segments (and the Golgi/RER regions of the inner segment) while after detachment in a normoxic animal, labeling spreads to the plasma membrane surrounding the whole cell (**B**). In hyperoxia the label is once again confined to the outer segment, and the outer segments approach normal length and appearance. **D,E,F.** Double-label images after labeling with an antibody to the short-wavelength sensitive cone-opsin (red), and an antibody to cytochrome oxidase (green) which labels the

Synaptic terminal withdrawal and regression

The synaptic endings of surviving rods are also affected strikingly by detachment. Structurally, the synaptic terminals of the rods appear to withdraw from their normal location on the border of the outer plexiform layer so that the synaptic structures now appear within the cell body, instead of at the end of the "axon," (Figs. 4J,K; 5A,B,E,F; Erickson et al., 1983). Thus, the layer of rod spherules becomes disrupted, no longer forming a compact zone at the interface of the outer nuclear and outer plexiform layers (ONL, OPL) (Figs. 4J, K; 5A–C; Lewis et al., 1998, 1999a; Mervin et al., 1999). Since the rod nuclei form many rows within the ONL, their terminals begin to assume a random scattering throughout that layer as they withdraw towards the cell body (Fig. 5C). Ultrastructurally, the distinctive invaginations with their complex array of postsynaptic processes disappear from these terminals (Fig. 5G). They now assume a configuration reminiscent of developing photoreceptors (Linberg and Fisher, 1990) where the ribbons and vesicles are located in a small rim of basal cytoplasm, often closely juxtaposed to the nucleus, and are apposed directly to the flattened presynaptic membrane (Fig. 5G; Erickson et al., 1983). Postsynaptic processes can still be clearly identified by electron microscopy, even

mitochondria. (The antibody to S-cone opsin was kindly provided by Dr. J. Nathans). Cone outer segments degenerate quickly, and labeling of the plasma membrane is not as dramatic as for rods. Hyperoxia maintains the cone outer segments and mitochondria. **G,H,I.** The tubulin cytoskeleton is labeled with an antibody to beta-tubulin. The labeling in the region marked OS represents labeling of the connecting cilium, and that labeling is virtually lost in the normoxic detached retina, while that in the inner segment region (IS) assumes a more diffuse and amorphous appearance. The inner segment labeling appears more organized in hyperoxia, and the connecting cilium labeling is maintained, although not as well oriented as in a normal retina. **J,K,L.** Double labeling with the antibody to cytochrome oxidase (red) and an antibody to synaptophysin (green). The latter shows the order and organization of the photoreceptor synaptic terminals in normal retina (**J**), the loss of this organization in detached retina (**K**), and its maintenance by oxygen therapy (**L**). Also note the loss of mitochondrial labeling (red) in detached retina and compare this to normal and oxygen-treated detached retina. Reprinted, with permission, from Mervin et al. (1999).

686

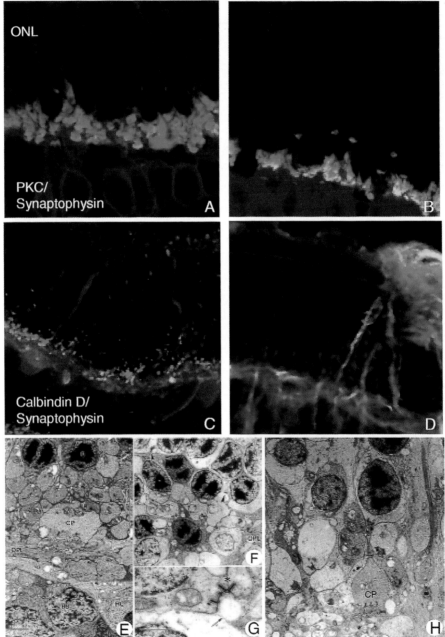

Photoreceptor Synapse/
2nd Order Neuron Responses

Fig. 5. The response of rod photoreceptor synaptic terminals and second-order neurons to detachment. **A,B**. Double-label images with antibodies to synaptophysin (green) that labels the photoreceptor terminals and protein kinase C (red) that labels the rod bipolar cells and their dendrites. Note the loss of synaptophysin labeling from the layer of terminals in the detached retina, the shift of this labeling into the ONL as rod terminals retract, and the extension of labeled neurites from the rod bipolar cells to the retracted rod terminals. **C**. Labeling of retracted rod terminals with an antibody to synaptophysin (green) and outgrowths from horizontal cells with an

when there is no invagination, and when the synaptic structures lie deep in the ONL, far from the original zone of synaptic terminals. The spatial relationship between these processes appears to be much different than that occurring within the invagination. Presumably the deep synaptic invagination into the rod terminal plays some role in the physiology of information processing at this, one of the most complex synapses in the whole central nervous system. What happens to the physiology of this synapse, and to information processing in the rod pathway when the postsynaptic processes are no longer within the confined space of an invagination?

Shifting the focus to cones

Rod degeneration has been studied in many animal models, although an emphasis on studying cones would seem highly compelling considering the devastating effects of foveal damage by trauma or diseases such as age-related macular degeneration. Presumably the reason for this is the ease with which rods are studied (being much more abundant than cones in most mammalian species), and the variety of naturally occurring mutations that affect rods, providing models for retinitis pigmentosa. There are, however, about 10 million people in the United States affected by age-related macular degeneration, compared with about 100,000 afflicted with retinitis pigmentosa. In both genetically induced retinal degenerations, and degeneration induced by constant light exposure, cone cells appear to survive until late in the degeneration. Data from the detachment model is providing a more detailed picture of the cones' responses. Many cones do, indeed, appear to survive the degeneration induced by detachment, but they

may do so utilizing a different mechanism than the rods. Certainly these two differ greatly in how they express various proteins during an episode of detachment. Using that as a criterion, cones appear more susceptible to degeneration than rods. The cell bodies of the cones in cat retina are arrayed among the cell bodies of rods in the outermost row of the ONL, and thus, they have long axons that traverse the ONL to terminate in large, elaborate synaptic pedicles in the OPL (Fig. 6A). These axons do not retract as do those of the rods, but the synaptic pedicles change their overall shape, generally losing the large number of invaginations that populate the pedicle base (Figs. 5, 6B), and losing their large, distinctive mitochondria as well. The cone nuclei often shift their location to deeper into the outer nuclear layer. Whether this is an active relocation, or passive movement due to remodeling of the ONL as large numbers of rods die is not known. However, the most distinctive differences between rods and cones emerge when the retina is labeled with various antibodies. For example, rods continue to label intensely with antibodies to rhodopsin even in very long-term detachments (Fig. 7A–C). Outer segments consisting of only a few discs continue to label at the same relative intensity as an intact outer segment, but at the same time there is a distinctive shift in the labeling pattern. Within a day of detachment there is a recognizable increase in labeling of the plasma membrane around the inner segment and cell body. With time this labeling increases in intensity, and extends into the plasma membrane around the synaptic terminal so that eventually the whole cell is outlined (Fig. 7B; Lewis et al., 1991; Fariss et al., 1997). This pattern continues in surviving rods as long as the retina remains detached. It is not known if it is reversed when the retina is reattached and the

---

antibody to calbindin D (red). Note how some of these stout outgrowths run the width of the ONL. **D.** Labeling of horizontal cell outgrowths in detached retina with an antibody to calbindin D (red) and Müller cell processes with an antibody to GFAP (green). Note how the outgrowths seem to follow the hypertrophied Müller cell processes. **E.** An electron micrograph of the layer of photoreceptor synaptic terminals and the outer plexiform layer (OPL) in normal cat retina. CP, a cone pedicle. HC, horizontal cell; R, rod nucleus; RS, rod spherules. **F.** An electron micrograph showing disruption of the OPL and retraction of rod terminals in detached retina. The arrowheads mark rod synapses within the ONL. **G.** A higher magnification electron micrograph of a rod synapse in a cell that has retracted its synaptic terminal. The asterisk marks synaptic ribbons and the arrow a post-synaptic process. Fig. E, F and G, reprinted, with permission, from Lewis et al., 1998. **H.** An electron micrograph of the OPL after detachment showing that cone pedicles (CP) change their shape but do not retract from their normal location on the border of the outer plexiform layer. Note the large mitochondria in the CP in **E**, and the tiny remnants of mitochondria in the CP in **H**. Also the cone terminal in **H** has ribbons along its base, but no deep invaginations.

Changes in Cone Terminals

Control   3 Day

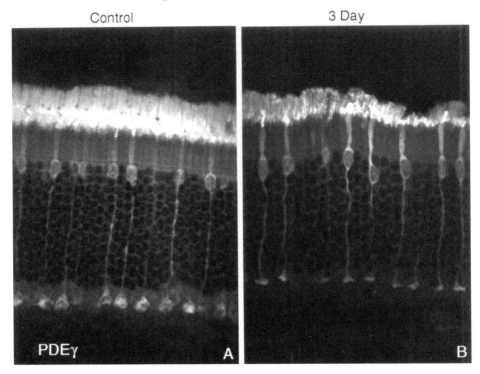

Fig. 6. An antibody to the γ subunit of phosphodiesterase (kindly provided by B. Fung) heavily labels the outer segments of the rods, but cone photoreceptors in their entirety. Note the significant change in the size and shape of the cone terminals when the retina has been detached for 3 days (**B**), and the fact that these terminals do not withdraw from their normal location along the OPL.

rods begin to regenerate an outer segment, or whether it represents some permanent change to the cell. It is still unknown how this opsin finds its way into the plasma membrane. Whether it is through some form of "reverse flow," from the degenerating outer segment, or whether it represents opsin that is inserted into the plasma membrane because it continues to be synthesized but cannot be used to construct an outer segment (Fariss et al., 1997) remains unresolved. There is evidence supporting the latter hypothesis, but there is also no obvious reason why both mechanisms could not be operating. Cones show a different pattern. There is a short time (about 3 days) during which the plasma membrane may show a slight increase in labeling intensity with a cone opsin antibody (Figs. 4E, K, 7E). This labeling rarely extends into the synaptic terminals, and disappears completely from the majority of surviving cones after about 1 week (Fig. 7F). Essentially the same trend

occurs when other photoreceptor-specific antibodies are used. Although the pattern and intensity of label will vary, rods continue to express all of the proteins studied to date even in detachments of a month's duration. Indeed, in the case of phosducin, there is actually an increase in the amount detected in the rods, while others such as opsin and peripherin/rds shift their pattern of expression (Fisher et al., 1996; Fariss et al., 1997). As derived from a variety of studies using quantitative ELISAs, immunohisto-chemistry, and in situ hybridization, proteins produced by rods continue to be expressed, even though their pattern and location may be significantly different from those in normal retina (Fisher et al., 1996; Fariss et al., 1997). In the cones, however, the expression of each protein studied to date declines to very near the limits of detection by immunocyto-chemistry within a few days (Rex et al., 1997, 2000), or their presence becomes so sporadic that only an

The Müller Cell Response

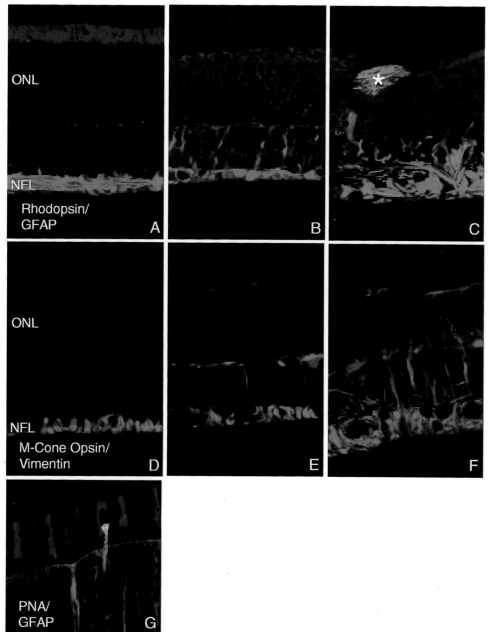

Fig. 7. The gliotic response of Müller cells to detachment demonstrated by immunolabeling with antibodies to intermediate filaments. ONL, outer nuclear layer; NFL, nerve fiber layer. **A,B,C**. Anti-GFAP (green) labels astrocytes in the optic nerve and faintly labels processes of Müller cells in normal retina. The rod outer segments are labeled with anti-rod opsin (red). Note the progressive labeling of the Müller cell processes with detachment time. In **C**, there is a large Müller cell scar (*) in the subretinal space. **D,E,F**. Labeling with anti-vimentin and an antibody to the M-cones. Anti-vimentin does not label astrocytes and shows the same Müller cell response as the anti-GFAP. **G**. Peanut agglutinin (PNA) is used to label all cones (red) in this section of retina detached for 3 days; the anti-GFAP (green) labeling shows how the leading edge of an expanding Müller cell process associates with a cone inner segment.

occasional, surviving cell shows immunolabeling. The data showing a dramatic increase in phosducin in the photoreceptors, and the fact that there is such a wide range of values for the expression of other rod-specific proteins indicates that these changes are almost certainly highly regulated, and not simply a "metabolic shut-down" of the rods as might be expected.

A logical interpretation of this data would be that individual rods continue producing opsin at near normal levels, and that they place much of this opsin into the plasma membrane because they cannot use it to construct an outer segment. The sharp decline in overall opsin levels comes from the combined loss of outer segments and rod cell death, and is not an indicator of the capacity of individual cells to synthesize the protein. This may position these cells favorably to begin re-constructing their outer segment as soon as favorable environmental conditions return, e.g. when the retina is reattached. Cones on the other hand, appear to enter a state where they stop expressing protein molecules, including their specific opsins. Why would the rods and cones differ so dramatically in their responses? Perhaps each has independently evolved mechanisms of self-protection and survival under "hostile" conditions. Rods far out-number cones in the feline (and primate) retina, so there may be enough redundancy in their numbers that even a significant loss of cells can be tolerated with relatively little effect on rod-mediated vision. Thus, some rods may be "culled" from the population when there is a lack of oxygen and nutrients from the RPE/choroid, allowing those that survive to continue synthesizing molecules used in transduction, and thus, be poised to regenerate rapidly. Because there are far-fewer cones, and because they tend to be concentrated in central retina and are critical to high-acuity vision, their loss, even in relatively small numbers may be visually significant. Thus, having all of the cones reduce their metabolic activities to a minimum level may be advantageous, and allow for survival of more of these cells.

If the metabolic effect on cones is indeed to stop their expression of various proteins as a means of survival, then it would be predicted that a greater percentage of the cone than rod population would survive, and that their recovery might be slower than that of the rods. Because of the loss of cone-specific markers, quantitating the number of cones that *survive* in the rod-dominated cat retina has proven exceptionally difficult (Linberg et al., 2000). We have two sets of studies underway that will help answer some of the questions of cone survival, and recovery. The first is a study of reattachment in the cat. In a retina detached for 7 days cone markers already provide an unreliable estimate of surviving cells. For example, the number of cones in the mid-periphery that label with an antibody to S-cone opsin is reduced to about 2.7% of the number in normal retina, and yet using another marker (anti-calbindin D) we would predict that 50% of the cones survive in this portion of the retina (Linberg et al., 2001). We can, however, detach the retina for 7 days and then reattach it for varying periods of time and use various cone markers to compare the number of cones at various reattachment intervals to those in normal and detached retina. If they are present in greater numbers after reattachment, than after detachment, they must have survived since new photoreceptors are not added in adult mammalian retina. The other study entails experimental detachments and reattachments in a retina that is cone-dominated (Linberg et al., 1999, 2000). With cones in the majority, do we find the same responses as in the rod-dominated retinas? Understanding the intriguing differences between rods and cones may be a significant step in conquering the sight-impairing diseases that affect the macula.

Photoreceptor cell death

It has been known now for over 15 years that significant numbers of photoreceptor cells die after detachment in both animal models (Erickson et al., 1983) and in humans (Wilson and Green, 1987). Apoptosis is probably the predominant mechanism of cell death (Cook et al., 1995; Chang et al., 1996). It appears that about 80% of the outer nuclear layer survives during 3 days of a detachment (Mervin et al., 1999). Since the cat retina is heavily rod-dominated, this is probably a good measure of rod survival. Quantitating the number of cones that die or survive has so far proven difficult as discussed above. Superficially, our data point to cones being lost more quickly than the rods. When anti-calbindin D labeling is used as a marker to count the number of cones there is a reduction from 7,000/mm² in the mid-peripheral retina of control eyes to 3,900/mm² in a comparable area of a 3-day detachment, a reduction to 56% of control values. When an antibody to the short-wavelength sensitive opsin is used to count the S-sensitive cones, they are reduced from 1,100 to 200/mm², a reduction to 18% of control values. Thus by either method it would *appear* that cones are lost much more rapidly than rods, and perhaps S-cones more quickly than the M-cones in this species (Linberg et al., 2001). But the fact is that we have no reliable marker for cones once they have been detached for as little as 3 days, and what we may well be describing is the loss of proteins, not the loss of cells. Thus, the important question of cone-survival remains a frustratingly unresolved one.

Effects on the inner retina

Plastic changes in second-order neurons

Initial ultrastructural observations showed the presence of post-synaptic processes at retracted rod photoreceptor terminals (Erickson et al., 1983), even those terminals that were deep in the ONL. Subsequent studies using antibodies that specifically label rod bipolar cells (anti-PKC), and horizontal cells (anti-calbindin D), showed that these observations were explained by the apparent growth of neurites from these cells (and presumably other second order neurons as well) (Lewis et al., 1998 and Fig. 5A–D). Indeed, these outgrowths appear to temporally accompany the retraction of the rod terminals, and by 3 days they are extensive across the zone of detachment. An interesting phenomenon occurs in longer-term detachments because the processes can often be identified growing past the layer of photoreceptors to the outer edge of the ONL where they appear to end "blindly." This latter effect was particularly prominent among the calbindin-D positive (horizontal cell) processes (Fig. 5C). Many of these growing processes also appear to run among or parallel to the processes of Müller cells. Whether they are in some way actively attracted to the Müller cells (Fig. 5D), which are undergoing many changes of

their own, or whether this is a passive phenomenon is unknown. Do third and fourth order neurons (amacrine and ganglion cells) react to detachment? Although detailed evidence is not yet available, preliminary evidence suggests that they do.

Müller cells and gliosis

In the brain and spinal cord, injury results in a rapidly mounted, stereotypical response by astrocytes known as gliosis. This can involve proliferation of these cells as well as their extensive hypertrophy to form glial scars in the region of the injury. In the feline (also rabbit, and probably primate) retinas, there is extensive proliferation of astrocytes after detachment, but the cells seem to remain relatively stable in terms of their size and location (Fisher et al., 1991; Geller et al., 1995). Müller cells, however, mount a robust astrocytic-like response. Indeed, their response is rapid, dramatic and can result in a complete remodeling of the structural appearance of the retina. They also play, along with the RPE cells, a serious role in proliferative diseases that can occur secondarily to detachment and cause blindness. One of these, proliferative vitreoretinopathy, or the proliferation and eventual contraction of cells on the vitreal surface of the retina, occurs in about 7–10% of successful reattachment surgeries. Basic structural changes can be recognized in Müller cells within a day or two as they increase the number of intermediate (GFAP and vimentin-containing) filaments in their cytoplasm. Within 3 days their processes can be seen growing into the subretinal space, and becoming thickened within the retina (Fig. 7). As detachment time proceeds, these changes become more exaggerated as their cytoplasm fills with newly synthesized intermediate filaments, and the processes enlarge within the retina and expand on the retinal surfaces (Fig. 7). Utilizing a variety of methods one can develop an appreciation for the complex response mounted by the Müller cells as they undergo significant transformations after detachment:

1. They proliferate. Normally quiescent, like the RPE, Müller cells begin to proliferate within a day, with the response reaching a peak at 3–4 days (Fig. 8J,K), but continuing at some low level

692

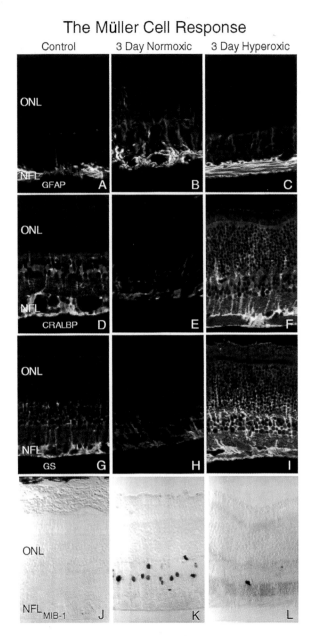

The Müller Cell Response

Control 3 Day Normoxic 3 Day Hyperoxic

as long as the retina remains detached (Fisher et al., 1991; Geller et al., 1995).

2. They expand in size. Müller cells normally have a fairly thin, sometimes branched, "trunk" that runs from the vitreal border to the level of the outer limiting membrane where their apical microvilli extend into the space between neural retina and RPE. The processes within the neural retina begin to grow in diameter until they can be fairly massive in size, cutting a huge swath through the retina (Figs. 7B; 8B). It might be thought that these expand to fill space left behind by dying neurons, except that they expand across the entire retina and neurons are lost only from the ONL. As mentioned above, they extend processes out of the neural retina (Fig. 2F). Antibodies to intermediate filament proteins clearly show this response (Fig. 7C). The processes that grow into the subretinal space seem to have a special affinity for cones cell bodies (Fig. 7G; Lewis and Fisher, 2000), perhaps due to the expression of the growth factor bFGF by these cells (Mervin et al., 1999). Growth of these processes on the photoreceptor surface interferes absolutely with outer segment regeneration in reattached retina (Fig. 2F). Growth occurs on the inner retinal surface as well, but only in detachments of long duration (28 days or more) in the feline model. As part of this response, their nuclei often migrate into the outer retina or even the subretinal space (Fig. 2F), but interestingly, never towards the inner retina.

3. They change their profile of protein expression. Besides the dramatic increase in GFAP and vimentin expression (Figs. 7; 8A,B), the expression of many other proteins change as well. Their cytoplasm rapidly becomes nearly devoid of such proteins as carbonic anhydrase C, cellular retinaldehyde binding protein (Fig. 8D,E), and

Fig. 8. Müller cell reactivity and responsiveness to hyperoxia. The left two columns are from animals (control or 3-day detached) kept in a normoxic environment, the right-hand column has data from 3-day detached retinas in which the animals were kept in an environment of 70% oxygen. **A,B,C.** Anti-GFAP labeling demonstrates the hypertrophy of Müller cells by 3-days in normoxia, and the significant lack of this response in animals kept in hyperoxia. **D,E,F.** Cellular retinaldehyde binding protein (CRALBP) is normally present throughout the Müller cell cytoplasm (**D**), and rapidly decreases when the retina is detached (**E**). Hyperoxia not only maintains but appears to increase the amount of CRALBP in the Müller cells after detachment (**F**). **G,H,I.** The pattern of labeling with anti-glutamine synthetase is remarkably similar to that of CRALBP. **J,K,L.** Labeling with the MIB-1 antibody to the Ki-67 antigen shows the presence of cells that have begun dividing. Routinely no labeled cells occur in normal retinae (**J**). The number of labeled cells is at its maximum at 3 days of detachment (**K**), and is greatly reduced by hyperoxia.

glutamine synthetase (Fig. 8G,H; Lewis et al., 1989; Lewis et al., 1994).

4. They change their amino acid profile. The loss of the glutamine synthetase correlates with a very large accumulation of glutamate (and a commensurate decline in glutamine) by these cells (Marc et al., 1998). The significance of this change is not known but the release or accumulation of glutamate during an episode of detachment may contribute to the overall responses of the retina, since glutamate is a powerful neurotoxin (Marc et al., 1998).

5. They react rapidly, with their response seemingly mediated through immediate early-response signaling pathways. The extracellular signaling kinase, ERK, becomes phosphorylated in Müller cells (and RPE cells) within 15 min of detachment. There is apparent de novo production of *c-fos* mRNA, and increased c-Fos and c-Jun (members of the AP-1 transcription factor) protein expression in both cell types within 2 h of a detachment (Geller et al., 2001).

Non-neuronal cells play an important part in the response to detachment

Thus, at least 2 non-neural cell types, the RPE and Müller cells have been demonstrated to play major roles in the retina's responses to detachment. They react quickly, transform their morphology, proliferate, and extensively change their metabolism (although data on the latter changes in RPE are scant), and these changes can have significant effects on the recovery process. A third cell type, the astrocytes that reside in the inner retinal layers also clearly react because they proliferate vigorously, but the significance of their response remains enigmatic. Understanding the role of the non-neuronal cells in maintaining the health of the normal and damaged retina remains an important challenge.

Mechanisms

We now have a few clues as to mechanisms that may be operating to produce the numerous changes that result from detachment:

1. Basic fibroblast growth factor (bFGF), probably plays a major role. When injected into the vitreous of normal eyes it causes Müller cells to divide (Fig. 9A), and to increase the number of intermediate filaments in their cytoplasm (Lewis et al., 1992). It also binds to Müller cells in what is most-likely a receptor mediated event (Fig. 9B; Lewis et al., 1996). Furthermore, there is an apparent release of bFGF from the inner retina after detachment (Fig. 9C,D), which is prevented by hyperoxia (Fig. 9E,F; Mervin et al., 1999). Hyperoxia also appears to increase the expression of bFGF by cones after detachment (Fig. 9E,F). The receptor for bFGF is phosphorylated rapidly after detachment (Geller et al., 2001).

2. Hypoxia of the outer nuclear layer may be responsible for many of the changes observed after detachment. Increasing the availability of environmental oxygen can both prevent photoreceptor cell deconstruction and the Müller cell gliotic response (see below; and Mervin et al., 1999; Lewis et al., 1999b). Modeling studies suggest that even relatively shallow detachments can produce significant hypoxia of the photoreceptors (Linsenmeier and Padnick-Silver, 2000).

Figure 10 shows proposed relationships between hypoxia, the inner retina, and bFGF that could result in the genesis of the changes that constitute the retinopathy resulting from a retinal detachment (Lewis et al., 1999b).

Preventing the retinopathy of detachment

Current experimental evidence suggests that the management of several different responses after detachment may be necessary to improve visual recovery above that obtained by the sophisticated procedures of modern retinal surgery: (1) preventing photoreceptor deconstruction and death, (2) improving the recovery capacity of photoreceptors after reattachment, and (3) preventing changes in non-neuronal (specifically the RPE and Müller cells) cells that may contribute to imperfect recovery or undesirable long-term side effects. There is now

bFGF and Retinal Detachment

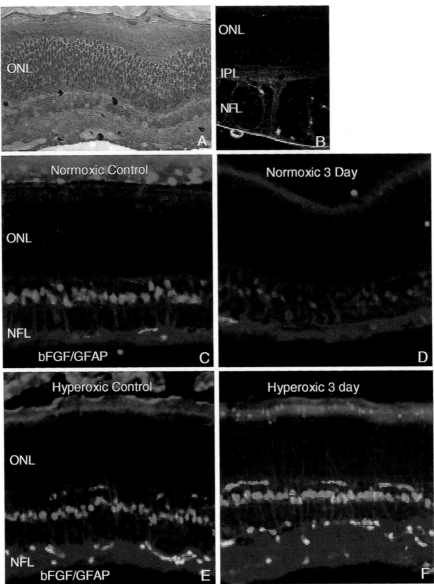

Fig. 9. Basic fibroblast growth factor bFGF and detachment. **A**. Labeling with the MIB-1 antibody 3 days after the injection of bFGF into the vitreous shows the presence of proliferating cells. **B**. When biotinylated bFGF is injected into the vitreous and detected with avidin-Cy3, it is first found associated mainly with the inner limiting membrane and within the extracellular space of the inner retina, 6 h later, it appears as punctate labeling associated with Müller cells, astrocytes, the RPE, and as a row in the OPL. At higher magnification the latter can be seen as within the synaptic invaginations of the photoreceptors. **C,D**. The localization of bFGF protein (green) and GFAP (red) in normal, normoxic retina (**C**), and normoxic 3-day detached retina (**D**). The protein appears to be rapidly lost from the inner retina after detachment. Note the faint labeling of cone outer segments in detached retina. **E,F**. The localization of bFGF protein (green) and GFAP (red) in normal hyperoxic retina (**E**), and hyperoxic 3-day detached retina (**F**). The hyperoxia may slightly increase the amount of bFGF in cells of the inner nuclear layer. In hyperoxic detached retina (**F**), the loss of bFGF from inner retina is prevented by the hyperoxia, and the labeling of cones is much more intense than in hyperoxic control retina.

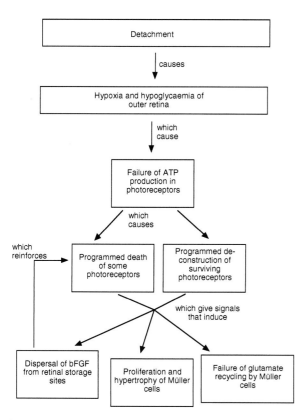

Fig. 10. An hypothesized scheme for the interactions of hypoxia and intracellular signaling to produce the retinopathy of detachment. Reprinted, with permission, from Lewis et al. (1999).

evidence that the neurotrophin BDNF (brain-derived neurotrophic factor) can slow the effects of detachment, and promote the production of remarkably well-formed outer segments in the absence of attachment to the RPE (Lewis et al., 1999a). BDNF treatment also reduces proliferation within the retina, and may prevent the long-term formation of glial scars. Keeping experimental animals in an atmosphere enriched with oxygen can have a similar effect including: preventing the loss of photoreceptor cells, preventing or slowing photoreceptor deconstruction (Fig. 4; Mervin et al., 1999), and mitigating the gliotic response of Müller cells (Fig. 8; Lewis et al., 1999b). Presently, the mechanisms through which the neurotrophin works is not well understood, especially since its effects on photoreceptors may be indirect, thus perhaps lessening its attractiveness as an adjunct to surgical therapy. Treatment of detachments with

hyperoxia though has considerable rationale and attraction. Modeling shows that detachments as shallow as 100 μm can create serious hypoxia of the photoreceptor layer, and that increasing environmental oxygen can have significant effects on oxygen available to the photoreceptor cells (Linsenmeier and Padnick-Silver, 2000). Short-term oxygen therapy is in use worldwide on a daily basis with essentially no adverse effects (Mervin et al., 1999).

Conclusions and future perspectives

While this research has specifically focused on retinal detachment, it is hoped that its outcome will be to produce a better understanding of retinal degenerations in general, and, perhaps lead us to clues that will be useful in preventing photoreceptor degeneration not just in cases of detachment, but in such diseases as age related macular degeneration, where millions suffer from a loss of sight with little hope for treatment. Clearly we must find ways to prevent photoreceptor cells from dying, and to stimulate those that survive to maintain the molecular machinery necessary for structural integrity, and visual transduction. We must also understand how rods and cones differ and how they are alike. These two subtypes of cells may react differently to degeneration induced by injury than to degeneration induced by genetic mutation. We have lagged significantly in our understanding of cone degenerations by comparison to those of rods. We must also determine if the primate fovea presents a specialized environment with its own set of rules and regulations by comparison to the rod-dominated periphery. We must seek to understand the role of non-neuronal cells in retinal degenerations, not only in the obvious proliferative diseases but also the role of these cells in maintaining the healthy and injured retina. New technologies such as gene array analysis will undoubtedly speed-up our understanding of the retina's response to injury, or its response to biological factors such as trophic molecules that may prove useful in treating degenerative diseases.

We have spent well over a decade studying retinal detachment as an "undesirable" condition, but as we enter the 21st Century, we find that retinal surgeons are now creating large retinal detachments as part of

696

experimental therapy to treat specific events in the subretinal space, especially in the neovascular changes that occur in age-related macular degeneration (Lewis et al., 1999). Therapies also are being proposed for diseases like retinitis pigmentosa that involve the injection of factors or biological vectors into the subretinal space, creating a temporary detachment (Flannery et al., 1997; Lewin et al., 1998; Lau et al., 2000). Will these detachments be sufficient to initiate the cascade leading to proliferative diseases months or years later? Will photoreceptors, already rendered fragile by an underlying pathological condition die in response to these treatments simply by virtue of their separation from the RPE? Can we treat these patients with something as simple as oxygen therapy and prevent these undesirable events? Although these are questions with specific clinical ramifications, their answers will come from the continued study and appreciation of basic retinal biology, through the continued study of the retina with the most modern methods available to biologists. It is the inspiration and dedication of scientists like John Dowling and his continuing, untiring advocacy for taking advantage of the most modern technology available to understand the retina that will lead us into a new era for the treatment of blinding diseases.

Acknowledgments

The research described in this chapter was supported by grant EY-00888 from the National Eye Insitute to SKF.

References

Anderson, D.H. and Fisher, S.K (1975) Disc shedding in rodlike and conelike photoreceptors of tree squirrels. *Science*, 187: 953–955.

Anderson, D.H. and Fisher, S.K. (1979) The relationship of primate foveal cones to the pigment epithelium. *J. Ultrastruct. Res.*, 67: 23–32.

Anderson, D.H., Fisher, S.K. and Steinberg, R.H. (1978) Mammalian cones: Disc shedding, phagocytosis, and renewal. *Invest. Ophthalmol. Vis. Sci.*, 17: 117–133.

Anderson, D.H., Stern, W.H., Fisher, S.K. Erickson, P.A. and Borgula, G.A. (1981) The onset of pigment epithelial proliferation after retinal detachment. *Invest. Ophthalmol. Vis. Sci.*, 21: 10–16.

Anderson, D.H., Stern, W.H., Fisher, S.K., Erickson, P.A. and Borgula, G.A. (1983) Retinal detachment in the cat: the pigment epithelial-photoreceptor interface. *Invest. Ophthalmol. Vis. Sci.*, 24: 906–926.

Anderson, D.H., Guerin, C.J., Erickson, P.A., Stern, W.H. and Fisher, S.K. (1986) Morphological recovery in the reattached retina. *Invest. Ophthalmol. Vis. Sci.*, 27: 168–183.

Chang, C., Lai, W., Edward, D. and Tso, M. (1996) Apoptotic photoreceptor cell death after traumatic retinal detachment in humans. *Arch. Ophthalmol.*, 114: 1158–1159.

Cook, B., Lewis, G.P., Fisher, S.K. and Adler, R. (1995) Apoptotic photoreceptor degeneration in experimental retinal detachment. *Invest. Ophthalmol. Vis. Sci.*, 36: 990–996.

Dowling, J.E. and Gibbons, I.R. (1961) The effect of vitamin A deficiency in the fine structure of the retina. In: Smelser, G.K. (Ed.), *Structure of the Eye.*, Academic Press, London, pp. 85–99.

Dowling, J.E. and Gibbons, I.R. (1962) The fine structure of the pigment epithelium in the albino rat. *J. Cell Biol.*, 14: 459–474.

Erickson, P., Fisher, S., Anderson, D., Stern, W. and Borgula, G. (1983) Retinal detachment in the cat: the outer nuclear and outer plexiform layers. *Invest. Ophthalmol. Vis. Sci.*, 24: 927–942.

Fariss, R.N., Molday, R.S., Fisher, S.K. and Matsumoto, B. (1997) Evidence from normal and degenerating photorectors that two outer segment integral membrane proteins have separate transport pathways. *J. Comp. Neurol.*, 387: 148–156.

Fisher, S.K. and Steinberg, R.H. (1982) Origin and organization of pigment epithelial apical projections to cones in cat retina. *J. Comp. Neurol.*, 206: 131–145.

Fisher, S.K., Pfeffer, B.A. and Anderson, D.H. (1983) Both rod and cone disc shedding are related to light onset in the cat. *Invest. Ophthalmol. Vis. Sci.*, 24: 844–856.

Fisher, S.K., Erickson, P.A., Lewis, G.P. and Anderson, D.H. (1991) Intraretinal proliferation induced by retinal detachment. *Invest. Ophthalmol. Vis. Sci.*, 32: 1739–1748.

Fisher, S.K., Lewis, G.P., Lo, G., Hussey, R.W. and Fariss, R.N. (1996) Changes in the expression of photoreceptor specific proteins after experimental retinal detachment. *Invest. Ophthalmol. Vis. Sci.*, 37: S1046.

Flannery, J.G., Zolotukhin, S., Vuero, M.I., LaVail, M.M., Muzyczka, N. and Hauswirth, W.W. (1997) Efficient photoreceptor-targeted gene expression in vivo by recombinant adeno-associated virus. *Proc. Natl. Acad. Sci. USA*, 94: 6916–6921.

Geller, S.C., Lewis, G.P., Anderson, D.H. and Fisher, S.K. (1995) The use of the MIB-1 antibody for detecting proliferating cells in the retina. *Invest. Ophthalmol. Vis. Sci.*, 36: 737–743.

Geller, S.F., Lewis, G.P. and Fisher, S.K. (2001) FGFR1, signalling, and AP-1 expression following retinal detachment: reactive Müller and RPE cells. *Invest. Ophthalmal. Vis. Sci.*, in press.

Hale, I.L., Fisher, S.K. and Matsumoto, B. (1991) Effects of retinal detachment on rod disc membrane assembly in cultured frog retinas. *Invest. Ophthalmol. Vis. Sci.*, 32: 2873–2881.

Hale, I.L., Fisher, S.K. and Matsumoto, B. (1996) The actin network in the ciliary stalk of photoreceptors functions in the generation of new outer segment discs. *J. Comp. Neurol.*, 376: 128–142.

Hay, A. and Landers, M.B. III. (1994) Types of pathogenetic mechanisms of retinal detachment. In: Glaser, B.M. (Ed.), *Retina, Surgical Retina*, Vol. 3, St. Louis, Mosby, pp. 1971–1977.

Hogan, M.J., Wood, I. and Steinberg, R.H. (1974) Phagocytosis by pigment epithelium of human retinal cones. *Nature (Lond.)*, 252: 305–307.

Kroll, A.J. and Machemer, R. (1968) Experimental detachment in the owl monkey. III. Electron microscopy of retina and pigment epithelium. *Am. J. Ophthal.*, 66: 410–427.

Kroll, A.J. and Machemer, R. (1969) Experimental retinal detachment in the owl monkey. V. Electron microscopy of the reattached retina. *Am. J. Ophthal*, 67: 117–130.

Lau, D., McGee, L., Zhou, S., Rendahl, K., Manning, W., Escobedo, J. and Flannery, J. (2000) Retinal degeneration is slowed in transgenic rats by AAV mediated delivery of FGF-2. *Invest. Ophthalmol. Vis. Sci.*, 41: 3622–3633.

Lewin, A.S., Drenser, K.A., Hauswirth, W.W., Nishikawa, S., Yasumura, D., Flannery, J.G. and LaVail, M.M. (1998) Ribozyme rescue of photoreceptor cells in a transgenic rat model of autosomal dominant retinitis pigmentosa. *Nat. Med.*, 4: 967–971.

Lewis, G.P., Erickson, P.A., Guerin, C.J., Anderson, D.H. and Fisher, S.K. (1989) Changes in the exprssion of specific Müller cell proteins during long-term retinal detachment. *Exp. Eye Res.*, 49: 93–111.

Lewis, G.P., Erickson, P.A., Anderson, D.H. and Fisher, S.K. (1991) Opsin distribution and protein incorporation in photoreceptors after experimental retinal detachment. *Exp. Eye Res.*, 53: 629–640.

Lewis, G.P., Erickson, P.A., Guerin, C.J., Anderson, D.H. and Fisher, S.K. (1992) Basic fibroblast growth factor: a potential regulator of proliferation and intermediate filament expression in the retina. *J. Neurosci.*, 12: 3968–3978.

Lewis, G.P., Guerin, C.J., Anderson, D.H., Matsumoto, B. and Fisher, S.K. (1994) Experimental retinal detachment causes rapid changes in the expression of glial cell proteins. *Am. J. Ophthalmol.*, 118: 368–376.

Lewis, B.P., Matsumoto, B. and Fisher, S.K. (1995) Changes in the organization and expression of cytoskeletal proteins during retinal degeneration induced by retinal detachment. *Invest. Ophthalmol. Vis. Sci.*, 36: 2404–2416.

Lewis, G.P., Erickson, P.A., Guerin, C.J., Anderson, D.H. and Fisher, S.K. (1996) Fate of biotinylated basic fibroblast growth factor in the retina following intravitreal injection. *Exp. Eye Res.*, 62: 309–324.

Lewis, G.P., Linberg, K.A. and Fisher, S.K. (1998) Neurite outgrowth from bipolar and horizontal cells after experimental retinal detachment. *Invest. Ophthalmol. Vis. Sci.*, 39: 424–434.

Lewis, G.P., Linberg, K.A., Geller, S.F., Guerin, C.J. and Fisher, S.K. (1999a) Effects of the neurotrophin brain-derived neurotrophic factor in an experimental model of retinal detachment. *Invest. Ophthalmol. Vis. Sci.*, 40: 1530–1544.

Lewis, G.P., Mervin, K., Valter, K., Maslim, J., Kappel, P.J., Stone, J. and Fisher, S. (1999b) Limiting the proliferation and reactivity of retinal Müller cells during experimental retinal detachment: The value of oxygen supplementation. *Am. J. Ophthalmol.*, 128: 165–172.

Lewis, G.P. and Fisher, S.K. (2000) Müller cell outgrowth after retinal detachment: association with cone photoreceptors. *Invest. Ophthalmol. Vis. Sci.*, 41: 1542–1545.

Lewis, H., Kaiser, P.K., Lewis, S. and Estafnaous, M. (1999) Macular translocation for subfoveal choroidal neovascularization in age-related macular degeneration: a prospective study. *Am. J. Ophthalmol.*, 128: 135–146.

Linberg, K.A. and Fisher, S.K. (1990) A burst of differentiation in the outer posterior retina of the eleven-week human fetus: an ultrastructural study. *Vis. Neurosci.*, 5: 43–60.

Linberg, K.A., Lewis, G.P., Charteris, D.G. and Fisher, S.K. (1999) Experimental detachment in cone dominant retina. *Invest. Ophthalmol. Vis. Sci.*, 40: S951.

Linberg, K.A., Lewis, G.P., Sakai, T., Leitner, W.P. and Fisher, S.K. (2000) A comparison of cellular responses to retinal detachment in cone- and rod-dominant species. *Invest. Ophthalmol. Vis. Sci.*, 41: S570.

Linberg, K.A., Lewis, G.P., Shaaw, C., Rex, T.S. and Fisher, S.K. (2001) The distribution of S- and M-cones in normal and experimentally detached cat retina. *J. Comp. Neurol.*, 430: 343–346.

Linsenmeier, R.A. and Padnick-Silver, L. (2000) Metabolic dependence of photoreceptors on the choroids in the normal and detached retina. *Invest. Ophthalmol. Vis. Sci.*, 41: 3117–3123.

Marc, R.E., Murry, R.F., Fisher, S.K., Linberg, K.A. and Lewis, G.P. (1998) Amino acid signatures in the detached cat retina. *Invest. Ophthalmol. Vis. Sci.*, 39: 1694–1702

Mervin, K., Valter, K., Maslim, J., Lewis, G., Fisher, S. and Stone, J. (1999) Limiting photoreceptor death and deconstruction during experimental retinal detachment: the value of oxygen supplementation. *Am. J. Ophthalmol.*, 128: 155–164.

Rex, T., Lewis, G. and Fisher, S. (1997) Rapid loss of blue and red/green opsin immunolabeling following experimental retinal detachment. *Invest. Ophthalmol. Vis. Sci.*, 38: S35.

Rex, T.S., Lewis, G.P., Yokoyama, S. and Fisher, S.K. (2000) Downregulation of cone opsin mRNA in surviving cones after retinal detachment. *Invest. Ophthalmol. Vis. Sci.*, 41: S599.

Steinberg, R.H. and Wood, I. (1974) Pigment epithelial cell ensheathment of cone outer segments in the retina of the domestic cat. *Proc. R. Soc. Lond. (Biol.)*, 187: 461–478.

Steinberg, R.H., Wood, I. and Hogan, M.J. (1977) Pigment epithelial ensheathment and phagocytosis of extrafoveal cones in human retina. *Philos. Trans. R. Soc. Lond. (Biol.)*, 277: 459–474.

Steinberg, R.H., Fisher, S.K. and Anderson, D.H. (1980) Disc morphogenesis in vertebrate photoreceptors. *J. Comp. Neurol.*, 190: 501–519.

Vaughan, D.K. and Fisher, S.K. (1987) The distribution of F-actin in cells isolated from vertebrate retinas. *Exp. Eye Res.*, 44: 393–406.

Williams, D.S. and Fisher, S.K. (1987) Prevention of rod disk shedding by detachment from the retinal pigment epithelium. *Invest. Ophthalmol. Vis. Sci.*, 28: 184–197.

Wilson, D.J. and Green, W.R. (1987) Histopathologic study of the effect of retinal detachment surgery on 49 eyes obtained post mortem. *Am. J. Ophthalmol.*, 103: 167–179.

Winkler, B. (1983) The intermediary metabolism of the retina: biochemical and functional aspects. In: Anderson, R.E. (Ed.), *Biochemistry of the Eye*. American Academy of Ophthalmol., San Francisco, pp. 227–242.

Young, R.W. (1967) The renewal of photoreceptor cell outer segments. *J. Cell Biol.*, 33: 61–72.

Young, R.W. and Bok, D. (1969) Participation of the retinal pigment epithelium in the rod outer segment renewal process. *J. Cell Biol.*, 42: 392–403.

Young, R.W. (1971) An hypothesis to account for a basic distinction between rods and cones. *Vision Res.*, 11: 1–5.

H. Kolb, H. Ripps and S. Wu (Eds.)
Progress in Brain Research, Vol. 131
© 2001 Elsevier Science B.V. All rights reserved

CHAPTER 50

The origin of photo-oxidative stress in the aging eye

Randolph D. Glickman*

*Department of Ophthalmology, University of Texas Health Science Center at San Antonio,
7703 Floyd Curl Drive, San Antonio, TX 78229-3900, USA*

Introduction

According to Harman's "free radical theory of aging" (Harman, 1956), many if not most age-related changes in biological organisms are due to the cumulative damage produced by free radical (oxidative) reactions. The effects of these reactions become more pronounced because of a decline in the aging organism's ability to resist oxidative damage, which in turn allows an increasing number of free radical reactive intermediates to be produced or released into the tissue matrix. The aging process then accelerates, leading ultimately to death. The eye, unfortunately, is not immune to these changes. Indeed many ocular disorders, including glaucoma, cataract, and retinal degenerations are age-related, and to some extent have been attributed to free radical processes (Zigman, 1985; Newsome et al., 1988; van Kuijk, 1991; Rice-Evans and Diplock, 1993; Linetsky and Ortwerth, 1996; Becquet et al., 1997). Among these disorders, the retinal degenerations, and more specifically age-related macular degeneration (ARMD), are the most relevant to the subject of this paper. In the work presented in this chapter, I have adopted a fundamentally "photo/biochemical" approach to understanding the origin of oxidative stress in the eye that might contribute to the onset of ARMD.

I think this approach—investigating visual problems at the cellular and molecular level—is a direct outgrowth of the training and experience I received in John Dowling's lab as a postdoctoral fellow in the late 1970s. At that time, much of the work in John's lab was directed at understanding phototransduction in terms of biochemical or molecular mechanisms. I would like to think that I adapted this biochemical methodology to my own area of interest, which was at that time retinal ganglion cell physiology, and that I have continued to do so throughout my career, so that the present work is a natural outgrowth of the experience received in John Dowling's laboratory.

ARMD is the leading cause of visual impairment among the population over the age of 60 (Rosen, 1979). Because there is no effective treatment for the disease, it presents a growing challenge for ophthalmology. Without a real understanding of the origins of ARMD, there has been little progress in developing effective treatments (although an experimental photodynamic therapy for some forms of ARMD involving subretinal neovascularization is showing some promise (Anonymous, 1999)). ARMD has been attributed to many factors, including metabolic disorders, toxic factors, nutritional deficiencies, smoking, and environmental stress including light damage (see Chan (1998); O'Shea (1998); and Smith et al., (1999) for recent reviews). While ARMD probably has a multifactorial etiology, the possibility that chronic light stress has a contributory role

* Tel.: 210-567-8420; Fax: 210-567-8413;
E-mail: glickman@uthscsa.edu

(Tso, 1988; Taylor et al., 1990) justifies investigating photochemical mechanisms of oxidative stress involving the RPE pigments, because the earliest signs of ARMD frequently occur in the RPE (Tso, 1988).

RPE pigments as chromophores

The basic premise of this chapter is that photo-oxidative stress in the eye is directly related to the light-induced reactions of the RPE pigments: melanin, lipofuscin, and melanolipofuscin. All of these pigment granules have been shown to possess photosensitizing properties, i.e. during irradiation with UV and visible wavelengths, they are excited to free radicals, and promote or participate in oxidative reactions. It has long been known that exposure to visible light excites melanin to a free radical (Mason et al., 1960; Cope et al., 1963). Lipofuscin and melanolipofuscin are pigments associated with age-related changes in the eye (Feeney-Burns and Eldred, 1983; Feeney-Burns et al., 1984, 1990), and are known to produce reactive molecular species (particularly oxygen radicals) during irradiation with visible and ultraviolet light (Gaillard et al., 1995; Reszka et al., 1995; Rozanowska et al., 1995). Recently, lipofuscin has been shown to cause oxidation of polyunsaturated fatty acids even in the absence of light (Dontsov et al., 1999). Melanin, on the other hand, is conventionally regarded as having a protective role against light damage (Rapp and Williams, 1980; Sanyal and Zeilmaker, 1988), but may also promote light damage under certain conditions because it is a photoinducible free radical (Cope et al., 1963), produces reactive oxygen radicals when irradiated (Sarna and Sealy, 1984; Korytowski et al., 1987), and promotes photochemical reactions with physiological substrates (Menon and Haberman, 1979; Glickman and Lam, 1992; Glickman et al., 1997; Rozanowska et al., 1997). An overview of the photochemistry of the RPE pigments and its relevance to oxidative stress in the eye will be presented below.

There is an extensive literature on ocular light damage and toxicity, much of which has been carried out in various rodent models. Because of the availability of diverse inbred strains of mice, it is now possible to investigate the contribution of specific genetic variations to mechanisms of retinal light toxicity (see, for example, LaVail et al. (1999)). Questions have been raised, however, regarding the extent to which the degenerative processes studied in rodents may be extrapolated to primates, including humans (Lawwill, 1982). Partly because of these questions, the experiments described here were designed to reconsider the issue of photo-oxidative damage in the eye at a basic level; namely, determining which chromophores are responsible for photochemical damage in the RPE, as well as the mechanisms by which these activated chromophores promote photo-oxidative damage.

Studies on isolated RPE melanosomes

Because of the difficulty of measuring directly in vivo the photoactivation of pigment molecules, e.g. excited triplet or free radical states, the general approach taken in these studies was to measure identifiable chemical products resulting from presumed photochemical reactions. A relatively simple assay of this type was developed that measured the oxidation of the nicotinamide cofactor, NADPH, caused by photoactivation of RPE pigment granules, primarily melanin (Glickman et al., 1996). The assay was based on the property of NADPH that, as it is oxidized, its optical density at 340 nm decreases. In practice, the extent of pigment photoactivation was quantified simply by measuring the change in optical density of a NADPH-melanin reaction mixture after a period of light exposure.

Melanin in the RPE is contained in structures called melanosomes that possess protein coats, but lack true membranes. The other RPE pigments, lipofuscin and melanolipofuscin, are present in less well-defined granules. For the initial in vitro experiments, relatively pure melanosomes were isolated from bovine eyes obtained from young, slaughterhouse animals. The anterior segments were dissected from these eyes, and the RPE cells and choroid were brushed from the posterior poles. After breaking the cells by ultrasonication, the melanosomes were purified by successive centrifugations through different concentrations of sucrose (Glickman et al., 1993; Dontsov et al., 1999).

Free radical activity was induced in reaction mixtures of melanosomes and NADPH by a 5 min exposure to the mixed 488 and 514.5 nm output of a Argon ion (Ar$^+$) continuous wave (CW) laser at a typical sample irradiance of 2 to 3 W/cm^2. Following the laser exposure, the samples were filtered to remove the melanosomes, and the optical density at 340 nm (A$_{340}$) read in a spectrophotometer. The results of such an experiment, using various durations of Ar$^+$ laser exposure to "pump" the melanosome reaction, are shown in Fig. 1. The decline in A$_{340}$ was linearly proportional to the laser exposure time (Glickman et al., 1996). In the dark, there was little NADPH oxidation indicating that melanin was quiescent in the absence of light irradiation.

An interesting finding made during the course of these investigations was that the reactivity of the RPE

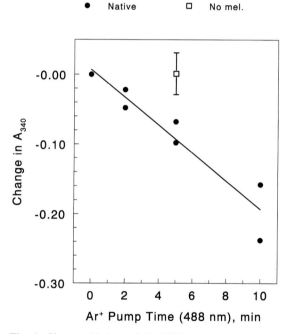

Fig. 1. Photo-oxidation of NADPH by laser-excited intact melanosomes. Reaction mixtures consisted of approximately 7500 bovine melanosomes and 7 mM β-NADPH in 80 mM Tris buffer (pH 7.2), in a volume of 25 μl. Samples were placed in clear plastic microcentrifuge tubes, and exposed to the 488 nm line of an Ar$^+$ laser CW for the indicated "pump" times. Following laser exposure, melanosomes were removed from the samples by filtration through a 0.45 μm pore nitrocellulose filter, and the optical density at 340 nm of the filtrates was measured. The drop in A$_{340}$ in the graph represents the difference between paired, laser-exposed and unexposed samples. (From Glickman et al., 1996)

melanosomes depended on their structural integrity. The reaction shown in Fig. 1 utilized "native" melanosomes, i.e. granules isolated only by the procedure outlined above. Melanosomes, however, could be photodisrupted by exposing them to the output of a pulsed source such as a Q-switched Neodymium:YAG laser with a typical output pulse duration of about 10 ns (10×10^{-9} s). Such short laser pulses, if they delivered a sufficient amount of energy per pulse, disrupted tissue explosively because the energy was delivered faster than the thermal relaxation time (about 1 μs for many biological structures in an aqueous medium), causing explosive vaporization of water contained in the internal structures. This type of laser damage mechanism has been termed "thermal confinement" (Jacques, 1992). Scanning electron micrographs of native and photodisrupted RPE melanosomes are shown in Fig. 2.

When photodisrupted melanosomes were used in the photoactivation assay, the amount of NADPH oxidized per unit CW laser pump time was increased about three-fold (Fig. 3). Whether this increase was due to a change induced by the YAG laser exposure in the number of reactive sites in the melanin heteropolymer, or simply because the effective surface area was increased by breaching the protein coats of the melanosomes, has not been established. Nevertheless, this observation suggested that when the melanosome degenerates, such as occurs in some age-related processes, the apparent inhibitory effect of the melanoproteins is diminished and the photochemical activity of the RPE melanin increases, contributing to an overall increase in oxidative stress to the retina-RPE complex.

Action spectrum of the melanin radical estimated from NADPH oxidation

The NADPH assay was also used to determine an effective action spectrum for melanin reactions in the visible range, using various visible wavelengths generated by Ar$^+$, Kr$^+$, and Helium-Cadmium (HeCd) CW lasers (Fig. 4). All the exposures with the exception of the 441.6 nm emission of the HeCd laser were adjusted to deliver 3.18×10^{21} photons/cm^2 during a 5 min exposure of the sample (see Fig. 4 for details). These measurements revealed that the

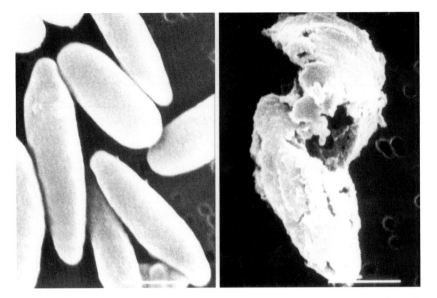

Fig. 2. Scanning electron micrographs of intact and laser-disrupted bovine RPE melanosomes. Left: native melanosomes. Right: melanosomes exposed to a train of 1800 pulses from a Nd:YAG laser (frequency-doubled output: 532 nm, nominal pulse width 10 ns) that delivered 214 mJ/cm^2 per pulse to the melanosomes. Scale bars in both images indicate 1 μm. (From Glickman et al., 1996)

efficiency for exciting the melanin radical is greatest for wavelengths between 450 and 500 nm, and decreased at shorter and longer wavelengths. Assuming that photoactivated melanin is a principal chromophore responsible for promoting oxidative damage in the RPE and retina, this action spectrum may point to the photophysical basis for so-called "blue light toxicity" to the primate retina (Harwerth and Sperling, 1971; Moon et al., 1978).

Melanosomes and photo-oxidative damage to proteins

Light-activated melanosomes also promote oxidative damage to biological macromolecules such as proteins. This was demonstrated by the detection of carbonyl adducts, a classic marker of protein oxidation (Levine et al., 1990; Stadtman, 1993), in a preparation of soluble retinal proteins containing bovine RPE melanosomes, following exposure to a monochromatic laser. The protein carbonyl adducts were detected with a sensitive western blot immunoassay using the technique of Shacter et al. (1994). The results of such a western blot assay is shown in Fig. 5. The horizontal bands in each vertical lane in the figure are the images of chemiluminescent proteins separated on the original polyacrylamide gel: the darker the image, the more oxidized the original protein.

In the absence of any light exposure (lane 1 of Fig. 5), the protein carbonyl signal was very low. Exposure of the proteins to a broadband light source (a Xenon arc lamp) without melanosomes present produced a large increase in the number of carbonyl adducts (dark bands in lane 2 of Fig. 5). The addition of melanosomes to the proteins appeared to confer some protection against the arc lamp exposure, as indicated by a reduced number of carbonyl adducts per unit quantity of protein (reduced band density in lanes 3 and 4 of Fig. 5). In distinction to the effects with the arc lamp exposure, the presence of melanosomes greatly enhanced protein oxidation produced by exposure to the Ar$^+$ laser emission. In the absence of any melanosomes, the laser radiation produced little oxidation of the proteins (lane 5 of Fig. 5). This is consistent with the low visible wavelength absorption of most proteins. When melanosomes were present, however, exposure of the proteins to the mixed, 488 and 514.5 nm laser wavelengths produced massive oxidation of virtually all of the proteins in the sample (lanes 6 and 7, Fig. 5). These experiments

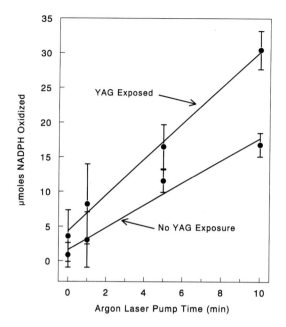

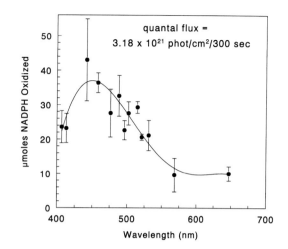

Fig. 3. YAG laser disruption of bovine RPE melanosomes enhances their photochemical activity (means ± 1 S.D.). Paired aliquots of bovine melanosomes were placed in separate microcentrifuge tubes. One member of each pair was exposed to a train of 1800 pulses from a Nd:YAG laser (fundamental output: 1064 nm, 10 ns pulse width, repetition rate of 10 Hz) so that the sample received a radiant exposure of 1900 mJ/cm^2/pulse. (A higher radiant exposure had to be used with the 1064 nm laser emission to achieve disruption because the internal absorption coefficient in melanin is lower at this wavelength than at 532 nm). Upon completion of photodisruption, both samples were mixed with the NADPH reaction mixture, "pumped" by exposure to the Ar$^+$ CW laser at 2 W/cm^2 for the times indicated on the graph, and the A_{340} measured as described in Fig. 1. The amount of NADPH oxidized was calculated from the optical absorbance change using the molar extinction coefficient for NADPH at 340 nm, which is ∼6100/cm/M. The photodisrupted melanosomes are about three times more reactive than their intact counterparts in the NADPH assay. (From Gerstman and Glickman, 1999)

Fig. 4. Action (or efficiency) spectrum of RPE melanosomes determined by the NADPH photo-oxidation assay. Photo-oxidation measurements, using the NADPH assay as described in Fig. 1, were made using different "pump" wavelengths in the range from 406.7 to 647.1 nm. The wavelengths were derived from several CW laser sources. All the exposures were set to deliver 3.18 × 10^{21} photons/cm^2/s, with the exception of the 441.6 nm line derived from a HeCd laser. The power available from this laser was insufficient to reach the required level, so the data obtained at this wavelength were scaled up, assuming a linear relationship between sample irradiance and NADPH oxidation. This manipulation, however, increased the variance in the data and resulted in the large error bars (means ± 1 S.D.) shown in Fig. 1 for the data point at 441.6 nm. The rest of the data, however, showed much less variability. (From Glickman et al., 1997)

wavelengths emitted by the Xe arc lamp. On the other hand, the Ar$^+$ laser emitted all of its light energy near the peak of the melanin action spectrum, and maximally excited the melanin radical resulting in widespread protein oxidation.

Other RPE pigments

The aging RPE contains other pigments besides melanin, notably lipofuscin and melanolipofuscin (Feeney-Burns et al., 1984). These pigments also exhibit photochemical activity. Lipofuscin and melanolipofuscin granules, as well as melanosomes, were prepared by a modification of the technique of Boulton and Marshall (1985). Specific details concerning the preparation of the pigment granules may be found in Dontsov et al. (1999). The isolated

not only revealed the broad effects of melanin photoactivation, but also indicated that an important factor governing whether melanin is photoprotective or photosensitizing is the spectral nature of the incident radiation. That is, the broadband light probably delivered an insufficient number of photons in the critical 450–500 nm region to excite the melanin oxidative reactions, and therefore the melanin actually served to screen and partially protect the proteins from phototoxic effects of the UVA

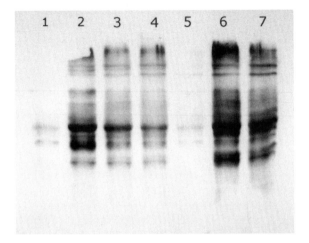

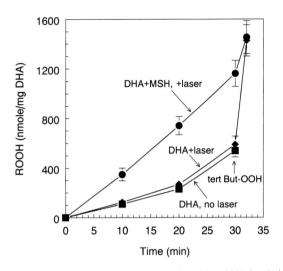

Fig. 5. Chemiluminescent assay of carbonyl adducts in laser-exposed soluble retinal proteins. Proteins were prepared by disrupting freshly obtained baboon retina in Tris buffered saline. Solid debris was removed by centrifugation at $14,000 \times g$ for 10 min at 4°C. The soluble retinal proteins in the supernatant were used for these experiments. Twenty-five-μl aliquots of the supernatant were placed in 1.5 ml plastic centrifuge tubes, either alone, or with 5-μl (lanes 3 and 6) or 10-μl (lanes 4 and 7) of a suspension of bovine melanosomes. The protein mixtures were then exposed for ten minutes to the broadband output of a 150 mW Xenon arc lamp at a sample irradiance of 1.17 W/cm^2 (lanes 2, 3 and 4), or to the mixed 488 and 514.5 nm output of an Ar$^+$ CW laser at a sample irradiance of 1.29 W/cm^2 (lanes 5, 6 and 7). Following irradiation, protein carbonyls were detected in a western blot using the Oxyblot® chemiluminescence assay. (See Glickman et al. (1997) for details)

Fig. 6. Peroxidation of docosahexaenoic acid (DHA) by Ar$^+$ laser exposure in the presence and absence of human melanosomes (MSH). The reaction mixtures consisted of 70–80 μg/ml DHA mixed with 0.1 M potassium phosphate buffer, pH 7.44, 1 mM EDTA, 1 mM glutathione (GSH), 0.7 units GSH reductase, 0.4 units of GSH peroxidase, 200 μM NADPH, and, in the condition testing the effect of MSH, 2.2×10^7 melanin granules/ml. The sample was divided into two equal parts, one exposed to light, and one maintained in the dark. Following laser exposure, the samples were placed in a spectrophotometer cuvette, and A_{340} was measured over time. After 30 min, tert-butyl-OOH was added to demonstrate activity of the enzyme assay system. The results were converted into nmol hydroperoxides, and plotted against time as shown here. Adding melanosomes greatly increased the amount of DHA hydroperoxides produced during the laser exposure. (From Dontsov et al., 1999)

human RPE pigment granules were used to study photoinduced peroxidation of the polyunsaturated fatty acid (PUFA), cis-4,7,10,13,16,19-docosahexaenoic acid (DHA) (Dontsov et al., 1999). DHA is an especially appropriate substrate in the context of ocular oxidative damage, because it is the most unsaturated physiological fatty acid, accounts for nearly 25% of the fatty acids in the retina, and is the most common PUFA in photoreceptors (van Kuijk and Buck, 1992).

DHA photo-oxidation by light-excited RPE pigment granules

Peroxidation of the PUFA, DHA, was demonstrated by irradiating mixtures of various RPE pigment granules and DHA with the blue-green emission of the Ar$^+$ CW laser. Sample irradiance was studied over the range of 50 to 1500 mW/cm^2, and the exposure duration was 10 min. The production of fatty acid hydroperoxides was determined enzymatically using the reaction of the resulting hydroperoxides with NADPH-dependent glutathione peroxidase (Organisciak and Noell, 1976). The results of such an experiment showing stimulation of DHA peroxidation in the presence of RPE melanosomes are shown in Fig. 6. Only when melanosomes were present, did laser exposure increase the oxidation of DHA above the ambient autoxidation level.

The photoreactivity towards DHA of all of the RPE pigment granule types was compared in similar experiments, the results of which are displayed in Fig. 7. The three panels of this figure show the

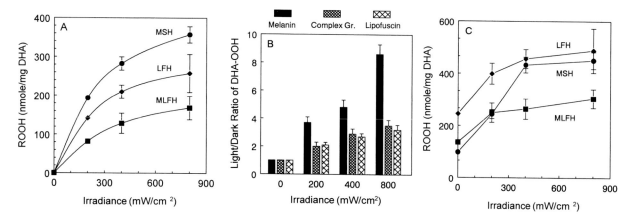

Fig. 7. Comparison of DHA peroxidation produced by photoactivation of the three types of RPE pigment granules. Abbreviations as follows: MSH, human RPE melanosomes; LFH, human lipofuscin granules; MLFH, human melanolipofuscin granules. Paired samples were used; one member of each pair was exposed to the blue-green output of an Ar$^+$ laser for 10 min at the indicated irradiance, while the other was kept as an unexposed control. Each point is the average of two measurements; the error bars show the range. Panel A (left): DHA hydroperoxides produced during light exposure minus the dark control level. Panel B (center): ratio of light to dark peroxidation. Panel C (right): total DHA hydroperoxides produced, i.e. light level plus dark level. (From Dontsov et al., 1999)

same data set, analyzed in different ways. Fig. 7A (left-hand panel) quantifies the production of DHA hydroperoxides as the laser-stimulated production minus the dark background (control) amount. Melanosome-containing samples exhibited the largest amount of light-stimulated peroxidation, followed by lipofuscin- and melanolipofuscin-containing samples, respectively. The center panel (Fig. 7B) shows the same data plotted as the ratio of laser-stimulated to dark control DHA hydroperoxides. Looking at the data in this way confirms that the melanosomes are the most photo-inducible of the three pigment types, generating over an eight-fold increase in DHA peroxidation at the highest sample irradiation studied, compared to three-fold or less for the other pigment types. A somewhat different conclusion, however, emerged when the data were plotted as the total production of DHA hydroperoxides, i.e. as laser-stimulated plus dark background activity (Fig. 7C, right hand panel). It is apparent that lipofuscin granules actually produced as much or more DHA hydroperoxidation than did the melanosomes, because lipofuscin was active even in the absence of light. The melanolipo-fuscin granules contributed the least to fatty acid peroxidation.

Measurement of photo-oxidative stress in intact RPE cells

The goal of these experiments was to demonstrate that the photochemical reactions observed with isolated, light-activated pigment granules also occur in intact RPE cells. Primary cultures of RPE cells were established in the laboratory using bovine eyes freshly obtained from a local slaughterhouse, and from baboon eyes generously provided by the Southwest Foundation for Biomedical Research in San Antonio. RPE cells were grown in Dulbecco's Minimum Essential Medium containing 10% fetal calf serum and maintained at 37°C in an atmosphere supplemented with 5% CO_2. To detect the presence of photo-oxidative reactions in the cells, we utilized two commercially available, oxidation-sensitive probes, 2'-7'-dichlorofluorescein (DCFH) and dihydrorhodamine 123 (DHR123). These probes are nonfluorescent when chemically reduced, but become highly fluorescent when oxidized. In use the probes are applied in the reduced form to the cells under study, which then take up the probe. Following some experimental manipulation, any fluorescence that develops in the cells is considered a marker of oxidative stress, and may be observed directly by fluorescence microscopy or quantified by instrumental fluorescence measurement (see, for example, Royall and Ischiropoulos (1993)). Both approaches were used to study photo-oxidative stress in the cultured RPE cells.

Direct visualization of oxidative processes in RPE cells

If a vital, fluorescent stain can be visualized with fluorescence microscopy, information about the spatial localization of oxidative reactions within the cell may be obtained. Fluorescence microscopy was used to image RPE cells loaded with DCFH or DHR123, following induction of photo-oxidative stress in the cells by exposure to a light source. A low-power Argon laser, or the blue FITC exciter lamp in the fluorescence microscope, was used as the light source. Initially, the results were encouraging, as an increase in cellular fluorescence after light exposure was observed (Glickman et al., 1999). Unexposed cells, or cells exposed to long-wavelength visible light, developed much less fluorescence. It proved impractical, however, to obtain quantitative data strictly with imaging, chiefly because of two factors. One was the difficulty in calibrating the fluorescence signal so that meaningful comparisons could be made between experiments. The second problem resulted from the cells' pigmentation. Many of the cells in the primary RPE cell cultures used in these studies were heavily pigmented, and the pigment itself tended to quench or block the fluorescence signal from the cells. In many cells, only a bright, fluorescent halo could be observed. Nevertheless, in those preparations in which intracellular fluorescence was clearly observed, the fluorescence was limited to the cytoplasm, and did not extend into the nucleus. This observation indicated that photo-oxidative reactions occurred in the vicinity of the melanosomes, which are only located in the cytoplasm, and is consistent with the pigment granules being involved with photo-oxidative stress in the cell. The limited, qualitative nature of the data yielded by fluorescence microscopy stimulated the development of a biochemical methodology for direct analysis of the probe.

Direct analysis of oxidation-sensitive probes

It proved possible to recover up to 80% of the intracellular probe by using solid phase extraction (SPE) to separate oxidized probe from soluble cellular lysates. SPE employs selective elution of analytes of interest from a sorbent material (usually a silica derivative) using a specific solvent, leaving unwanted material bound to the extraction cartridge. This technique worked quite well in recovering probe molecules from lysed RPE cells. The extract was then injected into a reverse phase HPLC column and the eluant passed through a fluorescence detector to measure the amount of probe oxidized in the cell.

Cellular uptake of fluorescent probe

To determine whether the probes were actually taken up by the cultured cells, RPE cells were incubated for various time periods in 10 μM DCFH or DHR123, and then the probes were extracted from the cells using SPE. The cell extracts were chemically oxidized by treatment with horseradish peroxidase and H_2O_2. This was done to make any probe contained in the extracts fluorescent and thus measureable with HPLC analysis with fluorescence detection. The time course of RPE cell probe uptake versus time determined by HPLC is shown in Fig. 8. DCFH generally was taken up quickly and reached a maximum in about 20 min, after which the intracellular content of the probe gradually declined (Fig. 8, left). DHR123 was accumulated more slowly, reaching a plateau at about 60 min which was maintained for up to another hour (Fig. 8, right) (Glickman et al., 1999).

Photo-oxidation of intracellular probe

If light exposure does in fact excite intracellular pigments, then the resulting photochemical reactions may be coupled to the oxidation of the probe molecules to an extent depending on the irradiation of the cells and the wavelength of the irradiating light (because of the action spectra of the responsible chromophore). The quantitative nature of the HPLC analysis made it possible to address this hypothesis (Glickman et al., 1999). RPE cell cultures were incubated with 10 μM DCFH or DHR123

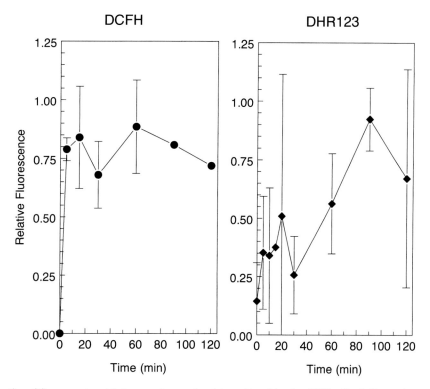

Fig. 8. Uptake kinetics of fluorescent, oxidation-sensing probes into cultured bovine RPE cells. Left panel: uptake of DCFH. Right panel: uptake of DHR123. Data are plotted as means ± 1 S.D. Method: Aliquots of 10^6 RPE cells were incubated in 10 μM probe for varying times, centrifuged, and the resulting pellet washed once in probe-free culture medium. Cells were lysed by incubation with 500 μl of 0.5% Triton X in Tris buffered saline for 10 min. The samples were centrifuged, and the supernatant containing the probe and soluble components of the cytosol were chemically oxidized and then processed with a Waters Oasis HLB SPE cartridge eluted with methanol. Aliquots of this eluant were injected into a Waters Bondapak-C$_{18}$ HPLC analytical column. The mobile phase for DCFH analysis was 8 mM ammonium phosphate (pH 8.0) in 60% methanol, and for DHR123 was 8 mM ammonium phosphate (pH 8.0) in 60% acetonitrile. The flow rate was 1 ml/min. Fluorescence detection was performed with excitation at 488 nm, and emission at 530 nm. (From Glickman et al., 1999)

for 1 h, and then either kept in the dark as a control or exposed for 10 min to one of the following laser emissions: 488 nm (Ar$^+$ laser), 514.5 nm (Ar$^+$ laser), or 647.1 nm (Kr$^+$ laser). All exposures were quantum-equivalent, delivering ~4.99 × 10^{18} photons/cm^2/s in the 10 min period. Following the laser exposure, the cells were lysed and the probe isolated from the lysates by SPE. Twenty-μl aliquots were injected into the HPLC column and the probe content quantified by fluorescence detection. DCFH exhibited a clear pattern of photo-oxidation by laser exposure, as shown in Fig. 9. In the dark, or with samples containing cell-free media, there was a low level of fluorescence detected, indicating that most of the probe remained in the reduced form. All of the three laser wavelengths resulted in DCFH oxidation,

but the degree to which the probe was oxidized was clearly wavelength-dependent. On a quantal basis, the Argon 488 nm output was the most efficient in producing photo-oxidation. In contrast, DHR123 was not consistently photo-oxidized. The amount of fluorescence recovered from exposed RPE cells labeled with DHR123 did not bear any clear relationship to the wavelength or intensity of the laser irradiation (data not shown).

Significance of the wavelength dependence of DCFH photo-oxidation

Although the intracellular photo-oxidative conversion of DCFH to DCF (the fluorescent form)

708

has been characterized for only three principal wavelengths, the results obtained were very consistent with the melanin action spectrum shown in Fig. 4. Both data sets have a peak in the wavelength range between 450 and 500 nm. It is interesting that if the data shown in Fig. 9 are normalized and super-imposed on the melanin action spectrum of Fig. 4, the two sets of data overlap closely, as shown in Fig. 10. Apparently, photo-oxidation of DCFH in laser-exposed RPE cells follows a very similar wavelength dependence as that of NADPH with isolated melanosomes. It is uncertain why DHR123 was not similarly photo-oxidized in the RPE cell, but recently we have found that this probe has a higher oxidation potential (0.490 V) than that of DCFH (0.411 V), relative to normal hydrogen electrode,

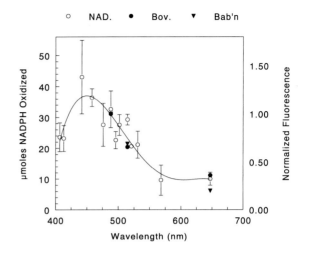

Fig. 10. Correspondence of photo-oxidative stress in intact RPE cells, measured by DCF fluorescence, with the action spectrum of isolated RPE melanosomes, as measured by the NADPH assay. Open circles (data from experiment shown in Fig. 4): photo-oxidation of NADPH. Filled symbols (data from experiment shown in Fig. 9): normalized DCFH fluorescence measurements in bovine (filled circles) and baboon (filled triangles) RPE cells. See text for additional discussion.

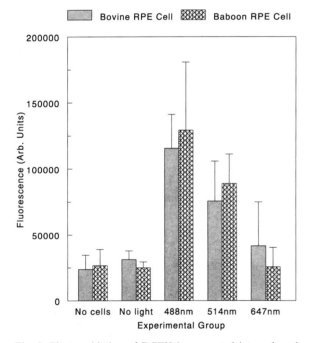

Fig. 9. Photo-oxidation of DCFH incorporated into cultured bovine and baboon RPE cells following exposure to the wavelengths indicated in the figure, which were derived from Ar$^+$ and Kr$^+$ laser sources. All exposures delivered 4.99×10^{18} photons/cm^2/s for 10 min. The probes were extracted from the cells using SPE, and fluorescence was assayed by HPLC by the method described in Fig. 8, except that the extracts were *not* chemically oxidized prior to HPLC analysis. Histogram bars show mean fluorescence in arbitrary units, plus 1 s.d. The 488 nm wavelength was the most quantum-efficient in producing oxidative conversion of the probes. (From Glickman et al., 1999)

and, too, the oxidation reaction kinetics differ (Glickman et al., 1998). The higher redox potential of DHR123 may prevent it from reacting with specific oxidizing species in the cell. Another possibility is that because DHR123 is more lipophilic than DCFH, the probe may be selectively taken up in membranous structures such as mito-chondria where it is inaccessible to the pigment granules.

The localization of DCF fluorescence only in the cytoplasm of the cell argues strongly that the chromophore responsible for this photochemical reaction is one of the RPE pigment granules. Melanin is the most likely candidate for two reasons. One, because the DCFH photo-oxidation data over-laps the melanin action spectrum as discussed above, and two, because lipofuscin and melanolipo-fuscin, the other two RPE pigment granules, are not found in appreciable quantities in the young bovine eyes used in these experiments (Dontsov et al., 1999). The baboon eyes that were also used were from older animals possibly containing larger amounts of lipofuscin, therefore the contribution of lipofuscin cannot be totally excluded. There was insufficient tissue available from the baboon eyes to analyze for lipofuscin. Nevertheless, because lipofuscin is capable of inducing oxidative reactions in the dark (Dontsov et al., 1999), the minimal amount of probe oxidation in the control conditions suggests that the involvement of lipofuscin granules was negligible. In vivo, however, oxidative stress from lipofuscin and melanolipofuscin granules accumulating in the aging RPE cell is likely to be significant.

Photochemical reaction mechanisms in the RPE

Based on the assumption that molecular oxygen is present in excess in the RPE, it is likely that the reaction of photoexcited melanin proceeds according to the mechanism(s) proposed by Rozanowska et al. (1997), and extended by Dontsov et al. (1999). The probable primary reactive species are the quinone (MQ), semiquinone (MSQ$^{\bullet-}$), and hydroquinone (MQH$_2$) groups of the hydroxyindole subunits of the melanin heteropolymer. The effect of visible light is to push the equilibrium between the quinone, hydroquinone, and semiquinone species to the right so that the occurrence of the semiquinone form is favored:

$$MQ + MQH_2 \overset{h\nu}{\rightleftharpoons} 2MSQ^{\bullet-} + 2H^+ \qquad (1)$$

This is presumably the only light-induced reaction. The semiquinones may react with suitable substrates, such as PUFA, directly in a Type I (free radical) reaction or through a Type II reaction involving an oxygen radical intermediate (Girotti, 1990; Holte et al., 1990) as follows:

Type I

$$MSQ^{\bullet-} + DHA\text{-}H + H^+ \rightleftharpoons DHA^{\bullet} + MQH_2 \quad (2)$$

where DHA-H represents the PUFA and DHA$^{\bullet}$ the alkyl radical, or

Type II

$$MSQ^{\bullet-} + O_2 \rightleftharpoons MQ + O_2^{\bullet-} \qquad (3)$$

where the reaction of the semiquinone radical with oxygen produces superoxide anion. Following this/these reaction(s), hydroperoxides of the fatty acids may be produced in the following reaction:

$$DHA\text{-}H + HOO^{\bullet} \rightarrow H_2O_2 + DHA^{\bullet} \qquad (4)$$

in which DHA$^{\bullet}$ is formed by abstraction of a hydrogen atom by the perhydroxyl radical, HOO$^{\bullet}$. Although this conjugate acid may only represent 1% of the total superoxide at physiological pH, it is relatively efficient at producing fatty acid hydroperoxides, especially if hydroperoxides are already present (Aikens and Dix, 1991). Interaction of the alkyl radical with oxygen forms a peroxyl radical:

$$DHA^{\bullet} + O_2 \rightarrow DHA\text{-}OO^{\bullet} \qquad (5)$$

A chain reaction between the peroxyl radical and the PUFA ensues, producing the hydroperoxide products:

$$DHA\text{-}OO^{\bullet} + DHA\text{-}H \rightarrow$$
$$DHA\text{-}OOH + DHA^{\bullet} \qquad (6)$$

Other physiological substrates may react in a similar fashion, undergoing oxidative damage by Type I or Type II reactions, depending on local conditions in the tissue. Lipofuscin probably undergoes a similar set of free radical reactions, except that because of the catalytic action of the divalent metal ions commonly associated with lipofuscin, Type II reaction mechanisms are likely to dominate.

Conclusions and future perspectives

The experimental findings reported here confirm previous reports of the photochemical reactivity of RPE pigments (Sarna and Sealy, 1984; Glickman et al., 1993; Gaillard et al., 1995; Rozanowska et al., 1995, 1997; Dontsov et al., 1999). The question may be raised, however, if the reactions of isolated pigment granules, easily demonstrated in vitro, are relevant to the more complex situation in vivo. In particular, the dual role of melanin is troubling, i.e. whether it serves to protect against, or to promote, phototoxicity. Classically regarded as a protective pigment on account of its presumed screening properties (Wolbarsht et al., 1981), ability to sequester heavy metals (Swartz et al., 1992), or trap free radicals (Sakina et al., 1990; Porebska-Budny et al., 1992), the results presented here indicate that under certain conditions melanin can function as a photosensitizer. For example, in highly oxygenated tissues such as the retina, RPE, and choroid, photoactivated melanin is likely to participate in free radical reactions, especially if cellular antioxidants are depleted. This may in fact be the case in the aging eye, when, because of insufficient supplies of anti-oxidants or a reduced capacity to maintain the energy-dependent recycling of antioxidant (i.e. from the oxidized to reduced forms as in the case of ascorbic acid (Rose and Bode, 1992)), melanin functions more as a photosensitizer than as a protective pigment. An additional oxidative burden in the aging RPE cell is the progressive accumulation of the degenerative pigments, lipofuscin and melanolipofuscin, both of which are photochemically reactive. Moreover, the ability of lipofuscin to promote oxidative damage to PUFA even in the dark supports the view that lipofuscin itself is a marker of oxidative stress. The other consequence of lipofuscin's basal oxidative activity is that simply eliminating the light activation of the RPE pigment reactions—for example by reducing the amount of blue light entering the eye—will not totally prevent, but only reduce, oxidative damage from occurring. The situation seems to call for a targeted antioxidant that will be able to cross the blood-retina barrier, accumulate in RPE cells, and directly quench the RPE pigment reactions regardless of whether those reactions are light-stimulated or constitutive.

Although the photochemical reactions described above generally proceed with relatively fast kinetics, i.e. with rate constants typically in excess of $10^4/\mathrm{M/s}$, the oxidative damage they produce contributes to the progressive accumulation of damaged material within the cell. Moreover, the constant oxidative stress presented by these reactions causes ongoing errors in the cell's reparative mechanisms that ultimately result in defective products expressed from the cell's genome. It is this cumulative load of free-radical induced damage occurring over the cell's lifetime that constitutes the aging process (Harman, 1956).

By adopting the "Dowling approach" to the problem of oxidative stress, that is by investigating the problem beyond a purely physiological level to gain an insight into relevant biochemical mechanisms, we have begun to appreciate the complex role in health and disease of the photoreactive pigments of the primate RPE. Unless the RPE cells have anti-oxidants that quench the reactive species produced directly or indirectly by these light-activated pigment granules, cellular damage will likely ensue. The cumulative effects of such damage over the course of a lifetime may be the basis of some of the age-related retinal degenerations. The RPE melanosome also breaks down in age, leading to the accumulation of melanolipofuscin granules along with the lipofuscin granules. The breakdown of the melanosome structure, particularly its melanoprotein coat, is associated with increased photochemical reactivity. All of these observations considered together lead to the general conclusion that the RPE pigments may play "Jekell and Hyde" roles in the eye: protecting against light damage as long as sufficient antioxidants are present to quench light-induced pigment radicals, but promoting light damage in the event of anti-oxidant depletion or inability to support antioxidant recycling. By understanding how the RPE cell utilizes antioxidant stores, mobilizes antioxidants and reparative enzymes, and disposes of oxidatively damaged molecules, we will finally have a basis for preventing oxidative stress in the retina and its supportive tissues, and for designing effective therapies against retinal degenerations.

Acknowledgments

I thank the following collaborators for their contributions to this research; it would not have been possible without their participation and intellectual stimulation: Drs. Alexander E. Dontsov, Bernard S. Gerstman, Steven L. Jacques, Kwok-Wai Lam, Mikhail A. Ostrovsky, and Benjamin A. Rockwell. Ms. Neeru Kumar provided excellent technical assistance. Drs. G. Buhr, M. Vendal, and M.A. Gonzalez performed research in my laboratory as Lions Summer Scholars. Research support was provided by Air Force Office of Scientific Research grants F49620-95-1-0332 and F49620-98-1-0210, the San Antonio Area Foundation, Lions Club Local 2A2, the Howard Hughes Medical Institute Research Resources Program grant to the UTHSCSA, the Helen Freeborn Kerr Foundation, and an unrestricted grant from Research to Prevent Blindness (RPB) to the UTHSCSA Department of Ophthalmology. I thank Drs. Glen Pu and Michael Zeldin for their constructive comments on this manuscript.

References

Aikens, J. and Dix, T.A. (1991) Perhydroxyl radical (HOO•) initiated lipid peroxidation. *J. Biol. Chem.*, 266: 15091–15098.

Anonymous (1999) Photodynamic therapy of subfoveal choroidal neovascularization in age-related macular degeneration with verteporfin: one-year results of 2 randomized clinical trials–TAP report. Treatment of Age-related macular degeneration with Photodynamic therapy (TAP) Study Group. *Arch. Ophthalmol.*, 117: 1329–1345.

Becquet, F., Courtois, Y. and Goureau, O. (1997) Nitric oxide in the eye: Multifaceted roles and diverse outcomes. *Surv. Ophthalmol.*, 42: 71–82.

Boulton, M. and Marshall, J. (1985) Repigmentation of human retinal pigment epithelial cells in vitro. *Exp. Eye Res.*, 41: 209–218.

Chan, D. (1998) Cigarette smoking and age-related macular degeneration. *Optom. Vis. Sci.*, 75: 476–484.

Cope, F.W., Sever, R.J. and Polis, B.D. (1963) Reversible free radical generation in the melanin granules of the eye by visible light. *Arch. Biochem.*, 100: 171–177.

Dontsov, A.E., Glickman, R.D. and Ostrovsky, M.A. (1999) Retinal pigment epithelium pigment granules stimulate the photo-oxidation of unsaturated fatty acids. *Free Rad. Biol. Med.*, 26: 1436–1446.

Feeney-Burns, L. and Eldred, G.E. (1983) The fate of the phagosome: conversion to 'age pigment' and impact in human retinal pigment epithelium. *Trans. Ophthalmol. Soc. UK*, 103(Pt 4): 416–421.

Feeney-Burns, L., Hilderbrand, E.S. and Eldridge, S. (1984) Aging human RPE: morphometric analysis of macular, equatorial and peripheral cells. *Invest. Ophthalmol. Vis. Sci.*, 25: 195–200.

Feeney-Burns, L., Burns, R.P. and Gao, C.L. (1990) Age-related macular changes in humans over 90 years old. *Am. J. Ophthalmol.*, 109: 265–278.

Gaillard, E.R., Atherton, S.J., Eldred, G. and Dillon, J. (1995) Photophysical studies on human retinal lipofuscin. *Photochem. Photobiol.*, 61: 448–453.

Gerstman, B.S. and Glickman, R.D. (1999) Activated rate processes and a specific biochemical mechanism for explaining delayed laser induced thermal damage to the retina. *J. Biomed. Opt.*, 4: 345–351.

Girotti, A.W. (1990) Photodynamic lipid peroxidation in biological systems. *Photochem. Photobiol.*, 51: 497–509.

Glickman, R.D. and Lam, K.-W. (1992) Oxidation of ascorbic acid as an indicator of photooxidative stress in the eye. *Photochem. Photobiol.*, 55: 191–196.

Glickman, R.D., Sowell, R. and Lam, K.-W. (1993) Kinetic properties of light-dependent ascorbic acid oxidation by melanin. *Free Rad. Biol. Med.*, 15: 453–457.

Glickman, R.D., Jacques, S.L., Schwartz, J.A., Rodriguez, T., Lam, K.-W. and Buhr, G. (1996) Photodisruption increases the free radical reactivity of melanosomes isolated from retinal pigment epithelium. In: Jacques, S.L. (Ed.), *Laser-Tissue Interaction VII, Proc. SPIE*, 2681, Bellingham (WA): SPIE, pp. 460–467.

Glickman, R.D., Rockwell, B.A. and Jacques, S.L. (1997) Action spectrum of oxidative reactions mediated by light-activated melanin. In: Jacques, S.L. (Ed.), *Laser-Tissue Interaction VIII, Proc. SPIE*, 2975, Bellingham (WA): SPIE, pp. 138–145.

Glickman, R.D., Gonzales, M.A., Kumar, N. and Vendal, M. (1998) Oxidative stress in retinal pigment epithelium. *Free Rad. Biol. Med.*, 25(suppl 1): S102.

Glickman, R.D., Vendal, M., Gonzales, M.A. and Kumar, N. (1999) Intracellular photochemical reactions in the RPE cell exhibit a wavelength dependence that resembles the action spectrum of melanin. In: Jacques, S.L., Müller, G.J., Roggan, A. and Sliney, D.H. (Eds.), *Laser-Tissue Interaction X: Photochemical, Photothermal, and Photomechanical, Proc. SPIE*, 3601, Bellingham (WA): SPIE, pp. 94–101.

Harman, D. (1956) Aging: a theory based on free radical and radiation chemistry. *J. Gerontol.*, 11: 298–300.

Harwerth, R.S. and Sperling, H.G. (1971) Prolonged color blindness induced by intense spectral lights in rhesus monkeys. *Science*, 174: 520–523.

Holte, L.L., van Kuijk, F.J.G.M. and Dratz, E.A. (1990) Preparative high-performance liquid chromatograpy purification of polyunsaturated phospholipids and characterization using ultraviolet derivative spectroscopy. *Anal. Biochem.*, 188: 136–141.

Jacques, S.L. (1992) Laser-tissue interactions: photochemical, photothermal, and photomechanical. *Surg. Clin. N. Am.*, 72: 531–558.

Korytowski, W., Pilas, B., Sarna, T. and Kalyanaraman, B. (1987) Photoinduced generation of hydrogen peroxide and hydroxyl radicals in melanins. *Photochem. Photobiol.*, 45: 185–190.

LaVail, M.M., Gorrin, G.M., Yasumura, D. and Matthes, M.T. (1999) Increased susceptibility to constant light in *nr* and *pcd* mice with inherited retinal degenerations. *Invest. Ophthalmol. Vis. Sci.*, 40: 1020–1024.

Lawwill, T. (1982) Three major pathologic processes caused by light in the primate retina: A search for mechanisms. *Trans. Am. Ophthal. Soc.*, 80: 517–579.

Levine, R.L., Garland, D., Oliver, C.N., Amici, A., Climent, I., Lenz, A.-G., Ahn, B.-W., Shaltiel, S. and Stadtman, E.R. (1990) Determination of carbonyl content in oxidatively modified proteins. *Methods Enzymol.*, 186: 464–478.

Linetsky, M. and Ortwerth, B.J. (1996) Quantitation of the reactive oxygen species generated by the UVA irradiation of ascorbic acid-glycated lens proteins. *Photochem. Photobiol.*, 63: 649–655.

Mason, H.S., Ingram, D.J.E. and Allen, B. (1960) The free radical property of melanins. *Arch. Biochem. Biophys.*, 86: 225–230.

Menon, I.A., and Haberman, H.F. (1979) Mechanisms of action of melanin in photosensitized reactions. In: Klaus, S.N. (Ed.), *Pigment Cell*, Basel: Karger, pp. 345–351.

Moon, M.E., Clarke, A.M., Ruffolo, J.J. Jr., Mueller, H.A. and Ham, W.T. Jr. (1978) Visual performance in the rhesus monkey after exposure to blue light. *Vis. Res.*, 18: 1573–1577.

Newsome, D.A., Swartz, M., Leone, N.C., Elston, R.C. and Miller, E. (1988) Oral zinc in macular degeneration. *Arch. Ophthalmol.*, 106: 192–198.

Organisciak, D.T. and Noell, W.K. (1976) Hereditary retinal dystrophy in the rat: lipid composition of debris. *Exp. Eye Res.*, 22: 101–113.

O'Shea, J.G. (1998) Age-related macular degeneration. *Postgr. Med. J.*, 74: 203–207.

Porebska-Budny, M., Sakina, N.L., Stepien, K.B., Dontsov, A.E. and Wilczok, T. (1992) Antioxidative activity of synthetic melanins. Cardiolipin liposome model. *Biochem. Biophys. Acta.*, 1116: 11–16.

Rapp, L.M. and Williams, T.P. (1980) A parametric study of retinal light damage in albino and pigmented rats. In: Williams, T.P. and Baker, B.N. (Eds.), *The Effects of Constant Light on Visual Processes*, New York: Plenum Press, pp. 135–159.

Reszka, K., Eldred, G.E., Wang, R.H., Chignell, C. and Dillon, J. (1995) The photochemistry of human retinal lipofuscin as studied by EPR. *Photochem. Photobiol.*, 62: 1005–1008.

Rice-Evans, C.A. and Diplock, A.T. (1993) Current status of antioxidant therapy. *Free Rad. Biol. Med.*, 15: 77–96.

Rose, R.C. and Bode, A.M. (1992) Tissue-mediated regeneration of ascorbic acid: Is the process enzymatic? *Enzyme*, 46: 196–203.

Rosen, E.S. (1979) Involutional macular degeneration. In: Yannuzzi, L.A. Gitter, K.A. and Schatz, H. (Eds.), *The Macula: A Comprehensive Text and Atlas*, Baltimore (MD): Williams & Wilkins Co, pp. 203–208.

Royall, J.A. and Ischiropoulos, H. (1993) Evaluation of 2',7'-dichlorofluorescin and dihydrorhodamine 123 as fluorescent probes for intracellular H_2O_2 in cultured endothelial cells. *Arch. Biochem. Biophys.*, 302: 348–355.

Rozanowska, M., Jarvis-Evans, J., Korytowski, W., Boulton, M.E., Burke, J.M. and Sarna, T. (1995) Blue light-induced reactivity of retinal age pigment. In vitro generation of oxygen-reactive species. *J. Biol. Chem.*, 270: 18825–18830.

Rozanowska, M., Bober, A., Burke, J.M. and Sarna, T. (1997) The role of retinal pigment epithelium melanin in photo-induced oxidation of ascorbate. *Photochem. Photobiol.*, 65: 472–479.

Sakina, N.L., Dontsov, A.E., Afanas'ev, G.G., Ostrovski, M.A. and Pelevina, I.I. (1990) The accumulation of lipid peroxidation products in the eye structures of mice under whole-body x-ray irradiation [Russian]. *Radiobiologia.*, 30: 28–31.

Sanyal, S. and Zeilmaker, G.H. (1988) Retinal damage by constant light in chimaeric mice: implications for the protective role of melanin. *Exp. Eye Res.*, 46: 731–743.

Sarna, T. and Sealy, R.C. (1984) Free radicals from eumelanin: quantum yields and wavelength dependence. *Arch. Biochem. Biophys.*, 232: 574–578.

Shacter, E., Williams, J.A., Lim, M. and Levine, R.L. (1994) Differential susceptibility of plasma proteins to oxidative modification. Examination by western blot immunoassay. *Free Rad. Biol. Med.*, 17: 429–437.

Smith, W., Mitchell, P., Webb, K. and Leeder, S.R. (1999) Dietary antioxidants and age-related maculopathy: the Blue Mountains Eye Study. *Ophthalmol.*, 106: 761–767.

Stadtman, E.R. (1993) Oxidation of free amino acids and amino acid residues by radiolysis and by metal-catalyzed reactions. *Ann. Rev. Biochem.*, 62: 797–821.

Swartz, H.M., Sarna, T. and Zecca, L. (1992) Modulation by neuromelanin of the availability and reactivity of metal ions. *Ann. Neurol.*, 32(Suppl): S69–S75.

Taylor, H.R., Munos, B., West, S., Bressler, N.M., Bressler, S.B. and Rosenthal, F.S. (1990) Visible light and risk of age-related macular degeneration. *Trans. Am. Ophthal. Soc.*, 88: 163–178.

Tso, M.O.M. (1988) Photic injury to the retina and pathogenesis of age-related macular degeneration. In: Tso, M.O.M. (Ed.), *Retinal Diseases*, Philadelphia: J.B. Lippincott, pp. 187–214.

van Kuijk, F.J.G.M. (1991) Effects of ultraviolet light on the eye: Role of protective glasses. *Environ. Health Perspect.*, 96: 177–184.

van Kuijk, F.J.G.M. and Buck, P. (1992) Fatty acid composition of the human macula and peripheral retina. *Invest. Ophthalmol. Vis. Sci.*, 33: 3493–3496.

Wolbarsht, M.L., Walsh, A.W. and George, G. (1981) Melanin, a unique biological absorber. *Appl. Opt.*, 20: 2184–2186.

Zigman, S. (1985) Photobiology of the lens. In: Maisel, H. (Ed.), *The Ocular Lens: Structure, Function, Pathology*, Marcel Dekker, Inc., New York, pp. 301–347.

H. Kolb, H. Ripps and S. Wu (Eds.)
Progress in Brain Research, Vol. 131
© 2001 Elsevier Science B.V. All rights reserved

CHAPTER 51

Retinal ganglion cells, glaucoma and neuroprotection

Stuart A. Lipton*

*Center for Neuroscience and Aging, The Burnham Institute, 10901 North Torrey Pines Road, La Jolla, CA 92037, USA
and The Scripps Research Institute; The Salk Institute for Biological Studies, La Jolla, CA 92037, USA
and University of California, San Diego, CA, USA*

Introduction

My own introduction to the retina came as a graduate student in John Dowling's laboratory beginning in the late summer of 1974. Along with Sandy Ostroy, who was on sabbatical, and with the help of another mentor, Howard Rasmussen, who was known for his seminal work relating the intertwined effects of Ca^{2+} and cyclic nucleotides, we began to study the electrophysiological effects of these agents on the rod photoresponse. Using sharp electrodes, this work was the first to describe the electrophysiological effects of cGMP on the light response of single photoreceptors (Lipton et al., 1977b). Our results paved the way for the later discovery of cGMP-activated ion channels in rod photoreceptors using the yet-to-be-invented patch-clamp technique (Fesenko et al., 1985). Additionally, we studied light and dark adaptation in rods, and the influence of Ca^{2+} on adaptation in vertebrate photoreceptors was characterized for the first time (Lipton et al., 1977a, 1979).

Little did I know at that time what a profound influence that work in the retina would have on my career, and also how indebted I was to John for his mentoring of students, insights into physiological processes, and ethical approach to science. Later, after I had become a neurologist at Harvard studying neuroprotection in the brain, I would return to the retina to show that glaucoma, the most common cause of blindness in the USA (and second worldwide), had a neurological basis and could be treated with the very neuroprotective agents that our group had found worked elsewhere in the brain for other neurodegenerative conditions. I never would have had this insight into retinal protection without John's teaching that "The Retina [is] an Approachable Part of the Brain." Below, I briefly outline the story of neuroprotection in the retina and how it grew out of more general neuroprotective studies deeper in the brain because of my earlier work with John.

Excitotoxic and free radical injury to retinal ganglion cells

In recent years, excitotoxic (glutamate-related) and free radical-mediated injury/cell death of neurons has been recognized as an important final common pathway in a variety of neurological disease, ranging from acute ischemic stroke and trauma, to chronic neurodegenerative conditions such as Huntington's Disease, amyotrophic lateral sclerosis, Alzheimer's disease, and HIV-associated dementia (Choi, 1988; Meldrum and Garthwaite, 1990; Dawson et al., 1991; Lipton et al., 1993; Lipton and Rosenberg, 1994;

---

* Tel.: 858-713-6261; Fax: 858-713-6262;
E-mail: slipton@burnham.org

714

Ankarcrona et al., 1995; Bonfoco et al., 1995). Although retinal ganglion cells have a variety of glutamate receptors (Aizenman et al., 1988) and were the first neurons to be demonstrated to be killed by glutamate (Lucas and Newhouse, 1957), relatively little had been done to relate this type of cell death to the major diseases of the retina until the last decade (Hahn et al., 1988; Olney, 1990). Retinal ganglion cells were known to die in a variety of ophthalmological disorders. My colleagues and I have shown that these maladies, which include such diverse entities as retinal artery occlusion (ischemia), glaucoma, and AIDS-associated damage due to the release of neurotoxins from HIV-infected macrophages and microglia, are all due at least in part to the excitotoxic and free radical nature of the insult. Moreover, the existence of a final common pathway for neuronal damage means that a similar therapeutic approach may possibly be effective for each of these varied insults.

An excitotoxic/free radical etiology for glaucoma

Glaucoma leads to a particularly enigmatic form of retinal ganglion cell death. We all think of glaucoma as a primarily anterior chamber disease mediated in most cases by high intraocular pressure. However, ophthalmologists have know for years that relief of high pressure in many cases does not cure the disease, and patients go on to become blind in the face of lowered pressures. About a dozen years ago, my colleagues and I realized that glaucomatous pressure, like trauma or ischemia in the nervous system, may be responsible for the release of excessive glutamate into the vitreous, to produce what John Olney has called for other regions of the central nervous system (CNS), excitotoxic damage. Such an insult could outstrip its protective neurotrophic factor supply and lead to retinal ganglion cell death, as observed in glaucoma. Indeed, we subsequently demonstrated that vitreal glutamate is elevated to levels that cause apoptosis of retinal ganglion cells over a prolonged period of time (Figs. 1 and 2) (Dreyer et al., 1996). We also showed that, in general, mild excitotoxic/free radical insults for prolonged periods can result in apoptosis, as observed in glaucoma, while more intense exposure can result in extreme energy

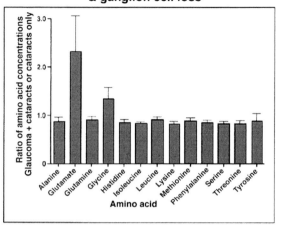

Fig. 1. Histograms to show elevated amino acids in the vitreous in glaucoma. Glutamate levels are elevated 2 to 3-fold in glaucomatous vitreous compared to other amino acids; this increase is highly statistically significant (Dreyer et al., 1996; Dreyer and Lipton, 1999). Glycine is modestly elevated but the increase did not reach statistical significance.

depletion with consequent failure of ionic homeostasis and cell lysis or necrosis, as seen at the focal point of an acute ischemic insult (Dreyer et al., 1994; Ankarcrona et al., 1995; Bonfoco et al., 1995; Dreyer et al., 1995). An additional theory to excitotoxicity in glaucomatous damage holds that deprivation of growth factors may result in the demise of retinal ganglion cells, and both excitotoxic and growth factor components may well exist (Dreyer and Lipton, 1999).

Therapeutic approaches to preventing retinal ganglion cell injury: glutamate receptor antagonists

The major type of glutamate receptor that leads to retinal ganglion cell injury in our experiments is due to overstimulation of the N-methyl-D-aspartate (NMDA) subtype of receptor (Hahn et al., 1988; Sucher et al., 1991). Although other glutamate receptors can contribute to excitotoxicity, the NMDA receptor is particularly important because of its extreme permeability to Ca^{2+}, which in excess can overload mitochondria, and lead to excessive enzyme activity and free radical formation. Previously, multiple attempts to develop clinically

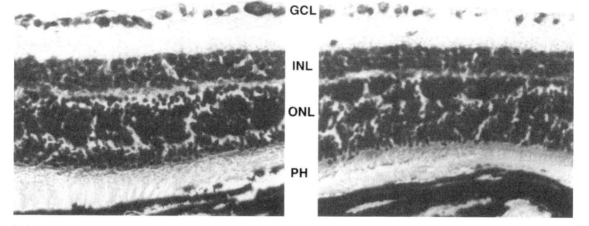

Fig. 2. A normal rodent retina (left) has a large number of cells in the ganglion cell layer (GCL) while mild chronic elevation of the glutamate level, as seen in glaucoma (right), has resulted in the loss of many of these cells. (From Vorwerk et al., 1996)

tolerated NMDA receptor antagonists have failed because of problems with side effects (Lipton, 1993; Lipton and Rosenberg, 1994). After all, the NMDA receptor is important in normal functioning of the nervous system, for example, in many CNS pathways mediating long-term potentiation, thought to represent a cellular correlate of learning and memory.

NMDA receptor antagonists: open-channel block and S-nitrosylation

We have developed a series drugs that interfere only with excessive activation of NMDA receptor-operated ion channels and leave relatively spared normal, physiological activity (Chen et al., 1992; Chen and Lipton, 1997; Chen et al., 1998). In this manner, side effects are avoided. Interestingly, one such agent that we have developed, the open-channel blocker memantine, is of relatively low affinity, and thus spares normal function. However, it is of high selectivity so it does not block the functioning of other receptor types. Our laboratory has used this therapeutic approach to prevent apoptosis and necrosis of various neuronal cell types bearing NMDA receptors, including retinal ganglion cells. In fact, memantine recently passed a series of five phase III (final) clinical trials for vascular dementia and Alzheimer's disease in both Europe and the USA. The drug is now marketed in Europe as a neuroprotectant and is being considered for approval by the Food and Drug

Administration in the US. Additionally, a very large phase III clinical trial for glaucomatous damage is currently underway on several continents with memantine, and the results of that trial are expected within the next couple of years.

We have also described redox modulatory sites, consisting of several critical cysteine residues on the NMDA receptor, that appear to act biophysically as the gain control of the receptor. In simple terms, these sites, similar to memantine blocking the NMDA receptor-operated ion channel only when it is open for excessively long (pathological) periods of time, act like a volume control on your television set. By turning down the volume, we can avoid excessive stimulation of the cell by NMDA receptors and thus avoid excitotoxic cell death. Redox related forms of nitric oxide (NO) can react with some of these cysteine residues by a novel chemical reaction that we and our colleagues have characterized, known as S-nitrosylation (representing transfer of the NO group to a cysteine sulfhydryl). This reaction affords neuroprotection to retinal ganglion cells as well as to other types of neurons (Lipton et al., 1993; Kim et al., 1999; Choi et al., 2000). We have also combined these redox-active drugs with channel blockers like memantine to produce new therapeutic agents, called nitro-memantines, that act as if they modulate two volume control knobs on your television set. In this manner, we can fine tune receptor activity and avoid side effects even more effectively while preventing neuronal cell damage. By combining structure–function information about the NMDA receptor in this manner and by obtaining crystal structure information at the sites of drug interaction, we hope to design even better and safer therapeutic reagents.

A new family of NMDA receptor subunits that act as modulatory agents

Recently, while studying drug-receptor interactions, we cloned and characterized a new family of NMDA receptor subunits, termed NR3. In the case of NR3A, the first family member that we cloned, the subunit acts in a novel manner somewhat akin to memantine and NO-related species to modulate NMDA receptor activity by acting as a "volume control." In this case, when expressed in conjunction with the previously known NR1 and NR2 subunits of the NMDA receptor, NR3A decreases the unitary current and the degree of Ca^{2+} permeability of the channels (Sucher et al., 1995; Das et al., 1998). Therefore may be of therapeutic importance, and indeed preliminary evidence suggests that NR3A protects the young nervous system from excitotoxic damage during development.

Events downstream to the NMDA receptor

Additional studies on our laboratory have characterized a series of downstream signaling pathways thatlead to apoptosis and are triggered by excessive stimulation of NMDA receptors in both retinal ganglion cells and cerebrocortical neurons (Fig. 3). These pathways include: (i) mitochondrial Ca^{2+} overload with subsequent cytochrome c release (Budd et al., 2000); (ii) free radical production (reactive nitrogen intermediates, such as nitric oxide, and reactive oxygen species, such as superoxide anion) (Lipton et al., 1993; Bonfoco et al., 1995); (iii) p38 mitogen activated protein kinase (MAPK)-induced phosphorylation/activation of MEF2 transcription factor (Leifer et al., 1993; Okamoto et al., 2000) and (iv) caspase activation with DNA fragmentation and apoptosis (Tenneti et al., 1998; Tenneti and Lipton, 2000). Interestingly, we have shown that NO-related species can react not only with critical cysteines on the NMDA receptor but also with a cysteine residue

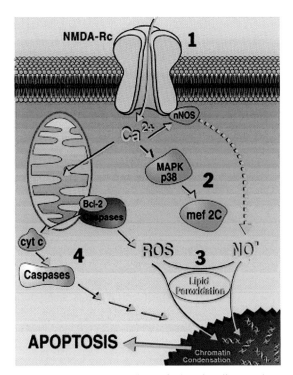

Fig. 3. Schematic illustration of the signaling pathways discovered or characterized in the Lipton laboratory that can be targeted to prevent neuronal apoptosis in a variety of neurologic diseases, including glaucoma. Drug or molecular therapies are being developed to (1) antagonize NMDA receptors (NMDA-Rc); (2) modulate activation of the p38 MAPK-MEF2 transcription factor pathway; (3) prevent toxic reactions of free radicals such as nitric oxide (NO·) and reactive oxygen species (ROS) including superoxide anion and (4) inhibit apoptosis-inducing enzymes including caspases.

in the active site of caspases to down-regulate excessive enzymatic activity and prevent neuronal apoptosis (Tenneti et al., 1997; Choi et al., 2000). As mentioned above, we have termed this reaction S-nitrosylation, and it consists of transfer of NO-related species (specifically NO^+, with one less electron than nitric oxide (NO) to the thiol group critical cysteine residues on proteins to control their function (Stamler et al., 1997).

MEF2C, the predominant form of the MEF2 transcription factor family in cerebral cortex and retina, was initially cloned in our laboratory (Leifer et al., 1993). Recently, it has been found that the stress-activated MAPK p38 can activate MEF2 in an apparently Ca^{2+} dependent manner, and that this pathway can lead to apoptosis. Preliminary data suggest that caspase activation can be both upstream (initiator caspases) and downstream (effector caspases) in the p38/MEF2 pathway. Interestingly, transfecting dominant interfering and constitutively active forms of p38 and MEF2C, we have recently demonstrated that activation of the p38/MEF2 pathway exerts the opposite effect during neuronal development, namely to prevent apoptosis. In fact, transfection with MEF2C can drive precursor cells into a neuronal phenotype, acting as a master switch in controlling neuronal differentiation (Okamoto et al., 2000). A better understanding of this pathway may well lead to new antiapoptotic drugs in the CNS in general and in the retina in particular. For example, p38 antagonists are already in advanced clinical trials for a variety of degenerative conditions such as arthritis, and our preliminary work suggests that they may well be useful in protecting retinal ganglion cells from excitotoxic and traumatic insults similar to those occurring in glaucoma (Kikuchi et al., 2000).

Conclusions and future perspectives

The realization of John Dowling that the retina is an approachable part of the brain led our group to apply neuroprotective principles to the retina. As a result, drugs that we have developed for other neurological disorders are now being tested in advanced clinical trials to prevent the apoptosis of retinal ganglion cells that occurs in glaucoma. Such drugs offer the potential for therapeutic intervention by interrupting apoptotic signaling in retinal ganglion cells at several levels, ranging from glutamate receptors to free radicals, MAP kinases, transcription factors, and caspase-mediated pathways. Clinical trials now underway for glaucoma and a variety of other insults will test this potential, and soon determine if these new neuroprotective strategies will become a reality for our patients.

References

Aizenman, E., Frosch, M.P. and Lipton, S.A. (1988) Responses mediated by excitatory amino acids in solitary retinal ganglion cells from rat. *J. Physiol. (Lond.)*, 396: 75–91.

Ankarcrona, M., Dypbukt, J.M., Bonfoco, E., Zhivotovsky, B., Orrenius, S., Lipton, S.A. and Nicotera, P. (1995) Glutamate-induced neuronal death: A succession of necrosis or apoptosis depending on mitochondrial function. *Neuron*, 15: 961–973.

Bonfoco, E., Krainc, D., Ankarcrona, M., Nicotera, P. and Lipton, S.A. (1995) Apoptosis and necrosis: two distinct events induced respectively by mild and intense insults with NMDA or nitric oxide/superoxide in cortical cell cultures. *Proc. Natl. Acad. Sci. USA*, 92: 7162–7166.

Budd, S.L., Tenneti, L., Lishnak, T. and Lipton, S.A. (2000) Mitochondrial and extramitochondrial apoptotic signaling pathways in cerebrocortical neurons. *Proc. Natl. Acad. Sci. USA*, 97: 6161–6166.

Chen, H.-S.V. and Lipton, S.A. (1997) Mechanism of memantine block of NMDA-activated channels in rat retinal ganglion cells: uncompetitive antagonism. *J. Physiol. (Lond.)*, 499: 27–46.

Chen, H.-S.V., Pellegrini, J.W., Aggarwal, S.K., Lei, S.Z., Warach, S., Jensen, F.E. and Lipton, S.A. (1992) Open-channel block of NMDA responses by memantine: therapeutic advantage against NMDA receptor-mediated neurotoxicity. *J. Neurosci.*, 12: 4427–4436.

Chen, H.-S.V., Wang, Y.F., Rayudu, P., Edgecomb, P., Neill, J.C., Segal, M.M., Lipton, S.A. and Jensen, F.E. (1998) Neuroprotective concentrations of the NMDA open-channel blocker memantine are effective without cytoplasmic vacuolation following post-ischemic administration and do not block maze learning or LTP. *Neuroscience*, 86: 1121–1132.

Choi, D.W. (1988) Glutamate neurotoxicity and diseases of the nervous system. *Neuron*, 1: 623–634.

Choi, Y.-B., Tenneti, L., Le, D.A., Ortiz, J., Bai, G., Chen, H.-S.V. and Lipton, S.A. (2000) Molecular basis of NMDA receptor-coupled ion channel modulation by *S*-nitrosylation. *Nat. Neurosci.*, 3: 15–21.

Das, S., Sasaki, Y.F., Rothe, T., Premkumar, L.S., Takasu, M., Crandall, J.E., Dikkes, P., Connor, D.A., Rayudu, P.V., Cheung, W., Chen, H.-S.V., Lipton, S.A. and Nakanishi, N. (1998) Increased NMDA current and spine density in mice lacking the NMDA receptor subunit NR3A. *Nature*, 393: 377–381.

Dawson, V.L., Dawson, T.M., London, E.D., Bredt, D.S. and Snyder, S.H. (1991) Nitric oxide mediates glutamate neurotoxicity in primary cortical cultures. *Proc. Natl. Acad. Sci. USA*, 88: 6368–6371.

Dreyer, E.B. and Lipton, S.A. (1999) New perspectives on glaucoma. *JAMA*, 281: 306–308.

Dreyer, E.B., Pan, Z.-H., Storm, S. and Lipton, S.A. (1994) Greater sensitivity of larger retinal ganglion cells to NMDA-mediated cell death. *NeuroReport*, 5: 629–631.

Dreyer, E.B., Zhang, D. and Lipton, S.A. (1995) Transcriptional or translational inhibition blocks low dose NMDA-mediated cell death. *NeuroReport*, 6: 942–944.

Dreyer, E.B., Zurakowsi, D., Schumer, R.A., Podos, S.M. and Lipton, S.A. (1996) Elevated glutamate in the vitreous body

718

of humans and monkeys with glaucoma. *Arch. Ophthalmol.*, 114: 299–205.

Fesenko, E.E., Kolesnikov, S.S., Lyubarsky, A.L. (1985) Induction by cyclic GMP of cationic conductance in plasma membrane of retinal rod outer segment. *Nature*, 313: 310–313.

Hahn, J.S., Aizenman, E. and Lipton, S.A. (1988) Central mammalian neurons normally resistant to glutamate toxicity are made sensitive by elevated extracellular Ca^{2+}: toxicity is blocked by the *N*-methyl-*D*-aspartate antagonist MK-801. *Proc. Natl. Acad. Sci. USA*, 85: 6556–6560.

Kikuchi, M., Tenneti, L. and Lipton, S.A. (2000) Role of p38 mitogen-activated protein kinase in axotomy-induced apoptosis of rat retinal ganglion cells. *J. Neurosci.*, 20: 5037–5044.

Kim, W.-K., Choi, Y.-B., Rayudu, P.V., Das, P., Asaad, W., Arnelle, D.R., Stamler, J.S. and Lipton, S.A. (1999) Attenuation of NMDA receptor activity and neurotoxicity by nitroxyl anion, NO^-. *Neuron*, 24: 461–469.

Leifer, D., Krainc, D., Yu, Y.-T., McDermott, J., Breitbart, R.E., Heng, J., Neve, R.L., Kosofsky, Nadal-Ginard, B. and Lipton, S.A. (1993) A novel MADS/MEF2-family transcription factor expressed in a laminar distribution in cerebral cortex. *Proc. Natl. Acad. Sci. USA*, 90: 1546–1550.

Lipton, S.A. (1993) Prospects for clinically tolerated NMDA antagonists: open-channel blockers and alternative redox states of nitric oxide. *Trends Neurosci.*, 16: 527–532.

Lipton, S.A., Choi, Y.-B., Pan, Z.-H., Lei, S.Z., Chen, H.-S.V., Sucher, N.J., Loscalzo, J., Singel, D.J. and Stamler, J.S. (1993) A redox-based mechanism for the neuroprotective and neurodestructive effects of nitric oxide and related nitroso-compounds. *Nature*, 364: 626–632.

Lipton, S.A., Ostroy, S.E. and Dowling, J.E. (1977a) Electrical and adaptive properties of rod photoreceptors in *Bufo marinus*. I. Effects of altered extracellular calcium. *J. Gen. Physiol.*, 70: 747–770.

Lipton, S.A., Ostroy, S.E. and Dowling, J.E. (1979) Calcium and photoreceptor adaptation. *Nature (Lond.)*,281: 407–408.

Lipton, S.A., Rasmussen, H. and Dowling, J.E. (1977b) Electrical and adaptive properties of rod photoreceptors in *Bufo marinus*. II. Effects of cyclic nucleotides and prostaglandins. *J. Gen. Physiol.*, 70: 771–791.

Lipton, S.A. and Rosenberg, P.A. (1994) Mechanisms of disease: Excitatory amino acids as a final common pathway for neurologic disorders. *N. Engl. J. Med.*, 330: 613–622.

Lucas, D.R. and Newhouse, J.P. (1957) The toxic effect of sodium L-glutamate on the inner layers of the retina. *Arch. Ophathalmol.*, 58: 193–201.

Meldrum, B. and Garthwaite, J. (1990) Excitatory amino acid neurotoxicity and neurodegenerative disease. *Trends Pharmacol. Sci.*, 11: 379–387.

Okamoto, S.-I., Krainc, D., Sherman, K. and Lipton, S.A. (2000) Antiapoptotic role of the p38 mitogen-activated protein kinase–myocyte enhancer factor 2 transcription factor pathway during neuronal differentiation. *Proc. Natl. Acad. Sci. USA*, 97: 7561–7566.

Olney, J.W. (1990) Excitotoxin-mediated neuron death in youth and old age. *Prog. Brain. Res.*, 86: 37–51.

Stamler, J.S., Toone, E.J., Lipton, S.A. and Sucher, N.J. (1997) (S)NO signals: Translocation, regulation, and a consensus motif. *Neuron*, 18: 691–696.

Sucher, N.J., Aizenman, E. and Lipton, S.A. (1991) NMDA antagonists prevent kainate neurotoxicity in rat retinal ganglion cells. *J. Neurosci.*, 11: 966–971.

Sucher, N.J., Akabarian, S., Chi, C.L., Leclerc, C.L., Awobuluyi, M., Deitcher, D.L., Wu, M.K., Yuan, J.P., Jones, E.G. and Lipton, S.A. (1995) Developmental and regional expression pattern of a novel NMDA receptor-like subunit (NMDAR-L) in the rodent brain. *J. Neurosci.*, 15: 6509–6520.

Tenneti, L., D'Emilia, D.M. and Lipton, S.A. (1997) Suppression of neuronal apoptosis by *S*-nitrosylation of caspases. *Neurosci. Lett.*, 236: 139–142.

Tenneti, L., D'Emilia, D.M., Troy, C.M. and Lipton, S.A. (1998) Role of caspases in *N*-methyl-*D*-aspartate-induced apoptosis of cerebrocortical neurons. *J. Neurochem.*, 71: 946–959.

Tenneti, L. and Lipton, S.A. (2000) Involvement of activated caspase-3-like proteases in *N*-methyl-*D*-aspartate-induced apoptosis in cerebrocortical neurons. *J. Neurochem.*, 74: 134–142.

Vorwerk, C.K., Lipton, S.A., Zurakowski, D., Hyman, B.T., Sabel, B.A. and Dreyer, E.B. (1996) Chronic low dose glutamate is toxic to retinal ganglion cells: toxicity blocked by memantine. *Invest. Ophthalmol. Vis. Sci.*, 37: 1618–1624.

SECTION VIII

Epilogue

H. Kolb, H. Ripps and S. Wu (Eds.)
Progress in Brain Research, Vol. 131
© 2001 Elsevier Science B.V. All rights reserved

CHAPTER 52

Reflections and comments

John E. Dowling*

Department of Molecular and Cellular Biology, Harvard University, 16 Divinity Avenue, Cambridge, MA 02138, USA

I remember clearly the day when as a student in George Wald's laboratory, Paul Brown, Wald's long-time collaborator, called me into his darkroom to look at a section of the mudpuppy retina he had just cut and stained. Paul was just beginning his microspectroscopic studies on individual photoreceptor cell outer segments and he wished to take advantage of the large mudpuppy cells. He was excited to show me the beauty of the rods and cones in that retina, but what impressed me more was the enormous size of the neurons and what then appeared to be the relative simplicity of this retina with its single layer of photoreceptor and ganglion cells and an inner nuclear layer just four cells thick. I recall sharing with Paul the exciting idea that this retina might be an ideal one to analyze—that if it were possible to record from individual retinal cells, this would be where to start. Eventually that came to pass, but not for several years.

My interests then were focused on vitamin A deficiency, photoreceptor mechanisms and visual adaptation, interests that have carried on to this day and are now reflected in the work of many students and colleagues. From undergraduate research on the effects of vitamin A deficiency on the rat retina came an interest in retinal degenerations, both inherited and induced and this has become an exploding field (see, for example, the papers in this volume by Brockerhoff, Aguirre, Fisher et al. and LaVail). The first manifestation of

vitamin A deficiency in an animal is, of course, night blindness and that led early on to studies of light and dark adaptation and the relation of visual pigment levels to visual sensitivity. Visual adaptation has turned out to be a most complex and fascinating area of inquiry involving both photoreceptor and non-photoreceptor cells as well as visual pigment and synaptic mechanisms (see, for example, the papers by Ripps, Fain, Hurley and Chen, Burkhardt, McMahon et al. and Baldridge).

What initially led me deeper into the retina and the quest for understanding retinal circuitry and its functional organization were some electron microscopic observations I made on the ground squirrel retina. I was studying cone structure in the ground squirrel retina and saw what appeared to be synapses between the photoreceptor and horizontal cells (Dowling, 1964). At that time, little was known about horizontal cells—indeed, some investigators believed they were glial cells. But finding photoreceptors synapsing on these cells clearly indicated to me that they were neurons. That naturally aroused a curiosity about other retinal synapses and their organization. My collaboration with Brian Boycott began at about this time and soon we identified the synapses made by many of the retinal cells (Dowling and Boycott, 1966). Brian's particular expertise was Golgi staining of the retina and when Helga Kolb joined the laboratory and began to combine Golgi-staining with electron microscopy, the possibility of unraveling retinal synaptic circuitry became a reality (Kolb, 1970). The progress made in this area has been remarkable and is well described in this

* Tel.: 617-495-2245; Fax: 617-496-3321;
E-mail: Dowling@fas.harvard.edu

volume (see, for example, the papers by Kolb et al., Linberg, et al., Meinertzhagen and Sorra, Marshak and Zucker and Ehinger).

As the first glimpses of retinal circuitry were revealed, it became clear that we needed to know the nature of the signals generated by the retinal neurons and their responses to light. Frank Werblin, an electrical engineering graduate student at Johns Hopkins, joined the laboratory and it was then I recalled the possibilities offered by the mudpuppy retina. We decided to analyze the mudpuppy retina both anatomically and physiologically, and that was the beginning of our attempts to understand the functional organization of the retina (Dowling and Werblin, 1969; Werblin and Dowling, 1969). Not in my wildest dreams did I expect this area of research would go so far. (See, for example, the papers by Wu et al., Yazulla et al., Connaughton, Bloomfield, Cohen and Werblin et al.)

What impresses me most today is the richness of neural mechanisms operating in the retina, and the papers in this volume describe and review many of these mechanisms. And we are likely still just scratching the surface of all that is going on. I said brashly in the early 1970s that I thought the retina would be pretty much understood within a decade. That was more than 25 years ago, and I couldn't have been more wrong. I was a "lumper" in those days, believing in simplifying the retina, what it does and how it does it, and I was very skeptical of the "splitters" who, it seemed to me, wanted to make things more complex than they need be, and less understandable. But today, I am joining the "splitters"—it is the complexity and richness of all that goes on in the retina that makes it the "genuine neural center" that Ramon y Cajal (1892) called it. If we are to understand the brain, we must come to grips with the complexity and variety of neural and glial interactions that exist in brains, and my guess is that they are all going on here in the retina—which is, of course, a true part of the brain pushed out into the eye during development.

We needed to start with a framework of the major pathways of information flow through the retina, some understanding of the electrical and chemical responses occurring in the cells, an identification of the major substances used to communicate information between neurons, and so forth. That has been accomplished for the most part, as the papers in this volume amply illustrate. Now we can get into the details of how it all really works—and it is getting exciting. This is not to say that we have answered all of the fundamental questions posed twenty-five or more years ago. For example, the photoreceptor synapses are still a puzzle. Why are there the invaginated ribbon synapses? The lateral elements are horizontal cell processes and the central elements are usually bipolar cell dendrites, but why are these synapses invaginated? One guess is that the invaginations facilitate interactions between the horizontal, bipolar and photoreceptor terminals, but how does this happen?

Synaptic transmitter release certainly occurs at the base of the synaptic ribbons in the photoreceptor terminals, but cones make a second type of synapse— the basal or flat junction. How do they work? No synaptic vesicles are associated with these contacts, so how is transmitter released there? Or is all the release at the ribbon synapse in photoreceptor terminals, and the transmitter somehow finds its way to the basal contacts. There is much interest in photoreceptor synapses in both vertebrate and invertebrate retinas (see, for example, the papers by Witkovsky et al., Nelson et al., and Meinertzhagen and Sorra). New data is showing us a variety of receptor molecules that are responsible for neurotransmission at both the ribbon synapses and at conventional synapses throughout the retina (see papers by Kolb et al., Qian and Ripps, and Miller et al., in this volume). Hopefully answers to these questions will soon be forthcoming.

How do horizontal cells work? They clearly form the surround responses observed in many bipolar cell recordings, and physiological recordings from photoreceptor cells show that the horizontal cells feed back onto the cone photoreceptors. Horizontal cells may now be the best understood of all retinal cells, and many papers in this volume discuss their properties. But the nature of how they exert their effects back onto photoreceptors—whether it is chemical or electrical—is still unclear. And it is still unclear whether they also can make feedforward synapses onto bipolar cells.

What has been recently established does seem a bit bewildering at times—a dozen or so types of bipolar cells in most retinas, two dozen amacrine and ganglion cells, ten strata in the IPL, but we are getting glimpses of what this all means (see, for example, the papers by Wu et al., Kolb et al. and Werblin et al., in this volume). There are at least twenty-five neuroactive substances released at retinal synapses and perhaps a hundred or more ligand-gated channels and receptor molecules there, and surprises all the time (see Zucker and Ehinger, Miller et al., Yang et al. and Qian and Ripps). Retinoic acid, a morphogen, acting also as a neuromodulatory substances? (see Weiler et al. and McMahon et al., this volume). Intriguing! Again, the retina is leading the way in understanding the subtleties of neural mechanisms.

There is an enormous amount of neuromodulation that is continually occurring in the retina as we go from light to dark and back again, or even as we go through the day and night and are influenced by circadian rhythms (see section on Circadian Rhythms). Elsewhere, particularly from studies on invertebrate nervous systems, we had indications that neuromodulatory substances, including the monoamines and neuropeptides, could change synaptic strengths and modify circuitry within an invertebrate ganglion. In the retina, we now see how this happens with both chemical and electrical synapses and begin to deduce the significance of this for visual processing under various lighting and stimulus conditions (see Yazulla et al., McMahon et al., Baldridge, Barlow and Mangel, this volume). The retina is clearly not a hard-wired computer!

Are there particular lessons to be learned from the collected papers in this volume? Where do we go from here in the year 2000—at the millenium? As the information on retinal anatomy, physiology, and pharmacology becomes richer and more detailed—which is happening all the time—I think there is need for more measurements of visual behavior in our experimental animals. Visual behavioral measurements have not kept pace with the advances in physiology and our understanding of function, and this needs to be done. Ultimately, it is visual behavior that we wish to explain, and we need to make sure that we know what and how well the animal is seeing while we are carrying out our experimental manipulations. I first illustrate this with an example involving dopamine, rod vision and zebrafish.

There has been a longstanding argument as to when dopamine is released in the retina—in the light or dark. There is evidence on both sides and many of us think it might be released under both conditions (see Marshak, this volume). The view most usually given is that dopamine is a light signal in the eye, but these studies are based almost exclusively on studies carried out on the outer retina.

A year or so ago Lei Li (see Li, this volume) did a simple behavioral experiment with zebrafish measuring dark adaptation in animals depleted of dopamine by 6-hydroxydopamine injections into the eye. Much to our surprise he found these animals had no rod function when dark adapted. Their behavioral responses were all photopic. If dopamine is a light signal, why is there no rod function in the absence of dopamine, and what might be going on? A few years ago, Heidleberger and Mathews (1994) found that Ca^{2+} influx into rod bipolar cell terminals in the goldfish was increased by dopamine, suggesting that the release of transmitter from these bipolar cells is under dopamine control (see also, Yazulla et al., this volume). Ethan Cohen, is now following up on these observations and has shown that excitatory postsynaptic currents (EPSC's) are greatly enhanced in certain ganglion cells when dopamine is added to the bathing medium (see Cohen, this volume). Can it be that some dopamine is required for rod transmission through the inner plexiform layer in zebrafish? The story is certainly not complete, but it makes the important point that our major goal is to understand the role of the retina in terms of what an animal sees, and knowing the visual behavior of our experimental animals is critical for attaining this goal and even pointing us in the right direction.

A prescient paper in this regard is that of Maturana et al., entitled "Anatomy and Physiology of Vision in the Frog (*Rana pipiens*)", published 40 years ago[1]. (A less complete version of this paper was published a year earlier with the provocative and now famous title of "What the frog's eye tells the frog's brain".) This paper did not measure visual behavior in frogs, but its thrust was to explain their visual behavior. They asked how this might be accomplished with the tools of the day—extracellular

---

[1]In the discussion period at the end of the Symposium, it was Mark Lurie who pointed out that the Maturana and Lettvin paper emphasized the need to explain retinal anatomy and physiology in terms of the behavior of an animal.

recordings from ganglion cells and methylene blue and silver staining of the retinal neurons.

To analyze the "analytic functions of the ganglion cells, [they] adopted a naturalistic approach and studied them in terms of their response to real objects of the natural environment". They make the point that: "Spots of light are not natural stimuli for the frog in the way that a fly or worm is". They described five classes of ganglion cells that perform different operations on the visual image and showed the five cell types project to different layers of the tectum. In trying to explain how the responses of the five ganglion cell types are established, they noted that the "ganglion cells form several morphologically discontinuous groups that differ in the pattern of branching and the level of stratification of their dendrites in the internal plexiform (layer)" so that "each type of ganglion cell can synapse only with certain types of bipolars and the converse is true".

This was written before we even knew what retinal synapses look like or the nature of the responses of any of the retinal cells save ganglion cells. Now 40 years later, we know much about the retinal circuitry and retinal cell physiology, and several papers in this volume address precisely a number of the questions posed then (see, for example, Kolb et al. and Wu et al.). The time is appropriate to revisit the notion they advanced—to discover how the retina analyzes the visual image in terms of what the animal's visual system is designed to do (see Werblin et al., this volume). Many common principles exist among the retinas of different species—this we know and take advantage of—but there are differences, too, and what do those differences mean in terms of visual performance and behavior of an animal? The frog's retina is especially designed to detect moving stimuli, and we know that the frog's retina is rich in amacrine cell synaptic interactions that we believe are important for the detection of movement (Dowling, 1968). But, how these amacrine cell interactions lead to the responses of movement and directional-selective ganglion cells in the frog or other animals is not completely understood (see, Zucker and Ehinger, this volume). As we explore these questions, it is essential to keep in mind what role a particular type of ganglion cell is playing in the animal's behavioral repertoire. And the same point can be made for the sub-types of all other retinal cells that we study. This is an enormous challenge, but one that is essential if we are to finally understand the retina. And it is not one retina that we need to understand, but the retinas of many, if not all, species.

I close with another example of the value of behavioral studies for understanding our physiological observations. We've known since Hartline's classic work in the late 1930s that there are ganglion cells that respond when the light is turned ON, and others that respond when the light is turned OFF (Hartline, 1938). By the late 1960s, it was shown that the bipolar cells respond to light either with ON (depolarizing) or OFF (hyperpolarizing) responses (Werblin and Dowling, 1969). Thus, the division of visual information into ON and OFF pathways begins in the outer plexiform layer, at the synapse between the photoreceptors and bipolar cells. But why are there both ON and OFF channels in the visual system? This was not made clear until Peter Schiller and his colleagues (1986) pharmacologically blocked the ON bipolar cell response selectively with 2-amino-4-phosphonobutyrate (APB) in monkeys, and then asked how the animal's vision was altered. They found under photopic conditions that the monkeys could not tell if a spot of light was intensifying or brighter than the background. On the other hand, the animals could readily distinguish a spot of light becoming weaker in intensity or a spot of light dimmer than the background illumination. They also showed there was a loss of contrast sensitivity in the animals. These data provided clear evidence that ON retinal pathways signal the brain about increments in illumination, whereas OFF retinal pathways signal decrements of illumination. I don't believe any physiological experiment could have provided such a crisp answer to the question of why there are ON and OFF channels in the visual system as did the behavioral one.

The future of retinal research seems as promising to me today as when I started in the field over forty years ago. I won't be so rash as to predict that we will soon understand the retina, but the progress that has been made, coupled with the enormous variety of cells, synapses and interactions that are present in retinas along with known species differences, suggest that there is much gold yet to be mined in the field. And new areas are emerging and flourishing. How retinas develop is fast moving from a descriptive field of study to a cellular and molecular one, and impressive progress in retinal genetics has recently been made (see, for example, the section on Retinal Development and Genetics). Virtually every topic on retinal biology is touched on in this volume, attesting to the vitality and imagination of the wonderful group of individuals I have had the opportunity of working with over the years. This volume is a tribute to me, but in reality it is a tribute to all those who have made my life and this field so rich.

References

Dowling, J.E. (1964) Structure and function in the all-cone retina of the ground squirrel. In: Riggs, L. (Ed.), *Proceedings of Form Discrimination Symposium*. Brown University, Providence, Rhode Island, pp. 17–23.

Dowling, J.E. (1968) Synaptic organization of the frog retina: An electron microscopic analysis comparing the retinas of frogs and primates. *Proc. Roy. Soc. B*, 170: 205–228.

Dowling, J.E. and Boycott, B.B. (1966) Organization of the primate retina: Electron Microscopy. *Proc. Roy. Soc. B*, 166: 80–111.

Dowling, J.E. and Werblin, F.S. (1969) Organization of the retina of the mudpuppy, *Necturus maculosus*: I. Synaptic structure. *J. Neurophysiol.*, 255: 315–338.

Hartline, H.K. (1938) The response of single optic nerve fibers of the vertebrate eye to illumination of the retina. *Am. J. Physiol.*, 121: 400–415.

Heidelberger, R. and Matthews, G. (1994) Dopamine enhances Ca^{2+} responses in synaptic terminals of retinal bipolar neurons. *Neuro Report*, 5: 729–732.

Kolb, H. (1970) Organization of the outer plexiform layer of the primate retina. Electron microscopy of Golgi-impregnated cells. *Phil. Trans.*, 258: 261–283.

Maturana, H. R., Lettvin, J. Y, McCulloch, W.S. and Pitts, W.H. (1960) Anatomy and physiology of vision in the frog (*Rana pipiens*). *J. Gen. Physiol.*, 43: 129–175.

Ramón y Cajal, S. (1892) La rétine des vertébrés. La céllule 9: 119–257. For English translation, see Thorpe, S.A. and Glickstein, M., Springfield, Ill.: Thomas, C.C., 1972, and Maguire, D. and Rodieck, R. W., in The Vertebrate Retina, San Francisco: W. H. Freeman, 1973, pp. 775–904.

Schiller, P.H., Sandell, J.H. and Maunsell, J.H.R. (1986) Functions of the ON and OFF channels of the visual system. *Nature*, 322: 824–825.

Werblin, F.S. and Dowling, J.E. (1969) Organization of the retina of the mudpuppy, *Necturus maculosus*. II. Intracellular recording, *J. Neurophysiol.*, 32: 339–355.

H. Kolb, H. Ripps and S. Wu (Eds.)
Progress in Brain Research, Vol. 131

APPENDIX I

Graduate students, postdoctoral fellows, visiting scholars, collaborators, staff and undergraduate senior thesis students of John Dowling's laboratory (*Numbers in bold italic correspond to the numbers in the photograph insert of Appendix II pages 730–731*).

(1) Graduate Students (year of obtaining Ph.D.)

Frank Werblin (1968) *(54)*
Mark Dubin (1969) *(34)*
Richard Chappell (1970) *(55)*
Ralph Nelson (1972) *(37)*
Gordon Fain (1973) *(25)*
Jochen Kleinschmidt (1974)
Willard Hedden (1975)
Stuart Lipton (1977) *(35)*
Geoffrey Gold (1977)
Glen Pu (1978) *(38)*
Samuel Wu (1979) *(15)*
Howard Harary (1983)
Judith Mosinger (1983) *(49)*
Robert Van Buskirk (1983)
Lucy Young (1984)
Nicholas Marsh-Armstrong (1994) *(20)*
Carl Fulwiler (1994)
Thomas Jordan (1998)
Brenda Allwardt (1999)
Kwoon Wong

(2) Postdoctoral Fellows (years in the lab)

George Weinstein (1964–1966)
Dwight Burkhardt (1965–1967) *(31)*
Robert Frank (1967–1968)
Helga Kolb (1966–1971) *(41)*
Robert Miller (1968–1970) *(12)*
Gustavo Aguirre (1969–1971) *(13)*
Leslie Fisher (1969–1971)
Steven Fisher (1969–1971) *(8)*
Roger West (1970–1973)
Stephen Yazulla (1972–1974) *(3)*
David Pepperberg (1973–1976) *(26)*
Jose Sobrino (l972)

Mark Lurie (1973–1975) *(16)*
Ian Meinertzhagen (1974–1976) *(10)*
Christine Armett-Kibel (1974–1976)
Roger Zimmerman (1976–1978) *(32)*
Richard Kline (1976–1978)
Lillemor Wachtmeister (1976–1977) *(18)*
Randolph Glickman (1977–1979) *(45)*
Geraldine Waloga (1975–1977)
Lindesay Harkness (1977–1980)
Ingrid Holmgren-Taylor (1980–1981)
Eric Lasater (1980–1985) *(17)*
Joel Cohen (1979–1982)
Keith Watling (1980–1983)
Stuart Mangel (1981–1984) *(14)*
Michael Ariel (1981–1984)
Stewart Bloomfield (1981–1983) *(21)*
David Marshak (1982–1984) *(57)*
Denis O'Brien (1982–1984) *(4)*
Patricia O'Connor (1982–1985)
Rita Kropf (1983–1986)
Charles Zucker (1984–1987) *(44)*
Kristina Tornqvist (1985–1986) *(64)*
Andrew Knapp (1985–1989)
Douglas McMahon (1985–1990) *(2)*
Paulo Rodrigues (1988–1990)
Karl Schmidt (1988–1989)
Ellen Schmitt (1988–present)
Huan-Ji Du (1990–1992)
George Hyatt (1991–1996)
George Grant (1993–1995)
Haohua Qian (1992–1996) *(52)*
Ulrike-Janssen-Bienhold (1994) *(51)*
Susan Brockerhoff (1994–1996) *(56)*
James Fadool (1994–1997) *(28)*
Lei Li (1995–1999) *(1)*
Clare Chung (1996–1998) *(61)*
Eileen Rounds (1997–2000) *(62)*

728

Brian Link (1998–)
Tristan Darland (1998–)
Deborah Stull (1998–)
Pamela Kainz (1998–) *(58)*
Brian Perkins (2000–) *(47)*

(3) Visiting Scholars

Alan Adolph *(59)*
Brian Boycott
Beth Burnside *(33)*
Ethan Cohen
Joaquin De Juan
Berndt Ehinger *(50)*
Daniel Green *(27)*
James Hurley *(22)*
Abner Lall *(29)*
Nicholas Leibovic *(46)*
Hai-Biao Li
Sanford Ostroy
Ido Perlman *(5)*
José Sahel *(43)*
Osamu Umino
Xiong-Li Yang *(11)*
Michael Zeldin

(4) Other Collaborators

William Baldridge *(6)*
Robert Barlow *(7)*
Vikki Connaughton *(9)*
Ursula Dräger *(60)*
Stephen Easter *(24)*
William Eldred *(42)*
Alan Laties *(53)*
Richard Masland
Harris Ripps *(30)*
Richard Sidman
Reto Weiler
Paul Witkovsky *(48)*
Jimin Zhou *(63)*

(5) Staff

Patricia Sheppard—Research Assistant
Stephanie Levinson—Secretary *(36)*

William McCarthy (Director of Zebrafish Lab)
Christian Lawrence—Zebrafish Facility
Salvatore Sciascia—Zebrafish Facility

(6) Undergraduates (year of senior thesis)

Cynthia N. Johnson (1964)
Nicholas Spitzer (1964)
Willard Hedden (1973)
Ann E. Randall (1973)
Marian Craighill (1975)
Craig McArdle (1976)
Henry D. Jampel (1977)
Steven M. Greenberg (1978)
Anthony Maranto (1978)
Steven M. Greenberg (1981)
Deborah S. Jacobs (1981)
Sara Dorison (1983)
Mami Iwamoto (1983)
Peggy Mason (1983)
Jang Ho Cha (1984)
Alan Crane (1986)
Eva Lin (1986)
Martin H. Reinke (1986)
Mark S. Weinfeld (1986)
Robert C. Lowe (1988)
Nancy K. Mayer (1988)
Michael R. Albert (1989)
Lisa Goodrich (1991)
Jennifer Linden (1991)
Abraham S. C. Chyung (1992)
Vanessa J. Parise (1992)
Richard Winakur (1992)
Laura C. Alonso (1993)
Katherine Cunningham (1993)
Jennie Kim (1993)
Richard C.-S. Lin (1993)
Amir Goldkorn (1994)
Lydia E. Matesic (1994)
Jessica L. Hanover (1995)
Laura Meeks (1996)
Jeremy Parise (1996)
Alberto Hazan (1999)
Thomas Ryou (2000)

APPENDIX II

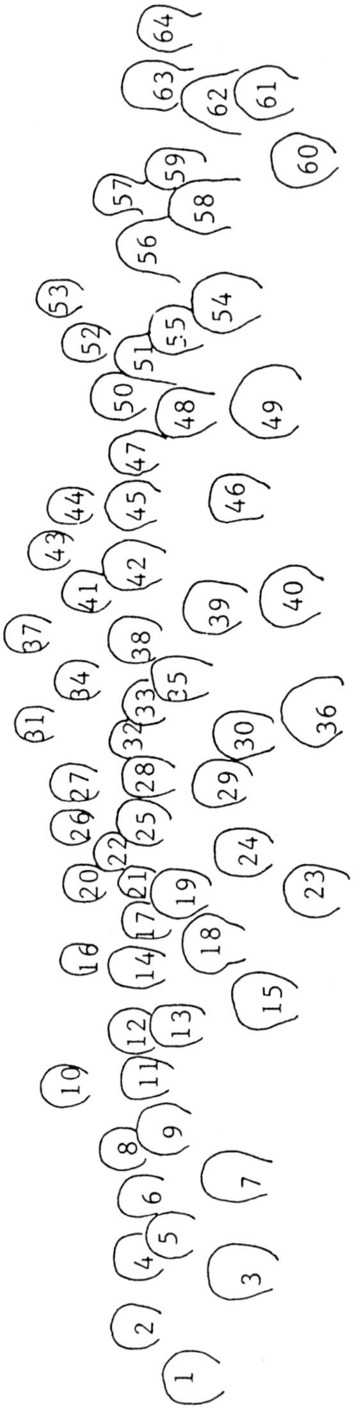
1
2
3
4
5
6
7
8
9
10
11
12
13
14
15
16
17
18
19
20
21
22
23
24
25
26
27
28
29
30
31
32
33
34
35
36
37
38
39
40
41
42
43
44
45
46
47
48
49
50
51
52
53
54
55
56
57
58
59
60
61
62
63
64

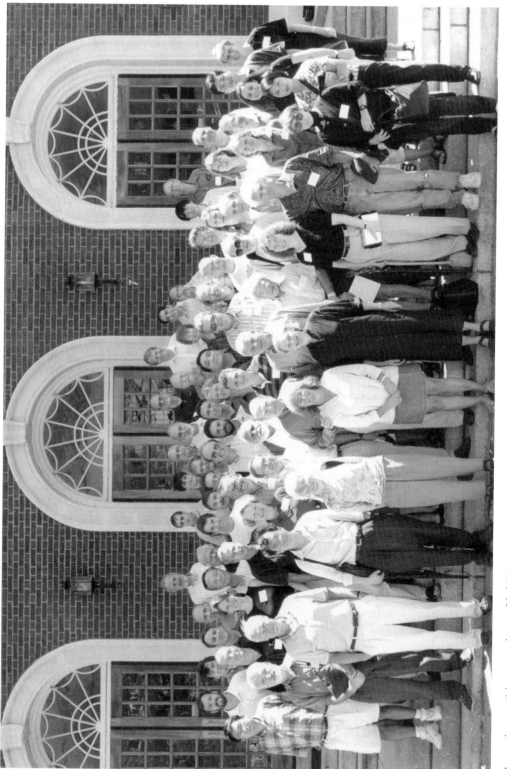

Symposium participants on August 25, 2000, at the Marine Biological Laboratory. *The names of the participants which correspond to the following numbers are given in Appendix 1. Names that are not in Appendix 1:* John Dowling *(39)*, Judith Dowling *(40)*, Ken Linberg *(19)*, Ruth Hubbard *(23)*.

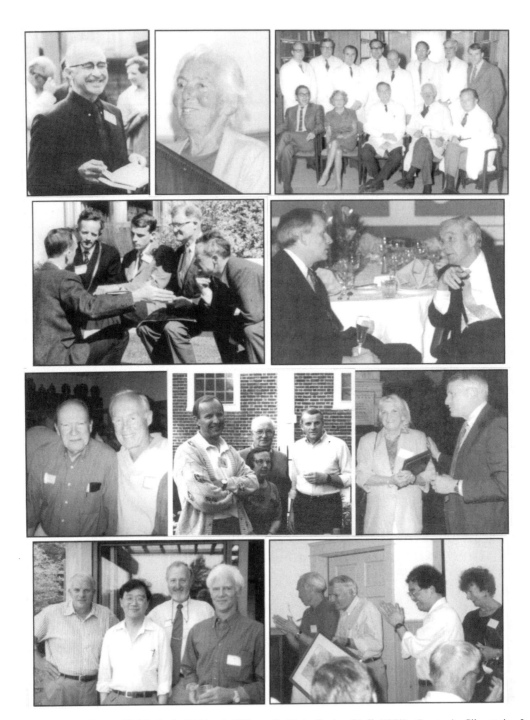

(left to right) Top row: George Wald; Ruth Hubbard; Wilmer Institute Senior Staff (1970): *Front*: A. Silverstein, L. Sloane, A. E. Maumenee, F. Walsh, G. von Noorden. *Back*: I. Pollack, W. Green, Maurice Langham, K. Greene, A. Patz, D. Knox, D. Paton J. Dowling.
2nd row: Ken Brown, Alexi Byzov, John Dowling, William Rushton and Alan Hodgkin; John Dowling and Alan Hodgkin.
3rd row: Harris Ripps and Bob Barlow; Heinz Wassle, Marjorie Boycott, Brian Boycott and John Dowling; Patricia Sheppard and John Dowling.
4th row: John Dowling, Sam Wu, Ian Meinertzhagen and Frank Werblin; Bob Barlow, John Dowling, Sam Wu and Helga Kolb.

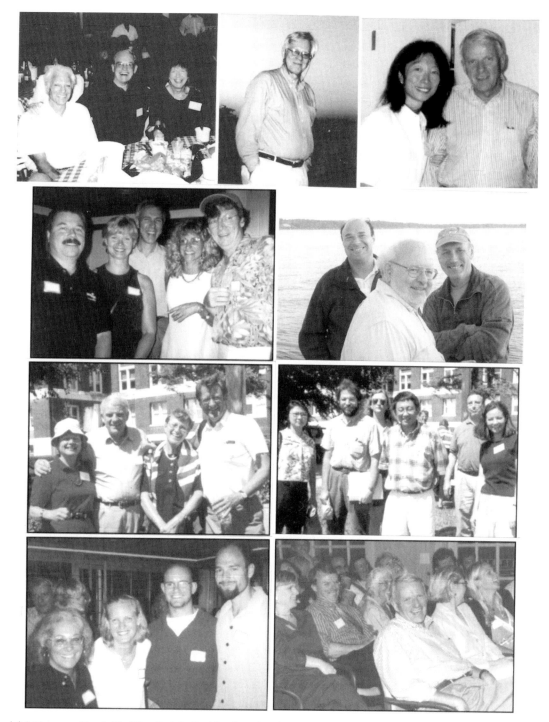

(left to right) Top row: Frank Werblin, Dwight Burkhardt and Helga Kolb; Bob Miller; Lucy Young and John Dowling.
2nd row: Rick Lasater, Jill Lasater, Keith Watling, A. Watling and Denis. O'Brien; David Marshak, Matt LaVail and Steve Fisher.
3rd row: Lillemor Wachtmeister, John Dowling, Kristina Tornqvist and Berndt Ehinger; Clare Chung, Ethan Cohen, Ulrike Janssen-Bienhold, Lei Li, Roger Zimmerman and Eileen Rounds.
4th row: Steffie Levinson, Pam. Kainz, Brian Perkins and Brian Link; *Front*: John Dowling, Judy Dowling, Alex Dowling, *Back*: J. Dowling, Nick Dowling, Ruth Hubbard and Dick Cone.

Subject Index